KEEP YOUR ENTIRE DRUG REFEREN☑ W9-BKB-248 COMPLETELY UP-TO-DATE WITH THESE KEY VOLUMES!

1996 PHYSICIANS' DESK REFERENCE®

Up-to-the-minute drug information is more crucial than ever. New medicines, new drug interaction data, the latest side effects findings, and certain drugs now removed from the market make it absolutely imperative that you update your reference material this year. The 1996 PDR guarantees you the security of having the latest FDA-approved data on over 7,000 prescription drugs. Published December, 1995. $69.95

1996 PDR® SUPPLEMENTS

Never again worry about missing the newest prescription drug developments during the year. PDR Supplements bring you every important update between annual editions of the PDR. 200 pgs total. Published May & September, 1996. $20.95.

1996 PDR GUIDE TO DRUG INTERACTIONS, SIDE EFFECTS, INDICATIONS™

Completely cross-referenced to your 1996 PDR. This newly-expanded directory is the most comprehensive and reliable publication of its kind! It gives you up-to-date information in three vital areas. **For interactions:** quick, accurate access to all the facts you need to identify potential problems with

Three of the most critical prescription checkpoints!

drug combinations by brand and generic names. **For indications:** a list of all drugs indicated for the precise clinical situation you face. **For side effects:** simply look up the specific sign, symptom or abnormality to determine if any drugs the patient is taking might be the problem. Published January, 1996. $48.95.

PDR® MEDICAL DICTIONARY

More than 100,000 entries. 1,900 pages include a complete Medical Etymology section to help the reader understand medical/scientific word formation. Includes a comprehensive cross reference table of generic and brand-name pharmaceuticals and manufacturers, plus a 31-page appendix containing useful charts on scales, temperatures, temperature equivalents, metric and SI units, weights and measures, laboratory and reference values, blood groups and much more. Published March, 1995. $44.95

FIRST EDITION!

1996 PDR® GENERICS™

The most comprehensive reference of its kind, providing complete prescribing and pricing information on every recognized prescription medication on the

The resource for today's healthcare environment!

market. Covers nearly 40,000 medications — both brand and generic. In-depth monographs on almost every brand and FDA-rated bio-equivalent prescription drug. Cost of drug therapy guide. Three indices, appendices, 1500 color photos and much more. Published February, 1996. $79.95

1996 PDR FOR NONPRESCRIPTION DRUGS®

The latest facts on OTC drugs and preparations!

More and more over-the-counter drugs and preparations enter the market every year. Stay fully informed with this easy-to-use reference of today's most dependable data on OTC pharmaceutical products, including ingredients, indications, interactions, dosage, administration, and more. Four complete indices, color photos. Published March, 1996. $43.95.

1996 PDR FOR OPHTHALMOLOGY®

Nowhere else can you find such a comprehensive guide to eyecare. This indispensable directory gives you in-depth drug and product information in the fields of optometry and ophthalmology, specialized instrumentation, equipment and lenses, color photos, color-blind test. Four indices. Published October, 1995. $44.95.

The definitive eye-care product reference!

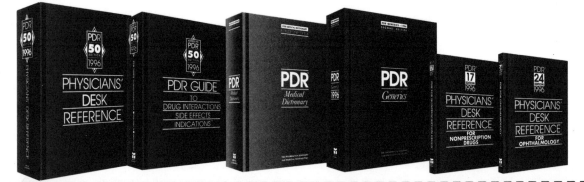

COMPLETE YOUR 1996 PDR LIBRARY NOW!

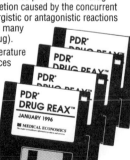

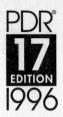

PHYSICIANS' DESK REFERENCE

FOR NONPRESCRIPTION DRUGS®

Medical Consultant
Ronald Arky, MD, Charles S. Davidson Professor of Medicine and Master, Francis Weld Peabody Society, Harvard Medical School

President and Chief Operating Officer, Drug Information Services Group: Thomas F. Rice

Director of Product Management: Stephen B. Greenberg
Senior Associate Product Manager: Cy S. Caine
Associate Product Manager: Howard N. Kanter
National Sales Manager: James R. Pantaleo
Senior Account Managers: Dikran N. Barsamian, Michael S. Sarajian
Account Managers: Donald V. Bruccoleri, Lawrence C. Keary, Jeffrey M. Keller, P. Anthony Pinsonault, Anthony Sorce
Trade Sales Manager: Robin B. Bartlett
Trade Sales Account Executive: Bill Gaffney
Direct Marketing Manager: Robert W. Chapman
Marketing Communications Manager: Maryann Malorgio
Vice President of Production: Steven R. Andreazza
Director, Professional Support Services: Mukesh Mehta, RPh
Drug Information Specialists: Thomas Fleming, RPh, Marion Gray, RPh

Manager, Database Administration: Lynne Handler
Contracts and Support Services Director: Marjorie A. Duffy
Production Managers: Kimberly Hiller-Vivas, Robert Loeser
Production Coordinators: Amy B. Brooks, Mary Ellen Hegarty, Dawn B. McCall
Senior Format Editor: Gregory J. Westley
Format Editor: Edna V. Berger
Index Editor: Jeffrey Schaefer
Art Associate: Joan K. Akerlind
Director of Corporate Communications: Gregory J. Thomas
Electronic Publishing Coordinator: Joanne M. Pearson
Art Director: Richard A. Weinstock
Electronic Publishing Designer: Kevin J. Leckner
Digital Photography: Shawn W. Cahill, Frank J. McElroy, III
Director, Circulation and Fulfillment: Marianne Clarke
Product Fulfillment Manager: Stephen Schweikhart
Editor, Special Projects: David W. Sifton

Officers of Medical Economics: *President and Chief Executive Officer:* Norman R. Snesil; *President and Chief Operating Officer:* Curtis B. Allen; *Executive Vice President and Chief Financial Officer:* J. Crispin Ashworth; *Senior Vice President—Corporate Operations:* John R. Ware; *Senior Vice President—Corporate Business Development:* Raymond M. Zoeller; *Vice President, Information Services and Chief Information Officer:* Edward J. Zecchini

ISBN: 1-56363-133-4

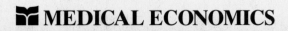
MEDICAL ECONOMICS

FOREWORD

Welcome to the seventeenth edition of *Physicians' Desk Reference For Nonprescription Drugs.* This companion volume to the main edition of PDR provides detailed information on 700 over-the-counter remedies, as well as a number of home diagnostic tests and other medical aids for consumers.

Once again we're pleased to present an up-to-the-minute status report on the burgeoning use of over-the-counter drugs and their growing impact on health-care. The popularity of the self-care movement among consumers, increasing cost pressures throughout the healthcare system, and the expanding number of Rx-to-OTC conversions have all conspired to make nonprescription drugs an ever more significant factor in the healthcare equation. Our detailed analysis, which can be found in Section 5, spells out the changes and examines their effect on medical therapy.

As the role of over-the-counter drugs continues to expand, we feel certain that you'll find *PDR For Nonprescription Drugs* to be an increasingly important part of your working reference library. In conjunction with *Physicians' Desk Reference®* and *PDR For Ophthalmology®*, it supplies you with America's most authoritative, comprehensive, and reliable database of product-specific drug information. In turn, this core database is fully indexed in the 1,500 page *PDR Guide to Drug Interactions • Side Effects • Indications™.* An invaluable addition to the PDR library of drug references, the *PDR Guide* permits fast, easy identification of an adverse reaction's probable source — and the approved alternatives for the problem medication.

All of these volumes are now available in electronic form as part of the remarkable new *PDR® Electronic Library™* on CD-ROM, released this year in commemoration of PDR's fiftieth anniversary. This Windows-compatible disc provides users with a complete database of PDR prescribing information, electronically searchable for instant retrieval. A standard subscription includes PDR's sophisticated prescription-screening program and an exhaustive file of chemical structures, illustrations, and full-color product photographs. Optional enhancements include the complete contents of *The Merck Manual* and *Stedman's Medical Dictionary,* as well as a handy file of patient handouts drawn from PDR's consumer handbook, *The PDR® Family Guide to Prescription Drugs®.* The disc is available for use on individual PCs and PC networks.

For facilities with large, mainframe-based information systems, PDR information is also available as a pre-formatted text file on magnetic tape. For practitioners who seek drug interaction information drawn from the peer-reviewed clinical literature, there's the new *PDR® DrugREAX™* system, available for Windows-based PCs. And for personal use—on rounds or on the go—there's *Pocket PDR®,* a unique handheld electronic database of prescribing information that literally fits in your pocket.

In the current cost-conscious healthcare environment, you should also be aware of another of the newest members of the PDR family of references. Entitled *PDR® Generics™,* this exhaustive pharmaceutical compendium includes generic monographs covering virtually all prescription drugs—plus brand/generic unit cost comparisons, average generic prices by package size for all therapeutically equivalent products, and average wholesale prices of all available supplies. Drugs in this volume are indexed by brand and generic name, international trade name, therapeutic category, and indication. Off-label indications are included, and the volume boasts a unique cost-of-therapy section comparing the daily cost of the major pharmaceutical alternatives for a variety of common indications.

Also new and noteworthy is the *PDR® Medical Dictionary,* an authoritative reference that combines a complete medical lexicon with PDR's unparalleled database of brand and generic drug names, and the brand new *PDR® Nurse's Handbook™,* with over 1,400 pages of specially tailored drug information, including full details of the nursing considerations associated with each product.

For more information on any of these important references, please call, toll-free, 1-800-232-7379 or fax 201-573-4956.

Physicians' Desk Reference For Nonprescription Drugs is published annually by Medical Economics Company in cooperation with participating manufacturers. The function of the publisher is the compilation, organization, and distribution of product information obtained from manufacturers. Each product description has been prepared by the manufacturer, and edited and approved by the manufacturer's medical department, medical director, and/or medical consultant. During compilation of this information, the publisher has emphasized the necessity of describing products comprehensively, in order to provide all the facts necessary for sound and intelligent decision making. The descriptions seen here include all information made available by the manufacturer.

In organizing and presenting this material in *Physicians' Desk Reference For Nonprescription Drugs,* the publisher does not warrant or guarantee any of the products described, or perform any independent analysis in connection with any of the product information contained herein. *Physicians' Desk Reference For Nonprescription Drugs* does not assume, and expressly disclaims, any obligation to obtain and include any information other than that provided to it by the manufacturer. It should be understood that by making this material available the publisher is not advocating the use of any product described herein, nor is the publisher responsible for misuse of a product due to typographical error. Additional information on any product may be obtained from the manufacturer.

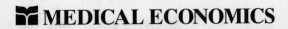
MEDICAL ECONOMICS

CONTENTS

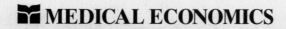

SECTION 1

MANUFACTURERS' INDEX

Listed in this index are all manufacturers that have supplied information in this edition. Each company's entry includes the address, phone, and fax number of its headquarters and regional offices, as well as contacts for inquiries, orders, and emergency information. A list of the company's major over-the-counter products is also included.

The ◆ symbol marks drugs shown in the Product Identification Guide. If a company has two page numbers, the first refers to its photographs in the "Product Identification Guide," the second to its prescribing information.

AK PHARMA **503, 602**
P.O. Box 111
Pleasantville, NJ 08232-0111
Direct Inquiries to:
Elizabeth Wexler
(609) 645-5100
FAX: (609) 645-0767
For Medical Emergencies Contact:
Leonard P. Smith
(609) 645-5100
FAX: (609) 645-0767

OTC Products Available:
◆ Beano

AMERICAN LIFELINE, INC. **602**
103 S. Second Street
Madison, WI 53704
Direct Inquiries to:
Dave Sullivan
(800) 257-5433
(608) 836-3477

OTC Products Available:
FLORAjen

AML LABORATORIES **602**
A Division of The Winning Combination
1753 Cloverfield Boulevard
Santa Monica, CA 90404
Direct Inquiries to:
(800) 800-1200

OTC Products Available:
Natural MD BASIC Rx
Breath + Plus
Complete Family Multi-Vitamin-Mineral Formulas

Common Sense Complete
Common Sense Complete with Extra Calcium and Iron
Complete for Men
Complete for Women
Natural MD Complete Rx
Fat Burning Factors
Fruit and Vegetable Safety Rinse
Stress Gum

B. F. ASCHER & **503, 606**
COMPANY, INC.
15501 West 109th Street
Lenexa, KS 66219
Mailing Address:
P.O. Box 717
Shawnee Mission, KS 66201-0717
Direct Inquiries to:
Joan F. Bowen
(913) 888-1880

OTC Products Available:
◆ Ayr Saline Nasal Drops
◆ Ayr Saline Nasal Gel
◆ Ayr Saline Nasal Mist
◆ Cough-X Lozenges
◆ Itch-X Gel
◆ Itch-X Spray
◆ Mobigesic Tablets
◆ Mobisyl Analgesic Creme

ASTRA USA, INC. **503, 608**
50 Otis Street
Westborough, MA 01581-4500
Direct Inquiries to:
Professional Information Department
(508) 366-1100
FAX: (508) 366-7406
For Medical Emergencies Contact:
Medical Information Services
(800) 262-0460

OTC Products Available:
◆ Xylocaine 2.5% Ointment

AYERST LABORATORIES
Division of American Home Products Corporation
685 Third Avenue
New York, NY 10017-4071
For information for Ayerst's consumer products, see product listings under Whitehall - Robins Healthcare.
Please turn to WHITEHALL - ROBINS HEALTHCARE

BAUSCH & LOMB **503, 608**
INCORPORATED
Personal Products Division
1400 North Goodman Street
P.O. Box 450
Rochester, NY 14692-0450
Direct Inquiries to:
Ronald M. Kline
(716) 338-5775
FAX: (716) 338-0184
For Medical Emergencies Contact:
Consumer Affairs
(800) 572-2931

OTC Products Available:
◆ Curel Lotion and Cream

BAYER CORPORATION **503, 608**
CONSUMER CARE DIVISION
36 Columbia Road
Morristown, NJ 07960-4518
Direct Inquiries to:
Consumer Affairs
(800) 331-4536

(◆) Shown in Product Identification Guide

BAYER CORPORATION
CONSUMER CARE DIVISION—*cont.*

For Medical Emergencies Contact:
Bayer Corporation
Consumer Care Division
(800) 331-4536

OTC Products Available:
- ◆ Actron Caplets and Tablets
- ◆ Alka-Mints Chewable Antacid
- ◆ Alka-Seltzer Cherry Effervescent Antacid and Pain Reliever
- ◆ Alka-Seltzer Extra Strength Effervescent Antacid and Pain Reliever
- ◆ Alka-Seltzer Fast Relief Caplets
- ◆ Alka-Seltzer Gold Effervescent Antacid
- ◆ Alka-Seltzer Lemon Lime Effervescent Antacid and Pain Reliever
- ◆ Alka-Seltzer Original Effervescent Antacid and Pain Reliever
- ◆ Alka-Seltzer Plus Cold Medicine
- ◆ Alka-Seltzer Plus Cold Medicine Liqui-Gels
- ◆ Alka-Seltzer Plus Cold & Cough Medicine
- ◆ Alka-Seltzer Plus Cold & Cough Medicine Liqui-Gels
- ◆ Alka-Seltzer Plus Flu & Body Aches Effervescent Tablets
- ◆ Alka-Seltzer Plus Flu & Body Aches Liqui-Gels Non-Drowsy Formula
- ◆ Alka-Seltzer Plus Night-Time Cold Medicine
- ◆ Alka-Seltzer Plus Night-Time Cold Medicine Liqui-Gels
- ◆ Alka-Seltzer Plus Sinus Medicine
- ◆ Bactine Antiseptic/Anesthetic First Aid Liquid
- Bactine First Aid Antibiotic Plus Anesthetic Ointment
- Bactine Hydrocortisone Anti-Itch Cream
- ◆ Extra Strength Bayer Arthritis Pain Regimen Formula
- ◆ Extra Strength Bayer Aspirin Caplets & Tablets
- ◆ Genuine Bayer Aspirin Tablets & Caplets
- ◆ Aspirin Regimen Bayer 81 mg Tablets with Calcium
- ◆ Aspirin Regimen Bayer Adult Low Strength 81 mg Tablets
- ◆ Aspirin Regimen Bayer Children's Chewable Aspirin
- ◆ Aspirin Regimen Bayer Regular Strength 325 mg Caplets
- ◆ Extended-Release Bayer 8-Hour Aspirin
- ◆ Extra Strength Bayer Plus Aspirin Caplets
- ◆ Extra Strength Bayer PM Aspirin Plus Sleep Aid
- Bayer Select Backache Pain Relief Formula
- Bayer Select Headache Pain Relief Formula
- Bayer Select Ibuprofen Pain Relief Formula
- Bayer Select Menstrual Multi-Symptom Formula
- Bayer Select Night Time Pain Relief Formula
- Bayer Select Sinus Pain Relief Formula
- Bronkaid Caplets
- Bronkaid Mist
- Bronkaid Mist Suspension
- ◆ Bugs Bunny Complete Children's Chewable Vitamins + Minerals with Iron and Calcium (Sugar Free)
- ◆ Bugs Bunny Plus Iron Children's Chewable Vitamins (Sugar Free)
- ◆ Bugs Bunny With Extra C Children's Chewable Vitamins (Sugar Free)
- Campho-Phenique Antiseptic Gel
- Campho-Phenique Cold Sore Gel
- Campho-Phenique Liquid
- Campho-Phenique Maximum Strength First Aid Antibiotic Plus Pain Reliever Ointment
- Dairy Ease Caplets and Tablets
- Dairy Ease Drops
- Dairy Ease Real Milk

- ◆ Domeboro Astringent Solution Effervescent Tablets
- ◆ Domeboro Astringent Solution Powder Packets
- ◆ Fergon Iron Supplement Tablets
- ◆ Flintstones Children's Chewable Vitamins
- ◆ Flintstones Children's Chewable Vitamins Plus Extra C
- ◆ Flintstones Children's Chewable Vitamins Plus Iron
- ◆ Flintstones Complete With Calcium, Iron & Minerals Children's Chewable Vitamins
- ◆ Flintstones Plus Calcium Children's Chewable Vitamins
- Haley's M-O, Regular & Flavored
- ◆ Maximum Strength Multi-Symptom Formula Midol
- Night Time Formula Midol PM
- ◆ PMS Multi-Symptom Formula Midol
- ◆ Maximum Strength Midol Teen Multi-Symptom Formula
- Miles Nervine Nighttime Sleep-Aid
- Mycelex OTC Cream Antifungal
- Mycelex OTC Solution Antifungal
- ◆ Mycelex-7 Vaginal Cream Antifungal
- ◆ Mycelex-7 Vaginal Antifungal Cream with 7 Disposable Applicators
- ◆ Mycelex-7 Vaginal Inserts Antifungal
- ◆ Mycelex-7 Combination-Pack Vaginal Inserts & External Vulvar Cream
- ◆ NāSal Moisturizer AF Nasal Drops
- ◆ NāSal Moisturizer AF Nasal Spray
- ◆ Neo-Synephrine Maximum Strength 12 Hour Nasal Spray
- ◆ Neo-Synephrine Maximum Strength 12 Hour Extra Moisturizing Nasal Spray
- ◆ Neo-Synephrine Maximum Strength 12 Hour Nasal Spray Pump
- ◆ Neo-Synephrine Nasal Drops, Pediatric, Mild, Regular & Extra Strength
- ◆ Neo-Synephrine Nasal Sprays, Pediatric, Mild, Regular & Extra Strength
- NTZ Long Acting Nasal Spray & Drops 0.05%
- ◆ One-A-Day Antioxidant Plus
- ◆ One-A-Day Calcium Plus
- ◆ One-A-Day Essential Vitamins with Beta Carotene
- ◆ One-A-Day Garlic Softgels
- ◆ One-A-Day Maximum
- ◆ One-A-Day Men's
- ◆ One-A-Day Women's
- ◆ One-A-Day 55 Plus
- ◆ Phillips' Gelcaps
- ◆ Phillips' Milk of Magnesia Liquid
- Stri-Dex Antibacterial Cleansing Bar
- Stri-Dex Antibacterial Face Wash
- Stri-Dex Clear Gel
- Stri-Dex Dual Textured Maximum Strength Pads
- Stri-Dex Maximum Strength Pads
- Stri-Dex Regular Strength Pads
- Stri-Dex Sensitive Skin Pads
- Stri-Dex Super Scrub Pads—Oil Fighting Formula
- ◆ Vanquish Analgesic Caplets

BEACH PHARMACEUTICALS 628
Division of Beach Products, Inc.
EXECUTIVE OFFICE:
5220 South Manhattan Avenue
Tampa, FL 33611
(813) 839-6565
Direct Inquiries to:
Victor De Oreo, R Ph, V.P., Sales:
(803) 277-7282
Richard Stephen Jenkins, Exec. V.P.:
(813) 839-6565
Manufacturing and Distribution:
Main Street at Perimeter Road
Conestee, SC 29605
(800) 845-8210

OTC Products Available:
Beelith Tablets

BEIERSDORF INC. 506, 628
360 Dr. Martin Luther King Dr.
Norwalk, CT 06856-5529
Direct Inquiries to:
Medical Division
(203) 853-8008
FAX: (203) 854-8180

OTC Products Available:
- ◆ Aquaphor Healing Ointment
- ◆ Aquaphor Healing Ointment, Original Formula
- Basis Facial Cleanser (Normal to Dry Skin)
- Basis Soap-Combination Skin
- Basis Soap-Extra Dry Skin
- Basis Soap-Normal to Dry Skin
- Basis Soap-Sensitive Skin
- ◆ Eucerin Cleansing Bar
- ◆ Eucerin Original Moisturizing Creme
- ◆ Eucerin Facial Moisturizing Lotion SPF 25
- ◆ Eucerin Original Moisturizing Lotion
- ◆ Eucerin Plus Alphahydroxy Moisturizing Creme
- ◆ Eucerin Plus Alphahydroxy Moisturizing Lotion
- Nivea Bath and Body Oil
- Nivea Creamy Conditioning Oil
- Nivea Moisturizing Body Wash
- Nivea Moisturizing Lotion (Extra Enriched)
- Nivea Moisturizing Lotion (Original Formula)
- Nivea Moisturizing Shower Gels
- Nivea Skin Oil
- Nivea Visage Facial Nourishing Creme
- Nivea Visage No Oil, All Moisture Hydrogel
- Nivea Visage Shine Control Matifying Fluid
- Nivea Visage UV Care Daily Moisture Lotion

BLAINE COMPANY, INC. 629
1465 Jamike Lane
Erlanger, KY 41018
Direct Inquiries to:
Mr. Alex M. Blaine
(800) 633-9353
FAX: (606) 283-9460

OTC Products Available:
Mag-Ox 400
Uro-Mag

BLAIREX LABORATORIES, INC. 630
3240 North Indianapolis Road
P.O. Box 2127
Columbus, IN 47202-2127
Direct Inquiries to:
Customer Service
(800) 252-4739
FAX: (812) 378-1033
For Medical Emergencies Contact:
Customer Service
(800) 252-4739
FAX: (812) 378-1033

OTC Products Available:
Broncho Saline
Nasal Moist
Pertussin Adult Extra Strength
Pertussin Children's Strength
Unit Dose Sterile Sodium Chloride Solutions

BLOCK DRUG 506, 631
COMPANY, INC.
257 Cornelison Avenue
Jersey City, NJ 07302
Direct Inquiries to:
Lori Hunt
(201) 434-3000, Ext. 1308

For Medical Emergencies Contact:
Consumer Service/Block
(201) 434-3000, Ext. 1308

OTC Products Available:
BC Powder
Arthritis Strength BC Powder
BC Cold Powder Multi-Symptom Formula
(Cold-Sinus-Allergy)
BC Cold Powder Non-Drowsy Formula
(Cold-Sinus)
Balmex Ointment
Goody's Extra Strength Headache
Powders
Goody's Extra Strength Pain Relief Tablets
Maximum Strength Nytol Caplets
Nytol QuickCaps Caplets
◆ Phazyme Drops
◆ Phazyme-95 Tablets
◆ Phazyme-125 Chewable Tablets
◆ Phazyme-125 Softgels Maximum Strength
Promise Sensitive Toothpaste
Cool Gel Sensodyne
Fresh Mint Sensodyne Toothpaste
Original Formula Sensodyne-SC
Toothpaste
Sensodyne with Baking Soda
Tegrin Dandruff Shampoo
Tegrin Skin Cream & Tegrin Medicated
Soap

BOIRON, THE WORLD LEADER ... 635 IN HOMEOPATHY

HEADQUARTERS AND EAST COAST
BRANCH:
6 Campus Blvd., Building A
Newtown Square, PA 19073
Direct Inquiries to:
John Durkin
East Coast Branch Manager
(800) 258-8823
For Medical Emergencies Contact:
Mark Land
Technical Services Manager
(610) 325-7464

WEST COAST BRANCH:
98C West Cochran Street
Simi Valley, CA 93065
Direct Inquiries to:
Ambroise Demonceaux
West Coast Branch Manager
(805) 582-9091

OTC Products Available:
Arnica & Calendula Gel
Arnicalm, the homeopathic bumps and
bruises medicine
Camilia, the homeopathic baby teething
medicine
Chestal, the homeopathic cough syrup
Cocyntal, the homeopathic baby colic
medicine
Coldcalm, the homeopathic cold medicine
Cyclease, the homeopathic cramp
medicine
Hayfever, the homeopathic pollen-allergy
medicine
Homeodent toothpaste
Natural Phases, the homeopathic PMS
medicine
Nervousness, the homeopathic stress
medicine
Optique 1, the homeopathic eye drop
Oscillococcinum
Quiétude the homeopathic sleep aid
Sinusitis, the homeopathic sinus
medicine
Sportenine, the homeopathic sports
medicine
Yeastaway, the homeopathic yeast
medicine

BRISTOL-MYERS .... 506, 635 PRODUCTS

A Bristol-Myers Squibb Company
345 Park Avenue
New York, NY 10154
Direct Inquiries to:
Bristol-Myers Products Division
Consumer Affairs Department
1350 Liberty Avenue
Hillside, NJ 07207
For Medical Emergencies Contact:
(800) 468-7746

OTC Products Available:
Alpha Keri Moisture Rich Body Oil
Alpha Keri Moisture Rich Cleansing Bar
Ammens Medicated Powder
Backache Caplets
BAN Antiperspirant Deodorant Cream
BAN Basic Non-Aerosol Antiperspirant
Spray
BAN Clear Antiperspirant
BAN Clear Roll-On
BAN for Men Clear Antiperspirant
BAN Roll-On Antiperspirant Deodorant
BAN Sensitive Touch Roll-On
Antiperspirant Deodorant
BAN Sensitive Touch Solid Antiperspirant
Deodorant
BAN Solid Antiperspirant Deodorant
◆ Bufferin Analgesic Tablets
◆ Arthritis Strength Bufferin Analgesic
Caplets
◆ Extra Strength Bufferin Analgesic Tablets
◆ Allergy-Sinus Comtrex Multi-Symptom
Allergy-Sinus Formula Tablets and
Caplets
Allergy-Sinus Comtrex Multi-Symptom
Day/Night Tablets and Caplets
Comtrex Multi-Symptom Cold Reliever
Liquid
◆ Comtrex Multi-Symptom Cold Reliever
Liqui-Gels
◆ Comtrex Multi-Symptom Cold Reliever
Tablets and Caplets
Comtrex Multi-Symptom Day/Night
Caplet-Tablet
◆ Comtrex Multi-Symptom Non-Drowsy
Caplets
Comtrex Multi-Symptom Non-Drowsy
Liqui-gels
◆ Aspirin Free Excedrin Analgesic Caplets
and Geltabs
◆ Excedrin Extra-Strength Analgesic Tablets
& Caplets
◆ Excedrin P.M. Analgesic/Sleeping Aid
Tablets, Caplets, Liquigels
Sinus Excedrin Analgesic, Decongestant
Tablets & Caplets
Fisherman's Friend Lozenges
Fostex 10% Benzoyl Peroxide Bar
Fostex 10% Benzoyl Peroxide (Vanish) Gel
Fostex 10% Benzoyl Peroxide Wash
Fostex Medicated Cleansing Bar
Fostex Medicated Cleansing Cream
◆ 4-Way Fast Acting Nasal Spray (regular &
mentholated)
◆ 4-Way 12 Hour Nasal Spray
KeriCort-10 Cream
◆ Keri Lotion - Original Formula
◆ Keri Lotion - Sensitive Skin
◆ Keri Lotion - Silky Smooth
Minit-Rub Analgesic Ointment
Mum Antiperspirant Cream Deodorant
Chewable NODOZ Tablets
No Doz Maximum Strength Caplets
Backache Caplets from Nuprin Analgesic
◆ Nuprin Ibuprofen/Analgesic Tablets &
Caplets
Pazo Hemorrhoid Ointment &
Suppositories
◆ Therapeutic Mineral Ice, Pain Relieving
Gel

Therapeutic Mineral Ice Exercise Formula,
Pain Relieving Gel

BURROUGHS WELLCOME CO
(See WARNER WELLCOME)

CAMPBELL LABORATORIES ..... 646 INC.

Direct Inquiries to:
James R. Stork, Vice President
P.O. Box 639
Deerfield Beach, FL 33443

OTC Products Available:
Herpecin-L Cold Sore Lip Balm

CARE-TECH LABORATORIES, ... 646 INC.

3224 South Kingshighway Boulevard
St. Louis, MO 63139
Direct Inquiries to:
Sherry L. Brereton
(314) 772-4610
FAX: (314) 772-4613
For Medical Emergencies Contact:
Customer Service
(800) 325-9681
FAX: (314) 772-4613

OTC Products Available:
Barri-Care Antimicrobial Barrier Ointment
Care Creme Antimicrobial Cream
CC-500 Antibacterial Skin Cleanser for
Dialysis Patient Care
Clinical Care Dermal Wound Cleanser
Concept Antimicrobial Skin Cleanser
Formula Magic Antibacterial Powder
Just Lotion - Highly Absorbent Aloe Vera
Glycerine Based Skin Lotion
Loving Lather II Antibacterial Skin
Cleanser
Loving Lotion Antibacterial Skin & Body
Lotion
Matrix Microclysmic Gel
Orchid Fresh II Perineal/Ostomy Cleanser
Satin Antimicrobial Skin Cleanser for
Diabetic/Cancer Patient Care
Skin Magic - Antimicrobial Body Rub &
Emollient
Soft Skin Non-greasy Bath Oil with Rich
Emollients for Severely Damaged
Dermal Tissue
Swirlsoft Whirlpool Emollient for Dry Skin
Conditions
Tech 2000 Antimicrobial Oral Rinse (No
Alcohol, No Sodium)
Techni-Care Surgical Scrub and Wound
Cleanser
Velvet Fresh Non-irritating Cornstarch
Baby Powder

J. R. CARLSON .... 647 LABORATORIES, INC.

15 College Drive
Arlington Heights, IL 60004-1985
Direct Inquiries to:
Customer Service
(708) 255-1600
FAX: (708) 255-1605
For Medical Emergencies Contact:
Customer Service
(708) 255-1600
FAX: (708) 255-1605

OTC Products Available:
ACES Antioxidant Soft Gels
E-Gems Soft Gels

CHURCH & DWIGHT CO., INC. 648

469 North Harrison Street
Princeton, NJ 08543-5297
Direct Inquiries to:
Cathy Marino
(609) 683-7015

(◆) Shown in Product Identification Guide

CHURCH & DWIGHT CO., INC.—*cont.*

For Medical Emergencies Contact:
HIS
(800) 228-5635
Extension 7

OTC Products Available:
Arm & Hammer Pure Baking Soda

**CIBA SELF-MEDICATION, ... 507, 648
INC.**
Division of CIBA-GEIGY Corporation
581 Main Street
Woodbridge, NJ 07095
Direct Inquiries to:
Nancy Casper
(908) 602-6000
FAX: (908) 602-6612
For Medical Emergencies Contact:
(908) 602-6780

OTC Products Available:
◆ Acutrim Late Day Strength Appetite
   Suppressant
◆ Acutrim Maximum Strength Appetite
   Suppressant
◆ Acutrim 16 Hour Steady Control Appetite
   Suppressant
   Allerest Eye Drops
   Allerest Maximum Strength
   Allerest No Drowsiness
   Allerest Sinus Pain Formula
   Americaine Hemorrhoidal Ointment
◆ Americaine Topical Anesthetic First Aid
   Ointment
◆ Americaine Topical Anesthetic Spray
◆ Arthritis Pain Ascriptin
◆ Maximum Strength Ascriptin
◆ Regular Strength Ascriptin Tablets
   Bacid Capsules
◆ Caldecort Anti-Itch Hydrocortisone Cream
◆ Caldecort Anti-Itch Hydrocortisone Spray
◆ Caldecort Light Cream
◆ Caldesene Medicated Ointment
◆ Caldesene Medicated Powder
◆ Cruex Antifungal Cream
◆ Cruex Antifungal Powder
◆ Cruex Antifungal Spray Powder
◆ Desenex Antifungal Ointment
◆ Desenex Antifungal Powder
◆ Desenex Antifungal Spray Powder
   Desenex Foot & Sneaker Deodorant
      Powder Plus
◆ Desenex Foot & Sneaker Deodorant
   Spray
◆ Prescription Strength Desenex AF Cream
◆ Prescription Strength Desenex Spray
   Powder and Spray Liquid
   Desenex Soap
◆ Doan's Extra-Strength Analgesic
◆ Doan's Regular Strength Analgesic
◆ Extra Strength Doan's P.M.
◆ Dulcolax Suppositories
◆ Dulcolax Tablets
◆ Efidac/24
◆ Efidac 24 Chlorpheniramine
◆ Eucalyptamint Arthritis Pain Reliever
   (External Analgesic)
◆ Eucalyptamint Muscle Pain Relief Formula
◆ Kondremul
◆ Maalox Antacid Caplets
◆ Maalox Antacid Plus Anti-Gas Tablets
◆ Maalox Anti-Diarrheal Caplets
◆ Maalox Anti-Gas Tablets, Regular Strength
◆ Maalox Anti-Gas Tablets, Extra Strength
   Maalox Heartburn Relief Suspension
◆ Maalox Magnesia and Alumina Oral
   Suspension
◆ Extra Strength Maalox Antacid Plus
      Antigas Liquid and Tablets
◆ Myoflex External Analgesic Creme
◆ 12 Hour Nöstrilla
◆ Nupercainal Hemorrhoidal and Anesthetic
   Ointment

◆ Nupercainal Hydrocortisone 1% Cream
◆ Nupercainal Pain Relief Cream
   Nupercainal Suppositories
◆ Otrivin Nasal Drops
◆ Otrivin Pediatric Nasal Drops
◆ Otrivin Nasal Spray
◆ Perdiem
◆ Perdiem Fiber
◆ Privine Nasal Drops
   Privine Nasal Spray
   Sinarest Tablets
   Sinarest Extra Strength Caplets
   Sinarest No Drowsiness Caplets
◆ Slow Fe Tablets
◆ Slow Fe with Folic Acid
◆ Sunkist Children's Chewable Multivitamins
      - Complete
◆ Sunkist Children's Chewable Multivitamins
      - Plus Extra C
◆ Sunkist Children's Chewable Multivitamins
      - Plus Iron
◆ Sunkist Children's Chewable Multivitamins
      - Regular
◆ Sunkist Vitamin C - Chewable
◆ Sunkist Vitamin C - Easy to Swallow
◆ Ting Antifungal Cream
◆ Ting Antifungal Powder
◆ Ting Antifungal Spray Liquid
   Ting Antifungal Spray Powder
   Vitron-C Tablets

**DEL PHARMACEUTICALS, .. 509, 667
INC.**
A Subsidiary of Del Laboratories, Inc.
163 East Bethpage Road
Plainview, NY 11803
Direct Inquiries to:
Charles J. Hinkaty, President
(516) 844-2020
FAX: (516) 293-9018
For Medical Emergencies Contact:
Serap Ozelkan,
Director of Pharmaceutical Development
(516) 844-2020

OTC Products Available:
◆ ArthriCare Odor Free Rub
◆ ArthriCare Triple Medicated Rub
   Auro-Dri Ear Water-Drying Aid
   Auro Ear Wax Removal Aid
   Boil-Ease Pain Relieving Ointment
   Dermarest DriCort Anti-Itch Creme
   Dermarest Plus Gel
   Detane Desensitizing Lubricant
   Diaper Guard Skin Rash Ointment
   Exocaine Analgesic Rubs
   Off-Ezy Wart Remover
   Baby Orajel Nighttime Formula
◆ Baby Orajel Teething Pain Medicine
◆ Baby Orajel Tooth & Gum Cleanser
◆ Orajel CoverMed Tinted Cold Sore
   Medicine
   Orajel Denture Pain Medicine
◆ Orajel Maximum Strength Toothache
   Medication
◆ Orajel Mouth-Aid for Canker and Cold
   Sores
◆ Orajel Perioseptic Oxygenating Liquid
◆ Pronto Lice Killing Shampoo &
   Conditioner in One Kit
◆ Pronto Lice Killing Spray
   Propa pH Acne Medications
   Skin Shield Liquid Bandage
   Stye Ophthalmic Ointment
◆ Tanac Medicated Gel
◆ Tanac No Sting Liquid
   Triptone for Motion Sickness

**EFFCON 510, 670
LABORATORIES, INC.**
P.O. Box 7499
Marietta, GA 30065-1499

Direct Inquiries to:
Customer Service
(800) 722-2428
FAX: (770) 428-6811
For Medical Emergencies Contact:
J. Kent Burklow
(800) 722-2428
FAX: (770) 428-6811

OTC Products Available:
◆ Pin-X Pinworm Treatment

**FISONS CORPORATION 670
PRESCRIPTION PRODUCTS**
755 Jefferson Road
Rochester, NY 14623
Mailing Address:
P.O. Box 1766
Rochester, NY 14603
Direct Inquiries to:
Medical Information Department
P.O. Box 1766
Rochester, NY 14603
(716) 475-9000

OTC Products Available:
Delsym Extended-Release Suspension

FLEMING & COMPANY........... 670
1600 Fenpark Dr.
Fenton, MO 63026
Direct Inquiries to:
John J. Roth, M.D.
(314) 343-8200
For Medical Emergencies Contact:
John R. Roth, M.D.
(314) 343-8200

OTC Products Available:
Chlor-3 Condiment
Impregon Concentrate
Magonate Tablets and Liquid
Marblen Suspension Peach/Apricot
Marblen Tablets
Nephrox Suspension
Nicotinex Elixir
Ocean Nasal Mist
Purge Concentrate

A. C. GRACE COMPANY 671
1100 Quitman Rd., P.O. Box 570
Big Sandy, TX 75755
Direct Inquiries To:
Roy Erickson
(903) 636-4368
FAX : (903) 636-4051
For Medical Emergencies Contact:
Roy Erickson
(903) 636-4368
FAX : (903) 636-4051

OTC Products Available:
Unique E Vitamin E Capsules

**HOGIL 510, 672
PHARMACEUTICAL CORP.**
Two Manhattanville Road
Purchase, NY 10577
Direct Inquiries To:
Tanya Castagna
(914) 696-7600
FAX: (914) 696-4600
For Medical Emergencies Contact:
Dr. Gilbert Spector
(914) 696-7600
FAX: (914) 696-4600

OTC Products Available:
◆ A-200 Lice Control Spray
◆ A-200 Lice Killing Gel
◆ A-200 Lice Killing Shampoo
   A-200 Lice Treatment Kit
◆ InnoGel Plus
   Innomed Lice Treatment Kit

(◆) Shown in Product Identification Guide

Psor-A-Set Liquid, Shampoo, & Soap
Sine-Off No Drowsiness Formula Caplets
Sine-Off Sinus Medicine Caplets
Teldrin 12 Hour Antihistamine/Nasal
   Decongestant Allergy Relief Caplets

INTER-CAL CORPORATION 673
533 Madison Avenue
Prescott, AZ 86301
Direct Inquiries to:
Dr. Jack Hegenauer
(520) 445-8063
FAX: (520) 778-7986
For Medical Emergencies Contact:
Dr. Jack Hegenauer
(520) 445-8063
FAX: (520) 778-7986

OTC Products Available:
Ester-C Mineral Ascorbates Powder

IYATA PHARMACEUTICAL, INC ... 674
735 North Water Street
Suite 612
Milwaukee, WI 53202
Direct Inquiries to:
Michael B. Adekunle, M.D.
(414) 272-1982
FAX: (414) 272-2919
For Medical Emergencies Contact:
Michael B. Adekunle, M.D.
(414) 272-1982
(800) 809-7918
FAX: (414) 272-2919

OTC Products Available:
Capsagel

JOHNSON & JOHNSON • 510, 675
MERCK CONSUMER
PHARMACEUTICALS CO.
Camp Hill Road
Fort Washington, PA 19034
Direct Inquiries to:
Consumer Affairs Department
(215) 233-7000
For Medical Emergencies Contact:
(215) 233-7000

OTC Products Available:
◆ ALternaGEL Liquid
◆ Dialose Tablets
◆ Dialose Plus Tablets
◆ Mylanta Gas Relief Gelcaps
◆ Mylanta Gas Relief Tablets
◆ Maximum Strength Mylanta Gas Relief
   Tablets
◆ Mylanta Gelcaps Antacid
◆ Mylanta Liquid
◆ Mylanta Soothing Lozenges
◆ Mylanta Tablets
◆ Mylanta Double Strength Liquid
◆ Mylanta Double Strength Tablets
◆ Infants' Mylicon Drops
◆ Pepcid AC Acid Controller

KONSYL PHARMACEUTICALS, ... 679
INC.
4200 South Hulen
Ft. Worth, TX 76109
Direct Inquiries to:
Bill Steiber
(817) 763-8011 Ext. 23
FAX: (817) 731-9389

OTC Products Available:
Konsyl Fiber Tablets
Konsyl Powder Sugar Free Unflavored

KYOLIC LTD., ... 523, 680
DIVISION OF
WAKUNAGA OF AMERICA
CO., LTD.
Subsidiary of Wakunaga Pharmaceutical
Co., Ltd.
23501 Madero
Mission Viejo, CA 92691
Direct Inquiries to:
(800) 421-2998

OTC Products Available:
Be Sure
Ginkgo Biloba Plus
Kyo-Chrome
Kyo-Dophilus
   Acidophilase Capsules: L. acidophilus,
     B. bifidum, amylase, protease, lipase
   Kyo-Dophilus Capsules: L. acidophilus,
     B. longum, B. bifidum
   Kyo-Dophilus Chewable Tablets: L.
     acidophilus
Kyo-Green Powder: Barley & wheat grass,
   chlorella, kelp, brown rice
◆ Kyolic Aged Garlic Extract Caplets
Kyolic Aged Garlic Extract Flavor and Odor
   Modified Plain Liquid
Kyolic Reserve Capsules: Aged garlic
   extract powder (600mg)
Kyolic—Super Formula 100 Tablets &
   Capsules: Aged garlic extract powder
   (300mg), whey
Kyolic—Super Formula 101 Garlic Plus:
   Tablets & Capsules: Aged garlic
   extract powder (270mg), whey,
   brewer's yeast, kelp, algin
Kyolic—Super Formula 102 Tablets &
   Capsules: Aged garlic extract powder
   (350mg), amylase, protease,
   cellulase, lipase
Kyolic—Super Formula 103 Capsules:
   Aged garlic extract powder (220mg),
   Ester C, astragalus, calcium
Kyolic—Super Formula 104 Capsules:
   Aged garlic extract powder (300mg),
   lecithin
Kyolic—Super Formula 105 Capsules:
   Aged garlic extract powder (200mg),
   beta carotene, vitamin C, vitamin E,
   selenium, green tea
Kyolic—Super Formula 106 Capsules:
   Aged garlic extract powder (300mg),
   hawthorne berry, vitamin E, cayenne
   pepper
Premium Kyolic-EPA Gel Caps: Aged garlic
   extract powder (120mg), fish oil [EPA
   (280mg), DHA (120mg)]
Pro Formula 1000 A.G.E./SGP: Aged
   Garlic Extract Powder (350mg)

LAVOPTIK COMPANY, INC........ 681
661 Western Avenue North
St. Paul, MN 55103
Direct Inquiries to:
661 Western Avenue North
St. Paul, MN 55103-1694
(612) 489-1351
For Medical Emergencies Contact:
B. C. Brainard
(612) 489-1351
FAX: (612) 489-0760

OTC Products Available:
Lavoptik Eye Cup
Lavoptik Eye Wash

LEDERLE CONSUMER 511, 681
HEALTH
A Division of Whitehall-Robins Healthcare
Five Giralda Farms
Madison, NJ 07940
Direct Inquiries to:
Lederle Consumer Product Information
(800) 282-8805

Distribution Centers:
GARDEN GROVE
   11700 Monarch Street
   Garden Grove, CA 92641
   (714) 891-3743
   Attn: Richard A. Benvenuti
DES PLAINS
   1908 S. Mount Prospect Road
   Des Plains, IL 60018
   (708) 299-2206
   Attn: James P. Smith
DALLAS
   4116 Bronze Way
   Dallas, TX 75237
   (214) 399-8361
   Attn: Thomas G. Culp
RICHMOND
   2300 Darbytown Road
   Richmond, VA 23231
   (804) 226-6700
   Attn: J. Stuart Smith
KINNESAW
   1000 Union Court
   Kennesaw, GA 30144
   (404) 421-0039
   Attn: E. Norman Blackwell
FRAZER
   31 Morehall Road
   Frazer, PA 19355
   (610) 644-8000
   Attn: Douglas M. Holste

OTC Products Available:
◆ Caltrate PLUS
Caltrate 600
Caltrate 600 + D
◆ Centrum
◆ Centrum, Jr. (Children's Chewable) +
   Extra C
Centrum, Jr. (Children's Chewable) +
   Extra Calcium
Centrum, Jr. (Children's Chewable) + Iron
◆ Centrum Silver
Ferro-Sequels
◆ FiberCon Caplets
◆ Protegra Antioxidant Vitamin & Mineral
   Supplement
Stresstabs
◆ Stresstabs + Iron
Stresstabs + Zinc

LENES PHARMACAL, ... 511, 686
INC.
1990 S.W. 27th Avenue
Miami, FL 33145
Direct Inquiries to:
P.O. Box 45-1350
(305) 858-8111
FAX: (305) 859-7227
For Medical Emergencies Contact:
Abdon S. Borges Jr., M.D.
(305) 858-8111
FAX: (305) 859-7227

OTC Products Available:
◆ Venolax

LEVER BROTHERS.......... 512, 686
390 Park Avenue
New York, NY 10022
Direct Inquiries to:
(212) 688-6000

OTC Products Available:
◆ Dove Bar (Original, Unscented, and
   Sensitive Skin Formula)
Dove Moisturizing Body Wash
Liquid Dove Beauty Wash
◆ Lever 2000 Antibacterial Bar and Liquid

(◆) Shown in Product Identification Guide

3M PERSONAL HEALTH CARE 512, 686

Bldg. 515-3N-02
St. Paul, MN 55144-1000
Direct Inquiries to:
Customer Service
(800) 537-2191
For Medical Emergencies Contact:
(612) 733-2882 (answered 24 hrs.)
Sales and Ordering or Returns:
(800) 832-2189

OTC Products Available:
◆ Titralac Antacid Regular
◆ Titralac Antacid Extra Strength
◆ Titralac Plus Liquid
◆ Titralac Plus Tablets

MARLYN NUTRACEUTICALS 687

14851 North Scottsdale Road
Scottsdale, AZ 85254 USA
(800) 462-7596
(602) 991-0200
Direct Inquiries to:
Kelly Easton
(602) 991-0200
FAX: (602) 991-0551

OTC Products Available:
4-Beauty
4-Hair, Internal
4-Hair, Topical
4-Nails, Internal
4-Nails, Topical
Hep-Forte Capsules
Marlyn Formula 50 Capsules
Marlyn PMS
Osteo Fem
Pro Skin, Internal
Pro Skin, Topical

McNEIL CONSUMER .... 512, 687 PRODUCTS CO.

Division of McNeil-PPC, Inc.
Camp Hill Road
Fort Washington, PA 19034
Direct Inquiries to:
Consumer Affairs Department
Fort Washington, PA 19034
(215) 233-7000
Manufacturing Divisions:
Fort Washington, PA 19034

Southwest Manufacturing Plant
4001 N. I-35
Round Rock, TX 78664

Road 183 KM 19.8
Barrios Montones
Las Piedras, Puerto Rico 00771

OTC Products Available:
◆ Children's Motrin Ibuprofen Oral
  Suspension
◆ Children's TYLENOL acetaminophen
  Chewable Tablets, Elixir, Suspension
  Liquid
◆ Children's TYLENOL Cold Multi Symptom
  Chewable Tablets and Liquid
◆ Children's TYLENOL Cold Plus Cough Multi
  Symptom Chewable Tablets and
  Liquid
◆ Imodium A-D Caplets and Liquid
◆ Infants' TYLENOL acetaminophen Drops
  and Suspension Drops
◆ Infants' TYLENOL Cold Decongestant &
  Fever Reducer Drops
◆ Junior Strength TYLENOL acetaminophen
  Coated Caplets and Chewable Tablets
◆ Lactaid Drops
◆ Lactaid Extra Strength Caplets
◆ Lactaid Original Strength Caplets
◆ PediaCare Cough-Cold Chewable Tablets
  and Liquid

◆ PediaCare Infants' Decongestant Drops
◆ PediaCare Infants' Drops Decongestant
  Plus Cough
◆ PediaCare Night Rest Cough-Cold Liquid
◆ Sine-Aid Maximum Strength Sinus
  Headache Gelcaps, Caplets and
  Tablets
◆ TYLENOL acetaminophen Extended Relief
  Caplets
  TYLENOL acetaminophen, Extra Strength
  Adult Liquid Pain Reliever
◆ TYLENOL acetaminophen, Extra Strength
  Gelcaps, Caplets, Tablets, Geltabs
◆ TYLENOL acetaminophen, Regular
  Strength, Caplets and Tablets
◆ TYLENOL Allergy Sinus Medication,
  Maximum Strength Caplets, Gelcaps,
  and Geltabs
◆ TYLENOL Allergy Sinus Medication
  NightTime, Maximum Strength Caplets
◆ TYLENOL Cold Medication, Multi Symptom
  Caplets and Tablets
◆ TYLENOL Cold Medication, Multi Symptom
  Hot Liquid Packets
◆ TYLENOL Cold Medication, No Drowsiness
  Formula Caplets and Gelcaps
◆ TYLENOL Cough Medication, Multi
  Symptom
◆ TYLENOL Cough Medication with
  Decongestant, Multi Symptom
◆ TYLENOL Flu NightTime, Maximum
  Strength Gelcaps
◆ TYLENOL Flu NightTime, Maximum
  Strength Hot Medication Packets
◆ TYLENOL Flu No Drowsiness Formula,
  Maximum Strength Gelcaps
◆ TYLENOL Headache Plus Pain Reliever
  with Antacid, Extra Strength Caplets
◆ TYLENOL PM Pain Reliever/Sleep Aid,
  Extra Strength Gelcaps, Caplets,
  Geltabs
◆ TYLENOL Severe Allergy Medication
  Caplets
◆ TYLENOL Sinus Medication, Maximum
  Strength Geltabs, Gelcaps, Caplets,
  Tablets

MEAD JOHNSON .... 708 NUTRITIONALS

Mead Johnson & Company
A Bristol-Myers Squibb Company
2400 W. Lloyd Expressway
Evansville, IN 47721
Direct Inquiries to:
Product Information Section
Medical Services Department
(812) 429-5599

OTC Products Available:
Enfamil Human Milk Fortifier
Enfamil Infant Formula
Enfamil With Iron Infant Formula
Enfamil Next Step Toddler Formula
Enfamil Next Step Soy Toddler Formula
Enfamil Premature Formula
Enfamil Premature Formula With Iron
Fer-In-Sol Iron Supplement Drops, Syrup,
  Capsules
Infalyle Oral Electrolyte Maintenance
  Solution made with Rice Syrup Solids
Kinderkal
Lactofree Milk-Based, Lactose-Free
  Formula
Lofenalac Iron Fortified Low Phenylalanine
  Diet Powder
Metabolic Modules, Special
  HIST 1
  HIST 2
  HOM 1
  HOM 2
  LYS 1
  LYS 2
  MSUD 1
  MSUD 2
  OS 1

  OS 2
  PKU 1
  PKU 2
  PKU 3
  Product 80056 Protein-Free Diet
    Powder
  TYR 1
  TYR 2
  UCD 1
  UCD 2
Moducal Dietary Carbohydrate Powder
MSUD Diet Powder
Nutramigen Hypoallergenic Protein
  Hydrolysate Formula
Phenyl-Free Phenylalanine-Free Diet
  Powder
Poly-Vi-Sol Vitamins, Chewable Tablets
  and Drops (without Iron)
Poly-Vi-Sol Vitamins, Peter Rabbit Shaped
  Chewable Tablets (without Iron)
Poly-Vi-Sol Vitamins with Iron, Peter Rabbit
  Shaped Chewable Tablets
Poly-Vi-Sol Vitamins with Iron, Drops
Portagen Iron Fortified Powder with
  Medium Chain Triglycerides
Pregestimil Iron Fortified Protein
  Hydrolysate Formula with Medium
  Chain Triglycerides
Product 3200AB Low PHE/TYR Diet
  Powder
Product 3200K Low Methionine Diet
  Powder
Product 3232A Mono and
  Disaccharide-Free Diet Powder
ProSobee Soy Formula
Theragran Tablets
Theragran-M Tablets
Tri-Vi-Sol Vitamin Drops
Tri-Vi-Sol Vitamin Drops with Iron

THE MENTHOLATUM .... 709 COMPANY, INC.

1360 Niagara Street
Buffalo, NY 14213
Direct Inquiries to:
Director of Consumer Affairs
(716) 882-7660
FAX: (716) 882-6563
For Medical Emergencies Contact:
Dr. Henry Chan
(716) 882-7660
FAX: (716) 882-6563

OTC Products Available:
Fletcher's Castoria
Fletcher's Cherry Flavor
Medi-Quik
Mentholatum Cherry Chest Rub for Kids
Mentholatum Deep Heating Extra
  Strength Formula Rub
Mentholatum Menthacin
Mentholatum Ointment
Red Cross Toothache Medication
Unguentine Plus

MILES INC. CONSUMER HEALTHCARE PRODUCTS

(See BAYER CORPORATION CONSUMER
CARE DIVISION)

MURO PHARMACEUTICAL, ... 712 INC.

890 East Street
Tewksbury, MA 01876-1496
Direct Inquiries to:
Professional Service Department
(800) 225-0974
(508) 851-5981

OTC Products Available:
Bromfed Syrup
Guaifed Syrup
Salinex Nasal Mist and Drops

(◆) Shown in Product Identification Guide

NICHE PHARMACEUTICALS, ... 713
INC.
200 N. Oak Street
P.O. Box 449
Roanoke, TX 76262
Direct Inquiries to:
Steve F. Brandon
(817) 491-2770
FAX: (817) 491-3533
For Medical Emergencies Contact:
Gerald L. Beckloff, M.D.
(817) 491-2770
FAX: (817) 491-3533

OTC Products Available:
MagTab SR Caplets
Unifiber

OHM LABORATORIES, INC........ 713
P.O. Box 7397
North Brunswick, NJ 08902
Direct Inquiries to:
Alan Korn
(800) 527-6481
FAX: (908) 247-0268

OTC Products Available:
Acetaminophen 325 mg White Bisected
  Tablets
Acetaminophen 500 mg Red/White
  Capsules
Acetaminophen 500 mg White Bisected
  Tablets
Acetaminophen 500 mg White Film
  Coated Caplets
Bisacodyl USP 5 mg Yellow Sugar Enteric
  Coated Tablets
Ibuprofen 200 mg USP White Sugar
  Coated Tablets
Ibuprofen 200 mg USP White Sugar
  Coated Tablets
Ibuprohm (Ibuprofen) Caplets, 200 mg
Ibuprohm (Ibuprofen) Tablets, 200 mg
Loperamide HCl 2.0 mg Light Green
  Caplets
Pseudoephedrine HCl 30 mg Red Sugar
  Coated Tablets
Pseudoephedrine HCl 60 mg White
  Bisected Tablets
Pseudoephedrine HCl 30 mg +
  Acetaminophen 500 mg Peach Caplets
Pseudoephedrine HCl 60 mg +
  Chlorpheniramine Maleate 4 mg White
  Bisected Tablets
Senna Concentrate Army Green Tablets
Yellow Phenolphthalein 90 mg Beige
  Sugar Coated Tablets

P & S LABORATORIES
(See STANDARD HOMEOPATHIC COMPANY)

PARKE-DAVIS
(See WARNER WELLCOME)

THE PARTHENON COMPANY, ... 714
INC.
3311 West 2400 South
Salt Lake City, UT 84119
Direct Inquiries to:
(801) 972-5184
FAX: (801) 972-4734
For Medical Emergencies Contact:
Nick G. Mihalopoulos
(801) 972-5184

OTC Products Available:
Devrom Chewable Tablets

PFIZER INC 515, 714
CONSUMER HEALTH
CARE GROUP
Division of Pfizer Inc.
235 E. 42nd Street
New York, NY 10017-5755

Direct Inquiries & Comments to:
Consumer Relations
(800) 723-7529
For Medical Emergencies/Information
Contact:
(800) 723-7529

OTC Products Available:
◆ BenGay External Analgesic Products
  Bonine Tablets
◆ Daily Care from DESITIN
◆ Desitin Cornstarch Baby Powder
◆ Desitin Ointment
  Rheaban Maximum Strength Fast Acting
    Caplets
  Rid Lice Control Spray
  Rid Lice Killing Shampoo
  Maximum Strength Unisom Sleepgels
  Unisom Nighttime Sleep Aid
  Unisom With Pain Relief-Nighttime Sleep
    Aid and Pain Reliever
◆ Visine Maximum Strength Allergy Relief
◆ Visine L.R. Eye Drops
◆ Visine Moisturizing Eye Drops
◆ Visine Original Eye Drops
  Wart-Off Wart Remover

PHARMATON NATURAL 515, 721
HEALTH PRODUCTS
A Division of Boehringer
Ingelheim Pharmaceutical
Inc.
900 Ridgebury Road
Ridgefield, CT 06877
Direct Inquiries to:
Customer Service
(800) 243-0127
FAX: (203) 798-5771
For Medical Emergencies Contact:
Marvin Wetter, M.D.
(203) 798-4361
FAX: (203) 798-5771

OTC Products Available:
◆ Ginkoba
◆ Ginsana

PLOUGH, INC.
(See SCHERING-PLOUGH HEALTHCARE
PRODUCTS)

PREMIER, INC. 722
Greenwich Office Park One
Greenwich, CT 06831
Direct Inquiries to:
Robert Albus
(203) 622-1211
FAX: (203) 622-0773
For Medical Emergencies Contact:
Sergio Nacht, Ph.D.
(415) 366-2626
FAX: (415) 368-4470
Subash J. Saxena, Ph.D.
(415) 366-2626
FAX: (415) 368-4470
Branch Office:
3696 Haven Avenue
Redwood City, CA 94063
(415) 366-2626
FAX: (415) 368-4470

OTC Products Available:
Exact Adult Acne Medication
Exact Cleansing Wipes
Exact Face Wash
Exact Pore Treatment Gel
Exact Vanishing and Tinted Creams

PROCTER & GAMBLE 515, 722
P.O. Box 5516
Cincinnati, OH 45201
Direct Inquiries to:
Charles Lambert
(800) 358-8707

For Medical Emergencies:
Call Collect: (513) 558-4422

OTC Products Available:
◆ Aleve
  Children's Vicks Chloraseptic Sore Throat
    Lozenges
  Children's Vicks Chloraseptic Sore Throat
    Spray
  Children's Vicks DayQuil Allergy Relief
  Children's Vicks NyQuil Cold/Cough Relief
  Crest Sensitivity Protection Toothpaste
  Head & Shoulders Intensive Treatment
    Dandruff and Seborrheic Dermatitis
    Shampoo
  Metamucil Effervescent Sugar-Free,
    Lemon-Lime Flavor
  Metamucil Effervescent Sugar-Free,
    Orange Flavor
  Metamucil Powder, Original Texture
    Orange Flavor
  Metamucil Powder, Original Texture
    Regular Flavor
◆ Metamucil Smooth Texture Powder,
    Orange Flavor
  Metamucil Smooth Texture Powder,
    Sugar-Free, Regular Flavor
  Metamucil Smooth Texture Powder,
    Sugar-Free, Orange Flavor
  Metamucil Smooth Texture, Citrus Flavor
  Metamucil Smooth Texture, Sugar-Free,
    Citrus Flavor
◆ Metamucil Wafers, Apple Crisp &
    Cinnamon Spice Flavors
  Oil of Olay Daily UV Protectant SPF 15
    Beauty Fluid-Original and Fragrance
    Free (Olay Co. Inc.)
  Original Vicks Cough Drops, Menthol and
    Cherry Flavors
  Pediatric Vicks 44d Cough & Head
    Congestion Relief
  Pediatric Vicks 44e Cough & Chest
    Congestion Relief
  Pediatric Vicks 44m Cough & Cold Relief
  Pepto Diarrhea Control
  Pepto-Bismol Original Liquid, Original and
    Cherry Tablets & Easy-to-Swallow
    Caplets
  Pepto-Bismol Maximum Strength Liquid
  Percogesic Analgesic Tablets
  Vicks 44 Cough Relief
  Vicks 44 LiquiCaps Cough, Cold & Flu
    Relief
  Vicks 44 LiquiCaps Non-Drowsy Cough &
    Cold Relief
  Vicks 44D Cough & Head Congestion
    Relief
  Vicks 44E Cough & Chest Congestion
    Relief
  Vicks 44M Cough, Cold & Flu Relief
  Vicks Chloraseptic Cough & Throat Drops,
    Menthol, Cherry and Honey Lemon
    Flavors
  Vicks Chloraseptic Sore Throat Lozenges,
    Menthol and Cherry Flavors
  Vicks Chloraspetic Sore Throat Spray,
    Gargle and Mouth Rinse, Menthol and
    Cherry Flavors
  Vicks Cough Drops, Menthol and Cherry
    Flavors
  Vicks DayQuil Allergy Relief 12-Hour
    Extended Release Tablets
  Vicks DayQuil Allergy Relief 4-Hour Tablets
  Vicks DayQuil LiquiCaps/Liquid
    Multi-Symptom Cold/Flu Relief
  Vicks DayQuil SINUS Pressure &
    CONGESTION Relief
  Vicks DayQuil SINUS Pressure & PAIN
    Relief with IBUPROFEN
  Vicks Nyquil Hot Therapy
  Vicks NyQuil LiquiCaps/Liquid
    Multi-Symptom Cold/Flu Relief,
    Original and Cherry Flavors
  Vicks Sinex 12-Hour Nasal Decongestant
    Spray and Ultra Fine Mist

(◆) Shown in Product Identification Guide

(◆) Shown in Product Identification Guide

SCHERING CORPORATION
(See SCHERING-PLOUGH HEALTHCARE PRODUCTS)

SCHERING-PLOUGH 518, 757
HEALTHCARE PRODUCTS
110 Allen Road
Liberty Corner, NJ 07938
Direct Product Requests to:
Public Relations
(908) 604-1836
For Medical Emergencies Contact:
Clinical Department
(901) 320-2998

OTC Products Available:
◆ A and D Medicated Diaper Rash Ointment
◆ A and D Ointment
Afrin Cherry Scented Nasal Spray 0.05%
◆ Afrin Extra Moisturizing Nasal Spray
Afrin Menthol Nasal Spray, 0.05%
◆ Afrin Nasal Spray 0.05% and Nasal Spray Pump
Afrin Nose Drops 0.05%
◆ Afrin Saline Mist
Afrin Sinus
◆ Chlor-Trimeton Allergy Decongestant Tablets
Chlor-Trimeton Allergy-Sinus Headache Caplets
◆ Chlor-Trimeton Allergy Tablets
◆ Coppertone Skin Selects Sunscreen Lotion SPF 15 For Dry Skin
◆ Coppertone Skin Selects Sunscreen Lotion SPF 15 For Oily Skin
◆ Coppertone Skin Selects Sunscreen Lotion SPF 15 For Sensitive Skin
◆ Coricidin Cold + Flu Tablets
◆ Coricidin Cough + Cold Tablets
◆ Coricidin 'D' Decongestant Tablets
◆ Correctol Extra Gentle Stool Softener
◆ Correctol Herbal Tea Laxative
◆ Correctol Laxative Tablets & Caplets
Di-Gel Antacid/Anti-Gas
◆ Drixoral Allergy/Sinus Extended Release Tablets
◆ Drixoral Cold and Allergy Sustained-Action Tablets
◆ Drixoral Cold and Flu Extended-Release Tablets
◆ Drixoral Cough Liquid Caps
◆ Drixoral Cough + Congestion Liquid Caps
◆ Drixoral Cough + Sore Throat Liquid Caps
◆ Drixoral Non-Drowsy Formula Extended-Release Tablets
◆ DuoFilm Liquid Wart Remover
◆ DuoFilm Patch Wart Remover
◆ DuoPlant Gel Plantar Wart Remover
Duration 12 Hour Nasal Spray
◆ Lotrimin AF Antifungal Cream, Lotion and Solution
◆ Lotrimin AF Antifungal Spray Liquid, Spray Powder, Spray Deodorant Powder, Powder and Jock Itch Spray Powder
◆ Shade Gel SPF 30 Sunblock
◆ Shade Lotion SPF 45 Sunblock
◆ Shade UVAGUARD SPF 15 Suncreen Lotion
◆ St. Joseph Adult Chewable Aspirin (81 mg.)

SIMILASAN CORPORATION 769
1321 S. Central Avenue
Kent, WA 98032
Direct Inquiries to:
Brian S. Banks
(800) 426-1644
(305) 859-9072
FAX: (305) 859-9102
For Medical Emergencies Contact:
Alfred Knaus
(800) 426-1644
(305) 859-9072
FAX: (305) 859-9102

OTC Products Available:
Similasan Cold Drops #1, 2 & 3
Similasan Colds and Influenza
Similasan Cough Drops #1, 2 & 3
Similasan Eye Drops #1
Similasan Eye Drops #2
Similasan Hayfever Drops #1
Similasan Nasal Spray
Similasan Sore Throat Drops #1 & 2

SMITHKLINE BEECHAM 519, 770
CONSUMER
HEALTHCARE, L.P.
Unit of SmithKline Beecham, Inc.
P.O. Box 1467
Pittsburgh, PA 15230
For Medical Information Contact:
(800) 245-1040 (Consumer Inquiries)
(800) 378-4055 (Healthcare Professional Inquiries)
Direct Healthcare Professional Sample Requests to:
(800) BEECHAM

OTC Products Available:
◆ CĒPASTAT Cherry Flavor Sore Throat Lozenges
◆ CĒPASTAT Extra Strength Sore Throat Lozenges
◆ CITRUCEL Orange Flavor
◆ CITRUCEL Sugar Free Orange Flavor
◆ Contac Allergy 12 Hour Tablets
◆ Contac Continuous Action Nasal Decongestant/Antihistamine 12 Hour Capsules
◆ Contac Day Allergy/Sinus Caplets
◆ Contac Day & Night Cold/Flu Caplets
◆ Contac Day & Night Cold/Flu Night Caplets
◆ Contac Maximum Strength Continuous Action Decongestant/Antihistamine 12 Hour Caplets
◆ Contac Night Allergy/Sinus Caplets
◆ Contac Severe Cold and Flu Formula Caplets
◆ Contac Severe Cold & Flu Non-Drowsy
◆ Debrox Drops
◆ Ecotrin Enteric Coated Aspirin Maximum Strength Tablets and Caplets
◆ Ecotrin Enteric Coated Aspirin Regular Strength and Adult Low Strength Tablets
◆ Feosol Capsules
◆ Feosol Elixir
◆ Feosol Tablets
◆ Gaviscon Antacid Tablets
◆ Gaviscon-2 Antacid Tablets
◆ Gaviscon Extra Strength Relief Formula Antacid Tablets
◆ Gaviscon Extra Strength Relief Formula Liquid Antacid
◆ Gaviscon Liquid Antacid
◆ Gly-Oxide Liquid
Massengill Disposable Douches
Massengill Feminine Cleansing Wash
Massengill Fragrance-Free and Baby Powder Scent Soft Cloth Towelettes
Massengill Liquid Concentrate
◆ Massengill Medicated Disposable Douche
Massengill Medicated Liquid Concentrate
Massengill Medicated Soft Cloth Towelette
Massengill Powder
N'ICE Medicated Sugarless Sore Throat and Cough Lozenges
◆ Novahistine DMX
◆ Novahistine Elixir
◆ Panodol Tablets and Caplets
◆ Children's Panodol Chewable Tablets, Liquid, Infant's Drops
Simron Capsules
◆ Sine-Off No Drowsiness Formula Caplets
◆ Sine-Off Sinus Medicine
Singlet Tablets

◆ Sucrets Children's Cherry Flavored Sore Throat Lozenges
◆ Sucrets Maximum Strength Wintergreen, Maximum Strength Vapor Black Cherry Sore Throat Lozenges
◆ Sucrets Regular Strength Wild Cherry, Regular Strength Original Mint, Regular Strength Vapor Lemon Sore Throat Lozenges
◆ Sucrets 4-Hour Cough Suppressant
◆ Tagamet HB Tablets
◆ Teldrin 12 Hour Antihistamine/Nasal Decongestant Allergy Relief Capsules
◆ Tums Antacid/Calcium Supplement Tablets
◆ Tums Anti-gas/Antacid Formula Tablets, Assorted Fruit
◆ Tums E-X Antacid/Calcium Supplement Tablets
Tums 500 Calcium Supplement
◆ Tums ULTRA Antacid/Calcium Supplement Tablets

SMITHKLINE CONSUMER PRODUCTS
(See SMITHKLINE BEECHAM CONSUMER HEALTHCARE, L.P.)

STANDARD HOMEOPATHIC 788
COMPANY
210 West 131st Street
Box 61067
Los Angeles, CA 90061
Direct Inquiries to:
Jay Borneman
(800) 624-9659

OTC Products Available:
Hyland's Arnicaid Tablets
Hyland's Bedwetting Tablets
Hyland's Calms Forté Tablets
Hyland's ClearAc
Hyland's Colic Tablets
Hyland's Cough Syrup with Honey
Hyland's C-Plus Cold Tablets
Hyland's EnurAid Tablets
Hyland's Headache Tablets
Hyland's Leg Cramps Tablets
Hyland's Teething Tablets

STELLAR PHARMACAL 790
CORPORATION
1990 N.W. 44th Street
Pompano Beach, FL 33064-8712
Direct Inquiries to:
Scott L. Davidson
(954) 972-6060
Customer Service & Order Department:
(800) 845-7827

OTC Products Available:
Star-Otic Ear Solution

STERLING HEALTH
(See BAYER CORPORATION CONSUMER CARE DIVISION)

SUNSOURCE 521, 791
INTERNATIONAL, INC.
535 Lipoa Parkway
Suite 110
Kihei, HI 96753
Direct Inquiries to:
Preston Zoller, Director of Marketing
(808) 874-6733, Ext. 277

OTC Products Available:
◆ Garlique
◆ Melatonex
◆ Rejuvex
◆ Sunsource Allergy Relief Tablets
◆ Sunsource Arthritis Relief Cream
◆ Sunsource Arthritis Relief Tablets
◆ Sunsource Cold Relief Tablets

(◆) Shown in Product Identification Guide

SUNSOURCE INTERNATIONAL, INC.
—*cont.*
◆ Sunsource Flu Relief Tablets
◆ Sunsource Insomnia Relief Tablets
◆ Sunsource Psoriasis/Eczema Relief
   Cream
◆ Sunsource Sinus Relief Tablets
◆ Sunsource Sports Injury Relief Cream

THOMPSON MEDICAL 522, 794
COMPANY, INC.
222 Lakeview Avenue
West Palm Beach, FL 33401
Direct Inquiries to:
Consumer Services
(407) 820-9900
FAX: (407) 832-2297

OTC Products Available:
Aqua-Ban Maximum Strength Tablets
Arthritis Hot
◆ Aspercreme Creme, Lotion Analgesic Rub
Breathe Free
◆ Capzasin-P
Control Caplets
◆ Cortizone for Kids
◆ Cortizone-5 Creme and Ointment
◆ Cortizone-10 Creme and Ointment
◆ Cortizone-10 External Anal Itch Relief
◆ Cortizone-10 Scalp Itch Formula
Dexatrim Maximum Strength
   Caffeine-Free Caplets
Dexatrim Maximum Strength Extended
   Duration Time Tablets
◆ Dexatrim Maximum Strength Plus Vitamin
   C/Caffeine-Free Caplets
◆ Dexatrim Plus Vitamins Caplets
Diar Aid Tablets
Encare Vaginal Contraceptive
   Suppositories
End Lice
Hemorid Creme
◆ Hemorid For Women Cleanser
◆ Hemorid Ointment
◆ Hemorid Suppositories
Ibuprin
NP-27 Cream, Solution & Spray Powder
◆ Sleepinal Night-time Sleep Aid Capsules
   and Softgels
Sportscreme External Analgesic Rub
   Cream & Lotion
◆ Tempo Soft Antacid
Tribiotic Plus

TISHCON CORPORATION 799
30 New York Avenue
Westbury, NY 11590
Direct Inquiries to:
Product Information Director
(516) 333-3050
FAX: (516) 997-1052

OTC Products Available:
Lumitene

TRITON CONSUMER 800
PRODUCTS, INC.
561 West Golf Road
Arlington Heights, IL 60005
Direct Inquiries to:
Karen Shrader
(800) 942-2009
For Medical Emergencies Contact:
(800) 942-2009

OTC Products Available:
MG 217 Medicated Tar Shampoo
MG 217 Medicated Tar-Free Shampoo
MG 217 Psoriasis Ointment and Lotion
MG 217 Sal-Acid Ointment
ProTech First-Aid Stik
Retre-Gel Medicated Cold Sore Gel
Skeeter Stik Insect Bite Medication

UAS LABORATORIES 800
5610 Rowland Road #110
Minnetonka, MN 55343
Direct Inquiries to:
Dr. S.K. Dash
(612) 935-1707
FAX: (612) 935-1650
For Medical Emergencies Contact:
Dr. S.K. Dash
(612) 935-1707
FAX: (612) 935-1650

OTC Products Available:
DDS-Acidophilus

THE UPJOHN COMPANY 522, 800
7000 Portage Road
Kalamazoo, MI 49001
**For Medical and Pharmaceutical
Information, Including Emergencies:**
(616) 329-8244
(616) 323-6615
Pharmaceutical Sales Areas:
Atlanta (Chamblee)
   GA 30341-2626
   (404) 452-4607
   (800) 426-4609
Chicago (Downers Grove)
   IL 60515
   (708) 663-9300
   (800) 253-1935
Cincinnati
   OH 45202
   (513) 723-1010
   (800) 543-0278
Dallas (Irving)
   TX 75062
   (214) 256-0022
Kansas City (Overland Park)
   AR 66210
   (913) 469-8863
   (800) 272-8702
Los Angeles (Simi Valley)
   CA 93065
   (805) 582-0188
   (800) 772-3011
Memphis
   TN 38183
   (901) 685-8192
   (800) 238-5970
New York (Valhalla)
   NY 10595
   (914) 245-8412
Orlando
   FL 32809
   (407) 859-4591
   (800) 432-4332
Philadelphia (Berwyn)
   PA 19312
   (215) 993-0100
   (800) 523-8686
Portland
   OR 97232
   (503) 232-2133
Washington (Falls Church)
   VA 22402
   (703) 849-1300
   (800) 852-5048
Distribution Centers:
Atlanta (Chamblee)
   GA 30341
   (404) 452-4612
   (800) 241-7117
Kalamazoo
   MI 49001
   (616) 384-9000
   (800) 253-9860
Los Angeles (Simi Valley)
   CA 93065
   (805) 582-0072
   (800) 821-7000

OTC Products Available:
Cortaid Sensitive Skin Cream with Aloe

◆ Cortaid Sensitive Skin Ointment with Aloe
◆ Maximum Strength Cortaid Cream
◆ Maximum Strength Cortaid FastStick
   Maximum Strength Cortaid Ointment
   Maximum Strength Cortaid Spray
◆ Doxidan Liqui-Gels
◆ Dramamine Chewable Tablets
◆ Children's Dramamine Liquid
◆ Dramamine Tablets
◆ Dramamine II Tablets
◆ Kaopectate Children's Liquid
◆ Kaopectate Concentrated Anti-Diarrheal,
   Peppermint Flavor
◆ Kaopectate Concentrated Anti-Diarrheal,
   Regular Flavor
◆ Kaopectate Maximum Strength Caplets
◆ Motrin IB Caplets, Tablets, and Gelcaps
◆ Mycitracin Plus Pain Reliever
◆ Maximum Strength Mycitracin Triple
   Antibiotic First Aid Ointment
◆ Surfak Liqui-Gels

WAKUNAGA OF AMERICA CO., LTD.
(See KYOLIC LTD.)

WALLACE 523, 803
LABORATORIES
Half Acre Road
Cranbury, NJ 08512
Direct Inquiries to:
Wallace Laboratories
Div. of Carter-Wallace, Inc..
P.O. Box 1001
Cranbury, NJ 08512
(609) 655-6000
For Medical Emergencies Contact:
(800) 526-3840

OTC Products Available:
◆ Maltsupex Liquid, Powder & Tablets
◆ Ryna Liquid
◆ Ryna-C Liquid
◆ Ryna-CX Liquid

WARNER-LAMBERT 523, 805
COMPANY
Consumer Health Products Group
201 Tabor Road
Morris Plains, NJ 07950
(See also Warner Wellcome)
Direct Inquiries to:
1-(800) 223-0182
For Consumer Product Information Call:
1-(800) 524-2854
1-(800) 223-0182

OTC Products Available:
◆ Celestial Seasonings Soothers Herbal
   Throat Drops
◆ Halls Juniors Sugar Free Cough
   Suppressant Drops
◆ Halls Mentho-Lyptus Cough Suppressant
   Drops
◆ Halls Plus Maximum Strength Cough
   Suppressant Drops
◆ Halls Sugar Free Mentho-Lyptus Cough
   Suppressant Drops
◆ Halls Vitamin C Drops
◆ Rolaids Antacid Tablets
◆ Rolaids Antacid Calcium Rich/Sodium
   Free Tablets

WARNER WELLCOME....... 524, 807
Consumer HealthCare Products
Warner-Lambert Company
201 Tabor Road
Morris Plains, NJ 07950
(See also Warner-Lambert)
For Product Information Call:
1-(800) 223-0182
1-(800) 524-2624
1-(800) 562-0266
1-(800) 378-1783

(◆) Shown in Product Identification Guide

1-(800) 337-7266
1-(800) 773-1554
1-(800) 547-8374

OTC Products Available:
- ◆ Actifed Allergy Daytime/Nighttime Caplets
- ◆ Actifed Cold & Allergy Tablets
- ◆ Actifed Cold & Sinus Caplets and Tablets
- ◆ Actifed Sinus Daytime/Nighttime Tablets and Caplets
- Agoral Liquid
- ◆ Anusol HC-1 Hydrocortisone Anti-Itch Ointment
- ◆ Anusol Hemorrhoidal Ointment
- ◆ Anusol Hemorrhoidal Suppositories
- ◆ Benadryl Allergy Chewables
- ◆ Benadryl Allergy/Cold Tablets
- ◆ Benadryl Allergy Decongestant Liquid Medication
- ◆ Benadryl Allergy Decongestant Tablets
- ◆ Benadryl Allergy Kapseals
- ◆ Benadryl Allergy Liquid Medication
- ◆ Benadryl Allergy Tablets
- ◆ Benadryl Allergy Sinus Headache Caplets
- ◆ Benadryl Dye-Free Allergy Liquid Medication
- ◆ Benadryl Dye-Free Allergy Liqui-gel Softgels
- ◆ Benadryl Itch Relief Stick Extra Strength
- ◆ Benadryl Itch Stopping Cream Extra Strength
- ◆ Benadryl Itch Stopping Cream Original Strength
- ◆ Benadryl Itch Stopping Gel Extra Strength
- ◆ Benadryl Itch Stopping Gel Original Strength
- ◆ Benadryl Itch Stopping Spray Extra Strength
- ◆ Benadryl Itch Stopping Spray Original Strength
- ◆ Benylin Adult Formula Cough Suppressant
- ◆ Benylin Expectorant
- ◆ Benylin Multisymptom
- ◆ Benylin Pediatric Cough Suppressant
- ◆ Borofax Skin Protectant Ointment
- ◆ Caladryl Clear Lotion
- ◆ Caladryl Cream For Kids
- ◆ Caladryl Lotion
- Corn Husker's Lotion
- Empirin Aspirin Tablets
- ◆ e.p.t. Pregnancy Test
- ◆ Gelusil Antacid-Anti-gas Liquid
- ◆ Gelusil Antacid-Anti-gas Tablets
- ◆ Listerine Antiseptic
- ◆ Cool Mint Listerine
- ◆ FreshBurst Listerine
- ◆ Listermint
- ◆ Lubriderm Bath and Shower Oil
- ◆ Lubriderm Dry Skin Care Lotion
- ◆ Lubriderm Moisture Recovery Alpha Hydroxy Cream and Lotion
- ◆ Lubriderm Moisture Recovery GelCreme
- ◆ Lubriderm Seriously Sensitive Lotion
- Myadec Tablets
- ◆ Neosporin Ointment
- ◆ Neosporin Plus Maximum Strength Cream
- ◆ Neosporin Plus Maximum Strength Ointment
- ◆ Nix Creme Rinse
- ◆ Polysporin Ointment
- ◆ Polysporin Powder
- ◆ Replens Vaginal Moisturizer
- ◆ Sinutab Non-Drying Liquid Caps
- ◆ Sinutab Sinus Allergy Medication, Maximum Strength Tablets and Caplets
- ◆ Sinutab Sinus Medication, Maximum Strength Without Drowsiness Formula, Tablets & Caplets
- ◆ Sudafed Children's Cold & Cough Liquid Medication
- ◆ Sudafed Children's Nasal Decongestant Liquid Medication
- ◆ Sudafed Cold & Allergy Tablets
- ◆ Sudafed Cold and Cough Liquid Caps

- ◆ Sudafed Nasal Decongestant Tablets, 30 mg
- ◆ Sudafed Nasal Decongestant Tablets, 60 mg
- ◆ Sudafed Non-Drying Sinus Liquid Caps
- ◆ Sudafed Pediatric Nasal Decongestant Liquid Oral Drops
- ◆ Sudafed Severe Cold Formula Caplets
- ◆ Sudafed Severe Cold Formula Tablets
- ◆ Sudafed Sinus Caplets
- ◆ Sudafed Sinus Tablets
- ◆ Sudafed 12 Hour Caplets
- ◆ Tucks Clear Hemorrhoidal Gel
- ◆ Tucks Premoistened Hemorrhoidal/Vaginal Pads
- Tucks Take-Alongs

WELLNESS INTERNATIONAL ..... 830 NETWORK, LTD.
1501 Luna Road, Bldg. 102
Carrollton, TX 75006
Direct Inquiries to:
Director of Product Development
(214) 245-1097
FAX: (214) 389-3060

OTC Products Available:
Bio-Complex 5000 Gentle Foaming Cleanser
Bio-Complex 5000 Revitalizing Conditioner
Bio-Complex 5000 Revitalizing Shampoo
BioLean
BioLean Accelerator
BioLean Free
BioLean LipoTrim
BioLean Meal
Food for Thought
Phyto-Vite
StePHan Bio-Nutritional Daytime Hydrating Creme
StePHan Bio-Nutritional Eye-Firming Concentrate
StePHan Bio-Nutritional Nightime Moisture Creme
StePHan Bio-Nutritional Refreshing Moisture Gel
StePHan Bio-Nutritional Ultra Hydrating Fluid
StePHan Clarity
StePHan Elasticity
StePHan Elixir
StePHan Essential
StePHan Feminine
StePHan Flexibility
StePHan Lovpil
StePHan Masculine
StePHan Protector
StePHan Relief
StePHan Tranquility
Winrgy

WHITEHALL LABORATORIES INC.
(See WHITEHALL-ROBINS HEALTHCARE)

WHITEHALL-ROBINS .... 528, 836 HEALTHCARE
American Home Products Corporation
Five Giralda Farms
Madison, NJ 07940-0871
Direct Inquiries to:
Whitehall Consumer Product Information:
(800) 322-3129
Robins Consumer Product Information:
(800) 762-4672
Professional Samples:
Whitehall - Robins
(800) 343-0856

OTC Products Available:
- ◆ Advil Cold and Sinus Caplets and Tablets
- ◆ Advil Ibuprofen Tablets, Caplets and Gel Caplets
- Anacin Caplets and Tablets

Aspirin Free Anacin Gel Caplets
Aspirin Free Anacin Maximum Strength
Baby Anbesol
Anbesol Gel and Liquid
Chapstick Lip Balm
Chapstick Sunblock 15 Lip Balm
- ◆ Clearblue Easy
- ◆ Clearplan Easy
Denorex Medicated Shampoo and Conditioner
Dermoplast Anesthetic Pain Relief Spray and Lotion
Dimetapp Dye-Free Allergy (Children's)
Dimetapp Allergy Dye-Free Elixir
Dimetapp Allergy Sinus Caplets
Dimetapp Cold & Allergy Chewable Tablets
Dimetapp Cold & Cough Liqui-Gels
Dimetapp Cold & Fever Suspension
Dimetapp Decongestant Pediatric Drops
Dimetapp DM Elixir
- ◆ Dimetapp Elixir
- ◆ Dimetapp Extentabs
Dimetapp Liqui-Gels
Dimetapp Tablets
Dristan Maximum Strength Cold Non-Drowsiness Gel Caplets
Dristan 12-hour Nasal Spray
- ◆ Orudis KT
Posture 600 mg
- ◆ Preparation H Hemorrhoidal Cream
- ◆ Preparation H Hemorrhoidal Ointment
- ◆ Preparation H Hemorrhoidal Suppositories
Preparation H Hydrocortisone 1% Cream
- ◆ Primatene Mist
- ◆ Primatene Tablets
Riopan Suspension
Robitussin
Robitussin Cold & Cough Liqui-Gels
Robitussin Cold, Cough & Flu Liqui-Gels
Robitussin Liquid Center Cough Drops
Robitussin Maximum Strength Cough Suppressant
Robitussin Maximum Strength Cough & Cold
Robitussin Night-Time Cold Formula
Robitussin Pediatric Cough & Cold Formula
Robitussin Pediatric Cough Suppressant
Robitussin Pediatric Drops
Robitussin Severe Congestion Liqui-Gels
Robitussin Sugar-Free Cough Drops
Robitussin-CF
- ◆ Robitussin-DM
Robitussin-PE

J.B. WILLIAMS .... 528, 849 COMPANY, INC.
65 Harristown Rd
Glen Rock, NJ 07452
Direct Inquiries to:
Consumer Affairs
(800) 254-8656
(201) 251-8100
FAX: (201) 251-8097
For Medical Emergencies Contact:
(800) 254-8656

OTC Products Available:
- ◆ Cēpacol/Cēpacol Mint Antiseptic Mouthwash/Gargle
- ◆ Cēpacol Maximum Strength Sore Throat Lozenges, Cherry Flavor
- ◆ Cēpacol Maximum Strength Sore Throat Lozenges, Original Mint Flavor
Cēpacol Regular Strength Sore Throat Lozenges, Cherry Flavor
Cēpacol Regular Strength Sore Throat Lozenges, Original Mint Flavor
- ◆ Cēpacol Maximum Strength Sore Throat Spray, Cherry Flavor
- ◆ Cēpacol Maximum Strength Sore Throat Spray, Cool Menthol Flavor

(◆) Shown in Product Identification Guide

THE WINNING COMBINATION
(See AML LABORATORIES)

WYETH-AYERST **528, 850**
LABORATORIES
Division of American Home Products
Corporation
P.O. Box 8299
Philadelphia, PA 19101
Direct Inquiries to:
Professional Service
(610) 688-4400
For EMERGENCY Medical Information
Contact:
Day: (800) 934-5556
Night: (610) 688-4400
For Medical/Pharmacy Inquiries on
Marketed Products Call:
(800) 934-5556
8:30 AM to 4:30 PM (Eastern Standard
Time)
WYETH-AYERST DISTRIBUTION
CENTERS
(Do not use freight addresses
for mailing orders.)
Atlanta, GA—P.O. Box 1773
Paoli, PA 19301-1773
(800) 666-7248

Freight Address:
100 Union Court
Kennesaw, GA 30144
Mail DEA order forms to:
P.O. Box 4365
Atlanta, GA 30302
Chicago, IL—P.O. Box 1773
Paoli, PA 19301-1773
(800) 666-7248

Freight Address:
284 Lies Road
Carol Stream, IL 60188
Mail DEA order forms to:
P.O. Box 140

Wheaton, IL 60189-0140
Dallas, TX—P.O. Box 1773
Paoli, PA 19301-1773
(800) 666-7248
Freight Address:
11240 Petal Street
Dallas, TX 75238
Mail DEA order forms to:
P.O. Box 650231
Dallas, TX 75265-0231
Hawaii—P.O. Box 1773
Paoli, PA 19301-1773
(800) 666-7248
Mail DEA order forms to:
96-1185 Waihona Street, Unit C1
Pearl City, HI 96782
Sparks, NV—1802 Briely Way
Sparks, NV 89431
(800) 666-7248
Freight Address
1802 Briely Way
Sparks, NV 89431
Mail DEA order forms to:
1802 Briely Way
Sparks, NV 89431
Philadelphia, PA—P.O. Box 1773
Paoli, PA 19301-1773
(800) 666-7248
Freight Address:
31 Morehall Road
Frazer, PA 19355
Mail DEA order forms to:
P.O. Box 61
Paoli, PA 19301
Seattle, WA—P.O. Box 1773
Paoli, PA 19301-1773
(800) 666-7248
Freight Address:
19255 80th Ave. South
Kent, WA 98032
Mail DEA order forms to:
P.O. Box 5609
Kent, WA 98064-5609

OTC Products Available:
- Aludrox Oral Suspension
- Amphojel Suspension (Mint Flavor)
- Amphojel Suspension without Flavor
- Amphojel Tablets
- Basaljel Capsules
- Basaljel Suspension
- Basaljel Tablets
- Bonamil Infant Formula, Concentrated
  Liquid, Ready-to-Feed Liquid, and
  Powder
- Cerose DM
- Collyrium for Fresh Eyes
- Collyrium Fresh
- Donnagel Liquid and Donnagel Chewable
  Tablets
- Nursoy, Soy Protein Isolate Formula for
  Infants, Concentrated Liquid,
  Ready-to-Feed Liquid, and Powder
- SMA Iron Fortified Infant Formula,
  Concentrated Liquid, Ready-to-Feed
  Liquid, and Powder
- SMA Lo-Iron Infant Formula,
  Concentrated, Ready-to-Feed, and
  Powder
- Wyanoids Relief Factor Hemorrhoidal
  Suppositories

ZILA **529, 856**
PHARMACEUTICALS, INC.
5227 North 7th Street
Phoenix, AZ 85014-2817

Direct Inquiries to:
Jerry Kaster
Director of Marketing
(602) 266-6700

OTC Products Available:
- Zilactin Medicated Gel
- Zilactin-B Medicated Gel with Benzocaine
- Zilactin-L Liquid

SECTION 2

PRODUCT NAME INDEX

This index includes all entries in the "Product Information" section. Products are listed alphabetically by brand name.

If two page numbers appear, the first refers to the product's photograph, the second to its prescribing information.

- **Bold page numbers** indicate full prescribing information.

- *Italic page numbers* signify partial information.

Italic Page Number Indicates Brief Listing

Italic Page Number Indicates Brief Listing

Italic Page Number Indicates Brief Listing

Italic Page Number Indicates Brief Listing

Italic Page Number Indicates Brief Listing

Italic Page Number Indicates Brief Listing

SECTION 3

PRODUCT CATEGORY INDEX

This index cross-references each brand by prescribing category. All entries in the "Product Information"section are included. In each category, all fully described products are listed first, followed by those with only partial descriptions.

If two page numbers appear, the first refers to the product's photograph, the second to its prescribing information.

- **Bold page numbers** indicate full prescribing information.

The categories employed in this index were established by the OTC Review process of the United States Food and Drug Administration. Classification of products within these categories has been determined in cooperation with the products' manufacturers or, when necessary, by the publisher alone.

Neosporin Plus Maximum
Strength Ointment
(WARNER WELLCOME) **526, 822**

Xylocaine 2.5% Ointment
(Astra) **503, 608**

Zilactin-L Liquid
(Zila Pharmaceuticals) **529, 856**

ANTIBACTERIALS

Barri-Care Antimicrobial Barrier
Ointment (Care-Tech) **646**

Care Creme Antimicrobial Cream
(Care-Tech) **646**

Clinical Care Dermal Wound Cleanser
(Care-Tech) **646**

Concept Antimicrobial Skin Cleanser
(Care-Tech) **646**

Formula Magic Antibacterial Powder
(Care-Tech) **647**

Mycitracin Plus Pain Reliever
(Upjohn) **523, 803**

Neosporin Ointment
(WARNER WELLCOME) **526, 821**

Orchid Fresh II Perineal/Ostomy
Cleanser (Care-Tech) **647**

Polysporin Ointment
(WARNER WELLCOME) **526, 822**

Polysporin Powder
(WARNER WELLCOME) **526, 823**

Satin Antimicrobial Skin Cleanser for
Diabetic/Cancer Patient Care
(Care-Tech) **647**

Techni-Care Surgical Scrub and Wound
Cleanser (Care-Tech) **647**

ANTIBIOTICS

Mycitracin Plus Pain Reliever
(Upjohn) **523, 803**

Maximum Strength Mycitracin
Triple Antibiotic First Aid
Ointment (Upjohn) **523, 803**

Neosporin Ointment
(WARNER WELLCOME) **526, 821**

Neosporin Plus Maximum
Strength Cream
(WARNER WELLCOME) **526, 821**

Neosporin Plus Maximum
Strength Ointment
(WARNER WELLCOME) **526, 822**

Polysporin Ointment
(WARNER WELLCOME) **526, 822**

Polysporin Powder
(WARNER WELLCOME) **526, 823**

ANTI-INFLAMMATORY AGENTS

Massengill Medicated Soft Cloth
Towelette
(SmithKline Beecham Consumer) ..**781**

ASTRINGENTS

Domeboro Astringent Solution
Effervescent Tablets
(Bayer Consumer) **504, 620**

Domeboro Astringent Solution
Powder Packets
(Bayer Consumer) **504, 620**

Tucks Clear Hemorrhoidal Gel
(WARNER WELLCOME) **528, 829**

Tucks Premoistened
Hemorrhoidal/Vaginal Pads
(WARNER WELLCOME) **527, 830**

Tucks Take-Alongs
(WARNER WELLCOME) **830**

BARRIER

Barri-Care Antimicrobial Barrier
Ointment (Care-Tech) **646**

BATH OILS

Alpha Keri Moisture Rich Body Oil
(Bristol-Myers Products) **635**

BURN RELIEF

A and D Ointment
(Schering-Plough HealthCare) **518, 757**

Americaine Topical Anesthetic
First Aid Ointment
(Ciba Self-Medication) **507, 649**

Americaine Topical Anesthetic
Spray (Ciba Self-Medication) .. **507, 649**

Aquaphor Healing Ointment
(Beiersdorf) **506, 628**

Barri-Care Antimicrobial Barrier
Ointment (Care-Tech) **646**

BiCozene Creme
(Sandoz Consumer) **516, 747**

Borofax Skin Protectant Ointment
(WARNER WELLCOME) **525, 817**

Care Creme Antimicrobial Cream
(Care-Tech) **646**

Desitin Ointment
(Pfizer Consumer) **515, 715**

Matrix Microclysmic Gel (Care-Tech)..... **647**

Mycitracin Plus Pain Reliever
(Upjohn) **523, 803**

Neosporin Ointment
(WARNER WELLCOME) **526, 821**

Neosporin Plus Maximum
Strength Cream
(WARNER WELLCOME) **526, 821**

Neosporin Plus Maximum
Strength Ointment
(WARNER WELLCOME) **526, 822**

Nupercainal Pain Relief Cream
(Ciba Self-Medication) **509, 661**

Polysporin Ointment
(WARNER WELLCOME) **526, 822**

Polysporin Powder
(WARNER WELLCOME) **526, 823**

CLEANSING AGENTS

Bio-Complex 5000 Gentle Foaming
Cleanser (Wellness International) ..**830**

Concept Antimicrobial Skin Cleanser
(Care-Tech) **646**

Dove Bar (Original, Unscented,
and Sensitive Skin Formula)
(Lever) **512, 686**

Dove Moisturizing Body Wash
(Lever) **686**

Liquid Dove Beauty Wash (Lever) **686**

Eucerin Cleansing Bar
(Beiersdorf) **506, 628**

Massengill Fragrance-Free and Baby
Powder Scent Soft Cloth
Towelettes (SmithKline Beecham
Consumer) **781**

Orchid Fresh II Perineal/Ostomy
Cleanser (Care-Tech) **647**

Satin Antimicrobial Skin Cleanser for
Diabetic/Cancer Patient Care
(Care-Tech) **647**

Techni-Care Surgical Scrub and Wound
Cleanser (Care-Tech) **647**

COAL TAR

MG 217 Medicated Tar Shampoo
(Triton Consumer) **800**

MG 217 Psoriasis Ointment and Lotion
(Triton Consumer) **800**

Tegrin Dandruff Shampoo (Block) **634**

Tegrin Skin Cream & Tegrin Medicated
Soap (Block) **634**

CONDITIONING RINSES

Bio-Complex 5000 Revitalizing
Conditioner (Wellness
International) **830**

CONTACT DERMATITIS

Care Creme Antimicrobial Cream
(Care-Tech) **646**

Maximum Strength Cortaid Cream
(Upjohn) **522, 800**

Maximum Strength Cortaid
FastStick (Upjohn) **522, 800**

Maximum Strength Cortaid Ointment
(Upjohn) **800**

Maximum Strength Cortaid Spray
(Upjohn) **800**

Satin Antimicrobial Skin Cleanser for
Diabetic/Cancer Patient Care
(Care-Tech) **647**

DANDRUFF MEDICATIONS

Head & Shoulders Intensive Treatment
Dandruff and Seborrheic Dermatitis
Shampoo (Procter & Gamble) **723**

MG 217 Medicated Tar Shampoo
(Triton Consumer) **800**

MG 217 Medicated Tar-Free Shampoo
(Triton Consumer) **800**

Selsun Blue Dandruff Shampoo 2-in-1
Treatment (Ross) **746**

Selsun Blue Dandruff Shampoo
Balanced Treatment (Ross) **746**

Selsun Blue Dandruff Shampoo
Medicated Treatment (Ross)..........**746**

Selsun Blue Dandruff Shampoo
Moisturizing Treatment (Ross)........**746**

Tegrin Dandruff Shampoo (Block) **634**

DEODORANTS

Desenex Foot & Sneaker
Deodorant Spray
(Ciba Self-Medication) **508, 653**

DERMATITIS RELIEF

A and D Ointment
(Schering-Plough HealthCare) **518, 757**

Alpha Keri Moisture Rich Body Oil
(Bristol-Myers Products) **635**

Balmex Ointment (Block) **631**

BiCozene Creme
(Sandoz Consumer) **516, 747**

Caladryl Clear Lotion
(WARNER WELLCOME) **525, 817**

Caladryl Cream For Kids
(WARNER WELLCOME) **525, 817**

Caladryl Lotion
(WARNER WELLCOME) **525, 817**

Caldecort Anti-Itch
Hydrocortisone Cream
(Ciba Self-Medication) **507, 651**

Caldesene Medicated Ointment
(Ciba Self-Medication) **507, 652**

Caldesene Medicated Powder
(Ciba Self-Medication) **507, 652**

Concept Antimicrobial Skin Cleanser
(Care-Tech) **646**

Cortaid Sensitive Skin Cream with Aloe
(Upjohn) **800**

Cortaid Sensitive Skin Ointment
with Aloe (Upjohn) **522, 800**

Maximum Strength Cortaid Cream
(Upjohn) **522, 800**

Maximum Strength Cortaid
FastStick (Upjohn) **522, 800**

Maximum Strength Cortaid Ointment
(Upjohn) **800**

Maximum Strength Cortaid Spray
(Upjohn) **800**

Cortizone for Kids
(Thompson Medical) **522, 795**

Cortizone-5 Creme and Ointment
(Thompson Medical) **522, 795**

Cortizone-10 Creme and
Ointment (Thompson
Medical) **522, 795**

Cortizone-10 External Anal Itch
Relief (Thompson Medical) **522, 795**

Cortizone-10 Scalp Itch Formula
(Thompson Medical) **522, 795**

Desitin Ointment
(Pfizer Consumer) **515, 715**

Domeboro Astringent Solution
Effervescent Tablets
(Bayer Consumer) **504, 620**

Domeboro Astringent Solution
Powder Packets
(Bayer Consumer) **504, 620**

Eucerin Facial Moisturizing Lotion
SPF 25 (Beiersdorf) **506, 629**

Massengill Medicated Soft Cloth
Towelette
(SmithKline Beecham Consumer) ..**781**

Nupercainal Hydrocortisone 1%
Cream
(Ciba Self-Medication) **509, 661**

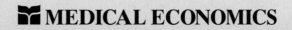
MEDICAL ECONOMICS

SECTION 4

ACTIVE INGREDIENTS INDEX

This index cross-references each brand by its generic ingredients. All entries in the "Product Information" section are included. Under each generic heading, all fully described products are listed first, followed by those with only partial descriptions.

If two page numbers appear, the first refers to the product's photograph, the second to its prescribing information.

- **Bold page numbers** indicate full prescribing information.

- *Italic page numbers* signify partial information.

Classification of products under these headings has been determined in cooperation with the products' manufacturers or, if necessary, by the publisher alone.

Italic Page Number **Indicates Brief Listing**

Italic Page Number **Indicates Brief Listing**

Italic Page Number **Indicates Brief Listing**

Italic Page Number **Indicates Brief Listing**

Italic Page Number **Indicates Brief Listing**

Italic Page Number **Indicates Brief Listing**

Italic Page Number **Indicates Brief Listing**

Italic Page Number **Indicates Brief Listing**

MAGNESIUM HYDROXIDE—cont.
Mylanta Double Strength Liquid
(J&J•Merck Consumer) **510, 676**
Mylanta Tablets
(J&J•Merck Consumer) **511, 677**
Mylanta Double Strength Tablets
(J&J•Merck Consumer) **511, 677**
Phillips' Milk of Magnesia Liquid
(Bayer Consumer) **506, 627**
Rolaids Antacid Tablets
(Warner-Lambert)................. **524, 807**
Tempo Soft Antacid
(Thompson Medical) **522, 799**

MAGNESIUM LACTATE
MagTab SR Caplets (Niché) **713**

MAGNESIUM OXIDE
Beelith Tablets (Beach) **628**
Bufferin Analgesic Tablets
(Bristol-Myers Products) **506, 636**
Arthritis Strength Bufferin
Analgesic Caplets
(Bristol-Myers Products) **506, 637**
Extra Strength Bufferin Analgesic
Tablets
(Bristol-Myers Products) **506, 637**
Caltrate PLUS
(Lederle Consumer) **511, 681**
Cama Arthritis Pain Reliever
(Sandoz Consumer) **748**
Mag-Ox 400 (Blaine) **629**
Uro-Mag (Blaine) **630**

MAGNESIUM SALICYLATE
Backache Caplets
(Bristol-Myers Products) **635**
Doan's Extra-Strength Analgesic
(Ciba Self-Medication) **508, 653**
Extra Strength Doan's P.M.
(Ciba Self-Medication) **508, 653**
Doan's Regular Strength
Analgesic (Ciba
Self-Medication) **508, 654**
Mobigesic Tablets (Ascher) **503, 607**

MAGNESIUM TRISILICATE
Gaviscon Antacid Tablets
(SmithKline Beecham
Consumer) **520, 778**
Gaviscon-2 Antacid Tablets
(SmithKline Beecham
Consumer) **520, 779**

MALIC ACID
Salix SST Lozenges Saliva Stimulant
(Scandinavian Natural) **757**

MALT SOUP EXTRACT
Maltsupex Liquid, Powder &
Tablets (Wallace) **523, 803**

MANGANESE SULFATE
Caltrate PLUS
(Lederle Consumer) **511, 681**

MECLIZINE HYDROCHLORIDE
Bonine Tablets (Pfizer Consumer) **715**
Dramamine II Tablets (Upjohn) **523, 801**

MELATONIN
Melatonex (Sunsource) **521, 791**

MENTHOL
ArthriCare Odor Free Rub (Del) **509, 667**
ArthriCare Triple Medicated Rub
(Del) **509, 667**
BenGay External Analgesic
Products (Pfizer Consumer) .. **515, 714**
Celestial Seasonings Soothers
Herbal Throat Drops
(Warner-Lambert)................. **523, 805**

Cēpacol Maximum Strength Sore
Throat Lozenges, Cherry
Flavor (J.B. Williams) **528, 850**
Cēpacol Maximum Strength Sore
Throat Lozenges, Original
Mint Flavor (J.B. Williams) **528, 850**
Cēpacol Regular Strength Sore Throat
Lozenges, Cherry Flavor
(J.B. Williams) **850**
Cēpacol Regular Strength Sore Throat
Lozenges, Original Mint Flavor
(J.B. Williams) **850**
Eucalyptamint Arthritis Pain
Reliever (External Analgesic)
(Ciba Self-Medication) **508, 656**
Eucalyptamint Muscle Pain Relief
Formula
(Ciba Self-Medication) **508, 656**
Halls Juniors Sugar Free Cough
Suppressant Drops
(Warner-Lambert)................. **523, 806**
Halls Mentho-Lyptus Cough
Suppressant Drops
(Warner-Lambert)................. **523, 806**
Halls Plus Maximum Strength
Cough Suppressant Drops
(Warner-Lambert)................. **524, 806**
Halls Sugar Free Mentho-Lyptus
Cough Suppressant Drops
(Warner-Lambert)................. **523, 806**
Listerine Antiseptic
(WARNER WELLCOME) **525, 820**
Cool Mint Listerine
(WARNER WELLCOME) **526, 820**
FreshBurst Listerine
(WARNER WELLCOME) **526, 820**
Mentholatum Cherry Chest Rub for
Kids (Mentholatum) **710**
Mentholatum Deep Heating Extra
Strength Formula Rub
(Mentholatum).......................... **710**
Mentholatum Menthacin
(Mentholatum).......................... **711**
Mentholatum Ointment
(Mentholatum).......................... **711**
N'ICE Medicated Sugarless Sore
Throat and Cough Lozenges
(SmithKline Beecham Consumer) .. **781**
Original Vicks Cough Drops, Menthol
and Cherry Flavors
(Procter & Gamble) **733**
Therapeutic Mineral Ice, Pain
Relieving Gel
(Bristol-Myers Products) **507, 645**
Vicks Chloraseptic Cough & Throat
Drops, Menthol, Cherry and Honey
Lemon Flavors (Procter & Gamble) **732**
Vicks Chloraseptic Sore Throat
Lozenges, Menthol and Cherry
Flavors
(Procter & Gamble) **732**
Vicks Cough Drops, Menthol and
Cherry Flavors (Procter & Gamble).. **732**
Vicks VapoRub Cream
(Procter & Gamble) **739**
Vicks VapoRub Ointment
(Procter & Gamble) **739**
Vicks VapoSteam
(Procter & Gamble) **739**

METHYL NICOTINATE
ArthriCare Odor Free Rub (Del) **509, 667**
ArthriCare Triple Medicated Rub
(Del) **509, 667**

METHYL SALICYLATE
ArthriCare Triple Medicated Rub
(Del) **509, 667**
BenGay External Analgesic
Products (Pfizer Consumer) .. **515, 714**
Listerine Antiseptic
(WARNER WELLCOME) **525, 820**

Cool Mint Listerine
(WARNER WELLCOME) **526, 820**
FreshBurst Listerine
(WARNER WELLCOME) **526, 820**
Mentholatum Deep Heating Extra
Strength Formula Rub
(Mentholatum).......................... **710**

METHYLCELLULOSE
Citrucel Orange Flavor
(SmithKline Beecham
Consumer) **519, 770**
Citrucel Sugar Free Orange Flavor
(SmithKline Beecham
Consumer) **519, 770**

MICONAZOLE NITRATE
Prescription Strength Desenex
Spray Powder and Spray
Liquid (Ciba Self-Medication) **508, 653**
Lotrimin AF Antifungal Spray
Liquid, Spray Powder, Spray
Deodorant Powder, Powder
and Jock Itch Spray Powder
(Schering-Plough HealthCare) **519, 766**
Ting Antifungal Spray Powder
(Ciba Self-Medication) **666**

MILK, LACTASE REDUCED
Dairy Ease Real Milk
(Bayer Consumer) *620*

MINERAL OIL
Alpha Keri Moisture Rich Body Oil
(Bristol-Myers Products) **635**
Anusol Hemorrhoidal Ointment
(WARNER WELLCOME) **524, 810**
Aquaphor Healing Ointment
(Beiersdorf)....................... **506, 628**
Aquaphor Healing Ointment,
Original Formula (Beiersdorf) **506, 628**
Eucerin Original Moisturizing
Creme (Beiersdorf) **506, 628**
Eucerin Original Moisturizing
Lotion (Beiersdorf)............... **506, 629**
Eucerin Plus Alphahydroxy
Moisturizing Lotion
(Beiersdorf)....................... **506, 629**
Eucerin Plus Alphahydroxy
Moisturizing Creme
(Beiersdorf)....................... **506, 629**
Hemorid Creme
(Thompson Medical) **797**
Hemorid Ointment
(Thompson Medical) **522, 797**
Keri Lotion - Original Formula
(Bristol-Myers Products) **507, 644**
Kondremul
(Ciba Self-Medication) **508, 656**
Lubriderm Bath and Shower Oil
(WARNER WELLCOME) **526, 821**
Nephrox Suspension (Fleming) **671**
Preparation H Hemorrhoidal
Ointment (Whitehall-Robins) .. **528, 842**
Replens Vaginal Moisturizer
(WARNER WELLCOME) **526, 823**

MINERAL WAX
Aquaphor Healing Ointment
(Beiersdorf).......................... **506, 628**
Aquaphor Healing Ointment,
Original Formula (Beiersdorf) **506, 628**

MONOCLONAL ANTIBODY
Clearplan Easy
(Whitehall-Robins) **528, 837**

MULTIMINERALS
(see VITAMINS WITH MINERALS)

MULTIVITAMINS
(see VITAMINS, MULTIPLE)

MULTIVITAMINS WITH MINERALS
(see VITAMINS WITH MINERALS)

Italic Page Number **Indicates Brief Listing**

N

NAPHAZOLINE HYDROCHLORIDE
Clear Eyes ACR Astringent/Lubricant
Redness Reliever Eye Drops
(Ross)..**743**
Clear Eyes Lubricant Eye Redness
Reliever Eye Drops (Ross)..............**743**
4-Way Fast Acting Nasal Spray
(regular & mentholated)
(Bristol-Myers Products) **506, 644**
Privine Nasal Drops
(Ciba Self-Medication) **509, 663**
Privine Nasal Spray
(Ciba Self-Medication) **663**

NAPROXEN SODIUM
Aleve (Procter & Gamble) **515, 722**

NEOMYCIN SULFATE
Mycitracin Plus Pain Reliever
(Upjohn) **523, 803**
Maximum Strength Mycitracin
Triple Antibiotic First Aid
Ointment (Upjohn) **523, 803**
Neosporin Ointment
(WARNER WELLCOME) **526, 821**
Neosporin Plus Maximum
Strength Cream
(WARNER WELLCOME) **526, 821**
Neosporin Plus Maximum
Strength Ointment
(WARNER WELLCOME) **526, 822**

NIACIN
Kyo-Chrome (Kyolic Ltd.) **680**
Nicotinex Elixir (Fleming) **671**

NONOXYNOL-9
Encare Vaginal Contraceptive
Suppositories (Thompson Medical) **797**

O

OCTOXYNOL-9
Massengill Liquid Concentrate
(SmithKline Beecham Consumer) ..**780**

OCTYL DIMETHYL PABA
(see PADIMATE O (OCTYL DIMETHYL PABA))

OCTYL METHOXYCINNAMATE
Eucerin Facial Moisturizing Lotion
SPF 25 (Beiersdorf) **506, 629**
Oil of Olay Daily UV Protectant SPF 15
Beauty Fluid-Original and Fragrance
Free (Olay Co. Inc.)
(Procter & Gamble) **725**
Shade UVAGUARD SPF 15
Suncreen Lotion
(Schering-Plough HealthCare) **519, 768**

OCTYL SALICYLATE
Eucerin Facial Moisturizing Lotion
SPF 25 (Beiersdorf) **506, 629**

OXYBENZONE
Coppertone Skin Selects
Sunscreen Lotion SPF 15 For
Dry Skin
(Schering-Plough HealthCare) **518, 759**
Coppertone Skin Selects
Sunscreen Lotion SPF 15 For
Oily Skin
(Schering-Plough HealthCare) **518, 760**
Shade Gel SPF 30 Sunblock
(Schering-Plough HealthCare) **519, 767**
Shade Lotion SPF 45 Sunblock
(Schering-Plough HealthCare) **519, 767**
Shade UVAGUARD SPF 15
Suncreen Lotion
(Schering-Plough HealthCare) **519, 768**

OXYMETAZOLINE HYDROCHLORIDE
Afrin Cherry Scented Nasal Spray
0.05% (Schering-Plough
HealthCare)..............................**757**
Afrin Extra Moisturizing Nasal
Spray
(Schering-Plough HealthCare) **518, 757**
Afrin Menthol Nasal Spray
(Schering-Plough HealthCare) **757**
Afrin Nasal Spray 0.05% and
Nasal Spray Pump
(Schering-Plough HealthCare) **518, 757**
Afrin Nose Drops 0.05%
(Schering-Plough HealthCare) **757**
Afrin Sinus
(Schering-Plough HealthCare) **757**
Duration 12 Hour Nasal Spray
(Schering-Plough HealthCare) **766**
4-Way 12 Hour Nasal Spray
(Bristol-Myers Products) **506, 644**
Neo-Synephrine Maximum
Strength 12 Hour Nasal Spray
(Bayer Consumer) **505, 624**
Neo-Synephrine Maximum
Strength 12 Hour Extra
Moisturizing Nasal Spray
(Bayer Consumer) **505, 624**
Neo-Synephrine Maximum
Strength 12 Hour Nasal Spray
Pump (Bayer Consumer) **505, 624**
12 Hour Nōstrilla
(Ciba Self-Medication) **509, 660**
Vicks Sinex 12-Hour Nasal
Decongestant Spray and Ultra Fine
Mist
(Procter & Gamble) **738**
Visine L.R. Eye Drops
(Pfizer Consumer) **515, 719**

P

PADIMATE O (OCTYL DIMETHYL PABA)
Herpecin-L Cold Sore Lip Balm
(Campbell) **646**

PAMABROM
PMS Multi-Symptom Formula
Midol (Bayer Consumer) **505, 622**
Maximum Strength Midol Teen
Multi-Symptom Formula
(Bayer Consumer) **505, 621**

PASSIFLORA
Hyland's Calms Forté Tablets
(Standard Homeopathic) **788**

PECTIN
Celestial Seasonings Soothers
Herbal Throat Drops
(Warner-Lambert).................. **523, 805**

PERMETHRIN
A-200 Lice Control Spray
(Hogil)................................. **510, 672**
Nix Creme Rinse
(WARNER WELLCOME) **526, 822**

PETROLATUM
A and D Ointment
(Schering-Plough HealthCare) **518, 757**
Aquaphor Healing Ointment
(Beiersdorf)......................... **506, 628**
Aquaphor Healing Ointment,
Original Formula (Beiersdorf) **506, 628**
Eucerin Original Moisturizing
Creme (Beiersdorf) **506, 628**
Keri Lotion - Sensitive Skin
(Bristol-Myers Products) **507, 644**
Keri Lotion - Silky Smooth
(Bristol-Myers Products) **507, 644**
Preparation H Hemorrhoidal
Cream (Whitehall-Robins) **528, 842**
Preparation H Hemorrhoidal
Ointment (Whitehall-Robins) .. **528, 842**

PETROLATUM, WHITE
A and D Medicated Diaper Rash
Ointment
(Schering-Plough HealthCare) **518, 757**
Borofax Skin Protectant Ointment
(WARNER WELLCOME) **525, 817**
Caldesene Medicated Ointment
(Ciba Self-Medication) **507, 652**
Hemorid Creme
(Thompson Medical) **797**
Hemorid Ointment
(Thompson Medical) **522, 797**

PHENOL
Cēpastat Cherry Flavor Sore
Throat Lozenges
(SmithKline Beecham
Consumer) **519, 770**
Cēpastat Extra Strength Sore
Throat Lozenges
(SmithKline Beecham
Consumer) **519, 770**
Children's Vicks Chloraseptic Sore
Throat Spray (Procter & Gamble) **730**
Vicks Chlorasptic Sore Throat Spray,
Gargle and Mouth Rinse, Menthol
and Cherry Flavors
(Procter & Gamble) **732**

PHENOLPHTHALEIN
Dialose Plus Tablets
(J&J•Merck Consumer) **510, 675**
Doxidan Liqui-Gels (Upjohn) **522, 801**
Ex-Lax Chocolated Laxative
Tablets (Sandoz Consumer) .. **516, 748**
Extra Gentle Ex-Lax Laxative Pills
(Sandoz Consumer) **516, 749**
Maximum Relief Formula Ex-Lax
Laxative Pills
(Sandoz Consumer) **516, 749**
Regular Strength Ex-Lax Laxative
Pills (Sandoz Consumer)........ **516, 749**
Fletcher's Cherry Flavor
(Mentholatum)............................**710**
Phillips' Gelcaps
(Bayer Consumer) **506, 627**

PHENYLBENZIMIDAZOLE SULFONIC ACID
Oil of Olay Daily UV Protectant SPF 15
Beauty Fluid-Original and Fragrance
Free (Olay Co. Inc.)
(Procter & Gamble) **725**

PHENYLEPHRINE HYDROCHLORIDE
Cerose DM (Wyeth-Ayerst) **529, 853**
4-Way Fast Acting Nasal Spray
(regular & mentholated)
(Bristol-Myers Products) **506, 644**
Hemorid Creme
(Thompson Medical) **797**
Hemorid Ointment
(Thompson Medical) **522, 797**
Hemorid Suppositories
(Thompson Medical) **522, 797**
Neo-Synephrine Nasal Drops,
Pediatric, Mild, Regular &
Extra Strength (Bayer
Consumer) **505, 624**
Neo-Synephrine Nasal Sprays,
Pediatric, Mild, Regular &
Extra Strength (Bayer
Consumer) **505, 624**
Novahistine Elixir
(SmithKline Beecham
Consumer) **521, 782**
Preparation H Hemorrhoidal
Cream (Whitehall-Robins) **528, 842**
Preparation H Hemorrhoidal
Ointment (Whitehall-Robins) .. **528, 842**
Vicks Sinex Nasal Spray and Ultra Fine
Mist (Procter & Gamble) **738**

PHENYLPROPANOLAMINE BITARTRATE
Alka-Seltzer Plus Cold Medicine
(Bayer Consumer) **504, 611**

Italic Page Number **Indicates Brief Listing**

Italic Page Number **Indicates Brief Listing**

NONPRESCRIPTION DRUGS IN 1996: THEIR IMPACT AND USE

Each year, Americans spend almost $14 billion on nonprescription drugs, an amount that increases by 8 percent to 10 percent annually. This growth is fueled in part by two important trends: the self-care movement and an increase in the number of OTC (over-the-counter) products, mainly through Rx-to-OTC switches and product line extensions. It's important for physicians and pharmacists to be aware of these trends, and to understand how and why patients use OTCs. Because consumers turn to you as a drug expert, you play a critical role in providing counseling on the safe and effective use of medications. The information and guidance you provide can help lead to positive outcomes and help prevent costly and potentially harmful drug misuse by your patients.

This chapter is designed to help you more thoroughly understand the nonprescription drug market and the drugs themselves.

The first section, "The Changing OTC Market," discusses the growth of the OTC marketplace and factors contributing to this increase, including:

■ the growing self-care movement among consumers;
■ the increasing availability of new products and categories of products, mainly due to Rx-to-OTC switches;
■ the cost effectiveness of OTCs in the face of rising health care costs.

The second part, "Consumer Perceptions and OTC Use," focuses on how consumers perceive and use OTCs, the effect of demographics on OTC utilization, and sales volumes by product category.

Section three, "Establishing Safety and Effectiveness," provides an overview of the approval process for OTC and switched products, as well as labeling, packaging, and marketing regulations.

"Patient Counseling: A Critical Role for Physicians and Pharmacists" outlines the growing need for patient counseling on OTC use, and explains how you can help fill this critical information gap. The effect of OTCs on physicians' and pharmacists' practices is also covered.

Finally, "The Future of OTCs" examines trends and issues that are likely to affect the nonprescription drug industry into the next century, as well as likely sources of future drugs and the kinds of new drugs that may soon become available over-the-counter.

Chapter 1: The Changing OTC Market

Most medications used in the United States today are nonprescription, or over-the-counter (OTC), drugs. In fact, six of every ten medications bought in the U.S. are nonprescription. Studies show that the rate of OTC use is steadily increasing, fueling market growth of eight percent to ten percent each year.

There are a number of factors propelling this growth, including a growing number of new products and classes of products, heightened interest among consumers in their own care, and a national health care agenda geared toward controlling costs. Indeed, the relatively low cost of OTCs contributes greatly to their success. For despite the wide use of nonprescription drugs (accounting for 30 percent of all drug expenditures), total spending for OTC medications takes less than two cents of the U.S. health care dollar. Over-the-counter drugs are thus one of the most cost-effective segments of health care.

These forces, combined with the overall safety and efficacy of the drugs, mean that OTC drugs will likely only increase in importance to consumers and manufacturers. U.S. and global sales figures support this.

Worldwide, OTC sales reached $37 billion in 1994. In the U.S. in 1994, nonprescription drugs were a $13.8 billion industry. Nonprescription drugs represent a growing market as well. Sales in the U.S. increased 40 percent between 1986 and 1991. In both 1993 and 1994, worldwide OTC sales increased by over $1 billion.

What Is an OTC?

Under current law, there are only two classes of drugs available on the market: OTC's—those safe for consumers to use on the basis of their labeling alone—and Rx—those that cannot be used safely without a physician's prescription.

To be marketed in the U.S., an OTC must be effective for its intended use and provide a margin of safety when used as directed.

Differences between OTC and Rx Drugs

Generally, OTC drugs pose minimum risk and possess a higher safety profile than Rx drugs, which are typically more toxic and defined as safe in the context of specific benefit-risk ratios. Another important distinction between the two classes of drugs is that OTCs are used to treat complaints or illnesses for which users recognize their own symptoms and level of relief; conditions treated by Rx drugs are usually more difficult to self-assess.

Nonprescription drugs differ from prescription drugs in other ways as well:

- Labeling for an OTC, unlike an Rx, must, by law, provide all the information a consumer needs for safe and effective use.
- OTC drugs are advertised directly to consumers, whereas Rx medications have traditionally been marketed to health professionals. This distinction is blurring, however, as drug companies make use of "institutional" advertising to alert consumers about prescription products with the recommendation to "ask your doctor." Common examples are advertisements for such Rx products as Rogaine and Seldane. These ads are strictly regulated and restricted in what they can tell consumers.
- OTCs are far more numerous than Rx drugs. There are about 300,000 OTC drugs (including different package sizes, dose strengths, and forms) currently on the market. Prescription drugs, on the other hand, number about 65,000.

A Brief History of the Two-Class System

The Federal Food, Drug, and Cosmetic Act (passed in 1938) is the primary law governing drugs sold in the U.S. The act prohibits the sale of drugs that are contaminated, misbranded, or otherwise dangerous to health; establishes minimum standards of strength, quality, and purity; and sets up specifications for labeling. According to this law, a drug is suitable for nonprescription use if it is not habit-forming and can be used safely by laymen without professional supervision.

The 1938 legislation, however, left it to drug manufacturers to make the distinction, and it wasn't until 1951 that federal law set up specific standards for determining whether or not a drug should be sold on a prescription-only basis. The 1951 Durham-Humphrey amendments established a consumer's right to self-treatment with safe and effective OTCs. It also stated that if a drug is safe and effective, and if labeling can be written so that a consumer may use it without professional supervision, it must be available over-the-counter.

Prescription drugs, on the other hand, were defined by the 1951 amendment as:

- certain habit-forming drugs (listed by name in the act);
- drugs not safe for use except under a physician's supervision because of toxicity or other potential harmful effects, the method of use, or other measures necessary for use;
- drugs limited to prescription use under a new drug application.

Today, the Food and Drug Administration (FDA) through its various divisions, review boards, and committees devoted to OTCs, reviews data required to establish safety, effectiveness, and proper labeling for OTCs, and approves proposed manufacturer labeling. (The approval process and safety and efficacy of OTCs are discussed in more detail later.)

Self-Care, Self-Medication

The self-care movement is one of the prime movers behind the rise of OTCs. Americans want more control over their own health, and studies show that they are more involved in their own care, a trend that is leading to better lifestyle choices and a growing awareness of preventive measures. Not surprisingly, today's consumer is also better informed about health issues than previous generations.

According to a survey published in the pharmacy news publication *Drug Topics,* nearly all consumers say they practice self-medication at some time; and over three-quarters do so frequently (see figure 1).

Figure 1
Frequency with which Americans Practice Self-Care

Frequency	% of Consumer
Frequently	76%
Occasionally	17%
Rarely	4%
Never	1%
No Response	2%

Source: Gannon, K., "Exclusive Consumer OTC Survey: Who's Buying What" *Drug Topics,* January 8, 1990.

And that trend is growing: A quarter of those polled said they self-medicate more now than in the past (see figure 2).

Figure 2
The Trend toward Self-Care

Increase in Self-Care	% of Consumers
Substantial Increase	13%
Increase	13%
No Change	66%
Decrease	5%
No Response	3%

Source: Gannon, K., "Exclusive Consumer OTC Survey: Who's Buying What" *Drug Topics,* January 8, 1990.

Over-the-counter medications play an important role in this self-care movement. A survey of over 1,500 Americans conducted by the Heller Research Group examined how consumers handle common health complaints. It revealed that the average person suffers six common health problems in any given two-week period, and over one-third (38 percent) of these are treated with an OTC (see figure 3).

Figure 3
Treatment of Common Health Complaints with OTCs

Treatment	1983	1992
Treated with an OTC	35%	38%
Not treated	37%	30%
Treated with home remedy	14%	16%
Treated with previous Rx	11%	13%
Sought professional help	9%	17%

Source: Heller Research Group. "Self-Medication in the 90s: Practices and Perceptions." New York, 1992.

Nonprescription drugs are therefore the most common alternative used by consumers to treat everyday ailments. The trend toward self-care may also be accelerated as the average age of the population increases. Certainly, the "aging of America" and a concomitant increase in chronic health problems will have an impact on OTC use. The elderly, in particular, rely on cost-effective treatment options as their incomes shrink and their health complaints proliferate with age.

The Heller study also showed that consumers are achieving healthier lifestyles. It said, for example, that Americans are changing the way they eat by adopting diets that are lower in fat and cholesterol. Consumers are also smoking less, exercising more and taking more vitamins and other dietary supplements.

Cost-Effectiveness of OTCs

One of the main benefits of over-the-counter drugs is their relatively low cost, a factor that has contributed greatly to their success and growing popularity in the marketplace. This relative low cost has also generated significant savings within the health care system. It's estimated, for example, that OTCs saved the nation $10.5 billion in health care costs in 1987 alone. This figure includes savings on prescription drugs, doctor visits, lost work time, insurance costs, and travel. Today, OTCs are estimated to save $20 billion each year. These numbers take on even greater significance when they are considered in the context of rising health care costs.

In 1991, total health care expenditures topped $750 billion or 13 percent of all national spending on goods and services (GNP) for that year. By 1994, health care costs reached an astounding $938 billion. Of that amount, however, over-the-counter drugs accounted for a tiny portion—$13.8 billion, or less than two cents of each U.S. health care dollar. And while other health care costs have risen dramatically year after year, OTC prices have increased by 4 percent or less each year since 1986 (excluding 1989, when prices jumped 5 percent).

The low cost of OTCs makes them very attractive to consumers, who are concerned with both costs and health. In fact, a typical OTC costs the consumer

Figure 4
The OTC Market in 1994, by Product Category

Category	Dollar Sales (in thousands)	% Change over previous year
Internal analgesics	$2,771,927	1.8
Cold/sinus/cough drops	2,081,162	0.0
Vitamins	1,830,858	9.7
Antacids	865,874	5.0
Miscellaneous remedies	849,738	2.3
Laxatives	729,156	(1.4)
Cold/allergy/sinus powder	477,812	(3.0)
Cough syrup	408,709	(11.6)
Nasal spray	342,521	(1.8)
Miscellaneous health treatments	217,816	18.0
External analgesic rubs	202,614	4.5
Miscellaneous remedy tablets	199,425	3.6
Miscellaneous health tablets	152,276	1.3

Source: Information Resources Inc., Chicago, 1995.

less than $4, compared with $25 for an average prescription drug. In addition, consumers spend only about $47 a year on OTCs. According to a Nielsen North America study done in 1995, it costs only 11 cents to treat a headache with one dose of an OTC, 12 cents to relieve an upset stomach, and 20 cents per dose to fight symptoms of a cold or cough. These economical alternatives give consumers a wide range of choice as they seek to control their own health and health-care decisions.

Increasing Number of OTCs

Increased use of OTCs by health- and cost-conscious consumers is not the only factor driving the OTC market. The number and variety of OTCs are also swelling.

Today, there are about 300,000 different OTC products being marketed in the United States. The array changes constantly in response to shifting demographics, outbreaks of flu and other communicable conditions, and consumer trends and perceptions.

Even though the market is subject to rapid change, the latest research gives some indication of how it is carved up (see figure 4). Internal analgesics lead the field in OTC sales, accounting for $2.8 billion in sales in 1994. Other high-volume product categories are cold/sinus/cough drops ($2.1 billion), vitamins ($1.8 billion), antacids ($865.9 million),

and laxatives ($729.2 million). Those product categories showing the greatest increase over the previous year include vitamins (9.7 percent) and antacids (5 percent).

One important sales trend gaining momentum—and providing consumers with even more OTC alternatives—is the private label. These are OTC products sold under a store name and generally offered at competitive prices. In 1991, private labels accounted for 10 percent of total drugstore Health and Beauty Care sales, and in some categories of products, up to 13 percent of sales.

Impact of Rx-to-OTC Switching

Another important trend in the growing OTC market is the fairly new practice of switching prescription drugs to OTC status. This process makes entire new categories of treatments available to consumers without a prescription.

Although many new drugs have been introduced since World War II, virtually all have been marketed as prescription drugs. Then, about a decade ago, the FDA adopted a policy of switching drugs from prescription to OTC status. This policy has had a tremendous impact on the OTC market, with 56 ingredients or dosages switched to OTC status and over 25 more pending. Today, more than 600 OTC products use ingredients and dosages available by prescription-only 20 years ago. And more than 70 petitions from manufacturers to switch ingredients are expected in the next five years.

Important recent switches include anti-ulcer medication, topical hydrocortisone, antihistamines, and analgesics. Figure 5 shows other products that are likely candidates for a future OTC switch.

Figure 5
CANDIDATES FOR FUTURE OTC SWITCH

Category: Cold, Allergy, Sinus, and Asthma

Active Ingredient	Description	Product Examples	Manufacturers
Cromolyn sodium	Anti-allergy	Intal Nasalcrom	Fisons Fisons
Loratadine	Non-sedating antihistamine	Claritin	Schering-Plough
Terfenadine	Antihistamine	Seldane	Hoechst Marion Roussel

Category: Analgesics

Active Ingredient	Description	Product Examples	Manufacturers
Diflunisal	NSAID	Dolobid	J&J-Merck
Indomethacin	NSAID	Indocin	J&J-Merck
Piroxicam	NSAID	Feldene	Pfizer
Sulindac	NSAID	Clinoril	J&J-Merck

Category: Gastrointestinal Drugs

Active Ingredient	Description	Product Examples	Manufacturers
Nizatidine	Anti-ulcer	Axid	Lilly/Whitehall Labs
Ranitidine (HCl)	Anti-ulcer	Zantac	Glaxo, Sandoz
Sucralfate	Anti-ulcer	Carafate	Hoechst Marion Roussel

Category: Antifungals and Antiinfectives

Active Ingredient	Description	Product Examples	Manufacturers
Acyclovir	Antiviral	Zovirax	Warner Wellcome
Econazole	Antifungal	Spectazole	Ortho
Ketoconazole	Antifungal	Nizoral	Janssen
Methenamine mandelate	Urinary tract infection	Mandelamine	Parke-Davis
Nystatin	Anti-fungal	Mycostatin	Bristol-Meyers Squibb

Category: Other

Active Ingredient	Description	Product Examples	Manufacturers
Carisoprodol	Muscle relaxant	Soma	Wallace Laboratories
Cyclobenzaprine HCl	Muscle relaxant	Flexeril	J&J-Merck
Cholestyramine	Cholesterol-lowering	Cholybar	Parke-Davis
Nicotine polacrilex	Smoking-cessation	Nicorette	SmithKline Beecham
Sulfacetamide sodium	Ocular anti-infective	Bleph-10 Sulamyd	Allergan Schering-Plough
Minoxidil	Hair loss treatment	Rogaine	Pharmacia & Upjohn

Source: FIND/SVP Inc. "The Market for Rx-to-OTC Switches." 1994.

Effect of Switching on Costs and Care

The range of health problems that can be treated with OTCs has grown dramatically in the last ten years, and switches have played an important role in this growth. Consumers are very aware of these newly available switched products. They perceive them as strong, cost-effective medications. According to the Heller survey, close to 60 percent of consumers say they believe switches make it possible for them to save money, and almost two-thirds (64 percent) say they favor the process of Rx to OTC switching. Consumers also said that they buy more switches, by a margin of two to one, when they are available.

The effect of switches on health care costs has also been tremendous. For example, the net annual savings from the switch of cough-cold medicines to OTC status is estimated at about three-quarters of a billion dollars. Another example is the 1979 switch of 1/2 percent hydrocortisone that saved American consumers more than $1 billion in the first three years after the change.

The Line Extension Strategy

Line extensions are another important strategy that drug makers are using to bring new products to the shelves of the nation's 750,000 OTC outlets, pharmacies, supermarkets, convenience stores, and mass merchandisers. This is the practice of extending an established brand name to an entire line of nonprescription products. Thus, an extra-strength or non-drowsy formulation may be marketed under a pre-existing product name. The success of this practice is based on the trust that consumers develop for specific brand names leading them to purchase other products with the same brand name.

The FDA has expressed concern about whether this proliferation of products confuses consumers. However, the Nonprescription Drug Manufacturers Association (NDMA), a Washington, DC-based trade association representing OTC makers, claims that line extensions are useful to consumers, since they offer new solutions and more choices for common complaints. It cites, for example, the use of clear labeling and explanatory advertising to prevent confusion about line extensions and other new products, and also points to a growing number of published guides to medications and self-care, such as *PDR for Nonprescription Drugs*.

Chapter 2: Consumer Perceptions and OTC Use

Studies that have explored the ways consumers use and perceive nonprescription medicines shed light on the following issues:

■ Americans' use of OTCs in comparison to other nationalities;
■ OTCs as serious medicine;
■ Safety and correctness of nonprescription drug use;
■ Effect of age, sex, and economic status on self-medication habits;
■ Product choice and availability;
■ Impact of the rise of managed care and the national movement toward health care reform.

Important and far-reaching trends in these areas may be changing the way nonprescription—and prescription—drugs are used. In addition, the role that physicians and pharmacists play in the use of OTCs is paramount, and is discussed in a separate section.

Use Highest in the U.S.

Americans use more OTCs than people in other countries, according to a study comparing 14 national surveys on self-medication (see figure 1). The review ascribes this usage to the fact that the U.S. is the only country lacking a national health care program. It concludes: "Many U.S. citizens must pay for both doctor visits and prescription medicines; others [U.S. citizens] must pay a percentage of these costs. As a result, for common conditions, many Americans consider self-treatment with over-the-counter medicines a cost-saving alternative to doctor visits and prescription drugs."

Figure 1
Use of OTCs for Common Health Complaints: A Worldwide Comparison

Country	Percent of Consumers Using OTCs
United States	33%
Australia	28%
Germany	28%
Spain	24%
United Kingdom	24%
Sweden	24%
Switzerland	22%
Mexico	21%
Italy	20%
Japan	16%

Source: World Federation of Proprietary Medicine Manufacturers. "Health Care, Self-Care and Self-Medication" 1991.

Other consumer surveys bear out the importance of cost. In a national Gallup poll, nearly half of those surveyed cited low cost as the greatest advantage to using an OTC. Other important features are convenience (cited by 29 percent) and the fact that OTCs eliminate the need for a doctor's visit (23 percent).

Conditions for which OTCs are used are similar throughout the world. In all countries surveyed, the common cold is the most frequently reported ailment for which OTCs are used, followed by headache, digestive problems, and body aches and pains.

Satisfied Customers

OTCs can treat or cure about 400 different common health complaints. The average consumer reports suffering from about six of these every two weeks, ranging from headaches, which are treatable with an OTC according to more than three-quarters of consumers (76 percent), to dry skin and sinus problems (56 percent and 54 percent respectively) (see figure 2). By category, respiratory and feminine complaints are most likely to be treated with a nonprescription medication (see figure 3).

Figure 2
Top Ten Problems Most Likely to be Treated with OTCs

Complaint	Percent Who Would Treat with OTCs
Headache	76%
Athlete's foot	69%
Lip problems	68%
Common cold	63%
Chronic dandruff	59%
Pre-menstrual	58%
Menstrual	57%
Upset Stomach	57%
Painful/dry skin	56%
Sinus problems	54%

Source: Heller Research Group. "Self-Medication in the 90s: Practices and Perceptions." New York, 1992.

Figure 3
Major Categories for which OTCs are used

Condition	Percent Treated with OTCs
Respiratory	50%
Feminine	50%
Pain	46%
Digestive	44%
Eye/ear/mouth	41%
Skin	33%
General well being	8%

Source: Heller Research Group. "Self Medication in the 90s: Practices and perceptions." New York, 1992.

American consumers also say that OTCs are effective treatment for these conditions. Americans are, in fact, more satisfied with OTCs than consumers in other countries (see figure 4). Of all 14 countries surveyed, the U.S. had the highest level of satisfaction with nonprescription drugs.

Figure 4
Percentage of Consumers, by Country, who are Satisfied with OTCs.

Country	%
United States	92%
Mexico	90%
United Kingdom	83%
Canada	80%
Australia	75%

Source: World Federation of Proprietary Medicine Manufacturers. "Health Care, Self-Care and Self-Medication" 1991.

In a survey conducted in the U.S., 94 percent of those surveyed said they would retake OTCs they've used previously, and more than nine out of ten reported that they were satisfied with the products they had used. Indeed, nearly three-quarters of Americans say they believe OTCs are as effective as prescription medications.

Finally, studies have also probed the reasons consumers stop taking an OTC. Ninety percent of those surveyed said they discontinued use because the problem went away. Only 3 percent said they used a medicine that did not work.

The Safe Use of OTCs

No drug is completely safe, and consumers have shown that they appreciate the potential risk of taking any medication. In one survey, 94 percent of American consumers said that care must be used when taking medications, even those that are not prescription drugs. Ninety-five percent disagreed with the statement that "it is safe to take as many OTCs as you wish."

Over-medication with nonprescription drugs is rare among consumers. According to the Heller study, seven out of ten respondents prefer to fight symptoms without taking medications at all, and nine out of ten said they know all medications should only be used when absolutely necessary. In the same survey, 85 percent said it is nonetheless important to have nonprescription medications available to help relieve minor medical problems.

Americans rate second only to residents of the UK when it comes to reading the label before using an OTC, according to national surveys. Ninety-six percent of U.S. consumers said they read OTC labels, compared with 97 percent in the U.K. Many U.S. studies have confirmed this fact, reporting percentages ranging from 88 percent to 93 percent.

National surveys also show that:

■ Americans generally take less than the maximum recommended daily dose when using OTC analgesics. (For colds, menstruation, and headache, the average number of tablets taken ranges from four to six; for arthritis, rheumatism, and backache, the average number taken each day of use is five);
■ Nearly all OTCs are used for considerably less time than the standard ten-day limit-of-use warning;
■ Consumer knowledge about OTCs is more accurate than consumer knowledge of many other areas, including banking, nutrition, and insurance. In comparative studies, consumers show a solid understanding, with scores of 75 percent or higher, for over half of the drug questions;
■ Consumers read labels more carefully now than in the past.

Demographics of OTC Use

The way consumers approach self-medication with a nonprescription drug is affected by age, sex, and economic status, among other factors.

For example, the level of OTC use remains fairly constant with age, although younger consumers tend to use OTCs for acute conditions, whereas the elderly turn to them more often for chronic conditions.

The level of usage and conditions for which OTCs are used do differ with gender. Women not only buy more OTCs than men, they also use them more and use them to treat different types of conditions. Women take OTCs for anxiety, indigestion and stom-

Figure 5
Recent Additions to the OTC Market

Ingredient	Category	Products
Cimetidine	Heartburn relief	Tagamet HB
Clemastine fumarate	Antihistamine	Tavist-1
Clemastine fumarate with phenylpropanolamine HCl	Antihistamine/decongestant	Tavist -D
Famotidine	Acid controller	Pepcid AC
Hydrocortisone acetate	Antipruritic	Anusol, Caldecort
Ketoprofen	Internal analgesic	Orudis KT, Actron
Miconazole nitrate	Anticandidal	Monistat 7
Naphazoline HCl with pheniramine maleate	Antihistamine/decongestant eye drop	Opcon A
Naproxen	Internal analgesic/antipyretic	Aleve, Naprosyn

Source: Nonprescription Drug Manufacturers Association, 1995.

ach complaints, headaches, fatigue, sleep problems, arthritis, lip and skin conditions, and weight control. Among men, OTCs are used predominantly for aches and pains, cuts, and colds.

Economic status also affects how OTCs are used. Americans covered by Medicaid, for example, are less likely to take an OTC. They are more likely to seek a physician's care or use a prescription medication that is already in the home.

Increasing Product Choices

New categories and forms of OTCs in the market also affect consumer's self-medication choices. New drugs and whole new categories of products provide consumers with a growing number of effective alternatives for self-care. These new entities also increase the importance of physicians and pharmacists as OTC counselors.

Most of today's new nonprescription drugs contain ingredients that have recently been switched to OTC status. (Examples of these new OTCs are listed in figure 5.) And as noted above, consumer acceptance of switches is exceptionally high. For example, two feminine antifungal ingredients—clotrimazole and miconazole nitrate—became available over-the-counter in 1991. These products, which provide women with an entirely new class of over-the-counter remedies for treating vaginal infections, accounted for about 90 percent of Health and Beauty Care new-

item sales volume in drugstores and other outlets in the year they appeared on the market.

The high use of switched products by consumers is also strongly demonstrated by a survey of top-selling OTCs. In 1992, 14 of the 15 best-selling OTCs introduced since 1975 were either switched brands or switch-related products, as shown in figure 6.

Figure 6
Consumer Preference for Switched Products

In 1992, 14 of the 15 best selling OTCs introduced since 1975 were either switched brands or switch-related products.

Product	1992 Sales (in millions)
Advil	$320
Monistat 7	114
Benadryl	92
Sudafed	92
Motrin IB*	87
Imodium AD	85
Dimetapp	77
Nuprin	67
Afrin	62
Gyne-Lotrimin	53
Oxy-line	52
Drixoral	49
Chlor-Trimeton	44
Actifed	44
Comtrex**	35

*Switch-related
**New proprietary product
Source: Sudler & Hennessy, New York, 1992.

Effects of Health Care Reform and Managed Care

Two trends that have affected every segment of health care delivery are health care reform and managed care. Since these trends are still evolving, their impact on the OTC market cannot yet be determined, but some outcomes can reasonably be projected.

Managed care probably has less of a direct effect on the use of OTCs than on other segments of health care since most third-party health care plans do not cover nonprescription drugs. By contrast, prescription drugs are often closely managed by the use of drug formularies; through financial incentives to members to use less expensive products, mail order pharmacies, and generics; and through drug utilization review. Nonetheless, because of the cost-effectiveness of OTCs, it is likely that their use will increase as health care costs rise and efforts to contain costs are exerted by payers and national reform programs. Self-medication will most likely be recognized as part of the solution to the problems of rising costs and limited access.

Managed care may also increase OTC use in another indirect way. Managed care typically uses capitated plans in which physicians and pharmacists are paid a flat rate per member by the managed care administrator, regardless of the amount of care provided. Plan members may also be given financial incentives to use fewer plan services. As a result, both providers and plan members often have an incentive to contain costs and use fewer of the medical services and products covered by the plan. Self-medication may therefore become more accepted and encouraged under this type of managed care reimbursement system.

By contrast, traditional fee-for-service health insurance plans provide reimbursement based on utilization rates. Under this system, self-care is, in effect, a form of competition for physicians and pharmacists since it decreases office visits and prescription drug use.

In addition, although most consumers are not reimbursed by health insurance companies for OTCs, nonprescription drugs nonetheless generally end up costing less than a prescription since the copay and/or deductible on an Rx drug usually exceeds the average price of an OTC.

Finally, health care reform, in an effort to make health care affordable and accessible, may also encourage the process of switching Rx products to over-the-counter status. In fact, experts predict that this trend may put a high number of new OTC products on the market in the near future.

Chapter 3: Establishing Safety and Effectiveness

Every over-the-counter medication marketed in the U.S. must meet rigorous safety and efficacy standards set by the Food and Drug Administration (FDA). Manufacturers are required by law to follow strict labeling, packaging, and advertising regulations. In addition, the industry has created voluntary standards and specific guidelines for many aspects of product safety and effective use. The high safety profile and effectiveness that consumers count on in OTC medicines are thus the result of a collaborative effort between the government and the pharmaceutical industry.

History of Government Regulation

The first U.S. drug law—the Food and Drugs Act of 1906—required only that drug products meet standards of purity and strength. Under this law, fraudulent labeling was the only basis for removing a product from the market and even in these cases, the burden of proof rested with the government.

In 1938, the more comprehensive Federal Food, Drug, and Cosmetic Act was passed. The legislation followed closely on the heels of a tragedy in which 107 people, mostly children, were poisoned by "elixir sulfanilamide," which contained ethylene glycol, a colorless syrupy alcohol used as an antifreeze in heating and cooling systems. The new law required drug companies to demonstrate the safety of all new products—before they were marketed. This was to be accomplished by making the drug meet the preapproval requirements of a new drug application (NDA). (Pre-existing drugs were grandfathered in under the new law.) The legislation also eliminated the need for the government to show intent to defraud in cases of mislabeling; provided tolerances for necessary poisonous substances; authorized factory inspections; and added court injunctions to existing seizure and prosecution provisions for violators.

It wasn't until 1951 that certain drugs were required to be labeled as prescription only. The Durham-Humphrey Amendments were added to federal law to provide for those medications that are unsafe to take without a physician's supervision. The amendments state that if a drug is safe and effective and can be labeled for use without professional supervision, it must be available over-the-counter.

OTC Drug Review

Providing evidence of safety prior to marketing was therefore required as early as 1938. However, it wasn't until 1962 that proof of efficacy was required as well. In that year, another amendment to the 1938 law required manufacturers to prove the effectiveness of a drug before it is marketed. Shortly thereafter, the FDA contracted for a review of all drugs, including OTCs that had been grandfathered in by the 1938 law. After 512 OTCs were evaluated, 75 percent were found to lack evidence of effectiveness. As a result, the FDA broadened its review to include all OTC products.

The FDA Division of OTC Evaluation chose to review the 700 or so active ingredients found in OTCs, rather than each of the 300,000 products on the market. This effort, which is still in progress, consists of classifying nonprescription drugs into 81 treatment categories (antacids, internal analgesics, etc.), and evaluating all the active ingredients in those categories in order to establish dosage and labeling regulations for each of them.

In the case of multiple indications or dosages, the ingredients are covered in more than one category. Diphenhydramine HCl, for example, has indications as a sleep aid, antitussive, antiemetic, and antihistamine, and is thus discussed in each of those categories.

The first phase of OTC review, which took place from 1972 to 1981, also established panels of outside experts to evaluate the OTC ingredients. Their review placed OTC products into one of three categories:

■ Category I: generally recognized as safe and effective for the therapeutic indication claimed;
■ Category II: not generally recognized as safe and effective, or having unacceptable indications;
■ Category III: insufficient data to permit final classification.

OTC Monographs and Nonmonographs

During the second phase of OTC review, which continues today, the FDA reviews the panels' findings and publishes in the Federal Register tentative monographs establishing dosage and labeling requirements. After considering objections and comments, a final monograph is published in the *Code of Federal Regulations*. Of the 85 product monographs to be published, 58 have been completed to date. Products that contain ingredients without a final monograph are marketed on a provisional basis and are subject to the requirements of a final monograph.

All OTC monographs consist of Subpart A, which includes regulations common to all OTCs, general warning labeling requirements, and a list of permissible inactive ingredients for the category. Subpart B identifies active ingredients that may be used within the category and acceptable combinations with other active ingredients. Subpart C contains indications, warnings and precautions, directions for use, dosages, dose frequency, and any specialized labeling requirements. Subpart D includes testing procedures, if any are required for the category, such as acid-neutralizing tests for antacids.

Once a monograph is final, any manufacturer may market a product without preapproval, provided the product meets the monograph's standards. Products that use new drug delivery systems or formulations, such as timed-release products, however, require a new drug application and separate approval.

In some cases, "nonmonographs" have been published following this stringent review process. A nonmonograph indicates that an ingredient or category of products fails to demonstrate safety and/or efficacy. The OTC review has resulted in nonmonographs—with concomitant removal of products from the market—in a number of product categories:

- anticholinergics;
- aphrodisiacs;
- camphorated oil;
- daytime sedatives;
- hair loss prevention products;
- halogenated salicylanilides;
- oral insect repellants;
- stomach acidifiers;
- sweet spirits of nitre;
- topical hormones;
- zirconium aerosols.

OTC Switching Procedures

The process of switching a prescription drug to nonprescription status also establishes its safety and efficacy as an OTC. (See figure 1 for a list of all 56 ingredients that have been switched to date.)

There are a number of mechanisms used to switch an Rx product.

- The FDA advisory panels for OTC drug review may recommend that a drug be switched. This type of review is responsible for about 40 of the switches to date, including hydrocortisone, diphenhydramine, nystatin, and oxymetazoline.
- A full NDA can be submitted for a current Rx drug in a new dosage or formulation. Since the FDA requires costly new studies for switches to be approved under a full NDA, it also grants the sponsor exclusive marketing rights for a period of years following approval. This mechanism, which deals with products rather than ingredients, is behind the approval of a number of new OTC products, including ibuprofen, loperamide, permethrin, micozole, and clotrimazole. Full NDAs will probably be preferred by manufacturers for future switches, since it gives them marketing exclusivity and thus an edge over their competition.
- A supplemental NDA may be filed by a holder of an approved original or abbreviated application for a closely related product.
- An abbreviated NDA may be submitted for products that are identical to an existing Rx product. This is used mainly for near duplicates of an Rx drug.
- The FDA can determine that an Rx is unnecessary for an existing drug. Requests for this type of switch can come from a company, or any interested party. However, there have been no switches resulting from this mechanism since 1971.

Drugs are switched to over-the-counter status on a case-by-case basis. General criteria that act as informal guidelines for the process include an acceptable margin of safety, lack of toxicity, adequate labeling, treatment of recognizable symptoms, a simple treatment regimen, and the potential savings that a switch might yield to consumers and to the health care system.

To ensure that OTCs receive the same level of regulatory priority as Rx drugs, the FDA restructured the Division of OTC Drug Evaluation to form the Office of OTC Drug Evaluation in 1991. This new office provides a forum for reviewing a drug's status. A committee of outside experts was established at the same time to advise the FDA on nonprescription drugs.

Industry Self Regulation

Federal regulation is just one aspect of OTC safety and effectiveness. Since 1934, member companies of the Nonprescription Drug Manufacturers Association (NDMA) have established voluntary guidelines covering a variety of marketing issues, including packaging, labeling, distribution, and advertising. Today, there are twelve voluntary guidelines used extensively by the industry. The most recently implemented are guidelines to improve readability of labels. Other areas of voluntary regulation include:

- advertising codes;
- package sizes of certain OTCs;
- "label flags" for those products with significant changes;
- complaint protocols;
- money-back guarantees;
- safety closures for products that may be harmful to children;
- standardization of children's aspirin products;
- disclosure of the quantities of active ingredients;
- disclosure of inactive ingredients;
- bulk mail sampling;
- expiration dates;
- product identification of solid dosage OTC products.

Labeling and Packaging: Issues and Regulations

Labeling for nonprescription drugs must either include all the required elements indicated in an OTC monograph or receive preapproval through an NDA. Labels are required by law to provide detailed information on ingredients, product use, dosages, dose frequencies, possible reactions, contraindications, and other warnings, if applicable (see figure 2).

Despite these regulations, some labeling issues, such as label clarity, continue to cause concern. Studies show that about 90 percent of consumers read OTC labels (96 percent in the case of children's medicine labels). Nonetheless, about 10 percent of consumers say that OTC labels are too difficult to understand. Although many OTC labels are written on a ninth-grade level, the average consumer reads at only the eighth grade level, and 20 percent of

Figure 1

Ingredients Switched from Rx Status to OTC

Ingredient	Adult Dosage	Product Category	Product Examples and Manufacturer
Acidulated phosphate fluoride rinse*	0.02% fluoride in aqueous solution (topical)	Dental rinse	
Brompheniramine maleate	4 mg/4-6 h (oral)	Antihistamine	Dimetane (A.H. Robins)
Chlorphedianol HCl	25 mg/6-8 h (oral)	Antitussive	
Chlorpheniramine maleate	4 mg/4-6 h (oral)	Antihistamine	Allerest (Pharmacraft), Chlor-Trimeton (Schering), Contac (Menley & James), Sudafed Plus (Burroughs Wellcome)
Chlorpheniramine maleate (NDA)	12 mg/12 h (oral timed-release)	Antihistamine	Triaminic 12 (Dorsey)
Cimetidine	200 mg up to twice a day	Heartburn relief	Tagamet HB (SKB)
Clemastine fumarate (NDA)	1.34 mg/12 h	Antihistamine	Tavist-1 (Sandoz)
Clemastine fumarate phenylpropanolamine HCl (NDA)	1.34 mg/12 h	Antihistamine with decongestant	Tavist D (Sandoz)
Clotrimazole (NDA)	1% lotion/cream 2x/day	Antifungal	Lotrimin AF (Schering)
Clotrimazole (NDA)	1% cream; 100 mg inserts	Anticandidal	Gyne-Lotrimin (Schering), Mycelex-7 (Miles)
Dexbrompheniramine maleate	2 mg/4-6 h (oral)	Antihistamine	
Dexbrompheniramine maleate (NDA)	3 mg/6-8 h (oral)	Antihistamine	Drixoral Plus (Schering)
Dexbrompheniramine maleate (NDA)	6 mg/12 h (oral timed-release)	Antihistamine	Drixoral (Schering)
Dexchlorpheniramine maleate	2 mg/4-6 h (oral)	Antihistamine	
Diphenhydramine HCl (NDA)	25 mg/4 hr (oral)	Antitussive	Benylin (Parke-Davis)
Diphenhydramine HCl	50 mg/single dose only (oral)	Sleep Aid	Sominex 2 (Beecham), Sleep-eze 3 (Whitehall)
Diphenhydramine HCl Diphenhydramine HCl	25-50 mg/4-6 h (oral) 25-50 mg/4-6 h (oral)	Antiemetic Antihistamine	Benadryl 25 (Parke-Davis)
Diphenhydramine monocitrate	76 mg/single dose only (oral)	Sleep Aid	
Doxylamine succinate (NDA)	25 mg/single dose only (oral)	Sleep Aid	Unisom (Pfizer)
Doxylamine succinate	7.5-12.5 mg/4-6 h (oral)	Antihistamine	Nyquil (Vicks)
Dyclonine HCl*	0.05-0.1% in rinse, mouthwash, gargle, or spray 3-4x/day; 1-3 mg as lozenge	Oral Anesthetic	Sucrets Maximum Strength Lozenges (Beecham)
Ephedrine sulfate	0.1-1.25% (topical)	Anorectal/Vaso-constrictor	
Epinephrine HCl	0.005 to 0.01% (topical)	Anorectal/Vaso-constrictor	
Famotidine	10 mg, up to 20 mg/day	Acid controller	Pepcid AC (J&J, Merck)
Haloprogin	1.0% (topical)	Antifungal	
Hydrocortisone*	0.25-0.50% (topical)	Antipruritic	Cortaid (Upjohn), Lanacort (Combe)
Hydrocortisone*	above 0.50-1.0% (topical)	Antipruritic	
Hydrocortisone acetate*	0.25-0.50% (topical)	Antipruritic	Bactine (Miles), Caldecort (Pharmacraft)
Hydrocortisone acetate*	above 0.50-1.0% (topical)	Antipruritic	
Ibuprofen (NDA)	200 mg/4-6 h (oral)	Internal analgesic	Advil (Whitehall), Nuprin (Bristol-Myers)

Figure 1

Ingredients Switched from Rx Status to OTC, continued

Ingredient	Adult Dosage	Product Category	Product Examples and Manufacturer
Ibuprofen solution	7.5 mg/kg up to 4 times-a-day	Internal analgesic/ antipyretic	Children's Motrin (McNeil)
Ketoprofen	12.5 mg every 4-6 hours	Internal analgesic	Orudis KT (Whitehall-Robins) Actron (Bayer)
Liposperse cholecystokinetic (hydrogenated soybean oil and lecithin)	12.4g powder dissolved in 2-3 oz. water 20 minutes before gall bladder x-ray		
Loperamide (NDA)	4 mg, then 2 mg; max. 8 mg/day (oral)	Antidiarrheal	Imodium A-D (Johnson & Johnson)
Miconazole nitrate	2.0% (topical)	Antifungal	Micatin (Ortho)
Miconazole nitrate (NDA)	2.0% cream; 100 mg inserts	Anticandidal	Monistat 7 (Ortho)
Naphazoline HCl with pheniramine maleate	0.027% naphazoline HCl/ 0.315% pheniramine maleate	Antihistamine/ decon-gestant, eye drop	Opcon A (Bausch &Lomb)
Naproxen (NDA)	200 mg/8-12 h (oral)	Internal analgesic; antipyretic	Aleve (Procter & Gamble) Naprosyn (Syntex)
Oxymetazoline HCl*	0.05% aqueous solution (topical)	Nasal decongestant	Afrin (Schering), Duration (Plough), Dristan Long Lasting (Whitehall), Neo-Synephrine 12 Hour (Winthrop)
Oxymetazoline HCl (NDA)	0.025% solution/drops (topical)	Ocular vasoconstrictor	Ocuclear (Schering)
Permethrin (NDA)	1% cream rinse	Pediculicide	Nix (Burroughs-Wellcome)
Phenylephrine HCl*	0.5 mg in aqueous solution (topical)	Anorectal vasoconstrictor	
Phenylpropanolamine HCl (NDA)	75 mg/12 h (oral timed-release)	Nasal decongestant	Triaminic 12 (Dorsey)
Povidone iodine (NDA)	10% sponge (new dosage form)	Antimicrobial	E-Z Scrub 241 (Deseret)
Pseudophedrine HCl*	60 mg/4 or 4-6 h (oral); 240 mg max./24 h	Nasal decongestant	Sudafed (Burroughs Wellcome), Neo-Synephrinol (Winthrop)
Pseudophedrine HCl (NDA)	120 mg/12 h (oral timed-release)	Nasal decongestant	Actifed (Burroughs Wellcome)
Pseudophedrine sulfate*	60 mg/4 or 4-6 h (oral)	Nasal decongestant	Afrinol (Schering), Chlor-Trimeton (Schering)
Pseudophedrine sulfate (NDA)	120 mg/12 h (oral timed-release)	Nasal decongestant	Afrinol Repetabs (Schering)
Pyrantel pamoate	11 mg/kilo body weight; max. dose 1g (oral)	Anthelmintic	Antiminth (Pfizer)
Sodium fluoride rinse*	0.05% aqueous solution (topical)	Dental rinse	Fluorigard (Colgate-Palmolive)
Stannous fluoride gel*	0.4% aqueous solution (topical)	Dental rinse	
Stannous fluoride rinse*	0.1% aqueous solution (topical)	Dental Rinse	Stan Care (Block)
Tioconazole (NDA)	1% cream	Antifungal	TZ-3 (Pfizer)
Triprolidine HCl*	2.5 mg/4-6 h	Antihistamine	Actifed Capsules (Burroughs Wellcome), Actidil Syrup and Capsules (Burroughs Wellcome)
Triprolidine HCl (NDA)	5 mg/12 h	Antihistamine	Actifed 12 Hour Capsules (Burroughs Wellcome)
Xylometazoline HCl*	0.01% aqueous solution (topical)	Nasal decongestant	Orrivin (CIBA)

* FDA approval for OTC marketing is on an interim basis pending adoption of a final monograph

(NDA) Denotes switched under a new drug application

Source: Nonprescription Drug Manufacturers Association, "Ingredients & Dosages Transferred from Rx to OTC Status as a Consequence of the U.S. Food and Drug Administration's Review of Nonprescription Drug Products." Washington, DC, 1995.

What's on the Label

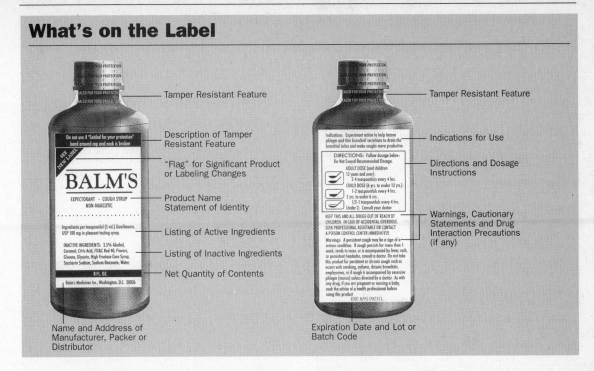

Tamper Resistant Feature

Description of Tamper Resistant Feature

"Flag" for Significant Product or Labeling Changes

Product Name Statement of Identity

Listing of Active Ingredients

Listing of Inactive Ingredients

Net Quantity of Contents

Name and Adddress of Manufacturer, Packer or Distributor

Tamper Resistant Feature

Indications for Use

Directions and Dosage Instructions

Warnings, Cautionary Statements and Drug Interaction Precautions (if any)

Expiration Date and Lot or Batch Code

Americans are functionally illiterate. Label readability can also be affected by such factors as poor vision and inadequate lighting in retail settings, particularly for the elderly.

The OTC industry has actively sought ways to help resolve readability issues. In 1990, the NDMA established a special task force to recommend label improvements. The resulting voluntary guidelines established specific requirements for layout, design, typography, and printing, to assist manufacturers in making labels as legible as possible.

Perhaps even more critical is product tampering. The first main incidence of OTC tampering occurred in Chicago in 1982, and led to swift enactment of tamper-resistant packaging regulations by the FDA. Federal laws also beefed up jail terms and fines for product tampering.

The OTC industry also responded vigorously to the Chicago poisonings and to subsequent tampering cases. In addition to designing tamper-resistant packaging at a cost of approximately $1 billion, individual companies offered large cash rewards for information, and the industry set up tampering hotlines for consumers and launched a massive public education campaign. The results have been positive, and OTC tampering has decreased significantly since 1982. In addition, consumers approve of the methods used to deter tampering. A national survey of 1,500 consumers indicated that tamper-resistant containers and consumer education were the best possible solutions to the tampering problem.

Marketing and Advertising OTCs

United States law allows OTC makers to advertise their products directly to consumers under the authority of the Federal Trade Commission (FTC). Reviews by this body are conducted for all OTC ads on a case-by-case basis after the ads are used, and are subject to the same truth in advertising guidelines as any other product.

An international study recently assessed the impact of advertising on OTC use. It indicated that use of nonprescription medicines is no greater in those countries that allow consumer advertising than in those that don't. Sweden and Switzerland, which restrict OTC advertising, for example, have the same level of OTC use as countries with consumer ads. The study concluded that advertising OTCs directly to consumers does not lead to overuse or misuse.

Some states have also proposed laws that would place new requirements on OTC makers. The pharmacy news magazine, *Drug Topics,* reported in 1994 that 68 such proposals had been made in the previous 18 months. These included a bill in New York requiring special label warnings for the elderly and a bill in Texas calling for bittering agents in topical OTCs. As a whole, the industry has criticized what it calls the evolution of 50 "mini-FDAs" that it believes individual state legislation would bring. According to industry leaders, present federal laws and regulation work effectively to protect consumers against unsafe, ineffective, or mislabeled medicines. They argue that state regulations are not only an unnecessary replication of FDA efforts, but would also mean chaos for the interstate commerce in OTCs.

Chapter 4: Patient Counseling:
A Critical Role for Physicians and Pharmacists

The Consumer's Self-Medication Bill of Rights, drafted by the Nonprescription Drug Manufacturers Association, states: "Next to safe and effective products, information is the most important commodity in self-care/self-medication." And as OTC use increases and the number of available products grows, consumers will require more information than ever to choose the right products and use them effectively and safely. For most consumers, that information comes from their health care providers. Physicians and pharmacists are in an ideal and unique position to provide patients with informed and up-to-date OTC advice. Through effective patient counseling on OTC use, physicians and phamacists can help improve medical outcomes and prevent costly incidents of drug misuse.

A Growing Need For Information

For most consumers, information on nonprescription drugs comes from product labels and advertising, but these can be confusing or incomplete. Consumers thus rely on the one-to-one relationship they possess with their doctors and pharmacists for additional information.

New products, line extensions, and OTC switches are just some of the factors that may overwhelm even the most well-informed patient. In 1993, for example, 97 percent of all pharmacists surveyed across the nation said that line extensions for adult cough/cold/flu preparations led to significant confusion among their customers. Switches for children's cough/cold preparations caused even more problems.

Such confusion, multiplied by the number of products on the market, can foster potential medical misadventures, including:

■ use of an inappropriate medication;
■ use of an inappropriate dosage;
■ use of an OTC that is contraindicated;
■ drug-drug interactions;
■ inappropriate duration of OTC use;
■ side effects.

In addition, although all consumers need counseling on OTCs, many have special needs. Groups requiring special attention include:

■ patients with comprehension problems (20 percent of consumers are illiterate and nearly 10 percent say they are sometimes confused by OTC labels);
■ blind and other visually impaired patients;
■ deaf and other hearing-impaired patients;
■ the elderly;
■ children;
■ patients with comprehension deficits;
■ pregnant or nursing patients.

For these patients, self-medicating safely may pose difficulties, and counseling from a physician or pharmacist is particularly important.

All consumers have occasional questions about nonprescription medications. These range from requests for product recommendations to questions about cost. (Figure 1 lists the most commonly asked questions.) According to one national survey, almost two-thirds (65 percent) of consumers ask their physician for OTC advice and over half (54 percent) consult their pharmacist. (The total exceed 100 percent, since many consumers consult both physicians and pharmacists.) Consumers place a high value on the advice they receive. The same study revealed that 58 percent of patients are extremely satisfied with their doctor's advice, and 61 percent give the same high grade to pharmacists.

Figure 1

Commonly Asked Questions About OTCs

Question	Percent of Pharmacists receiving the question
Recommendations for the best OTC product for a specific ailment	94%
Side effects	54%
Dosage/duration of therapy	37%
Information on medical conditions	36%
Cost of OTC	35%

Source: Cardinale, V. "Pharmacists as OTC Counselors," *Drug Topics* (suppl.), 1994.

OTCs and Physicians

Nearly all (97 percent) physicians recommend OTCs to their patients, according to a recent survey by the international business consulting firm Kline & Co. They do so, in fact, for 27 percent of all their patients. As the professionals that consumers count on most, physicians and pharmacists play an important role in how OTCs are used. In turn, physician and pharmacy practices are also affected by the wide availability and effectiveness of these medications.

Americans take about one-tenth of their health problems to physicians. For the remainder of injuries and illnesses, they resort to no treatment or self-treatment; and 70 percent say they self-medicate regularly. For physicians, OTCs have a direct impact on the number of patients they see and the reasons for those office visits.

One study found that MD visits for the common cold dropped by 110,000 a year between 1976 and 1989. The study attributed the decrease to the high number of switched drugs available for treating cold symptoms. The number of visits for other ailments, including serious respiratory conditions, did not decrease in the same period. Another survey revealed that over half (54 percent) of Americans believe that new, switched OTCs saved them trips to the doctor.

Self-medication and seeking out a health care professional are not mutually exclusive. In fact, both approaches are increasing in frequency. Apparently, as their awareness grows, consumers place more reliance on physicians, as well as OTCs. For physicians, OTCs may often serve to screen out those patients with minor, self-treatable conditions, and free up valuable practice time for conditions that do require professional attention.

Some over-the-counter products actually encourage consumers to seek medical care. The greater availability of self-diagnostic and self-monitoring products, for example, serve to increase office visits by alerting patients to the need for a doctor's attention.

Finally, the impact of OTCs on physicians' practices in the future may be even greater under managed care programs. Capitated reimbursement systems, in which providers are reimbursed per enrollee, encourage practitioners to contain costs, reduce unnecessary services, and write fewer and less costly prescriptions. Under managed care, therefore, self-medication may be seen as an important component of cost-containment.

OTCs and Pharmacists

Year after year in national Gallup polls, consumers vote pharmacists the most trusted professional. It's not surprising that 98 percent of pharmacists say their customers generally or always follow their advice on OTCs and purchase the products they recommend.

Pharmacists are also the most accessible health care provider for consumers, and many prefer buying

Figure 2
Product Categories Causing Confusion Among Consumers

Product Category	% of pharmacists asked for recommendation	Average number of recommendations per month
Allergy relief products	99.5	28.0
Adult cough medications	99.5	31.2
Adult cold preparations	99.0	28.3
Antidiarrheals	98.5	14.5
Stool softeners/ other laxatives	98.5	13.6
Sinus remedies	98.1	25.4
Children's cough medications	98.1	24.5
Ibuprofens	98.0	22.5
Antacids	98.0	16.4
Vitamins, adult	97.0	15.8
Throat lozenges	94.6	15.6
Athlete's foot remedies	94.5	8.1
Children's cold preparations	94.4	22.9
Canker/cold sore remedies	91.1	7.7
Hemorrhoidal preparations	90.7	8.0
Topical anti-infectives	88.6	14.8
Acetaminophens	88.3	24.5
Naproxen sodium products	88.3	12.7
Eyedrops	88.0	9.4
Aspirins	88.0	14.0
Bulk laxatives	87.9	8.7
Flu remedies	87.0	15.8
Poison ivy treatments	86.4	10.6
Throat sprays	85.7	10.6
Blood glucose monitors	85.1	6.6
Jock itch remedies	84.3	4.6
Sleep aids	84.0	6.5
Wart removers	83.7	3.8
Vitamins, children's	83.5	9.8
Vaginal antifungals	83.1	7.8
Suntan/sunscreen products	78.5	8.7

Source: Rosendahl, I. "OTC Recommendations By Pharmacists Hit New High," *Drug Topics*, suppl., September, 1995.

their OTCs in a pharmacy because a pharmacist is on hand to provide counseling. There are, for instance, over three-quarters of a million OTC outlets, and only about 10 percent of these are pharmacies. Yet, about 45 percent of all the nation's OTCs are bought in drugstores. Consumers clearly go out of their way to purchase OTCs in a pharmacy.

Consumers often rely on their pharmacist to provide counseling on an OTC until they can make an appointment with a physician, and nearly all pharmacists report that patients occasionally or frequently come to them for OTC advice as an alternative to consulting their physician. In fact, patient counseling by pharmacists is a growing practice. In one recent study, pharmacists were shown to have made an average of 450 more OTC recommendations than they had in the previous year. In 1994, the number of OTC consultations per pharmacist reached 7,781—or almost 846 million per year nationwide—and the level is still rising. In 1995, over half (55 percent) of all pharmacists polled said that they were providing more OTC counseling. In addition, consumers ask pharmacists for help with every category of OTC product. Figure 2 ranks the percentage of pharmacists who were asked to make a product recommendation in that category. It also shows the average number of recommendations made per month.

OTCs are a crucial element in pharmacy practice. About 30 percent of pharmacy revenues come from OTC sales, and for chain drugstores the number is even higher. In addition, pharmacy owners who report expanding OTC sales cite pharmacist counseling as the number one reason for the increase.

With the rise of interest in pharmaceutical care, in which pharmacists are part of a health care team that plans, implements, and monitors patient care, some pharmacists today receive reimbursement for the time they spend counseling a patient. And many pharmacy plans provide financial incentives to pharmacists who encourage use of less expensive Rx or OTC medications. All of these factors may work to encourage OTC counseling by pharmacists in the near future, and may certainly change the way they dispense medications.

Figure 3
What Physicians Want to Know About OTCs
Physicians indicate that they often need more information about an OTC before making a recommendation to their patients. These categories were ranked as most important.

Type of Information	% of Physicians
Side effects, contraindications, symptoms and treatment of overdose	89
Clinical data from an independent source	77
Dosing, directions for use, how supplied	73
Direct comparison to similar products	50
Patient acceptance, compliance	41
Unique physical characteristics	41
Consumer pricing information	37
Reputation of company marketing the product	30
Unique packaging features	19
Clinical data from manufacturer	15
Differences in consumer and professional labeling	9
Type of consumer promotion and support	7
Market share data	2

Source: Griffie, K.G. "How Healthcare Providers Influence Drug Use," Kline & Co., Fairfield, NJ 1993.

Counseling Obstacles
Despite the increase in OTC use, and in patient counseling, studies show that consumers do not always receive the help they need from their health care providers. Physicians, constrained by time and the amount of other information that must be exchanged during a phone consultation or office visit, may neglect to discuss the OTCs their patients use.

Pharmacists also face busy schedules, and studies show that they cite time constraints as the main barrier to OTC counseling. Other obstacles for pharmacists include lack of reimbursement for counseling services, a need for more education on OTCs, and the absence of a physical area that provides privacy. Pharmacists report that insufficient staff and lack of management support are further disincentives for counseling.

Poor communication skills on the part of physicians and pharmacists may also impede effective patient counseling. The following elements of good communication can enhance the counseling process:

■ Listen to patients, ask them for details and clarification, and repeat their answers to confirm your understanding.

■ Assess the knowledge level of your patient. This process can often uncover special problems, such as a reading disability.

■ Use nontechnical terms with patients, and ask them to repeat the instructions you've given them.

■ Provide clearly-written instructions whenever possible. Oral instructions are often quickly forgotten.

■ Stay up-to-date on OTC products, and use current reference books, journals, product information from manufacturers, and other necessary sources, for the most recent and complete information. (Physicians and pharmacists both indicate that they would like to know more about the OTC products they recommend for their patients. Figure 3, for example, shows the percentage of doctors who seek more information on particular OTC topics.)

Finally, one useful aspect of patient counseling is often underused by pharmacists and physicians alike. This is the practice of recommending a companion OTC when a prescription is written or dispensed. Despite the benefits that companion OTCs can provide a patient, half of all pharmacists say they never recommend them. Many nonprescription drugs, however, can help control side effects and improve the efficacy of Rx drugs. Companion OTC recommendations also provide a useful service to patients, help build loyalty, encourage communication, and, for pharmacies, boost OTC sales. (Figure 4 shows which categories of OTC drugs can be helpful with which categories of Rx drugs.)

Figure 4
OTC Companions

OTCs are often overlooked for the relief they can bring from Rx drug side effects, or the added effectiveness they can bring to prescription drugs. Some examples are:

OTC Category	Prescription Drug Category
Antacids	Gastrointestinal drugs
Antacids	Glucocorticoids
Diabetes testing products and supplies	Antidiabetics
Anti-infective agents	Antifungals
Laxatives and vitamins	Cholesterol-lowering drugs
Antacids and analgesics	Rx analgesics
Analgesics	Cardiovascular drugs

Chapter 5: The Future of OTCs

By 2010, OTC sales are expected to reach $28 billion, more than double today's volume. Sales and use will be driven by the development of new technologies and treatments and by ongoing changes in society and how we view and use health care.

New Treatments and New Technologies

Powerful new products, will be the driving force behind the growing popularity of OTCs and self-medication. These products will come from a number of sources. Switches, for example, have already added 56 ingredients to the market, and as many as 70 new applications are expected in the next five years. If approved, these will provide consumers with:

■ new combinations of existing ingredients, for example, hydrocortisone and an antifungal;
■ new formulations, for example, stronger dosages or time-released versions of existing drugs;
■ new ingredients, such as the NSAID, diflunisal;
■ entirely new classes of OTC medications, e.g., antivirals (acyclovir).

Many proposed switches are already in process and may be granted over-the-counter status in the near future. These include medications for treating sleep disorders, obesity, smoking, anxiety, arthritis, diabetes, ulcers, and cardiovascular conditions. Other medications pending approval are dermatological, ophthalmological, genitourinal, and cholesterol-lowering agents. The availability of these strong medications will give consumers an even greater degree of control over their own care, and at a low price. By the year 2000, in fact, it's estimated that switches will have saved the U.S. $34 billion in health care costs.

Another vital source of future medications is biotechnology. Since the first successful genetic engineering experiment took place in California in 1973, this method of drug development is being adopted in every biological research institution in the nation. In fact, the number of applications for approval of biotechnology drugs actually outstripped the number of applications for traditional drugs in the early 1990s. Although most of these genetically engineered medicines are designed to treat serious conditions that require a physician's care, refinements such as the development of peptides that can be taken orally will undoubtedly lead to new OTC drugs in the future. Promising leads for tomorrow's biotechnology drugs include breakthroughs in immunomodulators, anticancer drugs, antivirals, anti-inflammatories, hormones, tissue repair treatments, and antithrombotics.

Along with new ingredients and treatments, new ways to deliver medications are also the subject of intense research. Some of these innovative delivery systems, such as transdermal patches and aerosols, are already being used in prescription medications. Studies are also underway on specially coated molecules that are either more rapidly absorbed or designed to stay in the body longer. Molecular sponges and tiny pumps inserted under the skin may also be used some day, and researchers are experimenting with piggy-backing molecules on existing drugs, to produce products that are less toxic or more effective.

Certainly, other countries must also be counted as a potential source for future OTCs. Today, there are about 35 OTCs that are marketed only outside the U.S. Subject to FDA approval, however, they could eventually become available to American consumers.

Future Trends in the OTC Market

A number of societal trends will also shape the OTC market of tomorrow.

■ As the 58 million members of the baby boomer generation reach old age, their reliance on OTC treatments, especially for chronic conditions such as arthritis and diabetes, will undoubtedly grow significantly.
■ We can expect a continued emphasis on wellness and self-care with a heightened interest in prevention and in medications that enhance quality of life. Currently available and newly developed diagnostic and monitoring products will also play a large role in self-care.
■ The "information revolution" will lead to better-informed patients and more self-treatment and self-diagnosis.

Figure 1
A Surge in Biotech Drugs

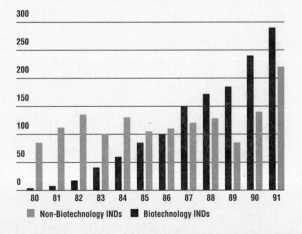

Non-Biotechnology INDs ■ Biotechnology INDs

■ The number of new nonprescription products, as well as their increasing strength and sophistication, will require greater understanding and increased education among consumers and continued reliance on health care providers for expertise and advice.

■ The OTC market could also be affected by a push from pharmacies and other groups to establish a third class of drugs that would be available only through pharmacies. Manufacturers strongly oppose the proposal as anticonsumer, anticompetitive, unnecessary, and a threat to the industry. The FDA has rejected the idea several times over the past two decades but in many other countries there are already three or more classes of drugs.

■ With or without health care reform legislation, the trend toward managed care, with its emphasis on cost containment, is already having an impact on OTC use. In this cost-conscious environment, we can expect to see an increasing emphasis on the approval and use of OTC products and self-treatment in general.

Conclusion

Whatever the source of future OTCs, one thing is certain: tomorrow's consumers will have a wide array of new nonprescription drug products from which to choose. They will play an increasingly important role in the self-treatment of your patients. Keeping abreast of these new therapeutic alternatives will become an ever more critical part of cost-effective patient care and counseling.

Sources

Chapter One

Heller Research Group. Self-medication in the '90s: Practices and perceptions. New York, 1992.

Nielsen North America, 1991.

Nonprescription Drug Manufacturers Association, 1995.

Gannon, K. Exclusive consumer OTC survey: Who's buying what. *Drug Topics,* Jan. 8, 1990.

Find/SVP Inc. The market for Rx-to-OTC switches. 1994.

Sudler & Hennessy. Switches vs. non-switches, Results and insights. New York, 1992.

Temin, P. Realized benefits from switching drugs. *J. Law Econ.* (25)2, 1992.

Information Resources, Inc. Chicago, 1995.

U.S. Bureau of Statistics, 1993.

Kline & Co. Economic benefit of self-medication. Fairfield, New Jersey, 1993.

Kline & Co. Fairfield, New Jersey, 1991.

Chapter Two

World Federation of Proprietary Medicine Manufacturers. Health Care, Self-Care and Self Medication, 1991.

Market Research Corporation of America. Health care remedies usage study. February, 1990.

Consumer Federation of America. September, 1990.

Gallup Organization. *American Health,* March, 1989.

Gallup Organization. *American Health,* 1991.

Heller Research Group. Self-Medication in the '90s: Practices and perceptions. New York, 1992.

Holt G.A., Beck D., Williams M.M. Interview analysis regarding health status, health needs and health care utilization of ambulatory elderly. 40th Annual Conference of the National Council of Aging, Washington, DC, April, 1990.

Shanas E., Maddox G. Aging, health, and the organization of health resources. In: Binstock R., Shanas E., eds. *Handbook of Aging and the Social Sciences.* Van Nostrand Reinhold, New York, 1985.

Princeton Survey Research Associates. *Prevention,* 1992.

Gannon K. The Rx-to-OTC switch race: Drugstores setting the pace. *Drug Topics,* November 22, 1993.

Sudler & Hennessy. New York, 1992.

Rosendahl I. The private label story. *Drug Topics* June 13, 1994.

Chapter Three

Gannon K. Shelf busters: Analyzing nonprescription drug trends. *Drug Topics* January 25, 1993.

Nonprescription Drug Manufacturers Association. Ingredients & dosages transferred from Rx to OTC status as a consequence of the U.S. Food and Drug Administration's Review of Nonprescription Drug Products. Washington DC, 1995.

Nonprescription Drug Manufacturers Association. *Voluntary Codes and Guidelines of the OTC Medicines Industry.* Washington DC.

Nonprescription Drug Manufacturers Association. *Self-Medication's Role in U.S. Health Care.* Washington DC.

Cardinale V. Self-medication: Trend to be reckoned with, not wrecked. *Drug Topics* April 5, 1993.

Gannon K. NDMA's Cope upholds consumer's 'rights' on OTCs. Drug Topics June 13, 1994.

Mercill A.W. Regulation of nonprescription drug products in the United States. Presented at the World Federation of Proprietary Medicine Manufacturers, March 6, 1990.

Princeton Survey Research Associates, 1992.

Code of Federal Regulations. April 1, 1994.

Heller Research Group. Self-medication in the '90s: Practices and perceptions. New York, 1992.

Farley D. Benefit vs. risk: How FDA approves new drugs. *The FDA Consumer.* 1989.

Walden J.T. Impact of tampering on the OTC industry. *The Nielsen Researcher.* Fall, 1986.

Epstein D. More counseling called for in medicating the illiterate. *Drug Topics* November, 1988.

Chapter Four

IMS America. National Disease and Therapeutic Index, 1990.

Temin, P. Realized benefits from switching drugs. *J. Law Econ.* (25)2, 1992.

Gannon K. Pharmacists step up level of counseling on OTCs. *Drug Topics*, September 20, 1993.

Cardinale V. Pharmacists as OTC Counselors, *Drug Topics* (suppl.). 1994.

Gannon K. What do patient want to know about OTCs? *Drug Topics*, August 21, 1989

Epstein D. More counseling called for in medicating the illiterate. *Drug Topics,* November, 1988.

Rosendahl, I. OTC recommendations by pharmacists hit new high. *Drug Topics,* suppl., September, 1995.

Schering Laboratories. *What's Right with Pharmacy.* The Schering Report VII, Kenilworth, New Jersey.

Griffie K.G. *How Healthcare Providers Influence Drug Use.* Kline & Co., Fairfield, New Jersey, 1993.

Chapter Five

Nonprescription Drug Manufacturers Association. The U.S. system of drug distribution. Washington, DC, 1994.

Kline & Co., Fairfield, New Jersey, 1993.

Nonprescription Drug Manufacturers Association. Self-Medication's Role in U.S. Health Care. Washington, DC, 1993.

Eckian A.G. *The Frontiers of Rx-to-OTC Switch.* Presented at the Research and Scientific Development Conference, Nonprescription Drug Manufacturers Association, December 12, 1986.

Nonprescription Drug Manufacturers Association. Rx-to-OTC switch: The right trend for the '90s. Washington DC, 1993.

Ringel M. Changing disease patterns, shifting demographics: Effects on laboratory practices. *Clin. Lab. Mgt. Rev.* September/October, 1994.

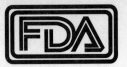

U.S. FOOD AND DRUG ADMINISTRATION

Medical Product Reporting Programs

MedWatch (24 hour service) **800-332-1088**
   Reporting of problems with drugs, devices, biologics (except vaccines), medical foods, dietary supplements.

Vaccine Adverse Event Reporting (24 hour service).....................................**800-822-7967**
   Reporting of vaccine-related problems.

Mandatory Medical Device Reporting...**301-427-7500**
   Reporting required from User facilities regarding device-related deaths and serious injuries.

Veterinary Adverse Drug Reaction Program (7:30 a.m. to 4:00 p.m., eastern time) **301-594-1751**
   Reporting of adverse drug events in animals (collect calls accepted).

Medical Advertising Information (24 hour service)......................................**800-238-7332**
   Inquiries from health professionals regarding product promotion.

Information for Health Professionals

Center for Drugs Executive Secretariat **301-594-1012**
   Information on human drugs including hormones.

Center for Biologics Executive Secretariat **301-594-1800**
   Information on biological products including vaccines and blood.

Center for Devices and Radiological Health..**301-443-4190**
   Automated request for information on medical devices and radiation-emitting products.

Office of Orphan Products Development **301-443-4718**
   Information on products for rare diseases.

Office of Health Affairs Medicine Staff **301-443-5470**
   Information for health professionals on FDA activities.

General Information

General Consumer Inquiries...**301-443-3170**
   Consumer information on regulated products/issues.

Freedom of Information **301-443-6310**
   Request for publicly available FDA documents.

Office of Public Affairs...**301-443-1130**
   Interviews/press inquiries on FDA activities.

Breast Implant Inquiries (24 hour service) **800-332-4440**
   Prerecorded message/request information.

Seafood Hotline (24 hour service)..**800-332-4010**
   Prerecorded message/request information (English/Spanish).

All numbers accessible 8:00 a.m. to 4:30 p.m. eastern time, except where otherwise noted.

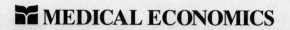

DRUG INFORMATION CENTERS

For additional information on overdosage, adverse reactions, drug interactions, and any other medication problem, specialized drug information centers are strategically located throughout the nation. Use the directory that follows to find the center nearest you. Listings are alphabetical by state and city.

ALABAMA

BIRMINGHAM

Drug Information Service
University of Alabama
Hospital
619 S. 19th St.
Birmingham, AL 35233
Mon.-Fri. 8 AM-5 PM
Tel: 205-934-2162
Fax: 205-934-3501

Global Drug
Information Center
Samford University
School of Pharmacy
800 Lakeshore Dr.
Birmingham, AL 35229
Mon.-Fri. 8 AM-4:30 PM
Tel: 205-870-2891
Fax: 205-870-2016

HUNTSVILLE

Huntsville Hospital
Drug Information Center
101 Sivley Rd.
Huntsville, AL 35801
Mon.-Fri. 8 AM-5 PM
Tel: 205-517-8288
Fax: 205-517-6558

ARIZONA

TUCSON

Arizona Poison and Drug
Information Center
Arizona Health
Sciences Center
University Medical Center
1501 N. Campbell Ave.
Room 1156
Tucson, AZ 85724
7 days/week, 24 hours
Tel: 602-626-6016
      800-362-0101 (AZ)
Fax: 602-626-2720

ARKANSAS

LITTLE ROCK

Arkansas Poison and Drug
Information Center
College of Pharmacy-UAMS
4301 W. Markham St.
Little Rock, AR 72205
7 days/week, 24 hours
Tel: 800-376-4766 (AR)
Fax: 501-686-7357

CALIFORNIA

LOS ANGELES

Los Angeles Regional
Drug and Poison
Information Center
LAC & USC Medical Center
1200 N. State St.
Room 1107 A & B
Los Angeles, CA 90033
7 days/week, 24 hours
Tel: 213-226-2622
      800-777-6476 (CA)
Fax: 213-226-4194

SAN DIEGO

Drug Information
Analysis Service
Veterans Administration
Medical Center
3350 La Jolla Village Dr.
San Diego, CA 92161
Mon-Fri. 8 AM-4:30 PM
Tel: 619-552-8585
Fax: 619-552-7582

Drug Information Center
U.S. Naval Hospital
34800 Bob Wilson Dr.
San Diego, CA 92134-5000
Mon.-Fri. 8 AM-4 PM
Tel: 619-532-8414

Drug Information Service
University of California
San Diego Medical Center
200 West Arbor Dr.
San Diego, CA 92103
Mon.-Fri. 9 AM-5 PM
Tel: 900-288-8273
Fax: 619-692-1867

SAN FRANCISCO

Drug Information
Analysis Service
Veterans Administration
Medical Center
University of California
P.O. Box 0622
San Francisco, CA 94143
Mon.-Fri. 8 AM-5 PM
Tel: 415-476-4346

STANFORD

Drug Information Center
Stanford University Hospital
Dept. of Pharmacy H0301
300 Pasteur Dr.
Stanford, CA 94305
Mon.-Fri. 9 AM-5 PM
Tel: 415-723-6422
Fax: 415-725-5028

COLORADO

DENVER

Rocky Mountain Drug
Consultation Center
88-02 E. 9th Ave.
Denver, CO 80220
Mon.-Fri. 8 AM-4 PM
Tel: 303-893-3784
Fax: 303-739-1119
Outside Denver County:
      900-370-3784
      $1.99 per minute

Drug Information Center
University of Colorado
Health Science Center
4200 E. 9th Ave.
Campus Box C239
Denver, CO 80262
Mon.-Fri. 8:30 AM-4:30 PM
Tel: 303-270-8489
Fax: 303-270-3353

CONNECTICUT

FARMINGTON

Drug Information Service
University of Connecticut
Health Center
263 Farmington Ave.
Farmington, CT 06030
Mon.-Fri. 8 AM-4:30 PM
Tel: 203-679-3783

HARTFORD

Drug Information Center
Hartford Hospital
P.O. Box 5037
80 Seymour St.
Hartford, CT 06102
Mon.-Fri. 8:30 AM-5 PM
Tel: 860-545-2221
      860-545-2961
      (main pharmacy)
      after hours
Fax: 860-545-2415

NEW HAVEN

Drug Information Center
Yale-New Haven Hospital
20 York St.
New Haven, CT 06504
Mon.-Fri. 8:15 AM-4:45 PM
Tel: 203-785-2248
Fax: 203-737-4229

DISTRICT OF COLUMBIA

Drug Information Center Washington Hospital Center
110 Irving St., NW
Washington, DC 20010
Mon.- Fri. 7:30 AM-4 PM
Tel: 202-877-6646
Fax: 202-877-5428

Drug Information Service Howard University Hospital
2041 Georgia Ave. NW
Washington, DC 20060
Mon.-Fri. 9 AM-5 PM
Tel: 202-865-1325
Fax: 202-745-3731

FLORIDA

GAINESVILLE
Drug Information & Pharmacy Resource Center Shands Hospital at University of Florida
P.O. Box 100316
Gainesville, FL 32610
Mon.-Fri. 9 AM- 5 PM
Tel: 904-395-0408
(for health-care professionals only)
Fax: 904-338-9860

JACKSONVILLE
Drug Information Service University Medical Center
655 W. 8th St.
Jacksonville, FL 32209
Mon.-Fri. 8 AM-5 PM
Tel: 904-549-4095
Fax: 904-549-4272

MIAMI
**Drug Information Center (119)
Miami VA Medical Center**
1201 NW 16th St.
Miami, FL 33125
Mon.-Fri. 7:30 AM-4:30 PM
Tel: 305-324-3237
Fax: 305-324-3394

NORTH MIAMI BEACH
Drug Information Service Nova Southeastern University College of Pharmacy
1750 NE 167th St.
N. Miami Beach, FL 33162
Mon.-Fri. 9 AM-5 PM
Tel: 305-948-8255

GEORGIA

ATLANTA
Emory University Hospital Dept. of Pharmaceutical Services
1364 Clifton Rd. NE
Atlanta, GA 30322
Mon.-Fri. 8:30 AM-5 PM
Tel: 404-712-4640
Fax: 404-712-7577

Drug Information Service Northside Hospital
1000 Johnson Ferry Rd.
Atlanta, GA 30342
Mon.-Fri. 9 AM-4 PM
Tel: 404-851-8676
Fax: 404-851-8682

Drug Information Center Grady Memorial Hospital and Mercer University
80 Butler St., SE
P.O. Box 26041
Atlanta, GA 30335-3801
Mon.-Fri. 8 AM-4 PM
Tel: 404-616-7725
Fax: 404-616-7727

AUGUSTA
Drug Information Center University of Georgia Medical College of GA
Room BIW201
1120 15th St.
Augusta, GA 30912-5600
Mon.-Fri. 8:30 AM-5 PM
Tel: 706-721-2887
Fax: 706-721-3827

IDAHO

POCATELLO
Idaho Drug Information Service
Box 8092
Pocatello, ID 83209
Mon.-Fri. 8 AM-5 PM
Tel: 208-236-4689
Fax: 208-236-4687

ILLINOIS

BLOOMINGTON
Drug Information Center BroMenn Life Care Center
807 N. Main St.
Bloomington, IL 61701
7 days/week, 24 hours
Tel: 309-829-0755
Fax: 309-829-0760

CHICAGO
Drug Information Center Northwestern Memorial Hospital
250 E. Superior St.
Wesley 153
Chicago, IL 60611
Tel: 312-908-7573
Fax: 312-908-7956

Dr. Carl Fraterrigo Director of Pharmacy Saint Joseph Hospital
2900 N. Lake Shore Dr.
Chicago, IL 60657
Tel: 312-665-3140

Drug Information Services University of Chicago
5841 S. Maryland Ave.
MC 0010
Chicago, IL 60637
Mon.-Fri. 8 AM-5 PM
Tel: 312-702-1388
Fax: 312-702-6631

Drug Information Center University of Illinois at Chicago
Room C300, MC 883
1740 W. Taylor St.
Chicago, IL 60612
Mon.-Fri. 8 AM-4 PM
Tel: 312-996-3681
Fax: 312-413-4146

HARVEY
Drug Information Center Ingalls Memorial Hospital
1 Ingalls Dr.
Harvey, IL 60426
Mon.-Fri. 8 AM-4:30 PM
Tel: 708-333-2300
Fax: 708-210-3108

HINES
Drug Information Service Hines Veterans Administration Hospital
Inpatient Pharmacy (119B)
Hines, IL 60141
Mon.-Fri. 8 AM-4:30 PM
Tel: 708-343-7200

PARK RIDGE
Drug Information Center Lutheran General Hospital
1775 Dempster St.
Park Ridge, IL 60068
Mon.-Fri. 7:30 AM-4 PM
Tel: 708-696-8128

ROCKFORD
Drug Information Center Swedish-American Hospital
1400 Charles St.
Rockford, IL 61104
7 days/week, 24 hours
Tel: 815-968-4400
     x 4577, 4800

INDIANA

INDIANAPOLIS
Drug Information Center St. Vincent Hospital and Health Services
2001 W. 86th St.
P.O. Box 40970
Indianapolis, IN 46240
Mon.-Fri. 8 AM-4 PM
Tel: 317-338-3200
Fax: 317-338-6547

Indiana University Medical Center/Pharmacy
Dept. UH1410
550 N. University Blvd.
Indianapolis, IN 46202
Mon.-Fri. 8 AM-4:30 PM
Tel: 317-274-3581
Fax: 317-274-2327

IOWA

DES MOINES
Regional Drug Information Center Mercy Hospital Medical Center
400 University Ave.
Des Moines, IA 50314
Mon.-Fri. 8 AM-4:30 PM
Tel: 515-247-3286
(answered 7 days/week, 24 hours)
Fax: 515-247-3966

Mid-Iowa Poison and Drug Information Center Iowa Methodist Medical Center
1200 Pleasant St.
Des Moines, IA 50309
7 days/week, 24 hours
Tel: 515-241-6254
     800-362-2327 (IA)
Fax: 515-241-5085

IOWA CITY
Drug Information Center University of Iowa Hospitals and Clinics
200 Hawkins Dr.
Iowa City, IA 52242
Mon.-Fri. 8 AM-5 PM
Tel: 319-356-2600

KANSAS

KANSAS CITY

Drug Information Center
University of Kansas
Medical Center
3901 Rainbow Blvd.
Kansas City, KS 66160
Mon.-Fri. 8:30 AM-4:30 PM
Tel: 913-588-2328

KENTUCKY

LEXINGTON

Drug Information Center
Chandler Medical Center,
College of Pharmacy
University of Kentucky
800 Rose St., C-117
Lexington, KY 40536
Mon.-Fri. 8 AM- 5 PM
Tel: 606-323-5320
Fax: 606-323-2049

LOUISIANA

MONROE

Drug Information Center
St. Francis Medical Center
309 Jackson St.
Monroe, LA 71201
7 days/week, 24 hours
Tel: 318-327-4250
Fax: 318-327-4125

NEW ORLEANS

Xavier University Drug
Information Center
Tulane University
Hospital and Clinic
Box HC-12
1415 Tulane Ave.
New Orleans, LA 70112
Mon.- Fri. 9 AM-5 PM
Tel: 504-588-5670
Fax: 504-588-5862

MARYLAND

ANDREWS AFB

Drug Information Services
89th Med Gp/SGSAP
1050 W. Perimeter Rd.
Suite B1-39
Andrews AFB, MD 20331
Mon.-Fri. 7:30 AM-6 PM
Tel: 301-981-4209
Fax: 301-981-4544

ANNAPOLIS

Drug Information Services
The Anne Arundel
Medical Center
Franklin & Cathedral Sts.
Annapolis, MD 21401
7 days/week, 24 hours
Tel: 410-267-1130
    410-267-1000
Fax: 410-267-1628

BALTIMORE

Drug Information Services
Franklin Square
Hospital Center
9000 Franklin Square Dr.
Baltimore, MD 21237
7 days/week, 24 hours
Tel: 410-682-7744
    410-267-1000
    (after hours)
Fax: 410-682-7374

Drug Information Service
John Hopkins
Medical Center
600 N. Wolfe St.
Halsted 503
Baltimore, MD 21287
Mon.-Fri. 8:30 AM-5 PM
Tel: 410-955-6348
Fax: 410-955-8283

Drug Information Center
University of Maryland at
Baltimore School of
Pharmacy
506 W. Fayette, 3rd Floor
Baltimore, MD 21201
Mon.-Fri. 8:30 AM-5 PM
Tel: 410-706-7568
Fax: 410-706-0897

BETHESDA

Drug Information Center
Pharmacy Dept.
Warren G. Magnuson
Clinic Center
National Institutes
of Health
9000 Rockville Pike
Bldg. 10, Room IN-257
Bethesda, MD 20892
Mon.-Fri. 8:30 AM-5 PM
Tel: 301-496-2407
Fax: 301-496-0210

EASTON

Drug Information Center
Memorial Hospital
219 S. Washington St.
Easton, MD 21601
7 days/week, 24 hours
Tel: 410-822-1000,
    x 5645
Fax: 410-820-9489

MASSACHUSETTS

BOSTON

Drug Information Service
Brigham and Women's
Hospital
75 Frances St.
Boston, MA 02115
Mon.-Fri. 7 AM-3:30 PM
Tel: 617-732-7166
Fax: 617-732-7497

Drug Information Service
New England Medical
Center Pharmacy
750 Washington St.
Box 420
Boston, MA 02111
Mon.-Fri. 8 AM-4:30 PM
Tel: 617-636-5380
Fax: 617-956-5638

WORCESTER

Drug Information Center
U.M.M.C. Hospital
55 Lake Ave. North
Worcester, MA 01655
Mon.-Fri. 8:30 AM-5 PM
Tel: 508-856-3456
    508-856-2775
Fax: 508-856-1850

MICHIGAN

ANN ARBOR

Drug Information Service
University of Michigan
Medical Center
1500 East Medical
Center Dr.
UHB2 D301 Box 0008
Ann Arbor, MI 48109
Mon.-Fri. 8 AM-5 PM
Tel: 313-936-8200
    313-936-8251
    (after hours)
Fax: 313-936-7027

DETROIT

Drug Information Services
Harper Hospital
3990 John R. St.
Detroit, MI 48201
Mon.-Fri. 8 AM-5 PM
Tel: 313-745-2006
    313-745-8216
    (after hours)
Fax: 313-745-1628

LANSING

Drug Information Center
Sparrow Hospital
1215 E. Michigan Ave.
Lansing, MI 48912
Mon.-Fri. 8 AM-4:30 PM
Tel: 517-483-2444
Fax: 517-483-2088

PONTIAC

Drug Information Center
St. Joseph Mercy Hospital
900 Woodward
Pontiac, MI 48341
Mon.-Fri. 8 AM-4:30 PM
Tel: 810-858-3055
Fax: 810-551-2426

ROYAL OAK

Drug Information Services
William Beaumont Hospital
3601 West 13 Mile Rd.
Royal Oak, MI 48073
Mon.-Fri. 8 AM-4:30 PM
Tel: 810-551-4077
Fax: 810-551-4046

SOUTHFIELD

Drug Information Service
Providence Hospital
16001 West 9 Mile Rd.
P.O. Box 2043
Southfield, MI 48075
Mon.-Fri. 8 AM-4 PM
Tel: 810-424-3125
Fax: 810-424-5364

MINNESOTA

ROCHESTER

Drug Information Service
Mayo Clinic
1216 2nd St., SW
Rochester, MN 55902
Mon.-Fri. 8 AM-5 PM
Tel: 507-255-5062
    507-255-5732
    (after hours)
Fax: 507-255-7556

ST. PAUL

Drug Information Service
United Hospital and
Children's Healthcare
— St. Paul
333 N. Smith Ave.
St. Paul, MN 55102
Mon.-Fri. 9 AM-5 PM
Tel: 612-220-8566
Fax: 612-220-5323

MISSISSIPPI

JACKSON

Drug Information Center
University of Mississippi
Medical Center
2500 N. State St.
Jackson, MS 39216
Mon.-Fri. 8 AM-5 PM
Tel: 601-984-2060
(on call 24 hours)
Fax: 601-984-2063

MISSOURI

SPRINGFIELD

St. John's Regional Health Center Drug Information & Clinical Research Services
1235 E. Cherokee
Springfield, MO 65804
Mon.-Fri. 7:30 AM-4:30 PM
Tel: 417-885-3488
Fax: 417-888-7788

ST. JOSEPH

Drug Information Service Heartland Hospital West
801 Faraon St.
St. Joseph, MO 64501
Mon.-Sat. 8 AM-8 PM
Tel: 816-271-7582
Fax: 816-271-7590

NEBRASKA

OMAHA

Drug Information Service School of Pharmacy Creighton University
2500 California Plaza
Omaha, NE 68178
Mon.-Fri. 8:30 AM-4:30 PM
Tel: 402-280-5101
Fax: 402-280-5149

Drug Information and Education Services University of Nebraska Medical Center
600 S. 42nd St.
Omaha, NE 68178
Mon.-Fri. 8 AM-4:30 PM
Tel: 402-559-4114
Fax: 402-559-4907

NEW MEXICO

ALBUQUERQUE

New Mexico Poison & Drug Information Center University of New Mexico
Albuquerque, NM 87131
7 days/week, 24 hours
Tel: 505-843-2551
    800-432-6866 (NM)
Fax: 505-277-5892

NEW YORK

BRONX

Drug Information Center
Dept. of Pharmacy
Room BN32
Jacobi Medical Center
Pelham Pkwy. South and Eastchester Rd.
Bronx, NY 10461
Mon.-Fri. 9 AM-5 PM
Tel: 718-918-4556
Fax: 718-918-7848

BROOKLYN

International Drug Information Center Long Island University Arnold & Marie Schwartz College of Pharmacy and Health Sciences
1 University Plaza
Brooklyn, NY 11201
Mon.-Fri. 9 AM-5 PM
Tel: 718-488-1064
Fax: 718-780-4056

COOPERSTOWN

Drug Information Center The Mary Imogene Bassett Hospital
1 Atwell Rd.
Cooperstown, NY 13326
Mon.-Fri 8:30 AM-5 PM
Tel: 607-547-3686
Fax: 607-547-3629

NEW HYDE PARK

Drug Information Center St. John's University at Long Island Jewish Medical Center
270-05 76th Ave.
New Hyde Park, NY 11042
Mon.-Fri. 9 AM-3 PM
Tel: 718-470-DRUG
Fax: 718-470-1742

NEW YORK

Drug Information Center Memorial Sloan-Kettering Cancer Center
1275 York Ave.
New York, NY 10021
Mon.-Fri. 9 AM-5 PM
Tel: 212-639-7552
Fax: 212-639-2171

Drug Information Center Mount Sinai Medical Center
1 Gustave Levy Place
New York, NY 10029
Mon.-Fri. 9 AM-5 PM
Tel: 212-241-6619
Fax: 212-348-7927

Drug Information Center Bellevue Hospital Center
462 1st Ave.
New York, NY 10016
Mon.-Fri. 9 AM-5 PM
Tel: 212-562-6504
Fax: 212-562-6503

Drug Information Service The New York Hospital
525 E. 68th St.
New York, NY 10021
Mon.-Fri. 9 AM-5 PM
Tel: 212-746-0741
Fax: 212-746-8506

ROCHESTER

Drug Information Service Dept. of Pharmacy University of Rochester
601 Elmwood Ave.
Rochester, NY 14642
Mon.-Fri. 8 AM-5 PM
Tel: 716-275-3718
    716-275-2681
    (after hours)
Fax: 716-473-9842

STONY BROOK

Suffolk Drug Information Center University Hospital S.U.N.Y. - Stony Brook
Room 3 - 559, Z7310
Stony Brook, NY 11794
Mon.-Fri. 8 AM-4:30 PM
Tel: 516-444-2672
    516-444-2680
    (after hours)
Fax: 516-444-7935

NORTH CAROLINA

BUIES CREEK

Drug Information Center School of Pharmacy Campbell University
P.O. Box 1090
Buies Creek, NC 27506
Mon.-Fri. 8:30 AM - 4:30 PM
Tel: 910-893-1200
    x 2701
    800-327-5467 (NC)
Fax: 910-893-1476

CHAPEL HILL

Drug Information Center University of North Carolina Hospitals
101 Manning Dr.
Chapel Hill, NC 27514
Mon.-Fri. 8 AM-5 PM
Tel: 919-966-2373
Fax: 919-966-1791

GREENSBORO

Triad Poison Center Moses H. Cone Memorial Hospital
1200 N. Elm St.
Greensboro, NC 27401
7 days/week, 24 hours
Tel: 910-574-8105
Fax: 910-574-7910

GREENVILLE

Eastern Carolina Drug Information Center Pitt County Memorial Hospital Dept. of Pharmacy Service
2100 Stantonsburg Rd.
Greenville, NC 27835
Mon.-Fri. 8 AM- 5 PM
Tel: 919-816-4257
Fax: 919-816-7425

WINSTON-SALEM

Drug Information Service Center NC Baptist Hospital Bowman-Gray Medical Center
Medical Center Blvd.
Winston-Salem, NC 27157
Mon.-Fri 8 AM-5 PM
Tel: 910-716-2037
Fax: 910-716-2186

OHIO

ADA

Drug Information Center Raabe College of Pharmacy
Ohio Northern University
Ada, OH 45810
Mon.-Fri. 9 AM - 5 PM
Tel: 419-772-2307
Fax: 419-772-2289

CLEVELAND

Drug Information Center Cleveland Clinic Foundation
9500 Euclid Ave.
Cleveland, OH 44195
Mon.-Fri. 8 AM - 4:30 PM
Tel: 216-444-6456
Fax: 216-445-6221

COLUMBUS

Central Ohio Poison Center
700 Children's Dr.
Columbus, OH 43205
Tel: 513-222-2227
Fax: 614-221-2672

Drug Information Center
Dept. of Pharmacy,
Ohio State University
Hospital
Doan Hall 368
410 W. 10th Ave.
Columbus, OH 43210
Mon.-Fri. 8 AM - 4 PM
Tel: 614-293-8679
Fax: 614-293-3264

Drug Information Center
Riverside Methodist
Hospital
3535 Olantangy River Rd.
Columbus, OH 43214
Tel: 614-566-5425
Fax: 614-566-5447

PARMA

Clinical Pharmacy
Services Regional Drug
Information Service
12301 Snow Rd.
Parma, OH 44130
Tel: 216-265-4400
       216-362-2727
       pager 3133

TOLEDO

Drug Information Center
The Toledo Hospital
2142 N. Cove Blvd.
Toledo, OH 43606
Mon.-Fri. 8 AM-4:30 PM
Tel: 419-471-2171
       419-471-5637
       (after hours)
Fax: 419-479-6926

ZANESVILLE

Drug Information/
Poison Center
Bethesda Hospital
2951 Maple Ave.
Zanesville, OH 43701
7 days/week, 24 hours
Tel: 614-454-4221
       800-686-4221 (OH)
Fax: 614-454-4059

OKLAHOMA

OKLAHOMA CITY

Drug Information Center
Baptist Medical Center
of Oklahoma
3300 Northwest Expwy
Oklahoma City, OK 73112
Mon.-Fri. 8 AM-4:30 PM
Tel: 405-949-3660
Fax: 405-945-5858

Drug Information Center
Presbyterian Hospital
700 NE 13th St.
Oklahoma City, OK 73104
Mon.-Fri. 7 AM-3:30 PM
Tel: 405-271-6226
Fax: 404-271-3460

Drug Information Service
University of Oklahoma
Health Sciences Ctr.
Rm LIB-380A
1000 S.L. Young Blvd.
Oklahoma City, OK 73117
Mon.-Fri. 8 AM-5 PM

TULSA

Drug Information Service
St. Francis Hospital
6161 S. Yale Ave.
Tulsa, OK 74136
Mon.-Fri. 9 AM-5:30 PM
Tel: 918-494-6339
Fax: 918-494-1893

OREGON

PORTLAND

University Drug
Consultation Service
Oregon Health Sciences
University
3181 SW Sam Jackson
  Park Rd.
Portland, OR 97201
Mon.-Fri. 8:30 AM-5 PM
Tel: 503-494-7530
Fax: 503-494-1096

PENNSYLVANIA

ERIE

Pharmacy and Drug
Information Services
Hamot Medical Center
201 State St.
Erie, PA 16550
7 days/week, 24 hours
Tel: 814-877-6022
Fax: 814-877-6108

PHILADELPHIA

Drug Information Center
Temple University
Hospital Dept. of
Pharmacy
Broad and Ontario Sts.
Philadelphia, PA 19140
Mon.-Fri. 8 AM-4:30 PM
Tel: 215-701-4644
Fax: 215-701-3463

Drug Information Center
Thomas Jefferson
University Hospital
111 S. 11th and Walnut Sts.
Philadelphia, PA 19107
Mon.-Fri. 8 AM-5 PM
Tel: 215-955-8877

PITTSBURGH

The Center for Drug
Information
The Mercy Hospital of
Pittsburgh
1400 Locust St.
Pittsburgh, PA 15219
Mon.-Fri. 8 AM-4:30 PM
Tel: 412-232-7903
       412-232-7907
Fax: 412-232-8422

Drug Information and
Pharmacoepidemiology
Center
University of Pittsburgh
Medical Center
137 Victoria Bldg.
Pittsburgh, PA 15261
Mon-Fri. 8 AM-6 PM
Tel: 412-624-3784
Fax: 412-642-6350

UPLAND

Drug Information Center
Crozer-Chester
Medical Center
1 Medical Center Blvd.
Upland, PA 19013
Mon.-Fri. 8 AM-4:30 PM
Tel: 610-447-2851
       610-447-2862
       (after hours)
Fax: 215-447-2820

WILLIAMSPORT

Drug Information Center
Susquehanna
Health System
Rural Ave. Campus
777 Rural Ave.
Williamsport, PA 17701
Mon.-Fri. 8 AM-4 PM
Tel: 717-321-3289
Fax: 717-321-3230

PUERTO RICO

SAN JUAN

Centro Informacion
Medicamentos
Escuela de Farmacia RCM
P.O. Box 365067
San Juan, PR 00936-
5067
Mon.-Fri. 8 AM-4 PM
Tel: 809-758-2525
       x 1516
Tel. & Fax: 809-763-0196

RHODE ISLAND

PROVIDENCE

Drug Information Service
Dept. of Pharmacy
Rhode Island Hospital
593 Eddy St.
Providence, RI 02903
7 days/week, 24 hours
Tel: 401-444-5547
Fax: 401-444-8062

Drug Information Service
University of Rhode Island
Roger Williams
Medical Center
825 Chalkstone Ave.
Providence, RI 02908
Mon.-Fri. 8 AM-4 PM
Tel: 401-456-2260
Fax: 401-456-2377

SOUTH CAROLINA

CHARLESTON

Drug Information Service
Medical University of
South Carolina
171 Ashley Ave.
Room 515-SFX
Charleston, SC 29425
Mon.- Fri. 8 AM-5:30 PM
Tel: 803-792-3896
       800-922-5250
Fax: 803-792-5532

SPARTANBURG

Drug Information Center
Spartanburg Regional
Medical Center
101 E. Wood St.
Spartanburg, SC 29303
Mon.-Fri. 8 AM-5 PM
Tel: 803-560-6910
Fax: 803-560-6017

SOUTH DAKOTA

BROOKINGS

South Dakota Drug
Information Center
300 22nd Ave.
Brookings, SD 57006
7 days/week, 8 AM-4:30 PM
Tel: 800-456-1004

SIOUX FALLS
Drug Information Center
McKennan Hospital
800 E. 21st St.
Sioux Falls, SD 57117
7 days/week, 24 hours
Tel: 605-336-3894
      800-952-0123 (SD)
      800-843-0505
      (MN, IA, NE)
Fax: 605-333-8206

TENNESSEE
KNOXVILLE
Drug Information Center
University of Tennessee
Medical Center
1924 Alcoa Hwy.
Knoxville, TN 37920
Mon.-Fri. 8 AM-4:30 PM
Tel: 423-544-9125

MEMPHIS
South East Regional Drug
Information Center
VA Medical Center
1030 Jefferson Ave.
Memphis, TN 38104
Mon.-Fri. 7:30 AM-4 PM
Tel: 901-523-8990

Drug Information Center
University of Tennessee
847 Monroe Ave.
Suite 238
Memphis, TN 38163
Mon.-Fri. 8:30 AM - 4:30 PM
Tel: 901-448-5555
Fax: 901-448-5419

TEXAS
GALVESTON
Drug Information Center
University of Texas
Medical Branch
301 University Blvd. - G01
Galveston, TX 77555
Mon.-Fri. 8 AM-5 PM
Tel: 409-772-2734
Fax: 409-772-8404

HOUSTON
Drug Information Center
Ben Taub General Hospital
Texas Southern
University/HCHD
1504 Taub Loop
Houston, TX 77030
Mon.-Fri. 8 AM-5 PM
Tel: 713-793-2920
Fax: 713-793-2937

Drug Information Center
Methodist Hospital
6565 Fannin (DB1-09)
Houston, TX 77030
Mon.-Fri. 8 AM-5 PM
Tel: 713-790-4190
Fax: 713-793-1224

LACKLAND AFB
Drug Information Center
Dept. of Pharmacy
Wilford Hall Medical
Center
2200 Berquist Dr., Suite 1
Lackland AFB, TX 78236
Mon.-Fri. 7:30 AM-5 PM
Tel: 210-670-6291
      210-670-5408

LUBBOCK
Methodist Hospital
Drug Information &
Consultation Service
3615 19th St.
Lubbock, TX 79410
Mon.-Fri. 8 AM-5 PM
Tel: 806-793-4012
Fax: 806-784-5323
  (Attn: Pharmacy)

TEMPLE
Drug Information Center
Scott and White
Memorial Hospital
2401 S. 31st St.
Temple, TX 76508
Mon.-Fri. 8 AM-6 PM
Tel: 817-724-4636
Fax: 817-724-1731

UTAH
SALT LAKE CITY
Drug Information Center
Dept. of Pharmacy
University of Utah
Hospital Services
Room A-050
50 N. Medical Dr.
Salt Lake City, UT 84132
Mon.-Fri. 8:30 AM-4:30 PM
Tel: 801-581-2073
Fax: 801-585-6688

VIRGINIA
HAMPTON
Drug Information Center
Sentara Hampton
General Hospital
3120 Victoria Blvd.
Hampton, VA 23669
7 days/week, 7 AM-
  Midnight
Tel: 804-727-7185
Fax: 804-727-7398

RICHMOND
Drug Information Center
St. Mary's Hospital
5801 Bremo Rd.
Richmond, VA 23226
7 days/week, 24 hours
Tel: 804-281-8058
Fax: 804-285-4411

WEST VIRGINIA
MORGANTOWN
West Virginia Drug
Information Center
West Virginia University-
Robert C. Byrd Health
Sciences Center
1124 HSN, P.O. Box 9520
Morgantown, WV 26506
Tel: 304-293-6640
      800-352-2501 (WV)
Fax: 304-293-5483

WISCONSIN
MADISON
Drug Information Center
University of Wisconsin
Hospital & Clinics
600 Highland Ave.
Madison, WI 53792
Voice mail/24 hrs a day,
responses in 3 days
Tel: 608-262-1315
Fax: 608-263-9424

WYOMING
LARAMIE
Drug Information Center
University of Wyoming
P.O. Box 3375
Laramie, WY 82071
Mon.-Fri. 8 AM-5 PM
Tel: 307-766-6128
Fax: 307-766-2953

PRODUCT IDENTIFICATION GUIDE

To aid in quick identification, this section provides full-color, actual-size photographs of tablets and capsules. A variety of other dosage forms and packages are shown at less than actual size. In all, the section contains a total of nearly 1,000 photos.

Products in this section are arranged alphabetically by manufacturer. In some instances, not all dosage forms and sizes are pictured. Letters or numbers representing the manufacturer's identification code are preceded by an asterisk.

For more information on any of the products in this section, please turn to the "Product Information" section, or check directly with the manufacturer. For easy reference, the page number of each product's text entry appears with its photographs.

While every effort has been made to guarantee faithful reproduction of the photos in this section, changes in size, color, and design are always a possibility. Be sure to confirm a product's identity with the manufacturer or your pharmacist.

MANUFACTURER'S INDEX

AKPHARMA INC.

AkPharma Inc.
P. 602

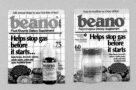

Food Enzyme Dietary Supplement
Drops and Tablets.

Beano®

ASCHER & CO., INC.

B.F. Ascher & Co., Inc.
P. 606

Available in 0.5 oz. Saline Nasal Gel,
50 mL Saline Nasal Drops and
50 mL Nasal Mist

Ayr®

B.F. Ascher & Co., Inc.
P. 606

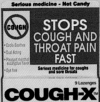

Cough Suppressant and
Sore Throat Relief Lozenges

COUGH-X®

B.F. Ascher & Co., Inc.
P. 607

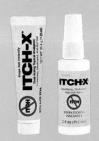

Available in: 35.4 g (1.25 oz) tube gel
and New 2 Fl. oz (59.1 mL) spray.

ITCH-X®

B.F. Ascher & Co., Inc.
P. 607

Analgesic Tablets
Available in: 18's, 50's & 100's

Mobigesic®

B.F. Ascher & Co., Inc.
P. 607

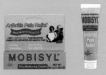

Analgesic Creme
Available in 1.25 oz., 3.5 oz.
and 8 oz. size

Mobisyl®

ASTRA USA

Astra USA, Inc.
P. 608

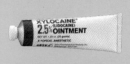

2.5% Ointment
Available in 35 gram Tube

Xylocaine®
(lidocaine)

BAUSCH & LOMB

Bausch & Lomb
P. 608

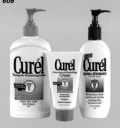

Therapeutic Moisturizing Lotion in
original and fragrance free (shown)
formulas, fragrance free cream,
and AlphaHydroxy formula.

Curél®

BAYER CORPORATION

Bayer Corporation
Consumer Care Division
P. 608

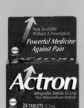

Ketoprofen Tablets and Caplets 12.5 mg

Actron™

Bayer Corporation
Consumer Care Division
P. 609

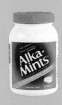

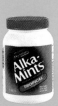

Spearmint, Cherry and Tropical
Chewable Antacid

Alka-Mints®

Bayer Corporation
Consumer Care Division
P. 611

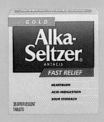

Effervescent Antacid

Alka-Seltzer® Gold

Bayer Corporation
Consumer Care Division
P. 609

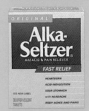

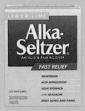
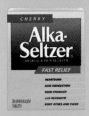

Original, Extra Strength,
Lemon Lime and Cherry
Effervescent Antacid and
Pain Reliever

Alka-Seltzer®

Bayer Corporation
Consumer Care Division
P. 610

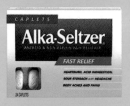

Antacid and
Non-Aspirin Pain Reliever

Alka-Seltzer® Caplets

Bayer Corporation
Consumer Care Division
P. 611

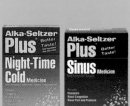

Cold, Cold & Cough,
Night-Time and Sinus
Effervescent Tablets

**Alka-Seltzer Plus®
Cold Medicine**

Bayer Corporation
Consumer Care Division
P. 612

Cold, Cold & Cough, Flu & Body Aches
and Night-Time.

**Alka-Seltzer Plus®
Cold Medicine
Liqui-Gels®**

Bayer Corporation
Consumer Care Division
P. 612

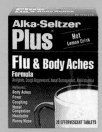

Effervescent Tablets

**Alka-Seltzer Plus®
Flu and Body Aches**

Bayer Corporation
Consumer Care Division

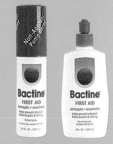

Antiseptic/Anesthetic
First Aid Spray and Liquid

Bactine®

Bayer Corporation
Consumer Care Division
P. 613

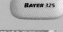

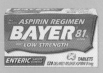

Genuine Bayer, Aspirin Regimen 81 mg,
Aspirin Regimen 325 mg

BAYER® Aspirin

Bayer Corporation
Consumer Care Division
P. 616

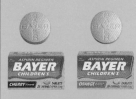

Low Strength, Chewable Aspirin
Orange and Cherry Flavors

**Aspirin Regimen
BAYER® Children's**

Bayer Corporation
Consumer Care Division
P. 615

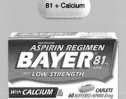

**Aspirin Regimen BAYER®
81 mg with Calcium**

Bayer Corporation
Consumer Care Division
P. 615

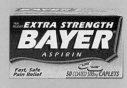

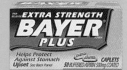

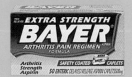

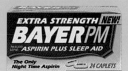

Extra Strength, Plus,
Arthritis Pain Regimen and PM

**Extra Strength
BAYER® Aspirin**

Bayer Corporation
Consumer Care Division
P. 616

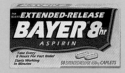

Only Extended-Release Aspirin

**Extended-Release BAYER®
8 Hour**

Bayer Corporation
Consumer Care Division
P. 619

Sugar Free Children's Chewable
Complete, with Extra C and Plus Iron

Bugs Bunny™ Vitamins

Bayer Corporation
Consumer Care Division
P. 620

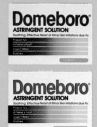

Astringent Solution
Effervescent Tablets and
Powder Packets

Domeboro®

Bayer Corporation
Consumer Care Division

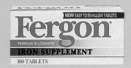

Ferrous Gluconate
Iron Supplement

Fergon®

Bayer Corporation
Consumer Care Division
P. 620

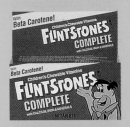

Children's Chewable Vitamins with
Iron, Calcium & Minerals

Flintstones® Complete

Bayer Corporation
Consumer Care Division
P. 621

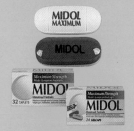

Caplets and Gelcaps

Midol® Maximum Strength

Bayer Corporation
Consumer Care Division

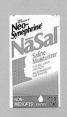

Nasal Moisturizer Spray and Drops

NaSal®

Bayer Corporation
Consumer Care Division
P. 625

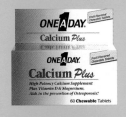

500 mg Calcium Carbonate
Plus Vitamin D and Magnesium

One-A-Day® Calcium Plus

Bayer Corporation
Consumer Care Division
P. 619

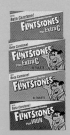

Children's Chewable Vitamins with
Extra C, Regular and Plus Iron

Flintstones®

Bayer Corporation
Consumer Care Division
P. 621

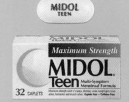

Maximum Strength Caplets

Midol® Teen

Bayer Corporation
Consumer Care Division
P. 624

Nasal Decongestant Drops, Spray
Pump or Spray Bottle
Available in Mild, Regular, Extra
Strength and Max 12-Hour Formula

Neo-Synephrine®

Bayer Corporation
Consumer Care Division
P. 624

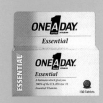

Bayer Corporation
Consumer Care Division
P. 620

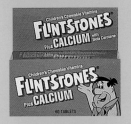

Children's Chewable Vitamins
with Calcium

Flintstones® Plus Calcium

Bayer Corporation
Consumer Care Division
P. 622

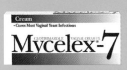

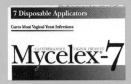

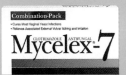

Vaginal Cream 1%
Vaginal Cream with 7
disposable applicators
Vaginal Inserts and
external vulvar cream

Mycelex®-7

Bayer Corporation
Consumer Care Division
P. 625

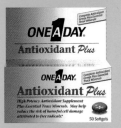

**One-A-Day®
Antioxidant Plus**

Bayer Corporation
Consumer Care Division
P. 626

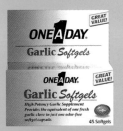

**One-A-Day®
Garlic Softgels**

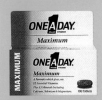

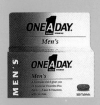

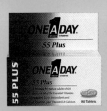

Essential, Maximum, Men's,
Women's and 55 Plus.

One-A-Day® Vitamins

Bayer Corporation
Consumer Care Division
P. 622

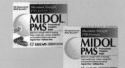

Gelcaps and Caplets

Midol® PMS

Bayer Corporation
Consumer Care Division
P. 627

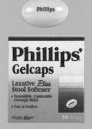

Laxative Plus Stool Softener
Avail. in 10, 30 and 60 count Gelcaps.

Phillips'® Gelcaps

Bayer Corporation
Consumer Care Division
P. 627

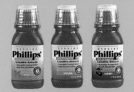

Available in Mint, Original,
and Cherry Flavors
4 oz, 12 oz and 26 oz Bottles

Phillips'®
Milk of Magnesia

Bayer Corporation
Consumer Care Division
P. 627

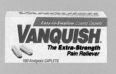

Extra-Strength Pain Formula

Vanquish®

BEIERSDORF

Beiersdorf Inc.
P. 628

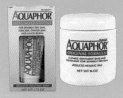

Healing Ointments For Dry Skin,
Minor Cuts and Burns

Aquaphor®

Beiersdorf Inc.
P. 628

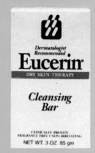

Cleansing Bar

Eucerin®

Beiersdorf Inc.
P. 629

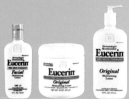

Sensitive Solutions For
Dry Skin Problems
Daily Facial Lotion SPF 25,
Moisturizing Creme and Lotion

Eucerin® Dry Skin Care

Beiersdorf Inc.
P. 629

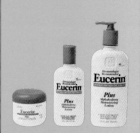

Severely Dry Skin Treatment

Eucerin® Plus

BLOCK DRUG

Block Drug
P. 633

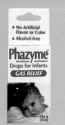

Available in 1 oz. and 1/2 oz. bottles
A liquid anti-gas that contains no
alcohol, and no artificial colors,
flavors or sweeteners

Phazyme® Drops for
Infants

Block Drug
P. 633

Fast dissolving tablets available in
boxes of 10, 30, 50 and 100.
Maximum strength softgels and
maximum strength chewable tablets
available in boxes of 10, 30 and 50.

Phazyme® Gas Relief

BRISTOL-MYERS PRODUCTS

Bristol-Myers Products
P. 644

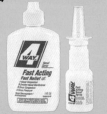

Regular available in:
1/2 oz. and 1 oz. Atomizers
Mentholated also available

4-Way® Fast Acting
Nasal Spray

Bristol-Myers Products
P. 644

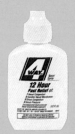

1/2 oz. Atomizers

4-Way® Long Acting
Nasal Spray

Bristol-Myers Products
P. 637

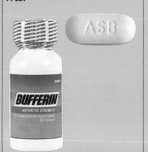

Bottles of 40 and 100 coated caplets

Bufferin®
Arthritis Strength

Bristol-Myers Products
P. 636

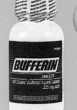

Bottles of 30, 50, 100, 200
and vials of 10 tablets

Bufferin®
Coated Analgesic

Bristol-Myers Products
P. 637

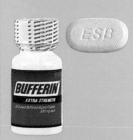

Bottles of 30, 50 and 100
coated tablets

Bufferin® Extra Strength

Bristol-Myers Products
P. 638

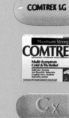

Liqui-Gels in blister packs
of 24 and 50
Coated caplets in blister packs
of 24 and bottles of 50
Coated tablets in blister packs
of 24 and bottles of 50

Comtrex® Multi-Symptom
Cold & Flu Relief

Bristol-Myers Products
P. 639

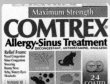

Available in blister packs of
24 and bottles of 50

Comtrex® Allergy-Sinus

Bristol-Myers Products
P. 640

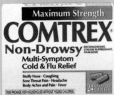

Multi-Symptom Cold Reliever Caplets
Blister packs of 24 and bottles of 50

**Comtrex® Non-Drowsy
Multi-Symptom
Cold & Flu Relief**

Bristol-Myers Products
P. 643

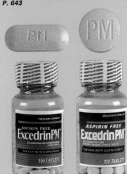

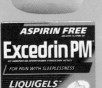

Tablets and Caplets in Bottles of 10,
24, 50 and 100
Liquigels Blisters of 20 and 40

Excedrin PM®

Bristol-Myers Products
P. 641

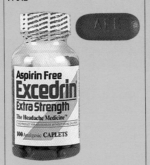

Bottles of 24, 50 and 100 caplets

Aspirin Free Excedrin®

Bristol-Myers Products
P. 642

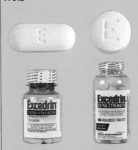

Bottles of 12, 24, 50, 100, 175
and 275, metal tins of 12
and vials of 10 tablets

Extra Strength Excedrin®

Bristol-Myers Products
P. 644

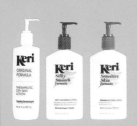

For Dry Skin Care
6.5, 11 and 15 oz. 20 oz. size
for Original Formula
Silky Smooth and Fragrance Free

Keri® Lotion

Bristol-Myers Products
P. 645

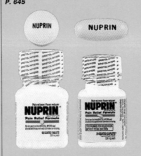

Bottles of 24, 50, 100, 150
and vials of 10 tablets

Nuprin®

Bristol-Myers Products
P. 645

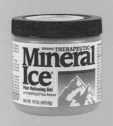

Available in: 3.5 oz., 8 oz.
and 16 oz. Pain Relieving Gel

Therapeutic Mineral Ice®

CIBA SELF-MEDICATION

Ciba Self-Medication, Inc.
P. 648

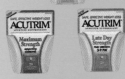

Appetite Suppressants
Caffeine Free/Works all Day

Acutrim®

Ciba Self-Medication, Inc.
P. 649

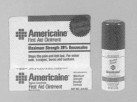

Ointment 3/4 oz. and Spray 2 oz.
Also available in
Hemorrhoidal Ointment 1 oz.

Americaine®

Ciba Self-Medication, Inc.
P. 650

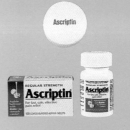

Bottles of 60, 100, 160,
225 & 500 Tablets

**Regular Strength
Ascriptin®**

Ciba Self-Medication, Inc.
P. 650

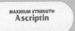

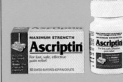

Bottles of 36, 50 & 85 Caplets

**Maximum Strength
Ascriptin®**

Ciba Self-Medication, Inc.
P. 650

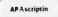

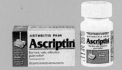

Bottles of 60, 100,
225 & 500 Caplets

**Arthritis Pain
Ascriptin®**

Ciba Self-Medication, Inc.
P. 651

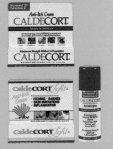

Caldecort and Caldecort Light® Cream
1.5 oz. Spray

Caldecort®

Ciba Self-Medication, Inc.
P. 652

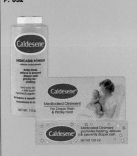

Medicated Powder and Ointment
Also available in 2 oz. and 4 oz. powder

Caldesene®

Ciba Self-Medication, Inc.
P. 652

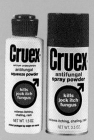

Antifungal Spray and Squeeze
Powder & Cream
Relieves Itching, Chafing, Rash
Cures Jock Itch

Cruex®

Ciba Self-Medication, Inc.
P. 652

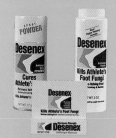

Spray Powder, Cream,
Ointment & Spray Liquid
Cures Athlete's Foot

Desenex®

Ciba Self-Medication, Inc.
P. 653

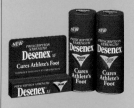

Spray Powder, Cream
& Liquid Spray
Cures Athlete's Foot

**Prescription Strength
Desenex®**

Ciba Self-Medication, Inc.
P. 653

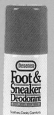

Foot & Sneaker Deodorant
Soothes, Cools, Comforts
and Absorbs Moisture

Desenex®

Ciba Self-Medication, Inc.
P. 653

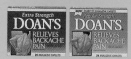

Backache Analgesic
Relieves Backache
Regular/Extra Strength/Nighttime

Doan's® & Doan's® P.M.

Ciba Self-Medication, Inc.
P. 654

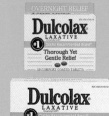

Tablets & Suppositories

Dulcolax® Laxative

Ciba Self-Medication, Inc.
P. 655

E ● 24

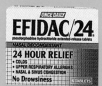

E

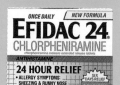

Nasal Decongestant

Efidac/24®

Ciba Self-Medication, Inc.
P. 656

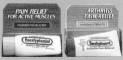

Alpine Breeze, Powder Fresh
and Arthritis Pain External Analgesics

Eucalyptamint®

Ciba Self-Medication, Inc.
P. 656

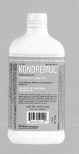

Plain (Mineral Oil)
Lubricant Laxative

Kondremul®

Ciba Self-Medication, Inc.
P. 657

Blister Packs of 24's and Bottles of
50's Antacid Caplets

Maalox® Antacid Caplets

Ciba Self-Medication, Inc.
P. 659

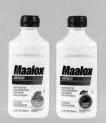

Mint & Cherry Creme
Available in 5 (Mint Only), 12 & 26 oz.

Maalox® Antacid

Ciba Self-Medication, Inc.
P. 659

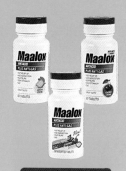

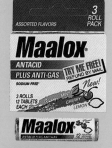

Lemon Assorted &
Cherry Flavors in Bottles
of 50 & 100 Tablets
Rollpacks in Assorted
and Lemon Flavors

**Maalox® Antacid
Plus Anti-Gas**

Ciba Self-Medication, Inc.
P. 657

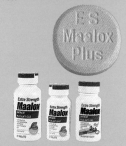

Cooling Mint Tablets and Assorted
Flavors in 38's, 75's

**Extra Strength Maalox®
Antacid Plus Anti-Gas**

Ciba Self-Medication, Inc.
P. 657

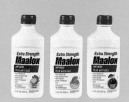

Cooling Mint, Smooth Cherry and
Refreshing Lemon
All available in 12 & 26 oz.
Refreshing Lemon also available in 5 oz.

**Extra Strength Maalox®
Antacid Plus Anti-Gas**

Ciba Self-Medication, Inc.
P. 658

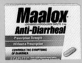

Available in 2 oz. and 4 oz. liquid
(cherry flavored) w/dosage cup
6 and 12 Caplets

Maalox® Anti-Diarrheal

Ciba Self-Medication, Inc.
P. 658

Peppermint and Sweet Lemon Flavor
Regular Strength 12's & 48's
Extra Strength 10's and 36's

Maalox® Anti-Gas

Ciba Self-Medication, Inc.
P. 660

External Analgesic Cream
Available in 2 oz. and 4 oz. tubes,
8 oz. and 16 oz. jars

Myoflex®

Ciba Self-Medication, Inc.
P. 660

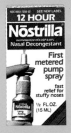

12 Hour Metered Pump Spray

Nostrilla®

Ciba Self-Medication, Inc.
P. 661

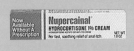

For fast, soothing relief of anal itch.

Nupercainal®

Ciba Self-Medication, Inc.
P. 661

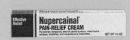

1 1/2 oz. Pain Relief Cream
Prompt, temporary relief of painful
sunburn, minor burns, scrapes, scratches,
and nonpoisonous insect bites.

Nupercainal®

Ciba Self-Medication, Inc.
P. 661

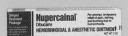

Hemmorhoidal & Anesthetic
Available in: Ointment 2 oz. & 1 oz.
Suppositories: boxes of 12 & 24

Nupercainal®

Ciba Self-Medication, Inc.
P. 662

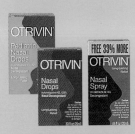

Nasal Decongestant Drops
Pediatric Drops and Nasal Spray

Otrivin®

Ciba Self-Medication, Inc.
P. 662

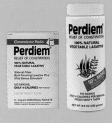

100% Natural Vegetable Laxative
250 gm and 6-6gm packets

Perdiem®

Ciba Self-Medication, Inc.
P. 662

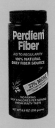

100% Natural
Daily Fiber Source
available in 250 gm only

Perdiem® Fiber

Ciba Self-Medication, Inc.
P. 663

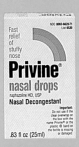

Also available in Nasal Spray

Privine®

Ciba Self-Medication, Inc.
P. 664

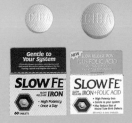

Slow Release Iron and Slow Release
Iron & Folic Acid

Slow Fe®

Ciba Self-Medication, Inc.
P. 664

Children's Multivitamins
Regular + Extra C + Iron Complete

Sunkist®

Ciba Self-Medication, Inc.
P. 666

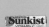

250 & 500 mg Chewable Tablets;
500 mg Easy to Swallow Caplets;
60 mg Chewable Tablets (11 Tablet Roll)

Sunkist® Vitamin C
Citrus Complex

Ciba Self-Medication, Inc.
P. 666

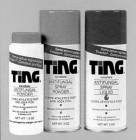

Cream, Powder, Spray Liquid & Powder
For Athlete's Foot & Jock Itch

Ting®

Del Pharmaceuticals
P. 667

Extra Strength Pain Relieving Rub
in Triple Medicated and Odor Free

ArthriCare®

Del Pharmaceuticals
P. 668

Sore Gums, Toothache Pain, and
Cold & Canker Sore Relief

Orajel®

Del Pharmaceuticals
P. 667

Teething Pain Medicine
Tooth & Gum Cleanser

Baby Orajel®

Del Pharmaceuticals
P. 669

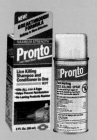

Maximum Strength
Lice Killing Shampoo
Household Spray

Pronto®

Del Pharmaceuticals
P. 669

Medicated Gel & No Sting Liquid

Tanac®

EFFCON

Effcon Laboratories
P. 670

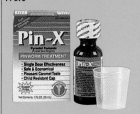

Oral Suspension 50 mg/mL
For the treatment of pinworm
infections.

Pin-X®
(pyrantel pamoate)

HOGIL PHARMACUETICAL

Hogil Pharmacuetical Corp.
P. 672

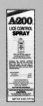
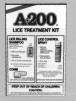

Lice Control Spray 6 oz.
Lice Treatment Kit (Kit includes
shampoo, spray, and comb)
Lice Killing Shampoo 2 & 4 oz. sizes
(Special comb included)
Lice Killing Gel

A 200®

Hogil Pharmacuetical Corp.
P. 673

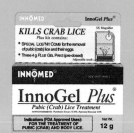

Pubic (Crab) Lice
Treatment Kit

InnoGel Plus™

J&J-MERCK CONSUMER

J&J-Merck Consumer
P. 675

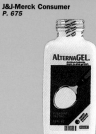

12 fl oz
High potency aluminum
hydroxide antacid

AlternaGel®

J&J-Merck Consumer
P. 675

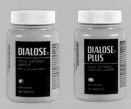

Bottles of 36 & 100 tablets

**Dialose® and
Dialose® Plus**

J&J-Merck Consumer
P. 677

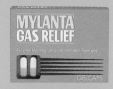
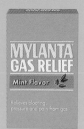

Gelcaps:
(2 tablets / 125 mg)

Chewable tablets:
RS Mint (80 mg) 12, 30, 60, 100;
Cherry 12

MS Mint (125 mg) 12, 24, 48

Mylanta® Gas Relief

J&J-Merck Consumer
P. 677

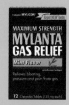

125 mg
12 & 24 tablet convenience packs
and bottles of 48.

**Maximum Strength
Mylanta® Gas Relief**

J&J-Merck Consumer
P. 678

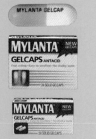

Available in boxes of 24 and
Bottles of 50 and 100
24 Gelcap convenience pack

Mylanta® Gelcaps

J&J-Merck Consumer
P. 676

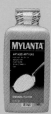

Available in Original, Cool Mint
Creme and Cherry Creme in bottles of
5, 12 and 24 oz.

Mylanta® Liquid

J&J-Merck Consumer
P. 676

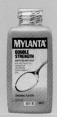

Available in Original, Cool Mint
Creme and Cherry Creme in bottles of
5, 12 and 24 oz.

**Mylanta® Double
Strength Liquid**

J&J-Merck Consumer
P. 678

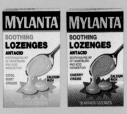

Available in Cool Mint Creme
and Cherry Creme
18 lozenges convenient packs
and bottles of 50

Mylanta® Lozenges

J&J-Merck Consumer
P. 677

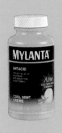

Available in Cool Mint Creme
and Cherry Creme in bottles of 50 and
100 and rollpacks of 12

Mylanta® Tablets

J&J-Merck Consumer
P. 677

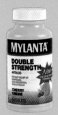

Tablets in bottles of 35, 70
and rollpacks of 8

Mylanta® Double
Strength Tablets

J&J-Merck Consumer
P. 676

Available in 0.5 oz. and 1.0 oz. bottles

Infants' Mylicon® Drops

J&J-Merck Consumer
P. 679

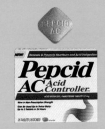

Available in 6's, 12's, 18's and 30's

Pepcid AC®

LEDERLE

***LEDERMARK®
Product
Identification Code**

Many Lederle tablets and capsules bear an identification code, and these codes are listed with each product pictured.

Lederle Laboratories
P. 681

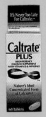

Also Available: Caltrate® 600 and
Caltrate® 600+D

Caltrate® Plus
(calcium carbonate)

Lederle Laboratories
P. 682

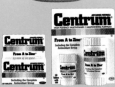

Bottles of 60 and 100 with 30
High Potency Multivitamin/
Multimineral Formula

Centrum®

Lederle Laboratories
P. 682

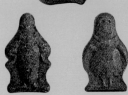

60 Tablets Children's
Chewable Vitamin/Mineral Formula
with beta carotene
Also Available: Centrum Jr.® Shamu and
his Crew® + Extra Calcium and Centrum
Jr.® Shamu and his Crew® + Iron

Centrum, Jr.® Shamu and
his Crew® + Extra C

Lederle Laboratories
P. 683

*CS11
Bottles of 60 and 100
Specially Formulated
Multivitamin/Multimineral
For Adults 50+

Centrum® SILVER®

Lederle Laboratories
P. 684

*F66
Available in boxes of
36 and 60 and bottles of 90

FiberCon®

Lederle Laboratories
P. 685

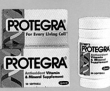

Bottles of 50 Softgels Antioxidant
Vitamin & Mineral Supplement

PROTEGRA®

Lederle Laboratories
P. 685

*S2
Bottles of 60
High Potency Stress Formula Vitamins
Also available: Stresstabs® and
Stresstabs® + Zinc

Stresstabs® + Iron

LENES PHARMACAL, INC.

Lenes Pharmacal, Inc.
P. 686

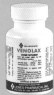

Venolax®

While every effort has
been made to reproduce
products faithfully, this
section is to be considered a Quick-Reference
Identification aid.

LEVER BROTHERS

Lever Brothers
P. 686

Available in Bar & Liquid

Dove®

Lever Brothers
P. 686

Antibacterial Soap
Available in Bar and Liquid

Lever 2000®

3M

3M
P. 686

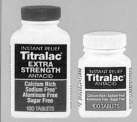

Available in: Regular Strength 40,
100, 1000 Tablets and Extra Strength
100 Tablets only

3M™ Titralac™ Antacid

3M
P. 687

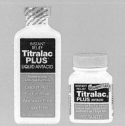

Antacid with Simethicone
Available in:
100 Tablets and 12 Fl. oz. liquid

3M™ Titralac™ Plus Antacid

MCNEIL

McNeil Consumer Products
P. 691

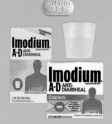

Available in 2 and 4 fl. oz. bottles
with a convenient dosage cup, and
caplets in 6's, 12's and 18's

Imodium® A-D

Lactaid Inc. Marked By
McNeil Consumer Products
P. 693

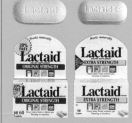

Original strength available
in bottles of 60
Extra strength available
in bottles of 24 and 50

Lactaid® Caplets

Lactaid Inc. Marked By
McNeil Consumer Products
P. 693

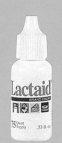

Available in 30 qt. supply

Lactaid® Drops

Lactaid Inc. Marked By
McNeil Consumer Products
P. 687

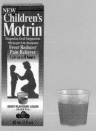

100 mg/5 mL

Children's Motrin Ibuprofen Oral Suspension

McNeil Consumer Products
P. 693

PediaCare® Cough-Cold Chewables

Blister Packs of 16 Chewable Tablets
Liquid available in 4 fl. oz. bottle
with child-resistant safety cap and
convenient dosage cup

PediaCare® Cough-Cold

McNeil Consumer Products
P. 693

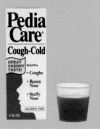

Available in ½ fl. oz.
bottle with child-resistant safety cap
and calibrated dropper

PediaCare® Infants' Drops Decongestant Plus Cough

McNeil Consumer Products
P. 693

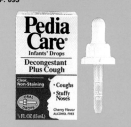

Available in 1/2 fl. oz. bottle with
child-resistant safety cap and
calibrated dropper

PediaCare® Infants' Decongestant Drops

McNeil Consumer Products
P. 693

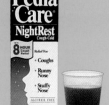

Available in 4 fl. oz. bottle with
child-resistant safety cap and
convenient dosage cup

PediaCare® NightRest Cough-Cold Liquid

McNeil Consumer Products
P. 695

Tablets and Caplets in blister packs
of 24 & bottles of 50
Gelcaps in blister packs
of 20 & bottles of 40

Maximum Strength Sine-Aid®

McNeil Consumer Products
P. 688

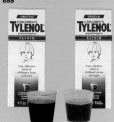

Available in cherry and grape flavors
in 2 and 4 fl. oz. bottles with
child-resistant safety cap and
convenient dosage cup. Alcohol
Free, 80 mg. per 1/2 teaspoon

Children's TYLENOL® Elixir

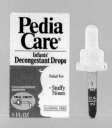

McNeil Consumer Products
P. 688

Fruit Flavor: bottles of 30 with child resistant safety cap and blister-packs of 48

Bubble Gum and Grape Flavor Bottles of 30 with child-resistant safety cap

**Children's TYLENOL®
80 mg Chewable Tablets**

McNeil Consumer Products
P. 688

Available in rich cherry flavor in 2 and 4 fl. oz. bottles and Bubble Gum Flavor in 4 fl. oz. with child-resistant safety cap and convenient dosage cup. Alcohol Free, 80 mg per 1/2 teaspoon

**Children's TYLENOL®
Suspension Liquid**

McNeil Consumer Products
P. 691

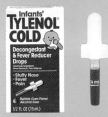

Available in 1/2 fl. oz. bottle with child-resistant safety cap and calibrated dropper. Bubble Gum Flavor, Alcohol-free.

**Infant's TYLENOL® Cold
Decongestant and Fever
Reducer Drops**

McNeil Consumer Products
P. 688

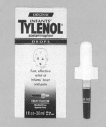

Available in 1/2 and 1 fl. oz. bottle with child-resistant safety cap and calibrated dropper. Fruit Flavor, Alcohol Free, 80 mg. per 0.8 mL

Infant's TYLENOL® Drops

McNeil Consumer Products
P. 688

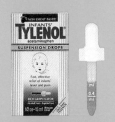

Available in 1/2 oz. bottle with child resistant safety cap and calibrated dropper. Rich Grape Flavor, Alcohol Free, 80 mg per 0.8 mL

**Infants' TYLENOL®
Suspension Drops**

McNeil Consumer Products
P. 692

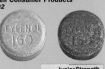

Available in Fruit and Grape Flavored Chewable tablets of 160 mg available in blister pack of 24

**Junior Strength
TYLENOL®**

McNeil Consumer Products
P. 692

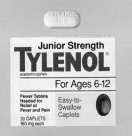

Swallowable Caplets: 160 mg blister packs of 30

**Junior Strength
TYLENOL®**

McNeil Consumer Products
P. 689

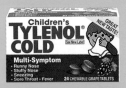

Available in bottles of 24 chewable tablets with child-resistant safety cap

Children's TYLENOL® Cold

McNeil Consumer Products
P. 689

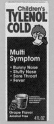

Multi-Symptom Formula
Available in 4 fl. oz. bottle with child-resistant safety cap and convenient dosage cup

**Children's TYLENOL®
Cold Liquid**

McNeil Consumer Products
P. 690

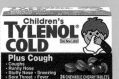

Available in bottles of 24 chewable tablets with child-resistant safety cap

**Children's TYLENOL® Cold
Plus Cough Chewable**

McNeil Consumer Products
P. 690

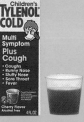

Multi-Symptom Plus Cough Formula
Available in 4 fl. oz. bottle with child-resistant safety cap and convenient dosage cup.

**Children's TYLENOL®
Cold Plus Cough Liquid**

McNeil Consumer Products
P. 697

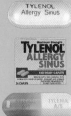

Caplets in blister packs of 24 & bottles of 60
Gelcaps in blister packs of 24 & bottles of 60
Geltabs in blister packs of 24 & bottles of 60

**Maximum Strength
TYLENOL® Allergy Sinus**

McNeil Consumer Products
P. 698

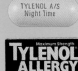

Caplets available in blister packs of 24's

**Maximum Strength
TYLENOL® Allergy Sinus
NightTime**

McNeil Consumer Products
P. 706

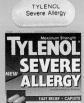

Caplets available in blister packs of 12's and 24's

**Maximum Strength
Tylenol® Severe Allergy**

McNeil Consumer Products
P. 699

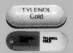
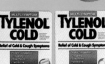

Caplets and Tablets available in
blister-packs of 24 and bottles of 50

**TYLENOL® Cold
Medication**

McNeil Consumer Products
P. 699

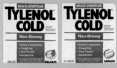

Gelcaps available in
blister-packs of 24 and bottles of 40
Caplets available in blister-packs
of 24 and bottles of 50
No Drowsiness Formula

**TYLENOL® Cold
Medication**

McNeil Consumer Products
P. 699

Available in cartons of 6 individual
packets. Hot Liquid Medication

**Multi-Symptom
TYLENOL® COLD**

For more detailed infor-
mation on the products
illustrated in this section,
consult the Product
Information Section or
manufacturers may be
contacted directly.

McNeil Consumer Products
P. 701

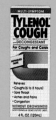

Available in 4 fl. oz. bottles

**Multi-Symptom
TYLENOL® Cough**

McNeil Consumer Products
P. 703

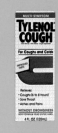

Gelcaps available in blister-packs of
10's, and 20's
No Drowsiness Formula

**Maximum Strength
TYLENOL® Flu**

McNeil Consumer Products
P. 703

Available in cartons of 6 individual
packets. Hot Liquid Medication

**Maximum Strength
TYLENOL® Flu NightTime**

McNeil Consumer Products
P. 703

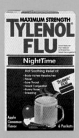

Gelcaps Available in
Blister Packs of 10's and 20's

**Maximum Strength
TYLENOL® Flu NightTime**

McNeil Consumer Products
P. 696

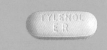
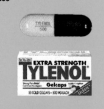

Caplets available in
24's, 50's and 100's

**TYLENOL® Extended
Relief**

McNeil Consumer Products
P. 696

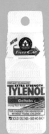

Geltabs available in tamper-resistant
bottles of 24's, 50's and 100's and
FastCap™ bottle of 72's "for households without children"
Gelcaps available in tamper-resistant
bottles of 24's, 50's, 100's,
150's and 225's and FastCap™ bottle
of 72's "for households
without children"

Extra Strength TYLENOL®

McNeil Consumer Products
P. 696

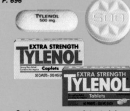

Caplets: tamper-resistant vials
of 10 and bottles of 24's, 50's,
100's, 175's and 250's
Tablets: tamper-resistant vials
of 10 and bottles of 30's,
60's, 100's and 200's
Liquid: tamper-resistant
bottles of 8 fl. oz.

Extra Strength TYLENOL®

McNeil Consumer Products
P. 696

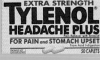
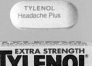

Tablets and Caplets available in:
24's, 50's, 100's and 200's and
Tins of 12's

**Regular Strength
TYLENOL®**

McNeil Consumer Products
P. 705

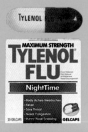

Caplets available in 24's and 50's

**Extra Strength TYLENOL®
Headache Plus**

McNeil Consumer Products
P. 705

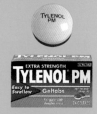

Geltabs and Gelcaps available
in tamper-resistant bottles of 24's
and 50's. Caplets available in
tamper-resistant bottles of 24's,
50's, 100's and 150's

TYLENOL® PM

McNeil Consumer Products
P. 707

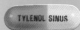

Caplets, Gelcaps and Geltabs
in blister packs of 24
& bottles of 60

**Maximum Strength
TYLENOL® Sinus**

PFIZER

Pfizer Consumer Health Care
P. 714

Arthritis Formula, Greaseless,
Original Formula, Ultra Strength
and Vanishing Scent.

BENGAY®

Pfizer Consumer Health Care
P. 715

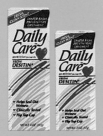

Diaper Rash Prevention Ointment

**Daily Care®
from DESITIN®**

Pfizer Consumer Health Care
P. 715

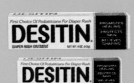

Diaper Rash Ointment

DESITIN®

Pfizer Consumer Health Care
P. 715

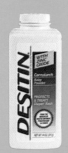

**DESITIN® Cornstarch
Baby Powder**

Pfizer Consumer Health Care
P. 719

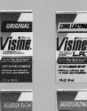

Original, Long Lasting,
Allergy Relief and Moisturizing

Visine®

PHARMATON

Pharmaton
P. 721

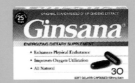

100 mg

Ginsana®

Pharmaton
P. 721

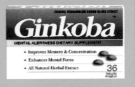

40 mg

Ginkoba®

PROCTER & GAMBLE

Procter & Gamble
P. 722

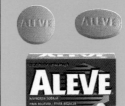

Tablets and caplets available
in 24, 50, 100 and 150 count.
Caplets also available in 200 count.

Aleve®

Procter & Gamble
P. 723

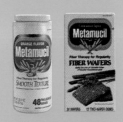

Available in 48, 72 and 114 dose
canisters and 30 one-dose packets.
Also available in sugar free.

Metamucil®

ROBERTS

Roberts Pharmaceutical Corp.
P. 740

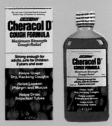

4 oz., 6 oz. Cough Formula
Also available Cheracol Plus
Head Cold/Cough Formula 4 oz., 6 oz.

Cheracol D®

Roberts Pharmaceutical Corp.
P. 741

Stool softener – 50mg/100mg
100 mg available:
Two tone color 30, 60, 100, 250, 1000
50 mg available: 30, 60, 100
Available in Liquid and Syrup

Colace®

Roberts Pharmaceutical Corp.

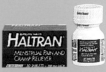

Bottles of 30: 200 mg Tablets

Haltran®

Roberts Pharmaceutical Corp.
P. 742

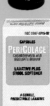

Bottles of 30, 60, 100, 250, 1000
Laxative and Stool Softener
Available in Syrup

Peri-Colace®

Roberts Pharmaceutical Corp.
P. 742

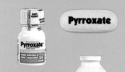

Nasal Decongestant/
Antihistamine/Analgesic
Bottles of 24 and 500 Caplets
Pyrroxate®

Roberts Pharmaceutical Corp.

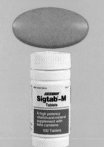

Bottles of 100 Tablets
High Potency Vitamin Supplement
Also Available in Sigtab
Sigtab®-M

ROSS

Ross Products
P. 744

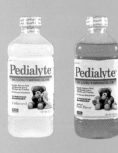

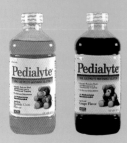

1-Liter Bottles
Oral Electrolyte
Maintenance Solution
Available in Unflavored, Fruit,
Bubble-Gum And Grape Flavors
Pedialyte®

Ross Products
P. 745

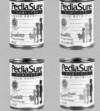

8-Fl-oz Cans
Complete Liquid Nutrition
Available in Strawberry, Vanilla,
Chocolate and Banana Cream Flavors
and Vanilla With Fiber Flavor
PediaSure®

Ross Products
P. 746

8-Fl-oz Drink Box
Nutritional Beverage with Iron
Available in Vanilla, Chocolate
and Berry Flavors
Similac® Toddler's Best™

SANDOZ

Sandoz Consumer Division
P. 747

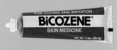

Cream 1 oz. (28.4 g)
Bicozene®

Sandoz Consumer Division
P. 748

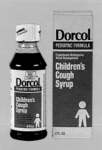

Children's Cough Syrup 4 oz.
Dorcol®

Sandoz Consumer Division
P. 749

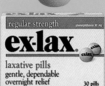

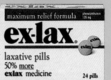

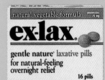

Regular Strength 8's, 30's, 60's
Maximum Relief Formula 24's, 48's
Extra Gentle 24's
Gentle Nature™ 16's
Ex-lax®

Sandoz Consumer Division
P. 748

Chocolated Laxative
Tablets 6's, 18's, 48's and 72's
Ex-lax®

Sandoz Consumer Division
P. 749

Extra-Strength Cherry 18's, 48's
Extra-Strength Peppermint 18's, 48's
(125 mg simethicone)
Gas-X®

Sandoz Consumer Division
P. 749

Cherry 12's, 36's
Peppermint 12's, 36's
(80 mg simethicone)
Gas-X®

Sandoz Consumer Division
P. 749

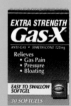

Extra Strength Softgels
in packs of 15's and 30's
Gas-X®

Sandoz Consumer Division
P. 749

8's, 16's, 32's
Tavist-1®

Sandoz Consumer Division
P. 750

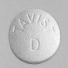

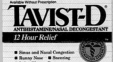

8's, 16's, 32's, 50's

Tavist-D®

Sandoz Consumer Division
P. 750

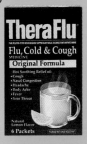

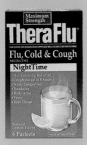

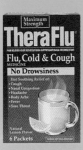

Flu, Cold & Cough Medicine

Maximum Strength Nighttime Flu, Cold & Cough Medicine

Maximum Strength, No Drowsiness Flu, Cold & Cough Medicine

In packs of 6 and 12 ct.

TheraFlu®

Sandoz Consumer Division
P. 750

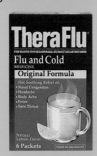

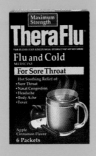

Flu and Cold Medicine

Maximum Strength Flu and Cold Medicine for Sore Throat

In packs of 6 and 12 ct.

TheraFlu®

Sandoz Consumer Division
P. 752

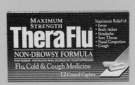

12's, 24's

Non-drowsy Flu, Cold and Cough Caplets

TheraFlu® Maximum Strength

Sandoz Consumer Division
P. 752

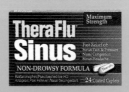

Maximum Strength Sinus Non-Drowsy Formula in packs of 24 caplets

TheraFlu® Sinus

Sandoz Consumer Division
P. 753

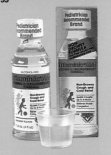

4 oz., 8 oz.

Triaminic® AM Cough & Decongestant Formula

Sandoz Consumer Division
P. 753

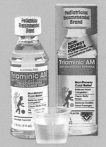

4 oz., 8 oz.

Triaminic® AM Decongestant Formula

Sandoz Consumer Division
P. 756

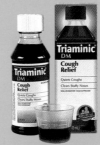

4 oz., 8 oz.

Triaminic® DM

Sandoz Consumer Division
P. 753

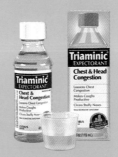

4 oz., 8 oz.

Triaminic® Expectorant

Sandoz Consumer Division
P. 754

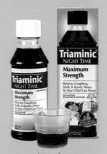

4 oz., 8 oz.

Triaminic® Nite Time®

Sandoz Consumer Division
P. 755

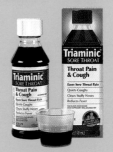

4 oz., 8 oz.

Triaminic® Sore Throat

Sandoz Consumer Division
P. 755

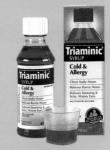

4 oz., 8 oz.

Triaminic® Syrup

Sandoz Consumer Division
P. 756

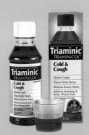

4 oz., 8 oz.

Triaminic® Triaminicol®

Sandoz Consumer Division
P. 756

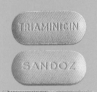

12's, 24's, 48's, 100's

Triaminicin®

SCHERING-PLOUGH

Schering-Plough HealthCare
P. 757

Regular and Medicated
A and D® Ointment

Schering-Plough HealthCare
P. 757

Extra-Moisturizing 12 Hour
**Afrin® Extra
Moisturizing Nasal Spray**

Schering-Plough HealthCare
P. 757

Regular 12 Hour
Safety Sealed
Afrin® Nasal Spray

Schering-Plough HealthCare
P. 758

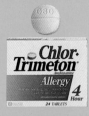

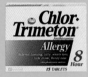

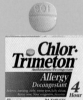

4 Hour Allergy Tablets
8 Hour Allergy Tablets
12 Hour Allergy Tablets
4 Hour Allergy Decongestant Tablets
12 Hour Allergy Decongestant Tablets

Chlor-Trimeton®

Schering-Plough HealthCare
P. 759

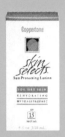

**Coppertone® Skin Selects™
Sunscreen Lotion SPF 15
For Dry Skin**

Schering-Plough HealthCare
P. 760

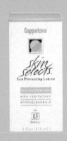

**Coppertone® Skin Selects™
Sunscreen Lotion SPF 15
For Sensitive Skin**

Schering-Plough HealthCare
P. 760

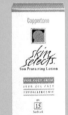

**Coppertone® Skin Selects™
Sunscreen Lotion SPF 15
For Oily Skin**

Schering-Plough HealthCare
P. 760

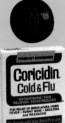

For Relief Of Cold & Flu Symptoms
Coricidin®

Schering-Plough HealthCare
P. 760

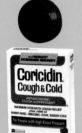

For Relief Of Cold & Cough Symptoms
Coricidin®

Schering-Plough HealthCare
P. 760

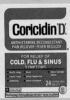

For Relief Of Cold, Flu
& Sinus Symptoms
Coricidin-D®

Schering-Plough HealthCare
P. 761

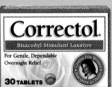

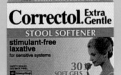

Laxative Tablets and Caplets
and Stool Softener Soft Gels
Correctol®

Schering-Plough HealthCare
P. 761

Cinnamon Spice and
Honey Lemon Flavors

Correctol®
Herbal Tea Laxative

Schering-Plough HealthCare
P. 763

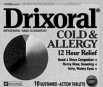

12 Hour Sustained-Action Tablets

Drixoral®
Cold & Allergy

Schering-Plough HealthCare
P. 764

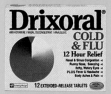

12 Hour Extended-Release Tablets

Drixoral® Cold & Flu

Schering-Plough HealthCare
P. 762

Cough & Sore Throat,
Cough & Congestion and Cough

Drixoral® Liquid Caps

Schering-Plough HealthCare
P. 764

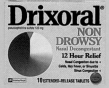

12 Hour
Extended-Release Tablets

Drixoral® Non-Drowsy

Schering-Plough HealthCare
P. 765

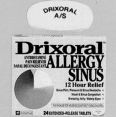

24 Hour Extended-Release Tablets

12 Hour Extended-Release Tablets

Drixoral® Allergy Sinus

Schering-Plough HealthCare
P. 765

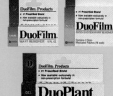

Wart Remover
and Plantar War Remover

DuoFilm®/DuoPlant®

Schering-Plough HealthCare
P. 768

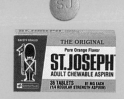

St. Joseph®
Adult Chewable Asprin

Schering-Plough HealthCare
P. 766

Antifungal for Athlete's Foot
and Jock Itch

Lotrimin® AF

Schering-Plough HealthCare
P. 766

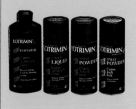

Shaker Powder, Spray Liquid, Spray
Powder and Jock Itch Spray Powder

Lotrimin® AF
(2% miconazole nitrate)

Schering-Plough HealthCare
P. 767

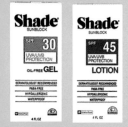

Also available:
SPF 30 Stick

Shade® Sunblock

Schering-Plough HealthCare
P. 768

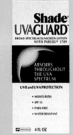

Broad Spectrum Sunscreen Lotion with
PARSOL® 1789

Shade® UVAGUARD™

**SmithKline Beecham
Consumer Healthcare, L.P.**
P. 770

Sore Throat Lozenges

Extra Strength and Cherry
18 lozenges per package

Cepastat®

**SmithKline Beecham
Consumer Healthcare, L.P.**
P. 770

Fiber Therapy for Regularity
Sugar Free Orange available in:
8.6 oz. and 16.9 oz.
Regular Orange available in:
16 oz. and 30 oz. containers

Citrucel®

**SmithKline BeechamConsumer
Healthcare, L.P.**
P. 773

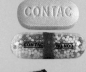

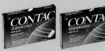

Continuous Action
Nasal Decongestant Antihistamine
Packages of 10 and 20
capsules and caplets

Contac® 12 Hour

**SmithKline Beecham
Consumer Healthcare, L.P.**

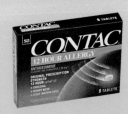

Contac® 12 Hour Allergy

SmithKline Beecham
Consumer Healthcare, L.P.
P. 771

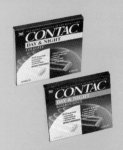

**Contac® Day & Night
Cold & Flu and
Allergy/Sinus**

SmithKline Beecham
Consumer Healthcare, L.P.
P. 775

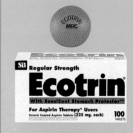

Regular Strength Tablets
in bottles of 100, 250
Ecotrin®

SmithKline Beecham
Consumer Healthcare, L.P.
P. 777

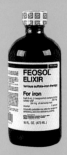

16 oz. bottle
Feosol® Elixir

SmithKline Beecham
Consumer Healthcare, L.P.
P. 779

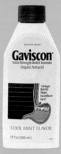

Extra Strength Relief Formula
**Gaviscon® Extra Strength
Liquid Antacid**

SmithKline Beecham
Consumer Healthcare, L.P.
P. 774

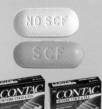

Non-Drowsy Formula
Packages of 16 caplets
**Contac® Severe
Cold & Flu**

SmithKline Beecham
Consumer Healthcare, L.P.
P. 775

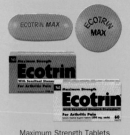

Maximum Strength Tablets
in bottles of 60, 150 and
Caplets in bottles of 60
Ecotrin®

SmithKline Beecham
Consumer Healthcare, L.P.
P. 778

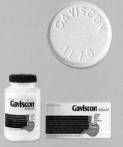

100-Tablet bottles
30-Tablet box (foil-wrapped 2s)
Gaviscon® Antacid

SmithKline Beecham
Consumer Healthcare, L.P.
P. 779

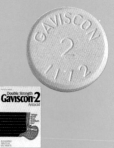

Box of 48 foil-wrapped tablets
Gaviscon®-2 Antacid

SmithKline Beecham
Consumer Healthcare, L.P.
P. 775

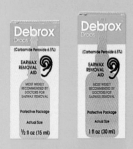

Drops
1/2 Fl. oz. 1 Fl. oz.
Debrox®

SmithKline Beecham
Consumer Healthcare, L.P.
P. 777

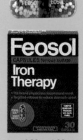

Packages of 30 and 60 capsules
Feosol®

SmithKline Beecham
Consumer Healthcare, L.P.
P. 779

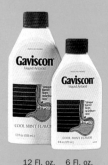

12 Fl. oz.   6 Fl. oz.
Gaviscon® Liquid Antacid

SmithKline Beecham
Consumer Healthcare, L.P.
P. 779

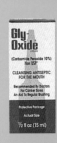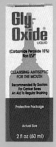

1/2 Fl. oz. 2 Fl. oz.
Gly-Oxide® Liquid

SmithKline Beecham
Consumer Healthcare, L.P.
P. 775

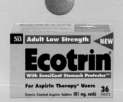

Adult Low Strength Tablets in Bottles
of 36
Ecotrin®

SmithKline Beecham
Consumer Healthcare, L.P.
P. 778

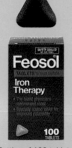

Bottles of 100 tablets
Feosol®

SmithKline Beecham
Consumer Healthcare, L.P.
P. 778

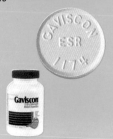

Extra Strength Relief Formula
100-Tablet bottles
**Gaviscon® Extra
Strength Antacid**

SmithKline Beecham
Consumer Healthcare, L.P.
P. 780

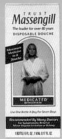

Medicated Disposable Douche
With Povidone-iodine
Available in single or twin packs
Massengill®

SmithKline Beecham
Consumer Healthcare, L.P.
P. 782

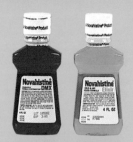

Cough/Cold Formula & Decongestant
and Cold & Hay Fever Formula

Novahistine®
DMX & Elixir

SmithKline Beecham
Consumer Healthcare, L.P.
P. 783

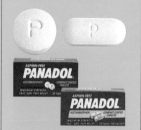

Asprin-Free Tablets and Caplets

Panadol®

SmithKline Beecham
Consumer Healthcare, L.P.
P. 783

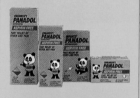

Chewable Tablets, Caplets,
Liquid and Drops

Children's Panadol®

SmithKline Beecham
Consumer Healthcare, L.P.
P. 784

No Drowsiness Formula Caplets

Sine®-Off

SmithKline Beecham
Consumer Healthcare, L.P.
P. 784

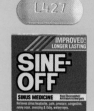

Packages of 24 and 100 Caplets

Sine®-Off

SmithKline Beecham
Consumer Healthcare, L.P.
P. 785

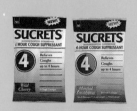

Available in Wild Cherry and
Menthol-Eucalyptus

Sucrets® 4-Hour Cough
Suppressant

SmithKline Beecham
Consumer Healthcare, L.P.
P. 785

Sore Throat Lozenges
Available in: Regular Strength
(Wild Cherry, Original Mint, Vapor
Lemon and Assorted)
Maximum Strength (Wintergreen,
Vapor Black Cherry) and
Childrens Cherry

Sucrets®

SmithKline Beecham
Consumer Healthcare, L.P.
P. 786

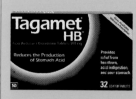

Acid Reducer
Packages of 16, 32, 48 and 64.

Tagamet® HB™

SmithKline Beecham
Consumer Healthcare, L.P.
P. 786

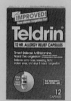

Timed-Release Capsules
Packages of 12, 24 and 48 capsules

Teldrin®

SmithKline Beecham
Consumer Healthcare, L.P.
P. 787

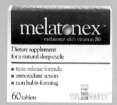

Peppermint and
Assorted Flavors

Tums®

SmithKline Beecham
Consumer Healthcare, L.P.
P. 787

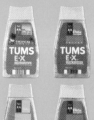

Tropical Fruit, Cherry,
Wintergreen and Assorted Flavors

Tums E-X®

SmithKline Beecham
Consumer Healthcare, L.P.
P. 787

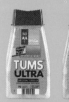

Assorted Mint and Fruit Flavors

Tums® Ultra™

Sunsource
P. 791

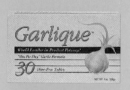

30 Odor-Free Tablets

Garlique™

Sunsource
P. 791

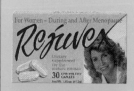

Available in boxes of 30 and
60 tablets

Melatonex™

Sunsource
P. 791

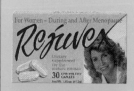

Available in boxes of 30 and 50
(economy pack) caplets

Rejuvex®

Sunsource
P. 792

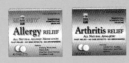

Allergy Relief, Arthritis Relief,
Cold Relief, Flu Relief,
Insomnia Relief and Sinus Relief

Sunsource™
All Natural Homeopathic Medicine

Sunsource
P. 793

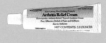

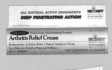

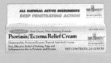

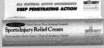

Arthritis Relief Cream,
Psoriasis/Eczema Relief Cream
and Sports Injury Relief Cream

Sunsource™
Traditional Homeopathic Medicine

THOMPSON

Thompson Medical Co., Inc.
P. 794

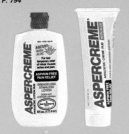

Available in 1 1/4 oz., 3 oz. and
5 oz. Creme and 6 oz. Lotion

Aspercreme® with Aloe

Thompson Medical Co., Inc.
P. 794

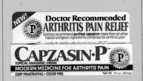

Tropical Analgesic Creme
Available in 1.5 oz Creme

Capzasin•P™

Thompson Medical Co., Inc.
P. 795

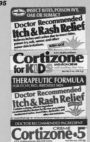

Available in 1 oz. and 2 oz. Creme
and 1 oz. Ointment
Kids available in 1/2 oz.
and 1 oz. Creme

Cortizone-5®

Thompson Medical Co., Inc.
P. 795

Available in 1 oz. and 2 oz. Creme
and Ointment; 1.5 fl. oz. Liquid.

Cortizone-10™

Thompson Medical Co., Inc.
P. 795

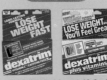

Available in 10, 20, and 40 Caplet
sizes also in 20 and 40 Tablet sizes.

Maximum
Strength Dexatrim®

Thompson Medical Co., Inc.
P. 797

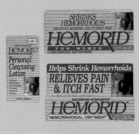

Available in 1 oz. Creme, 1 oz. Ointment,
12 ct. Suppositories and 4 oz. Cleanser

Hemoroid™ For Women

Thompson Medical Co., Inc.
P. 798

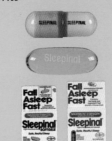

Available in 16 and 32 Capsule sizes
and 8 & 16 Softgel sizes

Sleepinal®

Thompson Medical Co., Inc.
P. 799

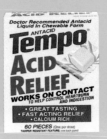

Soft Antacid
Available in 10, 30 and 60 Tablet sizes

Tempo®

UPJOHN

The Upjohn Company
P. 800

Maximum Strength (1% hydrocortisone)
is available in cream, ointment, and spray.
Sensitive Skin (1/2% hydrocortisone) is
available in cream and ointment.

Cortaid®

The Upjohn Company
P. 800

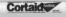

Roll-on relief for insect
bites, itches and rashes

Maximum Strength

Cortaid® FastStick™
(1% hydrocortisone)

The Upjohn Company
P. 801

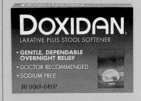

Stimulant/Stool Softener Laxative
Packages of 10, 30, 100 and 1,000

Doxidan® Liqui-Gels®
(docusate calcium 60 mg and
yellow phenolphthalein 65 mg)

The Upjohn Company
P. 801

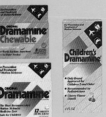

Tablets, Chewables and
Children's Liquid

Dramamine®
(dimenhydrinate)

Warner Wellcome
P. 814

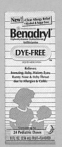

Available in 8 fl. oz. bottles

Benadryl® Dye-Free Allergy Liquid Medication

Warner Wellcome
P. 815

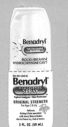

Original and Extra Strength

Benadryl® Itch Stopping Spray

Warner Wellcome
P. 816

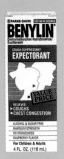

Available in 4 oz. bottles

Benylin® Expectorant

Warner Wellcome
P. 817

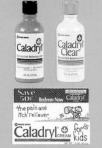

Itch Relief Plus Drying Action. Available in Lotion, Clear Lotion and Cream for Kids

Caladryl®

Warner Wellcome
P. 813

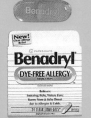

Available in Boxes of 24

Benadryl® Dye-Free Allergy Liqui-Gels® Softgels

Warner Wellcome
P. 814

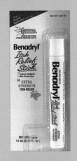

Extra Strength

Benadryl® Itch Relief Stick

Warner Wellcome
P. 816

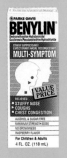

Available in 4 oz. bottles

Benylin® Multi-Symptom

Warner Wellcome
P. 818

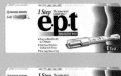
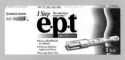

1 and 2 Pregnancy Test Kits Available One Step. Easy to read. Lab Accurate results.

e.p.t®

Warner Wellcome
P. 813

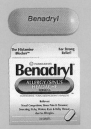

Available in boxes of 24 Caplets

Benadryl® Allergy Sinus Headache

Warner Wellcome
P. 815

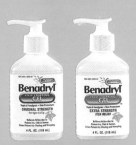

Original and Extra Strength

Benadryl® Itch Stopping Gel

Warner Wellcome
P. 817

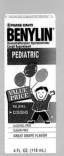

Available in 4 oz. bottles

Benylin® Pediatric

Warner Wellcome
P. 819

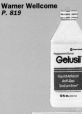

Antacid-Anti-gas Sodium Free Available in boxes of 100 and as a liquid in 12 Fl. oz. bottles

Gelusil®

Warner Wellcome
P. 814

Original and Extra Strength

Benadryl® Itch Stopping Cream

Warner Wellcome
P. 817

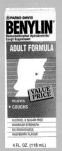

Available in 4 oz. bottles

Benylin® Adult

Warner Wellcome
P. 817

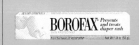

Skin Protectant Ointment Available in 1.8 oz (50g) tube

Borofax®

Warner Wellcome
P. 820

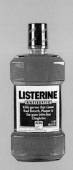

Listerine® Antiseptic

Warner Wellcome
P. 820

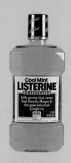

**Cool Mint
Listerine® Antiseptic**

Warner Wellcome
P. 821

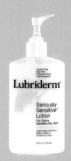

**Lubriderm® Seriously
Sensitive Lotion**

Warner Wellcome
P. 821

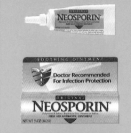

First Aid Antibiotic Ointment
Available in 1/2 oz. (14.2g) or 1 oz.
(28.4g) tubes; 1/32 oz. (0.9 g)

Neosporin®

Warner Wellcome
P. 822

Lice Treatment Creme Rinse
2 fl. oz. (59 mL)
Also available in:
2-bottle family pack

Nix®

Warner Wellcome
P. 820

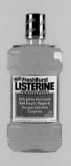

FreshBurst Listerine®

Warner Wellcome
P. 821

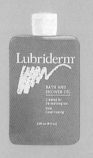

**Lubriderm® Bath &
Shower Oil**

Warner Wellcome
P. 821

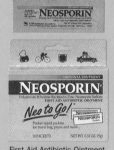

First Aid Antibiotic Ointment.
Available in Individual
Foil Packets. 0.31 oz. (9g)

Neosporin® Neo to Go!™

Warner Wellcome
P. 822

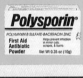

First Aid Antibiotic Powder & Ointment
Powder, 0.35 oz. (10g) Ointment,
1/2 oz. (14.2g) and 1 oz. (28.4g)

Polysporin®

Warner Wellcome
P. 820

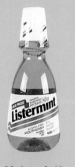

**Listermint®
Alcohol-Free Mouthwash**

Warner Wellcome
P. 821

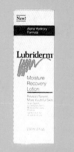

**Lubriderm® Moisture
Recovery Alpha Hydroxy
Cream & Lotion**

Warner Wellcome
P. 821

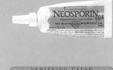
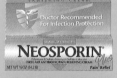

Maximum Strength Cream
Available in 1/2 oz. (14.2g) tubes

Neosporin® Plus

Warner Wellcome
P. 823

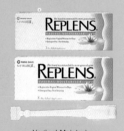

Vaginal Moisturizer
Available in boxes of 3 and 8
single-use applicators

Replens®

Warner Wellcome
P. 820

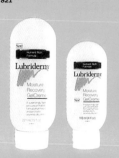

Scented and Fragrance Free Lotion
For Dry Skin Care
Lubriderm® Lotion

Warner Wellcome
P. 821

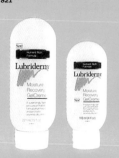

**Lubriderm® Moisture
Recovery GelCreme**

Warner Wellcome
P. 822

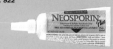
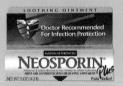

Maximum Strength Ointment
Available in 1/2 oz. (14.2g)
and 1 oz. (28.4g) tubes

Neosporin® Plus

Warner Wellcome
P. 823

Available in Boxes of 24

**Sinutab® Non-Drying
Liquid Caps**

Warner Wellcome
P. 824

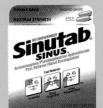

Maximum Strength
Without Drowsiness Formula
Available in 24 Caplets or Tablets

Sinutab® Sinus

Warner Wellcome
P. 823

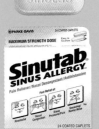

Maximum Strength Formula
Available in 24 Caplets or Tablets

Sinutab® Sinus Allergy

Warner Wellcome
P. 825

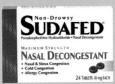

30 mg Tablets
Available in 24, 48 and 100

Sudafed® Nasal Decongestant

Warner Wellcome
P. 825

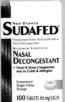

60 mg Tablets
Available in 100

Sudafed® Nasal Decongestant

Warner Wellcome
P. 824

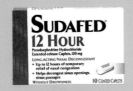

12 Hour Caplets
Available in 10 and 20 caplets

Sudafed® 12 Hour

Warner Wellcome
P. 825

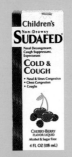

Available in 4 fl. oz. bottles

Sudafed® Children's Cold and Cough

Warner Wellcome
P. 826

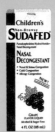

Available in 4 Fl. Oz. bottles

Sudafed® Children's Nasal Decongestant Liquid Medication

Warner Wellcome
P. 826

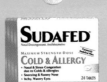

Available in boxes of 24 and 48 tablets.

Sudafed® Cold and Allergy

Warner Wellcome
P. 826

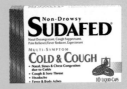

Available in 10's or 20's Liquid Caps

Sudafed® Cold & Cough

Warner Wellcome
P. 828

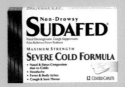

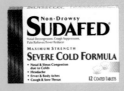

Available in 10 and 20 caplets and tablets

Sudafed® Severe Cold Formula

Warner Wellcome
P. 827

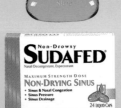

Available in 24 Liquid Caps

Sudafed® Non-Drying Sinus Liquid Caps

Warner Wellcome
P. 829

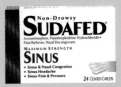

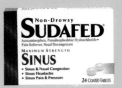

Available in 24 and 48 caplets and tablets

Sudafed® Sinus

Warner Wellcome
P. 827

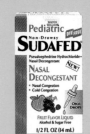

Available in ½ fl. oz. bottles

Sudafed® Pediatric Nasal Decongestant Liquid Oral Drops

Warner Wellcome
P. 830

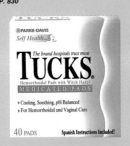

Pre-Moistened Pads
Available in 40 and 100 pad packages

Tucks®

Warner Wellcome
P. 829

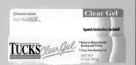

Available in 0.7 oz. (19.8 g) tubes

Tucks® Clear Gel

WHITEHALL-ROBINS

Whitehall-Robins
P. 836

Gel Caplets in Bottles of
4, 8, 24, 50, 100, 165 and 250.
Coated Tablets in Bottles of
4, 8, 24, 50, 72, 100, 165 and 250.
Coated Caplets in Blister Packs of
8 and bottles of 24, 50, 72, 100,
165 and 250.

Advil®

Whitehall-Robins
P. 837

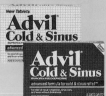

Coated Caplets and Tablets in
Packages of 20 and Bottles of 40

Advil® Cold & Sinus

Whitehall-Robins
P. 837

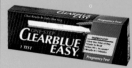

One-Step Pregnancy Test

CLEARBLUE EASY®

Whitehall-Robins
P. 837

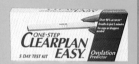

One-Step Ovulation Predictor

CLEARPLAN EASY™

Whitehall-Robins
P. 840

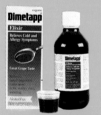

Available in 4 oz., 8 oz., 12 oz.,
16 oz. and 128 oz. bottles

Alcohol Free

Dimetapp® Elixir

Whitehall-Robins
P. 841

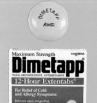

Available in blister packs of 12's, 24's
48's and bottles of 100's and 500's

Dimetapp® Extentabs®

Whitehall-Robins
P. 842

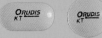

Coated tablets or caplets
available in bottles of
24, 50, and 100

Orudis® KT™

Whitehall-Robins
P. 842

Hemorrhoidal Ointment:
1 oz and 2 oz tubes
Cream: 0.9 oz and 1.8 oz
Suppositories: 12's, 24's and 48's

Preparation H®

Whitehall-Robins
P. 843

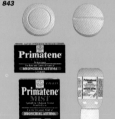

Available in 15 mL Inhaler
Units; 15 mL and 22.5 mL Refills;
Tablets in 24's, 60's

Primatene®

Whitehall-Robins
P. 846

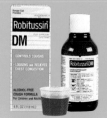

Available in single-dose 6's and 4 oz.,
8 oz., 12 oz. and 16 oz. bottles

Alcohol Free

Robitussin® DM Syrup

J.B WILLIAMS CO.

J.B Williams Co.
P. 849

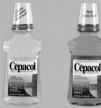

Original and Mint Antiseptic
Mouthwash/Gargle
Available in 4, 12, 24
and 32 Fl. oz. bottles

Cepacol®

J.B Williams Co.
P. 850

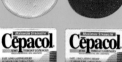

Maximum Strength Sore Throat
Lozenges
Original Mint and Cherry Flavors
Also Available in Regular Strength.
18 lozenges per pack

Cepacol®

J.B Williams Co.
P. 849

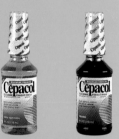

Maximum Strength Sore Throat Spray
Cool Menthol and Cherry Flavors.
4 Fl. oz. bottles

Cepacol®

WYETH-AYERST

**Tamper-Resistant/
Evident Packaging**

Statements alerting con-
sumers to the specific type
of Tamper-Resistant/Evident
Packaging appear on the bottle labels and cartons of all
over-the-counter products of
Wyeth-Ayerst. This includes
plastic cap seals on bottles,
individually wrapped tablets
or suppositories, and sealed
cartons. This packaging has
been developed to better
protect the consumer.

Wyeth-Ayerst Laboratories
P. 850

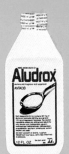

Suspension Antacid 12 Fl. oz.

Aludrox®

Wyeth-Ayerst Laboratories
P. 851

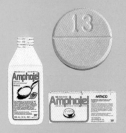

0.6 gram (10 gr.) Tablet shown above
12 Fl. oz. bottle and 100 tablets
Tablets and Suspension Antacid

Amphojel®

Wyeth-Ayerst Laboratories
P. 851

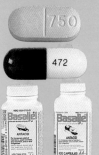

Antacid Tablets and Capsules

Basaljel®

Wyeth-Ayerst Laboratories
P. 851

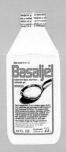

Suspension Antacid 12 Fl. oz.

Basaljel®

Wyeth-Ayerst Laboratories
P. 852

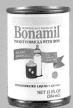

13 Fl. oz. Concentrated Liquid

Also available in Ready-to-Feed
Liquid and Powder

**Bonamil® Infant
Formula with Iron**

Wyeth-Ayerst Laboratories
P. 853

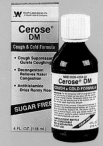

4 Fl. oz. Cough/Cold Formula
with Dextromethorphan
Also available in 1 pint bottles

Cerose® DM

Wyeth-Ayerst Laboratories
P. 853

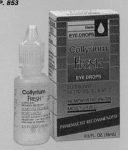

1/2 Fl. oz. (15 mL)
Eye drops with tetrahydrozoline HCl
plus glycerin

Collyrium Fresh™

Wyeth-Ayerst Laboratories
P. 853

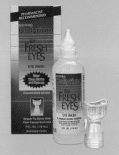

Eye Wash 4 Fl. oz. (118 mL)
with separate eyecup bottle cap

Collyrium for Fresh Eyes

Wyeth-Ayerst Laboratories
P. 854

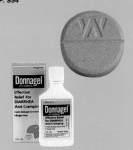

Available in bottles of 4 and 8 Fl. oz.
Chewable tablets
available in cartons of 18

Donnagel®

Wyeth-Ayerst Laboratories
P. 854

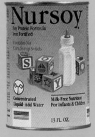

13 Fl. oz. Iron Fortified
Soy Protein Formula Concentrated Liquid
Also available in
Ready-to-Feed Liquid and Powder

Nursoy®

Wyeth-Ayerst Laboratories
P. 855

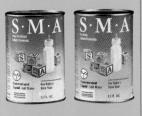

Iron Fortified Concentrated Liquid and
Lo-Iron Concentrated Liquid
Also available in Ready-to-Feed
Liquid and Powder

S·M·A·® Infant Formula

Wyeth-Ayerst Laboratories
P. 856

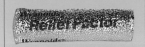

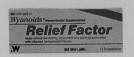

Box of 12 suppositories

Wyanoids® Relief Factor

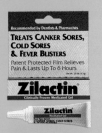
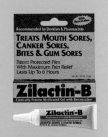
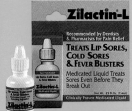
While every effort has
been made to reproduce
products faithfully, this
section is to be consid-
ered a Quick-Reference
Identification aid.

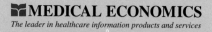

PRODUCT INFORMATION

This section provides information on medications, testing kits, and other medical products designed for home use by consumers. It is made possible through the courtesy of the manufacturers whose products appear on the following pages. The information concerning each product has been prepared, edited, and approved by the medical department, medical director, and/or medical counsel of each manufacturer.

The product descriptions in this section comply with labeling regulations. They are designed to provide all information necessary for informed use, including, when applicable, active ingredients, indications, actions, warnings, cautions, drug interactions, symptoms and treatment of oral overdosage, dosage and directions for use, professional labeling, and how supplied. In some cases, additional information has been supplied to complement the standard labeling.

In compiling this section, the publisher has emphasized the necessity of describing products comprehensively. The descriptions seen here include all information made available by the manufacturer. The publisher does not warrant or guarantee any product described here, and does not perform any independent analysis of the information provided. Inclusion of a product in this book does not represent an endorsement, and the publisher does not necessarily advocate the use of any product listed.

AkPharma Inc.
P.O. BOX 111
PLEASANTVILLE, NJ
08232-0111

Direct Inquiries To:
Elizabeth Wexler: (609) 645-5100
FAX: (609) 645-0767

Medical Emergency Contact:
Leonard P. Smith: (609) 645-5100

BEANO®

PRODUCT OVERVIEW

Key Facts: Beano® alpha-galactosidase enzyme hydrolyzes raffinose, verbascose and stachyose into the digestible sugars—sucrose, fructose, glucose and galactose. Beano drops are added to food and Beano tablets are swallowed, chewed, or crumbled onto food immediately prior to eating, for *in vivo* treatment of the food during digestion.

Major Uses: Helps stop gas before it starts. Beano® enzyme has been shown to be effective in both clinical and anecdotal studies with humans when consuming foods with high alpha-linked sugars content. Use of Beano results in substantially reduced breath hydrogen emissions and marked reduction or elimination of symptoms, compared with identical challenges without Beano.

Safety Information: Beano® enzyme should be discontinued in anyone who develops hypersensitivity to the enzyme.

PRODUCT INFORMATION

BEANO®

Description: Beano drops: each 5 drop dosage follows Food Chemical Codex (FCC) standards for activity and contains not less than 150 GalU (galactosidase units) of alpha-D-galactosidase derived from *Aspergillus niger* mold. The enzyme is in a liquid carrier of water and sorbitol. Add about 5 drops on the first bite of food serving, but remember a normal meal has 2–3 servings of the problem foods. Beano tablets: each tablet follows Food Chemical Codex (FCC) standards for activity and contains not less than 150 GalU (galactosidase units) of alpha-D-galactosidase derived from *Aspergillus niger* mold. The enzyme is in a carrier of corn starch, sorbitol, mannitol, and hydrogenated cottonseed oil. 2–3 tablets, swallowed, chewed, or crumbled onto food, should be enough for a normal meal of 2 or 3 servings of problem foods. Beano will hydrolyze complex sugars, raffinose, stachyose and verbascose, into the simple sugars—glucose, galactose and fructose, and the easily digestible disaccharide, sucrose. (Sucrose hydrolysis happens simultaneously with normal digestion.) In some cases, more enzyme than 5 drops or 3 tablets will be required, and this is a function of the quantity of food eaten, the levels of alpha-linked sugars in the food and the gas-producing propensity of the person.

Action: Hydrolysis converts raffinose, stachyose and verbascose into their monosaccharide components: glucose, galactose, fructose and sucrose. Raffinose yields sucrose + galactose; stachyose yields sucrose + galactose; verbascose yields glucose + fructose + galactose.

Indications: Flatulence and/or bloat as a result of eating a variety of grains, cereals, nuts, seeds, and vegetables containing the sugars raffinose, stachyose and/or verbascose. This includes all or most legumes and all or most cruciferous vegetables. Examples of such foods are oats, wheat, beans of all kinds, chickpeas, peas, lentils, peanuts, soy-content foods, broccoli, brussels sprouts, cabbage, carrots, corn, leeks, onions, parsnips, squash. Note: Most vegetables and beans also contain fiber, which is gas productive in some people, but usually far less so than the alpha-linked sugars. Beano® has no effect on fiber.

Usage: About 5 drops per food serving or 2–3 tablets per meal of 2 or 3 servings of problem foods; higher levels depending on symptoms.

How Supplied: Beano® is supplied in both a stable liquid form (12, 30 and 75-serving sizes, at 5 drops per serving), and a stable tablet form (12, 30, 60, 100 tablet sizes and 24 tablets in packets of 2).

Toxicity: None known

Adverse Reactions: None known; enzyme is derived from *Aspergillus niger*, a mold, and it is conceivable that mold-sensitive persons could react.

Drug Interactions: None known but because Beano is derived from a fermentation, it is advisable to avoid use with an MAO inhibitor. Beano® is classified as a dietary supplement, not a drug.

Precautions: Diabetics should be aware that the sugars in these vegetables will now be metabolically available and must be taken into account. No reports received of any diabetics' reactions. Galactosemics should not use without physician's advice, since one of the breakdown sugars is galactose.
For more information and samples, please write or call toll-free 1-800-257-8650.

Shown in Product Identification Guide, page 503

UNKNOWN DRUG?
Consult the
Product Identification Guide
(Gray Pages)
for full-color photos of
leading over-the-counter
medications

American Lifeline, Inc.
103 S. SECOND STREET
MADISON, WI 53704

Direct Inquiries to:
Dave Sullivan
1-800-257-5433

**FLORAjen® Acidophilus
Extra Strength
Non-Dairy Capsule form Refrigerated**

Ingredients: Active—Over ten (10) billion viable freeze dried *Lactobacillus acidophilus* cells per capsule. Equal to the *L. acidophilus* in six (6) cups of fresh yogurt. Potency guaranteed through expiration date on label.
Inactive—Rice maltodextrin gelatin capsule.

Directions: One capsule daily on an empty stomach with non-chlorinated water, fruit juice or preferably milk if not lactose intolerant. If taking antibiotics take FLORAjen 1–2 hours after antibiotic. While traveling, OK at room temperature for two weeks, otherwise must refrigerate.

How Supplied: 30 capsule bottle
60 capsule bottle

AML Laboratories
A Winning Combination Company
1753 CLOVERFIELD
BOULEVARD
SANTA MONICA, CA 90404

TELEPHONE INFO:

For Customer Service or For Additional Product Information Call Toll Free 1 (800) 800-1200

**Natural MD
BASIC Rx™
Multi-Vitamin Phytonutrient Formula**

Description: Natural MD BASIC Rx™ is a high potency selected nutrient multivitamin formula designed to meet the needs of those individuals seeking the maximum potencies of those vitamins and phytonutrient-containing botanicals cited by the scientific literature as potentially possessing a role in the possible reduction of certain degenerative diseases.

Ingredients: Calcium ascorbate, garlic concentrate, d-alpha tochopheryl succinate, citrus bioflavonoids, green tea extract, beta carotene, red wine concentrate, pyridoxine, selenomethionine, cyanocobalamin, folic acid.
CONTAINS NO ADDED INGREDIENTS.

Four capsules of **Natural MD BASIC Rx™** provide the following:

	Quantity	US RDA
Vitamin A		
Beta Carotene	20,000 IU	400%
Vitamine E	400 IU	1,333%
Vitamin C	1,000 mg	1,666%
Vitamin B6	40 mg	2,000%
Vitamin B12	100 mcg	1,666%
Folic Acid	400 mcg	100%
Selenium	100 mcg	*
Garlic Concentrate	600 mg	*
Citrus Bioflavonoids	200 mg	*
Green Tea Extract	160 mg	*
Red Wine Concentrate	80 mg	*

* No US RDA established

Suggested Use: As a dietary supplement, consume one or more capsules daily with a complete meal.

How Supplied: HDPE bottle containing 30, 90 or 180 capsules.

BREATH + PLUS™
Natural Breath Freshener

Description: Each small softgel capsule contains a concentrated, balanced blend of three powerful natural breath fresheners and antioxidant vitamins.

Actions: Bad breath (halitosis) is a condition generally treated by intensive oral hygiene; however, bad breath will not respond to oral hygiene treatment when the source of bad breath is the stomach or digestive system. BREATH+PLUS ™ is designed to work in the digestive system where oral hygiene has no impact. BREATH+PLUS™ is not a temporary "cover-up" like mouthwash and mints. It is a longlasting breath treatment that goes beyond brushing and flossing to neutralize unpleasant breath odors at their source—in the stomach. BREATH+PLUS™ is most effective against odors caused by spicy or pungent foods, such as garlic, onions and peppers. BREATH+PLUS™ has also been reported to be effective against tobacco, alcohol, morning breath and other odors stemming from the stomach and digestive tract. In addition to its natural breath freshening agents, BREATH+PLUS™ also contains the antioxidant nutrients Beta Carotene and Vitamin E.

Indications: For use with bad breath (halitosis) stemming from the stomach or digestive system. Effective against odors from spicy foods and can also be used immediately before bed or upon awakening for morning breath. Also reported to be effective against tobacco and alcohol odors emanating from the gastrointestinal tract.

Active Ingredients: Sunflower Oil, Parsley Seed Oil, Peppermint Oil, Chlorophyll, Vitamin E and Beta Carotene in a soft gelatin capsule.
CONTAINS NO ADDED INGREDIENTS.

Three capsules of **BREATH+PLUS™** contain the following vitamins:

	Quantity	US RDA
Vitamin A		
Beta Carotene	1,500 IU	30%
Vitamin E	15 IU	50%

Suggested Use: For odors stemming from food or beverages, SWALLOW (do not chew) 2 or 3 capsules with liquid immediately after eating. For morning breath, SWALLOW (do not chew) 2 or 3 capsules with liquid immediately before bed or upon awakening.

How Supplied: HDPE bottles of 200 softgels, or small 40-softgel dispensers, or single use 3-softgel packets.

COMPLETE FAMILY
High Antioxidant Stress Multi-Vitamin-Mineral Formulas

Description: There are five different COMPLETE™ Multi-Vitamin-Mineral formulas of varying potency and/or gender specificity. Each is a comprehensive multi-vitamin multi-mineral formula delivering over twenty essential vitamins and minerals with particular focus on providing high potencies of the antioxidant nutrients (Beta Carotene, Vitamin C and Vitamin E), as well as the B-Complex vitamins. The COMPLETE™ family of products conveniently and economically provides high levels of antioxidant protection previously only available by combining numerous separate supplement formulas.

Actions: The COMPLETE™ multivitamin multi-mineral product line is specially formulated to meet the widest range of requirements for a high potency anti-oxidant supplement while also providing a full complement of other essential vitamins, minerals, and cofactors. Antioxidants have become important because scientists and researchers now believe that antioxidant nutrients like Vitamin E, Vitamin C and Beta Carotene may neutralize the cellular damaging effects of free radicals (oxidizers). It is this potential ability of antioxidants to prevent cellular damage caused by free radicals that scientists and researchers believe may be associated with antioxidants' possible role in reducing the risk of certain degenerative diseases.

COMPLETE FOR MEN™
High Antioxidant Stress Multi-Vitamin-Mineral Formula

Description: COMPLETE FOR MEN™ is a high potency complete multi-vitamin multi-mineral formula specifically designed to meet the needs of active men and to insure optimum intake of twenty-five essential nutrients, particularly all of the antioxidant nutrients and the B-Complex vitamins. These key nutrients are provided at potencies far higher than conventional multi-vitamins in order to be consistent with the current research

and therefore offer the possibility of delivering their potential health benefits.

Ingredients: Calcium ascorbate, calcium aspartate, d-alpha tocopheryl succinate, magnesium oxide, calcium carbonate, beta carotene, ascorbyl palmitate, zinc aspartate, zinc histidine, inositol hexaniacinate, zinc glycinate, iron glycinate, calcium pantothenate, riboflavin, copper glycinate, thiamine, selenomethionine, pyridoxine, chromium polynicotinate, manganese glycinate, molybdenum glycinate, boron aspartate, cyanocobalamin, vanadium glycinate, cholecalciferol, folic acid, potassium iodide, phytonadione, biotin.
CONTAINS NO ADDED INGREDIENTS

Three capsules of **COMPLETE FOR MEN™** provide the following:

Vitamins	Quantity	US RDA
Vitamin A		
Beta Carotene	20,000 IU	400%
Vitamin D	400 IU	100%
Vitamin E	270 IU	900%
Vitamin K-1	80 mcg	*
Vitamin C	720 mg	1,200%
Vitamin B1	13.5 mg	900%
Vitamin B2	15.3 mg	900%
Vitamin B3	37 mg	185%
Vitamin B5	14 mg	140%
Vitamin B6	12 mg	600%
Vitain B12	19.5 mcg	325%
Folic Acid	400 mcg	100%
Biotin	60 mcg	20%

Minerals	Quantity	US RDA
Calcium	200 mg	20%
Magnesium	100 mg	25%
Iron	5 mg	27%
Zinc	30 mg	200%
Iodine	150 mcg	100%
Selenium	140 mcg	*
Chromium	100 mcg	*
Copper	1.5 mg	75%
Manganese	2 mg	*
Molybdenum	75 mcg	*
Vanadium	10 mcg	*
Boron	200 mcg	*

* No US RDA established

Suggested Use: As a dietary supplement, consume the contents of one packet with your first substantial meal of the day. SEE OWNERS MANUAL FOR MORE DETAILED INSTRUCTIONS.

How Supplied: HDPE bottle of 90 Perma-Fresh foil-mylar packets containing 3 capsules each for a total supply of 270 capsules. Also available as a 30-day supply.

COMPLETE FOR WOMEN™
High Anitoxidant Stress Multi-Vitamin-Mineral Formula

Description: COMPLETE FOR WOMEN™ is a high potency complete multi-vitamin multi-mineral formula

Continued on next page

AML Laboratories—Cont.

specifically designed to meet the needs of active women and to insure optimum intake of twenty-five essential nutrients, particularly all of the antioxidant nutrients and the B-Complex vitamins. These key nutrients are provided at potencies far higher than conventional multi-vitamins in order to be consistent with the current research and therefore offer the possibility of delivering their potential health benefits. COMPLETE FOR WOMEN™ also supplies significantly higher levels of Calcium than ordinary mass market multi-vitamins, including those designed specifically for women.

Ingredients: Calcium aspartate, calcium ascorbate, calcium carbonate, magnesium oxide, d-alpha tocopheryl succinate, beta carotene, ascorbyl palmitate, zinc aspartate, zinc histidine, inositol hexaniacinate, zinc glycinate, iron glycinate, calcium pantothenate, pyridoxine, riboflavin, boron aspartate, copper glycinate, thiamine, selenomethionine, chromium polynicotinate, manganese glycinate, molybdenum glycinate, cyanocobalamin, vanadium glycinate, cholecalciferol, folic acid, potassium iodide, phytonadione, biotin.

CONTAINS NO ADDED INGREDIENTS.

Five capsules of **COMPLETE FOR WOMEN™** provide the following:

Vitamins	Quantity	US RDA
Vitamin A		
Beta Carotene	20,000 IU	400%
Vitamin D	400 IU	100%
Vitamin E	270 IU	900%
Vitamin K-1	80 mcg	*
Vitamin C	720 mg	1,200%
Vitamin B1	13.5 mg	900%
Vitamin B2	15.3 mg	900%
Vitamin B3	37 mg	185%
Vitamin B5	20 mg	200%
Vitamin B6	14 mg	700%
Vitamin B12	19.5 mcg	325%
Folic Acid	400 mcg	100%
Biotin	60 mcg	20%

Minerals	Quantity	US RDA
Calcium	600 mg	60%
Magnesium	200 mg	50%
Iron	10 mg	55%
Zinc	30 mg	200%
Iodine	150 mcg	100%
Selenium	140 mcg	*
Chromium	100 mcg	*
Copper	1.5 mg	75%
Manganese	2 mg	*
Molybdenum	75 mcg	*
Vanadium	10 mcg	*
Boron	800 mcg	*

*No US RDA establised

Suggested Use: As a dietary supplement, consume the contents of one packet with your first substantial meal of the day. SEE OWNERS MANUAL FOR MORE DETAILED INSTRUCTIONS.

How Supplied: HDPE bottle of 90 Perma-Fresh foil-mylar packets containing 5 capsules each for a total supply of 450 capsules. Also available as a 30-day supply.

Common Sense™ COMPLETE™
High Antioxidant Stress Multi-Vitamin-Mineral Formula

Description: Common Sense™ COMPLETE™ is a high potency complete multi-vitamin-mineral formula specifically designed to deliver the precise amounts of antioxidant nutrients demanded by individuals choosing high antioxidant supplements. Specifically, it contains 400 I.U. of Vitamin E, 20,000 I.U. of Beta Carotene and 1,000 milligrams of Vitamin C, along with proportionately higher potencies of twenty other essential nutrients. Common Sense™ COMPLETE™ does not contain iron since many individuals choosing a high antioxidant regimen avoid supplementing additional iron.

Ingredients: Calcium ascorbate, d-alpha tocopheryl succinate, calcium carbonate, ascorbyl palmitate, magnesium oxide, beta carotene, zinc aspartate, zinc histidine, inositol hexaniacinate, iron glycinate, pyridoxine, calcium pantothenate, riboflavin, thiamine, copper glycinate, selenomethionine, manganese glycinate, molybdenum glycinate, boron aspartate, cyanocobalamin, chromium polynicotinate, vanadium glycinate, cholecalciferol, folic acid, potassium iodide, biotin.

CONTAINS NO ADDED INGREDIENTS.

Four capsules of **Common Sense™ COMPLETE™** provide the following:

Vitamins	Quantity	US RDA
Vitamin A		
Beta Carotene	20,000 IU	400%
Vitamin D	400 IU	100%
Vitamin E	400 IU	1,333%
Vitamin C	1,000 mg	1,666%
Vitamin B1	15 mg	1,000%
Vitamin B2	17 mg	1,000%
Vitamin B3	38 mg	190%
Vitamin B5	16 mg	160%
Vitamin B6	16 mg	800%
Vitamin B12	20 mcg	333%
Folic Acid	400 mcg	100%
Biotin	100 mcg	33%

Minerals	Quantity	US RDA
Calcium	350 mg	35%
Magnesium	100 mg	25%
Zinc	30 mg	200%
Iodine	150 mcg	100%
Selenium	150 mcg	*
Chromium	150 mcg	*
Copper	1.5 mg	75%
Manganese	2 mg	*
Molybdenum	75 mcg	*
Vanadium	10 mcg	*
Boron	200 mcg	*

*No US RDA established

Suggested Use: As a dietary supplement, consume the contents of one packet with your first substantial meal of the day. SEE OWNERS MANUAL FOR MORE DETAILED INSTRUCTIONS.

How Supplied: HDPE bottle of 90 Perma-Fresh foil-mylar packets containing 4 capsules each for a total supply of 360 capsules. Also available as 30-day supply.

Common Sense™ COMPLETE™
High Antioxidant Stress Multi-Vitamin-Mineral Formula with extra Calcium and Iron

Description: Identical to Common Sense™ COMPLETE™ above, plus extra Calcium (600 milligrams) and Iron (10 milligrams).

Ingredients: Calcium aspartate, calcium ascorbate, calcium carbonate, magnesium oxide, d-alpha tocopheryl succinate, beta carotene, ascorbyl palmitate, zinc aspartate, zinc histidine, inositol hexaniacinate, zinc glycinate, iron glycinate, calcium pantothenate, pyridoxine, riboflavin, boron aspartate, copper glycinate, thiamine, selenomethionine, chromium polynicotinate, manganese glycinate, molybdenum glycinate, cyanocobalamin, vanadium glycinate, cholecalciferol, folic acid, potassium iodine, phytonadione, biotin.

CONTAINS NO ADDED INGREDIENTS.

Five capsules of **Common Sense™ COMPLETE with extra Calcium and Iron™** provide the following:

Vitamins	Quantity	US RDA
Vitamin A		
Beta Carotene	20,000 IU	400%
Vitamin D	400 IU	100%
Vitamin E	400 IU	1,333%
Vitamin C	1,000 mg	1,667%
Vitamin B1	15 mg	1,000%
Vitamin B2	17 mg	1,000%
Vitamin B3	38 mg	190%
Vitamin B5	16 mg	160%
Vitamin B6	16 mg	800%
Vitamin B12	20 mcg	333%
Folic Acid	400 mcg	100%
Biotin	100 mcg	33%

Minerals	Quantity	US RDA
Calcium	600 mg	60%
Magnesium	100 mg	25%
Iron	10 mg	55%
Zinc	30 mg	200%
Iodine	150 mcg	100%
Selenium	150 mcg	*
Chromium	150 mcg	*
Copper	1.5 mg	75%
Manganese	2 mg	*
Molybdenum	75 mcg	*
Vanadium	10 mcg	*
Boron	200 mcg	*

* No US RDA established

Suggested Use: As a dietary supplement, consume the contents of one packet with your first substantial meal of the day. SEE OWNERS MANUAL FOR MORE DETAILED INSTRUCTIONS.

How Supplied: HDPE bottle of 90 Perma-Fresh foil mylar packets containing 5 capsules each for a total supply of 450 capsules. Also available as 30-day supply.

Natural MD™ COMPLETE Rx™
Ultra-High Potency Antioxidant Stress Multi-Vitamin-Mineral Phytonutrient Formula

Description: Natural MD™ COMPLETE Rx™ is an ultra-high potency complete multi-vitamin-mineral formula designed to meet the needs of those individuals seeking the maximum potencies of antioxidant nutrients, B-Complex vitamins, along with several important nutritional cofactors and phytonutrient-containing botanicals. Its contents are selected from those nutrients and ingredients cited by the scientifc literature as potentially possessing a role in the possible reduction of certain degenerative diseases.

Ingredients: Potassium-magnesium aspartate, magnesium ascorbate, potassium ascorbate, garlic concentrate, ascorbyl palmitate, d-alpha tocopheryl succinate, L-carnitine tartrate, calcium carbonate, citrus bioflavonoid complex, N-acetylcysteine, beta carotene, green tea extract, co-enzyme Q-10, zinc glycinate, pyridoxine, red wine concentrate, calcium pantothenate, cranberry extract, inositol hexaniacinate, grape seed extract, thiamine, riboflavin, mixed carotenoids, copper glycinate, magnesium oxide, selenomethionine, cyanocobalamin, magnesium niacinate, pyridoxyl-5'-phosphate, pyconogenol, pine bark extract, manganese glycinate, riboflavin-5'-phosphate, boron aspartate, chromium niacinate, folic acid, cholecalciferol, biotin.
CONTAINS NO ADDED INGREDIENTS.

Thirty capsules (3 packets) of **Natural MD™ COMPLETE Rx™** provide the following:

Vitamins	Quantity	US RDA
Vitamin A		
Total Carotenoids	75,000 IU	1,500%
Vitamin D	300 IU	75%
Vitamin E	1,200 IU	4,000%
Vitamin C	7,500 mg	12,500%
Vitamin B1	100 mg	6,750%
Vitamin B2	100 mg	6,000%
Vitamin B3	150 mg	750%
Vitamin B5	120 mg	1,200%
Vitamin B6	150 mg	7,500%
Vitamin B12	600 mcg	10,000%
Folic Acid	800 mcg	200%
Biotin	150 mcg	50%

Minerals	Quantity	US RDA
Potassium	750 mg	*
Magnesium	750 mg	187%
Calcium	300 mg	30%
Copper	9 mg	450%
Zinc	45 mg	300%
Manganese	3 mg	*
Selenium	300 mcg	*
Chromium	300 mcg	*
Boron	300 mcg	*

Co-Factors and Botanicals	Quantity
Co-Enzyme Q-10	180 mg*
L-Carnitine	600 mg*
N-Acetylcysteine	600 mg*
Garlic Concentrate	2,250 mg*
Citrus Bioflavonoids	600 mg*
Green Tea Extract	300 mg*
Red Wine Concentrate	150 mg*
Cranberry Extract	150 mg*
Grape Seed Extract	150 mg*
Pine Bark Extract	20 mg*
Pycnogenol®	20 mg*

*No US RDA established

Suggested Use: As a dietary supplement consume one, two or three packets daily as needed or as directed by a physician. A three packet per day regimen is intended to be taken one packet with each of three complete meals throughout the day. For best results, always consume with a substantial meal. SEE OWNERS MANUAL FOR MORE DETAILED INSTRUCTIONS.

How Supplied: HDPE bottle of 90 Perma-Fresh foil-mylar packets containing 10 capsules each for a total supply of 900 capsules.

FAT BURNING FACTORS™
Lipotropic and Fat Metabolizing Formula

Description: FAT BURNING FACTORS™ is a dietary supplement containing lipotropics and other nutrients essential for and/or related to fat metabolism and weight loss which is offered as part of the Fat Burning Factors Lean Lifestyle Program.

Actions: FAT BURNING FACTORS™ is specifically designed for those individuals engaging in a program of physical activity designed to achieve fat loss. FAT BURNING FACTORS™ is not a stand alone weight loss product, but a dietary supplement containing all the nutrients and co-factors established by research to be essential and/or related to fat metabolism which is a necessary condition for weight loss.

Ingredients: L-carnitine tartrate, calcium ascorbate, choline bitartrate, lysine, arginine, leucine, inositol, valine, isoleucince, pyridoxine, calcium pantothenate, inositol hexaniacinate, riboflavin, thiamine, cyanocobalamin, chromium polynicotinate, folic acid, biotin.
CONTAINS NO ADDED INGREDIENTS.

Two capsules of **FAT BURNING FACTORS™** provide the following:

Vitamins	Quantity	US RDA
L-Carnitine	200 mg	*
Vitamin C	200 mg	333%
Lysine	200 mg	*
Arginine	100 mg	*
Leucine	100 mg	*
Isoleucine	25 mg	*
Valine	50 mg	*
Chromium	200 mcg	*
Vitamin B1	7.5 mg	500%
Vitamin B2	8.5 mg	500%
Vitamin B3	19 mg	95%
Vitamin B5	20 mg	200%
Vitamin B6	20 mg	1,000%
Vitamin B12	40 mcg	666%
Folic Acid	200 mcg	50%
Biotin	30 mcg	10%
Choline Bitartrate	100 mg	*
Inositol	100 mg	*

*No US RDA established

Suggested Use: As a dietary supplement to be used in conjunction with a program of regular physical activity targeted for fat loss, consume a total of two capsules daily, preferably one each with the morning and evening meal. As many as six capsules daily can be consumed divided equally over the day's meals.

How Supplied: HDPE bottle containing 180 capsules, or 90 capsules.

Fruit and Vegetable SAFETY RINSE™
Fruit and Vegetable Cleansing Product

Description: Fruit And Vegetable SAFETY RINSE™ is a cleansing solution containing a natural blend of food grade surfactants, and emulsifiers to assist in the removal of water soluble and water insoluble topical residues such as pesticides, fungicides, herbicides, waxes and other substances from fruits, vegetables and edible produce.

Indications: Fruit And Vegetable SAFETY RINSE™ is specifically designed for those individuals who seek to remove topical residues such as pesticides, fungicides, herbicides, waxes and other substances from fruits, vegetables and edible produce. It can be used by those individuals who possess sensitivities to many of the chemicals employed in the agricultural industry, several of which can evoke mild to severe allergic reactions. It is also intended for those individuals who are concerned about the potential long-term health risks posed by exposure to these agricultural chemicals in our food supply.

Actions: The surface active agents (surfactants) and emulsifiers present in Fruit And Vegetable SAFETY RINSE™ help remove topical residues, particularly the more persistent water insoluble pesticide, fungicide and waxy residues

Continued on next page

AML Laboratories—Cont.

that do not respond to ordinary rinsing or cleansing from the surface of fruits, vegetables and edible produce.

Ingredients: Purified water and a blend of non-toxic, biodegradeable, 100% natural food grade surface active (surfactants), emulsifying and chelating agents.

Suggested Use: Soak and/or generously spray on the surface of fruits, vegetables, and edible produce. Scrub with brush or massage by hand and then rinse thoroughly with water. SEE OWNERS MANUAL FOR MORE DETAILED INSTRUCTIONS.

Warning: Individuals with severe sensitivities to topical agricultural residues should seek the approval of their physician before using this product.

How Supplied: Sixteen ounce HDPE sprayer bottle. Thirty-two ounce HDPE concentrate for refilling sprayer bottle and/or for use with produce bath.

STRESS GUM™
Complete Multivitamin Chewing Gum

Description: STRESS GUM™ is a natural mint-flavored chewing gum that freshens breath while also providing a healthy, nutrient-rich alternative to ordinary chewing gum. It is a convenient complete source of additional vitamins, particularly for those individuals who have difficulty swallowing ordinary vitamin pills or for those who do not consume a conventional multi-vitamin supplement. It contains all thirteen essential vitamins, plus two essential minerals. It supplies higher potencies of the antioxidant nutrients (Beta Carotene, Vitamin C and Vitamin E).

Actions: STRESS GUM™ is specially formulated to provide complete balanced multi-vitamin supplementation in a mint-flavored breath freshening gum. STRESS GUM™ contains higher levels of antioxidants because scientists and researchers now believe that antioxidant nutrients like Vitamin E, Vitamin C and Beta Carotene may neutralize the cellular damaging effects of free radicals (oxidizers). It is this potential ability of antioxidants to prevent cellular damage caused by free radicals that scientists believe may be associated with antioxidants' possible role in reducing the risk of certain degenerative diseases.

Ingredients: Pure natural gum base, natural spearmint flavor, natural sugars; fructose, sorbitol, and mannitol, calcium ascorbate, d-alpha tocopheryl acetate, beta carotene, niacinamide, calcium pantothenate, pyridoxine, riboflavin, thiamine, cyanocobalamin, cholecalciferol, chromium niacinate, folic acid, sodium selenate, biotin, phytonadione, **Does not contain the preservative BHT.**

CONTAINS NO ADDED INGREDIENTS.

Two pieces of **STRESS GUM™** supply the following:

	Quantity	US RDA
Vitamin A		
Beta Carotene	1,667 IU	33%
Vitamin D	20 IU	5%
Vitamin E	30 IU	100%
Vitamin K-1	8 mcg	*
Vitamin C	60 mg	100%
Vitamin B1	500 mcg	33%
Vitamin B2	566 mcg	33%
Vitamin B3	6.6 mg	33%
Vitamin B5	1.3 mg	13%
Vitamin B6	666 mcg	33%
Vitamin B12	2 mcg	33%
Folic Acid	40 mcg	10%
Biotin	10 mcg	3%
Selenium	5 mcg	*
Chromium	5 mcg	*

*No US RDA established

Suggested Use: Chew STRESS GUM™ anytime throughout the day, particularly following meals. Do not exceed 20 pieces per day.

How Supplied: HDPE bottle containing 150 pieces of gum.

B.F. Ascher & Company, Inc.
15501 WEST 109th STREET
LENEXA, KS 66219
Mailing address:
P.O. BOX 717
SHAWNEE MISSION, KS
66201-0717

Direct Inquiries to:
Joan F. Bowen
(913) 888-1880

AYR® Saline Nasal Mist, Drops, and Gel
[ār]

AYR Mist, Drops or Gel restores vital moisture to provide prompt relief for dry, crusted and inflamed nasal membranes due to chronic sinusitis, colds, low humidity, overuse of nasal decongestant drops and sprays, allergies, minor nose bleeds and other minor nasal irritations. AYR provides a soothing way to thin thick secretions and aid their removal from the nose and sinuses. AYR can be used as often as needed without the side effects associated with overuse of decongestant nose drops and sprays.

SAFE AND GENTLE ENOUGH FOR CHILDREN AND INFANTS

AYR Drops are particularly convenient for easy application with infants and children. AYR is formulated to prevent stinging, burning and irritation of delicate nasal tissue, even that of babies.

Directions For Use: SPRAY—Squeeze twice in each nostril as often as needed. Hold bottle upright. To spray, give the bottle short, firm squeezes. Take care not

to aspirate nasal contents back into bottle. DROPS—Two to four drops in each nostril every two hours as needed, or as directed by your physician. GEL—Apply around nostrils and under nose. AYR Gel may be placed in nostrils to help relieve discomfort. Use at bedtime to prevent drying and crusting. Use as often as needed.

AYR is a specially formulated, buffered, isotonic saline solution containing sodium chloride 0.65% adjusted to the proper tonicity and pH with monobasic potassium phosphate/sodium hydroxide buffer to prevent nasal irritation. AYR also contains the non-irritating antibacterial and antifungal preservatives thimerosal and benzalkonium chloride and is formulated with deionized water.

How Supplied: AYR Mist in 50 ml spray bottles, AYR Drops in 50 ml dropper bottles, AYR Gel in 0.5 oz tube.
Shown in Product Identification Guide, page 503

COUGH-X®

Active Ingredients: Each lozenge contains dextromethorphan hydrobromide 5 mg and benzocaine 2 mg. Also contains: Corn syrup, eucalyptus oil, menthol, propylene glycol and sucrose.

Indications: Temporarily suppresses cough due to minor throat and bronchial irritants. Also, for the temporary relief of occasional minor irritation and sore throat.

Warnings: A persistent cough may be a sign of a serious condition. If cough persists for more than 1 week, tends to recur or if sore throat is severe, persists for more than 2 days or if cough and/or sore throat is accompanied or followed by fever, persistent headache, rash, swelling, nausea or vomiting, consult a physician. Do not take this product for persistent or chronic cough such as occurs with smoking, asthma, emphysema or if cough is accompanied by excessive phlegm (mucus) unless directed by a physician. Do not exceed recommended dosage. Do not use this product if you have a history of allergy to local anesthetics such as procaine, butacaine, benzocaine or other "caine" anesthetics. As with any drug, if you are pregnant or nursing a baby, seek the advice of a health professional before using this product. KEEP THIS AND ALL DRUGS OUT OF REACH OF CHILDREN. In case of accidental overdose, seek professional assistance or contact a Poison Control Center immediately.

Drug Interaction Precaution: Do not use this product if you are now taking a prescription monoamine oxidase inhibitor (MAOI) (certain drugs for depression, psychiatric or emotional conditions, or Parkinson's disease), or for 2 weeks after stopping the MAOI drug. If you are uncertain whether your prescription drug contains an MAOI, consult a health professional before taking this product.

Directions: Allow lozenge to dissolve slowly in the mouth. Adults and children 6 years of age and older: One lozenge every 2 hours as needed not to exceed 12 lozenges in 24 hours or as directed by a physician. Children 2 to 6 years of age: One lozenge every 4 hours not to exceed 6 lozenges in 24 hours or as directed by a physician. Children under 2 years of age: Consult a physician.

How Supplied: Available in pleasant-tasting menthol eucalyptus flavor. 9 individually-wrapped lozenges come packaged in a carton.
Shown in Product Identification Guide, page 503

ITCH–X® Gel & Spray
Dual-acting, itch-relieving gel and spray with aloe vera

Active Ingredients: Benzyl alcohol 10% and pramoxine HCl 1%.

Inactive Ingredients: Gel: aloe vera gel, carbomer 934, diaolidinyl urea, FD&C blue #1, methylparaben, propylene glycol, propylparaben, SD alcohol 40, styrene/acrylate copolymer, triethanolamine, and water.
Spray: Aloe vera gel, SD alcohol 40 and water.

Indications: For the temporary relief of pain and itching associated with minor skin irritations, allergic itches, rashes, hives, minor burns, insect bites, poison ivy, poison oak, and poison sumac.

Warnings: For external use only. Avoid contact with the eyes. Do not apply to open wounds or damaged skin. If condition worsens, or if symptoms persist for more than 7 days or clear up and occur again within a few days, discontinue use of this product and consult a physician. KEEP THIS AND ALL DRUGS OUT OF THE REACH OF CHILDREN. In case of accidental ingestion, seek professional assistance or contact a Poison Control Center immediately.
Additional Warning for Spray: Flammable, keep away from fire or flame.

Directions: Adults and children 2 years of age and older: Apply to affected area not more than 3 to 4 times daily. Children under 2 years of age: consult a physician.

How Supplied: Gel: 35.4g (1.25 oz) tube
Spray: 59.1 mL (2 fl oz) pump spray bottle.
Shown in Product Identification Guide, page 503

MOBIGESIC® Tablets
[mō′bĭ-jē′zĭk]
Pain reliever–Fever reducer

Indications: For the temporary relief of minor aches and pains associated with headache, muscular aches, backache, toothache, colds, premenstrual and menstrual cramps and for the minor pain from arthritis, and to reduce fever.

Directions: Adults and children 12 years of age and older: Oral dosage is 1 or 2 tablets every 4 hours while symptoms persist, not to exceed 10 tablets in 24 hours. Drink a full glass of water with each dose. Children 6 to under 12 years of age: Oral dosage is 1 tablet every 4 hours while symptoms persist, not to exceed 5 tablets in 24 hours. Drink water with each dose. Children under 6 years of age: Consult a physician.

Warnings: Do not take this product for pain for more than 10 days (5 days for children 6 to under 12 years of age) or for fever for more than 3 days unless directed by a physician. If pain or fever persists or gets worse, if new symptoms occur, or if redness or swelling is present, consult a physician because these could be signs of a serious condition. Children and teenagers who have or are recovering from chicken pox, flu symptoms or flu should NOT use this product. If nausea, vomiting or fever occur, consult a physician because these sysmptoms could be an early sigm of Reye syndrome, a rare but serious illness. If ringing in the ears or a loss of hearing occurs, consult a physician before taking any more of this product. Do not take this product if you have stomach problems (such as hearburn, upset stomach or stomach pain) that persist or recur, or if you have ulcers or bleeding problems, unless directed by a physician.

Drug Interaction Precaution: Do not take this product if you are taking a prescription drug for anticoagulation (thinning of the blood), diabetes, gout or arthritis unless directed by a physician. Do not take this product if you are allergic to salicylates (including aspirin) unless directed by a physician. May cause excitability especially in children. Do not take this product, unless directed by a physician, if you have a breathing problem such as emphysema or chronic bronchitis, or if you have glaucoma or difficulty in urination due to enlargement of the prostate gland. May cause drowsiness; alcohol, sedatives and tranquilizers may increase the drowsiness effect. Avoid alcoholic beverages while taking this product. Do not take this product if you are taking sedatives or tranquilizers, without first consulting your physician. Use caution when driving a motor vehicle or operating machinery. KEEP THIS AND ALL DRUGS OUT OF THE REACH OF CHILDREN. In case of accidental overdose, seek professional assistance or contact a Poison Control Center immediately. As with any drug, if you are pregnant or nursing a baby, seek the advice of a health professional before using this product.

Active Ingredients: Each tablet contains magnesium salicylate 325 mg and phenyltonaloxamine citrate 30 mg. Also contains: Micro crystalline cellulose, magnesium stearate and colloidal silicon dioxide.

How Supplied: Packages of 18's; bottles of 50's and 100's.
Shown in Product Identification Guide, page 503

MOBISYL® Analgesic Creme
[mō′bǐ-sǐl]
Penetrates to the site of pain to bring relief.

Active Ingredient: Trolamine salicylate 10%. Also Contains: Allantoin, aloe vera gel, carbomer, cetyl alcohol, diazolidinyl urea, glycerin, glyceryl stearate, isopropyl palmitate, lecithin, methylparaben, mineral oil, propylene glycol, propylparaben, stearic acid, sweet almond oil, tetrasodium EDTA, triethanolamine and water.

Description: MOBISYL is a greaseless, odorless, penetrating, non-burning, non-irritating analgesic creme.

Indications: For adults and children, 12 years of age and older, MOBISYL is indicated for the temporary relief of minor aches and pains of muscles and joints, such as simple backache, lumbago, arthritis, neuralgia, strains, bruises and sprains.

Actions: MOBISYL penetrates fast into sore, tender joints and muscles where pain originates. It works to reduce inflammation. Helps soothe stiff joints and muscles and gets you going again.

Warnings: For external use only. Avoid contact with the eyes. If condition worsens, or if symptoms persist for more than 7 days or clear up and occur again within a few days, discontinue use of this product and consult a physician. Do not use on children under 12 years of age except under the advice and supervision of a physician. In case of accidental ingestion, seek professional assistance or contact a Poison Control Center immediately. Store at room temperature (59–86°F). Close cap tightly. KEEP THIS AND ALL DRUGS OUT OF THE REACH OF CHILDREN.

Dosage and Administration: Place a liberal amount of MOBISYL Creme in your palm and massage into the area of pain and soreness three or four times a day, especially before retiring. MOBISYL may be worn under clothing or bandages.

How Supplied: MOBISYL is available in 35.4g (1.25 oz) tubes, 100g (3.5 oz) tubes, 226.8g (8 oz) jars.
Shown in Product Identification Guide, page 503

IF YOU SUSPECT AN INTERACTION...
The 1,500-page
PDR Guide to Drug Interactions •
Side Effects • *Indications*
can help.
Use the order form
in the front of this book.

Astra USA, Inc.
50 OTIS ST.
WESTBOROUGH, MA
01581-4500

Direct Inquiries to:
Professional Information Department:
(508) 366-1100
FAX: (508) 366-7406

For Medical Emergencies Contact:
Medical Information Services
(800) 262-0460

XYLOCAINE® 2.5% Ointment (lidocaine)

For temporary relief of pain and itching due to minor burns, sunburn, minor cuts, abrasions, insect bites and minor skin irritations.
Xylocaine® 2.5% Ointment should be applied liberally over the affected areas. Use enough to provide temporary relief and reapply Xylocaine 2.5% Ointment as needed for continued relief.

Warning: Use only as directed by a physician in persistent, severe or extensive skin disorders. In case of accidental ingestion, seek professional assistance or contact a poison control center immediately.
KEEP OUT OF REACH OF CHILDREN.
FOR EXTERNAL USE ONLY.
Xylocaine 2.5% Ointment is non-staining and is easily removed with water from skin or clothing.
Xylocaine 2.5% Ointment belongs in your home medicine chest and first aid kit.

Caution: Do not use in the eyes. Not for prolonged use. If the condition for which this preparation is used persists, or if a rash or irritation develops, discontinue use and consult a physician.

How Supplied: 1.25 ounce tubes containing 2.5% lidocaine base in water soluble carbowaxes.
ASTRA®
Astra USA, Inc.   021658R01
Westborough, MA 01581   11/93
Shown in Product Identification Guide, page 503

UNKNOWN DRUG?
Consult the
Product Identification Guide
(Gray Pages)
for full-color photos of
leading over-the-counter
medications

Ayerst Laboratories
Division of American Home
Products Corporation
685 THIRD AVE.
NEW YORK, NY 10017-4071

For information for Ayerst's consumer products, see product listings under Whitehall Laboratories.
Please turn to Whitehall Laboratories, page 836.

Bausch & Lomb Incorporated
Personal Products Division
ROCHESTER, NY 14692-0450

Direct Inquiries to:
Ronald M. Kline: (716) 338-5775
FAX: (716) 338-0184

For Medical Emergency Contact:
Consumer Affairs: (800) 572-2931

CUREL® Therapeutic Moisturizing Lotion and Cream

Indications: For control of dry skin symptoms, Curél delivers extra effective moisturization that with regular use, ends dry skin for most people.

Actions: Curél's unique cationic emulsion base enables it to be faster absorbing and more substantive to dry skin, all without a greasy after-feel. Curél is rich in humectant and occlusive ingredients, which help skin retain natural moisture and help heal dry skin problems like chapping, soreness, cracking, and erythema. Clinical skin hydration studies have shown that Curél moisturizes better than other leading therapeutic lotions, giving extra effective moisturization for softer, healthier skin.
Dermatologist tested and recommended, Curél contains no mineral oil or lanolin and all ingredients are non-comedogenic. Available in lightly fragranced original lotion, fragrance free lotion, fragrance free cream and alpha hydroxy fragrance free lotion.

Contents: Original Formula: Deionized Water, Glycerin, Distearyldimonium Chloride, Petrolatum, Isopropyl Palmitate, 1-Hexadecanol, Dimethicone, Sodium Chloride, Fragrance, Methyl Paraben, Propyl Paraben.
Fragrance Free: Deionized Water, Glycerin, Distearyldimonium Chloride, Petrolatum, Isopropyl Palmitate, 1-Hexadecanol, Dimethicone, Sodium Chloride, Methyl Paraben, Propyl Paraben.
Alpha Hydroxy: Deionized Water, Glycerin, Distearyldimonium Chloride, Petrolatum, Lactic Acid, Isopropyl Palmitate, 1-Hexadecanol, Glycolic Acid, Dimethicone, Ammonium Hydroxide, Methyl Paraben, Propyl Paraben.
Directions for Use: All products except Alpha Hydroxy lotion: Apply as

often as needed. Especially effective when applied after bathing while skin is still damp. For external use only.
Alpha Hydroxy lotion: For best results, apply to skin twice a day. For external use only.

How Supplied: Original Formula:
Lotion— 2.5 oz., 6 oz. and 10 oz. fliptop bottles
13 oz. pump bottle
Fragrance Free:
Cream— 4 oz. tube:
Lotion— 2.5 oz., 6 oz. and 10 oz. fliptop bottle
13 oz. pump bottle
Alpha Hydroxy—3.5 oz. bottle
7 oz. pump bottle
For Toll-Free Product Information: Call 1-800-572-2931
Shown in Product Identification Guide, page 503

Bayer Corporation Consumer Care Division
36 Columbia Road
Morristown, NJ 07960-4518

Direct Inquiries to:
Consumer Affairs
(800) 331-4536

For Medical Emergency Contact:
Bayer Corporation
Consumer Care Division
(800) 331-4536

ACTRON™
Ketoprofen Tablets and Caplets, 12.5 mg

Active Ingredient: Each tablet or caplet contains 12.5 mg Ketoprofen.

Inactive Ingredients: Corn Starch, Croscarmellose Sodium, Hydroxypropyl Methylcellulose, Lactose, Magnesium Stearate, Microcrystalline Cellulose, Polyethylene Gylcol, Titanium Dioxide.

Directions: Take with a full glass of water or other fluid. ADULTS: Take 1 tablet or caplet every 4–6 hours. If pain or fever does not get better in 1 hour, you may take 1 more tablet or caplet. With experience, some people may find they need 2 tablets or caplets for the first dose. The smallest effective dose should be used.
Do not take more than: 2 tablets or caplets in any 4–6 hour period.
6 tablets or caplets in any 24 hour period.
Children: Do not give to children under age 16 unless directed by a doctor.

Indications: For the temporary relief of minor aches and pains associated with: common cold, headache, toothache, muscular aches, backache, minor arthritis, menstrual cramps. For the temporary reduction of fever.

WARNINGS: Do not take this product if you have asthma, hives or any other allergic reaction after taking any pain reliever/fever reducer. Ketoprofen could cause similar reactions. As with any drug, if you are pregnant or nursing a baby, seek the advise of a health professional before using this product. **IT IS ESPECIALLY IMPORTANT NOT TO USE KETOPROFEN DURING THE LAST 3 MONTHS OF PREGNANCY UNLESS SPECIFICALLY DIRECTED TO DO SO BY A DOCTOR BECAUSE IT MAY CAUSE PROBLEMS IN THE UNBORN CHILD OR COMPLICATIONS DURING DELIVERY.** If you generally consume 3 or more alcohol-containing drinks per day you should talk to your doctor for advise on when and how you should take Actron or other pain relievers.

DO NOT USE: With any other pain reliever/fever reducer, with any other product containing ketoprofen, for more than 3 days for fever, for more than 10 days for pain.

ASK A DOCTOR BEFORE USE IF: The painful area is red or swollen, you take other drugs on a regular basis, you are under a doctor's care for any continuing medical condition, you have had problems or side effects with any pain reliever/fever reducer.

ASK A DOCTOR AFTER USE IF: Symptoms continue or worsen, new or unexpected symptoms occur, stomach pain occurs with use of this product. Keep this and all drugs out of the reach of children. In case of accidental overdose, seek professional assistance or contact a Poison Control Center immediately.

How Supplied: Tablets and caplets in bottles of 24's, 50's and 100's.
Shown in Product Identification Guide, page 503

ALKA–MINTS® Chewable Antacid Rich in Calcium

Active Ingredient: Each ALKA-MINTS Chewable Antacid tablet contains calcium carbonate 850 mg (340 mg of elemental calcium). Each tablet contains less than .5 mg sodium per tablet, and is dietarily sodium free.

Inactive Ingredients: Dioctyl sodium sulfosuccinate, flavor, hydrolyzed cereal solids, magnesium stearate, polyethylene glycol, sorbitol, sugar (compressible).

Indications: ALKA-MINTS is an antacid for occasional use for relief of acid indigestion, heartburn and sour stomach.

Actions: ALKA-MINTS has a natural, clean, spearmint taste that leaves the mouth feeling refreshed. Measured by the in-vitro standard established by the Food and Drug Administration, one ALKA-MINTS tablet neutralizes 15.9 mEq of acid.

Warnings: Do not take more than 9 tablets in a 24 hour period, or use the maximum dosage of this product for more than 2 weeks, except under the advice and supervision of a physician. May

cause constipation. As with any drug, if you are pregnant or nursing a baby, seek the advice of a health professional before using this product. Keep this and all drugs out of the reach of children.

Drug Interaction Precaution: Antacids may interact with certain prescription drugs. If you are presently taking a prescription drug, do not take this product without checking with your doctor or other health professional.

Dosage and Administration: Chew 1 or 2 tablets every 2 hours or as directed by a physician.

How Supplied: Bottles of 75's and 150's.

Product Identification Mark: ALKA-MINTS embossed on each tablet.
Shown in Product Identification Guide, page 503

ALKA-SELTZER® Original
ALKA-SELTZER® Extra Strength
ALKA-SELTZER® Lemon Lime
ALKA-SELTZER® Cherry
Effervescent Antacid Pain Reliever

Active ingredients:
ALKA-SELTZER® Original:
Aspirin 325 mg, Heat Treated Sodium Bicarbonate 1916 mg, Citric acid 1000 mg.
ALKA-SELTZER® Extra Strength:
Aspirin 500 mg, Heat Treated Sodium Bicarbonate 1985 mg, Citric acid 1000 mg.
ALKA-SELTZER® Lemon Lime and Cherry:
Aspirin 325 mg, Heat Treated Sodium Bicarbonate 1700 mg, Citric acid 1000 mg.

Inactive Ingredients:
ALKA-SELTZER® Original:
none.
ALKA-SELTZER® Extra Strength:
Flavor:
ALKA-SELTZER® Lemon Lime:
Aspartame, Dimethyl Poly Siloxane Powder, Docusate Sodium, Flavor, Povidine, Sodium Benzoate.
Phenylketonurics: Contains Phenylalanine 9 mg per tablet.
ALKA-SELTZER Cherry:
Aspartame, Dimethyl Poly Siloxane Powder, Docusate Sodium, Flavor, Povidone, Sodium Benzoate.
Phenylketonurics: Contains Phenylalanine 12.3 mg per tablet.

Indications: For fast relief of heartburn, acid indigestion, sour stomach with headache, or body aches and pain. Also for fast relief of upset stomach with headache from overindulgence in food and drink—especially recommended for taking before bed and again on arising. Effective for pain relief alone: headache, or body and muscular aches and pains.

Directions:
Alka-Seltzer® Original, Cherry and Lemon Lime.
Alka-Seltzer must be dissolved in water before taking. Adults: Dissolve 2 tablets

in 4 oz. of water every 4 hours not to exceed 8 tablets in 24 hours. (60 years or older, 4 tablets in a 24-hour period).
Alka-Seltzer® Extra Strength.
Adults: Dissolve 2 tablets in 4 oz. of water every 6 hours not to exceed 7 tablets in 24 hours. (60 years or older, 4 tablets in a 24-hour period).
Caution: If symptoms persist or recur frequently, or if you are under treatment for ulcer, consult your doctor.

Warnings: Children and teenagers should not use this medicine for chicken pox or flu symptoms before a doctor is consulted about Reye syndrome, a rare but serious illness reported to be associated with aspirin. As with any drug, if you are pregnant or nursing a baby, seek the advice of a health professional before using this product. IT IS ESPECIALLY IMPORTANT NOT TO USE ASPIRIN DURING THE LAST 3 MONTHS OF PREGNANCY UNLESS SPECIFICALLY DIRECTED TO DO SO BY A DOCTOR BECAUSE IT MAY CAUSE PROBLEMS IN THE UNBORN CHILD OR COMPLICATIONS DURING DELIVERY.
Except under the advice and supervision of a doctor. Do not take more than, ADULTS: 8 tablets in a 24-hour period, (60 years of age or older: 4 tablets in a 24-hour period), or use the daily maximum dosage for more than 10 days. Do not take this product if you are allergic to aspirin or have asthma, if you have bleeding problems, or if you are on a sodium restricted diet.
If ringing in the ears or a loss of hearing occurs, consult a doctor before taking any more of this product.
Do not take this product for pain for more than 10 days unless directed by a doctor. If pain persists or gets worse, if new symptoms occur, or if redness or swelling is present, consult a doctor because these could be signs of a serious condition.
Keep this and all drugs out of the reach of children.

Drug Interaction Precaution: Do not take this product if you are taking a prescription drug for anticoagulation (thinning the blood), diabetes, gout, or arthritis unless directed by a doctor. Antacids any interact with certain prescription drugs. If you are presently taking a prescription drug, do not take this product without checking with your doctor or other health professional.

Sodium Content per tablet:
Alka-Seltzer® Original: 567 mg
Alka-Seltzer® Extra Strength: 588 mg
Alka-Seltzer® Lemon Lime: 506 mg.
Alka-Seltzer® Cherry: 503 mg

Professional Labeling:
ASPIRIN FOR MYOCARDIAL INFARCTION

Indications: The Aspirin contained in Alka-Seltzer is indicated to reduce the

Continued on next page

Bayer—Cont.

risk of death and/or non-fatal myocardial infarction in patients

Clinical Trials: The indication is supported by the results of six, large randomized multicenter, placebo-controlled studies [1-7] involving 10,816, predominantly male, post-myocardial infarction (MI) patients and one randomized placebo-controlled study of 1,266 men with unstable angina. Therapy with aspirin was begun at intervals after the onset of acute MI varying from less than 3 days to more than 5 years and continued for periods of from less than one year to four years. In the unstable angina study, treatment was started within 1 month after the onset of unstable angina and continued for 12 weeks and complicating conditions such as congestive heart failure were not included in the study.

Aspirin therapy in MI patients was associated with about a 20 percent reduction in the risk of subsequent death and/or nonfatal reinfarction, a median absolute decrease of 3 percent from the 12 to 22 percent event rates in the placebo groups. In aspirin-treated unstable angina patients the reduction in risk was about 50 percent, a reduction in event rate of 5 percent from the 10 percent rate in the placebo group over the 12 weeks of study.

Daily dosage of aspirin in the post-myocardial infarction studies was 300 mg in one study and 900 to 1500 mg in five studies. A dose of 325 mg was used in the study of unstable angina.

Adverse Reactions: Gastrointestinal Reactions: Symptoms and signs of gastrointestinal irritation were not significantly increased in subjects treated for unstable angina with buffered aspirin in solution (ALKA-SELTZER®). Doses of 1000 mg per day of aspirin tablets caused gastrointestinal symptoms and bleeding that in some cases were clinically significant. In the largest post-infarction study (the Aspirin Myocardial Infarction Study (AMIS) with 4,500 people), the percentage incidences of gastrointestinal symptoms for the aspirin (1000 mg of a standard, solid-tablet formulation) and placebo-treated subjects, respectively, were: stomach pain (14.5%; 4.4%); heartburn (11.9%; 4.8%); nausea and/or vomiting (7.6%; 2.1%); hospitalization for gastrointestinal disorder (4.9%; 3.5%). In the AMIS and other trials, aspirin treated patients had increased rates of gross gastrointestinal bleeding. As with all aspirin products Alka-Seltzer is contra-indicated in patients with aspirin sensitivity, with asthma, or with coagulation disease.

Cardiovascular and Biochemical: In the AMIS trial, the dosage of 1000 mg per day of aspirin was associated with small increases in systolic blood pressure (BP) (average 1.5 to 2.1 mm) and diastolic BP (0.5 to 0.6 mm), depending upon whether maximal or last available readings were used. Blood urea nitrogen and uric acid levels were also increased, but by less than 1.0 mg%. Subjects with marked hypertension or renal insufficiency had been excluded from the trial so that the clinical importance of these observations for such subjects or for any subjects treated over more prolonged periods is not known. It is recommended that patients placed on long-term aspirin treatment, even at doses of 300 mg per day, be seen at regular intervals to assess changes in these measurements.

Sodium in Buffered Aspirin for Solution Formulations: One tablet daily of flavored buffered aspirin in solution adds 506 mg of sodium to that in the diet and may not be tolerated by patients with active sodium-retaining states such as congestive heart or renal failure. This amount of sodium adds about 30 percent to the 70 to 90 meq intake suggested as appropriate for dietary treatment of essential hypertension in the 1984 Report of the Joint National Committee on Detection, Evaluation, and Treatment of High Blood Pressure[8].

Dosage and Administration: Although most of the studies used dosages exceeding 300 mg, daily, two trials used only 300 mg and pharmacologic data indicate that this dose inhibits platelet function fully. Therefore, 300 mg or a conventional 325 mg aspirin dose daily is a reasonable, routine dose that would minimize gastrointestinal adverse reactions. This use of aspirin applies to both solid, oral dosage forms (buffered and plain aspirin) and buffered aspirin in solution.

References:
(1) Elwood, P.C., et al., A Randomized Controlled Trial of Acetysalicylic Acid in the Secondary Prevention of Mortality from Myocardial Infarction," *British Medical Journal* 1:436–440, 1974.
(2) The Coronary Drug Project Research Group, "Aspirin in Coronary Heart Disease," *Journal of Chronic Disease*, 29:625–642, 1976.
(3) Breddin K., et al,. "Secondary Prevention of Myocardial Infarction: A Comparison of Acetylsalicylic Acid, Phenprocoumon or Placebo," *International Congress Series* 470:263–268, 1979.
(4) Aspirin Myocardial Infarction Study Research Group, "A Randomized, Controlled Trial of Aspirin in Persons Recovered from Myocardial Infarction," *Journal American Medical Association* 245:661–669, 1980.
(5) Elwood, P.C., and P.M. Sweetnam, "Aspirin and Secondary Mortality after Myocardial Infarction," *Lancet* pp. 1313–1315, December 22–29, 1979.
(6) The Persantine-Aspirin Reinfarction Study Research Group, "Persantine and Aspirin in Coronary Heart Disease," *Circulation*, 62:449–460, 1980.
(7) Lewis, II. D., et al., "Protective Effects of Aspirin Against Acute Myocardial Infarction and Death in Men with Unstable Angina, Results of a Veterans Administration Cooperative Study," *New England Journal of Medicine* 309: 396–403, 1983.
(8) "1984 Report of the Joint National Committee on Detection, Evaluation, Treatment of High Blood Pressure," U.S. Department of Health and Human Services and United States Public Health Service, National Institutes of Health.

How Supplied: Foil sealed effervescent tablets in cartons of 12's in 6 foil twin pacts; 24's in 12 foil twin packs; 36's in 18 foil twin packs.

Shown in Product Identification Guide, page 503

ALKA-SELTZER®
Fast Relief Caplets

New ALKA-SELTZER CAPLETS provide fast, effective relief in convenient, easy to swallow caplets.

Indications: For the temporary relief of headache, minor aches and pains accompanied by heartburn, sour stomach, acid indigestion and upset stomach associated with these symptoms.

Directions For Use: Adults: 2 caplets every 6 hours. No more than a total of 8 caplets in any 24-hour period or as directed by a doctor.
Children (under 12): consult a doctor.

Warnings: Keep this and all other medications out of the reach of children. In case of accidental overdose, seek professional assistance or contact a Poison Control Center immediately. Prompt medical attention is critical for adults as well as for children even if you do not notice any signs or symptoms. As with any drug, if you are pregnant or nursing a baby, seek the advice of a health professional before using this product. Do not take more than 8 caplets in a 24-hour period or use the maximum dosage for more than 2 weeks except under the advice and supervision of a physician. Do not take this product for pain for more than 10 days unless directed by a doctor. If pain persists or gets worse, if new symptoms occur, or if redness or swelling is present, consult a doctor because these could be signs of a serious condition. May cause constipation.

Drug Interaction Precaution: Antacids may interact with certain prescription drugs. If you are presently taking a prescription drug, do not take this product without checking with your doctor or other health professional.

Active Ingredients: Each caplet contains: Acetaminophen 500 mg, Calcium Carbonate 380 mg.

Inactive Ingredient: Crospovidone, Docusate Sodium, Hydroxypropyl Methylcellulose, Lecithin, Magnesium Stearate, Polyvinylpyrrolidone, Sodium Benzoate, Sodium Hexamethaphosphate, Sodium Starch Glycolate, Starch, Stearic Acid.

How Supplied: ALKA-SELTZER® Fast Relief Caplets are available in 24 count blisters and 50 count bottles.

Shown in Product Identification Guide, page 503

ALKA–SELTZER® GOLD
Effervescent Antacid

Active Ingredients: Each tablet contains heat treated sodium bicarbonate 958 mg, citric acid 832 mg, potassium bicarbonate 312 mg. ALKA-SELTZER® Effervescent Antacid in water contains principally the antacids sodium citrate and potassium citrate.

Inactive Ingredient: A tableting aid. Does not contain aspirin.

Indications: ALKA-SELTZER® Effervescent Antacid is indicated for relief of acid indigestion, sour stomach or heartburn.

Actions: The ALKA-SELTZER® Effervescent Antacid solution provides quick and effective neutralization of gastric acid. Measured by the in vitro standard established by the Food and Drug Administration, one tablet will neutralize 10.6 mEq of acid.

Warnings: Except under the advice and supervision of a physician, do not take more than: Adults: 8 tablets in a 24-hour period (60 years of age or older: 7 tablets in a 24-hour period), Children: 4 tablets in a 24-hour period; or use the maximum dosage of this product for more than 2 weeks.
Do not use this product if you are on a sodium restricted diet. Each tablet contains 311 mg of sodium.
Keep this and all drugs out of the reach of children. As with any drug, if you are pregnant or nursing a baby, seek the advice of a health professional before using this product.

Drug Interaction Precaution: Antacids may interact with certain prescription drugs. If you are presently taking a prescription drug, do not take this product without checking with your doctor or other health professional.

Dosage and Administration: Adults: Take 2 tablets fully dissolved in water every 4 hours. Children: ½ the adult dosage or as directed by a doctor.

How Supplied: Boxes of 20 tablets in 10 foil twin packs; 36 tablets in 18 foil twin packs.

Shown in Product Identification Guide, page 503

ALKA-SELTZER PLUS®
Cold & Cough Medicine,
ALKA-SELTZER PLUS®
Nigh-Time Cold Medicine,
ALKA-SELTZER PLUS®
Cold Medicine,
ALKA-SELTZER PLUS®
Sinus Medicine

Active Ingredients:
ALKA-SELTZER PLUS® Cold & Cough Medicine: Aspirin 325 mg*, Chlorpheniramine Maleate 2 mg, Phenylpropanolamine Bitartrate 20 mg, Dextromethorphan Hydrobromine 10 mg.
ALKA-SELTZER PLUS® Night-Time Cold Medicine: Aspirin 500 mg* Doxylamine Succinate 6.25 mg, Phenylpropanolamine Bitartrate 20 mg, Dextromethorphan Hydrochloride 15 mg.
ALKA-SELTZER PLUS® Cold Medicine: Aspirin 325 mg*, Phenylpropanolamine Bitartrate 24.08 mg, Chlorpheniramine Maleate 2 mg.
ALKA-SELTZER PLUS® Sinus Medicine: Aspirin 500 mg*, Phenylpropanolamine Bitartrate 24.08 mg, Brompheniramine Maleate 2 mg.
*In water the aspirin is converted into its soluble ionic form, sodium acetylsalicylate.

Inactive Ingredients:
ALKA-SELTZER PLUS® Cold & Cough Medicine: Aspartame, Citric Acid, Flavor, Sodium Bicarbonate, Tableting aids.

Phenylketonurics: Contains Phenylalanine 11.2 mg per tablet.
ALKA-SELTZER PLUS® Night-Time Cold Medicine: Aspartame, Citric Acid, Flavor, Sodium Bicarbonate, Tableting aids.

Phenylketonurics: Contains Phenylalanine 16.2 mg per tablet.
ALKA-SELTZER PLUS® Cold Medicine: Citric Acid, Flavors, Sodium Bicarbonate.
ALKA-SELTZER® Sinus Medicine: Aspartame, Citric Acid, Flavors, Heat-treated Sodium Bicarbonate, Tableting aids.
PHENYLKETONURICS: Contains Phenylalanine 8.98 mg per tablet.

Indications: For the temporary relief of these major cold and flu symptoms: **coughing, nasal and sinus congestion, body aches and pains, runny nose, headaches and pains, sneezing, fever, *scratchy sore throat, so you can get the rest you need.

Directions for Use: Adults: Dissolve 2 tablets in approximately 4 oz. of water every 4 hours. Do not exceed 8 tablets in any 24-hour period.

Warning: Children and teenagers should not use this medicine for chicken pox or flu symptoms before a doctor is consulted about Reye syndrome, a rare but serious illness reported to be associated with aspirin. (If sore throat is severe, persists for more than 2 days, is accompanied by high fever, headache, nausea or vomiting, consult a physician promptly.)* As with any drug, if you are pregnant or nursing a baby, seek the advice of a health professional before using this product. **IT IS ESPECIALLY IMPORTANT NOT TO USE ASPIRIN DURING THE LAST 3 MONTHS OF PREGNANCY UNLESS SPECIFICALLY DIRECTED TO DO SO BY A DOCTOR BECAUSE IT MAY CAUSE PROBLEMS IN THE UNBORN CHILD OR COMPLICATIONS DURING DELIVERY.**

Do not exceed recommended dosage because at higher doses nervousness, dizziness or sleeplessness may occur. May cause excitability, especially in children. Do not take this product unless directed by a doctor if you are allergic to aspirin, have a breathing problem such as emphysema or chronic bronchitis, asthma, glaucoma, difficulty in urination due to enlargement of the prostate gland, heart disease, high blood pressure, diabetes, thyroid disease, bleeding problems or on a sodium restricted diet. Each tablet contains 506 mg of sodium. (ALKA-Seltzer Plus Cold & Cough Medicine 507 mg). May cause marked drowsiness; alcohol, sedatives and tranquilizers may increase drowsiness effect. Avoid alcoholic beverages while taking this product. Do not take this product if you are taking sedatives or tranquilizers without first consulting your doctor. Use caution when driving a motor vehicle or operating machinery. [Do not take this product for persistent or chronic cough such as occurs with smoking, asthma, emphysema, or if cough is accompanied by excessive phlegm (muscus), unless directed by a doctor. A persistent cough may be a sign of a serious condition. If cough persists for more than 1 week, tends to recur or is accompanied by fever, rash, or persistent headache, consult a doctor.**] Do not take this product for more than 7 days. If symptoms do not improve or are accompanied by fever or if fever persists for more than 3 days, consult a doctor. Keep this and all drugs out of the reach of children.

Drug Interaction Precaution: Do not take this product if you are presently taking a prescription drug for anticoagulation (thinning the bood), diabetes, gout, arthritis, high blood pressure or are presently taking a monoamine oxidase inhibitor (MAOI) (certain drugs for depression, psychiatric or emotional conditions, or Parkinson's disease), or for 2 weeks after stopping the MAOI drug. If you are uncertain whether your prescription drug contains an MAOI, consult a health professional before taking this product.
*Does not apply to ALKA-SELTZER PLUS Sinus Medicine.
**Applies only to ALKA-SELTZER PLUS Cold & Cough Medicine and Night-Time Cold Medicine.

How Supplied: ALKA-SELTZERPLUS Cold & Cough Medicine, and Night-Time Cold Medicine: Carton of 36 tablets in 18 foil twin packs; carton of 20 tablets in 10 foil twin packs; carton of 12 tablets in 6 foil packs.
ALKA-SELTZER PLUS Cold Medicine: Also available in the above sizes, plus carton of 48 in 24 foil twin packs.
ALKA-SELTZER PLUS Sinus: Carton of 20 tablets in 10 foil twin packs
Product Identification Mark:
A/S PLUS NIGHT-TIME etched on each tablet.

Shown in Product Identification Guide, page 504

Continued on next page

Bayer—Cont.

ALKA-SELTZER PLUS® NIGHT-TIME COLD MEDICINE LIQUI-GELS, ALKA-SELTZER PLUS® COLD & COUGH MEDICINE LIQUI-GELS, ALKA-SELTZER PLUS® COLD MEDICINE: LIQUI-GELS

Active Ingredients:
ALKA-SELTZER PLUS® NIGHT-TIME COLD MEDICINE:
Dextromethorphan Hydrobromide 10 mg, Doxylamine Succinate 6.25 mg, Pseudoephedrine HCl 30 mg, Acetaminophen 250 mg.
ALKA-SELTZER PLUS® COLD & COUGH MEDICINE:
Dextromethorphan Hydrobromide 10 mg, Chlorpheniramine Maleate 2 mg, Pseudoephedrine HCl 30 mg, Acetaminophen 250 mg.
ALKA-SELTZER PLUS® COLD MEDICINE:
Chlorpheniramine Maleate 2 mg, Pseudoephedrine HCl 30 mg, Acetaminophen 250 mg.

Inactive Ingredients: Artificial Colors, Gelatin, Glycerin, Polyethylene Glycol, Povidone, Propylene Glycol, Purified Water, Sorbitol, Titanium Dioxide.

Indications: Provides temporary relief of these major symptoms of cold and flu: *coughing, runny nose, nasal and sinus congestion, headache, body aches and pains, sneezing, fever and scratchy sore throat.

Direction for Use: ALKA-SELTZER PLUS® COLD MEDICINE, and COLD & COUGH MEDICINE:
ADULTS: Swallow 2 softgels with water. CHILDREN (6–12 YEARS): Swallow 1 softgel with water.
CHILDREN (under 6 years): Consult a doctor: Repeat every 4 hours, not to exceed 4 doses per day, or as directed by a doctor.
ALKA-SELTZER PLUS® NIGHT-TIME COLD MEDICINE:
Adults: Swallow 2 softgels with water, once daily, at bedtime. Not recommended for children.

Warnings: Do not exceed recommended dosage because at higher doses nervousness, dizziness or sleeplessness may occur. Do not take this product for more than 7 days or for fever for more than 3 days unless directed by a doctor. If symptoms do not improve or are accompanied by fever, consult a doctor.
If sore throat is severe, persists for more than 2 days, is accompanied by or followed by fever, headache, nausea or vomiting, consult a doctor promptly. May cause excitability especially in children. Do not take this product, unless directed by a doctor, if you have a breathing problem such as emphysema or chronic bronchitis, or glaucoma, difficulty in urination due to enlargement of the prostate gland or heart disease, high blood pressure, diabetes, or thyroid disease. May cause marked drowsiness; alcohol, sedatives and tranquilizers may increase drowsiness effect. Avoid alcoholic beverages while taking this product. Do not take this product if you are taking sedatives or tranquilizers without first consulting your doctor. Use caution when driving a motor vehicle or operating machinery. As with any drug, if you are pregnant or nursing a baby seek the advice of a health professional before using this product. Keep this and all medication out of the reach of children. In case of accidental overdose, contact a physician or Poison Control Center immediately. Prompt medical attention is critical for adults as well as children even if you do not notice any signs or symptoms. (A persistent cough may be a sign of a serious condition. If cough persists for more than 1 week, tends to recur or is accompanied by fever, rash or persistent headache, consult a doctor. Do not take this product for persistent for chronic cough such as occurs with smoking, asthma, emphysema or if cough is accompanied by excessive phlegm (muscus) unless directed by a doctor.)*

Drug Interaction Precaution: Do not take this product if you are taking a prescription drug for high blood pressure without first consulting your doctor or if you are now taking a prescription monoamine oxidase inhibitor (MAOI) (certain drugs for depression, psychiatric or emotional conditions, or Parkinson's disease), or for 2 weeks after stopping the MAOI drug. If you are uncertain whether your prescription drug contains an MAOI, consult a health professional before taking this product.
*Does not apply to Alka-Seltzer Plus Cold Medicine.

How Supplied: Carton of 12 and 20 softgels.
Shown in Product Identification Guide, page 504

ALKA-SELTZER® PLUS Flu and Body Aches Formula

Active Ingredients: Acetaminophen 325 mg, Dextromethorphan, Hydrobromide 10 mg, Phenylpropanolamine Bitartrate 20 mg, Chlorpheniramine, Maleate 2 mg.

Inactive Ingredients: Aspartame, Calcium Carbonate, Citric Acid, Croscarmellose Sodium, D&C Yellow #10, Flavor, Maltodextrin, Mannitol, Polyvinylpyrrolidone, Sodium Bicarbonate, Sodium Saccharin, Sorbitol, Starch, Stearic Acid, Tableting Aids.

Indications: Provides temporary relief of these symptoms associated with flu and common cold: headache, body aches, fever, coughing, minor sore throat pain, nasal and sinus congestion, runny nose and sneezing.

Recommended Dosage: ADULTS: Dissolve 2 tablets in 4 oz. of hot (not boiling) water. Sip while hot. Repeat every 4 hours, but not to exceed 4 doses per day, or as directed by a doctor. Children under 12 years of age: consult a doctor.

Warnings: Not recommended for children under 12. **Do not exceed recommended dosage.** If nervousness, dizziness or sleeplessness occur, discontinue use and consult a doctor. If symptoms do not improve within 7 days or are accompanied by fever, consult a doctor. A persistent cough may be a sign of a serious condition. If cough persists for more than 1 week, tends to recur or is accompanied by fever, rash or persistent headache, consult a doctor. Do not take this product for persistent or chronic cough such as occurs with smoking, asthma, emphysema, or if cough is accompanied by excessive phlegm (mucus) unless directed by a doctor. If sore throat is severe, persists for more than two days, is accompanied by or followed by fever, headache, rash, nausea, or vomiting, consult a doctor promptly. May cause excitability, especially in children. Do not take this product unless directed by a doctor, if you have a breathing problem such as emphysema or chronic bronchitis or glaucoma, difficulty in urination due to enlargement of the prostate gland or heart disease, high blood pressure, diabetes or thyroid disease.
May cause marked drowsiness; alcohol, sedatives and tranquilizers may increase drowsiness effect. Avoid alcoholic beverage while taking this product. Do not take this product if you are taking sedatives or tranquilizers without first consulting your doctor. Use caution when driving a motor vehicle or operating machinery. Each tablet contains 111 mg sodium. As with any drug, if you are pregnant or nursing a baby, seek the advice of a health professional before using this product. Keep this and all medication out of the reach of children. In case of accidental overdose, contact a physician or Poison Control Center immediately. Prompt medical attention is critical for adults as well as children even if you do not notice any signs or symptoms.

Phenylketonurics: Contains Phenylalanine 11.2 mg per tablet.

Drug Interaction Precaution: Do not use this product if you are taking a prescription drug for high blood pressure without first consulting your doctor or if you are now taking a prescription monoamine oxidase inhibitor (MAOI) (certain drugs for depression, psychiatric or emotional conditions, or Parkinson's disease) or for 2 weeks after stopping the MAOI drug. If you are uncertain whether your prescription drug contains an MAOI, consult a health professional before taking this product.

How Supplied: ALKA-SELTZER® Plus Flu and Body Aches is available in carton of 20 tablets in 10 foil twin packs; carton of 36 tablets in 18 foil twin packs.
Shown in Product Identification Guide, page 504

ALKA-SELTZER® PLUS Flu & Body Aches Liqui-Gels®
Non-Drowsy Formula

Indications: Provides temporary relief of these symptoms associated with flu and common cold including: headache, body aches, fever, coughing, minor sore throat pain, nasal and sinus congestion.

Directions For Use: ADULTS: Swallow 2 softgels with water. CHILDREN (6–12 years): Swallow 1 softgel with water. CHILDREN (under 6 years): Consult a doctor. Repeat every 4 hours, but not to exceed 4 doses per day, or as directed by a doctor.

Active Ingredients: Acetaminophen 250 mg, Pseudoephedrine Hydrochloride 30 mg, Dextromethorphan, Hydrobromide 10 mg.

Inactive Ingredients: FD&C Red #40, Gelatin, Glycerin, Polyethylene Glycol, Povidone, Propylene Glycol, Purified Water, Sorbitol, Titanium Dioxide.

Warnings: Do not exceed recommended dosage. If nervousness, dizziness or sleeplessness occur, discontinue use and consult a doctor. If symptoms do not improve within 7 days or are accompanied by fever, consult a doctor. A persistent cough may be a sign of a serious condition. If cough persists for more than 1 week, tends to recur or is accompanied by fever, rash, or persistent headache, consult a doctor. Do not take this product for persistent or chronic cough such as occurs with smoking, asthma, emphysema, or if cough is accompanied by excessive phlegm (mucus) unless directed by a doctor. If sore throat is severe, persists for more than two days, is accompanied by or followed by fever, headache, rash, nausea, or vomiting, consult a doctor promptly. Do not take this product if you have heart disease, high blood pressure, thyroid disease, diabetes or difficulty in urination due to enlargement of the prostate gland unless directed by a doctor. As with any drug, if you are pregnant or nursing a baby, seek the advise of a health professional before using this product. Keep this and all medication out of the reach of children. In case of accidental overdose, contact a physician or Poison Control Center immediately. Prompt medical attention is critical for adults as well as children even if you do not notice any signs or symptoms.

Drug Interaction Precaution: Do not use this product if you are taking a prescription drug for high blood pressure without first consulting your doctor or if you are now taking a prescription monoamine oxidase inhibitor (MAOI) (certain drugs for depression, psychiatric or emotional conditions, or Parkinson's disease), or for 2 weeks after stopping the MAOI drug. If you are uncertain whether your prescription drug contains an MAOI, consult a health professional before taking this product.

How Supplied: ALKA-SELTZER® PLUS Flu and Body Aches Liqui-Gels® are available in blisters of 12 and 20 count.

Shown in Product Identification Guide, page 504

ASPIRIN REGIMEN BAYER® 81 mg
ASPIRIN REGIMEN BAYER® 325 mg
Delayed Release Enteric Aspirin Adult Low Strength 81 mg Tablets and Regular Strength 325 mg Caplets

Composition: Active Ingredient: ASPIRIN REGIMEN BAYER® is an enteric-coated aspirin available in 81 mg tablet and 325 mg caplet forms. The enteric coating prevents disintegration in the stomach and promotes dissolution in the duodenum, where there is a more neutral to alkaline environment. This action aids in protecting the stomach against injuries that may occur as a result of ingesting non-enteric coated aspirin.

Safety: The safety of enteric-coated aspirin has been demonstrated in a number of endoscopic studies comparing enteric-coated aspirin and plain aspirin, as well as buffered aspirin and "arthritis strength" preparations. In these studies, endoscopies were performed in healthy volunteers before and after either 2-day or 14-day administration of aspirin doses of 3,900 or 4,000 mg per day. Compared to all the other preparations, the enteric-coated aspirin produced signficantly less damage to the gastric mucosa. There was also statistically less duodenal damage when compared with the plain, i.e., non-enteric-coated aspirin.

Bioavailability: The bioavailability of aspirin from **ASPIRIN REGIMEN BAYER®** has been confirmed. In single-dose studies[1] in which plasma acetylsalicylic acid and salicylic acid levels were measured, maximum concentrations were achieved at approximately 5 hours postdosing. **ASPIRIN REGIMEN BAYER®**, when compared with plain aspirin, achieves maximum plasma salicylate levels not significantly different from plain, i.e., non-enteric-coated, aspirin. Dissolution of the enteric coating occurs at a neutral to basic pH and is therefore dependent on gastric emptying into the duodenum. With continued dosing, appropriate therapeutic plasma levels are maintained.

Regular Strength 325mg—D&C Yellow #10, FD&C Yellow #6, Hydroxypropyl Methylcellulose, Methacrylic Acid Copolymer, Starch, Titanium Dioxide, Triacetin.
Adult Low Strength 81mg—Croscarmellose Sodium, D&C Yellow #10, FD&C Yellow #6, Hydroxypropyl Methylcellulose, Iron Oxides, Lactose, Methacrylic Acid, Microcrystalline Cellulose, Polysorbate 80, Sodium Lauryl Sulfate, Starch, Titanium Dioxide, Triacetin.

Indications: ASPIRIN REGIMEN BAYER® is an anti-inflammatory, analgesic, and antiplatelet agent indicated for the relief of painful discomfort and muscular aches and pains associated with conditions requiring long-term aspirin therapy, e.g., arthritis or rheumatism, and for situations where compliance with aspirin usage may be hindered by gastrointestinal side effects of non-enteric-coated or buffered aspirin. For additional **Anti-inflammatory, Antiarthritic,** and **Antiplatelet** indications, see the **PROFESSIONAL LABELING** section.

Directions: The following dosages are provided as appropriate for self-medication:
For analgesic indications the maximum adult nonprescription dosage of aspirin is 4,000 mg per day in divided doses, i.e., two 325 mg caplets or eight 81 mg tablets every 4 hours or three 325 mg caplets or twelve 81 mg tablets every 6 hours. Under a physician's recommendation, the dosage or frequency may be modified as appropriate for the clinical situation.

Consumer Warnings: Children and teenagers should not use this medicine for chicken pox or flu symptoms before a doctor is consulted about Reye Syndrome, a rare but serious illness reported to be associated with aspirin. Do not take for pain for more than 10 days or for fever for more than 3 days unless directed by a doctor. If pain or fever persists or gets worse, if new symptoms occur, or if redness or swelling is present, consult a doctor because these could be signs of a serious condition. Do not take this product if you are allergic to aspirin, have asthma, have stomach problems (such as heartburn, upset stomach or stomach pain) that persist or recur, or have gastric ulcers or bleeding problems unless directed by a doctor. If ringing in the ears or loss of hearing occurs, consult a doctor before taking any more of this product. Keep this and all drugs out of the reach of children. In case of accidental overdose, seek professional assistance or contact a poison control center immediately. As with any drug, if you are pregnant or nursing a baby, seek the advice of a health professional before using this product. **IT IS ESPECIALLY IMPORTANT NOT TO USE ASPIRIN DURING THE LAST 3 MONTHS OF PREGNANCY UNLESS SPECIFICALLY DIRECTED TO DO SO BY A DOCTOR BECAUSE IT MAY CAUSE PROBLEMS IN THE UNBORN CHILD OR COMPLICATIONS DURING DELIVERY.**

Drug Interaction Precaution: Do not take this product if you are taking a prescription drug for anticoagulation (thinning the blood), diabetes, gout, or arthritis unless directed by a doctor.

Professional Labeling:

Antiarthritic and Anti-inflammatory Effect

Indications: For conditions requiring chronic or long-term aspirin therapy for

Continued on next page

Bayer—Cont.

pain and/or inflammation, e.g., rheumatoid arthritis, juvenile rheumatoid arthritis, systemic lupus erythematosus, osteoarthritis (degenerative joint disease), ankylosing spondylitis, psoriatic arthritis, Reiter's syndrome, and fibrositis.

Antiplatelet Effect
Aspirin for Myocardial Infarction

Indication: Aspirin is indicated to reduce the risk of death and/or nonfatal myocardial infarction in patients with a previous infarction or unstable angina pectoris.

Clinical Trials: The indication is supported by the results of six large, randomized, multicenter, placebo-controlled studies involving 10,816 predominantly male, post-myocardial infarction (MI) patients and one randomized placebo-controlled study of 1,266 men with unstable angina.[2,8] Therapy wih aspirin was begun at intervals after the onset of acute MI varying from less than 3 days to more than 5 years and continued for periods of from less than 1 year to 4 years. In the unstable angina study, treatment was started within 1 month after onset of unstable angina and continued for 12 weeks, and patients with complicating conditions, such as congestive heart failure, were not included in the study.

Aspirin therapy in MI patients was associated with about a 20 percent reduction in the risk of subsequent death and/or nonfatal reinfarction, a median absolute decrease of 3 percent from the 12 to 22 percent event rates in the placebo groups. In aspirin-treated unstable angina patients, the reduction in risk was about 50 percent, a reduction in the event rate of 5 percent from the 10 percent rate in the placebo group over the 12 weeks of the study.

Daily dosage of aspirin in the post-myocardial infarction studies was 300 mg in one study and 900 to 1,500 mg in five studies. A dose of 325 mg was used in the study of unstable angina.

Adverse Reactions: Gastrointestinal Reactions: Doses of 1,000 mg per day of aspirin caused gastrointestinal symptoms and bleeding that in some cases were clinically significant. In the largest post-infarction study (the Aspirin Myocardial Infarction Study [AMIS] with 4,500 people), the percentage incidence of gastrointestinal symptoms for the aspirin- (1,000 mg of a standard, solid tablet formulation) and placebo-treated subjects, respectively, were: stomach pain (14.5 percent, 4.4 percent); heartburn (11.9 percent, 4.8 percent), nausea and/or vomiting (7.6 percent, 2.1 percent); hospitalization for gastrointestinal disorder (4.8 percent, 3.5 percent). In the AMIS and other trials, aspirin-treated patients had increased rates of gross gastrointestinal bleeding. Symptoms and signs of gastrointestinal irritation were not significantly increased in subjects treated for unstable angina with buffered aspirin in solution.

Cardiovascular and Biochemical: In the AMIS trial the dosage of 1,000 mg per day of aspirin was associated with small increases in systolic blood pressure (BP) (average 1.5 to 2.1 mm) and diastolic BP (0.5 to 2.1 mm), depending upon whether maximal or last available readings were used. Blood urea nitrogen and uric acid levels were also increased, but by less than 1.0 mg%. Subjects with marked hypertension or renal insufficiency had been excluded from trial so that the clinical importance of these observations for such subjects or for any subject treated over more prolonged periods is not known. It is recommended that patients placed on long-term aspirin treatment, even at doses of 300 mg per day, be seen at regular intervals to assess changes in these measurements.

Dosage and Administration: Although most of the studies used dosages exceeding 300 mg, two trials used only 300 mg and pharmacological data indicate that this dose inhibits platelet function fully. Therefore, 300 mg or a conventional 325 mg aspirin dose is a reasonable, routine dose that would minimize gastrointestinal adverse reactions. This use of aspirin applies to both solid oral dosage forms (buffered and plain aspirin) and buffered aspirin in solution.

Aspirin for Transient Ischemic Attacks

Indications: For reducing the risk of recurrent Transient Ischemic Attacks (TIAs) or storke in men who have transient ischemia of the brain due to fibrin emboli. There is inadequate evidence that aspirin or buffered aspirin is effective in reducing TIAs in women at the recommended dosage. There is no evidence that aspirin or buffered aspirin is of benefit in the treatment of completed strokes in men or women.

Clinical Trials: The indication is supported by the result of a Canadian study[9] in which 585 patients with threatened stroke followed in a randomized clinical trial for an average of 28 months to determine whether aspirin or sulfinpyrazone, singly or in combination, was superior to placebo in preventing transient ischemic attacks, stroke, or death. The study showed that although sulfinpyrazone had no statistically significant effect, aspirin reduced the risk of continuing transient ischemic attacks, stroke or death by 19 percent and reduced the risk of stroke or death by 31 percent. Another aspirin study trial carried out in the United States with 178 patients showed a statistically significant number of "favorable outcomes" including reduced transient ischemic attacks, stroke, and death.[10]

Precautions: Patients presenting with signs and symptoms of a TIA should have a complete medical and neurological evaluation. Consideration should be given to other disorders that resemble TIAs. Attention should be given to risk factors; it is important to evaluate and treat, if appropriate, other diseases associated with TIAs and stroke, such as hypertension and diabetes.

Other Precautions: Concurrent administration of absorbable antacids at therapeutic doses may increase the clearance of salicylates in some individuals. The concurrent administration of nonabsorbable antacids may alter the rate of absorption of aspirin, resulting in a decreased acetylsalicylic acid/salicylate ratio in plasma. The clinical significance of these decreases in available aspirin is unknown.

Dosage and Administration: Adult oral dosage for men is 1,300 mg a day, in divided doses of 650 mg twice a day or 325 mg four times daily.

Occasional reports have documented individuals with impaired gastric emptying in whom there may be retention of one or more enteric-coated tablets over time. This phenomenon may occur as a result of outlet obstruction from ulcer disease alone or combined with hypotonic gastric peristalsis. Because of the integrity of the enteric coating in an acidic environment, these tablets may accumulate and form a bezoar in the stomach. Individuals with this condition may present with complaints of early satiety or of vague upper abdominal distress. Diagnosis may be made by endoscopy or by abdominal films, which show opacities suggestive of a mass of small tablets.[11] Management may vary according to the condition of the patient. Options include gastrotomy and alternating slightly basic and neutral lavage.[12] While there have been no clinical reports, it has been suggested that such individuals may also be treated with parenteral cimetidine (to reduce acid secretion) and then given sips of slightly basic liquids to effect gradual dissolution of the enteric coating. Progress may be followed with plasma salicylate levels or via recognition of tinnitus by the patient. **It should be kept in mind that individuals with a history of partial or complete gastrectomy may produce reduced amounts of acid and therefore have less acidic gastric pH. Under these circumstances, the benefits offered by the acid-resistant enteric coating may not exist.**

References: 1. Data on file, Sterling Health. 2. Elwood PC, et al: A randomized controlled trial of acetylsalicylic acid in the secondary preventive of mortality from myocardial infarction. *Br Med J* 1974;1:436–440. 3. The Coronary Drug Project Research Group: Aspirin in coronary heart disease. *J Chronic Dis* 1976;29:625–642. 4. Breddin K, et al: Secondary prevention of myocardial infarction: A comparison of acetylsalicylic acid, phenprocoumon or placebo. *Homeostasis* 1979;470:263–268. 5. Aspirin Myocardial Infarction Study Research Group: A randomized, controlled trial of aspirin in persons recovered from myocardial infarction. *JAMA* 1980;245:661–669. 6. Elwood PC, Sweetnam PM: Aspirin and secondary mortality after myocardial infarction. *Lancet*, December 22–29, 1979, pp 1313–1315. 7. The Persantine-Aspirin Reinfarction Study Research Group: Persantine and aspirin in coronary heart disease. *Circulation* 1980;62:449–460. 8. Lewis HD, et al: Protective effects of aspirin against acute myocardial infarction and death in men with unstable angina: Results of a Veterans Administration Cooperative Study. *N Engl J Med* 1983;309:396–403. 9. The Canadian Cooperative Study Group: A randomized trial of aspirin and sulfinpyrazone in threatened stroke. *N Eng J Med* 1978;299:53–59. 10. Fields WS, et al: Controlled trial of aspirin in cerebral ischemia. *Stroke* 1977;8:301–316. 11. Bogacz K, Caldron P: Enteric-coated aspirin bezoar: Elevation of serum salicylate level by barium study. *Am J Med* 1987;83:783–786. 12. Baum J: Enteric-coated aspirin and the problem of gastric retention. *J Rheumatol* 1984;11:250–251.

How Supplied: ASPIRIN REGIMEN BAYER 325 mg—Regular strength 325 mg caplets in bottles of 100 with child-resistant safety closure.
ASPIRIN REGIMEN BAYER 81 mg—Adult Low Strenth 81 mg tablets in bottles of 120 with child-resistant safety closure.

REV. 11/94
Shown in Product Identification Guide, page 504

ASPIRIN REGIMEN BAYER® 81 mg WITH CALCIUM

Each caplet provides 81 mg of aspirin and 10% (100 mg) of the Daily Value of Calcium as part of the buffered base of Calcium Carbonate.

Indications. For the temporary relief of minor aches and pains or as recommended by your doctor. Ask your doctor about new uses for Aspirin Regimen BAYER® 81 mg With Calcium.

Directions: Adults and Children 12 years and over, take 4 to 8 caplets with water every 4 hours, as needed, up to a maximum of 32 caplets per 24 hours or as directed by a doctor.

Warnings: Children and teenagers should not use this medicine for chicken pox or flu symptoms before a doctor is consulted about Reye Syndrome, a rare but serious illness reported to be associated with aspirin. Do not take for pain for more than 10 days or for fever for more than 3 days unless directed by a doctor. If pain or fever persists or gets worse, if new symptoms occur or if redness or swelling is present, consult a doctor because these could be signs of a serious condition. Do not take this product if you are allergic to aspirin, have asthma, have stomach problems (such as heartburn, upset stomach or stomach pain) that persist or recur, gastric ulcers or bleeding problems unless directed by a doctor. If ringing in the ears or loss of hearing occurs, consult a doctor before taking any more of this product. Keep this and all drugs out of the reach of children. In case of accidental overdose, seek professional assistance or contact a poison control center immediately. As with any drug, if you are pregnant or nursing a baby, seek the advice of a health professional before using this product. IT IS ESPECIALLY IMPORTANT NOT TO USE ASPIRIN DURING THE LAST 3 MONTHS OF PREGNANCY UNLESS DIRECTED TO DO SO BY A DOCTOR BECAUSE IT MAY CAUSE PROBLEMS IN THE UNBORN CHILD OR COMPLICATIONS DURING DELIVERY.

Drug Interaction Precaution: Do not take this product if you are taking any prescription drug including those for anticoagulation (thinning the blood), diabetes, gout or arthritis unless directed by a doctor.

Active Ingredients: 81 mg Aspirin per caplet in a buffered base of Calcium Carbonate (250 mg = 100 mg of elemental calcium).

Inactive Ingredients: Colloidal Silicon Dioxide, FD&C Blue #2 Lake, Hydroxypropyl Methylcellulose, Microcrystalline Cellulose, Propylene Glycol, Sodium Starch Glycolate, Starch, Titanium Dioxide, Zinc Stearate.

How Supplied: ASPIRIN REGIMEN BAYER® 81 mg WITH CALCIUM is available in 60 count bottles.
Shown in Product Identification Guide, page 504

Extra Strength BAYER® Aspirin Arthritis Pain Regimen Formula [aspirin, 500 mg]

Enteric Coated Caplets
- Specifically designed for people on a regimen of aspirin, or as directed by your doctor.
- Contains the strongest dose of pain reliever you can buy.
- Safety coated to help protect your stomach.
- Pure BAYER® Aspirin inside.
- Caffeine free and very low sodium.
- Easy-to-swallow caplet shape.

The enteric coating on BAYER® Aspirin Arthritis Pain Regimen Formula is designed to allow the caplet to pass through the stomach to the intestine before it dissolves, providing protection against stomach upset.

Indications: For the temporary relief of minor aches and pains of arthritis or as recommended by your doctor.
For rheumatoid arthritis, juvenile rheumatoid arthritis, systemic lupus erythematosus, osteoarthritis (degenerative joint disease), ankylosing spondylitis, psoriatic arthritis, Reiter's syndrome, and fibrositis.
Because of its delayed action, BAYER® Aspirin Arthritis Pain Regimen Formula will not provide fast relief of headaches, fever or other symptoms needing immediate relief.

Direction: Adults and Children 12 years and over, take 2 caplets with water every 6 hours, as needed, up to a maximum of 8 caplets per 24 hours. Ask your doctor about recommended dosages for other indications.

Warnings: Children and teenagers should not use this medicine for chicken pox or flu symptoms before a doctor is consulted about Reye Syndrome, a rare but serious illness reported to be associated with aspirin. Do not take for pain for more than 10 days or for fever for more than 3 days unless directed by a doctor. If pain or fever persists or gets worse, if new symptoms occur or if redness or swelling is present, consult a doctor because these could be signs of a serious condition. Do not take this product if you are allergic to aspirin, have asthma, have stomach problems (such as heartburn, upset stomach or stomach pain) that persist or recur, gastric ulcers or bleeding problems unless directed by a doctor. If ringing in the ears or loss of hearing occurs, consult a doctor before taking any more of this product. Keep this and all drugs out of the reach of children. In case of accidental overdose, seek professional assistance or contact a poison control center immediately. As with any drug, if you are pregnant or nursing a baby, seek the advice of a health professional before using this product. IT IS ESPECIALLY IMPORTANT NOT TO USE ASPIRIN DURING THE LAST 3 MONTHS OF PREGNANCY UNLESS SPECIFICALLY DIRECTED TO DO SO BY A DOCTOR BECAUSE IT MAY CAUSE PROBLEMS IN THE UNBORN CHILD OR COMPLICATIONS DURING DELIVERY.

Drug Interaction Precaution: Do not take this product if you are taking a prescription drug for anticoagulation (thinning the blood), diabetes, gout or arthritis unless directed by a doctor.

Active Ingredient: 500 mg Aspirin per caplet.

Inactive Ingredients: D&C Yellow #10 FD&C Yellow #6. Hydroxypropyl Methylcellulose, Iron Oxide, Methacrylic Acid Copolymer, Starch, Titanium Dioxide, Triacetin.
Store at room temperature.

How Supplied: Extra Strength BAYER® Aspirin Arthritis Pain Regimen Formula is supplied in bottles of 50 caplets with a child-resistant safety closure.

Shown in Product Identification Guide, page 504

Continued on next page

Bayer—Cont.

Aspirin Regimen
BAYER® Children's Chewable
81 mg Aspirin

Active Ingredients: Aspirin Regimen Bayer Children's Chewable Aspirin—Aspirin 81 mg (1¼ grains) per orange flavored chewable tablet. Also available in cherry flavor.

Inactive Ingredients: Orange Flavored: Dextrose Excipient, FD&C Yellow #6, Flavor, Saccharin Sodium, Starch. Cherry Flavored: D&C Red #27, Dextrose Excipient, FD&C Red #40, Flavor, Saccharin Sodium, Starch.

Indications: For the temporary relief of minor aches, pains and headaches, and to reduce fever associated with colds, sore throats and teething.

Directions: The following dosages are those provided in the packaging, as appropriate for self-medication.
Children's Dose: To be administered only under adult supervision.

Age (Years)	Weight (lb)	Dosage
2 to under 4	32 to 35	2 tablets
4 to under 6	36 to 45	3 tablets
6 to under 9	46 to 65	4 tablets
9 to under 11	66 to 76	4–5 tablets
11 to under 12	77 to 83	4–6 tablets
Adults and Children 12 yrs and over		5–8 tablets

Indicated dosage may be repeated every four hours, while symptoms persist, up to a maximum of five doses per 24 hours or as directed by a doctor. For larger or more frequent doses or for children under 2, consult your doctor before taking.
Ways to Administer: CHEW, then follow with a half a glass of water, milk or fruit juice.
SWALLOW WHOLE with a half a glass of water, milk or fruit juice.
DISSOLVE ON TONGUE, followed with a half a glass of water, milk or fruit juice.
DISSOLVE TABLET in a little water, milk or fruit juice and drink the solution.
CRUSH in a teaspoonful of water—followed with a half a glass of water.

Warnings: Children and teenagers should not use this medicine for chicken pox or flu symptoms before a doctor is consulted about Reye syndrome, a rare but serious illness reported to be associated with aspirin.
Do not take this product for pain for more than 10 days (for adults) or 5 days (for children), and do not take for fever for more than 3 days unless directed by a doctor. If pain or fever persists or gets worse, if new symptoms occur, or if redness or swelling is present, consult a doctor because these could be signs of a serious condition. Do not give this product to children for the pain of arthritis unless directed by a doctor. If sore throat is severe, persists for more than 2 days, is accompanied or followed by fever, headache, rash, nausea, or vomiting, consult a doctor promptly. Do not take this product for at least 7 days after tonsillectomy or oral surgery unless directed by a doctor. Do not take this product if you are allergic to aspirin, have asthma, have stomach problems (such as heartburn, upset stomach or stomach pain) that persist or recur or have gastric ulcers or bleeding problems unless directed by a doctor. If ringing in the ears or loss of hearing occurs, consult a doctor before taking any more of this product.
KEEP THIS AND ALL DRUGS OUT OF THE REACH OF CHILDREN. IN CASE OF ACCIDENTAL OVERDOSE, SEEK PROFESSIONAL ASSISTANCE OR CONTACT A POISON CONTROL CENTER IMMEDIATELY. AS WITH ANY DRUG, IF YOU ARE PREGNANT OR NURSING A BABY, SEEK THE ADVICE OF A HEALTH PROFESSIONAL BEFORE USING THIS PRODUCT. **IT IS ESPECIALLY IMPORTANT NOT TO USE ASPIRIN DURING THE LAST 3 MONTHS OF PREGNANCY UNLESS SPECIFICALLY DIRECTED TO DO SO BY A DOCTOR BECAUSE IT MAY CAUSE PROBLEMS IN THE UNBORN CHILD OR COMPLICATIONS DURING DELIVERY.**

Drug Interaction Precaution: Do not take this product if taking a prescription drug for anticoagulation (thinning the blood), diabetes, gout or arthritis unless directed by a doctor.

How Supplied: Aspirin Regimen Bayer Children's Chewable Aspirin 81 mg (1¼ grains) is available in orange and cherry flavors in bottles of 36 tablets with child-resistant safety closure.
Store at room temperature.
Shown in Product Identification Guide, page 504

Extended-Release
BAYER® 8-Hour Aspirin
Aspirin (acetylsalicylic acid)

Active Ingredients: Each oblong white scored caplet contains 650 mg (10-grains) of aspirin in microencapsulated form.

Inactive Ingredients: Guar Gum, Microcrystalline Cellulose, Starch and other ingredients.

Indications: Extended-Release BAYER 8-Hour Aspirin is indicated for the temporary relief of nagging, recurring pain of backache, bursitis, minor pain and stiffness of arthritis and rheumatism, sprains, headaches, sinusitis pain, and painful discomfort and fever due to colds and flu.

Directions: Two Extended-Release BAYER 8-Hour Aspirin caplets every 8 hours provide effective long-lasting pain relief. This two-caplet 1300 mg or (20-grain) dose of extended-release aspirin promptly produces salicylate blood levels greater than those achieved by a 650 mg (10-grain) dose of regular aspirin, and in the second 4-hour period produces a salicylate blood level curve which approximates that of two successive 650 mg (10-grain) doses of regular aspirin at 4-hour intervals. The 650 mg (10-grain) scored Extended-Release BAYER 8-Hour Aspirin caplets permit administration of aspirin in multiples of 325 mg (5-grains) allowing individualization of dosage to meet the specific needs of the patient. For the convenience of patients on a regular aspirin dosage schedule, two 650 mg (10-grain) Extended-Release BAYER 8-Hour Aspirin caplets may be administered with water every 8 hours. Whenever necessary, two caplets 1300 mg or (20 grains) should be given before retiring to provide effective analgesic and anti-inflammatory action—for relief of pain throughout the night and lessening of stiffness upon arising. Do not exceed 6 caplets in 24 hours. Extended-Release BAYER 8-Hour Aspirin has been made in a special caplet to permit easy swallowing. However, for patients who do have difficulty, Extended-Release BAYER 8-Hour Aspirin caplets may be gently crumbled in the mouth and swallowed with water without loss of timed-release effect. There is no bitter "aspirin" taste. For children under 12, consult physician.

Warnings: Children and teenagers should not use this medicine for chicken pox or flu symptoms before a doctor is consulted about Reye syndrome, a rare but serious illness reported to be associated with aspirin.
Do not take for pain for more than 10 days or for fever for more than 3 days unless directed by a doctor. If pain or fever persists or gets worse, if new symptoms occur, or if redness or swelling is present consult a doctor because these could be signs of a serious condition. Do not take this product if you are allergic to aspirin, have asthma, stomach problems that persist or recur, gastric ulcers or bleeding problems unless directed by a doctor. If ringing in the ears or loss of hearing occurs, consult a doctor before taking any more of this product. Keep this and all drugs out of the reach of children. In case of accidental overdose, seek professional assistance or contact a poison control center immediately. As with any drug, if you are pregnant or nursing a baby, seek the advice of a health professional before using this product. **IT IS ESPECIALLY IMPORTANT NOT TO USE ASPIRIN DURING THE LAST 3 MONTHS OF PREGNANCY UNLESS SPECIFICALLY DIRECTED TO DO SO BY A DOCTOR BECAUSE IT MAY CAUSE PROBLEMS IN THE UNBORN CHILD OR COMPLICATIONS DURING DELIVERY.**

Drug Interaction Precaution: Do not take this product if you are taking a prescription drug for anticoagulation (thinning of the blood), diabetes, gout, or arthritis unless directed by a doctor.

How Supplied: Extended-Release Bayer 8-Hour Aspirin 650 mg (10 grains) is supplied in bottles of 50 caplets with a child-resistant safety closure.
Shown in Product Identification Guide, page 504

Extra Strength BAYER® Aspirin
Aspirin (Acetylsalicylic Acid)
Caplets and Tablets

Active Ingredients: Extra Strength Bayer Aspirin—Aspirin 500 mg (7.7 grains) contains a thin, inert, Hydroxypropyl Methylcellulose coating for easier swallowing. This is not an enteric coating and does not alter the onset of action of Bayer Aspirin.

Inactive Ingredients: Starch and Triacetin.

Indications: Analgesic, antipyretic, anti-inflammatory. For relief of headache; painful discomfort and fever of colds; muscular aches and pains; temporary relief of minor pains of arthritis; toothache, and pain following dental procedures; menstrual pain.

Directions: The following dosages are those provided on the packaging, as appropriate for self- medication. Larger or more frequent dosage may be necessary as appropriate for the condition or needs of the patient. The hydroxypropyl methylcellulose coating makes Extra Strength Bayer Aspirin particularly appropriate for those who have difficulty in swallowing uncoated tablets/caplets.
Usual Adult Dose: One or two tablets/caplets with water. May be repeated every four hours as necessary up to 8 caplets/tablets a day. Do not give to children under 12 unless directed by a doctor.

Warnings: Children and teenagers should not use this medicine for chicken pox or flu symptoms before a doctor is consulted about Reye syndrome, a rare but serious illness reported to be associated with aspirin. Do not take this product for pain for more than 10 days or for fever for more than 3 days unless directed by a doctor. If pain or fever persists or gets worse, if new symptoms occur, or if redness or swelling is present consult a doctor because these could be signs of a serious condition. Do not take this product if you are allergic to aspirin, have asthma, stomach problems that persist or recur, gastric ulcers or bleeding problems unless directed by a doctor. If ringing in the ears or loss of hearing occurs, consult a doctor before taking any more of this product. Keep this and all drugs out of the reach of children. In case of accidental overdose, seek professional assistance or contact a poison control center immediately. As with any drug, if you are pregnant or nursing a baby, seek the advice of a health professional before using this product. **IT IS ESPECIALLY IMPORTANT NOT TO USE ASPIRIN DURING THE LAST 3 MONTHS OF PREGNANCY UNLESS SPECIFICALLY DIRECTED TO DO SO BY A DOCTOR BECAUSE IT MAY CAUSE PROBLEMS IN THE UNBORN CHILD OR COMPLICATIONS DURING DELIVERY.**

Drug Interaction Precaution: Do not take this product if you are taking a prescription drug for anticoagulation (thinning the blood), diabetes, gout, or arthritis unless directed by a doctor.

How Supplied: Extra Strength Bayer Aspirin 500 mg (7.7 grains) is available in bottles of 24, 50 and 100 caplets, and bottles of 50 tablets.
Child-resistant safety closures on 50s bottles of caplets and tablets, 24s bottles of caplets. Bottle of 100s caplets available without safety closure for households without young children.
Shown in Product Identification Guide, page 504

Extra Strength BAYER® PLUS
Buffered Aspirin

Active Ingredients: Each Extra Strength Bayer Plus contains Aspirin (500 mg), in a buffered base of Calcium Carbonate.

Inactive Ingredients: Colloidal Silicon Dioxide, D&C Red #7 Lake, FD&C Blue #2 Lake, FD&C Red #40 Lake, Hydroxypropyl Methylcellulose, Microcrystalline Cellulose, Propylene Glycol, Sodium Starch Glycolate, Starch, Titanium Dioxide, Zinc Stearate.

Indications: Analgesic, antipyretic, anti-inflammatory. For the temporary relief of headache; painful discomfort and fever of colds; muscular aches and pains; temporary relief of minor pains of arthritis; toothache, and pain following dental procedures; menstrual pain.

Directions: The following dosages are those provided in the packaging, as appropriate for self-medication. Larger or more frequent dosage may be necessary as appropriate to the condition or needs of the patient. The addition of buffering agents makes Extra Strength Bayer® Plus particularly appropriate for those who must take frequent doses of aspirin. The hydroxypropyl methylcellulose coating benefits aspirin users who have difficulty in swallowing uncoated caplets.
Usual Adult Dose: Adults and Children 12 years & over; One or two caplets with water. May be repeated every 4 to 6 hours as necessary up to 8 caplets a day, or as directed by a doctor. Do not give to children under 12 unless directed by a doctor.

Warnings: Children and teenagers should not use this medicine for chicken pox or flu symptoms before a doctor is consulted about Reye syndrome, a rare but serious illness reported to be associated with aspirin. Do not take this product for pain for more than 10 days or for fever for more than 3 days unless directed by a doctor. If pain or fever persists or gets worse, if new symptoms occur, or if redness or swelling is present consult a doctor because these could be signs of a serious condition. Do not take this product if you are allergic to aspirin, have asthma, stomach problems that persist or recur, gastric ulcers or bleeding problems unless directed by a doctor. If ringing in the ears or loss of hearing occurs, consult a doctor before taking any more of this product. Keep this and all drugs out of the reach of children. In case of accidental overdose, seek professional assistance or contact a poison control center immediately. As with any drug, if you are pregnant or nursing a baby, seek the advice of a health professional before using this product. **IT IS ESPECIALLY IMPORTANT NOT TO USE ASPIRIN DURING THE LAST 3 MONTHS OF PREGNANCY UNLESS SPECIFICALLY DIRECTED TO DO SO BY A DOCTOR BECAUSE IT MAY CAUSE PROBLEMS IN THE UNBORN CHILD OR COMPLICATIONS DURING DELIVERY.**

Drug Interaction Precaution: Do not take this product if you are taking a prescription drug for anticoagulation (thinning the blood), diabetes, gout, or arthritis unless directed by a doctor.

How Supplied: Extra Strength Bayer® Plus Aspirin (500 mg) is available in bottles of 50 caplets. Child resistant closure on 50s caplets.
Shown in Product Identification Guide, page 504

Extra Strength BAYER® PM
Aspirin Plus Sleep Aid
[500 mg aspirin/diphenhydramine HCl]

Indications: For the temporary relief of occasional headaches and minor aches and pains with accompanying sleeplessness.

Directions: Adults and Children 12 years of age and over, take 2 caplets with water at bedtime, if needed, or as directed by a doctor.

Warnings: Do not give to children under 12 years of age. **Children and teenagers should not use this medicine for chicken pox or flu symptoms before a doctor is consulted about Reye Syndrome, a rare but serious illness reported to be associated with aspirin.** Do not take this product for pain for more than 10 days or for fever for more than 3 days unless directed by a doctor. If pain or fever persists or gets worse, if new symptoms occur, or if redness or swelling is present, consult a doctor because these could be signs of a serious condition. Do not take this product if you are allergic to aspirin or if you have asthma unless directed by a doctor. If ringing in the ears or a loss of hearing occurs, consult a doctor before taking any more of this product. Do not take this product if you have stomach problems (such as heartburn, upset stomach, or stomach pain) that persist or recur, or if you have ulcers or bleeding problems, unless directed by a doctor. If sleeplessness persists continuously for more than 2 weeks, consult your doctor. Insomnia

Continued on next page

Bayer—Cont.

may be a symptom of serious underlying medical illness. Do not take this product, unless directed by a doctor, if you have a breathing problem such as emphysema or chronic bronchitis, or if you have glaucoma or difficulty in urination due to enlargement of the prostate gland. Avoid alcoholic beverages while taking this product. Do not take this product if you are taking sedatives or tranquilizers, without first consulting your doctor. Keep this and all drugs out of the reach of children. In case of accidental overdose, seek professional assistance or contact a poison control center immediately. As with any drug, if you are pregnant or nursing a baby, seek the advice of a health professional before using this product. IT IS ESPECIALLY IMPORTANT NOT TO USE ASPIRIN DURING THE LAST 3 MONTHS OF PREGNANCY UNLESS SPECIFICALLY DIRECTED TO DO SO BY A DOCTOR BECAUSE IT MAY CAUSE PROBLEMS IN THE UNBORN CHILD OR COMPLICATIONS DURING DELIVERY.

Drug Interaction Precaution: Do not take this product if you are taking a prescription drug for anticoagulation (thinning the blood), diabetes, gout, or arthritis unless directed by a doctor.

Active Ingredients: 500 mg Aspirin, 25 mg Diphenhydramine Hydrochloride per caplet.

Inactive Ingredients: Colloidal Silicon Dioxide, Dibasic Calcium Phosphate, Dibutyl Sebacate, Ethylcellulose, FD&C Blue #1 Lake, FD&C Blue #2 Lake, Hydroxypropyl Methylcellulose, Microcrystalline Cellulose, Oleic Acid, Propylene Glycol, Starch, Titanium Dioxide, Zinc Stearate.
Store at room temperature.

How Supplied: Extra Strength BAYER® PM Aspirin is supplied in bottles of 24 caplets with a child-resistant safety closure.

Shown in Product Identification Guide, page 504

Genuine BAYER® Aspirin
Aspirin (Acetylsalicylic Acid)
Tablets and Caplets

Active Ingredients: Each Genuine Bayer Aspirin contains aspirin 325 mg (5 grains) in a thin, inert, hydroxypropyl methylcellulose coating for easier swallowing. This is not an enteric coating and does not alter the onset of action of Genuine Bayer Aspirin.

Inactive Ingredients: Starch and Triacetin.

Indications: Analgesic, antipyretic, anti-inflammatory. For the temporary relief of headache; painful discomfort and fever of colds; muscular aches and pains; temporary relief of minor pains of arthritis; toothache, and pain following dental procedures; menstrual pain.

Directions: The following dosages are those provided in the packaging, as appropriate for self-medication. Larger or more frequent dosage may be necessary as appropriate to the condition or needs of the patient. The hydroxypropyl methylcellulose coating makes Genuine Bayer Aspirin particularly appropriate for those who have difficulty in swallowing uncoated tablets and caplets.
Usual Adult Dose: Adults and Children 12 years and over One or two tablets/caplets with water. May be repeated every four hours as necessary up to 12 tablets/caplets a day or as directed by a doctor. Do not give to children under 12 unless directed by a doctor.

Warnings: Children and teenagers should not use this medicine for chicken pox or flu symptoms before a doctor is consulted about Reye syndrome, a rare but serious illness reported to be associated with aspirin. Do not take this product for pain for more than 10 days or for fever for more than 3 days unless directed by a doctor. If pain or fever persists or gets worse, if new symptoms occur, or if redness or swelling is present consult a doctor because these could be signs of a serious condition. Do not take this product if you are allergic to aspirin, have asthma, stomach problems that persist or recur, gastric ulcers or bleeding problems unless directed by a doctor. If ringing in the ears or loss of hearing occurs, consult a doctor before taking any more of this product. Keep this and all drugs out of the reach of children. In case of accidental overdose, seek professional assistance or contact a poison control center immediately. As with any drug, if you are pregnant or nursing a baby, seek the advice of a health professional before using this product. **IT IS ESPECIALLY IMPORTANT NOT TO USE ASPIRIN DURING THE LAST 3 MONTHS OF PREGNANCY UNLESS SPECIFICALLY DIRECTED TO DO SO BY A DOCTOR BECAUSE IT MAY CAUSE PROBLEMS IN THE UNBORN CHILD OR COMPLICATIONS DURING DELIVERY.**

Drug Interaction Precaution: Do not take this product if you are taking a prescription drug for anticoagulation (thinning the blood), diabetes, gout, or arthritis unless directed by doctor.

Professional Labeling:
ANTIARTHRITIC EFFECT
Indication: Conditions requiring chronic or long-term aspirin therapy for pain and/or inflammation, e.g., rheumatoid arthritis, juvenile rheumatoid arthritis, systemic lupus erythematosus, osteoarthritis (degenerative joint disease), ankylosing spondylitis, psoriatic arthritis, Reiter's syndrome, and fibrositis.

ANTIPLATELET EFFECT
In MI Prophylaxis:
Indication: Aspirin is indicated to reduce the risk of death and/or nonfatal myocardial infarction in patients with a previous infarction or unstable angina pectoris.
Clinical Trials: The indication is supported by the results of six large randomized, multicenter, placebo-controlled studies[1-7] involving 10,816 predominantly male post-myocardial infarction (MI) patients and one randomized placebo-controlled study of 1,266 men with unstable angina. Therapy with aspirin was begun at intervals after the onset of acute MI varying from less than three days to more than five years and continuing for periods of from less than one year to four years. In the unstable angina study, treatment was started within one month after the onset of unstable angina and continued for 12 weeks, and complicating conditions, such as congestive heart failure, were not included in the study.
Aspirin therapy in MI patients was associated with about a 20% reduction in the risk of subsequent death and/or nonfatal reinfarction, a median absolute decrease of 3% from the 12% to 22% event rates in the placebo groups. In the aspirin-treated unstable angina patients, the reduction in risk was about 50%, a reduction in the event rate of 5% from the 10% rate in the placebo group over the 12 weeks of study.
Daily dosage of aspirin in the post-myocardial infarction studies was 300 mg in one study and 900–1,500 mg in five studies. A dose of 325 mg was used in the study of unstable angina.
Adverse Reactions: Gastrointestinal reactions: Doses of 1,000 mg per day of aspirin caused gastrointestinal symptoms and bleeding that, in some cases, were clinically significant. In the largest postinfarction study (the Aspirin Myocardial Infarction Study [AMIS] with 4,500 people), the percentage of incidences of gastrointestinal symptoms for the aspirin (1,000 mg of a standard, solid-tablet formulation) and placebo-treated subjects, respectively, were stomach pain (14.5%, 4.4%), heartburn (11.9%, 4.8%), nausea and/or vomiting (7.6%, 2.1%), hospitalization for GI disorder (4.9%, 3.5%). In the AMIS and other trials, aspirin-treated patients had increased rates of gross gastrointestinal bleeding. Symptoms and signs of gastrointestinal irritation were not significantly increased in subjects treated for unstable angina with buffered aspirin in solution.
Cardiovascular and Biochemical: In the AMIS trial, the dosage of 1,000 mg per day of aspirin was associated with small increases in systolic blood pressure (BP) (average 1.5 to 2.1 mm) and diastolic BP (0.5 to 0.6 mm), depending upon whether maximal or last available readings were used. Blood urea nitrogen and uric acid levels were also increased but by less than 1.0 mg percent.

Subjects with marked hypertension or renal insufficiency had been excluded from the trial so that the clinical importance of these observations for such subjects or for any subjects treated over more prolonged periods is not known. It is recommended that patients placed on long-term aspirin treatment, even at doses of 300 mg per day, be seen at regular intervals to assess changes in these measurements.

Dosage and Administration: Although most of the studies used dosages exceeding 300 mg, two trials used only 300 mg daily and pharmacologic data indicate that this dose inhibits platelet function fully. Therefore, 300 mg or a conventional 325 mg aspirin dose daily is a reasonable routine dose that would minimize gastrointestinal adverse reactions. This use of aspirin applies to both solid oral dosage forms (buffered and plain aspirin) and buffered aspirin in solution.

In Transient Ischemic Attacks:
Indication: Aspririn is indicated for reducing the risk of recurrent transient ischemic attacks (TIAs) or stroke in men who have transient ischemia of the brain due to fibrin emboli. There is no evidence that aspirin is effective in reducing TIAs in women, or is of benefit in the treatment of completed strokes in men or women.

Clinical Trials: The indication is supported by the results of a Canadian study[8] in which 585 patients with threatened stroke were followed in a randomized clinical trial for an average of 28 months to determine whether aspirin or sulfinpyrazone, singly or in combination, was superior to placebo in preventing transient ischemic attacks, stroke, or death. The study showed that, although sulfinpyrazone had no statistically significant effect, aspirin reduced the risk of continuing transient ischemic attacks, stroke, or death by 19 percent and reduced the risk of stroke or death by 31 percent. Another aspirin study carried out in the United States with 178 patients showed a statistically significant number of "favorable outcomes," including reduced transient ischemic attacks, stroke, and death.[9]

Precautions: Patients presenting with signs and/or symptoms of TIAs should have a complete medical and neurologic evaluation. Consideration should be given to other disorders which may resemble TIAs. It is important to evaluate and treat, if appropriate, diseases associated with TIAs and stroke, such as hypertension and diabetes.
Concurrent administration of absorbable antacids at therapeutic doses may increase the clearance of salicylates in some individuals. The concurrent administration of nonabsorbable antacids may alter the rate of absorption of aspirin, thereby resulting in a decreased acetylsalicylic acid/salicylate ratio in plasma. The clinical significance of these decreases in available aspirin is unknown. Aspirin at dosages of 1,000 milligrams per day has been associated with small increases in blood pressure, blood urea nitrogen, and serum uric acid levels. It is recommended that patients placed on long-term aspirin treatment be seen at regular intervals to assess changes in these measurements.

Adverse Reactions: At dosages of 1,000 milligrams or higher of aspirin per day, gastrointestinal side effects include stomach pain, heartburn, nausea and/or vomiting, as well as increased rates of gross gastrointestinal bleeding.

Dosage and Administration: Adult oral dosage for men is 1,300 milligrams a day, in divided doses of 650 milligrams twice a day or 325 milligrams four times a day.

References: 1. Elwood PC, et al: A randomized controlled trial of acetylsalicylic acid in the secondary prevention of mortality from myocardial infarction. *Br Med J* 1974;1:436–440. 2. The Coronary Drug Project Research Group: Aspirin in coronary heart disease. *J Chronic Dis* 1976;29:625–642. 3. Breddin K, et al: Secondary prevention of myocardial infarction: A comparison of acetylsalicylic acid, phenprocoumon or placebo. *Homeostasis* 1979;470:263–268. 4. Aspirin Myocardial Infarction Study Research Group: A randomized, controlled trial of aspirin in persons recovered from myocardial infarction. *JAMA* 1980;245:661–669. 5. Elwood PC, Sweetnam PM: Aspirin and secondary mortality after myocardial infarction. *Lancet*, December 22–29, 1979, pp 1313–1315. 6. The Persantine-Aspirin Reinfarction Study Research Group: Persantine and aspirin in coronary heart disease. *Circulation* 1980;62:449–460. 7. Lewis, HD, et al: Protective effects of aspirin against acute myocardial infarction and death in men with unstable angina: Results of a Veterans Administration Cooperative Study. *N Engl J Med* 1983;309:396–403. 8. The Canadian Cooperative Study Group: A randomized trial of aspirin and sulfinpyrazone in threatened stroke. *N Engl J Med* 1978;299:53–59. 9. Fields WS, et al: Controlled trial of aspirin in cerebral ischemia. *Stroke* 1977;8:301–316.

How Supplied:
Genuine Bayer Aspirin 325 mg (5 grains) is supplied in packs of 12 tablets, bottles of 24, 50, 100, 200, 300, and 365 tablets, and bottles of 50 and 100 caplets. Child-resistant safety closures on 12s, 24s, 50s, 200s, 300s, 365s tablets and 50s caplets. Bottles of 100s tablets and caplets available without safety closure for households without small children.
Shown in Product Identification Guide, page 504

BUGS BUNNY™ Children's Chewable Vitamins Plus Iron (Sugar Free)
FLINTSTONES® Children's Chewable Vitamins
FLINTSTONES® Children's Chewable Vitamins Plus Iron

Vitamin Ingredients: Each multivitamin supplement with iron contains the ingredients listed in the chart below:

BUGS BUNNY™ Children's Chewable Vitamins Plus Iron (Sugar Free)
FLINTSTONES® Children's Chewable Vitamins Plus Iron

Vitamins	Quantity per Tablet	% Daily Value for Children 2–4 Years of Age	% Daily Value for Adults/ Children 4 or More Years of Age
Vitamin A 50% as Beta Carotene	2500 I.U.	100%	50%
Vitamin C	60 mg	150%	100%
Vitamin D	400 I.U.	100%	100%
Vitamin E	15 I.U.	150%	50%
Thiamin	1.05 mg	150%	70%
Riboflavin	1.2 mg	150%	70%
Niacin	13.5 mg	150%	67%
Vitamin B_6	1.05 mg	150%	52%
Folate	300 mcg	150%	75%
Vitamin B_{12}	4.5 mcg.	150%	75%
Iron (Elemental)	15 mg	150%	83%

FLINTSTONES® Children's Chewable Vitamins provide the same quantities of vitamins, but do not provide iron.

Indication: Dietary supplementation.

Dosage and Administration: One chewable tablet daily. For adults and children two years and older; tablet must be chewed.

Warning For Bugs Bunny Only: Phenylketonurics: Contains Phenylalanine.

Precaution:
IRON SUPPLEMENTS ONLY.
Close tightly and keep out of reach of children. Contains iron, which can be harmful or fatal to children in large doses. In case of accidental overdose, seek professional assistance or contact a Poison Control Center immediately.

Continued on next page

Bayer—Cont.

How Supplied: Flintstones are supplied in bottles of 60 and 100, Bugs Bunny in bottles of 60 with child-resistant caps.

Shown in Product Identification Guide, page 504 and 505

DAIRY EASE® Real Milk
Lactose Reduced Milk

Dairy Ease is also available in Real Milk which is 70% lactose reduced and contains vitamins A & D. A one quart size in three varieties is available: Nonfat, 1% lowfat, and 2% lowfat. Dairy Ease Real Milk can be used for cooking, on cereal or directly from the carton.

DOMEBORO® Astringent Solution (Powder Packets)
DOMEBORO® Astringent Solution (Effervescent Tablets)

Active Ingredients: When dissolved in water, the active ingredient is aluminum acetate resulting from the reaction of calcium acetate (938 mg) and aluminum sulfate (1191 mg) for powder packets, and calcium acetate (604 mg) and aluminum sulfate (878 mg) for the effervescent tablets. The resulting astringent solution is buffered to an acid pH.

Inactive Ingredients: DOMEBORO Astringent Solution (Powder Packets) Dextrin
DOMEBORO Astringent Solution (Effervescent Tablets) Dextrin, Polyethylene Glycol, Sodium Bicarbonate

Directions: For powder packets dissolve 1 or 2 packets, or for effervescent tablets 1 or 2 tablets in water and stir the solution until fully dissolved. Do not strain or filter the solution. Can be used as a compress, wet dressing or as a soak. AS A COMPRESS OR WET DRESSING: Saturate a clean, soft, white cloth (such as a diaper or torn sheet) in the solution; gently squeeze and apply loosely to the affected area. Saturate the cloth in the solution every 15 to 30 minutes and apply to the affected area. Discard solution after each use. Repeat as often as necessary. AS A SOAK: Soak affected area in the solution for 15 to 30 minutes. Discard solution after each use. Repeat 3 times a day.

Indications: For temporary relief of minor skin irritations due to poison ivy, poison oak, poison sumac, insect bites, athlete's foot or rashes caused by soaps, detergents, cosmetics or jewelry.

Warnings: If condition worsens or symptoms persist for more than 7 days discontinue use of the product and consult a doctor. For external use only. Avoid contact with eyes. Do not cover compress or wet dressing with plastic to prevent evaporation. Keep this and all drugs out of the reach of children. In case of accidental ingestion, seek professional assistance or contact a Poison Control Center immediately.

How Supplied: Boxes of 12 or 100 effervescent tablets or powder packets.

Shown in Product Identification Guide, page 504

FLINTSTONES® COMPLETE
With Iron, Calcium & Minerals Children's Chewable Vitamins

BUGS BUNNY™ COMPLETE
Children's Chewable Vitamins + Minerals With Iron and Calcium (Sugar Free)

Ingredients: Each supplement provides the ingredients listed in the chart below:

FLINTSTONES® COMPLETE
Children's Chewable Vitamins
BUGS BUNNY™ COMPLETE
Children's Chewable Vitamins + Minerals (Sugar Free)

Vitamins	Quantity per Tablet	% Daily Value for Children 2–4 Years of Age	Adults/Children 4 or More Years of Age
Vitamin A	5000 I.U. 50% as Beta Carotene	100%	100%
Vitamin C	60 mg	75%	100%
Vitamin D	400 I.U.	50%	100%
Vitamin E	30 I.U.	150%	100%
Thiamin	1.5 mg	107%	100%
Riboflavin	1.7 mg	106%	100%
Niacin	20 mg	111%	100%
Vitamin B₆	2 mg	143%	100%
Folate	400 mcg	100%	100%
Vitamin B₁₂	6 mcg	100%	100%
Biotin	40 mcg	13%	13%
Pantothenic Acid	10 mg	100%	100%
Calcium	100 mg	6%	10%
Iron (Elemental)	18 mg	90%	100%
Phosphorus	100 mg	6%	10%
Iodine	150 mcg	107%	100%
Magnesium	20 mg	5%	5%
Zinc	15 mg	94%	100%
Copper	2 mg	100%	100%

Indication: Dietary Supplementation.

Dosage and Administration: 2–4 years of age: Chew one-half tablet daily. Over 4 years of age: Chew one tablet daily.

Warning for Bugs Bunny only: Phenylketonurics: Contains Phenylalanine.

Precaution: Close tightly and keep out of reach of children. Contains iron, which can be harmful or fatal to children in large doses. In case of accidental overdose, seek professional assistance or contact a Poison Control Center immediately.

How Supplied: Bottles of 60's with child-resistant caps.

Shown in Product Identification Guide, page 504 and 505

FLINTSTONES® PLUS CALCIUM
with Beta Carotene
Children's Chewable Vitamins

Ingredients: Calcium Carbonate, Sorbitol, Starch, Sodium Ascorbate, Gelatin, Stearic Acid, Magnesium Stearate, Natural and Artificial Flavors. Vitamin E Acetate, Artificial Colors (including Yellow 6), Silica, Glycerides of Stearic and Palmitic Acids, Malic Acid, Aspartame* (a sweetener), Pyridoxine Hydrochloride, Riboflavin, Thiamine Mononitrate, Vitamin A Acetate, Beta Carotene, Monoammonium Glycyrrhizinate, Folic Acid, Vitamin D, Vitamin B12.
*****Phenylketonurics: Contains Phenylalanine**

CHEW ONE TABLET DAILY

One Tablet Daily Provides: Vitamins	Quantity Per Tablet	Percent U.S. RDA For Children 2 to 4 Years of Age	For Adults and Children Over 4 Years of Age
Vitamin A (as Acetate and Beta Carotene)	2500 I.U.	100	50
Vitamin D	400 I.U.	100	100
Vitamin E	15 I.U.	150	50
Vitamin C	60 mg	150	100
Folic Acid	0.3 mg	150	75
Thiamine	1.05 mg	150	70
Riboflavin	1.20 mg	150	70

Niacin	13.50 mg	150	67
Vitamin B-6	1.05 mg	150	52
Vitamin B-12	4.5 mcg	150	75

Minerals	Quantity	Percent U.S. RDA	
Calcium	200 mg	25	20

FOR ADULTS AND CHILDREN 2 YEARS AND OLDER; TABLET MUST BE CHEWED

KEEP OUT OF REACH OF CHILDREN.

Do not use this product if safety seal bearing Miles logo under cap is torn or missing.
Child Resistant Cap

How Supplied: Bottle of 60 Tablets
Shown in Product Identification Guide, page 505

FLINTSTONES® Plus Extra C
Children's Chewable Vitamins
BUGS BUNNY™ With Extra C
Children's Chewable Vitamins
(Sugar Free)

Vitamin Ingredients: Each multivitamin supplement contains the ingredients listed in the chart below:

BUGS BUNNY™ With Extra C
Children's Chewable Vitamins
(Sugar Free)
FLINTSTONES® Plus Extra C
Children's Chewable Vitamins

Vitamins	Quantity per Tablet	% Daily Value for Children 2–4 Years of Age	Adults/ Children 4 or More Years of Age
Vitamin A 50% as Beta Carotene	2500 I.U.	100%	50%
Vitamin C	60 mg	150%	100%
Vitamin D	400 I.U.	100%	100%
Vitamin E	15 I.U.	150%	50%
Thiamin	1.05 mg	150%	70%
Riboflavin	1.2 mg	150%	70%
Niacin	13.5 mg	150%	67%
Vitamin B_6	1.05 mg	150%	52%
Folate	300 mcg	150%	75%
Vitamin B_{12}	4.5 mcg	150%	75%
Iron (Elemental)	15 mg	150%	83%

Indication: Dietary supplementation.

Dosage and Administration: One tablet daily for adults and children two years and older; tablet must be chewed.

Warning For Bugs Bunny Only: Phenylketonurics: Contains Phenylalanine.

How Supplied: Flintstones in bottles of 60's & 100's, Bugs Bunny in bottles of 60 with child-resistant caps.
Shown in Product Identification Guide, page 504 and 505

Maximum Strength
MIDOL® Teen
Menstrual Formula
Multi-Symptom Formula

Active Ingredients: Each caplet contains Acetaminophen 500 mg and Pamabrom 25 mg.

Inactive Ingredients: Croscarmellose Sodium, D&C Red #7 Lake, FD&C Blue #2 Lake, Hydroxpropyl Methylcellulose, Magnesium Stearate, Microcrystaline Cellulose, Starch, Titanium Dioxide and Triacetin.

Indications: Relieves cramps, bloating, water-weight gain, headaches, backaches and muscular aches and pains.
● Provides effective relief of painful menstrual symptoms so you can get on with your life.
● Contains a special combination of safe, aspirin-free, caffeine-free ingredients which is not found in any ordinary pain reliever.
● Non-drowsy formula won't slow you down!

Directions: Adults and children 12 years and over: Take 2 caplets with water. Repeat every 4–6 hours, as needed, up to a maximum of 8 caplets per day. Under age 12: Consult your doctor.

Warnings: Do not use for more than 10 days unless directed by a doctor. If pain persists for more than 10 days, consult a doctor immediately. Keep this and all drugs out of reach of children. In case of accidental overdose, immediate medical attention is essential for adults as well as for children even if you do not notice any signs or symptoms. As with any drug, if you are pregnant or nursing a baby, seek the advice of a health professional before using this product.

How Supplied: White capsule-shaped caplets available in packages of 2 blisters of 8 caplets each and bottles of 32 caplets. Child-resistant safety closure on bottles of 32 caplets.
Shown in Product Identification Guide, page 505

Maximum Strength
Multi-Symptom Formula
MIDOL®
Menstrual Formula

Active Ingredients: Each caplet or gelcap contains Acetaminophen 500 mg, Caffeine 60 mg and Pyrilamine Maleate 15 mg.

Inactive Ingredients: Caplets—Croscarmellose Sodium, FD&C Blue #2, Hydroxypropyl Methylcellulose, Magnesium Stearate, Microcrystalline Cellulose, Pregelatinized Starch and Triacetin.
Gelcaps—Croscarmellose Sodium, D&C Red #33 Lake, EDTA Sodium, FD&C Blue #1 Lake, Gelatin, Glycerin, Hydroxypropyl Methylcellulose, Iron Oxide, Magnesium Stearate, Microcrystalline Cellulose, Starch, Stearic Acid, Titanium Dioxide, Triacetin.

Indications: Relieves all of these physical menstrual symptoms: cramps, bloating, water-weight gain, headaches, backaches, muscular aches and fatigue.
● Provides maximum strength relief of painful physical symptoms suffered during your menstrual cycle.
● Contains a combination of maximum strength, aspirin-free ingredients which is not found in any ordinary pain reliever.

Directions: Adults and children 12 years and over: Take 2 caplets with water. Repeat every 4–6 hours, as needed, up to a maximum of 8 caplets per day. Under age 12: Consult your doctor.

Warnings: Do not use for more than 10 days unless directed by a doctor. If pain persists for more than 10 days, consult a doctor immediately. May cause drowsiness; alcohol, sedatives or tranquilizers may increase drowsiness. Avoid alcoholic beverages while taking this product. Do not take this product if you are taking sedatives or tranquilizers without first consulting your doctor. Use caution when driving or operating machinery. May cause excitability, especially in children. The recommended dose of this product contains about as much caffeine as a cup of coffee. Limit the use of caffeine-containing medications, foods, or beverages while taking this product because too much caffeine may cause nervousness, irritability, sleeplessness, and occasionally, rapid heartbeat. Do not take this product, unless diected by a doctor, if you have a breathing problem such as emphysema or chronic bronchitis or if you have glaucoma or difficulty in urination due to enlargement of the prostate gland. Keep this and all drugs out of reach of children. In case of accidental overdose, immediate medical attention is essential for adults as well as for children even if you do not notice any signs or symptoms. As with any drug, if you are pregnant or nursing a baby, seek the advice of a health professional before using this product.

How Supplied: Caplets—White capsule-shaped caplets available in bottles of 8 and 32 caplets, and packages of 2 blisters of 8 caplets each. Child-resistant safety closures on bottles of 8 and 32 caplets.

Continued on next page

Bayer—Cont.

Gelcaps—Dark/light blue capsule-shaped gelcaps available in bottles of 24 gelcaps and packages of 2 blisters of 6 gelcaps each. Child-resistant safety closure on bottle of 24 gelcaps.

Shown in Product Identification Guide, page 505

Multi-Symptom Formula
PMS Formula
MIDOL®
Premenstrual Symptom Relief

Active Ingredients: Each caplet or gelcap contains Acetaminophen 500 mg, Pamabrom 25 mg and Pyrilamine Maleate 15 mg.

Inactive Ingredients: Caplets—Croscarmellose Sodium, D&C Red #30, D&C Yellow #10, Hydroxypropyl Methylcellulose, Magnesium Stearate, Microcrystalline Cellulose, Pregelatinized Starch and Triacetin.
Gelcaps—Croscarmellose Sodium, D&C Red #27 Lake, EDTA Disodium, FD&C Blue #1, FD&C Red #40 Lake, Gelatin, Glycerin, Hydroxypropyl Methylcellulose, Iron Oxide, Magnesium Stearate, Microcrystalline Cellulose, Starch, Stearic Acid, Titanium Dioxide, Triacetin.

Indications: Contains maximum strength medication for all these premenstrual symptoms: bloating, water-weight gain, cramps, headaches and backaches.
• Provides maximum strength relief of the physical symptoms of Premenstrual Syndrome so you can feel like yourself again.
• Contains a combination of aspirin-free ingredients which is not found in any ordinary pain reliever: a diuretic to alleviate water retention and an analgesic for pain.

Directions: Adults and children 12 years and over: Take 2 caplets with water. Repeat every 4–6 hours, as needed, up to a maximum of 8 caplets per day. Under age 12: Consult your doctor.

Warnings: Do not use for more than 10 days unless directed by doctor. If pain persists for more than 10 days, consult a doctor immediately. May cause drowsiness; alcohol, sedatives and tranquilizers may increase drowsiness. Avoid alcoholic beverages while taking this product. Do not take this product if you are taking sedatives or tranquilizers without first consulting your doctor. Use caution when driving or operating machinery. May cause excitability especially in children. Do not take this product, unless directed by a doctor, if you have a breathing problem such as emphysema or chronic bronchitis or if you have glaucoma or difficulty in urination due to enlargement of the prostate gland. Keep this and all drugs out of the reach of children. In case of accidental overdose, immediate medical attention is essential for adults as well as for children even if you do not notice any signs or symptoms. As with any drug, if you are pregnant or nursing a baby, seek the advice of a health professional before using this product.

How Supplied: Caplets—White capsule-shaped caplets available in packages of 2 blisters of 8 caplets each and bottles of 32 caplets. Child-resistant safety closure on bottles of 32 caplets. Gelcaps—Dark/light pink capsule-shaped gelcaps available in bottles of 24 gelcaps and packages of 2 blisters of 6 gelcaps each. Child-resistant safety closure on bottle of 24 gelcaps.

Shown in Product Identification Guide, page 505

MYCELEX® OTC CREAM ANTIFUNGAL

Active Ingredient: Clotrimazole 1%

Inactive Ingredients: Benzyl alcohol (1%) as a preservative, cetostearyl alcohol, cetyl esters wax, octyldodecanol, polysorbate 60, purified water, sorbitan monostearate.
Store between 2°–30°C (36°–86°F).

Indications: Cures athlete's foot (tinea pedis), jock itch (tinea cruris), and ringworm (tinea corporis). For effective relief of the itching, cracking, burning and discomfort which can accompany these conditions.

Warnings: For external use only. Do not use on children under 2 years of age except under the advice and supervision of a doctor. If irritation occurs or if there is no improvement within 4 weeks (for athlete's foot or ringworm) or within 2 weeks (for jock itch) discontinue use and consult a doctor or pharmacist. Keep this and all drugs out of the reach of children. In case of accidental ingestion seek professional assistance or contact a Poison Control Center immediately. Use only as directed.

Directions: Cleanse skin with soap and water and dry thoroughly. Apply a thin layer and gently massage over affected area morning and evening or as directed by a doctor. For athlete's foot, pay special attention to the spaces between the toes. It is also helpful to wear well-fitting, ventilated shoes and to change shoes and socks at least once daily. Best results in athlete's foot and ringworm are usually obtained with 4 weeks' use of this product and in jock itch with 2 weeks' use. If satisfactory results have not occurred within these times, consult a doctor or pharmacist. Children under 12 years of age should be supervised in the use of this product. This product is not effective on the scalp or nails.

FOR BEST RESULTS, FOLLOW DIRECTIONS AND CONTINUE TREATMENT FOR LENGTH OF TIME INDICATED.

How Supplied: Cream Tube 15 g (½ oz.)

MYCELEX-7®
VAGINAL CREAM ANTIFUNGAL

Active Ingredient: Clotrimazole 1%

Inactive Ingredients: Benzyl alcohol, cetostearyl alcohol, cetyl esters wax, octyldodecanol, polysorbate 60, purified water, sorbitan monostearate

Indications: For treatment of vaginal yeast (Candida) infection.

Actions: Cures most vaginal yeast infections. MYCELEX®-7 Antifungal Vaginal Cream can kill the yeast that may cause vaginal infection. It is greaseless and does not stain clothes.

Precautions: IF THIS IS THE **FIRST** TIME YOU HAVE HAD VAGINAL ITCH AND DISCOMFORT, CONSULT YOUR DOCTOR. IF YOU HAVE HAD A DOCTOR DIAGNOSE A VAGINAL YEAST INFECTION BEFORE AND HAVE THE SAME SYMPTOMS NOW, USE THIS CREAM AS DIRECTED FOR 7 CONSECUTIVE DAYS.

WARNING: DO NOT USE IF YOU HAVE ABDOMINAL PAIN, FEVER, OR FOUL-SMELLING DISCHARGE. CONTACT YOUR DOCTOR IMMEDIATELY.
IF YOU DO NOT IMPROVE IN 3 DAYS OR IF YOU DO NOT GET WELL IN 7 DAYS, YOU MAY HAVE A CONDITION OTHER THAN A YEAST INFECTION. CONSULT YOUR DOCTOR. If your symptoms return within two months or if you have infections that do not clear up easily with proper treatment, consult your doctor. You could be pregnant or there could be a serious underlying medical cause for your infections, including diabetes or a damaged immune system (including damage from infection with HIV-the virus that causes AIDS). (PLEASE READ PATIENT PACKAGE PAMPHLET.)
Do not use during pregnancy except under the advice and supervision of a doctor. Do not use tampons while using this medication. Keep this and all drugs out of the reach of children. In case of accidental ingestion, seek professional assistance or contact a Poison Control Center immediately. NOT FOR USE IN CHILDREN LESS THAN 12 YEARS OF AGE.

Dosage and Administration: Before using, read the enclosed pamphlet.
Directions: Fill the applicator and insert one applicatorful of cream into the vagina, preferably at bedtime. Repeat this procedure daily for 7 consecutive days.

How Supplied: 1.5 oz. (45 g) tube and applicator. (7-Day Therapy)

Shown in Product Identification Guide, page 505

MYCELEX-7 VAGINAL ANTIFUNGAL CREAM WITH 7 DISPOSABLE APPLICATORS

Description: MYCELEX®-7 Antifungal Vaginal Cream can kill the yeast that may cause vaginal infection. It is greaseless and does not stain clothes.

Indications: For treatment of vaginal yeast (Candida) infection.
IF THIS IS THE FIRST TIME YOU HAVE HAD VAGINAL ITCH AND DISCOMFORT, CONSULT YOUR DOCTOR. IF YOU HAVE HAD A DOCTOR DIAGNOSE A VAGINAL YEAST INFECTION BEFORE AND HAVE THE SAME SYMPTOMS NOW, USE THIS CREAM AS DIRECTED FOR 7 CONSECUTIVE DAYS.

WARNING: DO NOT USE IF YOU HAVE ABDOMINAL PAIN, FEVER, OR FOUL-SMELLING DISCHARGE. CONTACT YOUR DOCTOR IMMEDIATELY.

Before using, read the enclosed pamphlet.
Directions: Fill the applicator and insert one applicatorful of cream into the vagina, preferably at bedtime. Dispose of each applicator after use. Do not flush in toilet. Repeat this procedure daily with a new applicator for 7 consecutive days.

WARNING: IF YOU DO NOT IMPROVE IN 3 DAYS OR IF YOU DO NOT GET WELL IN 7 DAYS, YOU MAY HAVE A CONDITION OTHER THAN A YEAST INFECTION. CONSULT YOUR DOCTOR. If your symptoms return within two months or if you have infections that do not clear up easily with proper treatment, consult your doctor. You could be pregnant or there could be a serious underlying medical cause for your infections, including diabetes or a damaged immune system (including damage from infection with HIV—the virus that causes AIDS). (PLEASE READ PATIENT PACKAGE PAMPHLET.)
Do not use during pregnancy except under the advice and supervision of a doctor. Do not use tampons while using this medication. Keep this and all drugs out of the reach of children.
In case of accidental ingestion, seek professional assistance or contact a Poison Control Center immediately. NOT FOR USE IN CHILDREN LESS THAN 12 YEARS OF AGE.

If you have any questions about MYCELEX®-7 or vaginal yeast infection, contact your physician.
Store at room temperature between 2° and 30°C (36° and 86°F).
See end panel of carton and tube crimp for lot number and expiration date.

Active Ingredient: Clotrimazole 1%.

Inactive Ingredients: Benzyl alcohol, cetostearyl alcohol, cetyl esters wax, octyldodecanol, polysorbate 60, purified water, sorbitan monostearate.

How Supplied: One 45g (1.5 oz.) tube of vaginal cream and 7 applicators (7 day therapy)
Consumer Questions or Comments
Call 1-800-800-4793
8:30–5:00 EST M–F
Shown in Product Identification Guide, page 505

MYCELEX-7® VAGINAL INSERTS ANTIFUNGAL

Active Ingredient: Each insert contains 100 mg clotrimazole.

Inactive Ingredients: Corn starch, lactose, magnesium stearate, povidone.

Indications: For treatment of vaginal yeast (Candida) infection.

Actions: Cures most vaginal yeast infections. MYCELEX-7 Antifungal Vaginal Inserts can kill the yeast that may cause vaginal infection. They do not stain clothes.

Precautions: IF THIS IS THE FIRST TIME YOU HAVE HAD VAGINAL ITCH AND DISCOMFORT, CONSULT YOUR DOCTOR. IF YOU HAVE HAD A DOCTOR DIAGNOSE A VAGINAL YEAST INFECTION BEFORE AND HAVE THE SAME SYMPTOMS NOW, USE THESE INSERTS AS DIRECTED FOR 7 CONSECUTIVE DAYS.

WARNING: DO NOT USE IF YOU HAVE ABDOMINAL PAIN, FEVER, OR FOUL-SMELLING DISCHARGE. CONTACT YOUR DOCTOR IMMEDIATELY.
IF YOU DO NOT IMPROVE IN 3 DAYS OR IF YOU DO NOT GET WELL IN 7 DAYS, YOU MAY HAVE A CONDITION OTHER THAN A YEAST INFECTION. CONSULT YOUR DOCTOR. If your symptoms return within two months or if you have infections that do not clear up easily with proper treatment, consult your doctor. You could be pregnant or there could be a serious underlying medical cause for your infections, including diabetes or a damaged immune system (including damage from infection with HIV-the virus that causes AIDS). (PLEASE READ PATIENT PACKAGE PAMPHLET) Do not use during pregnancy except under the advice and supervision of a doctor. Do not use tampons while using this medication. Keep this and all drugs out of the reach of children. In case of accidental ingestion, seek professional assistance or contact a Poison Control Center immediately. NOT FOR USE IN CHILDREN LESS THAN 12 YEARS OF AGE.

Dosage and Administration: Before using, read the enclosed pamphlet.
Directions: Unwrap one insert, place it in the applicator, and use the applicator to place the insert into the vagina, preferably at bedtime. Repeat this procedure daily for 7 consecutive days.

How Supplied: 7 vaginal inserts and applicator. (7-Day Therapy)

MYCELEX-7 Combination-Pack VAGINAL INSERTS & EXTERNAL VULVAR CREAM
- Cures Most Vaginal Yeast Infections
- Relieves Associated External Vulvar Itching and Irritation

MYCELEX®-7 Antifungal Vaginal Inserts and External Vulvar Cream can kill the yeast that may cause vaginal infection. They do not stain clothes.

Indications: For treatment of vaginal yeast (Candida) infection and the relief of external vulvar itching and irritation associated with vaginal yeast infection.
IF THIS IS THE FIRST TIME YOU HAVE HAD VAGINAL OR VULVAR ITCH AND DISCOMFORT, CONSULT YOUR DOCTOR. IF YOU HAVE HAD A DOCTOR DIAGNOSE A VAGINAL YEAST INFECTION BEFORE AND HAVE THE SAME SYMPTOMS NOW, USE THESE INSERTS AND CREAM AS DIRECTED.
WARNING: DO NOT USE IF YOU HAVE ABDOMINAL PAIN, FEVER, OR FOUL-SMELLING DISCHARGE. CONTACT YOUR DOCTOR IMMEDIATELY.
Before using, read the enclosed pamphlet.

Directions:
Inserts: Unwrap one insert, place it in the applicator, and use the applicator to place the insert into the vagina, preferably at bedtime. Repeat this procedure daily for 7 consecutive days to treat vaginal (Candida) yeast infection.
Cream: Squeeze a small amount of cream onto your finger and gently spread the cream onto the irritated area of the vulva. Use once or twice daily for up to 7 days as needed to relieve external vulvar itching. THE CREAM SHOULD NOT BE USED FOR VULVAR ITCHING DUE TO CAUSES OTHER THAN A YEAST INFECTION.
WARNING: IF YOU DO NOT IMPROVE IN 3 DAYS OR IF YOU DO NOT GET WELL IN 7 DAYS, YOU MAY HAVE A CONDITION OTHER THAN A YEAST INFECTION. CONSULT YOUR DOCTOR. If your symptoms return within two months or if you have infections that do not clear up easily with proper treatment, consult your doctor. You could be pregnant or there could be a serious underlying medical cause for your infections, including diabetes or a

Continued on next page

Bayer—Cont.

damaged immune system (including damage from infection with HIV— the virus that causes AIDS). (PLEASE READ ENCLOSED PATIENT PACKAGE PAMPHLET.)

Do not use during pregnancy except under the advice and supervision of a doctor.

Do not use tampons while using this medication.

Keep this and all drugs out of the reach of children. In case of accidental ingestion, seek professional assistance or contact a Poison Control Center immediately.

NOT FOR USE IN CHILDREN LESS THAN 12 YEARS OF AGE.

If you have any questions about MYCE-LEX®-7 Combination-Pack or vaginal yeast infection, contact your physician.

Active Ingredient:
Inserts: Each insert contains 100 mg clotrimazole
Cream: Clotrimazole 1%

Inactive Ingredients:
Inserts: Corn starch, lactose, magnesium stearate, povidone
Cream: Benzyl alcohol, cetostearyl alcohol, cetyl esters wax, octyldodecanol, polysorbate 60, purified water, sorbitan monostearate

How Supplied: 7 vaginal inserts and applicator (7-day therapy) and one 7g. (.25 oz.) tube of external vulvar cream. **Store at room temperature between 2° and 30°C (36° and 86°F).**
See end panel of carton, foil wrappers and tube crimp for lot number and expiration date.
Consumer Questions or Comments call 1-800-800-4793
8:30–5:00 EST M-F
Shown in Product Identification Guide, page 505

NEO-SYNEPHRINE®
Pediatric Formula, Mild Formula, Regular Strength, and Extra Strength.

Description: This line of Nasal Sprays, Drops and Spray Pumps contains Phenylephrine Hydrochloride in strengths ranging from 0.125% (drops only) to 1%. Also contains: Benzalkonium Chloride and Thimerosal 0.001% as preservatives, Citric Acid, Purified Water, Sodium Chloride, Sodium Citrate.

Action: Rapid-acting nasal decongestant.

Directions: For a 0.125% solution: Children 2 to under 6 years of age (with adult supervision): 2 or 3 drops or sprays in each nostril not more often than every 4 hours. **Use only recommended amount.** Children under 2 years of age: consult a doctor.
For a 0.25% solution (Mild):
Adults and children 6 to under 12 years of age (with adult supervision): 2 or 3

drops or sprays in each nostril not more often than every 4 hours. Children under 6 years of age: consult a doctor.
For a 0.5% solution (Regular):
Adults and children 12 years of age and over: 2 or 3 drops or sprays in each nostril not more often than every 4 hours. Do not give to children under 12 years of age unless directed by a doctor.
For a 1% solution (Extra):
Adults and children 12 years of age and over: 2 or 3 drops or sprays in each nostril not more often than every 4 hours. Do not give to children under 12 years of age unless directed by a doctor.

Indications: For temporary relief of nasal congestion due to common cold, hay fever, sinusitis, or other upper respiratory allergies.

Warnings: For adults:
Do not exceed recommended dosage. This product may cause temporary discomfort such as burning, stinging, sneezing, or an increase in nasal discharge. The use of this container by more than one person may spread infection. Do not use this product for more than 3 days. Use only as directed. Frequent or prolonged use may cause nasal congestion to recur or worsen. If symptoms persist, consult a doctor. Do not use this product if you have heart disease, high blood pressure, thyroid disease, diabetes, or difficulty in urination due to enlargement of the prostate gland unless directed by a doctor.
For children under 12 years of age:
Do not exceed recommended dosage. This product may cause temporary discomfort such as burning, stinging, sneezing, or an increase in nasal discharge. The use if this container by more than one person may spread infection. Do not use this product for more than 3 days. Use only as directed. Frequent or prolonged use may cause nasal congestion to recur or worsen. If symptoms persist, consult a doctor. Do not use this product in a child who has heart disease, high blood pressure, thyroid disease, or diabetes unless directed by a doctor.
Prolonged exposure to air or strong light will cause oxidation and some loss of potency.
Keep these and all drugs out of the reach of children. In case of accidental ingestion seek professional assistance or contact a poison control center immediately. Do not use if brown in color or contains a precipitate.

How Supplied: Pediatric Formula (0.125%) in 15 mL drops. Mild Formula (0.25%) in 15 mL drops and spray. Regular Strength (0.5%) in 15 mL drops and spray. Extra Strength (1.0%) in 15 mL drops and spray.
Shown in Product Identification Guide, page 505

NEO-SYNEPHRINE®
Maximum Strength 12 Hour (nasal spray and spray pump)
Maximum Strength 12 Hour Extra Moisturizing (nasal spray)

Active Ingredient: Oxymetazoline Hydrochloride 0.05%.

Inactive Ingredients: Benzalkonium Chloride and Phenylmercuric Acetate 0.002% as preservatives, Glycine, Purified Water, Sorbitol.

Indications: For temporary relief, up to 12 HOURS, of nasal congestion due to a cold, hay fever, or other upper respiratory allergies or associated with sinusitis. Temporarily relieves stuffy nose. Temporarily restores freer breathing through the nose. Helps decongest sinus openings and passages; temporarily relieves sinus congestion and pressure.

Directions: Adults and children 6 to under 12 years of age (with adult supervision): 2 or 3 sprays in each nostril not more often than every 10 to 12 hours. Do not exceed 2 doses in any 24-hour period. Children under 6 years of age: consult a doctor.

Warnings: Do not exceed recommended dosage. This product may cause temporary discomfort such as burning, stinging, sneezing, or an increase in nasal discharge. The use of the container by more than one person may spread infection. Do not use this product for more than 3 days. Use only as directed. Frequent or prolonged use may cause nasal congestion to recur or worsen. If symptoms persist, consult a doctor. Do not use this product if you have heart disease, high blood pressure, thyroid disease, diabetes, or difficulty in urination due to enlargement of the prostate gland unless directed by a doctor. Keep this and all drugs out of the reach of children. In case of accidental ingestion, seek professional assistance or contact a Poison Control Center immediately. As with any drug, if you are pregnant or nursing a baby, seek the advice of a health professional before using this product.

How Supplied: *Nasal Spray Maximum Strength* — plastic squeeze bottles of 15 ml (½ fl. oz.); *Nasal Spray Pump* —15 ml bottle (½ fl. oz.). Maximum Strength 12 Hour Extra Moisturizing Nasal Spray — 15 ml (½ fl. oz.).
Shown in Product Identification Guide, page 505

ONE-A-DAY® 55 PLUS

Description: *ONE-A-DAY 55 Plus is specially formulated for mature adults with more Vitamin C, B-1, B-2, B-6, and E. ONE-A-DAY continues to apply the latest and best nutritional knowledge to help keep nutrition understandable and help protect your health. Trust ONE-A-DAY to be your partner in nutrition.*
MULTIVITAMIN/MULTIMINERAL SUPPLEMENT

Directions For Use: Adults take one tablet daily with food.

VITAMINS	QUANTITY	% U.S. RDA
Vitamin A (as Acetate) and Beta Carotene	6000 I.U.	120
Vitamin C	120 mg	200
Thiamine (B-1)	4.5 mg	300
Riboflavin (B-2)	3.4 mg	200
Niacin	20 mg	100
Vitamin D	400 I.U.	100
Vitamin E	60 I.U.	200
Vitamin B-6	6 mg	300
Folic Acid	0.4 mg	100
Vitamin B-12	25 mcg	417
Biotin	30 mcg	10
Pantothenic Acid	20 mg	200
Vitamin K	25 mcg	*

MINERALS	QUANTITY	% U.S. RDA
Calcium (elemental)	220 mg	22
Iodine	150 mcg	100
Magnesium	100 mg	25
Copper	2 mg	100
Zinc	15 mg	100
Chromium	10 mcg	*
Selenium	10 mcg	*
Molybdenum	10 mcg	*
Manganese	2.5 mg	*
Potassium	37.5 mg	*
Chloride	34 mg	*

*No U.S. RDA established.

Nutrient Information: Vitamin A is essential for the normal function of vision. **Niacin** plays a role in synthesis of DNA. **Vitamin D** helps properly utilize calcium and phosphorus necessary for strong bones and teeth. **Folic Acid** is essential to the formation of red blood cells. **Biotin** is essential in the metabolism of fat, sugar and some amino acids. **Pantothenic Acid** is essential for the metabolism of fat and sugar.

Ingredients: Calcium Carbonate, Magnesium Hydroxide, Ascorbic Acid, Potassium Chloride, Cellulose, Gelatin, Vitamin E Acetate, Zinc Sulfate, Acacia, Hydroxypropyl Methylcellulose, Modified Cellulose Gum, Calcium Pantothenate, Niacinamide, Citric Acid, Magnesium Stearate, Hydroxypropyl Cellulose, Selenium Yeast, Povidone, Artificial Colors (including Yellow 6), Pyridoxine Hydrochloride, Manganese Sulfate, Starch, Thiamine Mononitrate, Cupric Sulfate, Chromium Yeast, Molybdenum Yeast, Riboflavin, Dicalcium Phosphate, Dextrose, Vitamin A Acetate, Beta Carotene, Folic Acid, Potassium Iodide, Lecithin, Sodium, Haxametaphosphate, Vitamin K, Biotin, Vitamin B-12, Vitamin D.

How Supplied: Bottles of 50's and 80's with child-resistant caps.
Shown in Product Identification Guide, page 505

ONE–A–DAY® Essential Vitamins
11 Essential Vitamins

Ingredients: Calcium Carbonate, Ascorbic Acid, Gelatin, Vitamin E Acetate, Starch, Niacinamide, Calcium Pantothenate, Calcium Silicate, Hydroxypropyl Methylcellulose, Artificial Color, Hydroxypropylcellulose, Vitamin A Acetate, Pyridoxine Hydrochloride, Riboflavin, Thiamine Mononitrate, Magnesium Stearate, Folic Acid, Beta Carotene, Sodium Hexametaphosphate, Vitamin D, Vitamin B-12, Lecithin.

Vitamins	Quantity	U.S. RDA
Vitamin A (as Acetate and Beta Carotene)	5000 I. U.	100
Vitamin C	60 mg	100
Thiamine (B₁)	1.5 mg	100
Riboflavin (B₂)	1.7 mg	100
Niacin	20 mg	100
Vitamin D	400 I.U.	100
Vitamin E	30 I.U.	100
Vitamin B₆	2 mg	100
Folic Acid	0.4 mg	100
Vitamin B₁₂	6 mcg	100
Pantothenic Acid	10 mg	100

Indication: Dietary supplementation.

Dosage and Administration: Adults take one tablet daily.

How Supplied: Bottles of 75's and 130's with child-resistant caps.
Shown in Product Identification Guide, page 505

ONE-A-DAY® ANTIOXIDANT PLUS

Ingredients: Ascorbic Acid, Vitamin E Acetate, Gelatin, Glycerin, Soybean Oil, Selenium Yeast, Lecithin, Zinc Oxide, Vegetable Oil (Partially Hydrogenated Cottonseed and Soybean Oils), Yellow Wax (Beeswax, Yellow) Manganese Sulfate, Beta Carotene, Cupric Oxide, Titanium Dioxide, Artificial Colors including FD&C Yellow #5 (Tartrazine). Individual supplements can be taken alone or with your everyday multivitamin.

Directions for Use: Adults take one softgel capsule daily. To preserve quality and freshness, keep bottle tightly closed.

VITAMINS	QUANTITY	% US RDA
Vitamin E	200 I.U.	667
Vitamin C	250 mg	417
Vitamin A (as Beta Carotene)	5000 I.U.	100

MINERALS	QUANTITY	% US RDA
Zinc	7.5 mg	50
Copper	1.0 mg	50
Selenium	15.0 mcg	*
Manganese	1.5 mg	*

*No U.S. RDA established

Indications: **ONE-A-DAY ANTIOXIDANT PLUS** is specially formulated to create a *high potency* **antioxidant supplement that meets a wide range of dietary needs. Antioxidants** may neutralize the effects of free radicals (oxidants) which many scientists believe can be a cause of cell damage.
ONE-A-DAY PLUS ANTIOXIDANT formula combines the antioxidant nutrients with the essential trace minerals necessary for antioxidant enzyme activity.
Easy to swallow softgel capsule.
CHILD RESISTANT CAP
Do not use this product if safety seal bearing Bayer logo under cap is torn or missing.

How Supplied: Bottle of 50 softgels.
Shown in Product Identification Guide, page 505

ONE-A-DAY® CALCIUM Plus

Ingredients: Calcium Carbonate, Sorbitol, Magnesium Carbonate, Maltodextrin, Xylitol, Starch, Stearic Acid, Aspartame* (a sweetener), Natural and Artificial Flavors, Magnesium Stearate, Polyethylene Glycol, Gelatin, Polydextrose, Poloxamer 407, Docusate Sodium, Vitamin D3
*PHENYLKETONURICS: CONTAINS PHENYLALANINE.

Directions For Use: Adults and children 12 years of age or older take one to two chewable tablets daily (with food), or as recommended by your doctor, to supplement your normal dietary intake.
Two tablets provide 1,000 mg of elemental calcium, 100% of the Recommended Daily Value for adults and children 12 years of age or older.
Special Note for Pregnant and Lactating Women: Three tablets provide 1,500 mg of elemental calcium (125% of the Recommended Daily Value).

VITAMINS:

Each Tablet Contains	Quantity	RDA
Vitamin D	100 IU	25%

MINERALS:

Each Tablet Contains	Quantity	RDA
Calcium (elemental)	500 mg	50%
Magnesium (elemental)	50 mg	12.5%

Actions: ONE-A-DAY Calcium Plus aids in the prevention of the bone disease osteoporosis.
This high potency formula contains 500 mg of the most concentrated form of Calcium, plus Vitamin D and Magnesium, in a pleasant tasting chewable tablet.
Calcium is essential for building and maintaining strong and healthy bones. Vitamin D is necessary for optimal absorption and utilization of calcium by the body. Magnesium is necessary for strong teeth and bones.

Continued on next page

Bayer—Cont.

How Supplied: ONE-A-DAY® CALCIUM is available in bottles of 60 Chewable Tablets.
Shown in Product Identification Guide, page 505

ONE-A-DAY® GARLIC SOFTGELS

Ingredients: Garlic Oil Macerate, Gelatin, Glycerin, Sorbitol, Xylose.
Individual supplements can be taken alone or with your everyday multivitamin.

Directions For Use: Adults take one softgel capsule daily. Do not chew. Swallow whole to ensure maximum strength and breath freshness. To preserve quality and freshness, keep bottle tightly closed.
KEEP OUT OF REACH OF CHILDREN

Indications: ONE-A-DAY GARLIC SOFTGELS contains 600 mg of concentrated garlic which is equivalent to one garlic clove. Provides the benefits of fresh garlic in one softgel capsule. Easy to swallow high potency softgel capsule.
CHILD RESISTANT CAP
Do not use this product if safety seal bearing Bayer logo under cap is torn or missing.

How Supplied: Bottles of 45 softgels
Shown in Product Identification Guide, page 505

ONE-A-DAY® Maximum Multivitamin/Multimineral Supplement for Adults

Ingredients: Dicalcium Phosphate, Magnesium Hydroxide, Cellulose, Potassium Chloride, Ascorbic Acid, Gelatin, Ferrous Fumarate, Zinc Sulfate, Modified Cellulose Gum, Vitamin E Acetate, Citric Acid, Niacinamide, Hydroxypropyl Methylcellulose, Magnesium Stearate, Calcium Pantothenate, Selenium Yeast, Artifical Color, Polyvinylpyrrolidone, Hydroxypropylcellulose, Manganese Sulfate, Silica, Copper Sulfate, Chromium Yeast, Molybdenum Yeast, Pyridoxine Hydrochloride, Riboflavin, Thiamine Mononitrate, Beta Carotene, Vitamin A Acetate, Folic Acid, Potassium Iodide, Sodium Hexametaphosphate, Biotin, Vitamin D, Vitamin B-12, Lecithin.
One tablet daily of ONE-A-DAY® Maximum provides:

Vitamins	Quantity	% of U.S. RDA
Vitamin A (as Acetate and Beta Carotene)	5000 I.U.	100
Vitamin C	60 mg	100
Thiamine (B₁)	1.5 mg	100
Riboflavin (B₂)	1.7 mg	100
Niacin	20 mg	100
Vitamin D	400 I.U.	100
Vitamin E	30 I.U.	100
Vitamin B₆	2 mg	100
Folic Acid	0.4 mg	100
Vitamin B₁₂	6 mcg	100
Biotin	30 mcg	10
Pantothenic Acid	10 mg	100

Minerals	Quantity	% of U.S. RDA
Iron (Elemental)	18 mg	100
Calcium (Elemental)	130 mg	13
Phosphorus	100 mg	10
Iodine	150 mcg	100
Magnesium	100 mg	25
Copper	2 mg	100
Zinc	15 mg	100
Chromium	10 mcg	*
Selenium	10 mcg	*
Molybdenum	10 mcg	*
Manganese	2.5 mg	*
Potassium	37.5 mg	*
Chloride	34 mg	*

*No U.S. RDA established

Indication: Dietary supplementation.

Dosage and Administration: Adults take one tablet daily with food.

Precaution: Contains iron, which can be harmful in large doses. Close tightly and keep out of reach of children. In case of overdose, contact a physician or Poison Control Center immediately.

How Supplied: Bottles of 60 and 100 with child-resistant caps.
Shown in Product Identification Guide, page 505

ONE-A-DAY® MEN'S MULTIVITAMIN SUPPLEMENT

Ingredients: Ascorbic Acid, Calcium Carbonate, Gelatin, Vitamin E Acetate, Starch, Niacinamide, Cellulose, Calcium Silicate, Calcium Pantothenate, Hydroxypropyl Methylcellulose, Artificial Color (FD&C Yellow #6), Hydroxypropylcellulose, Magnesium Stearate, Pyridoxine Hydrochloride, Riboflavin, Thiamine Mononitrate, Vitamin A Acetate, Beta Carotene, Folic Acid, Sodium Hexametaphosphate, Vitamin D, Vitamin B-12, Lecithin.

Directions for Use: Adults take one tablet daily.

Vitamins	Quantity	% U.S. RDA
Vitamin A (as Acetate and Beta Carotene)	5000 I.U.	100
Vitamin C	200 mg	333
Thiamine (B-1)	2.25 mg	150
Riboflavin (B-2)	2.55 mg	150
Niacin	20 mg	100
Vitamin D	400 I.U.	100
Vitamin E	45 I.U.	150
Vitamin B-6	3 mg	150
Folic Acid	0.4 mg	100
Vitamin B-12	9 mcg	150
Pantothenic Acid	10 mg	100

KEEP OUT OF REACH OF CHILDREN

Indications: Dietary Supplementation.
CHILD RESISTANT CAP
Do not use this product if safety seal bearing Bayer logo under cap is torn or missing.

How Supplied: Bottles of 60's & 100's with child-resistant caps.
Shown in Product Identification Guide, page 505

ONE-A-DAY® WOMEN'S
**Multivitamin/Mineral Supplement
A formula which gives
you 11 essential vitamins plus
extra iron, and calcium & zinc.**

Ingredients: Calcium Carbonate, Acacia, Ferrous Fumarate, Ascorbic Acid, Gelatin, Vitamin E Acetate, Microcrystalline Cellulose, Hydroxypropyl Methylcellulose, Modified Cellulose Gum, Niacinamide, Zinc Oxide, Magnesium Stearate, Calcium Pantothenate, Artificial Colors including FD&C Yellow #5 (Tartrazine) and #6, Hydroxypropylcellulose, Starch, Pyridoxine Hydrochloride, Riboflavin, Thiamine Mononitrate, Beta Carotene, Vitamin A Acetate, Folic Acid, Sodium Hexametaphosphate, Lecithin, Vitamin D, Vitamin B-12.

Vitamins	Quantity	% of U.S. RDA
Vitamin A (as Acetate and Beta Carotene)	5000 I.U.	100
Vitamin C	60 mg	100
Thiamine (B₁)	1.5 mg	100
Riboflavin (B₂)	1.7 mg	100
Niacin	20 mg	100
Vitamin D	400 I.U.	100
Vitamin E	30 I.U.	100
Vitamin B₆	2 mg	100
Folic Acid	0.4 mg	100
Vitamin B₁₂	6 mcg	100
Pantothenic Acid	10 mg	100

Minerals	Quantity	% of U.S. RDA
Iron (Elemental)	27 mg	150
Calcium (Elemental)	450 mg	45
Zinc	15 mg	100

Indication: Dietary supplementation.

Dosage and Administration: Adults take one tablet daily with food.

Precaution: Contains iron, which can be harmful in large doses. Close tightly and keep out of reach of children. In case of overdose, contact a physician or Poison Control Center immediately.

How Supplied: Bottles of 60 and 100 with child-resistant caps.
Shown in Product Identification Guide, page 505

PHILLIPS'® GELCAPS
Laxative plus Stool Softener

Active Ingredients: A combination of phenolphthalein (90 mg) and docusate sodium (83 mg) per gelcap.

Inactive Ingredients: FD&C Blue # 2, gelatin, glycerin, PEG 400 and 3350, propylene glycol, sorbitol, and titanium dioxide.

Indications: For relief of occasional constipation (irregularity). This product generally produces bowel movement in 6 to 12 hours.

Action: Phenolphthalein is a stimulant laxative which increases the peristaltic activity of the intestine. Docusate sodium is a stool softener which allows easier passage of the stool.

Directions: Adults and children 12 and over take one (1) or two (2) gelcaps daily with a full glass (8 oz) of liquid, or as directed by a doctor. For children under 12, consult your doctor.

Drug Interaction Precaution: Do not take this product if you are presently taking mineral oil, unless directed by a doctor.

Warnings: Do not take any laxative if abdominal pain, nausea or vomiting are present unless directed by a doctor. If you have noticed a sudden change in bowel habits persisting for over 2 weeks, consult a doctor before using a laxative. Laxative products should not be used for a period longer than 1 week, unless directed by a doctor. Rectal bleeding or failure to have a bowel movement after use of a laxative may indicate a serious condition. Discontinue use and consult your doctor. If skin rash appears, do not use this product or any other preparation containing phenolphthalein. Keep this and all drugs out of the reach of children. In case of accidental overdose, seek professional assistance or contact a poison control center immediately. As with any drug, if you are pregnant or nursing a baby, seek the advice of a health professional before using this product.

How Supplied: Blister packs of 30 and 60 gelcaps.
Shown in Product Identification Guide, page 506

PHILLIPS'® MILK OF MAGNESIA
Laxative/Antacid

Active Ingredients: A suspension of magnesium hydroxide in purified water meeting all USP specifications. Phillips' Milk of Magnesia contains 400 mg per teaspoon (5 mL) of magnesium hydroxide.

Inactive Ingredients: Original—Purified water. Mint—Flavor, Mineral Oil, Purified water, Saccharin Sodium. Cherry—Carboxymethylcellulose Sodium, Citric Acid, D&C Red #28, Flavor, Glycerine, Microcrystalline Cellulose, Propylene Glycol, Purified water, Sorbitol, Sugar, Xantham Gum.

Indications: For relief of occasional constipation (irregularity), relief of acid indigestion, sour stomach and heartburn. The laxative dosage generally produces bowel movement in ½ to 6 hours.

Action at Laxative Dosage: Phillips' Milk of Magnesia is a mild saline laxative which acts by drawing water into the gut, increasing intraluminal pressure, and increasing intestinal motility.

Action at Antacid Dosage: Phillips' Milk of Magnesia is an effective acid neutralizer.

Directions: As a laxative, adults and children 12 years and older, 2–4 tbsp followed by a full glass (8 oz) of liquid; children 6–11 years, 1–2 tbsp followed by a full glass (8 oz) of liquid; children 2–5 years, 1–3 tsp followed by a full glass (8 oz) of liquid. Children under 2, consult a doctor.
As an antacid, adults & children 12 & older, 1–3 tsp with a little water, up to four times a day, or as directed by a doctor.

Drug Interaction Precaution: Antacids may interact with certain prescription drugs. If you are presently taking a prescription drug do not take this product without checking with your doctor or other health professional.

Laxative Warnings: Do not take any laxative if abdominal pain, nausea, vomiting or kidney disease are present unless directed by a doctor. If you have noticed a sudden change in bowel habits persisting for over 2 weeks, consult a doctor before using a laxative. Laxative products should not be used for a period longer than 1 week, unless directed by a doctor. Rectal bleeding or failure to have a bowel movement after use of a laxative may indicate a serious condition. Discontinue use and consult your doctor. Phillips® Milk of Magnesia is a saline laxative.

Antacid Warnings: Do not take more than the maximum recommended daily dosage in a 24-hour period (see Directions), or use the maximum dosage of this product for more than two weeks, or use this product if you have kidney disease, except under the advice and supervision of a doctor. May have laxative effect.

General Warnings: As with any drug, if you are pregnant or nursing a baby, seek the advice of a health professional before using this product. Keep this and all drugs out of reach of children. In case of accidental overdose, seek professional assistance or contact a poison control center immediately.

How Supplied: Phillips' Milk of Magnesia is available in original, mint and cherry flavor in 4, 12 and 26 fl oz bottles. Also available in tablet form and concentrated liquid form.
Shown in Product Identification Guide, page 506

VANQUISH® Analgesic Caplets

Active Ingredients: Each caplet contains aspirin 227 mg, acetaminophen 194 mg, caffeine 33 mg, dried aluminum hydroxide gel 25 mg, magnesium hydroxide 50 mg in a thin, inert hydroxypropyl methylcellulose coating for easier swallowing.

Inactive Ingredients: Microcrystalline Cellulose, Polyethylene Glycol, Polysorbate 80, Silicon Dioxide, Starch, Titanium Dioxide, Zinc Stearate.

Indications: A buffered analgesic, antipyretic for relief of headache; muscular aches and pains; neuralgia and neuritic pain; toothache; pain following dental procedures; for painful discomforts and fever of colds; functional menstrual pain, headache and pain due to cramps; temporary relief from minor pains of arthritis, rheumatism, bursitis, lumbago, sciatica.

Directions: Adults and children 12 years and over: Two caplets with water. May be repeated every four hours if necessary up to 12 caplets per day. Larger or more frequent doses may be prescribed by doctor if necessary.

Warnings: Children and teenagers should not use this medicine for chicken pox or flu symptoms before a doctor is consulted about Reye syndrome, a rare but serious illness reported to be associated with aspirin. Do not take this product for pain for more than 10 days or for fever for more than 3 days unless directed by a doctor. If pain or fever persists or gets worse, if new symptoms occur, or if redness or swelling is present consult a doctor immediately. Do not take this product if you are allergic to aspirin, have asthma, stomach problems that persist or recur, gastric ulcers or bleeding problems unless directed by a doctor. If ringing in the ears or loss of hearing occurs, consult a doctor before taking any more of this product. Keep this and all drugs out of the reach of children. In case of accidental overdose, immediate medical attention is essential for adults as well as for children even if you do not notice any sign or symptoms. As with any drug, if you are pregnant or nursing a baby, seek the advice of a health professional before using this product. **IT IS ESPECIALLY IMPORTANT NOT TO USE ASPIRIN DURING THE LAST 3 MONTHS OF PREGNANCY UNLESS SPECIFICALLY DIRECTED TO DO SO BY A DOCTOR BECAUSE IT MAY CAUSE PROBLEMS IN THE UNBORN CHILD OR COMPLICATIONS DURING DELIVERY.**

Drug Interaction Precaution: Do not take this product if you are taking a prescription drug for anticoagulation (thinning of the blood), diabetes, gout, or arthritis unless directed by a doctor.

Continued on next page

Bayer—Cont.

How Supplied:
White, capsule-shaped caplets in bottles of 30, 60 and 100 caplets. Child-resistant safety closures on bottles of 30 and 60 caplets. Bottle of 100 caplets available without safety closure for households without young children.

Shown in Product Identification Guide, page 506

Beach Pharmaceuticals
Division of Beach Products, Inc.
5220 SOUTH MANHATTAN AVE.
TAMPA, FL 33611

Direct Inquiries to:
Richard Stephen Jenkins, Exec. V.P.: (813) 839-6565

BEELITH Tablets
MAGNESIUM SUPPLEMENT
WITH PYRIDOXINE HCl
Each tablet supplies 362 mg (30 mEq) of magnesium and 25 mg of pyridoxine HCL.

Description: Each tablet contains magnesium oxide 600 mg and pyridoxine hydrochloride (Vitamin B_6) 25 mg equivalent to B_6 20 mg. Each tablet yields 362 mg of magnesium and supplies 90% of the Adult U.S. Recommended Daily Allowance (RDA) for magnesium and 1000% of the Adult RDA for vitamin B_6.

Indications: As a dietary supplement for patients with magnesium and/or Vitamin B_6 deficiencies resulting from malnutrition, alcoholism, magnesium depleting drugs, chemotherapy and inadequate nutritional intake or absorption. Also, increases urinary magnesium levels.

Dosage: One tablet daily or as directed by a physician.

Drug Interaction Precautions: Do not take this product if you are presently taking a prescription drug without consulting your physician or other health professional.

Warnings: If you have kidney disease, take only under the supervision of a physician. Excessive dosage may cause laxation. **KEEP OUT OF THE REACH OF CHILDREN.** As with any drug, if your are pregnant or nursing a baby, seek the advice of a health professional before using this product.

How Supplied: Golden yellow, film coated tablet with the name **BEACH** and the number **1132** printed on each tablet. Packaged in bottles of 100 (NDC 0486-1132-01) tablets.

Beiersdorf Inc.
360 Dr. Martin Luther King Dr.
NORWALK, CT 06856-5529

Direct Inquiries To:
Medical Division: (203) 853-8008
FAX: (203) 854-8180

AQUAPHOR®—
Original Formula Ointment
NDC Numbers— 10356-020-01
10356-020-02

Composition: Petrolatum, mineral oil, mineral wax and wool wax alcohol.

Actions and Uses: Aquaphor is a stable, neutral, odorless, anhydrous ointment base. Miscible with water or aqueous solutions, Aquaphor will absorb several times its own weight, forming smooth, creamy water-in-oil emulsions. In its pure form, Aquaphor is recommended for use as a topical preparation to help heal severely dry skin. Aquaphor contains no preservatives, fragrances or known irritants.

Administration and Dosages: Use Aquaphor alone or in compounding virtually any ointment using aqueous solutions or in combination with other oil-based substances and all common topical medications. Apply Aquaphor liberally to affected area.

Precautions: For external use only. Avoid contact with eyes. Not to be applied over third degree burns, deep or puncture wounds, infections or lacerations. If condition worsens or does not improve within 7 days, patient should consult a doctor.

How Supplied: 16 oz. jar—List No. 45585
5 lb. jar—List. No. 45586

Shown in Product Identification Guide, page 506

AQUAPHOR
Healing Ointment
NDC Number—10356-021-01

Composition: Petrolatum, Mineral Oil, Mineral Wax, Wool Wax Alcohol, Panthenol, Bisabolol, Glycerin.

Actions and Uses: Aquaphor Healing Ointment is specially formulated for faster healing of severely dry skin, cracked skin and minor burns. It is recommended for patients suffering from severe skin chapping and from skin disorders that result in severely dry skin. This formula is also indicated as a follow-up skin treatment for patients undergoing radiation therapy or other drying/burning medical therapies. It is preservative-free, fragrance-free and hypoallergenic.[1]

Administration and Dosage: Use Aquaphor Healing Ointment whenever a mild healing agent is needed. Apply liberally to affected areas two to three times

a day. In the case of minor wounds, clean area prior to application.

Precautions: For external use only. Avoid contact with the eyes. Not to be applied over third degree burns, deep or puncture wounds, infections or lacerations. If condition worsens or does not improve within seven days, patient should consult a physician.

How Supplied: 1.75 oz. tube
1.Data on file, BDF Inc

Shown in Product Identification Guide, page 506

EUCERIN® BAR
[ū'sir-in]
Cleansing Bar

Indications: Use with warm water to cleanse skin.

Contains: Disodium Lauryl Sulfosuccinate, Sodium Cocoyl Isethionate, Cetearyl Alcohol, Corn Starch, Glyceryl Stearate, Paraffin, Water, Titanium Dioxide, Octyldodecanol, Cyclopentadecanolide, Lanolin Alcohol, Bisabolol.

Actions and Uses: Eucerin® Cleansing Bar has been specially formulated for use on sensitive skin. The formulation contains Eucerite®, a special blend of ingredients that closely resemble the natural oils of the skin, thus providing excellent moisturizing properties. This formulation is fragrance-free and noncomedogenic. Additionally, the pH value of Eucerin Cleansing Bar is neutral so as not to affect the skin's normal acid mantle.

Directions: Use during shower, bath, or regular cleansing.

How Supplied: 3 ounce bar.
List number 3852

Shown in Product Identification Guide, page 506

EUCERIN® Creme
[ū'sir-in]
Original Moisturizing Creme
NDC Numbers—10356-090-01
10356-090-05
10356-090-04
10356-090-07

Indications: Use daily to help relieve dry and very dry skin conditions.

Composition: Triple Purified Water, Petrolatum, Mineral Oil, Ceresin, Lanolin Alcohol, Methylchloroisothiazolinone, Methylisothiazolinone.

Actions and Uses: A gentle, noncomedogenic, fragrance-free water-in-oil emulsion. Eucerin can be used for treating dry skin conditions associated with eczema, psoriasis, chapped or chafed skin, sunburn, windburn and itching associated with dryness.[1]

Administration and Dosages: Apply freely to affected areas of the skin as often as necessary or as directed by a physician.

Precautions: For external use only. Discontinue use if signs of irritation occur.

How Supplied: 16 oz. jar—List Number 0090
8 oz. jar—List Number 3774
4 oz. jar—List Number 3797
2 oz. tube—List Number 3868
1.Data on File.
Shown in Product Identification Guide, page 506

EUCERIN®
FACIAL MOISTURIZING LOTION
SPF 25
NDC Number—10356-972-01

Indications: Use daily to help relieve dry skin and provide broad spectrum sun protection.

Composition:
Active Ingredients: Octyl Methoxycinnamate, Octyl Salicylate, Titanium Dioxide.
Other Ingredients: Water, Octyldodecyl Neopentanoate, Dioctyl Malate, Glycerin, Petrolatum, Zinc Oxide, Cetearyl Alcohol, DEA-Cetyl Phosphate, PEG-40 Castor Oil, Glyceryl Stearate, Sodium Hyaluronate, Lactic Acid, Lanolin Alcohol, Sodium Cetearyl Sulfate, Xanthan Gum, Methicone, Dimethicone, EDTA, Sodium Hydroxide, Methylchloroisothiazolinone, Methylisothiazolinone.

Actions and Uses: Eucerin Facial Moisturizing Lotion SPF 25 is fragrance-free and non-comedogenic, with a unique sun screen (titanium dioxide) to protect skin from UVA and UVB light. It is specially formulated for dry, sensitive skin or for those undergoing therapies which irritate delicate facial skin. This light, oil-in-water formula is non-greasy and is easily absorbed into the skin.

Administration and Dosage: Apply Eucerin Facial Moisturizing Lotion SPF 25 twice a day or as directed by a physician (especially in the morning), to nourish and moisture skin and protect it from harmful UVA and UVB rays.

Precautions: For external use only. Avoid contact with eyes. Keep out of the reach of children. Discontinue use if signs of irritation occur.

How Supplied: 4-oz. bottle.—List No. 03972
Shown in Product Identification Guide, page 506

EUCERIN® Lotion
[ū'sir-in]
Original Moisturizing Lotion
NDC Numbers—10356-793-01
10356-793-04

Indications: Use daily to help relieve dry skin.

Composition: Water, Mineral Oil, Isopropyl Myristate, PEG-40 Sorbitan Peroleate, Glyceryl Lanoleate, Sorbitol, Propylene Glycol, Cetyl Palmitate, Magnesium Sulfate, Aluminum Stearate, Lanolin Alcohol, BHT, Methylchloroisothiazolinone, Methylisothiazolinone.

Actions and Uses: Eucerin Lotion is a non-comedogenic, fragrance-free, unique water-in-oil formulation that will help to alleviate and soothe dry skin, and provide long-lasting moisturization.

Administration and Dosage: Use daily on dry skin.

Precautions: For external use only. Discontinue use if signs of irritation occur.

How Supplied: 8 fluid oz. plastic bottle—List Number 3793
16 fluid oz. plastic bottle—List number 3794
Shown in Product Identification Guide, page 506

EUCERIN PLUS CREME
Moisturizing Alphahydroxy Creme
NDC 10356-036-01

Indications: Use daily to help relieve severely dry, flaky skin.

Composition: Water, Mineral Oil, Urea, Magnesium Stearate, Ceresin, Polyglyceryl-3 Diisostearate, Sodium Lactate, Isopropyl Palmitate, Benzyl Alcohol, Panthenol, Bisabolol, Lanolin Alcohol, Magnesium Sulfate.

Caution: For external use only. Avoid contact with eyes and areas where skin is inflamed or cracked. Discontinue use if signs of irritation occur. Keep out of reach of children.

Action and Uses: Eucerin Plus Creme is a unique alpha-hydroxy acid moisturizing creme (2.5% sodium lactate, 10% urea) that is clinically proven to relieve severely dry, flaky skin conditions[1]. Unlike other alpha-hydroxy acid moisturizers, Eucerin Plus Creme has low irritation potential, is fragrance-free and non-comedogenic.

Administration and Dosage: Use daily on severely dry, scaly skin.

Precautions: Avoid contact with eyes or areas where skin is inflamed or cracked. Discontinue use if signs of irritation occur. For external use only. Keep out of reach of children.

How Supplied: 4 oz. jar—List No. 03611
1.Data on file.
Shown in Product Identification Guide, page 506

EUCERIN PLUS LOTION
Alphahydroxy Moisturizing Lotion
NDC 10356-967-01
10356-967-03

Indications: Use daily to help relieve severely dry, flaky skin.

Composition: Water, Mineral Oil, PEG-7 Hydrogenated Castor Oil, Isohexadecane, Sodium Lactate 5%, Urea 5%, Glycerin, Isopropyl Palmitate, Panthenol, Ozokerite, Magnesium Sulfate, Lanolin Alcohol, Bisabolol, Methylchloroisothiazolinone, Methylisothiazolinone.

Action and Uses: Eucerin Plus Lotion in a unique alpha-hydroxy acid moisturizing lotion (5% Sodium Lactate, 5% Urea) that is clinically proven to relieve severely dry, flaky skin conditions.[1] Unlike other alpha-hydroxy acid moisturizing lotions, Eucerin Plus has low irritation potential, is fragrance free and non-comedogenic.

Administration and Dosage: Use daily on severely dry, flaky skin.

Precautions: Avoid contact with eyes or areas where skin is inflamed or cracked. Discontinue use if signs of irritation occur. For external use only. Keep out of reach of children.

How Supplied: 6 oz bottle—List No. 03967
12 oz bottle—List No. 03321
1. Data on File.
Shown in Product Identification Guide, page 506

Blaine Company, Inc.
1465 JAMIKE LANE
ERLANGER, KY 41018

Direct Inquiries to:
Mr. Alex M. Blaine
(800) 633-9353
FAX: (606) 283-9460

MAG–OX 400

Description: Each tablet contains Magnesium Oxide 400 mg. U.S.P. (Heavy), or 241.3 mg. Elemental Magnesium (19.86 mEq.)

Indications and Usage: Hypomagnesemia, magnesium deficiencies and/or magnesium depletion during therapy with diuretics and/or digitalis, aminoglycosides, amphotericin B, cyclosporin, chemotherapy, and during pregnancy, PMS, menopause, diabetes, hyperoxaluria, malnutrition, weight/strength training, restricted diet, or alcoholism.

Warnings: Do not use this product except under the advice and supervision of a physician if you have a kidney disease. May have laxative effect.

Dosage: Adult dose 1 or 2 tablets daily with meals or as directed by a physician.

Professional Labeling: Serum magnesium levels do not accurately represent total body, tissue, or bone magnesium levels.

How Supplied: Bottles of 100, 1000, and hospital unit dose (U.D. 100s)

Continued on next page

Blaine—Cont.

URO–MAG

Description: Each capsule contains Magnesium Oxide 140 mg. U.S.P. (Heavy), or 84.5 mg. Elemental Magnesium (6.93 mEq.)

Indications and Usage: Hypomagnesemia, magnesium deficiencies and/or magnesium depletion during therapy with diuretics and/or digitalis, aminoglycosides, amphotericin B, cyclosporin, chemotherapy, and during pregnancy, PMS, menopause, diabetes, hyperoxaluria, malnutrition, weight/strength training, restricted diet, or alcoholism.

Warnings: Do not use this product except under the advice and supervision of a physician if you have a kidney disease. May have laxative effect.

Dosage: Adult dose 3–4 capsules daily with meals or as directed by a physician.

Professional Labeling: Serum magnesium levels do not accurately represent total body, tissue, or bone magnesium levels.

How Supplied: Bottles of 100 and 1000.

EDUCATIONAL MATERIAL

Cardiovascular system charts, female reproductive system charts, samples, and literature available to physicians upon request.

Blairex Laboratories, Inc.
3240 NORTH INDIANAPOLIS ROAD
P.O. BOX 2127
COLUMBUS, IN 47202-2127

Direct Inquiries to:
Customer Service
(800) 252-4739
FAX (812) 378-1033

For Medical Emergency Contact:
Customer Service
(800) 252-4739
FAX (812) 378-1033

BRONCHO SALINE®
0.9% Sodium Chloride Aerosol for the dilution of bronchodilator inhalation solutions. Sterile normal saline for diluting bronchodilator solutions for oral inhalation.

Description: Broncho Saline® is for patients using bronchodilator solutions for oral inhalation that require dilution with sterile normal saline solution. Broncho Saline is a sterile liquid solution consisting of 0.9% sodium chloride for oral inhalation with a pH of 4.5 to 7.5. Not to be used for injection.

How Supplied: Broncho Saline® comes in 90cc (mL) and 240cc (mL) Pressurized Containers.
Store between 15–25°C (59–77°F). Keep out of reach of children. See WARNINGS.

NASAL MOIST®
Sodium Chloride 0.65%

Description: Isotonic saline solution buffered with sodium bicarbonate. Preserved with Benzyl alcohol.

Actions and Uses: Use for dry nasal membranes caused by chronic sinusitis, allergy, asthma, dry air, oxygen therapy. May be used as often as needed.

Directions: Squeeze twice into each nostril as needed.

How Supplied: 45 mL (1.5 oz.) plastic squeeze bottle, 15 mL (.5 oz.) plastic squeeze bottle with drop capability, and 15 mL (.5 oz.) fine mist metered pump.

PERTUSSIN® ADULT EXTRA STRENGTH
Cough Suppressant

Description: Each 5mL (one teaspoonful) contains:
Dextromethorphan Hydrobromide, USP 15mg

Inactive Ingredients: Carmel, Carboxymethylcellulose Sodium, Citric Acid, D&C Red No. 33, Flavor, Sorbic Acid, Sorbitol, Sugar, Purified Water. Contains 9.5% alcohol.

Indications: Temporarily relieves cough due to minor bronchial irritation associated with a cold.

Warnings: A persistent cough may be a sign of a serious condition. If cough persists more than 1 week, tends to recur, or is accompanied by a fever, rash, or persistent headache, consult a doctor. Do not take this product for persistent or chronic cough such as occurs with smoking, asthma, chronic bronchitis, emphysema, or cough is accompanied by excessive phlegm (mucus) unless directed by a doctor. As with any drug, if you are pregnant or nursing a baby, seek the advise of a health professional before using this product.
KEEP THIS AND ALL DRUGS OUT OF THE REACH OF CHILDREN, IN CASE OF ACCIDENTAL OVERDOSE, SEEK PROFESSIONAL ASSISTANCE OR CONTACT A POISON CONTROL CENTER IMMEDIATELY.

Drug Interaction Precaution: Do not use this product if you are taking a prescription drug containing a monoamine oxidase inhibitor (MAOI) (certain drugs for depression or psychiatric or emotional conditions), without first consulting your doctor. If you are uncertain whether your prescription drug contains an MAOI, consult a health professional before taking this product.

Directions: Adults and children 12 years of age and older: 2 teaspoonfuls every 6–8 hours as needed. Not to exceed 8 teaspoonfuls in 24 hours. Children 6 to under 12 years of age: One teaspoonful every 6–8 hours as needed. Not to exceed 4 teaspoonfuls in 24 hours. Do not administer to children under 6 years of age: Consult a doctor.

How Supplied: Available in shatter-resistant bottles of 4 fl. oz. (NDC 50486-048-20).

PERTUSSIN® CHILDREN'S STRENGTH
Cough Suppressant

Description: Each 5mL (one teaspoonful) contains:
Dextromethorphan Hydrobromide, USP 3.5mg

Inactive Ingredients: Citric Acid, Colors, Flavor, Sorbic Acid, Sorbitol, Sucrose, Purified Water. Alcohol-free.

Indications: Temporarily relieves cough due to minor bronchial irritation associated with a cold.

Warnings: A persistent cough may be a sign of a serious condition. If cough persists more than 1 week, tends to recur, or is accompanied by a fever, rash, or persistent headache, consult a doctor. Do not take this product for persistent or chronic cough such as occurs with smoking, asthma, chronic bronchitis, emphysema, or cough is accompanied by excessive phlegm (mucus) unless directed by a doctor. As with any drug, if you are pregnant or nursing a baby, seek the advise of a health professional before using this product.
KEEP THIS AND ALL DRUGS OUT OF THE REACH OF CHILDREN, IN CASE OF ACCIDENTAL OVERDOSE, SEEK PROFESSIONAL ASSISTANCE OR CONTACT A POISON CONTROL CENTER IMMEDIATELY.

Drug Interaction Precaution: Do not give this product to a child who is taking a prescription drug containing a monoamine oxidase inhibitor (MAOI) (certain drugs for depression or psychiatric or emotional conditions), without first consulting the child's doctor. If you are uncertain whether your child's prescription drug contains an MAOI, consult a health professional before giving this product.

Directions: Children 2 to under 6 years of age: 1 teaspoonful. Children 6 to under 12 years of age: 2 teaspoonfuls. Adults and children 12 years of age and older: 4 teaspoonfuls. Repeat every 4 hours as needed. Do not exceed 6 doses in a 24 hour period. Children under 2 years of age: Consult a doctor.

How Supplied: Available in shatter-resistant bottles of 4 fl. oz. (NDC 50486-048-40).

UNIT DOSE STERILE SODIUM CHLORIDE SOLUTIONS
0.9% Sodium Chloride
0.45% Sodium Chloride

Description: Unit dose sterile 0.9% Sodium Chloride and 0.45% Sodium Chloride solution. For patients using bronchodilator solutions for oral inhalation that require dilution with sterile saline solution. Prefilled sterile in unit dose vials. No bacteriostatic agent or other preservative added. Not to be used for injection. Not for parenteral administration.

How Supplied: 0.9% Sodium Chloride solution comes in 3mL and 5 mL plastic vial, 0.45% Sodium Chloride solution comes in 3mL unit dose vial.

Block Drug Company, Inc.
257 CORNELISON AVENUE
JERSEY CITY, NJ 07302

Direct Inquiries to:
Lori Hunt
(201) 434-3000 Ext. 1308

For Medical Emergencies Contact:
Consumer Service/Block
(201) 434-3000 Ext. 1308

BALMEX® OINTMENT
for diaper rash

Description: Balmex® contains Zinc Oxide (11.3%) in a unique formulation including Peruvian Balsam suitable for topical application for the treatment and prevention of diaper rash.

Indications and Uses: Balmex helps treat and prevent diaper rash in four ways: 1. Soothes irritation. 2. Provides protection. 3. Promotes healing. 4. Reduces inflammation.
The zinc oxide based formulation provides a protective barrier on the skin against the natural causes of irritation. Balmex spreads on smooth and wipes off the baby easily, without causing irritation to the affected area. Balmex tactile properties promote compliance amongst mothers, and clinical studies have demonstrated that Balmex is effective in treating diaper rash.

Directions: At the first sign of diaper rash or redness apply Balmex three or more times daily as needed. To help prevent diaper rash, apply Balmex liberally as often as necessary, with each diaper change, especially at bedtime or anytime when exposure to wet diapers may be prolonged.

Warnings: Avoid contact with the eyes. For external use only. If condition worsens or does not improve within 7 days, contact a physician. Keep out of reach of children.

Active Ingredient: Zinc Oxide.

Inactive Ingredients: Balsam (Specially Purified Balsam Peru), Beeswax, Benzoic Acid, Bismuth Subnitrate, Mineral Oil, Purified Water, Silicone, Synthetic White Wax, and other ingredients.

How Supplied: 2 oz. (57 g.) and 4 oz. (113 g.) tubes and 16 oz. (454 g.) jars.

BC® POWDER
ARTHRITIS STRENGTH BC® POWDER
BC® COLD POWDER

Description: BC® POWDER: Active Ingredients: Each powder contains Aspirin 650 mg, Salicylamide 195 mg and Caffeine 32 mg. ARTHRITIS STRENGTH BC® POWDER: Active Ingredients: Each powder contains Aspirin 742 mg, Salicylamide 222 mg and Caffeine 36 mg. BC® COLD POWDER MULTI-SYMPTOM FORMULA (COLD-SINUS ALLERGY)
BC® COLD POWDER NON-DROWSY FORMULA (COLD-SINUS)
BC Cold Powder Multi-Symptom Formula (Cold-Sinus-Allergy) Active Ingredients: Aspirin 650 mg, Phenylpropanolamine Hydrochloride 25 mg, and Chlorpheniramine Maleate 4 mg per powder. BC Cold Powder Non-Drowsy Formula (Cold-Sinus) Active Ingredients: Aspirin 650 mg and Phenylpropanolamine Hydrochloride 25 mg per powder.

Indications: BC Powder is for relief of simple headache; for temporary relief of minor arthritic pain, neuralgia, neuritis and sciatica; for relief of muscular aches, discomfort and fever of colds; and for relief of normal menstrual pain and pain of tooth extraction.
Arthritis Strength BC Powder is specially formulated to fight occasional minor pain and inflammation of arthritis. Like original formula BC, Arthritis Strength BC provides fast temporary relief of minor arthritis pain and inflammation, neuralgia, neuritis and sciatica; relief of muscular aches, discomfort and fever of colds; and pain of tooth extraction.
BC Cold Powder Multi-Symptom (Cold-Sinus-Allergy) is for relief of cold symptoms such as body aches, fever, nasal congestion, sneezing, running nose, and watery itchy eyes. BC Cold Powder Non-Drowsy Formula (Cold-Sinus) is for relief of such symptoms as body aches, fever, and nasal congestions.

BC Powder®, Arthritis Strength BC® Powder:

Warnings: BC Powder and Arthritis Strength BC® Powder: Children and teenagers should not use this medicine for chicken pox or flu symptoms before a doctor is consulted about Reye Syndrome, a rare but serious illness reported to be associated with aspirin. Do not take this product if you are allergic to aspirin. If pain persists for more than 10 days or redness is present, discontinue use of this

product and consult a physician immediately. Keep this and all medication out of children's reach. As with any drug, if you are pregnant or nursing a baby, consult your physician before using this product. IT IS ESPECIALLY IMPORTANT NOT TO USE ASPIRIN DURING THE LAST 3 MONTHS OF PREGNANCY UNLESS SPECIFICALLY DIRECTED TO DO SO BY A DOCTOR BECAUSE IT MAY CAUSE PROBLEMS IN THE UNBORN CHILD OR COMPLICATIONS DURING DELIVERY.

BC Cold Powder Line:

Warnings: Children and teenagers should not use BC for chicken pox or flu symptoms before a doctor is consulted about Reye Syndrome, a rare but serious illness reported to be associated with aspirin. Keep BC and all medicines out of children's reach. In case of accidental overdose, contact a physician immediately.
As with any drug, if you are pregnant or nursing a baby seek the advice of a health professional before using BC.
IT IS ESPECIALLY IMPORTANT NOT TO USE ASPIRIN DURING THE LAST 3 MONTHS OF PREGNANCY UNLESS SPECIFICALLY DIRECTED TO DO SO BY A DOCTOR BECAUSE IT MAY CAUSE PROBLEMS IN THE UNBORN CHILD OR COMPLICATIONS DURING DELIVERY.
Nervousness, dizziness or sleeplessness may occur if recommended dosage is exceeded. If symptoms do not improve within 7 days, or are accompanied by fever that lasts more than 3 days, or if new symptoms occur, consult a physician before continuing use. Do not take BC if you are sensitive to aspirin, or have heart disease, high blood pressure, thyroid disease, diabetes, asthma, glaucoma, emphysema, chronic pulmonary disease, shortness of breath, difficulty in breathing or difficulty in urination due to enlargement of the prostrate gland, or if you are presently taking a prescription antihypertensive or antidepressant drug containing a monoamine oxidase inhibitor unless directed by a doctor. BC Cold Powder Multi-Symptom with antihistamine may cause drowsiness. Avoid alcoholic beverages while taking this product. Use caution when driving a motor vehicle or operating machinery.

Overdosage: In case of accidental overdosage, contact a physician or poison control center immediately.

Dosage and Administration: BC® Powder, Arthritis Strength BC® Powder, BC® Cold Powder Line:
Place one powder on tongue and follow with liquid. If you prefer, stir powder into glass of water or other liquid. May be used every three to four hours, up to 4 powders each 24 hours. For children under 12, consult a physician.

How Supplied: BC Powder: Available in tamper resistant overwrapped envelopes of 2 or 6 powders, as well as

Continued on next page

Block Drug—Cont.

tamper resistant boxes of 24 and 50 powders.
Arthritis Strength BC Powder: Available in tamper resistant over wrapped envelopes of 6 powders, and tamper resistant overwrapped boxes of 24 and 50 powders.
BC Cold Powder Line:
Available in tamper-resistant over-wrapped envelopes of 6 powders, as well as tamper-resistant boxes of 24 powders.

GOODY'S
Extra Strength Headache Powders

Indications: For Temporary Relief of Minor Aches & Pain Due to Headaches, Arthritis, Colds & Fever

Directions: Adults: Place one powder on tongue and follow with liquid or stir powder into a glass of water or other liquid. May be repeated in 4 to 6 hours. Do not take more than 4 powders in any 24-hour period. Children under 12 years of age: Consult a doctor.

Warnings: Children and teenagers should not use this medicine for chicken pox or flu symptoms before a doctor is consulted about Reye Syndrome, a rare but serious illness reported to be associated with aspirin. As with any drug, if you are pregnant, or nursing a baby, seek the advice of a health professional before using this product.
IT IS ESPECIALLY IMPORTANT NOT TO USE ASPIRIN DURING THE LAST 3 MONTHS OF PREGNANCY UNLESS SPECIFICALLY DIRECTED TO DO SO BY A DOCTOR BECAUSE IT MAY CAUSE PROBLEMS IN THE UNBORN CHILD OR COMPLICATIONS DURING DELIVERY. Keep this and all medicine out of the reach of children. In case of accidental overdose, contact a doctor or poison control center immediately.
This product contains aspirin and should not be taken by individuals who are sensitive to aspirin. If pain persists for more than 10 days or redness is present, consult a physician immediately.

Active Ingredients: Each Powder contains 520 mg. aspirin in combination with 260 mg. acetaminophen and 32.5 mg. caffeine.

Inactive Ingredients: Lactose and Potassium Chloride.
Dist. By: GOODY'S PHARMACEUTICALS
Memphis, TN 38113

GOODY'S®
Extra Strength Pain Relief Tablets

Indications: Goody's EXTRA STRENGTH tablets are a specially developed pain reliever that provide fast & effective temporary relief from minor aches & pain due to headaches, arthritis, colds or "flu," muscle strain, sinusitis, backache & menstrual discomfort. It is recommended for temporary relief of toothaches and to reduce fever.

Directions: Adults: Two tablets with water or other liquid. May be repeated in 4 to 6 hours. Do not take more than 8 tablets in any 24-hour period. Children under 12 years of age: Consult a doctor.

Caution: Do not take more than the recommended dosage or take regularly for more than 10 days without consulting your doctor.

Warning: Children and teenagers should not use this medicine for chicken pox or flu symptoms before a doctor is consulted about Reye Syndrome, a rare but serious illness reported to be associated with aspirin. As with any drug, if you are pregnant, or nursing a baby, seek the advice of a health professional before using this product. IT IS ESPECIALLY IMPORTANT NOT TO USE ASPIRIN DURING THE LAST 3 MONTHS OF PREGNANCY UNLESS SPECIFICALLY DIRECTED TO DO SO BY A DOCTOR BECAUSE IT MAY CAUSE PROBLEMS IN THE UNBORN CHILD OR COMPLICATIONS DURING DELIVERY. Keep this and all medicine out of the reach of children. In case of accidental overdose, contact a doctor or poison control center immediately.

Active Ingredients: Each tablet contains 260 mg. aspirin in combination with 130 mg. acetaminophen and 16.25 mg. caffeine. **Inactive Ingredients:** Corn Starch, Modified Starch, Polyvinylpyrrolidone and Stearic Acid.
Dist. By: GOODY'S PHARMACEUTICALS
Memphis, TN 38113

Maximum Strength
NYTOL® Caplets

Active Ingredient: Doxylamine succinate, 25 mg per caplet.

Indications: Helps to reduce difficulty in falling asleep.

Warnings: DO NOT TAKE THIS PRODUCT IF YOU HAVE ASTHMA, GLAUCOMA, OR ENLARGEMENT OF THE PROSTATE GLAND EXCEPT UNDER THE ADVICE AND SUPERVISION OF A PHYSICIAN. If sleeplessness persists continuously for more than two weeks, consult your physician. Insomnia may be a symptom of serious underlying medical illness. Do not take this product if presently taking any other drug, without consulting your physician or pharmacist. Take this product with caution if alcohol is being consumed. As with any drug, if you are pregnant or nursing a baby, seek the advice of a health professional before using this product. For adults only. Do not give to children under 12 years of age.

Keep this and all drugs out of the reach of children. In case of accidental overdose, seek professional assistance or contact a Poison Control Center immediately.

Caution: This product contains an antihistamine and will cause drowsiness. It should be used only at bedtime.

Dosage and Administration: Adults and children 12 years of age and over, take 1 Maximum Strength NYTOL caplet 30 minutes before going to bed. Take once daily or as directed by a physician.

How Supplied: Available in packages of 8 and 16 caplets.

NYTOL® QUICK CAPS™ CAPLETS

Active Ingredient: Diphenhydramine Hydrochloride, 25 mg per caplet.

Indications: For relief of occasional sleeplessness. Diphenhydramine Hydrochloride is an antihistamine with anticholinergic and sedative effects which induces drowsiness and helps in falling asleep.

Warnings: Do not give children under 12 years of age. If sleeplessness persists continuously for more than 2 weeks, consult your doctor. Insomnia may be a symptom of serious underlying medical illness. Do not take this product, unless directed by a doctor, if you have a breathing problem such as emphysema or chronic bronchitis, or if you have glaucoma or difficulty in urination due to enlargement of the prostate gland. Avoid alcoholic beverages while taking this product. Do not take this product if you are taking tranquilizers or sedatives, without first consulting your doctor. In case of accidental overdose seek professional assistance or contact a poison control center immediately. As with any drug, if you are pregnant or nursing a baby, seek the advice of a health professional before using this product. Keep this and all drugs out of the reach of children.

Drug Interaction: Alcohol and other drugs which cause CNS depression will heighten the depressant effect of this product. Monoamine oxidase (MAO) inhibitors will prolong and intensify the anticholinergic effects of antihistamines.

Symptoms and Treatment of Oral Overdosage: In adults overdose may cause CNS depression resulting in hypnosis and coma. In children CNS hyperexcitability may follow sedation; the stimulant phase may bring tremor, delirium and convulsions. Gastrointestinal reactions may include dry mouth, appetite loss, nausea and vomiting. Respiratory distress and cardiovascular complications (hypotension) may be evident. Treatment includes inducing emesis, and controlling symptoms.

Dosage and Administration: Adults and children 12 years of age and over, take 2 NYTOL with DPH at bedtime if needed, or as directed by a physician.

How Supplied: Available in tamper resistant packages of 16, 32, and 72 caplets NYTOL with DPH.

PHAZYME®-95
[fay-zime]
Tablets

Description: Contains simethicone, an antiflatulent to alleviate or relieve the symptoms of gas. It has no known side effects or drug interactions.

Actions: Simethicone minimizes gas formation and relieves gas entrapment in both the stomach and the lower G.I. tract. This action combats the distress due to gastrointestinal gas.

Indication: To alleviate or relieve the symptoms of gas. May also be used for postoperative gas pain.

Warnings: Keep this and all drugs out of the reach of children. If condition persists, consult your physician.

Store at controlled room temperature 59°–86°F (15°–30°C).

Active Ingredient: Each tablet contains simethicone 95 mg.

Inactive Ingredients: Acacia, carnauba wax, compressible sugar, crosscarmellose sodium, FD&C red No. 40 aluminum lake, FD&C yellow No. 6 aluminum lake, hydroxypropyl methylcellulose, microcrystalline cellulose, polyoxyl 40 stearate, povidone, sodium benzoate, sucrose, talc, titanium dioxide, white wax.

Dosage: One tablet four times a day after meals and at bedtime. Do not exceed 5 tablets per day unless directed by a physician.

How Supplied: Red coated tablet imprinted "Phazyme 95" in 10 pack, 30 pack and bottles of 50's and 100's.
Shown in Product Identification Guide, page 506

PHAZYME® DROPS
[fay-zime]

Description: Contains simethicone, an antiflatulent to alleviate or relieve the symptoms of gas. It has no known side effects or drug interactions.

Active Ingredients: Each 0.6 mL contains simethicone, 40 mg.
Inactive Ingredients: Carbomer 934 P, citric acid, flavor (natural orange), hydroxypropyl methylcellulose, PEG-8 stearate, potassium sorbate, sodium citrate, sodium saccharin, water.

Actions: Simethicone minimizes gas formation and relieves gas entrapment in both the stomach and the lower G.I. tract. This action combats the distress due to gastrointestinal gas.

Indication: To alleviate or relieve the symptoms of gas. May also be used for postoperative gas pain or endoscopic examination.

Warnings: Keep this and all drugs out of the reach of children. If condition persists, consult your physician.

Store at controlled room temperature 59°–86°F (15°–30°C).

Dosage/Administration: Shake well before using.
Infants (under 2 years):
0.3 ml four times daily after meals and at bedtime or as directed by a physician. Can also be mixed with liquids for easier administration.
Children (2 to 12 years):
0.6 ml four times daily after meals and at bedtime or as directed by a physician.
Adults: 1.2 ml (take two 0.6 ml doses) four times daily after meals and at bedtime. Do not take more than six times per day unless directed by a physician.

How Supplied: Dropper bottles of 15 mL (0.5 fl oz) and 30 mL (1 fl oz).
Shown in Product Identification Guide, page 506

Maximum Strength
PHAZYME®-125 Chewable Tablets
[fayzime]

Description: Phazyme Chewables contain the highest dose of simethicone available in a single clean, fresh mint tasting chewable tablet. It has no known side effects or drug interactions.

Active Ingredient: Each tablet contains simethicone 125 mg.

Inactive Ingredients: Citric acid, D&C Yellow #10, dextrates, FD&C Blue #1, peppermint flavor, sorbitol, starch, sucrose, talc, tribasic calcium phosphate.

Actions: Simethicone minimizes gas formation and relieves gas entrapment in both the stomach and the lower G.I. tract. This action combats the distress due to gastrointestinal gas.

Indication: To alleviate or relieve the symptoms of gas. May also be used for postoperative gas pain.

Warnings: Keep this and all drugs out of the reach of children. If condition persists, consult your physician.

Store at controlled room temperature 59°–89°F (15°–30°C).

Dosage: One tablet, chewed thoroughly, four times a day after meals and at bedtime. Do not exceed 4 chewable tablets per day unless directed by a physician.

How Supplied: White, bevel-edged tablets with green speckles and imprinted with "Phazyme 125" in 10 pack, 30 pack and 50 pack.
Shown in Product Identification Guide, page 506

Maximum Strength
PHAZYME®-125 Softgel Capsules
[fayzime]

Description: A red softgel containing the highest dose of simethicone available in a single capsule. It has no known side effects or drug interactions.
Active Ingredient: Each capsule contains simethicone, 125 mg.
Inactive Ingredients: FD&C red No. 40, gelatin, glycerin, hydrogenated soybean oil, lecithin, methylparaben, polysorbate 80, propylparaben, soybean oil, titanium dioxide, vegetable shortening, yellow wax.

Actions: Simethicone minimizes gas formation and relieves gas entrapment in both the stomach and the lower G.I. tract. This action combats the distress due to gastrointestinal gas.

Indication: To alleviate or relieve the symptoms of gas. May also be used for postoperative gas pain.

Warnings: Keep this and all drugs out of the reach of children. If condition persists, consult your physician.

Store at controlled room temperature 59°–86°F (15°–30°C).

Dosage: One softgel capsule four times a day after meals and at bedtime. Do not exceed 4 softgel capsules per day unless directed by a physician.

How Supplied: Red softgel capsule imprinted Phazyme 125 in 10 pack, 30 pack and 50 count bottle.
Shown in Product Identification Guide, page 506

PROMISE® SENSITIVE TOOTHPASTE
For Sensitive Teeth and Cavity Prevention

Active Ingredients: Potassium Nitrate and Sodium Monofluorophosphate in a pleasantly mint-flavored dentifrice.

Promise contains Potassium Nitrate for relief of dentinal hypersensitivity resulting from the exposure of tooth dentin due to periodontal surgery, cervical (gumline) erosion, abrasion or recession which causes pain on contact with hot, cold, or tactile stimuli. Promise also contains Sodium Monofluorophosphate for cavity prevention.

Indications: Promise builds increasing protection against painful sensitivity of the teeth to cold, heat, acids, sweets or contact and aids in the prevention of dental cavities.

Actions: Promise significantly reduces tooth hypersensitivity, with response to therapy evident after two weeks of use. Controlled double-blind clinical studies provide substantial evidence of the safety and effectiveness of Promise. The current theory on mechanism of action is that the potassium nitrate in Promise

Continued on next page

Block Drug—Cont.

has an effect on neural transmission, interrupting the signal which would result in the sensation of pain. Sodium Monofluorophosphate protects the tooth surfaces to prevent cavities.

Warning: Sensitive teeth may indicate a serious problem that may need prompt care by a dentist. See your dentist if the problem persists or worsens. Do not use this product longer than 4 weeks unless recommended by a dentist or physician. **Keep this and all drugs out of the reach of children.**

Directions: Adults and children 12 years of age and older:
Apply at least a 1-inch strip of the product onto a soft bristle toothbrush. Brush teeth thoroughly for at least 1 minute twice a day (morning and evening) or as recommended by a dentist or doctor. Make sure to brush all sensitive areas of the teeth. Children under 12 years of age: Consult a dentist or physician.

How Supplied: Promise Sensitive is supplied in 1.6 oz. (46 g), 3.0 oz. (85 g) and 4.5 oz. (128 g) tubes.

**ORIGINAL FORMULA
SENSODYNE® –SC**
Toothpaste for Sensitive Teeth

Description: Each tube contains strontium chloride hexahydrate (10%) in a pleasantly flavored cleansing/polishing desensitizing dentifrice.

Actions/Indications: Tooth hypersensitivity is a condition in which individuals experience pain from exposure to hot, cold stimuli, from chewing fibrous foods, or from tactile stimuli (e.g. toothbrushing.) Hypersensitivity may also be caused by a reaction to sweet or acidic foods (OSMOTIC) stimuli. Hypersensitivity usually occurs when the protective enamel covering on teeth wears away (which happens most often at the gum line) or if gum tissue recedes and exposes the dentin underneath.
Running through the dentin are microscopic small "tubules" which, according to many authorities, carry the pain impulses to the nerve of the tooth.
Sensodyne–SC provides a unique ingredient—strontium chloride—which is believed to be deposited in the tubules where it blocks the pain. The longer Sensodyne–SC is used, the more of a barrier it helps build against pain.
The effect of Sensodyne–SC may not be manifested immediately and may require a few weeks or longer of use for relief to be obtained. A number of clinical studies in the U.S. and other countries have provided substantial evidence of the performance attributes of Sensodyne–SC. Complete relief of hypersensitivity has been reported in approximately 65% of users and measurable relief or reduction in hypersensitivity in approximately 90%. The Original Formula has been commercially available for over 30 years. The ADA Council on Dental Therapeutics has given Sensodyne–SC the Seal of Acceptance as an effective desensitizing dentifrice in otherwise normal teeth.

Contraindications: Subjects with severe dental erosion should brush properly and lightly with any dentifrice to avoid further removal of tooth structure.

Dosage and Administration: Adults and children 12 years of age and older: Apply at least a 1-inch strip of the product onto a soft bristle toothbrush. Brush teeth thoroughly for at least 1 minute twice a day (morning and evening) or as recommended by a dentist or physician. Make sure to brush all sensitive areas of the teeth. Children under 12 years of age: consult a dentist or physician.

Warnings: Sensitive teeth may indicate a serious problem that may need prompt care by a dentist. See your dentist if the problem persists or worsens. Do not use this product longer than 4 weeks unless recommended by a dentist or doctor.
Keep this and all drugs out of the reach of children.

How Supplied: SENSODYNE–SC Toothpaste is supplied in 2.1 oz. (60 g), 4.0 oz. (113 g), and 6.0 oz. (170 g).

**FRESH MINT SENSODYNE®
COOL GEL SENSODYNE®
SENSODYNE® WITH
BAKING SODA**
Toothpaste for Sensitive Teeth and Cavity Prevention
Desensitizing Dentrifice

Active Ingredients: 5% Potassium Nitrate and Sodium Monofluorophosphate (Fresh Mint) or Sodium Fluoride (Cool Gel and Baking Soda) in a pleasantly mint-flavored dentifrice.
Fresh Mint Sensodyne, Cool Gel Sensodyne and Sensodyne with Baking Soda contain Potassium Nitrate for relief of dentinal hypersensitivity resulting from the exposure of tooth dentin due to periodontal surgery, cervical (gum line) erosion, abrasion or recession which causes pain on contact with hot, cold, or tactile stimuli and fluoride for cavity prevention. Fresh Mint Sensodyne has been given the Seal of Acceptance by the ADA Council on Dental Therapeutics as an effective desensitizing dentifrice for otherwise normal teeth.

Actions: Fresh Mint Sensodyne, Cool Gel Sensodyne and Sensodyne with Baking Soda significantly reduce tooth hypersensitivity, with response to therapy evident after two weeks of use. Controlled double-blind clinical studies provide substantial evidence of the safety and effectiveness of potassium nitrate. The current theory on mechanism of action is that potassium nitrate has an effect on neural transmission, interrupting the signal which would result in the sensation of pain. Fluorides are anticariogenic, forming fluoroapatite in the outer surface of the dental enamel which is resistant to acids and caries.

Warnings: Sensitive teeth may indicate a serious problem that may need prompt care by a dentist. See your dentist if the problem persists or worsens. Do not use this product longer than 4 weeks unless recommended by a dentist or physician. Keep this and all drugs out of the reach of children.

Dosage and Administration: Adults and children 12 years of age and older: Apply at least a 1-inch strip of the product onto a soft bristle toothbrush. Brush teeth thoroughly for at least 1 minute twice a day (morning and evening) or as recommended by a dentist or doctor. Make sure to brush all sensitive areas of the teeth. Children under 12 years of age: consult a dentist or physician.

How Supplied: Fresh Mint Sensodyne is supplied in 2.1 (60 g), 4.0 (113 g) and 6.0 oz. (170 g) tubes and in 4.0 oz. pumps. Cool Gel and Sensodyne with Baking Soda are available in 2.1 (60 g), 4.0 (113 g) and 6.0 oz. (170 g) tubes.

**TEGRIN® DANDRUFF SHAMPOO
TEGRIN® FOR PSORIASIS
SKIN CREAM AND
MEDICATED SOAP**

Description: Tegrin® Dandruff Shampoo contains 7% coal tar solution equivalent to 1.1% coal tar, in a pleasantly scented, high-foaming, cleansing shampoo base with emollients, conditioners and other formula components.
Tegrin® for Psoriasis Skin Cream and Medicated Soap each contain 5% coal tar solution, equivalent to 0.8% coal tar. The Cream also contains alcohol (4.9% and 4.7%, respectively).

Actions/Indications: Coal Tar is obtained in the destructive distillation of bituminous coal and is a highly effective agent for controlling the flaking and itching of the scalp associated with dandruff, seborrheic dermatitis and psoriasis. The action of coal tar is believed to be keratolytic, antiseptic, antipruritic and astringent. The coal tar solution used in Tegrin Dandruff Shampoo is prepared in such a way as to reduce the pitch and other irritant components found in crude coal tar without reduction in therapeutic potency.
Coal tar solution has been used clincially for many years as a remedy for dandruff and for scaling associated with scalp disorders such as seborrhea and psoriasis. Its mechanism of action has not been fully established, but it is believed to retard the rate of turnover of epidermal cells with regular use. A number of clinical studies have demonstrated the performance attributes of Tegrin Dandruff Shampoo against dandruff and seborrheic dermatitis. In addition to relieving the above symptoms, Tegrin shampoo, used regularly, maintains scalp and hair

cleanliness and leaves the hair lustrous and manageable.

Warnings: *All Tegrin® products:* For external use only. Avoid contact with eyes. If contact occurs, rinse eyes thoroughly with water. If condition worsens or does not improve after regular use of this product as directed, consult a doctor. Use caution in exposing skin to sunlight after applying this product. It may increase tendency to sunburn for up to 24 hours after application. Do not use for prolonged periods without consulting a doctor. Do not use this product with other forms of psoriasis therapy, such as ultraviolet radiation or prescription drugs, unless directed by a doctor. Keep out of reach of children. In case of accidental ingestion, seek professional assistance or contact a Poison Control Center immediately.
Tegrin® for Psoriasis Skin Cream and Medicated Soap: If the condition covers a large area of the body, consult a doctor before using this product. (See other Warnings above).

Directions: Shake Tegrin Dandruff Shampoo well. Wet hair thoroughly. Rub Tegrin liberally into hair and scalp. Rinse thoroughly. Briskly massage a second application of the shampoo into a rich lather. Rinse thoroughly. For best results use at least twice a week or as directed by a doctor.
Apply Tegrin for Psoriasis cream to affected areas one to four times daily or as directed by a doctor. Use Tegrin Soap on affected areas in place of your regular soap.

How Supplied: Tegrin Dandruff Shampoo is supplied in 7 fl. oz. (207 ml) plastic bottles.
Tegrin Cream 2 oz. (57 g) and 4.4 oz. (124 g) tubes, Tegrin Soap 4.5 oz. (127 g) bars.

Boiron, The World Leader In Homeopathy
6 CAMPUS BLVD.
BUILDING A
NEWTOWN SQUARE, PA 19073

HEADQUARTERS AND EAST COAST BRANCH:
6 Campus Blvd., Building A
Newtown Square, PA 19073
(610) 325-7464

Direct Inquiries to:
John Durkin
East Coast Branch Manager
(800) 258-8823

For Medical Emergencies Contact:
Mark Land
Technical Services Manager
(610) 325-7464

WEST COAST BRANCH:
98C West Cochran Street
Simi Valley, CA 93065

Direct Inquiries to:
Ambroise Demonceaux
West Coast Branch Manager
(805) 582-9091

OSCILLOCOCCINUM®
[*ah-sill 'o-cox-see 'num '*]

Active Ingredient: Anas barbariae hepatis et cordis extractum HPUS 200CK

Indications: For the relief of symptoms of flu such as fever, chills, body aches and pains.

Actions: Like most homeopathic medicine, Oscillococcinum® acts gently by stimulating the patient's natural defense mechanisms.

Dosage and Administration: (Adults and Children over 2 years of age):
At the onset of symptoms, place the entire contents of one tube in the mouth and allow to dissolve under the tongue. Repeat for 2 more doses at 6 hour intervals. For maximum results, Oscillococcinum® should be taken early, at the onset of symptoms, and at least 15 minutes before or 1 hour after meals.

Warnings: If symptoms persist for more than three days or worsen, consult your physician. Keep this and all medication out of reach of children. As with any drug if you are pregnant or nursing a baby, seek professional advice before using this product. Diabetics: this product contains sugar (0.85 g sucrose, 0.15 g lactose per unit dose).

How Supplied: boxes of 3 unit doses or 6 unit doses of 0.04 oz. (1 gram) each (NDC #0220-9280-32 and NDC #0220-9288-33) Tamper resistant package.
Manufactured by Boiron, France.
Distributor: Boiron, Newtown Square, PA 19073

EDUCATIONAL MATERIAL

Boiron Product Catalogue
General description of the most popular Boiron products.
Oscillococcinum ® *Brochure*
Brochure describing clinical research on the product.
"What Is Homeopathy?"
Booklet describing the basic principles of homeopathy.
"An Introduction to Homeopathy for the Practicing Pharmacist"
An ACPE-approved continuing education booklet for pharmacists (0.2 CEUs).

Bristol-Myers Products
(A Bristol-Myers Squibb Company)
345 PARK AVENUE
NEW YORK, NY 10154

For Medical Information Contact:
Generally:
Bristol-Myers Products Division
Consumer Affairs Department
1350 Liberty Avenue
Hillside, NJ 07207

In Emergencies:
(800) 468-7746

ALPHA KERI®
Moisture Rich Body Oil

Composition: Contains mineral oil, Hydroloc™ brand of Westwood's PEG-4 dilaurate, lanolin oil, fragrance, benzophenone-3, D&C green 6.

Indications: ALPHA KERI is a water-dispersible oil for the care of dry skin. ALPHA KERI effectively deposits a thin, uniform, emulsified film of oil over the skin. This film lubricates and softens the skin. ALPHA KERI Moisture Rich Body Oil is an all-over skin moisturizer. Only Alpha Keri contains Hydroloc™—the unique emulsifier that provides a more uniform distribution of the therapeutic oils to moisturize dry skin. ALPHA KERI is valuable as an aid for dry skin and mild skin irritations.

Directions for Use: ALPHA KERI *should always be used with water, either added to water or rubbed on to wet skin.* Because of its inherent cleansing properties it is not necessary to use soap when ALPHA KERI is being used.
For external use only.
Label directions should be followed for use in shower, bath and cleansing.

Precaution: The patient should be warned to guard against slipping in tub or shower.

How Supplied: 4 fl. oz., 8 fl. oz., and 16 fl. oz., plastic bottles.

BACKACHE CAPLETS

Composition: Each caplet contains Magnesium Salicylate Tetrahydrate 580 mg (equivalent to 467 mg of anhydrous Magnesium Salicylate)
Other Ingredients: Carnauba Wax, Hydrogenated Vegetable Oil, Hydroxypropyl Methylcellulose, Magnesium Stearate, Microcrystalline Cellulose, Polyethylene Glycol, Polysorbate 80, Titanium Dioxide

Indications: For the temporary relief of minor aches and pains associated with backache and muscular aches (e.g., sprains and strains).

Directions: Adults: 2 caplets with water every 6 hours while symptoms persist, not to exceed 8 caplets in 24 hours or

Continued on next page

Bristol-Myers—Cont.

as directed by a doctor. Children under 12: Consult a doctor.

Warnings: Children and teenagers should not use this medicine for chicken pox or flu symptoms before a doctor is consulted about Reye syndrome, a rate but serious illness. **KEEP THIS AND ALL OTHER MEDICATIONS OUT OF THE REACH OF CHILDREN. IN CASE OF ACCIDENTAL OVERDOSE, SEEK PROFESSIONAL ASSISTANCE OR CONTACT A POISON CONTROL CENTER IMMEDIATELY.** As with any drug, if you are pregnant or nursing a baby, seek the advice of a health professional before using this product. Do not take this product for more than 10 days unless directed by a doctor. If pain persists or gets worse, if new symptoms occur, or if redness or swelling is present, consult a doctor because these could be signs of a serious condition. Do not take this product if you are allergic to salicylates (including aspirin), have asthma, have stomach problems (such as heartburn, upset stomach or stomach pain) that persists or recur, or if you have ulcers or bleeding problems, unless directed by a doctor. If ringing in the ears or loss of hearing occurs, consult a doctor before taking any more of this product.

Drug Interaction Precaution: Do not take this product if you are taking a prescription drug for anticoagulation (thinning of blood), diabetes, gout or arthritis unless directed by a doctor.

How Supplied: BACKACHE is a white caplet with the logo "N-BACK" debossed on one side.
NDC 19810–0579–1 Blister cards of 24's
The bottles of 50's are packaged in child resistant closures; the blister cards of 24's are recommended for households without young children and are packaged without a child resistant closure. Store at room temperature.

BUFFERIN®
[*bŭf′fĕr-ĭn*]
Analgesic

Composition:
Active Ingredient: Each coated tablet contains Aspirin 325 mg in a formulation buffered with Calcium Carbonate, Magnesium Oxide and Magnesium Carbonate.
Other Ingredients: Benzoic Acid, Citric Acid, Corn Starch, FD&C Blue No. 1, Hydroxypropyl Methylcellulose, Magnesium Stearate, Mineral Oil, Polysorbate 20, Povidone, Propylene Glycol, Simethicone Emulsion, Sodium Phosphate, Sorbitan Monolaurate, Titanium Dioxide. May also contain: Carnauba Wax, Zinc Stearate.

Indications: For fast temporary relief of headaches, minor arthritis pain and inflammation, muscle aches, pain and fever of colds, menstrual pain and toothaches.

Directions: Adults and chldren 12 years of age and over: 2 tablets with water every 4 hours while symptoms persist, not to exceed 12 tablets in 24 hours, or as directed by a doctor. Children under 12: Consult a doctor.

Warnings: Children and teenagers should not use this medicine for chicken pox or flu symptoms before a doctor is consulted about Reye syndrome, a rare but serious illness reported to be associated with aspirin. Keep this and all other medications out of the reach of children. In case of accidental overdose, seek professional assistance or contact a poison control center immediately. As with any drug, if you are pregnant or nursing a baby, seek the advice of a health professional before using this product. **IT IS ESPECIALLY IMPORTANT NOT TO USE ASPIRIN DURING THE LAST 3 MONTHS OF PREGNANCY UNLESS SPECIFICALLY DIRECTED TO DO SO BY A DOCTOR BECAUSE IT MAY CAUSE PROBLEMS IN THE UNBORN CHILD OR COMPLICATIONS DURING DELIVERY.** Do not take this product for pain for more than 10 days or for fever for more than 3 days unless directed by a doctor. If pain or fever persists or gets worse, if new symptoms occur, or if redness or swelling is present, consult a doctor because these could be signs of a serious condition. Do not take this product if you are allergic to aspirin, have asthma, have stomach problems (such as heartburn, upset stomach or stomach pain) that persist or recur, or if you have ulcers or bleeding problems, unless directed by a doctor. If ringing in the ears or loss of hearing occurs, consult a doctor before taking or giving any more of this product.

Drug Interaction Precaution: Do not take this product if you are taking a prescription drug for anticoagulation (thinning of blood), diabetes, gout or arthritis unless directed by a doctor.

How Supplied: BUFFERIN is supplied as:
Coated circular white tablet with letter "B" debossed on one surface.
NDC 19810-0093-3 Bottle of 30's
NDC 19810-0093-4 Bottle of 50's
NDC 19810-0073-5 Bottle of 100's
NDC 19810-0073-6 Bottle of 200's
All consumer sizes have child resistant closures except 100's for tablets which are sizes recommended for households without young children. Store at room temperature.

Professional Labeling

1. BUFFERIN® FOR RECURRENT TRANSIENT ISCHEMIC ATTACKS

Indication: For reducing the risk of recurrent transient ischemic attacks (TIA's) or stroke in men who have had transient ischemia of the brain due to fibrin platelet emboli. There is inadequate evidence that aspirin or buffered aspirin is effective in reducing TIA's in women at the recommended dosage. There is no evidence that aspirin or buffered aspirin is of benefit in the treatment of completed strokes in men or women.

Clinical Trials: The indication is supported by the results of a Canadian study (1) in which 585 patients with threatened stroke were followed in a randomized clinical trial for an average of 26 months to determine whether aspirin or sulfinpyrazone, singly or in combination, was superior to placebo in preventing transient ischemic attacks, stroke, or death. The study showed that, although sulfinpyrazone had no statistically significant effect, aspirin reduced the risk of continuing transient ischemic attacks, stroke, or death by 19 percent and reduced the risk of stroke or death by 31 percent. Another aspirin study carried out in the United States with 178 patients, showed a statistically significant number of "favorable outcomes," including reduced transient ischemic attacks, stroke, and death (2).

Precautions: Patients presenting with signs and symptoms of TIA's should have a complete medical and neurologic evaluation. Consideration should be given to other disorders that resemble TIA's. Attention should be given to risk factors: it is important to evaluate and treat, if appropriate, other diseases associated with TIA's and stroke, such as hypertension and diabetes.
Concurrent administration of absorbable antacids at therapeutic doses may increase the clearance of salicylates in some individuals. The concurrent administration of nonabsorbable antacids may alter the rate of absorption of aspirin, thereby resulting in a decreased acetylsalicylic acid/salicylate ratio in plasma. The clinical significance of these decreases in available aspirin is unknown. Aspirin at dosages of 1,000 milligrams per day has been associated with small increases in blood pressure, blood urea nitrogen, and serum uric acid levels. It is recommended that patients placed on long-term aspirin treatment be seen at regular intervals to assess changes in these measurements.

Adverse Reactions: At dosages of 1,000 milligrams or higher of aspirin per day, gastrointestinal side effects include stomach pain, heartburn, nausea and/or vomiting, as well as increased rates of gross gastrointestinal bleeding.

Dosage and Administration: Adult oral dosage for men is 1,300 milligrams a day, in divided doses of 650 milligrams twice a day or 325 milligrams four times a day.

References:
(1) The Canadian Cooperative Study Group. "A Randomized Trial of Aspirin and Sulfinpyrazone in Threatened Stroke," *New England Journal of Medicine*, 299:53–59, 1978.
(2) Fields, W.S., et al., "Controlled Trial of Aspirin in Cerebral Ischemia," *Stroke* 8:301–316, 1977.

2. BUFFERIN® FOR MYOCARDIAL INFARCTION

Indication: Aspirin is indicated to reduce the risk of death and/or nonfatal myocardial infarction in patients with a previous infarction or unstable angina pectoris.

Clinical Trials: The indication is supported by the results of six, large, randomized multicenter, placebo-controlled studies[1-7] involving 10,816, predominantly male, post-myocardial infarction (MI) patients and one randomized placebo-controlled study of 1,266 men with unstable angina. Therapy with aspirin was begun at intervals after the onset of acute MI varying from less than 3 days to more than 5 years and continued for periods of from less than one year to four years. In the unstable angina study, treatment was started within 1 month after the onset of unstable angina and continued for 12 weeks and complicating conditions such as congestive heart failure were not included in the study.

Aspirin therapy in MI patients was associated with about a 20 percent reduction in the risk of subsequent death and/or nonfatal reinfarction, a median absolute decrease of 3 percent from the 12 to 22 percent event rates in the placebo groups. In the aspirin-treated unstable angina patients the reduction in risk was about 50 percent, a reduction in the event rate of 5% from the 10% rate in the placebo group over the 12 weeks of the study.

Daily dosage of aspirin in the post-myocardial infarction studies was 300 mg. in one study and 900 and 1500 mg. in five studies. A dose of 325 mg. was used in the study of unstable angina.

Adverse Reactions: Gastrointestinal Reactions: Doses of 1000 mg. per day of aspirin caused gastrointestinal symptoms and bleeding that in some cases were clinically significant. In the largest post-infarction study (The Aspirin Myocardial Infaraction Study (AMIS) with 4,500 people), the percentage incidences of gastrointestinal symptoms for the aspirin (1000 mg. of a standard, solid-tablet formulation) and placebo-treated subjects, respectively, were: stomach pain (14.5%; 4.4%); heartburn (11.9%; 4.8%); nausea and/or vomiting (7.6%; 2.1%); hospitalization for gastrointestinal disorder (4.8%; 3.5%). In the AMIS and other trials, aspirin treated patients had increased rates of gross gastrointestinal bleeding. Symptoms and signs of gastrointestinal irritation were not significantly increased in subjects treated for unstable angina with buffered aspirin in solution.

Cardiovascular and Biochemical:
In the AMIS trial, the dosage of 1000 mg. per day of aspirin was associated with small increases in systolic blood pressure (BP) (average 1.5 to 2.1 mm) and diastolic BP (0.5 to 0.6 mm), depending upon whether maximal or last available readings were used. Blood urea nitrogen and uric acid levels were also increased, but by less than 1.0 mg%.

Subjects with marked hypertension or renal insufficiency had been excluded from the trial so that the clinical importance of these observations for such subjects or for any subjects treated over more prolonged periods is not known. It is recommended that patients placed on long-term aspirin treatment, even at doses of 300 mg. per day, be seen at regular intervals to assess changes in these measurements.

Administration and Dosage: Although most of the studies used dosages exceeding 300 mg., two trials used only 300 mg. and pharmacologic data indicate that this dose inhibits platelet function fully. Therefore, 300 mg. or a conventional 325 mg. aspirin dose is a reasonable, routine dose that would minimize gastrointestinal adverse reactions.

References: 1. Elwood P.C., et al., "A Randomized Controlled Trial of Acetylsalicylic Acid in the Secondary Prevention of Mortality from Myocardial Infarction," *British Medical Journal,* 1:436–440, 1974. 2. The Coronary Drug Project Research Group, "Aspirin in Coronary Heart Disease," *Journal of Chronic Disease,* 29:625–642, 1976. 3. Breddin K, et al., "Secondary Prevention of Myocardial Infarction; Comparison of Acetylsalicylic Acid Phenprocoumon and Placebo," *Thromb. Haemost.,* 41:225–236, 1979. 4. Aspirin Myocardial Infarction Study Research Group, "A Randomized, Controlled Trial of Aspirin in Persons Recovered from Myocardial Infarction," *Journal American Medical Association,* 243:661–669, 1980. 5. Elwood P.C., and Sweetnam, P.M., "Aspirin and Secondary Mortality after Myocardial Infarction," *Lancet,* pp. 1313–1315, December 22–29, 1979. 6. The Persantine-Aspirin Reinfarction Study Research Group. "Persantine and Aspirin in Coronary Heart Disease," *Circulation* 62;449–460, 1980. 7. Lewis H.D., et al., "Protective Effects of Aspirin Against Acute Myocardial Infarction and Death in Men with Unstable Angina, Results of a Veterans Administration Cooperative Study," *New England Journal of Medicine,* 309;396–403, 1983.

Shown in Product Identification Guide, page 506

Arthritis Strength BUFFERIN®
[bŭf'fĕr-ĭn]
Analgesic

Composition:
Active Ingredient: Aspirin (500 mg) in a formulation buffered with Calcium Carbonate, Magnesium Oxide and Magnesium Carbonate.
Other Ingredients: Benzoic Acid, Citric Acid, Corn Starch, FD&C Blue No. 1, Hydroxypropyl Methylcellulose, Magnesium Stearate, Mineral Oil, Polysorbate 20, Povidone, Propylene Glycol, Simethicone Emulsion, Sodium Phosphate, Sorbitan Monolaurate, Titanium Dioxide.

May also contain: Carnauba Wax, Zinc Stearate.

Indications: For fast temporary relief of the minor aches and pains, stiffness, swelling and inflammation of arthritis.

Directions: Adults: 2 caplets with water every 6 hours as needed, not to exceed 8 caplets a day. Children under 12: Consult a doctor.

Warnings: Children and teenagers should not use this medicine for chicken pox or flu symptoms before a doctor is consulted about Reye syndrome, a rare but serious illness reported to be associated with aspirin. KEEP THIS AND ALL OTHER MEDICATIONS OUT OF THE REACH OF CHILDREN. IN CASE OF ACCIDENTAL OVERDOSE, SEEK PROFESSIONAL ASSISTANCE OR CONTACT A POISON CONTROL CENTER IMMEDIATELY. As with any drug, if you are pregnant or nursing a baby, seek the advice of a health professional before using this product. **IT IS ESPECIALLY IMPORTANT NOT TO USE ASPIRIN DURING THE LAST 3 MONTHS OF PREGNANCY UNLESS SPECIFICALLY DIRECTED TO DO SO BY A DOCTOR BECAUSE IT MAY CAUSE PROBLEMS IN THE UNBORN CHILD OR COMPLICATIONS DURING DELIVERY.** Do not take this product for pain for more than 10 days or for fever for more than 3 days unless directed by a doctor. If pain or fever persists or gets worse, if new symptoms occur, or if redness or swelling is present, consult a doctor because these could be signs of a serious condition. Do not take this product if you are allergic to aspirin, have asthma, have stomach problems (such as heartburn, upset stomach or stomach pain) that persist or recur, or if you have ulcers or bleeding problems, unless directed by a doctor. If ringing in the ears or loss of hearing occurs, consult a doctor before taking any more of this product.

Drug Interaction Precaution: Do not take this product if you are taking a prescription drug for anticoagulation (thinning of blood), diabetes, gout or arthritis unless directed by a doctor.

How Supplied: Arthritis Strength BUFFERIN® is supplied as:
Plain white coated caplet "ASB" debossed on one side.
NDC 19810-0051-2 Bottle of 100's
Store at room temperature.
Shown in Product Identification Guide, page 506

Extra Strength BUFFERIN®
[bŭf'fĕr-ĭn]
Analgesic

Composition:
Active Ingredient: Aspirin (500 mg) in a formulation buffered with Calcium Carbonate, Magnesium Oxide and Magnesium Carbonate.

Continued on next page

Bristol-Myers—Cont.

Other Ingredients: Benzoic Acid, Citric Acid, Corn Starch, FD&C Blue No. 1, Hydroxypropyl Methylcellulose, Magnesium Stearate, Mineral Oil, Polysorbate 20, Povidone, Propylene Glycol, Simethicone Emulsion, Sodium Phosphate, Sorbitan Monolaurate, Titanium Dioxide. May also contain: Carnauba Wax, Zinc Stearate.

Indications: For fast temporary relief of headaches, minor arthritis pain and inflammation, muscle aches, pain and fever of colds, menstrual pain and toothaches.

Directions: Adults: 2 tablets with water every 6 hours as needed, not to exceed 8 tablets a day. Children under 12: Consult a doctor.

Warnings: Children and teenagers should not use this medicine for chicken pox or flu symptoms before a doctor is consulted about Reye syndrome, a rare but serious illness reported to be associated with aspirin. KEEP THIS AND ALL OTHER MEDICATIONS OUT OF THE REACH OF CHILDREN. IN CASE OF ACCIDENTAL OVERDOSE, SEEK PROFESSIONAL ASSISTANCE OR CONTACT A POISON CONTROL CENTER IMMEDIATELY. As with any drug, if your are pregnant or nursing a baby, seek the advice of a health professional before using this product. **IT IS ESPECIALLY IMPORTANT NOT TO USE ASPIRIN DURING THE LAST 3 MONTHS OF PREGNANCY UNLESS SPECIFICALLY DIRECTED TO DO SO BY A DOCTOR BECAUSE IT MAY CAUSE PROBLEMS IN THE UNBORN CHILD OR COMPLICATIONS DURING DELIVERY.** Do not take this product for more than 10 days or for fever for more than 3 days unless directed by a doctor. If pain or fever persists or gets worse, if new symptoms occur, or if redness or swelling is present, consult a doctor because these could be signs of a serious condition. Do not take this product if you are allergic to aspirin, have asthma, have stomach problems (such as heartburn, upset stomach or stomach pain) that persist or recur, or if you have ulcers or bleeding problems, unless directed by a doctor. If ringing in the ears or loss of hearing occurs, consult a doctor before taking any more of this product.

Drug Interaction Precaution: Do not take this product if you are taking a prescription drug for anticoagulation (thinning of blood), diabetes, gout or arthritis unless directed by a doctor.

How Supplied: Extra Strength BUFFERIN® is supplied as:
White elongated coated tablet with "ESB" debossed on one side.
NDC 19810-0074-1 Bottle of 30's
NDC 19810-0074-4 Bottle of 50's
NDC 19810-0074-3 Bottle of 100's
All sizes have child resistant closures except 50's which is recommended for households without young children.
Store at room temperature.

Shown in Product Identification Guide, page 506

COMTREX® Maximum Strength
[cŏm ′trĕx]
Multi-Symptom Cold Reliever

Composition: Each tablet, caplet, liqui-gel and fluidounce (30 ml.) contains: [See table below.]

Indications: For the temporary relief of the following symptoms associated with the common cold and flu: minor aches, pains, headache, muscular aches, and fever; cough; nasal congestion; runny nose and sneezing.

Directions:
Tablets or Caplets: Adults and children 12 years and over: 2 tablets or caplets every 6 hours while symptoms persist, not to exceed 8 tablets or caplets in 24 hours, or as directed by a doctor. Children under 12: Consult a doctor.
Liqui-Gel: Adults: 2 liqui-gels every 6 hours while symptoms persist, not to exceed 8 liqui-gels in 24 hours, or as directed by a doctor. Children under 12: Consult a doctor.
Liquid: Adults: One fluidounce (30 ml) in medicine cup provided or 2 tablespoons every 6 hours while symptoms persist, not to exceed 4 doses in 24 hours. Children under 12: Consult a doctor.

Warnings: Keep this and all drugs out of the reach of children. In case of accidental overdose, seek professional assistance or contact a poison control center immediately. Prompt medical attention is critical for adults as well as children even if you do not notice any signs or symptoms. As with any drug, if you are pregnant or nursing a baby, seek the advice of a health professional before using this product. Do not take this product for more than 7 days. A persistent cough

	COMTREX Per Tablet or Caplet	COMTREX Liquid-Gel per Liqui-Gel	COMTREX Liquid Per Fl. Ounce
Acetaminophen:	500 mg.	500 mg.	1000 mg.
Pseudoephedrine HCl:	30 mg.	—	60 mg.
Phenylpropanolamine HCl:	—	12.5 mg.	—
Chlorpheniramine Maleate:	2 mg.	2 mg.	4 mg.
Dextromethorphan HBr:	15 mg.	15 mg.	30 mg.

Tablet/Caplet	Liqui-Gels	Liquid
Benzoic Acid	D&C Yellow No. 10	Alcohol (10% by volume)
Carnauba Wax	FD&C Red No. 40	Benzoic acid
Corn Starch	Gelatin	D&C Yellow No. 10
D&C Yellow No. 10 Lake	Glycerin	FD&C Blue No. 1
FD&C Red No. 40 Lake	Polyethylene Glycol	FD&C Red No. 40
Hydroxypropyl Methylcellulose	Povidone	Flavors
Magnesium Stearate	Propylene Glycol	Glycerin
		Polyethylene Glycol
Methylparaben	Silicon Dioxide	Povidone
		Saccharin Sodium
Mineral Oil	Sorbitol	Sodium Citrate
Polysorbate 20	Titanium Dioxide	Sucrose
Povidone	Water	Water
Propylene Glycol		
Propylparaben		
Simethicone Emulsion		
Sorbitan Monolaurate		
Stearic Acid		
Titanium Dioxide		
May also contain:		
Carnauba wax		
D&C Yellow No. 10		
FD&C Red No. 4		

may be a sign of a serious condition. If cough persists for more than 7 days, tends to recur, or is accompanied by rash, persistent headache, fever that lasts for more than 3 days, or if new symptoms occur, consult a doctor. Do not take this product for persistent or chronic cough such as occurs with smoking, asthma, emphysema, or if cough is accompanied by excessive phlegm (mucus) unless directed by a doctor. **Do not exceed recommended dosage.** If nervousness, dizziness, or sleeplessness occur, discontinue use and consult a doctor. If symptoms do not improve within 7 days or are accompanied by fever, consult a doctor. Do not take this product unless directed by a doctor, if you have a breathing problem such as emphysema or chronic bronchitis, heart disease, high blood pressure, thyroid disease, diabetes, glaucoma, or difficulty in urination due to enlargement of the prostate gland. May cause excitability especially in children. May cause marked drowsiness; alcohol, sedatives, and tranquilizers may increase the drowsiness effect. Avoid alcoholic beverages while taking this product. Do not take this product if you are taking sedatives or tranquilizers, without first consulting your doctor. Use caution when driving a motor vehicle or operating machinery.

Drug Interaction Precaution: Do not use this product if you are now taking a prescription monoamine oxidase inhibitor (MAOI) (certain drugs for depression, psychiatric or emotional conditions, or Parkinson's disease), or for 2 weeks after stopping the MAOI drug. If you are uncertain whether your prescription drug contains an MAOI, consult a health professional before taking this product.

Overdose:
MUCOMYST (acetylcysteine) As An Antidote For Acetaminophen Overdose)
Acetaminophen is rapidly absorbed from the upper gastrointestinal tract with peak plasma levels occurring between 30 and 60 minutes after therapeutic doses and usually within 4 hours following an overdose. The parent compound, which is nontoxic, is extensively metabolized in the liver to principally the sulfate and glucuronide conjugates which are also nontoxic and are rapidly excreted in the urine. A small fraction of an ingested dose is metabolized in the liver by the cytochrome P-450 mixed function oxidase enzyme system to form a reactive, potentially toxic, intermediate metabolite which preferentially conjugates with hepatic glutathione to form the nontoxic cysteine and mercapturic acid derivatives which are then excreted by the kidney. Therapeutic doses of acetaminophen do not saturate the glucuronide and sulfate conjugation pathways and do not result in the formation of sufficient reactive metabolite to deplete glutathione stores. However, following ingestion of a large overdose (150 mg/kg or greater) the glucuronide and sulfate conjugation pathways are saturated resulting in a

larger fraction of the drug being metabolized via the P-450 pathway. The increased formation of reactive metabolite may deplete the hepatic stores of glutathione with subsequent binding of the metabolite to protein molecules within the hepatocyte resulting in cellular necrosis. Acetylcysteine has been shown to reduce the extent of liver injury following acetaminophen overdose. Early symptoms following a potentially hepatotoxic overdose may include: nausea, vomiting, diaphoresis and general malaise. Clinical and laboratory evidence of hepatic toxicity may not be apparent until 48 to 72 hours postingestion. In adults and adolescents, regardless of the quantity of acetaminophen reported to have been ingested, administer MUCO-MYST® acetylcysteine immediately. MUCOMYST acetylcysteine therapy should be initiated and continued for a full course of therapy. Its effectiveness depends on early administration, with benefit seen principally in patients treated within 16 hours of the overdose. If acetaminophen plasma assay capability is not available, and the estimated acetaminophen ingestion exceeds 150 mg/kg., MUCOMYST acetylcysteine therapy should be initiated and continued for a full course of therapy.
For full prescribing information, refer to the MUCOMYST package insert. Do not await the results of assays for acetaminophen level before initiating treatment with MUCOMYST acetylcysteine. The following additional procedures are recommended: The stomach should be emptied promptly by lavage or by induction of emesis with syrup of ipecac. A serum acetaminophen assay should be obtained as early as possible, but no sooner than four hours following ingestion. Liver function studies should be obtained initially and repeated at 24-hour intervals.
For additional emergency information call your regional poison center or toll-free (1-800-525-6115) to the Rocky Mountain Poison Center for assistance in diagnosis and for directions in the use of MUCOMYST acetylcysteine as an antidote.

How Supplied:
COMTREX® is supplied as:
Coated yellow tablet with letters "Cx" debossed on one surface.
NDC 19810-0092-1 Blister packages of 24's
NDC 19810-0092-2 Bottles of 50's
Coated yellow caplet with "Cx" debossed on one side.
NDC 19810-0055-1 Blister packages of 24's
NDC 19810-0055-2 Bottles of 50's
Yellow Liqui-Gel with "COMTREX LG" printed in red on one side.
NDC 19810-0431-1 Blister packages of 24's
NDC 19810-0431-2 Blister packages of 50's

Clear Red Cherry Flavored liquid:
NDC 19810-0527-1 6 oz. plastic bottles.
All sizes packaged in child resistant closures except for 24's for tablets, caplets and liqui-gels which are sizes recommended for households without young children. Store caplets, tablets and liquid at room temperature.
Store liqui-gels below 86° F. (30° C.). Keep from freezing.
Shown in Product Identification Guide, page 506

ALLERGY–SINUS COMTREX
Maximum Strength
[cŏm 'trĕx]
Multi-Symptom Allergy/Sinus Formula

Composition:
Active Ingredients: Each coated tablet or caplet contains 500 mg acetaminophen, 30 mg pseudoephedrine HCl, 2 mg chlorpheniramine maleate.
Other Ingredients: Benzoic acid, carnauba wax, corn starch, D&C yellow No. 10 lake, FD&C blue No. 1 lake, FD&C Red No. 40 lake, hydroxypropyl methylcellulose, mineral oil, polysorbate 20, povidone, propylene glycol, simethicone emulsion, sodium citrate, sorbitan monolaurate, stearic acid, titanium dioxide. May also contain: crospovidone, D&C yellow No. 10, erythorbic acid, FD&C blue No. 1, magnesium stearate, methylparaben, microcrystalline cellulose, polysorbate 80, propylparaben, silicon dioxide, wood cellulose.

Indications:
ALLERGY-SINUS COMTREX provides temporary relief of these upper respiratory allergy, hay fever, and sinusitis symptoms: sneezing, itchy watery eyes, runny nose, headache, nasal and sinus pressure and congestion.

Directions: Adults: 2 tablets or caplets every 6 hours while symptoms persist, not to exceed 8 tablets or caplets in 24 hours, or as directed by a doctor. Children under 12 years of age: Consult a doctor.

Warnings: KEEP THIS AND ALL OTHER MEDICATIONS OUT OF THE REACH OF CHILDREN. IN CASE OF ACCIDENTAL OVERDOSE, SEEK PROFESSIONAL ASSISTANCE OR CONTACT A POISON CONTROL CENTER IMMEDIATELY. PROMPT MEDICAL ATTENTION IS CRITICAL FOR ADULTS AS WELL AS FOR CHILDREN EVEN IF YOU DO NOT NOTICE ANY SIGNS OR SYMPTOMS. As with any drug, if you are pregnant or nursing a baby, seek the advice of a health professional before using this product. Do not take this product for more than 7 days unless directed by a doctor. If symptoms do not improve or are accompanied by a fever that lasts for more than 3 days, or if new symptoms occur, consult a doctor. Do not exceed recommended dosage because at higher doses nervousness, dizzi-

Continued on next page

Bristol-Myers—Cont.

ness or sleeplessness may occur. May cause excitability especially in children. Do not take this product unless directed by a doctor if you have a breathing problem such as emphysema, or chronic bronchitis, or if you have heart disease, high blood pressure, thyroid disease, diabetes, shortness of breath, or difficulty in urination due to enlargement of the prostate gland. May cause drowsiness; alcohol, sedatives and tranquilizers may increase the drowsiness effect. Avoid alcoholic beverages, while taking this product. Do not take this product if you are taking sedatives or tranquilizers without first consulting your doctor. Use caution when driving a motor vehicle or operating machinery.

Drug Interaction Precaution: Do not use this product if you are now taking a prescription monoamine oxidase inhibitor (MAOI) (certain drugs for depression, psychiatric or emotional conditions, or Parkinson's disease), or for 2 weeks after stopping the MAOI drug. If you are uncertain whether your prescription drug contains an MAOI, consult a health professional before taking this product.

Overdose:
MUCOMYST (acetylcysteine) As An Antidote For Acetaminophen Overdose)

Acetaminophen is rapidly absorbed from the upper gastrointestinal tract with peak plasma levels occurring between 30 and 60 minutes after therapeutic doses and usually within 4 hours following an overdose. The parent compound, which is nontoxic, is extensively metabolized in the liver to form principally the sulfate and glucuronide conjugates which are also nontoxic and are rapidly excreted in the urine. A small fraction of an ingested dose is metabolized in the liver by the cytochrome P-450 mixed function oxidase enzyme system to form a reactive, potentially toxic, intermediate metabolite which preferentially conjugates with hepatic glutathione to form the nontoxic cysteine and mercapturic acid derivatives which are then excreted by the kidney. Therapeutic doses of acetaminophen do not saturate the glucuronide and sulfate conjugation pathways and do not result in the formation of sufficient reactive metabolite to deplete glutathione stores. However, following ingestion of a large overdose (150 mg/kg or greater) the glucuronide and sulfate conjugation pathways are saturated resulting in a larger fraction of the drug being metabolized via the P-450 pathway. The increased formation of reactive metabolite may deplete the hepatic stores of glutathione with subsequent binding of the metabolite to protein molecules within the hepatocyte resulting in cellular necrosis. Acetylcysteine has been shown to reduce the extent of liver injury following acetaminophen overdose. Early symptoms following a potentially hepatotoxic overdose may include: nausea, vomiting, diaphoresis and general malaise. Clinical and laboratory evidence of hepatic toxicity may not be apparent until 48 to 72 hours postingestion. In adults and adolescents, regardless of the quantity of acetaminophen reported to have been ingested, administer MUCOMYST® acetylcysteine immediately. MUCOMYST acetylcysteine therapy should be initiated and continued for a full course of therapy. Its effectiveness depends on early administration, with benefit seen principally in patients treated within 16 hours of the overdose. If acetaminophen plasma assay capability is not available, and the estimated acetaminophen ingestion exceeds 150 mg/kg, MUCOMYST acetylcysteine therapy should be initiated and continued for a full course of therapy.

For full prescribing information, refer to the MUCOMYST package insert. Do not await the results of assays for acetaminophen level before initiating treatment with MUCOMYST acetylcysteine. The following additional procedures are recommended: The stomach should be emptied promptly by lavage or by induction of emesis with syrup of ipecac. A serum acetaminophen assay should be obtained as early as possible, but no sooner than four hours following ingestion. Liver function studies should be obtained initially and repeated at 24-hour intervals.

For additional emergency information call your regional poison center or toll-free (1-800-525-6115) to the Rocky Mountain Poison Center for assistance in diagnosis and for directions in the use of MUCOMYST acetylcysteine as an antidote.

How Supplied: Allergy-Sinus COMTREX® is supplied as:
Coated green tablets or caplets with "A/S" debossed on one side.
NDC 19810-0774-1 Blister packages of 24's
NDC 19810-0774-2 Bottles of 50's
All sizes packaged in child resistant closures except 24's which are sizes recommended for households without young children.
Store at room temperature.
Shown in Product Identification Guide, page 507

Non-Drowsy COMTREX® Maximum Strength

Each caplet or liqui-gel contains:
[See table below.]
Other Ingredients (Caplet): Benzoic acid, Corn starch, D&C Yellow No. 10 Lake, FD&C Red No. 40 Lake, Hydroxypropyl methylcellulose, Magnesium Stearate, Methylparaben, Mineral Oil, Polysorbate 20, Povidone, Propylene Glycol, Propylparaben, Simethicone Emulsion, Sorbitan Monolaurate, Stearic Acid, Titanium Dioxide.
May also contain: Carnauba Wax, D&C Yellow No. 10, FD&C Red No. 40

Other Ingredients (Liqui-gel): FD&C Yellow No. 6, Gelatin, Glycerin, Polyethylene Glycol, Povidone, Propylene Glycol, Silicon Dioxide, Sorbitol, Titanium Dioxide, Water

Indications: For the temporary relief of the following symptoms associated with the common cold and flu: minor aches, pains, headache, muscular aches, and fever; cough; and nasal congestion.

Warnings: Keep this and all drugs out of the reach of children. In case of accidental overdose, seek professional assistance or contact a poison control center immediately. Prompt medical attention is critical for adults as well as children even if you do not notice any signs or symptoms. As with any drug, if you are pregnant or nursing a baby, seek the advice of a health professional before using this product. Do not take this product for more than 7 days. A persistent cough may be a sign of a serious condition. If cough persists for more than 7 days, tends to recur, or is accompanied by rash, persistent headache, fever that lasts for more than 3 days, or if new symptoms occur, consult a doctor. Do not take this product for persistent or chronic cough such as occurs with smoking, asthma or emphysema, or if cough is accompanied by excessive phlegm (mucus) unless directed by a doctor. **Do not exceed recommended dosage.** If nervousness, dizziness, or sleeplessness occur, discontinue use and consult a doctor. If symptoms do not improve within 7 days or are accompanied by fever, consult a doctor. Do not take this product if you have heart disease, high blood pressure, thyroid disease, diabetes, or difficulty in urination due to enlargement of the prostate gland unless directed by a doctor.
DRUG INTERACTION PRECAUTION: Do not use this product if you are now taking a prescription monoamine oxidase inhibitor (MAOI) (certain drugs for depression, psychiatric or emotional conditions, or Parkinson's disease), or for 2 weeks after stopping the MAOI drug. If you are uncertain whether your prescription drug contains an MAOI, consult a health professional before taking this product.

Directions: Adults and children 12 years of age and over: 2 caplets every 6 hours, while symptoms persist, not to exceed 8 caplets in 24 hours, or as di-

Active:	Comtrex Non-Drowsy per caplet	Comtrex Non-Drowsy per liqui-gel
Acetaminophen	500 mg	500 mg
Pseudoephedrine HCL	30 mg	—
Dextromethorphan HBr	15 mg	15 mg
Phenylpropanolamine HCL	—	12.5 mg

rected by your doctor. Children under 12 years of age: consult a doctor.

Overdose: MUCOMYST (acetylcysteine) As An Antidote For Acetaminophen Overdose)

Acetaminophen is rapidly absorbed from the upper gastrointestinal tract with peak plasma levels occurring between 30 and 60 minutes after therapeutic doses and usually within 4 hours following an overdose. The parent compound, which is nontoxic, is extensively metabolized in the liver to form principally the sulfate and glucuronide conjugates which are also nontoxic and are rapidly excreted in the urine. A small fraction of an ingested dose is metabolized in the liver by the cytochrome P-450 mixed function oxidase enzyme system to form a reactive, potentially toxic, intermediate metabolite which preferentially conjugates with hepatic glutathione to form the nontoxic cysteine and mercapturic acid derivatives which are then excreted by the kidney. Therapeutic doses of acetaminophen do not saturate the glucuronide and sulfate conjugation pathways and do not result in the formation of sufficient reactive metabolite to deplete glutathione stores. However, following ingestion of a large overdose (150 mg/kg or greater) the glucuronide and sulfate conjugation pathways are saturated resulting in a larger fraction of the drug being metabolized via the P-450 pathway. The increased formation of reactive metabolite may deplete the hepatic stores of glutathione with subsequent binding of the metabolite to protein molecules within the hepatocyte resulting in cellular necrosis. Acetylcysteine has been shown to reduce the extent of liver injury following acetaminophen overdose. Early symptoms following a potentially hepatotoxic overdose may include: nausea, vomiting, diaphoresis and general malaise. Clinical and laboratory evidence of hepatic toxicity may not be apparent until 48 to 72 hours postingestion. In adults and adolescents, regardless of the quantity of acetaminophen reported to have been ingested, administer MUCOMYST® acetylcysteine immediately. MUCOMYST acetylcysteine therapy should be initiated and continued for a full course of therapy. Its effectiveness depends on early administration, with benefit seen principally in patients treated within 16 hours of the overdose. If acetaminophen plasma assay capability is not available, and the estimated acetaminophen ingestion exceeds 150 mg/kg, MUCOMYST acetylcysteine therapy should be initiated and continued for a full course of therapy.

For full prescribing information, refer to the MUCOMYST package insert. Do not await the results of assays for acetaminophen level before initiating treatment with MUCOMYST acetylcysteine. The following additional procedures are recommended: The stomach should be emptied promptly by lavage or by induction of emesis with syrup of ipecac. A serum acetaminophen assay should be obtained as early as possible, but no sooner than four hours following ingestion. Liver function studies should be obtained initially and repeated at 24-hour intervals.

For additional emergency information call your regional poison center or toll-free (1-800-525-6115) to the Rocky Mountain Poison Center for assistance in diagnosis and for directions in the use of MUCOMYST acetylcysteine as an antidote.

How Supplied: Non-Drowsy Comtrex® is supplied as:
Coated orange caplet with "CX-D" debossed on one surface.
NDC 19810-0046-1 Blister packages of 24's
NDC 19810-0046-2 Bottles of 50's
Liquigel printed with "COMTREX DAY"
NDC 19810-0008-1 Blister packages of 24's
NDC 19810-0008-2 Blister packages of 50's
The 24 size does not have a child resistant closure and is recommended for households without young children.
Store at room temperature.

Shown in Product Identification Guide, page 507

Aspirin Free EXCEDRIN®

Composition: Each caplet and geltab contains Acetaminophen 500 mg. and Caffeine 65 mg. Other Ingredients: (caplet) Benzoic Acid, Carnauba Wax, Corn starch, D&C Red No. 27 Lake, D&C Yellow No. 10 Lake, FD&C Blue No. 1 Lake, Hydroxypropyl methylcellulose, Magnesium stearate, Methylparaben, Microcrystalline Cellulose, Mineral Oil, Polysorbate 20, Povidone, Propylene Glycol, Propylparaben, Simethicone Emulsion, Sorbitan Monolaurate, Stearic Acid, Titanium Dioxide.
May also contain: Croscarmellose sodium, FD&C Red No. 40, Saccharin sodium, Sodium starch glycolate
Other Ingredients: (geltab) Benzoic Acid, Corn Starch, FD&C Blue No. 1, FD&C Red No. 40, FD&C Yellow No. 6, Gelatin, Glycerin, Hydroxypropyl methylcellulose, Magnesium stearate, Methylparaben, Microcrystalline cellulose, Mineral oil, Polysorbate 20, Povidone, Propylene glycol, Propylparaben, Simethicone emulsion, Sorbitan monolaurate, Stearic acid, Titanium dioxide.
May also contain: Croscarmellose sodium, Sodium starch glycolate

Indications: For temporary relief of the pain of headache, sinusitis, colds, muscular aches, menstrual discomfort, toothaches and minor arthritis pain.

Directions: Adults: 2 caplets or geltabs every 6 hours while symptoms persist, not to exceed 8 caplets or geltabs in 24 hours, or as directed by a doctor. Children under 12 years of age: Consult a doctor.

Warnings: Keep this and all other medications out of the reach of children.
In case of accidental overdose, seek professional assistance or contact a poison control center immediately. Prompt medical attention is critical for adults as well as for children even if you do not notice any signs or symptoms. As with any drug, if you are pregnant or nursing a baby, seek the advice of a health professional before using this product. Do not take this product for pain for more than 10 days or for fever for more than 3 days unless directed by a doctor. If pain or fever persists or gets worse, if new symptoms occur, of if redness or swelling is present, consult a doctor because these could be signs of a serious condition. Consult a dentist promptly for toothache.

Overdose: MUCOMYST (acetylcysteine) As An Antidote For Acetaminophen Overdose)

Acetaminophen is rapidly absorbed from the upper gastrointestinal tract with peak plasma levels occurring between 30 and 60 minutes after therapeutic doses and usually within 4 hours following an overdose. The parent compound, which is nontoxic, is extensively metabolized in the liver to form principally the sulfate and glucuronide conjugates which are also nontoxic and are rapidly excreted in the urine. A small fraction of an ingested dose is metabolized in the liver by the cytochrome P-450 mixed function oxidase enzyme system to form a reactive, potentially toxic, intermediate metabolite which preferentially conjugates with hepatic glutathione to form the nontoxic cysteine and mercapturic acid derivatives which are then excreted by the kidney. Therapeutic doses of acetaminophen do not saturate the glucuronide and sulfate conjugation pathways and do not result in the formation of sufficient reactive metabolite to deplete glutathione stores. However, following ingestion of a large overdose (150 mg/kg or greater) the glucuronide and sulfate conjugation pathways are saturated resulting in a larger fraction of the drug being metabolized via the P-450 pathway. The increased formation of reactive metabolite may deplete the hepatic stores of glutathione with subsequent binding of the metabolite to protein molecules within the hepatocyte resulting in cellular necrosis. Acetylcysteine has been shown to reduce the extent of liver injury following acetaminophen overdose. Early symptoms following a potentially hepatotoxic overdose may include: nausea, vomiting, diaphoresis and general malaise. Clinical and laboratory evidence of hepatic toxicity may not be apparent until 48 to 72 hours postingestion. In adults and adolescents, regardless of the quantity of acetaminophen reported to have been ingested, administer MUCOMYST® acetylcysteine immediately. MUCOMYST acetylcysteine therapy should be initiated and continued for a full course of therapy. Its effectiveness depends on early administration, with

Continued on next page

Bristol-Myers—Cont.

benefit seen principally in patients treated within 16 hours of the overdose. If acetaminophen plasma assay capability is not available, and the estimated acetaminophen ingestion exceeds 150 mg/kg, MUCOMYST acetylcysteine therapy should be initiated and continued for a full course of therapy.

For full prescribing information, refer to the MUCOMYST package insert. Do not await the results of assays for acetaminophen level before initiating treatment with MUCOMYST acetylcysteine. The following additional procedures are recommended: The stomach should be emptied promptly by lavage or by induction of emesis with syrup of ipecac. A serum acetaminophen assay should be obtained as early as possible, but no sooner than four hours following ingestion. Liver function studies should be obtained initially and repeated at 24-hour intervals.

For additional emergency information call your regional poison center or toll-free (1-800-525-6115) to the Rocky Mountain Poison Center for assistance in diagnosis and for directions in the use of MUCOMYST acetylcysteine as an antidote.

How Supplied: Aspirin Free EXCEDRIN® is supplied as: Coated red caplets with AFE debossed on one side
NDC 19810-0089-1 Bottles of 24's
NDC 19810-0089-2 Bottles of 50's
NDC 19810-0089-3 Bottles of 100's
All sizes packaged in child resistant closures except 100's size for caplets and 40's size for geltabs which is recommended for households without young children.
Easy to swallow red geltabs with "AF Excedrin" printed in white on one side
NDC 19810-0029-1 Bottles of 20's
NDC 19810-0029-2 Bottles of 40's
NDC 19810-0029-3 Bottles of 80's
All sizes packaged in child resistant closures except 40's which is recommended for households without young children. Store at room temperature.
Shown in Product Identification Guide, page 507

EXCEDRIN® Extra-Strength Analgesic
[ĕx "cĕd 'rĭn]

Composition: Each tablet or caplet contains Acetaminophen 250 mg.; Aspirin 250 mg.; and Caffeine 65 mg. Other Ingredients: Benzoic acid, Hydroxypropylcellulose, Hydroxypropyl methylcellulose, Microcrystalline Cellulose, Mineral Oil, Polysorbate 20, Povidone, Propylene Glycol, Simethicone Emulsion, Sorbitan Monolaurate, Stearic Acid,
May also contain: Carnauba wax, FD&C Blue No. 1, Saccharin Sodium, Titanium Dioxide

Indications: For temporary relief of the pain of headache, sinusitis, colds, muscular aches, menstrual discomfort, toothaches and minor arthritis pain.

Warnings: Children and teenagers should not use this medicine for chicken pox or flu symptoms before a doctor is consulted about Reye syndrome, a rare but serious illness reported to be associated with aspirin. Keep this and all other medications out of the reach of children. In case of accidental overdose, seek professional assistance or contact a physician or poison control center immediately. Prompt medical attention is critical for adults as well as for children even if you do not notice any signs or symptoms. As with any drug, if you are pregnant or nursing a baby, seek the advice of a health professional before using this product. IT IS ESPECIALLY IMPORTANT NOT TO USE ASPIRIN DURING THE LAST 3 MONTHS OF PREGNANCY UNLESS SPECIFICALLY DIRECTED TO DO SO BY A DOCTOR BECAUSE IT MAY CAUSE PROBLEMS IN THE UNBORN CHILD OR COMPLICATIONS DURING DELIVERY. Do not take this product for pain for more than 10 days or for fever for more than 3 days unless directed by a doctor. If pain or fever persists or gets worse, if new symptoms occur, or if redness or swelling is present, consult a doctor because these could be signs of a serious condition. Consult a dentist promptly for toothache. Do not take this product if you are allergic to aspirin, have asthma, have stomach problems (such as heartburn, upset stomach or stomach pain) that persist or recur, or if you have ulcers or bleeding problems, unless directed by a doctor. If ringing in the ears or loss of hearing occurs, consult a doctor before taking any more of this product.

Drug Interaction Precaution: Do not take this product if you are taking a prescription drug for anticoagulation (thinning of blood), diabetes, gout or arthritis unless directed by a doctor.

Directions: Adults: 2 tablets or caplets with water every 6 hours while symptoms persist, not to exceed 8 tablets or caplets in 24 hours, or as directed by a doctor. Children under 12 years of age: Consult a doctor.

Overdose: MUCOMYST (acetylcysteine) As An Antidote For Acetaminophen Overdose)
Acetaminophen is rapidly absorbed from the upper gastrointestinal tract with peak plasma levels occurring between 30 and 60 minutes after therapeutic doses and usually within 4 hours following an overdose. The parent compound, which is nontoxic, is extensively metabolized in the liver to form principally the sulfate and glucuronide conjugates which are also nontoxic and are rapidly excreted in the urine. A small fraction of an ingested dose is metabolized in the liver by the cytochrome P-450 mixed function oxidase enzyme system to form a reactive,

potentially toxic, intermediate metabolite which preferentially conjugates with hepatic glutathione to form the nontoxic cysteine and mercapturic acid derivatives which are then excreted by the kidney. Therapeutic doses of acetaminophen do not saturate the glucuronide and sulfate conjugation pathways and do not result in the formation of sufficient reactive metabolite to deplete glutathione stores. However, following ingestion of a large overdose (150 mg/kg or greater) the glucuronide and sulfate conjugation pathways are saturated resulting in a larger fraction of the drug being metabolized via the P-450 pathway. The increased formation of reactive metabolite may deplete the hepatic stores of glutathione with subsequent binding of the metabolite to protein molecules within the hepatocyte resulting in cellular necrosis. Acetylcysteine has been shown to reduce the extent of liver injury following acetaminophen overdose. Early symptoms following a potentially hepatotoxic overdose may include: nausea, vomiting, diaphoresis and general malaise. Clinical and laboratory evidence of hepatic toxicity may not be apparent until 48 to 72 hours postingestion. In adults and adolescents, regardless of the quantity of acetaminophen reported to have been ingested, administer MUCOMYST® acetylcysteine immediately. MUCOMYST acetylcysteine therapy should be initiated and continued for a full course of therapy. Its effectiveness depends on early administration, with benefit seen principally in patients treated within 16 hours of the overdose. If acetaminophen plasma assay capability is not available, and the estimated acetaminophen ingestion exceeds 150 mg/kg, MUCOMYST acetylcysteine therapy should be initiated and continued for a full course of therapy.

For full prescribing information, refer to the MUCOMYST package insert. Do not await the results of assays for acetaminophen level before initiating treatment with MUCOMYST acetylcysteine. The following additional procedures are recommended: The stomach should be emptied promptly by lavage or by induction of emesis with syrup of ipecac. A serum acetaminophen assay should be obtained as early as possible, but no sooner than four hours following ingestion. Liver function studies should be obtained initially and repeated at 24-hour intervals.

For additional emergency information call your regional poison center or toll-free (1-800-525-6115) to the Rocky Mountain Poison Center for assistance in diagnosis and for directions in the use of MUCOMYST acetylcysteine as an antidote.

How Supplied: Extra Strength EXCEDRIN® is supplied as:
White circular tablet with letter "E" debossed on one side.
NDC 19810-0700-2 Bottles of 12's
NDC 19810-0782-3 Bottles of 24's
NDC 19810-0782-4 Bottles of 50's

NDC 19810-0700-5 Bottles of 100's
NDC 19810-0061-9 Bottles of 175's
NDC 19810-0700-1 A metal tin of 12's
Coated while caplets with "E" debossed
on one side.
NDC 19810-0002-1 Bottles of 24's
NDC 19810-0002-2 Bottles of 50's
NDC 19810-0002-8 Bottles of 100's
NDC 19810-0091-1 Bottles of 175's
All sizes packaged in child resistant closures except 100's for tablets, 50's for caplets which are sizes recommended for households without young children.

Shown in Product Identification Guide, page 507

EXCEDRIN P.M.®
[ĕx "cĕd 'rĭn]
Analgesic Sleeping Aid

Composition: Each tablet, caplet or liquigel contains:

	EXCEDRIN®PM Per Tablet or Caplet
Acetaminophen	500 mg.
Diphenhydramine Citrate:	38 mg.

Other Ingredients: —
Tablet or Caplet
  benzoic acid
  carnauba wax
  corn starch
  D&C yellow no. 10
  D&C yellow no. 10 aluminum lake
  FD&C blue no. 1
  FD&C blue no. 1 aluminum lake
  hydroxypropyl methylcellulose
  magnesium stearate
  methylparaben
  pregelatinized starch
  propylene glycol
  propylparaben
  simethicone emulsion
  stearic acid
  titanium dioxide
May also contain:
  mineral oil
  polysorbate 20
  povidone
  sodium citrate
  sorbitan monolaurate .

	EXCEDRIN®PM Per Liquigel
Acetaminophen	500 mg.
Diphenhydramine HCL	25 mg.

Other Ingredients:
  D & C Red No. 33
  FD&C Blue No. 1
  FD&C Green No. 3
  Gelatin
  Glycerin
  Polyethlene Glycol
  Povidone
  Propylene Glycol
  Silicon Dioxide
  Sorbitol
  Titanium Dioxide
  Water

Indications: For temporary relief of occasional headaches and minor aches and pains with accompanying sleeplessness.

Warnings: KEEP THIS AND ALL OTHER MEDICATIONS OUT OF THE REACH OF CHILDREN. IN CASE OF ACCIDENTAL OVERDOSE, SEEK PROFESSIONAL ASSISTANCE OR CONTACT A POISON CONTROL CENTER IMMEDIATELY. PROMPT MEDICAL ATTENTION IS CRITICAL FOR ADULTS AS WELL AS FOR CHILDREN EVEN IF YOU DO NOT NOTICE ANY SIGNS OR SYMPTOMS. As with any drug, if you are pregnant or nursing a baby, seek the advice of a health professional before using this product. Do not give this product to children under 12 years of age or use for more than 10 days unless directed by a doctor. Consult a doctor if symptoms persist or get worse or if new ones occur, or if sleeplessness persists continuously for more than 2 weeks because these may be symptoms of serious underlying medical illnesses. Do not take this product if you have asthma, glaucoma, emphysema, chronic pulmonary disease, shortness of breath, difficulty in breathing, or difficulty in urination due to enlargement of the prostate gland unless directed by a doctor. Avoid alcoholic beverages while taking this product. Do not take this product if you are taking sedatives or tranquilizers, without first consulting your doctor.

Directions:
Adults, 2 tablets, caplets, or liquigels at bedtime if needed or as directed by a doctor.

Overdose: MUCOMYST (acetylcysteine) As An Antidote For Acetaminophen Overdose)
Acetaminophen is rapidly absorbed from the upper gastrointestinal tract with peak plasma levels occurring between 30 and 60 minutes after therapeutic doses and usually within 4 hours following an overdose. The parent compound, which is nontoxic, is extensively metabolized in the liver to form principally the sulfate and glucuronide conjugates which are also nontoxic and are rapidly excreted in the urine. A small fraction of an ingested dose is metabolized in the liver by the cytochrome P-450 mixed function oxidase enzyme system to form a reactive, potentially toxic, intermediate metabolite which preferentially conjugates with hepatic glutathione to form the nontoxic cysteine and mercapturic acid derivatives which are then excreted by the kidney. Therapeutic doses of acetaminophen do not saturate the glucuronide and sulfate conjugation pathways and do not result in the formation of sufficient reactive metabolite to deplete glutathione stores. However, following ingestion of a large overdose (150 mg/kg or greater) the glucuronide and sulfate conjugation pathways are saturated resulting in a larger fraction of the drug being metabolized via the P-450 pathway. The increased formation of reactive metabolite may deplete the hepatic stores of glutathione with subsequent binding of the metabolite to protein molecules within the hepatocyte resulting in cellular necrosis. Acetylcysteine has been shown to reduce the extent of liver injury following acetaminophen overdose. Early symptoms following a potentially hepatotoxic overdose may include: nausea, vomiting, diaphoresis and general malaise. Clinical and laboratory evidence of hepatic toxicity may not be apparent until 48 to 72 hours postingestion. In adults and adolescents, regardless of the quantity of acetaminophen reported to have been ingested, administer MUCOMYST® acetylcysteine immediately. MUCOMYST acetylcysteine therapy should be initiated and continued for a full course of therapy. Its effectiveness depends on early administration, with benefit seen principally in patients treated within 16 hours of the overdose. If acetaminophen plasma assay capability is not available, and the estimated acetaminophen ingestion exceeds 150 mg/kg, MUCOMYST acetylcysteine therapy should be initiated and continued for a full course of therapy.
For full prescribing information, refer to the MUCOMYST package insert. Do not await the results of assays for acetaminophen level before initiating treatment with MUCOMYST acetylcysteine. The following additional procedures are recommended: The stomach should be emptied promptly by lavage or by induction of emesis with syrup of ipecac. A serum acetaminophen assay should be obtained as early as possible, but no sooner than four hours following ingestion. Liver function studies should be obtained initially and repeated at 24-hour intervals.
For additional emergency information call your regional poison center or toll-free (1-800-525-6115) to the Rocky Mountain Poison Center for assistance in diagnosis and for directions in the use of MUCOMYST acetylcysteine as an antidote.
For overdose treatment information, consult a regional poison control center.

How Supplied: EXCEDRIN P.M.® is supplied as:

Light blue circular coated tablets with "PM" debossed on one side.
NDC 19810-0763-6 Bottles of 10's
NDC 19810-0764-3 Bottles of 24's
NDC 19810-0763-4 Bottles of 50's
NDC 19810-0764-4 Bottles of 100's
Light blue coated caplet with "PM" debossed on one side.
NDC 19810-0032-5 Bottles of 24's
NDC 19810-0032-3 Bottles of 50's
NDC 19810-0032-6 Bottles of 100's
Light blue liquigels with "Excedrin PM" printed on one side.
NDC 19810-0071-5 Bottles of 20's
NDC 19810-0071-6 Bottles of 40's
All sizes packaged in child resistant closures except 50's tablets and caplets and

Continued on next page

Bristol-Myers—Cont.

20's liquigels, which are recommended for households without young children. Store at room temperature.

Shown in Product Identification Guide, page 507

4-WAY® Fast Acting Nasal Spray

Composition:
Phenylephrine hydrochloride 0.5%, naphazoline hydrochloride 0.05%, pyrilamine maleate 0.2%, in a buffered solution. Also Contains: Benzalkonium Chloride, Boric Acid, Sodium Borate, Water. Also available in a mentholated formula containing Phenylephrine hydrochloride 0.5%, naphazoline hydrochloride 0.05%, pyrilamine maleate 0.2%, in a buffered solution. Also Contains: Benzalkonium Chloride, Boric Acid, Camphor, Eucalyptol, Menthol, Poloxamer 188, Polysorbate 80, Sodium Borate, Water.

Indications: For prompt, temporary relief of nasal congestion due to the common cold, sinusitis, hay fever or other upper respiratory allergies.

Directions and Use Instructions:
Directions: Adults: Spray twice into each nostril not more often than every 6 hours. Do not give to children under 12 years of age unless directed by a doctor.
Use Instructions: For Metered Pump— Remove protective cap. Hold bottle with thumb at base and nozzle between first and second fingers. With head upright, insert metered pump spray nozzle into nostril. Depress pump all the way down, with a firm even stroke and sniff deeply. Repeat in other nostril. Do not tilt head backward while spraying. Wipe tip clean after each use. Note: This bottle is filled to correct level for proper pump action. Before using the first time, remove the protective cap from the tip and prime the metered pump by depressing pump firmly several times.
Use Instructions: For Atomizer— With head in a normal upright position, put atomizer tip into nostril. Squeeze bottle with firm, quick pressure while inhaling.

Warnings: KEEP THIS AND ALL OTHER MEDICATIONS OUT OF THE REACH OF CHILDREN. IN CASE OF ACCIDENTAL OVERDOSE OR INGESTION, SEEK PROFESSIONAL ASSISTANCE OR CONTACT A POISON CONTROL CENTER IMMEDIATELY. Do not exceed recommended dosage because burning, stinging, sneezing, or increase of nasal discharge may occur. The use of this container by more than one person may spread infection. Do not use this product for more than 3 days. If symptoms persist, consult a doctor. Do not use this product in children under 12 years of age because it may cause sedation if swallowed. Do not use this product if you have heart disease, high blood pressure, thyroid disease, diabetes, or difficulty in urination due to enlargement of the prostate gland should not use this product unless directed by a doctor.

How Supplied:
Regular formula:
NDC 19810-0047-1 Atomizer of ½ fluid ounce.
NDC 19810-0047-2 Atomizer of 1 fluid ounce.
NDC 19810-0047-3 Metered pump of ½ fluid ounce.
Mentholated formula:
NDC 19810-0049-1 Atomizer of ½ fluid ounce.
Store at room temperature.

Shown in Product Identification Guide, page 506

4-WAY® 12 Hour Nasal Spray

Composition: Oxymetazoline Hydrochloride 0.05% in a buffered isotonic aqueous solution. Phenylmercuric Acetate 0.002% added as a preservative.
Also Contains: Benzalkonium Chloride, Glycine, Sorbitol, Water.

Indications: Temporarily relieves nasal congestion due to the common cold, hay fever or other upper respiratory allergies associated with sinusitis.

Directions and Use Instructions:
Directions: Adults and children 6 to under 12 years of age (with adult supervision): 2 or 3 sprays in each nostril not more often than every 10 to 12 hours. Do not exceed 2 applications in any 24-hour period. Children under 6 years of age: Consult a doctor.
Use Instructions:
With head in a normal, upright position, put atomizer tip into nostril. Squeeze bottle with firm, quick pressure while inhaling. Wipe nozzle clean after each use.

Warnings: Keep this and all drugs out of the reach of children. In case of accidental overdose or ingestion, seek professional assistance or contact a poison control center immediately. **Do not exceed recommended dosage.** This product may cause temporary discomfort such as burning, stinging, sneezing, or an increase in nasal discharge. The use of this container by more than one person may spread infection. Do not use this product for more than 3 days. Use only as directed. Frequent or prolonged use may cause nasal congestion or recur or worsen. If symptoms persist, consult a doctor. Do not use this product if you have heart disease, high blood pressure, thyroid disease, or diabetes or difficulty in urination due to enlargement of the prostate gland unless directed by a doctor. Do not use this product in a child who has heart disease, high blood pressure, thyroid disease, or diabetes unless directed by a doctor.

How Supplied: 4-WAY 12 Hour Nasal Spray is supplied as:
NDC 19810-0728-1 Atomizer of ½ fluid ounce.

Store at room temperature.
Shown in Product Identification Guide, page 506

KERI LOTION
Skin Lubricant—Moisturizer

Available in three formulations:
KERI Original

Composition: Water, mineral oil, propylene glycol, PEG-40 stearate, glyceryl stearate/PEG-100 stearate, PEG-4 dilaurate, laureth-4, lanolin oil, methyl paraben, carbomer , propylparaben, fragrance triethanolamine, dioctyl sodium sulfosuccinate, quaternium-15.

Direction for Use: Apply wherever skin feels dry, rough or irritated. For external use only.

KERI Silky Smooth recommended for daily use on dry skin.

Composition: Water, petrolatum, glycerin, dimethicone, stereth-2, cetyl alcohol, benzyl alcohol, laureth-23, magnesium aluminum silicate, carbomer, fragrance, sodium hydroxide, quaternium-15.

Directions for Use: Apply liberally after bathing, before bed or whenever skin feels dry. Use daily on hands, arms, legs, or anywhere skin feels dry for softer, smoother, healthier-looking skin. For external use only.

KERI Sensitive Skin

Composition: Water, petrolatum, glycerin, dimethicone, stereth-2, cetyl alcohol, benzyl alcohol, laureth-23, magnesium aluminum silicate, tocopheryl linoleate, carbomer, BHT, sodium hydroxide, disodium EDTA, quaternium-15.

Directions for Use: Apply liberally after bathing, before bed or whenever skin feels dry. Use daily on hands, arms, legs, or anywhere skin feels dry for softer, smoother, healthier-looking skin. For external use only.

How Supplied: KERI Lotion Original 6½ oz., 11 oz., 15 oz. and 20 oz. plastic bottles. KERI Silky Smooth 6½ oz., 11 oz. and 15 oz. plastic bottles. KERI Sensitive Skin 6½ oz., 11 oz. and 15 oz. plastic bottles.

Shown in Product Identification Guide, page 507

NO DOZ® Maximum Strength Caplets

Composition: Each caplet contains 200 mg. Caffeine. Other ingredients: Benzoic Acid, Corn Starch, FD&C Blue No. 1, Flavors, Hydroxypropyl Methylcellulose, Microcrystalline Cellulose, Propylene Glycol, Simethicone Emulsion, Stearic Acid, Sucrose, Titanium Dioxide. May also contain: Carnauba Wax, Mineral Oil, Polysorbate 20, Povidone, Sorbitan Monolaurate.

Indications: Helps restore mental alertness or wakefulness when experiencing fatigue or drowsiness.

Directions: Adults: one-half to one caplet not more often than every 3 to 4 hours.

Warnings: KEEP THIS AND ALL OTHER MEDICATIONS OUT OF THE REACH OF CHILDREN. IN CASE OF ACCIDENTAL OVERDOSE, SEEK PROFESSIONAL ASSISTANCE OR CONTACT A POISON CONTROL CENTER IMMEDIATELY. As with any drug, if you are pregnant or nursing a baby, seek the advice of a health professional before using this product. Do not give to children under 12 years of age. For occasional use only. Not intended for use as a substitute for sleep. If fatigue or drowsiness persists or continues to occur, consult a doctor. The recommended dose of this product contains about as much caffeine as a cup of coffee. Limit the use of caffeine-containing medications, foods, or beverages while taking this product because too much caffeine may cause nervousness, irritability, sleeplessness and, occasionally, rapid heart beat.

How Supplied: NO DOZ® Maximum Strength is supplied as: White coated caplets with "NO DOZ" debossed on one side. The opposite side is scored.
19810-0064-4 Bottles of 16's
19810-0064-5 Bottles of 36's
19810-0064-6 Bottles of 60's
Store at room temperature.

NUPRIN®
(ibuprofen)
Analgesic

Warning: ASPIRIN SENSITIVE PATIENTS. Do not take this product if you have had a severe allergic reaction to aspirin, e.g.—asthma, swelling, shock or hives, because even though this product contains no aspirin or salicylates, cross-reactions may occur in patients allergic to aspirin.

Composition: Each tablet or caplet contains ibuprofen USP, 200 mg. **Other Ingredients:** Carnauba wax, cornstarch, D&C Yellow No. 10, FD&C Yellow No. 6, hydroxypropyl methylcellulose, propylene glycol, silicon dioxide, stearic acid, titanium dioxide.

Indications: For the temporary relief of minor aches and pains associated with the common cold, headache, toothache, muscular aches, backache, for the minor pain of arthritis, for the pain of menstrual cramps and for reduction of fever.

Warnings: Do not take for pain for more than 10 days or for fever for more than 3 days unless directed by a doctor. If pain or fever persists or gets worse, if new symptoms occur, or if the painful area is red or swollen, consult a doctor. These could be signs of serious illness. If you are under a doctor's care for any serious condition, consult a doctor before taking this product. As with aspirin and

acetaminophen, if you have any condition which requires you to take prescription drugs or if you have had any problems or serious side effects from taking any non-prescription pain reliever, do not take NUPRIN without first discussing it with your doctor. If you experience any symptoms which are unusual or seem unrelated to the condition for which you took ibuprofen, consult a doctor before taking any more of it. Although ibuprofen is indicated for the same conditions as aspirin and acetaminophen, it should not be taken with them except under a doctor's direction. Do not combine this product with any other ibuprofen-containing product. As with any drug, if you are pregnant or nursing a baby, seek the advice of a health professional before using this product. IT IS ESPECIALLY IMPORTANT NOT TO USE IBUPROFEN DURING THE LAST 3 MONTHS OF PREGNANCY UNLESS SPECIFICALLY DIRECTED TO DO SO BY A DOCTOR BECAUSE IT MAY CAUSE PROBLEMS IN THE UNBORN CHILD OR COMPLICATIONS DURING DELIVERY. Keep this and all drugs out of the reach of children. In case of accidental overdose, seek professional assistance or contact a poison control center immediately.

Caution: Store at room temperature. Avoid excessive heat 40°C (104°F).

Directions: Adults: Take 1 tablet or caplet every 4 to 6 hours while symptoms persist. If pain or fever does not respond to 1 tablet or caplet, 2 tablets or caplets may be used but do not exceed 6 tablets or caplets in 24 hours, unless directed by a doctor. The smallest effective dose should be used. Take with food or milk if occasional and mild heartburn, upset stomach, or stomach pain occurs with use. Consult a doctor if these symptoms are more than mild or if they persist. Children: Do not give this product to children under 12 except under the advice and supervision of a doctor.

Overdose: For overdose treatment information, consult a regional poison control center.

How Supplied:
NUPRIN® is supplied as:
Golden yellow round tablets with "NUPRIN" printed in black on one side.
NDC 19810-0767-2 Bottles of 24's
NDC 19810-0767-3 Bottles of 50's
NDC 19810-0767-4 Bottles of 100's
NDC 19810-0767-9 Vials of 10's
Golden yellow caplets with "NUPRIN" printed in black on one side.
NDC 19810-0796-1 Bottles of 24's
NDC 19810-0796-2 Bottles of 50's
NDC 19810-0796-3 Bottles of 100's
All sizes packaged in child resistant closures except 24's for tablets and 24's for caplets, which are sizes recommended for households without young children.
Store at room temperature. Avoid excessive heat 40°C. (104°F.).
Distributed by Bristol-Myers Company
Shown in Product Identification Guide, page 507

THERAPEUTIC MINERAL ICE®

Composition:
Active Ingredient: Menthol 2%
Other Ingredients: Ammonium Hydroxide, Carbomer 934, Cupric Sulfate, FD&C Blue No. 1, Isopropyl Alcohol, Magnesium Sulfate, Sodium Hydroxide, Thymol, Water.

Indications: For the temporary relief of minor aches and pains of muscles and joints associated with arthritis, simple backache, strains, bruises, sprains and sports injuries. **USE ONLY AS DIRECTED. Read all warnings before use.**

Warnings: **KEEP OUT OF THE REACH OF CHILDREN.** For external use only. Not for internal use. Avoid contact with eyes and mucous membranes. Do not use with other ointments, creams, sprays, or liniments. **Do not use with Heating Pads or Heating Devices.** If condition worsens, or if symptoms persist for more than 7 days, or clear up and occur again within a few days, discontinue use of this product and consult your doctor. Do not apply to wounds or damaged skin. Do not bandage tightly. If you have sensitive skin, consult doctor **before** use. If skin irritation develops, discontinue use and consult your doctor. As with any drug, if you are pregnant or nursing a baby, seek the advice of a health professional before using this product. Keep cap tightly closed. Do not use, pour, spill or store near heat or open flame. **Note:** You can always use Mineral Ice as directed, but its use is never intended to replace your doctor's advice.

Directions: Adults and children 2 years of age and older: Clean skin of all other ointments, creams, sprays, or liniments. Apply to affected areas not more than 3 to 4 times daily. May be used with wet or dry bandages or with ice packs. No protective cover needed. Children under 2 years of age: Consult a doctor.

How Supplied:
NDC 19810-0034-4 3.5 oz.
NDC 19810-0034-2 8 oz.
NDC 19810-0034-3 16 oz.
Store at room temperature.
Shown in Product Identification Guide, page 507

UNKNOWN DRUG?
Consult the
Product Identification Guide
(Gray Pages)
for full-color photos of
leading over-the-counter
medications

Campbell Laboratories Inc.
700 W. HILLSBORO BLVD.
(#2-107)
DEERFIELD BEACH, FL 33441

Direct Inquiries to:
James R. Stork, Vice President
P.O. Box 639
Deerfield Bch Fl 33443

HERPECIN–L® Cold Sore Lip Balm
[*her "puh-sin-el "*]

PRODUCT OVERVIEW

Key Facts: HERPECIN-L Lip Balm is a convenient, easy-to-use treatment for perioral <u>herpes simplex</u> infections. Sunscreens provide an SPF of 15.

Major Uses: HERPECIN-L not only treats cold sores, sun and fever blisters, but with prophylactic use, its sunscreens also protect to help prevent them. Users report early use at the <u>prodromal stages</u> of an attack will often abort the lesions and prevent scabbing. Prescribe: Apply "early, often and liberally."

Safety Information: For topical use only. A rare sensitivity may occur.

PRESCRIBING INFORMATION
HERPECIN–L® Cold Sore Lip Balm

Composition: A soothing, emollient, lip balm incorporating the sunscreen, Padimate O, and allantoin, in a balanced, slightly acidic lipid base that includes petrolatum and titanium dioxide at a cosmetically acceptable level. (Does not contain any caines, antibiotics, phenol or camphor.) (NDC 38083-777-31)

Actions and Uses: HERPECIN-L relieves dryness and chapping by providing a lipid barrier to help restore normal moisture balance to the lips. Skin protectants help to soften the crusts and scabs of "cold sores." The sunscreen is effective in 2900-3200 AU range while titanium dioxide, though at low levels, helps to block, scatter and reflect the sun's rays. Applied as a lip balm, SPF is 15. Reapply often during sun exposure.

Administration: (1) *Recurrent "cold sores, sun and fever blisters"*: Simply put, use **soon** and **often**. Frequent sufferers report that with *prophylactic* use (BID/PRN), attacks are fewer and less severe. Most recurrent <u>herpes labialis</u> patients are aware of the <u>prodromal</u> symptoms: tingling, itching, burning. At this stage, or if the lesion has already developed, HERPECIN-L should be applied liberally as often as convenient —at least *every hour*. (2) *Outdoor protection:* Apply before and during sun exposure, after swimming and again at bedtime (h.s.). (3) *Dry, chapped lips:* Apply as needed.

Adverse Reactions: If sensitive to any of the ingredients, discontinue use.

Contraindications: None.

How Supplied: 2.8 gm. swivel tubes.

Samples Available: Yes. (Request on professional letterhead or Rx pad.)

Care-Tech Laboratories, Inc.
Div. of Consolidated Chemical, Inc.
3224 SOUTH KINGSHIGHWAY BOULEVARD
ST. LOUIS, MO 63139

Direct Inquiries to:
Sherry L. Brereton
(314) 772-4610
FAX: (314) 772-4613

For Medical Emergencies Contact:
Customer Service
(800) 325-9681
FAX: (314) 772-4613

BARRI–CARE®

Composition: Active Ingredient: Chloroxylenol
Inactive Ingredients: Petrolatum, Water, Paraffin, Propylene Glycol, Milk Protein, Cod Liver Oil, Aloe Vera Gel, Fragrance, Potassium Hydroxide, Methyl Paraben, Propyl Paraben, Vitamin A & D₃, (E) dl Alpha-Tocopheryl Acetate, (E) dl-Alpha-Tocopherol, D&C Yellow #11 and D&C Red #17.

Actions and Uses: Barri-Care is an antimicrobial ointment formulated to provide a moisture proof barrier against urine, detergent irritants, feces and drainage from wounds or skin lesions. Proven antimicrobial action against E. coli, MRSA, S. aureus and Pseudomonas aeruginosa. Protects perineal area of the incontinent patient from painful skin rashes and relieves irritation around stoma sites. Utilize on Grades I–IV pressure ulcers to halt skin breakdown. Can be used also on minor burns. Will not melt under feverish conditions.

Precautions: External Use Only. Non-Toxic. Avoid eye contact.

Directions: Cleanse affected area with Satin thoroughly. Apply ointment topically to affected area. Reapply 2–3 times daily or as directed by physician.

How Supplied: 1 ounce tubes, 4 oz. tubes, 8 oz. jar. NDC #46706-206

CARE CREME®

Composition: Active Ingredient: Chloroxylenol
Inactive Ingredients: Water, Cetyl Alcohol, Lanolin Oil, Cod Liver Oil, Sodium Laureth Sulfate, Triethanolamine, Propylene Glycol, Petrolatum, Lanolin Alcohol, Methyl Gluceth 20 Distearate, Beeswax, Citric Acid, Methyl Paraben, Fragrance, Propyl Paraben, Vitamins A, D₃ and E-dl Alpha-Tocopherol.

Actions and Uses: Care Creme is an antimicrobial skin care creme specially formulated for use on severely dry skin such as Sjogren's Syndrome, atopic dermatitis, psoriasis, minor burns, urine or fecal exposure, scaling and inter-tissue ammonia related rash. Extremely effective on oncology radiation burns. Use at first sign of reddened skin or initial breakdown. Vitamin and oil enriched to promote skin integrity. Contains no metallic ions. Provides moisture and vitamin enriched wound treatment.

Precautions: Non-toxic, External Use Only. Avoid use around eye area.

Directions: Cleanse affected area with Satin and gently massage Care Creme into skin until completely absorbed or as directed by physician.

How Supplied: 1 ounce tubes, 4 oz. tubes, 9 oz. jar. NDC #46706-205

CLINICAL CARE® WOUND CLEANSER

Composition: Active Ingredient: Benzethonium Chloride
Inactive Ingredients: Water, Amphoteric 2, Aloe Vera Gel, DMDM Hydantoin, Citric Acid.

Actions and Uses: Clinical Care is an antimicrobial, emulsifying solution which aids in removing debris and particulate matter from open, dermal wounds. Clinical Care inhibits the growth of pathogenic organisms. Proven effective at eliminating S. aureus, P. aeruginosa, S. typhimurium, Aspergillus, E. coli, MRSA, S. pyogenes and K. pneumonia. Will not produce dermal irritation.

Precautions: External Use Only. Non-Toxic. No contra-indicators.

Directions: Spray affected area as necessary to debride. Use sterile gauze to gently remove debris and necrotic tissue at dermal surface.

How Supplied: 4 oz. spray, 12 oz. spray

CONCEPT®

Composition: Active Ingredient: Chloroxylenol
Inactive Ingredients: Water, Amphoteric 9, Polysorbate 20, PEG-150 Distearate, Cocamide DEA, Cocoyl Sarcosine, Fragrance, D&C Green #5.

Actions and Uses: Concept is a geriatric shampoo and body wash for patients whose skin is irritated by soaps and harsh detergents. Concept is non-eye irritating and reduces bacteria on the skin. Excellent for replenishing moisture in dry, flaky dermal tissues and eliminating body odors. Utilize on children over 6 months of age to address rashing or atopic dermatitis. Excellent for use on HIV and oncology patients.

Precautions: External Use Only. Non-Toxic.

Directions: Use in normal manner of bathing and shampooing. Rinse thoroughly.

How Supplied: 8 oz., Gallons

FORMULA MAGIC®

Composition: Active Ingredient: Benzethonium Chloride
Inactive Ingredients: Talc, Mineral Oil, Magnesium Carbonate, Fragrance, DMDM Hydantoin.

Actions and Uses: Formula Magic is primarily a geriatric care powder and nursing lubricant. Aids in preventing excoriation, friction chafing and eliminating odor. Antibacterial action proven effective at 99.9% inhibition where Formula Magic is applied. Excellent for use on diabetic patients, feet and under breasts to relieve redness and skin irritation.

Precautions: Non-irritating to skin, non-toxic, slightly irritating to eyes.

Directions: Apply liberally to body and rub gently into skin.

How Supplied: 4 oz. and 12 oz. NDC #46706-202

MATRIX® MICROCLYSMIC GEL
Burn/Wound Healing Gel

Composition: Water, Propylene Glycol, Glycerine, Hydrolyzed Collagen, Citric Acid, Carbomer, Triethanolamine, Chondroitin Sulfate, Preservatives.

Actions and Uses: Provides endothernic and biomimetic properties to cool traumatized tissue and aid in the homeostasis of healing. Matrix® provides the ultimate moisturization for burns, autograft procedures, radiation irritation, glycolic acid peel irritation, mechanical injuries, laser treatment, and chronic wound therapy.

Precautions: External use only. Non-toxic. No contra-indications.

Directions: Cleanse the area with Techni-Care® Surgical Scrub, Prep. and Wound Cleanser, Rinse thoroughly with Clinical Care® Antimicrobial Wound Cleanser. Do not pat dry. Apply a layer of Matrix® Microclysmic Gel approximately 4mm. thick. Cover the wound with a non-occlusive dressing. Re-apply at every dressing change to maintain a moist wound environment.

How Supplied: 50 ml jars, NDC# 46706-440-2; 120 ml tubes NDC# 46706-440-4

ORCHID FRESH II®
Perineal/Ostomy Cleanser

Composition: Active Ingredient: Benzethonium Chloride

Inactive Ingredients: Water, Amphoteric 2, DMDM Hydantoin, Fragrance, Citric Acid.

Actions and Uses: Orchid Fresh II is an amphoteric, topical antimicrobial cleansing solution which gently cleans and emulsifies feces and urine on the incontinent patient. Use also on stoma sites and ostomy bags to deodorize and eliminate odor. Outstanding antimicrobial action on Pseudomonas, E. coli, Staphylococcus aureus, MRSA, etc. Orchid Fresh II will aid in reducing skin breakdown.

Precautions: External Use Only, Non-Toxic—Non-Dermal Irritating

Directions: Spray topically and remove feces and urine with warm, moist washcloth. Spray directly on peristomal skin areas, clean gently and pat dry. Utilize Care Creme on reddened skin areas.

How Supplied: 4 oz., 8 oz., 16 oz. and Gallons NDC #46706-115

SATIN® ANTIMICROBIAL SKIN CLEANSER

Composition: Active Ingredient: Chloroxylenol
Inactive Ingredients: Water, Sodium Laureth Sulfate, Cocamidopropyl Betaine, PEG-8, Cocamide DEA, Glycol Stearate, Lanolin Oil, Tetrasodium EDTA, D&C Yellow #10.

Actions and Uses: Satin has been specially formulated for use on sensitive or aging dermal tissue, atopic dermatitis and psoriasis. Effective in eliminating gram-positive and gram-negative pathogens such as E. coli, S. aureus, Pseudomonas, etc. Contains emollients to replenish natural oils and proteins. Satin also eliminates skin odor and dry, itchy skin.

Precautions: No contra-indicators. External use only. Non-Toxic.

Directions: Use during shower, bath or regular cleansing or as directed by physician.

How Supplied: 4 oz., 8 oz., 12 oz. 16 oz., 1 Gallon NDC #46706-101

TECHNI–CARE® SURGICAL SCRUB

Composition: Active Ingredient: Chloroxylenol 3%
Inactive Ingredients: Water, Sodium Lauryl Sulfate, Cocamide DEA, Propylene Glycol, Cocamidopropyl Betaine, Cocamidopropyl PG-Dimonium Chloride Phosphate, Citric Acid, Tetrasodium EDTA, Aloe Vera Gel, Hydrolyzed Animal Protein, D&C Yellow #10.

Actions and Uses: Techni-Care represents entirely new technology in a broad-spectrum, topical, antiseptic microbicide for skin degerming. 99.99% Bacterial reduction in 30 second contact usage. Techni-Care may be used for disinfection of wounds, for pre-op and post-op along with surgical scrub applications. Non-staining and non-irritating to dermal tissue. Techni-Care conditions dermal tissue and promotes more rapid rate of healing.

Precautions: Non-Toxic, Non-Irritating, External Use Only. Can be used safely around ears and eyes or as directed by a physician.

Directions: Apply, lather and rinse well. For pre-op, apply and let dry, no rinsing required.

How Supplied: 20 mL packets, 8 oz., 16 oz., 32 oz., Gallons and peel paks

---

J. R. Carlson Laboratories, Inc.
15 COLLEGE DR.
ARLINGTON HEIGHTS, IL 60004

Direct Inquiries to:
Customer Service
(708) 255-1600
FAX: (708) 255-1605

For Medical Emergency Contact:
Customer Service
(708) 255-1600
FAX: (708) 255-1605

ACES®
Vitamin, Antioxidants

Description: ACES provides four natural antioxidant nutrients.

Two Soft Gels Contain:	% U.S. RDA
Beta-Carotene (Pro-Vitamin A) 10,000 IU	200%
Vitamin C (Calcium Ascorbate) 1,000 mg	1667%
Vitamin E (d-Alpha Tocopherol) 400 IU	1333%
Selenium (L-Selenomethionine) 100 mcg	*

RDA: Recommended Daily Allowance - Adults
*U.S. RDA not determined

The nutrients in ACES are: Beta-Carotene (Pro-vitamin A) derived from tiny sea plants or algae (D. salina) grown in the fresh ocean waters off southern Australia; Vitamin C provided as the gentle, buffered calcium ascorbate; Vitamin E 100% natural-source from soy, the most biologically active form; and Selenium, organically bound with the essential nutrient methionine to promote assimilation.

Suggested Use: For dietary supplementation, take two soft gels daily, preferably at mealtime.
CORN-Free, WHEAT-Free, MILK-Free, SUGAR-Free, YEAST-Free, PRESERVATIVE-Free, Soft Gel Contents: Nutrients listed above, soybean oil, vegetable stearin, lecithin, beeswax, Soft Gel Shell: Beef gelatin, glycerin, water, carob.

How Supplied: In bottles of 50, 90, 200, and 360.
Also available as ACES (R) plus ZINC.

Continued on next page

J.R. Carlson—Cont.

E-GEMS®
Vitamins, Antioxidants

Description: 100% natural-source vitamin E (d-alpha tocopheryl acetate) soft gels. Available in 8 strengths: 30IU, 100IU, 200IU, 400IU, 600IU, 800IU, 1000IU, 1200IU.

How Supplied: Supplied in a variety of bottle sizes. Also in creams, ointments, spray, and more.

Church & Dwight Co., Inc.
469 N. HARRISON STREET
PRINCETON, NJ 08543-5297

Direct Inquiries to:
Cathy Marino
(609) 683-7015

For Medical Emergencies Contact:
HIS (800) 228-5635
Extension 7

ARM & HAMMER®
Pure Baking Soda

Active Ingredient: Sodium Bicarbonate U.S.P.

Indications: For alleviation of acid indigestion, also known as heartburn or sour stomach. Not a remedy for other types of stomach complaints such as nausea, stomachache, abdominal cramps, gas pains, or stomach distention caused by overeating and/or overdrinking. In the latter case, one should not ingest solids, liquids or antacid but rather refrain from all physical activity and—if uncomfortable—call a physician.

Actions: ARM & HAMMER® Pure Baking Soda provides fast-acting, effective neutralization of stomach acids. Each level ½ teaspoon dose will neutralize 20.9 mEq of acid.

Warnings: Except under the advice and supervision of a physician: (1) do not administer to children under five years of age, (2) do not take more than eight level ½ teaspoons per person up to 60 years old or four level ½ teaspoons per person 60 years or older in a 24-hour period, (3) do not use this product if you are on a sodium restricted diet, (4) do not use the maximum dose for more than two weeks.

Stomach Warning: To avoid serious injury, do not take until powder is completely dissolved. It is very important not to take this product when overly full from food or drink. Consult a physician if severe stomach pain occurs after taking this product.

Drug Interaction Precaution: Antacids may interact with certain prescription drugs. If you are presently taking a prescription drug, do not take this product without checking with your physician or other health professional.

Dosage and Administration: Level ½ teaspoon in ½ glass (4 fl. oz.) of water every two hours up to maximum dosage or as directed by a physician. Accurately measure level ½ teaspoon. Each level ½ teaspoon contains 20.9 mEq (.476 gm) sodium.

How Supplied: Available in 8 oz., 16 oz., 32 oz., 64 oz., and 160 oz. boxes.

Ciba Self-Medication, Inc.
MACK WOODBRIDGE II
581 MAIN STREET
WOODBRIDGE, NJ 07095

Direct Inquiries to:
Nancy Casper
(908) 602-6000
FAX: (908) 602-6612

For Medical Emergencies Contact:
(908) 602-6780

ACUTRIM® 16 HOUR*
STEADY CONTROL
APPETITE SUPPRESSANT
TABLETS
Caffeine Free
ACUTRIM® MAXIMUM STRENGTH
APPETITE SUPPRESSANT
TABLETS
Caffeine Free
ACUTRIM LATE DAY®
STRENGTH*
APPETITE SUPPRESSANT
TABLETS
Caffeine Free

Description: ACUTRIM® tablets are an aid to appetite control in conjunction with a sensible weight loss program. ACUTRIM® tablets deliver their maximum strength dosage of appetite suppressant at a precisely controlled rate. This timed release is scientifically targeted to effectively distribute the appetite suppressant all day.*
ACUTRIM makes it easier to follow the kind of reduced calorie diet needed for best weight control results.
A diet plan developed by an expert dietician is included in the package for your personal use as a further aid.

Formula: Each ACUTRIM® tablet contains: Active Ingredient—phenylpropanolamine HCl 75 mg (appetite suppressant, time release).
Inactive Ingredients—ACUTRIM® 16 HOUR Steady Control: Cellulose Acetate, Hydroxypropyl Methylcellulose, Stearic Acid—ACUTRIM® MAXIMUM STRENGTH: Cellulose Acetate, D&C Yellow #10, FD&C Blue #1, FD&C Yellow #6, Hydroxypropyl Methylcellulose, Povidone, Propylene Glycol, Stearic Acid, Titanium Dioxide—ACUTRIM LATE DAY® Strength: Cellulose Acetate, FD&C Yellow #6, Hydroxypropyl Methylcellulose, Isopropyl Alcohol, Propylene Glycol, Riboflavin, Stearic Acid, Titanium Dioxide.

Directions: Adult oral dosage is **one tablet** at mid-morning with a full glass of water. SWALLOW EACH TABLET WHOLE; DO NOT DIVIDE, CRUSH, CHEW, OR DISSOLVE THE TABLET. Exceeding the recommended dose has not been shown to result in greater weight loss. This product's effectiveness is directly related to the degree to which you reduce your usual daily food intake. Attempts at weight reduction which involve the use of this product should be limited to periods not exceeding 3 months, because this should be enough time to establish new eating habits. Read and follow important Diet Plan enclosed.
WARNINGS: FOR ADULT USE ONLY. Do not take more than one tablet per day (24 hours). Exceeding the recommended dose may cause serious health problems. Do not give this product to children under 12 years of age. Persons between 12 and 18 are advised to consult their physician before using this product. If nervousness, dizziness, sleeplessness, palpitations or headache occurs, stop taking this medication and consult your physician. If you are being treated for high blood pressure, depression, or an eating disorder or have heart disease, diabetes, or thyroid disease, do not take this product except under the supervision of a physician. As with any drug, if you are pregnant or nursing a baby, seek the advice of a health professional before using this product.
DRUG INTERACTION PRECAUTION: If you are taking a cough/cold or allergy medication containing any form of phenylpropanolamine, or any type of nasal decongestant, do not take this product. Do not take this product if you are taking any prescription drug, except under the advice and supervision of a physician. Do not use this product if you are presently taking a prescription monoamine oxidase inhibitor (MAOI) for depression or for two weeks after stopping use of a MAOI without first consulting a physician.
KEEP THIS AND ALL MEDICATION OUT OF THE REACH OF CHILDREN. In case of accidental overdose, seek professional assistance or contact a Poison Control Center immediately.

How Supplied: Tamper-evident blister packages of 20 and 40 tablets. Do not use if individual seals are broken.
DO NOT STORE ABOVE 30°C (86°F). PROTECT FROM MOISTURE.
*Peak strength and extent of duration relate solely to blood levels.
Shown in Product Identification Guide, page 507

ALLEREST® MAXIMUM STRENGTH, NO DROWSINESS, AND SINUS PAIN FORMULA

Active Ingredients: *Maximum Strength*—Chlorpheniramine maleate 2 mg, pseudoephedrine HCl 30 mg *No Drowsiness*—Acetaminophen 325 mg, pseudoephedrine HCl 30 mg *Sinus Pain Formula*—Acetaminophen 500 mg, chlorpheniramine maleate 2 mg, pseudoephedrine HCl 30 mg

Other Ingredients: *Maximum Strength* —Corn starch, FD&C Blue No. 1, hydroxypropyl methylcellulose, lactose, microcrystalline cellulose, polyethylene glycol, polysorbate 80, stearic acid, titanium dioxide. *No Drowsiness*—Corn starch, hydroxypropyl methylcellulose, microcrystalline cellulose, polyethylene glycol, polysorbate 80, stearic acid, titanium dioxide. *Sinus Pain Formula*—Corn starch, hydroxypropyl methylcellulose, microcrystalline cellulose, polyethylene glycol, polysorbate 80, polyvinylpyrrolidone, stearic acid, titanium dioxide.

Indications: *Maximum Strength*—For the temporary relief of runny nose, sneezing, itching of the nose or throat, and itchy, watery eyes due to hay fever or other upper respiratory allergies. For the temporary relief of nasal and sinus congestion. *No Drowsiness*—Temporarily relieves nasal congestion due to hay fever or other upper respiratory allergies, or associated with sinusitis. For temporary relief of minor aches, pains and headache. *Sinus Pain Formula*—Temporarily relieves nasal congestion, runny nose, sneezing, itching of the nose or throat, and itchy, watery eyes due to hay fever or other upper respiratory allergies. For temporary relief of minor aches, pains and headache.

Warnings: *All Products*—**Do not exceed recommended dosage.** If nervousness, dizziness, or sleeplessness occur, discontinue use and consult a physician. Do not take this product if you have heart disease, high blood pressure, thyroid disease, diabetes, or difficulty in urination due to enlargement of the prostate gland unless directed by a physician. As with any drug, if you are pregnant or nursing a baby, seek the advice of a health professional before using this product. Keep this and all drugs out of the reach of children. In case of accidental overdose, seek professional assistance or contact a Poison Control Center immediately. *Maximum Strength*—If symptoms do not improve within 7 days or are accompanied by fever, consult a physician. Do not take this product, unless directed by a physician, if you have a breathing problem such as emphysema or chronic bronchitis, or glaucoma. May cause excitability, especially in children. May cause drowsiness; alcohol, sedatives, and tranquilizers may increase the drowsiness effect. Avoid alcoholic beverages while taking this product. Do not take this product if you are taking sedatives or tranquilizers, without first consulting your physician. Use caution when driving a motor vehicle, or operating machinery. *No Drowsiness and Sinus Pain Formula*—Do not take this product for more than 10 days (for adults) or 5 days (for children). If symptoms do not improve or are accompanied by fever that lasts for more than 3 days, or if new symptoms occur, consult a physician. In case of accidental overdose, seek professional assistance or contact a Poison Control Center immediately. Prompt medical attention is critical for adults as well as for children even if you do not notice any signs or symptoms.

Drug Interaction Precaution: *All Products*—Do not use this product if you are now taking a prescription monoamine oxidase inhibitor (MAOI) (certain drugs for depression, psychiatric or emotional conditions, or Parkinson's disease), or for 2 weeks after stopping the MAOI drug. If you are uncertain whether your prescription drug contains an MAOI, consult a health professional before taking this product.

Directions: *Maximum Strength*—Dose as follows or as directed by a physician. Adults and children 12 years of age and over: 2 tablets every 4 to 6 hours, not to exceed 8 tablets in 24 hours. Children 6 to under 12 years of age: 1 tablet every 4 to 6 hours, not to exceed 4 tablets in 24 hours. Children under 6 years of age: Consult a physician. *No Drowsiness*—Dose as follows while symptoms persist, or as directed by a physician. Adults and children 12 years of age and over: 2 caplets every 4 to 6 hours, not to exceed 8 caplets in 24 hours. Children 6 to under 12 years of age: 1 caplet every 4 to 6 hours, not to exceed 4 caplets in 24 hours. Children under 6 years of age: Consult a physician. *Sinus Pain Formula*—Dose as follows while symptoms persist, or as directed by a physician. Adults and children 12 years of age and over: 2 caplets every 6 hours, not to exceed 8 caplets in 24 hours. Children under 12 years of age: Consult a physician.

How Supplied: *Maximum Strength* —Boxes of 24 tablets. *No Drowsiness*—Boxes of 20 caplets. *Sinus Pain Formula*—Boxes of 20 caplets. Allerest is a registered trademark of Ciba Self-Medication, Inc.

AMERICAINE® HEMORRHOIDAL OINTMENT
[a-mer 'i-kān]

Active Ingredient: Benzocaine 20%.

Other Ingredients: Benzethonium chloride, polyethylene glycol 300, polyethylene glycol 3350.

Indications: For the temporary relief of local pain, itching and soreness associated with hemorrhoids and anorectal inflammation.

Warnings: If condition worsens, or does not improve within 7 days, consult a physician. Do not exceed the recommended daily dosage unless directed by a physician. In case of bleeding, consult a physician promptly. Do not put this product into the rectum by using fingers or any mechanical device or applicator. Certain persons can develop allergic reactions to ingredients in this product. If the symptom being treated does not subside or if redness, irritation, swelling, pain, or other symptoms develop or increase, discontinue use and consult a physician. **Keep this and all drugs out of the reach of children.** In case of accidental ingestion, seek professional assistance or contact a Poison Control Center immediately.

Directions: *Adults:* When practical, cleanse the affected area with mild soap and warm water and rinse thoroughly. Gently dry by patting or blotting with toilet tissue or a soft cloth before application of this product. Apply externally to the affected area up to 6 times daily. *Children under 12 years of age:* Consult a physician.

How Supplied: *Hemorrhoidal Ointment*—1 oz. tube.
Store at 15°–30°C (59°–86°F).
AMERICAINE is a registered trademark of Ciba Self-Medication, Inc.

AMERICAINE® TOPICAL ANESTHETIC SPRAY AND FIRST AID OINTMENT
[a-mer 'i-kān]

Active Ingredient: Benzocaine 20%.

Other Ingredients: *Spray*—isobutane (propellant), polyethylene glycol 300, propane (propellant). *Ointment*—Benzethonium chloride, polyethylene glycol 300, polyethylene glycol 3350.

Indications: For the temporary relief of pain and itching associated with minor cuts, scrapes, burns, sunburn, insect bites, or minor skin irritations.

Continued on next page

The full prescribing information for each Ciba Self-Medication, Inc., product is contained herein and is that in effect as of December 15, 1995

Ciba Self-Medication, Inc.—Cont.

Warnings: "For external use only." Avoid contact with the eyes. If condition worsens, or if symptoms persist for more than 7 days or clear up and occur again within a few days, discontinue use of this product and consult a physician. **Keep this and all drugs out of the reach of children.** In case of accidental ingestion, seek professional assistance or contact a Poison Control Center immediately. *For Spray only*—Contents under pressure. Do not puncture or incinerate. Flammable mixture; do not use near fire or flame. Do not store at temperature above 49°C. Use only as directed. Intentional misuse by deliberately concentrating and inhaling the contents can be harmful or fatal.

Directions: Adults and children 2 years of age and older: Apply liberally to affected area not more than 3 to 4 times daily. Children under 2 years of age: Consult a physician.

How Supplied: *Topical Anesthetic Spray*—2 oz. aerosol container. *First Aid Ointment*—¾ oz. tube, which is a clear, fragrance-free gel formula that is non-staining, easy to apply, and is easily removed with soap and water.
Store at 15°–30°C (59°–86°F).
AMERICAINE is a registered trademark of Ciba Self-Medication, Inc.
Shown in Product Identification Guide, page 507

ASCRIPTIN®
[ă″skrĭp′tin]
Regular Strength
Maximum Strength
Arthritis Pain

Analgesic
Aspirin buffered with Maalox® for stomach comfort

Active Ingredients: Regular Strength and Arthritis Pain Ascriptin®:
Each tablet/caplet contains Aspirin (325 mg), buffered with Maalox® (Alumina-Magnesia) and Calcium Carbonate.
Maximum Strength Ascriptin®:
Each caplet contains Aspirin (500 mg), buffered with Maalox® (Alumina-Magnesia) and Calcium Carbonate.

Inactive Ingredients: Hydroxypropyl Methylcellulose, Magnesium Stearate, Microcrystalline Cellulose, Propylene Glycol, Starch, Talc, Titanium Dioxide, and other ingredients.

Description: Ascriptin is an excellent analgesic, antipyretic, and anti-inflammatory agent for general use, and is buffered with Maalox® for stomach comfort. Coated tablets/caplets make swallowing easy.

Indications: Regular Strength/Maximum Strength Ascriptin®: For the temporary relief of minor aches and pains associated with headaches, muscle aches, toothaches, menstrual cramps, and dis-comfort and fever of the common cold. Also provides relief from the minor aches and pains of arthritis.
Arthritis Pain Ascriptin®: For effective temporary relief of minor aches and pains associated with arthritis, osteoarthritis, and other arthritic conditions. Also provides relief from the minor aches and pains associated with headaches, muscle aches. toothaches, menstrual cramps and discomfort and fever of the common cold.

Directions: Regular Strength and Arthritis Pain Ascriptin®:
Adults: Two tablets/caplets with water every 4 hours while symptoms persist, not to exceed 12 tablets/caplets in 24 hours, or as your doctor directs. **Children under 12 years of age:** Consult a doctor.
Maximum Strength Ascription®:
Adults: Two caplets with water every 6 hours while symptoms persist, not to exceed 8 caplets in 24 hours, or as directed by a doctor. **Children under 12 years of age:** Consult a doctor.

Warnings: Children and teenagers should not use this medicine for chicken pox or flu symptoms before a doctor is consulted about Reye Syndrome, a rare but serious illness reported to be associated with aspirin. Keep this and all drugs out of the reach of children. Do not take this product for pain for more than 10 days or for fever for more than 3 days unless directed by a doctor. If pain or fever persists or gets worse, if new symptoms occur, or if redness or swelling is present, consult a doctor because these could be signs of a serious condition. Do not take this product if you are allergic to aspirin or if you have asthma unless directed by a doctor. Do not take this product if you have stomach problems (such as heartburn, upset stomach, or stomach pain) that persist or recur, or if you have ulcers or bleeding problems, unless directed by a doctor. As with any drug, if you are pregnant or nursing a baby, seek the advice of a health professional before using this product. **IT IS ESPECIALLY IMPORTANT NOT TO USE ASPIRIN DURING THE LAST 3 MONTHS OF PREGNANCY UNLESS SPECIFICALLY DIRECTED TO DO SO BY A DOCTOR BECAUSE IT MAY CAUSE PROBLEMS IN THE UNBORN CHILD OR COMPLICATIONS DURING DELIVERY.** If ringing in the ears or loss of hearing occurs, consult a doctor before taking any more of this product. **In case of accidental overdose, seek professional assistance or contact a poison control center immediately.**

Drug Interaction Precaution: Do not use if taking a prescription drug for anticoagulation (blood thinning), diabetes, gout or arthritis unless directed by a doctor. Antacids may interact with certain prescription drugs. If you are presently taking a prescription drug, do not take this product without checking with your doctor or other health professional.

Professional Labeling
ASCRIPTIN FOR MYOCARDIAL INFARCTION

Indication: Aspirin is indicated to reduce the risk of death and/or non-fatal myocardial infarction in patients with a previous infarction or unstable angina pectoris.

Clinical Trials: The indication is supported by the results of six large, randomized multicenter, placebo-controlled studies involving 10,816, predominantly male, post-myocardial infarction (MI) patients and one randomized placebo-controlled study of 1,266 men with unstable angina [1-7]. Therapy with aspirin was begun at intervals after the onset of acute MI varying from less than 3 days to more than 5 years and continued for periods of from less than one year to four years. In the unstable angina study, treatment was started within 1 month after the onset of unstable angina and continued for 12 weeks and patients with complicating conditions such as congestive heart failure were not included in the study.
Aspirin therapy in MI patients was associated with about a 20 percent reduction in the risk of subsequent death and/or nonfatal reinfarction, a median absolute decrease of 3 percent from the 12 to 22 percent event rates in the placebo groups. In the aspirin-treated unstable angina patients the reduction in risk was about 50 percent, a reduction in the event rate of 5% from the 10% rate in the placebo group over the 12 weeks of the study.
Daily dosage of aspirin in the post-myocardial infarction studies was 300 mg in one study and 900 to 1500 mg in five studies. A dose of 325 mg was used in the study of unstable angina.

Adverse Reactions: Gastrointestinal Reactions: Doses of 1000 mg per day of aspirin caused gastrointestinal symptoms and bleeding that in some cases were clinically significant. In the largest post-infarction study (The Aspirin Myocardial Infarction Study (AMIS) with 4,500 people), the percentage incidences of gastrointestinal symptoms for the aspirin (1000 mg of a standard, solid-tablet formulation) and placebo-treated subjects, respectively, were: stomach pain (14.5%; 4.4%); heartburn (11.9%; 4.8%); nausea and/or vomiting (7.6%; 2.1%); hospitalization for gastrointestinal disorder (4.8%; 3.5%). In the AMIS and other trials, aspirin treated patients had increased rates of gross gastrointestinal bleeding. Symptoms and signs of gastrointestinal irritation were not significantly increased in subjects treated for unstable angina with buffered aspirin in solution.
Cardiovascular and Biochemical:
In the AMIS trial, the dosage of 1000 mg per day of aspirin was associated with small increases in systolic blood pressure (BP) (average 1.5 to 2.1 mm) and diastolic BP (0.5 to 0.6 mm), depending upon whether maximal or last available read-

ings were used. Blood urea nitrogen and uric acid levels were also increased, but by less than 1.0 mg%.

Subjects with marked hypertension or renal insufficiency had been excluded from the trial so that the clinical importance of these observations for such subjects or for any subjects treated over more prolonged periods is not known. It is recommended that patients placed on long-term aspirin treatment, even at doses of 300 mg per day, be seen at regular intervals to assess changes in these measurements.

Dosage and Administration: Although most of the studies used dosages exceeding 300 mg, two trials used only 300 mg, and pharmacologic data indicate that this dose inhibits platelet function fully. Therefore, 300 mg or a conventional 325-mg aspirin dose is a reasonable, routine dose that would minimize gastrointestinal adverse reactions. This use of aspirin applies to both solid, oral dosage forms (buffered and plain aspirin), and buffered aspirin in solution.

References: 1. Elwood P.C., et al., "A Randomized Controlled Trial of Acetylsalicylic Acid in the Secondary Prevention of Mortality from Myocardial Infarction," *British Medical Journal*, 1:436–440, 1974. 2. The Coronary Drug Project Research Group, "Aspirin in Coronary Heart Disease," *Journal of Chronic Disease*, 29:625–642, 1976. 3. Breddin K. et al., "Secondary Prevention of Myocardial Infarction; Comparison of Acetylsalicylic Acid Phenprocoumon and Placebo," *Thromb, Haemost.*, 41:225–236. 1979. 4. Aspirin Myocardial Infarction Study Research Group, "A Randomized. Controlled Trial of Aspirin in Persons Recovered from Myocardial Infarction." *Journal American Medical Association*, 243:661–669, 1980. 5. Elwood P.C., and Sweetnam, P.M., "Aspirin and Secondary Mortality after Myocardial Infarction," *Lancet*, pp. 1313–1315, December 22–29, 1979. 6. The Persantine-Aspirin Reinfarction Study Research Group "Persantine and Aspirin in Coronary Heart Disease," *Circulation* 62;449–460. 1980. 7. Lewis H.D., et al., "Protective Effects of Aspirin Against Acute Myocardial Infarction and Death in Men with Unstable Angina, Results of a Veterans Administration Cooperative Study." *New England Journal of Medicine*, 309;396–403, 1983.

ASCRIPTIN FOR RECURRENT TIA's IN MEN

Indications: For reducing the risk of recurrent transient ischemic attacks (TIA's) or stroke in men who have had transient ischemia of the brain due to fibrin platelet emboli. There is inadequate evidence that aspirin or buffered aspirin is effective in reducing TIA's in women at the recommended dosage. There is no evidence that aspirin or buffered aspirin is of benefit in the treatment of completed strokes in men or women.

Clinical Trials: The indication is supported by the results of a Canadian

study[1] in which 585 patients with threatened stroke were followed in a randomized clinical trial for an average of 26 months to determine whether aspirin or sulfinpyrazone, singly or in combination was superior to placebo in preventing transient ischemic attacks, stroke, or death. The study showed that, although sulfinpyrazone had no statistically significant effect, aspirin reduced the risk of continuing transient ischemic attacks, stroke, or death by 19 percent and reduced the risk of stroke or death by 31 percent. Another aspirin study carried out in the United States with 178 patients, showed a statistically significant number of "favorable outcomes" including reduced transient ischemic attacks, stroke, and death[2].

Precautions: (1) Patients presenting with signs and symptoms of TIA's should have a complete medical and neurologic evaluation. Consideration should be given to other disorders which resemble TIA's. **(2)** Attention should be given to risk factors; it is important to evaluate and treat, if appropriate, other diseases associated with TIA's and stroke such as hypertension and diabetes. **(3)** Concurrent administration of absorbable antacids at therapeutic doses may increase the clearance of salicylates in some individuals. The concurrent administration of nonabsorbable antacids may alter the rate of absorption of aspirin, thereby resulting in a decreased acetylsalicylic acid/salicylate ratio in plasma. The clinical significance on TIA's of these decreases in available aspirin is unknown.

Aspirin at dosages of 1,000 milligrams per day has been associated with small increases in blood pressure, blood urea nitrogen, and serum uric acid levels. It is recommended that patients placed on long-term aspirin treatment be seen at regular intervals to assess changes in these measurements.

Adverse Reactions: At dosages of 1,000 milligrams or higher of aspirin per day, gastrointestinal side effects include stomach pain, heartburn, nausea and/or vomiting, as well as increased rates of gross gastrointestinal bleeding.

Dosage: Adults dosage for men is 1300 mg a day, in divided doses of 650 mg twice a day or 325 mg four times a day.

References: 1. The Canadian Cooperative Study Group. "A Randomized Trial of Aspirin and Sulfinpyrazone in Threatened Stroke," *New England Journal of Medicine*,299:53–59, 1978. 2. Fields, W.S., et al., "Controlled Trial of Aspirin in Cerebral Ischemia," *Stroke* 8:301–316, 1977.

How Supplied: Regular Strength: Bottles of 60 tablets (0067-0145-60), 100 tablets (0067-0145-68), 160 (0067-0145-30), 225 tablets (0067-0145-77) and 250 foil packet samples–2 tablets each (0067-0145-02). Bottles of 500 tablets (0067-0145-74) without child-resistant closures. Maximum Strength: Bottles of 36 caplets (0067-0146-63), 50 caplets (0067-0146-50), and 85 caplets (0067-0146-85).

Arthritis Pain: Bottles of 60 caplets (0067-0147-60), 100 caplets (0067-0147-68), and 225 caplets (0067-0147-77). Bottles of 500 caplets (0067-0147-74) without child-resistant closures.

Shown in Product Identification Guide, page 507

CALDECORT® ANTI-ITCH CREAM
1/2 oz + 1 oz
[kal 'de-kort]

Active Ingredient: Hydrocortisone acetate (equivalent to hydrocortisone free base 1%).

Other Ingredients: Cetostearyl alcohol, sodium lauryl sulfate, white petrolatum, propylene glycol, purified water, sorbitan monostearate, sorbitol solution, stearic acid.

Indications: For the temporary relief of itching associated with minor skin irritations, inflammation, and rashes due to eczema, insect bites, poison ivy, poison oak, poison sumac, soaps, detergents, cosmetics, jewelry, seborrheic dermatitis, psoriasis, and for external feminine itching. Other uses of this product should be only under the advice and supervision of a doctor.

Warnings: For external use only. Avoid contact with the eyes. If condition worsens, or if symptoms persist for more than 7 days or clear up and occur again within a few days, stop use of this product and do not begin use of any other hydrocortisone product unless you have consulted a doctor. Do not use for the treatment of diaper rash. Consult a doctor. Do not use if you have a vaginal discharge. Consult a doctor. **Keep this and all drugs out of the reach of children.** In case of accidental ingestion, seek professional assistance or contact a Poison Control Center immediately.

Directions: Adults and children 2 years of age and older: Apply to affected area not more than 3 or 4 times daily. Children under 2 years of age: Do not use, consult a doctor.

How Supplied: ½ oz. and 1 oz. tubes. CALDECORT is a registered trademark of Ciba Self-Medication, Inc.
581 Main St.
Woodbridge, NJ 07095

Shown in Product Identification Guide, page 507

Continued on next page

The full prescribing information for each Ciba Self-Medication, Inc., product is contained herein and is that in effect as of December 15, 1995

Ciba Self-Medication, Inc.—Cont.

CALDESENE® MEDICATED POWDER AND OINTMENT
[kal 'de-sēn]

Active Ingredients: *Powder* —Calcium undecylenate 10%. *Ointment* —White petrolatum 53.9%; zinc oxide 15%.

Other Ingredients: *Powder* — Fragrance, talc. *Ointment* —Cod liver oil, fragrance, lanolin, methylparaben, propylparaben, talc.

Indications: Caldesene Powder is medicated with calcium undecylenate to kill harmful bacteria while forming a protective barrier that repels moisture and helps keep sensitive skin dry. Only Caldesene has this special formula with two way action. Used regularly, Caldesene helps prevent skin infections and protects sensitive skin for both adults and children. Caldesene Medicated Ointment is specially formulated to soothe and treat diaper rash while protecting sensitive skin against wetness.

Actions: Caldesene Medicated Powder helps relieve, treat and prevent diaper rash, prickly heat, chafing, with two way action:
• kills bacteria
• protects against wetness.
Caldesene Medicated Ointment helps relieve, treat and prevent diaper rash; the high quality ingredients in Caldesene provide a water repellent barrier that protects the skin and allows it to heal.

Warnings: For external use only. Avoid contact with eyes. If condition worsens or does not improve within 7 days, consult a physician. **Keep this and all drugs out of the reach of children.** In case of accidental ingestion, seek professional assistance or contact a Poison Control Center immediately.
Powder only: Keep powder away from child's face to avoid inhalation, which can cause breathing problems. Do not use on broken skin.
Ointment only: Do not apply over deep or puncture wounds, infections or lacerations.

Directions: Use on baby after every bath or diaper change or as directed by a pediatrician.
Powder only: Apply powder close to the body away from child's face. (Shake bottle—don't squeeze—to apply powder to your hand or directly into the diaper.) For prickly heat, chafing—Smooth on Caldesene 3 or 4 times a day, or as recommended by your physician, to soothe and comfort sensitive skin and relieve minor irritation.
Ointment only: Cleanse and thoroughly dry baby's skin, then smooth an even layer of Caldesene Ointment over the diaper area.

How Supplied: *Medicated Powder* — 2 oz (57 g) and 4 oz (113 g) shaker containers. *Medicated Ointment* —1.25 oz (35 g).

CALDESENE is a registered trademark of Ciba Self-Medication, Inc.
Shown in Product Identification Guide, page 507

CRUEX® ANTIFUNGAL POWDER, SPRAY POWDER AND CREAM
[kru 'ex]

Active Ingredients: *Powder* —Undecylenate 10%, as calcium undecylenate. *Spray Powder* —Total undecylenate 19%, as undecylenic acid and zinc undecylenate. *Cream*—Total undecylenate 20%, as undecylenic acid and zinc undecylenate.

Other Ingredients: *Powder* —Colloidal silicon dioxide, fragrance, isopropyl myristate, talc. *Spray Powder* —Fragrance, isobutane (propellant), isopropyl myristate, menthol, talc, trolamine. *Cream* —Fragrance, glycol stearate SE, lanolin, methylparaben, PEG-8 laurate, PEG-6 stearate, propylparaben, sorbitol solution, stearic acid, trolamine, purified water, white petrolatum.

Indications: Cures jock itch. Relieves itching, chafing, and burning. Soothes irritation. Cruex powders also absorb perspiration.

Warnings: Do not use on children under 2 years of age unless directed by a doctor. For external use only. Avoid contact with the eyes. If irritation occurs, or if there is no improvement within 2 weeks, discontinue use and consult a doctor. **Keep this and all drugs out of the reach of children.** In case of accidental ingestion, seek professional assistance or contact a Poison Control Center immediately. *For Spray Powder only*—Avoid inhaling. Avoid contact with the eyes or other mucous membranes. Contents under pressure. Do not puncture or incinerate. Flammable mixture, do not use near fire or flame. Do not expose to heat or temperatures above 49°C (120°F.) Use only as directed. Intentional misuse by deliberately concentrating and inhaling the contents can be harmful or fatal.

Directions: Clean the affected area and dry thoroughly. Apply a thin layer of the product over affected area twice daily (morning and night) or as directed by a doctor. Supervise children in the use of this product. Use daily for 2 weeks. If condition persists longer, consult a doctor. This product is not effective on the scalp or nails.

How Supplied: *Powder* —1.5 oz (43 g) plastic squeeze bottle. *Spray Powder* —1.8 oz (51 g), 3.5 oz (99 g) and 5.5 oz (156 g) aerosol containers. *Cream* —½ oz (14 g) tube.
CRUEX is a registered trademark of Ciba Self-Medication, Inc.
Shown in Product Identification Guide, page 508

DESENEX® ANTIFUNGAL POWDER, SPRAY POWDER, AND OINTMENT
[dess 'i-nex]

Active Ingredients: *Ointment, Powder, and Spray Powder* —Total undecylenate 25%, as undecylenic acid and zinc undecylenate.

Other Ingredients: *Ointment* —Fragrance, glycol stearate SE, lanolin, methylparaben, PEG-8 laurate, PEG-6 stearate, propylparaben, purified water, sorbitol solution, stearic acid, trolamine, white petrolatum. *Powder* —Fragrance, talc. *Spray Powder* —Fragrance, isobutane (propellant), isopropyl myristate, menthol, talc, trolamine.

Indications: Proven clinically effective in the treatment of athlete's foot (tinea pedis). Relieves the painful itching, burning, cracking and discomfort associated with athlete's foot.

Warnings: Do not use on children under 2 years of age unless directed by a doctor. For external use only. Avoid contact with the eyes. If irritation occurs, or if there is no improvement within 4 weeks, discontinue use and consult a doctor. **Keep this and all drugs out of the reach of children.** In case of accidental ingestion, seek professional assistance or contact a Poison Control Center immediately. *For Spray Powder*, avoid inhaling. Avoid contact with the eyes or other mucous membranes. Contents under pressure. Do not puncture or incinerate. Flammable mixture, do not use near fire or flame. Do not expose to heat or temperatures above 49°C (120°F). Use only as directed. Intentional misuse by deliberately concentrating and inhaling the contents can be harmful or fatal.

Directions: Clean the affected area and dry thoroughly. Apply a thin layer of the product over affected area twice daily (morning and night) or as directed by a doctor. Supervise children in the use of this product. Pay special attention to the spaces between the toes. Wear well-fitting, ventilated shoes and change shoes and socks at least once daily. Use daily for 4 weeks. If condition persists longer, consult a doctor. This product is not effective on the scalp or nails. For persistent cases of athlete's foot, use Maximum Strength Desenex Ointment at night and Maximum Strength Desenex Spray Powder during the day.

How Supplied: *Ointment* —½ oz (14 g) and 1 oz (28 g) tubes. *Powder* —1.5 oz (43 g) and 3 oz (85 g) shaker containers. *Spray Powder* —2.7 oz (77 g) aerosol container.
DESENEX is a registered trademark of Ciba Self-Medication, Inc.
Shown in Product Identification Guide, page 508

DESENEX® FOOT & SNEAKER DEODORANT SPRAY

[dess'i-nex]

Ingredients: Isobutane (propellant), SD alcohol 40-B, talc, aluminum chlorohydrex, silica, diisopropyl adipate, fragrance, menthol, tartaric acid.

Description: Foot & Sneaker Deodorant Spray cools and comforts feet, helping them feel clean and refreshed. Helps foster good foot hygiene with regular use. Specially formulated to absorb wetness, deodorize and relieve the discomfort of hot, perspiring, active feet. Sprays on like a liquid—dries quickly to a fine powder.

Directions: **Shake well,** hold 6 inches from area and spray onto soles of your feet and between your toes daily. Also, spray liberally over entire area of shoes or sneakers before wearing.

Warnings: Avoid spraying in eyes or other mucous membranes. Contents under pressure. Do not puncture or incinerate. Flammable mixture, do not use near fire or flame. Do not expose to heat or temperatures above 49°C (120°F). Use only as directed. Intentional misuse by deliberately concentrating and inhaling the contents can be harmful or fatal. **Keep out of reach of children.**

How Supplied: *Desenex Foot & Sneaker Deodorant Spray Powder* —3 oz (85 g) aerosol container. Also available, Desenex Foot & Sneaker Deodorant Powder Plus with an antifungal—2 oz (57 g) shaker container.
DESENEX is a registered trademark of Ciba Self-Medication, Inc.
Shown in Product Identification Guide, page 508

PRESCRIPTION STRENGTH DESENEX® AF ANTIFUNGAL CREAM, PRESCRIPTION STRENGTH DESENEX® SPRAY POWDER AND SPRAY LIQUID

Active Ingredients: *Cream* —Clotrimazole 1%. *Spray Powder and Spray Liquid* —Miconazole Nitrate 2%.

Inactive Ingredients: *Cream* —Cetostearyl alcohol, cetyl esters wax, 2-octyldodecanol, polysorbate-60, sorbitan monostearate, purified water and, as a preservative, benzyl alcohol (1%). *Spray Powder* —Aloe vera gel, aluminum starch octenylsuccinate, isopropyl myristate, propylene carbonate, SD alcohol 40-B (10% w/w), sorbitan monooleate, stearalkonium hectorite. *Spray Liquid* —Polyethylene glycol 300, polysorbate 20, SD alcohol 40-B (15% w/w).

Propellant: *Spray Powder* —Isobutane/propane. *Spray Liquid* —Dimethyl ether.

Indications: *Cream* —Cures athlete's foot (tinea pedis), jock itch (tinea cruris), and ringworm (tinea corporis). For effective relief of the itching, cracking, burning, and discomfort which can accompany these conditions. *Spray Powder and Spray Liquid* —Proven clinically effective in the treatment of athlete's foot (tinea pedis) and ringworm (tinea corporis). Relieves the itching, scaling, burning, and discomfort that can accompany athlete's foot. Prescription Strength Desenex® Spray Powder is specially formulated to aid the drying of moist areas of the feet.

Warnings: Do not use on children under 2 years of age unless directed by a doctor. For external use only. Avoid contact with the eyes. If irritation occurs, or if there is no improvement within 4 weeks (for athlete's foot or ringworm) or within 2 weeks (for jock itch), discontinue use and consult a doctor. **Keep this and all drugs out of the reach of children.** In case of accidental ingestion, seek professional assistance or contact a Poison Control Center immediately. Use only as directed. *For Spray Powder and Spray Liquid* —Avoid inhaling. Avoid contact with the eyes or other mucous membranes. Contents under pressure. Do not puncture or incinerate. Flammable mixture, do not use near fire or flame. Do not expose to heat or temperatures above 49°C (120°F). Use only as directed. Intentional misuse by deliberately concentrating and inhaling the contents can be harmful or fatal.

Directions: Clean the affected area and dry thoroughly. Apply a thin layer of the product over affected area twice daily (morning and night) or as directed by a doctor. Supervise children in the use of this product. For athlete's foot, pay special attention to the spaces between the toes. Wear well-fitting, ventilated shoes and change shoes and socks at least once daily. Use daily for 4 weeks, (*Spray Powder* and *Spray Liquid*; when using the *Cream*, best results in athlete's foot and ringworm are usually obtained within 4 weeks use of this product, and, in jock itch, within 2 weeks' use). If condition persists longer, consult a doctor. This product is not effective on the scalp or nails.

How Supplied: *Cream* —15 g (½ oz). *Spray Powder* —85 g (3 oz). *Spray Liquid* —100 g (3.5 oz).
DESENEX is a registered trademark of Ciba Self-Medication, Inc.
Shown in Product Identification Guide, page 508

EXTRA STRENGTH DOAN'S® Analgesic Caplets

Indications: For temporary relief of minor backache pain.

Directions: Adults—Two caplets with water every 6 hours while symptoms persist, not to exceed 8 caplets during a 24-hour period or as directed by a doctor. Children under 12: consult a doctor.

Warnings: Children and teenagers should not use this medicine for chicken pox or flu symptoms before a doctor is consulted about Reye syndrome, a rare but serious illness. As with any drug, if you are pregnant or nursing a baby, seek the advice of a health professional before using this product. Do not take this product for pain for more than 10 days unless directed by a doctor. If pain or fever persists or gets worse, if new symptoms occur, or if redness or swelling is present, consult a doctor because these could be signs of a serious condition. Do not take this product if you are allergic to salicylates (including aspirin), have stomach problems (such as heartburn, upset stomach, or stomach pain) that persist or recur, or if you have ulcers or bleeding problems, unless directed by a doctor. If ringing in the ears or a loss of hearing occurs, consult a doctor before taking any more of this product.
KEEP THIS AND ALL DRUGS OUT OF THE REACH OF CHILDREN. In case of accidental overdose, seek professional assistance or contact a Poison Control Center immediately.

Drug Interaction Precaution: Do not take this product if you are taking a prescription drug for anticoagulation (thinning of the blood), diabetes, gout, or arthritis unless directed by a doctor.

Active Ingredient: Each caplet contains Magnesium Salicylate Tetrahydrate 580 mg. (equivalent to 467.2 mg. of anhydrous Magnesium Salicylate).

Also Contains: Magnesium Stearate, Microcrystalline Cellulose, Opadry White, Polyethylene Glycol, Stearic Acid.
Store at 15°–30°C (59°–86°F).
PROTECT FROM MOISTURE.
Shown in Product Identification Guide, page 508

Extra Strength DOAN'S® P.M. Magnesium Salicylate/ Diphenhydramine Analgesic/Sleep Aid Caplets

Indications: For temporary relief of minor back pain accompanied by sleeplessness.

Directions: Adults and children 12 years of age or older: Take 2 caplets with water at bedtime if needed, or as directed by a doctor.

Warnings: Children and teenagers should not use this medicine for chicken pox or flu symptoms before a doctor is consulted about Reye syndrome, a rare

Continued on next page

The full prescribing information for each Ciba Self-Medication, Inc., product is contained herein and is that in effect as of December 15, 1995

Ciba Self-Medication, Inc.—Cont.

but serious illness. **KEEP THIS AND ALL DRUGS OUT OF THE REACH OF CHILDREN.** IN CASE OF ACCIDENTAL OVERDOSE, SEEK PROFESSIONAL ASSISTANCE OR CONTACT A POISON CONTROL CENTER IMMEDIATELY. DO NOT GIVE THIS PRODUCT TO CHILDREN UNDER 12 YEARS OF AGE. As with any drug, if you are pregnant or nursing a baby, seek the advice of a health professional before using this product. Do not take this product for pain for more than 10 days unless directed by a doctor. If pain or fever persists or gets worse, if new symptoms occur, or if redness or swelling is present, consult a doctor because these could be signs of a serious condition. If sleeplessness persists continuously for more than 2 weeks, consult your doctor. Insomnia may be a symptom of serious underlying medical illness. Do not take this product, unless directed by a doctor, if you have a breathing problem such as emphysema or chronic bronchitis, or if you have glaucoma, difficulty in urination due to enlargement of the prostate gland, stomach problems (such as heartburn, upset stomach, or stomach pain) that persist or recur, ulcers or bleeding problems, or if you are allergic to aspirin or salicylates. If ringing in the ears or a loss of hearing occurs, consult a doctor before taking any more of this product. Avoid alcoholic beverages while taking this product. Do not take this product if you are taking sedatives or tranquilizers without first consulting your doctor.

Drug Interaction Precaution: Do not take this product if you are taking a prescription drug for anticoagulation (thinning of the blood), diabetes, gout, or arthritis unless directed by a doctor.

Active Ingredients: Each caplet contains Magnesium Salicylate Tetrahydrate 580mg. (equivalent to 467.2mg. of anhydrous Magnesium Salicylate) and Diphenydramine HCl 25mg.

Also Contains: Carnauba Wax, Colloidal Silicon Dioxide, Croscarmellose Sodium, Microcrystalline Cellulose, Magnesium Stearate, Opadry Blue, Stearic Acid, Talc.
Store at 15°–30°C (59°–86°F).
PROTECT FROM MOISTURE.
Shown in Product Identification Guide, page 508

REGULAR STRENGTH DOAN'S®
Analgesic Caplets

Indications: For temporary relief of minor backache pain.

Directions: Adults—Two caplets with water every 4 hours while symptoms persist, not to exceed 12 caplets during a 24-hour period or as directed by a doctor. Children under 12: consult a doctor.

Warnings: Children and teenagers should not use this medicine for chicken pox or flu symptoms before a doctor is consulted about Reye syndrome, a rare but serious illness. As with any drug, if you are pregnant or nursing a baby, seek the advice of a health professional before using this product. Do not take this product for pain for more than 10 days unless directed by a doctor. If pain or fever persists or gets worse, if new symptoms occur, or if redness or swelling is present, consult a doctor because these could be signs of a serious condition. Do not take this product if you are allergic to salicylates (including aspirin), have stomach problems (such as heartburn, upset stomach, or stomach pain) that persist or recur, or if you have ulcers or bleeding problems, unless directed by a doctor. If ringing in the ears or a loss of hearing occurs, consult a doctor before taking any more of this product.

KEEP THIS AND ALL DRUGS OUT OF THE REACH OF CHILDREN. In case of accidental overdose, seek professional assistance or contact a Poison Control Center immediately.

Drug Interaction Precaution: Do not take this product if you are taking a prescription drug for anticoagulation (thinning of the blood), diabetes, gout, or arthritis unless directed by a doctor.

Active Ingredient: Each caplet contains Magnesium Salicylate Tetrahydrate 377 mg. (equivalent to 303.7 mg. of anhydrous Magnesium Salicylate).

Also Contains: FD&C Yellow #6, Magnesium Stearate, Microcrystalline Cellulose, Opadry Light Green, Polyethylene Glycol, Stearic Acid.
Store at 15°–30°C (59°–86°F). PROTECT FROM MOISTURE.
Shown in Product Identification Guide, page 508

DULCOLAX®
[*dul'co-lax*]
brand of bisacodyl USP
Tablets of 5 mg
Suppositories of 10 mg
Laxative

Ingredients: Each enteric coated tablet contains: Active: Bisacodyl USP 5 mg. Also contains: Acacia, acetylated monoglyceride, carnauba wax, cellulose acetate phthalate, corn starch, D&C Red No. 30 aluminum lake, D&C Yellow No. 10 aluminum lake, dibutyl phthalate, docusate sodium, gelatin, glycerin, iron oxides, kaolin, lactose, magnesium stearate, methylparaben, pharmaceutical glaze, polyethylene glycol, povidone, propylparaben, sodium benzoate, sorbitan monooleate, sucrose, talc, titanium dioxide, white wax.
Each suppository contains: Active: Bisacodyl USP 10 mg. Also contains: Hydrogenated vegetable oil.
SODIUM CONTENT: Tablets and suppositories contain less than 0.2 mg per dosage unit and are thus dietetically sodium free.

Indications: For the relief of occasional constipation and irregularity. Physicians should refer to the "Professional Labeling" section for additional indications and information.

Directions:
Tablets
Adults and children 12 years of age and over: Take 2 or 3 tablets (usually 2) in a single dose once daily.
Children 6 to under 12 years of age: Take 1 tablet once daily.
Children under 6 years of age: Consult a physician.
Expect results in 8–12 hours if taken at bedtime or within 6 hours if taken before breakfast.
Suppositories
Adults and children 12 years of age and over: 1 suppository once daily. Remove foil wrapper. Lie on your side and, with pointed end first, push suppository high into the rectum so it will not slip out. Retain it for 15 to 20 minutes. If you feel the suppository must come out immediately, it was not inserted high enough and should be pushed higher.
Children 6 to under 12 years of age: ½ suppository once daily.
Children under 6 years of age: Consult a physician.
If the suppository seems soft, hold in foil wrapper under cold water for one or two minutes. In the presence of anal fissures or hemorrhoids, suppository may be coated at the tip with petroleum jelly before insertion.

Warnings: Do not use laxative products when abdominal pain, nausea, or vomiting are present unless directed by a physician. Restoration of normal bowel function by using this product may cause abdominal discomfort including cramps. Laxative products should not be used for a period longer than 1 week unless directed by a physician. Rectal bleeding or failure to have a bowel movement after use of a laxative may indicate a serious condition. If this occurs, discontinue use and consult your physician. As with any drug, if you are pregnant or nursing a baby, seek the advice of a health care professional before using this product. KEEP THIS AND ALL MEDICATION OUT OF THE REACH OF CHILDREN. In case of accidental overdose or ingestion, seek professional assistance or contact a poison control center immediately. For tablets: Do not chew or crush. Do not give to children under 6 years of age unless directed by a physician. Do not take this product within 1 hour after taking an antacid or milk.

How Supplied: Dulcolax, brand of bisacodyl: Yellow, enteric-coated tablets of 5 mg in boxes of 10, 25, 50 and 100; suppositories of 10 mg in boxes of 4, 8, 16 and 50.
NDC 0083-6200 or 0067-6200 (tablets)
NDC 0083-6100 or 0067-6100 (suppositories)

Note: Store Dulcolax suppositories and tablets at temperatures below 77°F (25°C). Avoid excessive humidity.

Also Available: Dulcolax® Bowel Prep Kit. Each kit contains:
 1 Dulcolax suppository of 10 mg bisacodyl;
 4 Dulcolax tablets of 5 mg bisacodyl;
 Complete patient instructions.

PROFESSIONAL LABELING:

Description and Clinical Pharmacology: Dulcolax is a contact stimulant laxative, administered either orally or rectally, which acts directly on the colonic mucosa to produce normal peristalsis throughout the large intestine. The active ingredient in Dulcolax, bisacodyl, is a colorless, tasteless compound that is practically insoluble in water or alkaline solution. Its chemical name is: bis(p-acetoxyphenyl)-2-pyridylmethane. Bisacodyl is very poorly absorbed, if at all, in the small intestine following oral administration, nor in the large intestine following rectal administration. On contact with the mucosa or submucosal plexi of the large intestine, bisacodyl stimulates sensory nerve endings to produce parasympathetic reflexes resulting in increased peristaltic contractions of the colon. It has also been shown to promote fluid and ion accumulation in the colon, which increases the laxative effect. A bowel movement is usually produced approximately 6 hours after oral administration (8–12 hours if taken at bedtime), and approximately 15 minutes to 1 hour after rectal administration, providing satisfactory cleansing of the bowel which may, under certain circumstances, obviate the need for colonic irrigation.

Indications and Usage: For use as part of a bowel cleansing regimen in preparing the patient for surgery or for preparing the colon for x-ray endoscopic examination. Dulcolax will not replace the colonic irrigations usually given patients before intracolonic surgery, but is useful in the preliminary emptying of the colon prior to these procedures.
Also for use as a laxative in postoperative care (i.e., restoration of normal bowel hygiene), antepartum care, postpartum care, and in preparation for delivery.

Contraindications: Stimulant laxatives, such as Dulcolax, are contraindicated for patients with acute surgical abdomen, appendicitis, rectal bleeding, or intestinal obstruction.

Precautions: Long-term administration of Dulcolax is not recommended in the treatment of chronic constipation.

Dosage and Administration:
Preparation for x-ray endoscopy: For barium enemas, no food should be given following oral administration to prevent reaccumulation of material in the cecum, and a suppository should be administered one to two hours prior to examination.
Children under 6 years of age: Oral administration is not recommended due to the requirement to swallow tablets whole. For rectal administration, the

suppository dosage is 5 mg (½ of 10 mg suppository) in a single daily dose.
Shown in Product Identification Guide, page 508

EFIDAC/24
Nasal decongestant

Indications: Provides temporary relief of nasal congestion due to the common cold, hay fever, or other upper respiratory allergies, and nasal congestion associated with sinusitis; reduces swelling of nasal passages; shrinks swollen membranes; relieves sinus pressure; and temporarily restores freer breathing through the nose.

Directions: Adults and children 12 years and over: Take just one tablet with fluid every 24 hours. DO NOT EXCEED ONE TABLET IN 24 HOURS. SWALLOW EACH TABLET WHOLE; DO NOT DIVIDE, CRUSH, CHEW, OR DISSOLVE THE TABLET. The tablet does not completely dissolve and may be seen in the stool (this is normal). Not for use in children under 12 years of age.

Warnings: DO NOT EXCEED RECOMMENDED DOSAGE because at higher doses nervousness, dizziness, or sleeplessness may occur. Do not take this product for more than 7 days. If symptoms do not improve or are accompanied by fever, consult a physician. Do not take this product if you have heart disease, high blood pressure, thyroid disease, diabetes, or difficulty in urination due to enlargement of the prostate gland, unless directed by a physician.
Rarely, tablets of this kind may cause bowel obstruction (blockage), usually in people with severe narrowing of the bowel (esophagus, stomach or intestine). If you have had obstruction or narrowing of the bowel, do not take this product without consulting your physician. Contact your physician if you experience persistent abdominal pain or vomiting. As with any drug, if you are pregnant or nursing a baby, seek the advice of a health professional before using this product.
KEEP THIS AND ALL DRUGS OUT OF THE REACH OF CHILDREN. In case of accidental overdose, seek professional assistance or contact a Poison Control Center immediately.

Drug Interaction Precaution: Do not use this product if you are now taking a prescription monoamine oxidase inhibitor (MAOI) (certain drugs for depression, psychiatric or emotional conditions, or Parkinson's disease), or for 2 weeks after stopping the MAOI drug. If you are uncertain whether your prescription drug contains an MAOI, consult a health professional before taking this product.
Store in a dry place between 4°–30°C (39°–86°F).
QUESTIONS? Please write Consumer Affairs at the address below.

Distributed by: Ciba Self-Medication, Inc., 581 Main Street, Woodbridge, NJ 07095

Active Ingredient: Each Efidac 24 tablet contains 240 mg Pseudoephedrine Hydrochloride

Inactive Ingredients: Cellulose, cellulose acetate, FD&C Blue #1, hydroxypropl cellulose, hydroxypropl methylcellulose, magnesium stearate, polyethylene glycol, polysorbate 80, povidone, sodium chloride, and titanium dioxide.
Shown in Product Identification Guide, page 508

EFIDAC 24 CHLORPHENIRAMINE
EFIDAC 24 is a line of products specially formulated to provide relief for 24 hours with a one tablet, once daily dosage. Each EFIDAC 24 tablet releases an outer coating of medication immediately and then continues to work by releasing medication at a precisely controlled rate for 24 hours of relief. EFIDAC 24 CHLORPHENIRAMINE contains an antihistamine to relieve allergy symptoms.

Active Ingredient: Each EFIDAC 24 CHLORPHENIRAMINE tablet contains a total of 16 mg chlorpheniramine maleate: 4 mg immediate release and 12 mg controlled release.

Inactive Ingredients: Cellulose, cellulose acetate, hydroxypropyl cellulose, hydroxypropyl methylcellulose, magnesium stearate, mannitol, polyethylene glycol, polysorbate 80, povidone, and titanium dioxide.

Indications: Provides temporary relief of runny nose, sneezing, itching of the nose or throat, and itchy, watery eyes due to hay fever or other upper respiratory allergies (allergic rhinitis); temporarily relieves runny nose and sneezing associated with the common cold.

Directions: Adults and children 12 years of age and over: Take just one tablet with fluid every 24 hours. **DO NOT EXCEED ONE TABLET IN 24 HOURS.** SWALLOW EACH TABLET WHOLE; DO NOT DIVIDE, CRUSH, CHEW, OR DISSOLVE THE TABLET. The tablet does not completely dissolve and may be seen in the stool (this is normal). Not for use in children under 12 years of age.

Warnings: DO NOT EXCEED RECOMMENDED DOSAGE. May cause excitability, especially in children. Do not take this product, unless directed by a physician, if you have a breathing problem such as emphysema or chronic bronchitis, or if you have glaucoma or

Continued on next page

The full prescribing information for each Ciba Self-Medication, Inc., product is contained herein and is that in effect as of December 15, 1995

Ciba Self-Medication, Inc.—Cont.

difficulty in urination due to enlargement of the prostate gland. May cause drowsiness; alcohol, sedatives, and tranquilizers may increase the drowsiness effect. Avoid alcoholic beverages while taking this product.

Do not take this product if you are taking sedatives or tranquilizers, without first consulting your physician. Use caution when driving a motor vehicle or operating machinery.

Rarely, tablets of this kind may cause bowel obstruction (blockage), usually in people with severe narrowing of the bowel (esophagus, stomach or intestine). If you have had obstruction or narrowing of the bowel, do not take this product without consulting your physician. Contact your physician if you experience persistent abdominal pain or vomiting.

As with any drug, if you are pregnant or nursing a baby, seek the advice of a health professional before using this product. **KEEP THIS AND ALL DRUGS OUT OF THE REACH OF CHILDREN.** In case of accidental overdose, seek professional assistance or contact a Poison Control Center immediately.

Store in a dry place between 4° and 30°C (39° and 86°F).

BLISTER PACKAGED FOR YOUR PROTECTION. DO NOT USE IF INDIVIDUAL SEALS ARE BROKEN. QUESTIONS ABOUT EFIDAC 24? Please write Consumer Affairs at the address below.

Distributed by: CIBA Consumer Pharmaceuticals,

581 Main St., Woodbridge, NJ 07095
©1994 CIBA CONSUMER PHARMACEUTICALS
NDC 0083-0255-93   LIST 5206
Shown in Product Identification Guide, page 508

EUCALYPTAMINT®
Arthritis Pain Reliever
Maximum Strength
External Analgesic

Description: Maximum Strength topical analgesic that provides hours of effective relief from minor arthritis pain.

Active Ingredient: Natural Menthol (16%).

Inactive Ingredients: Lanolin and Eucalyptus Oil.

Indications: For the temporary relief of minor aches and pains of muscles and joints associated with arthritis.

Directions: Adults and children 2 years of age and older: Gently massage a conservative amount into affected area not more than 3 to 4 times daily. Children under 2 years of age: Consult a physician.

Warning: FOR EXTERNAL USE ONLY. Avoid contact with eyes. Do not apply to wounds or damaged skin. Do not bandage tightly. Do not use with heating pads or heating devices. If condition

worsens, or if symptoms persist for more than 7 days, discontinue use of this product and consult a physician. Keep this and all drugs out of the reach of children. In case of accidental ingestion, seek professional assistance or contact a Poison Control Center immediately. Store at room temperature 15°–30°C (59°–86°F). Do not freeze. It is normal for the consistency of Eucalyptamint to vary with temperature changes. If thickening does occur, warm the tube in the palms of your hands or run under warm water.

Distributed By:
Ciba Self-Medication, Inc.
581 Main St.
Woodbridge, NJ 07095

How Supplied: Eucalyptamint Ointment is supplied in a 2 oz. easy to squeeze tube.

Shown in Product Identification Guide, page 508

EUCALYPTAMINT®
Muscle Pain Relief Formula
External Analgesic

Description: A uniquely scented gel creme formulation providing hours of effective pain relief for overworked muscles.

Active Ingredient: Menthol 8%.

Other Ingredients: Carbomer 980, Eucalyptus Oil, Fragrance, Propylene Glycol, SD 3A Alcohol, Triethanolamine, TWEEN 80, Water.

Indications: For the temporary relief of minor aches and pains of muscles associated with simple backache, strains, sprains and sports injuries.

Directions: Adults and children 2 years of age and older. Shake tube with cap facing downward. Gently massage a conservative amount into affected area not more than 3 to 4 times daily. Store on cap. Children under 2 years of age: Consult a physician.

Warning: FOR EXTERNAL USE ONLY. Avoid contact with eyes. Do not apply to wounds or damaged skin. Do not bandage tightly. Do not use with heating pads or heating devices. If condition worsens, or if symptoms persist for more than 7 days, discontinue use of this product and consult a physician. Keep this and all drugs out of the reach of children. In case of accidental ingestion, seek professional assistance or contact a Poison Control Center immediately. Store at room temperature 15°–30°C (59°–86°F). DO NOT FREEZE.

How Supplied: Eucalyptamint Muscle Pain Relief Formula is supplied in 2.25 oz. tubes and is available in two scents: Alpine Breeze and Powder Fresh. *Eucalyptamint is a registered trademark of Ciba Self-Medication, Inc.*
Distributed By:
Ciba Self-Medication, Inc.
581 Main St.
Woodbridge, NJ 07095

Shown in Product Identification Guide, page 508

KONDREMUL®

Active Ingredient: Mineral Oil (55%).

Inactive Ingredients: Acacia, benzoic acid, carrageenan (Irish Moss), ethyl vanillin, glycerin, mapliene triple oil, purified water, vanillin.

Indications: For relief of occasional constipation. This product generally produces bowel movement in 6–8 hours.

Actions: Promotes gentle, predicatable regularity of normal bowel movement. Pleasant tasting and smooth acting, it passes through stomach and upper intestine without upset or dehydration. Assures soft stool by retaining moisture balance and mixing thoroughly with bowel content. Permits passage of stool without straining. This product generally produces bowel movement in 6–8 hours.

Warning: Do not take with meals. Do not administer to children under 6 years of age, to pregnant women, to bedridden patients or to persons with difficulty swallowing. Do not use this product when abdominal pain, nausea or vomiting are present, unless directed by a physician. Laxative products should not be used for a period longer than 1 week unless directed by a physician. If you have noticed a sudden change in bowel habits that persists over a period of 2 weeks, consult a physician before using a laxative. Rectal bleeding or failure to have a bowel movement after use of a laxative may indicate a serious condition. Discontinue use and consult a physican. As with any drug, if you are pregnant or nursing a baby, seek the advice of a health care professional before using this product. KEEP THIS AND ALL DRUGS OUT OF THE REACH OF CHILDREN. In case of accidental overdose, seek professional assistance or contact a poison control center immediately.

Drug Interaction Precaution: Do not take this product if you are presently taking a stool softener laxative.

Directions: Shake well before using. Adults and children over 12 years of age: two to five tablespoonsful (30–75ml). Children 6 to under 12 years of age: two to five teaspoonful (10–25ml). The dose may be taken as a single dose or in divided doses.
Children under 6 years of age: consult a physician.
Store at room temperature 15°–30°C (59°–86°F).
Kondremul is a registered trademark of Ciba Self-Medication, Inc.
Distributed by:
Ciba Self-Medication, Inc.
581 Main St.
Woodbridge, NJ 07095

Shown in Product Identification Guide, page 508

MAALOX® Antacid Caplets

Description: Maalox® antacid caplets provide fast, effective relief of acid indigestion, heartburn, and sour stomach. Because they are easy-to-swallow caplets, there is no chalky aftertaste.

Active Ingredients: Each caplet contains 311 mg calcium carbonate and 232 mg magnesium carbonate.

Inactive Ingredients: Corn starch, hydroxypropyl methylcellulose, magnesium stearate, sodium croscarmellose, sodium lauryl sulfate, titanium dioxide, and other ingredients.

Minimum Recommended Dosage: Maalox Antacid Caplets		
Acid neutralizing capacity	NLT 20.5 mEq/ 2 caplets	
Sodium content	NMT 3 mg/ caplet	

Indications: For the relief of acid indigestion, heartburn, sour stomach and upset stomach.

Directions for Use: Swallow 2–4 caplets with liquid as needed or as directed by physician.

CAPLETS SHOULD NOT BE CHEWED.

Patient Warnings: Do not take more than 24 caplets in a 24-hour period or use the maximum dosage for more than 2 weeks or use if you have kidney disease, except under the advice and supervision of a physician. Keep this and all drugs out of the reach of children.

Drug Interaction Precaution: Antacids may interact with certain prescription drugs. If you are presently taking a prescription drug, do not take this product without checking with your physician or other health professional.

How Supplied: Maalox® Antacid Caplets are available in blister packages of 24 (0067-0183-24) and bottles of 50 (0067-0183-50).

Shown in Product Identification Guide, page 508

EXTRA STRENGTH MAALOX® ANTACID PLUS ANTI-GAS
Alumina, Magnesia and Simethicone Oral Suspensions and Tablets, Antacid/Anti-Gas

Suspensions and Tablets
☐ Refreshing Lemon
   Smooth Cherry
   Cooling Mint
☐ Physician-proven Maalox® formula for antacid effectiveness.
☐ Simethicone, at a recognized clinical dose, for antiflatulent action.

Description: Extra Strength Maalox® Antacid Plus Anti-Gas, a balanced combination of magnesium and aluminum hydroxides plus simethicone, is a non-constipating antacid/anti-gas product to provide symptomatic relief of acid indigestion, heartburn, and gas and upset stomach associated with these symptoms. Available in suspensions in Refreshing Lemon, Smooth Cherry, and Cooling Mint flavors and in tablets in Cooling Mint and assorted (Refreshing Lemon/Smooth Cherry/Cooling Mint) flavors.

Composition: To provide symptomatic relief of hyperacidity plus alleviation of gas symptoms, each teaspoonful/tablet contains:

Active Ingredients	Extra Strength Maalox® Antacid Plus Anti-Gas	
	Per Tsp. (5 mL)	Per Tablet
Magnesium Hydroxide	450 mg	350 mg
Aluminum Hydroxide (equivalent to dried gel, USP)	500 mg	350 mg
Simethicone	40 mg	30 mg

Inactive Ingredients: Suspensions: Calcium Saccharin, FD&C Red No. 40 (Smooth Cherry only), Flavors, Methylparaben, Propylparaben, Purified Water, Sorbitol & other ingredients.
Tablets: D&C Red No. 30, D&C Yellow No. 10, Dextrose, FD&C Blue No. 1, Flavors, Magnesium Stearate, Mannitol, Saccharin Sodium, Sorbitol, Starch, Sugar.

Directions for Use: Suspensions; 2 to 4 teaspoonfuls, 4 times per day, or as directed by a physician. Tablets; chew 1 to 3 tablets, 4 times per day, or as directed by a physician.

Patient Warnings: Do not take more than 12 teaspoonfuls or 12 tablets in a 24-hour period or use the maximum dosage for more than 2 weeks or use if you have kidney disease except under the advice and supervision of a physician. Keep this and all drugs out of the reach of children.

Drug Interaction Precaution: Antacids may interact with certain prescription drugs. If you are presently taking a prescription drug, do not take this product without checking with your physician or other health professional.
To aid in establishing proper dosage schedules, the following information is provided:

Minimum Recommended Dosage: Extra Strength Maalox® Antacid Plus Anti-Gas		
	Per 2 Tsp. (10 mL)	Per Tablet
Acid neutralizing capacity	52.2 mEq	NLT 16.7 mEq
Sodium content*	< 2 mg	< 1.7 mg

*Dietetically insignificant.

Professional Labeling

Indications: As an antacid for symptomatic relief of hyperacidity associated with the diagnosis of peptic ulcer, gastritis, peptic esophagitis, gastric hyperacidity, heartburn, or hiatal hernia. As an antiflatulent to alleviate the symptoms of gas, including postoperative gas pain.

Advantages: Among antacids, Extra Strength Maalox® Antacid Plus Anti-Gas Suspension and Extra Strength Maalox® Antacid Plus Anti-Gas Tablets are uniquely palatable—an important feature which encourages patients to follow your dosage directions. Extra Strength Maalox® Antacid Plus Anti-Gas Suspension and Extra Strength Maalox® Antacid Plus Anti-Gas Tablets have the time-proven, nonconstipating, sodium-free* Maalox® formula—useful for those patients suffering from the problems associated with hyperacidity. Additionally, Extra Strength Maalox® Antacid Plus Anti-Gas Suspension and Extra Strength Maalox® Antacid Plus Anti-Gas Tablets contain simethicone to alleviate discomfort associated with entrapped gas.
*Dietetically insignificant.

Warnings: Prolonged use of aluminum-containing antacids in patients with renal failure may result in or worsen dialysis osteomalacia. Elevated tissue aluminum levels contribute to the development of the dialysis encephalopathy and osteomalacia syndromes. Small amounts of aluminum are absorbed from the gastrointestinal tract and renal excretion of aluminum is impaired in renal failure. Aluminum is not well removed by dialysis because it is bound to albumin and transferrin, which do not cross dialysis membranes. As a result, aluminum is deposited in bone, and dialysis osteomalacia may develop when large amounts of aluminum are ingested orally by patients with impaired renal function. Aluminum forms insoluble complexes with phosphate in the gastrointestinal tract, thus decreasing phosphate absorption. Prolonged use of aluminum-containing antacids by normophosphatemic patients may result in hypophosphate-

Continued on next page

The full prescribing information for each Ciba Self-Medication, Inc., product is contained herein and is that in effect as of December 15, 1995

Ciba Self-Medication, Inc.—Cont.

mia if phosphate intake is not adequate. In its more severe forms, hypophosphatemia can lead to anorexia, malaise, muscle weakness, and osteomalacia.

How Supplied:
Extra Strength Maalox® Antacid Plus Anti-Gas Suspensions
Available in Refreshing Lemon in the following sizes: 5 fl. oz. (148 mL) (0067-0333-62), 12 fl. oz. (355 mL) (0067-0333-71), and 26 fl. oz. (769 mL) (0067-0333-44). Smooth Cherry is available in plastic bottles of 12 fl. oz. (355 mL) (0067-0336-71), and 26 fl. oz. (769 mL) (0067-0336-44). Cooling Mint is available in plastic bottles of 12 fl. oz. (355 mL) (0067-0338-71) and 26 fl. oz. (769 mL) (0067-0338-44).
Extra Strength Maalox® Antacid Plus Anti-Gas Cooling Mint Tablets are available in bottles of 38 tablets (0067-0345-38) and 75 tablets (0067-0345-75).
Extra Strength Maalox® Antacid Plus Anti-Gas assorted flavors tablets are available in bottles of 38 tablets (0067-7214-38) and 75 tablets (0067-7214-75).

Shown in Product Identification Guide, page 508

MAALOX® ANTI-DIARRHEAL
Loperamide Hydrochloride
Caplets, 2mg

Description: Maalox® Anti-Diarrheal relieves diarrhea for both adults and children 6 years of age and older, in many cases with just one dose. Maalox Anti-Diarrheal contains loperamide hydrochloride, previously available only in a prescription product. Loperamide hydrochloride has been prescribed for millions of people, and has proven to be an exceptionally safe and effective antidiarrheal medication.

Indications: Maalox Anti-Diarrheal controls the symptoms of diarrhea.

Active Ingredient: Loperamide hydrochloride 2 mg per caplet.

Inactive Ingredients: Corn starch, lactose, magnesium stearate, microcrystalline cellulose, FD&C Blue #1 and D&C Yellow #10.

Directions for Use: Follow specific dosing information below, and drink plenty of clear fluids to help prevent dehydration, which may accompany diarrhea.
Adults and children 12 years of age and older—
Take 2 caplets after the first loose bowel movement and 1 caplet after each subsequent loose bowel movement, but no more than 4 caplets a day for no more than 2 days.
Children 9–11 years (60–95 lbs.)—Take 1 caplet after the first loose bowel movement and ½ caplet after each subsequent loose bowel movement, but no

more than 3 caplets a day for no more than 2 days.
Children 6–8 years (48–59 lbs.)—Take 1 caplet after the first loose bowel movement and ½ caplet after each subsequent loose bowel movement, but no more than 2 caplets a day for no more than 2 days.
Children under 6 years (up to 47 lbs.)—Consult a physician. Not intended for use in children under 6 years old.

Warnings: DO NOT USE FOR MORE THAN TWO DAYS UNLESS DIRECTED BY A PHYSICIAN. Do not use if diarrhea is accompanied by high fever (greater than 101°), or if blood or mucus is present in the stool, or if you have had a rash or other allergic reaction to loperamide hydrochloride. If you are taking antibiotics or have a history of liver disease, consult a physician before using this product. As with any drug, if you are pregnant or nursing a baby, seek the advice of a health professional before using this product. Keep this and all drugs out of the reach of children. In case of accidental overdose, seek professional assistance or contact poison control center immediately.

How Supplied: Cartons of 6 and 12 caplets.

Shown in Product Identification Guide, page 509

MAALOX® ANTI-GAS
(Simethicone)
Tablets (Regular Strength)
Peppermint and Sweet Lemon Flavors

Description: Maalox Anti-Gas relieves the painful symptoms of bloating, pressure, and fullness, commonly referred to as gas. It is formulated with the active ingredient that diffuses the excess gas in the stomach and digestive tract.

Active Ingredient: Simethicone (80 mg per tablet).

Inactive Ingredients: Corn starch, flavor, gelatin, mannitol, sucrose, and tribasic calcium phosphate. Peppermint: D&C red no. 27 aluminum lake. Sweet Lemon: D&C red no. 30 aluminum lake, D&C yellow no. 10 aluminum lake.

Indications: For relief of painful symptoms of excess gas in the digestive tract.
Such gas is frequently caused by excessive swallowing of air or by eating foods that disagree.
Maalox® Anti-Gas acts in the stomach and intestines to change the surface tension of gas bubbles enabling them to coalesce: thus, the gas is freed and is eliminated more easily by belching or passing flatus.

Directions for Use: Chew 1 to 2 tablets thoroughly. Use after meals or at bedtime, or as directed by a physician. May also be taken as needed, up to 6 tablets daily. If symptoms persist, contact your physician. **DO NOT EXCEED**

6 TABLETS A DAY UNLESS DIRECTED BY A PHYSICIAN.

Warnings: Keep this and all drugs out of the reach of children.

How Supplied: Peppermint: Cartons of 12 and 48 tablets. Sweet Lemon: Cartons of 12 tablets.

Shown in Product Identification Guide, page 509

EXTRA STRENGTH MAALOX®
ANTI-GAS
(Simethicone) Tablets
Peppermint and Sweet Lemon Flavors

Description: Maalox Anti-Gas relieves the painful symptoms of bloating, pressure, and fullness commonly referred to as gas. It is formulated with the active ingredient that diffuses the excess gas in the stomach and digestive tract.

Active Ingredient: Simethicone (150 mg per tablet).

Inactive Ingredients: Corn starch, flavor, gelatin, mannitol, sucrose, and tribasic calcium phosphate. Peppermint: D&C red no. 27 aluminum lake. Sweet Lemon: D&C red no. 30 aluminum lake, D&C yellow no. 10 aluminum lake.

Indications: For relief of painful symptoms of bloating, pressure, and fullness, commonly referred to as gas.
Such gas is frequently caused by excessive swallowing of air or by eating foods that disagree.
Maalox® Anti-Gas acts in the stomach and intestines to change the surface tension of gas bubbles enabling them to coalesce: thus, the gas is freed and is eliminated more easily by belching or passing flatus.

Directions for Use: Chew 1 to 2 tablets thoroughly. Use after meals or at bedtime, or as directed by a physician. May also be taken as needed, up to 3 tablets daily. If symptoms persist, contact your physician. DO NOT EXCEED 3 TABLETS A DAY UNLESS DIRECTED BY A PHYSICIAN.

Warnings: Keep this and all drugs out of the reach of children.

How Supplied: Peppermint: Cartons of 10 tablets and 36 tablets. Sweet Lemon: Cartons of 10 tablets.
Shown in Product Identification Guide, page 509

MAALOX® HEARTBURN RELIEF
Suspension (Antacid)

Description: Maalox® Heartburn Relief provides symptomatic relief of heartburn, acid indigestion and/or sour stomach.

Active Ingredients: Each 5 ml (1 teaspoonful) contains aluminum hydroxide-magnesium carbonate codried gel 140 mg and magnesium carbonate USP 175 mg. It is formulated in a pleasant, cool mint flavor to help provide a cooling and soothing sensation as it goes down the esophagus.

Inactive Ingredients: Calcium carbonate, calcium saccharin, FD&C Blue No. 1, FD&C Yellow No. 5 (tartrazine) as a color additive, flavors, magnesium alginate, methyl and propyl parabens, potassium bicarbonate, purified water, sorbitol and other ingredients.

Minimum Recommended Dosage: Maalox Heartburn Relief Suspension Per 2 tsp. (10 mL)	
Acid neutralizing capacity	NLT 17 mEq
Sodium content	NMT 5 mg

Directions for Use: Two to four teaspoonfuls 4 times a day or as directed by a physician.

Patient Warnings: Do not take more than 16 teaspoonfuls in a 24-hour period or use the maximum dosage for more than 2 weeks or use if you have kidney disease except under the advice and supervision of a physician. Keep this and all drugs out of the reach of children.

Drug Interaction Precaution: Antacids may interact with certain prescription drugs. If you are presently taking a prescription drug, do not take this product without checking with your physician or other health professional.

Professional Labeling:

Warnings:
Prolonged use of aluminum-containing antacids in patients with renal failure may result in or worsen dialysis osteomalacia. Elevated tissue aluminum levels contribute to the development of the dialysis encephalopathy and osteomalacia syndromes. Small amounts of aluminum are absorbed from the gastrointestinal tract and renal excretion of aluminum is impaired in renal failure. Aluminum is not well removed by dialysis because it is bound to albumin and transferrin, which do not cross dialysis membranes. As a result, aluminum is deposited in bone, and dialysis osteomalacia may develop when large amounts of aluminum are ingested orally by patients with impaired renal function.
Aluminum forms insoluble complexes with phosphate in the gastrointestinal tract, thus decreasing phosphate absorption. Prolonged use of antacids containing aluminum by normophosphatemic patients may result in hypophosphatemia if phosphate intake is not adequate. In its more severe forms, hypophosphatemia can lead to anorexia, malaise, muscle weakness, and osteomalacia.

How Supplied: Maalox® Heartburn Relief is available in a 10 fl oz plastic bottle (0067-0350-71).

MAALOX®
Magnesia and Alumina
Oral Suspension
Antacid
Liquids
Mint Flavored
Cherry Creme

Description: Maalox® Antacid is used for the relief of acid indigestion, heartburn, sour stomach and upset stomach associated with these symptoms.

Active Ingredients	Maalox Suspension 5 mL teaspoon
Magnesium Hydroxide	200 mg
Aluminum Hydroxide (equivalent to dried gel, USP)	225 mg

Inactive Ingredients: Calcium saccharin, flavors, methylparaben, propylparaben, sorbitol, purified water and other ingredients.

Minimum Recommended Dosage: Maalox Suspension Per 2 Tsp. (10 mL)	
Acid neutralizing capacity	NLT 26.6 mEq
Sodium content	NMT 2 mg

Directions for Use: Two to four teaspoonfuls, four times a day or as directed by a physician.

Patient Warnings: Do not take more than 16 teaspoonfuls in a 24-hour period or use the maximum dosage for more than 2 weeks or use if you have kidney disease except under the advice and supervision of a physician. Keep this and all drugs out of the reach of children.

Drug Interaction Precaution: Antacids may interact with certain prescription drugs. If you are presently taking a prescription drug, do not take this product without checking with your physician or other health professional.

Professional Labeling:

Indications: As an antacid for symptomatic relief of hyperacidity associated with the diagnosis of peptic ulcer, gastritis, peptic esophagitis, gastric hyperacidity, heartburn, or hiatal hernia.

Warnings: Prolonged use of aluminum-containing antacids in patients with renal failure may result in or worsen dialysis osteomalacia. Elevated tissue aluminum levels contribute to the development of the dialysis encephalopathy and osteomalacia syndromes. Small amounts of aluminum are absorbed from the gastrointestinal tract and renal excretion of aluminum is impaired in renal failure. Aluminum is not well removed

by dialysis because it is bound to albumin and transferrin, which do not cross dialysis membranes. As a result, aluminum is deposited in bone, and dialysis osteomalacia may develop when large amounts of aluminum are ingested orally by patients with impaired renal function.
Aluminum forms insoluble complexes with phosphate in the gastrointestinal tract, thus decreasing phosphate absorption. Prolonged use of aluminum-containing antacids by normophosphatemic patients may result in hypophosphatemia if phosphate intake is not adequate. In its more severe forms, hypophosphatemia can lead to anorexia, malaise, muscle weakness, and osteomalacia.

How Supplied:
Maalox® Mint Flavored Suspension is available in plastic bottles of 5 oz (0067-0330-62), 12 oz (0067-0330-71) and 26 oz (0067-0330-44).
Maalox® Cherry Creme Flavored Suspension is available in plastic bottles of 12 oz (0067-0331-71) and 26 oz (0067-0331-44).

Shown in Product Identification Guide, page 508

MAALOX® Antacid Plus Anti-Gas
Alumina, Magnesia and Simethicone
Tablets
Antacid/Anti-Gas

Tablets
Lemon, Cherry, and Mint Flavors

☐ **Physician-proven Maalox® formula for antacid effectiveness.**
☐ **Simethicone, at a recognized clinical dose, for antiflatulent action.**

Description: Maalox® Antacid Plus Anti-Gas, a balanced combination of magnesium and aluminum hydroxides plus simethicone, is a non-constipating antacid/anti-gas product which comes in pleasant tasting flavors.

Composition: To provide symptomatic relief of hyperacidity plus alleviation of gas symptoms, each tablet contains:

Active Ingredients	Maalox® Antacid Plus Anti-Gas Per Tablet
Magnesium Hydroxide	200 mg
Aluminum Hydroxide (equivalent to dried gel, USP)	200 mg
Simethicone	25 mg

Continued on next page

The full prescribing information for each Ciba Self-Medication, Inc., product is contained herein and is that in effect as of December 15, 1995

Ciba Self-Medication, Inc.—Cont.

Inactive Ingredients: Maalox® Antacid Plus Anti-Gas Tablets: Confectioners' sugar, D&C Red No. 30, D&C Yellow No. 10, FD&C Blue No. 1, dextrose, flavors, glycerin, magnesium stearate, mannitol, saccharin sodium, sorbitol, starch, talc. May also contain citric acid. To aid in establishing proper dosage schedules, the following information is provided:

Minimum Recommended Dosage:	
	Per Tablet
Acid neutralizing capacity	NLT 10.65 mEq
Sodium content*	NMT 1 mg
Sugar content	0.54 g
Lactose content	None

*Dietetically insignificant.

Directions for Use: Chew 1 to 4 tablets 4 times a day or as directed by a physician.

Patient Warnings: Do not take more than 16 tablets in a 24-hour period or use the maximum dosage for more than 2 weeks or use if you have kidney disease except under the advice and supervision of a physician. Keep this and all drugs out of the reach of children.

Drug Interaction Precaution: Antacids may interact with certain prescription drugs. If you are presently taking a prescription drug, do not take this product without checking with your physician or other health professional.

Professional Labeling:

Indications: As an antacid for symptomatic relief of hyperacidity associated with the diagnosis of peptic ulcer, gastritis, peptic esophagitis, gastric hyperacidity, heartburn, or hiatal hernia. As an antiflatulent to alleviate the symptoms of gas, including postoperative gas pain.

Warnings: Prolonged use of aluminum-containing antacids in patients with renal failure may result in or worsen dialysis osteomalacia. Elevated tissue aluminum levels contribute to the development of the dialysis encephalopathy and osteomalacia syndromes. Small amounts of aluminum are absorbed from the gastrointestinal tract and renal excretion of aluminum is impaired in renal failure. Aluminum is not well removed by dialysis because it is bound to albumin and transferrin, which do not cross dialysis membranes. As a result, aluminum is deposited in bone, and dialysis osteomalacia may develop when large amounts of aluminum are ingested orally by patients with impaired renal function.

Aluminum forms insoluble complexes with phosphate in the gastrointestinal tract, thus decreasing phosphate absorption. Prolonged use of aluminum-containing antacids by normophosphatemic patients may result in hypophosphatemia if phosphate intake is not adequate. In its more severe forms, hypophosphatemia can lead to anorexia, malaise, muscle weakness, and osteomalacia.

Advantages: Maalox® Antacid Plus Anti-Gas Tablets are uniquely palatable—an important feature which encourages patients to follow your dosage directions. Maalox® Antacid Plus Anti-Gas Tablets have the time-proven, nonconstipating, sodium-free* Maalox® formula—useful for those patients suffering from the problems associated with hyperacidity. Additionally, Maalox® Antacid Plus Anti-Gas Tablets contain simethicone to alleviate discomfort associated with entrapped gas.

How Supplied: Maalox® Antacid Plus Anti-Gas Lemon Tablets are available in plastic bottles of 50 tablets (0067-0339-50) and 100 tablets (0067-0339-68), convenience packs of 12 tablets (0067-0339-19), tray of 12 rolls (0067-0339-23), and 3 roll packs of 36 tablets (0067-0339-33).

Maalox® Antacid Plus Anti-Gas Cherry Tablets are available in plastic bottles of 50 tablets (0067-0341-50) and 100 tablets (0067-0341-68).

Maalox® Antacid Plus Anti-Gas Tablets are also available in **assorted flavor** bottles of 50 tablets (0067-7346-50) and 100 tablets (0067-7346-68), tray of 12 rolls (0067-7346-23) and 3 roll packs of 36 tablets (0067-7346-33).

Shown in Product Identification Guide, page 508

MYOFLEX® EXTERNAL ANALGESIC CREME
[mī'ō-flex]

Description: Odorless, stainless and non-burning topical pain reliever.

Active Ingredient: Trolamine salicylate 10%.

Other Ingredients: Cetyl alcohol, disodium EDTA, fragrance, propylene glycol, purified water, sodium lauryl sulfate, stearyl alcohol, white wax.

Indications: For the temporary relief of minor aches and pains of muscles and joints associated with arthritis, strains and sprains, and simple backache.

Warning: FOR EXTERNAL USE ONLY. Do not apply to irritated skin or if excessive irritation develops. Avoid contact with eyes. If condition worsens, or if symptoms persist for more than 7 days or clear up and occur again within a few days, discontinue use of this product and consult a physician. Keep this and all drugs out of the reach of children. In case of accidental ingestion, seek professional

assistance or contact a Poison Control Center immediately. As with any drug, if you are pregnant or nursing a baby, seek the advice of a health professional before using this product.

Directions: Use only as directed. **Adults and children 2 years of age and older:** Apply to affected area not more than three to four times daily. Affected areas may be wrapped loosely with two- or three-inch elastic bandage. **Children under 2 years of age:** Consult a physician.
Protect from freezing or excessive heat. Store at controlled room temperature 15°–30°C (59°–86°F).

How Supplied: Myoflex Creme is supplied in 2 oz. and 4 oz. easy-squeeze tubes, and 8 oz. and 16 oz. jars.
MYOFLEX is a registered trademark of Ciba-Geigy Corporation.
Shown in Product Identification Guide, page 509

---

12 Hour NŌSTRILLA®
[nō-stril 'a]
Nasal Decongestant
oxymetazoline HCl, USP

Active Ingredient: oxymetazoline hydrochloride 0.05%.

Inactive Ingredients: benzalkonium chloride 0.02% as a preservative, glycerine, sorbitol solution, water.

Indications: For the temporary relief of nasal congestion due to the common cold, hay fever, or other upper respiratory allergies, or associated with sinusitis.

Actions: NŌSTRILLA metered pump spray for nasal decongestion delivers a measured dose of medication every time. Helps clear your stuffy nose fast so you can breathe easier all day or night.

Warnings: Do not exceed recommended dosage. This product may cause temporary discomfort such as burning, stinging, sneezing, or an increase in nasal discharge. The use of this container by more than one person may spread infection. Do not use this product for more than 3 days. Frequent or prolonged use may cause nasal congestion to recur or worsen. Use only as directed. If symptoms persist, consult a doctor. Do not use this product if you have heart disease, high blood pressure, thyroid disease, diabetes or difficulty in urination due to enlargement of the prostate gland unless directed by a doctor. Keep this and all drugs out of the reach of children. In case of accidental ingestion, seek professional assistance or contact a poison control center immediately.

Directions: Adults and children 6 to under 12 years of age (with adult supervision): 2 or 3 sprays in each nostril not more often than every 10 to 12 hours. Do not exceed 2 applications in any 24-hour period. Children under 6 years of age: consult a doctor.

To use pump: Remove protective cap and prime pump by depressing it firmly several times. Hold bottle with thumb at base and nozzle between first and second fingers. With head upright, insert nozzle into nostril. Depress pump two or three times, all the way down, and sniff deeply.

How Supplied: Metered nasal pump spray in white plastic bottles of ½ fl. oz. (15 ml) packaged in tamper-resistant outer cartons.

Shown in Product Identification Guide, page 509

NUPERCAINAL®
Dibucaine
Hemorrhoidal and Anesthetic Ointment

Ingredient: 1% dibucaine USP. Also contains: acetone sodium bisulfite, lanolin, light mineral oil, purified water, and white petrolatum.

Indications: For prompt, temporary relief of pain, itching and burning due to hemorrhoids or other anorectal disorders. May also be used topically for temporary relief of pain and itching associated with sunburn, minor burns, cuts, scrapes, insect bites, or minor skin irritation.

Directions: Adults: When practical, cleanse the affected area with mild soap and warm water and rinse thoroughly. Gently dry by patting or blotting with toilet tissue or a soft cloth before application of this product. Puncture tube seal with cap or sharp object. Apply externally to the affected area up to 3 or 4 times daily. Children 2–12: Do not use except under the advice and supervision of a physician. DO NOT USE IN INFANTS UNDER 2 YEARS OF AGE OR LESS THAN 35 LBS. WEIGHT.

Warnings: IF SWALLOWED, CONSULT A PHYSICIAN OR POISON CONTROL CENTER IMMEDIATELY. **Do not use in or near the eyes.** If condition worsens or does not improve within 7 days, consult a physician. Do not put this product into the rectum by using fingers or any mechanical device. Do not exceed recommended daily dosage unless directed by a physician. Certain persons can develop allergic reactions to ingredients in this product. If the symptom being treated does not subside or if redness, irritation, swelling, pain, bleeding or other symptoms develop or increase, discontinue use and consult a physician promptly. As with any drug, if you are pregnant or nursing a baby, seek the advice of a health care professional before using this product. KEEP THIS AND ALL MEDICATION OUT OF REACH OF CHILDREN.

How Supplied: Nupercainal Hemorrhoidal and Anesthetic Ointment is available in tubes of 1 and 2 ounces. See crimp of tube for lot number and expiration date. Store between 15°–30°C (59°–86°F).
NDC 0083-5812.

Nupercainal is a registered trademark of Ciba Self-Medication, Inc.
Distributed by: Ciba Self-Medicaton, Inc., 581 Main Street, Woodbridge, NJ 07095
Made in Canada
Shown in Product Identification Guide, page 509

NUPERCAINAL
HYDROCORTISONE 1% CREAM
Anti-Itch Cream

Indications: For the temporary relief of external anal itching. May also be used for the temporary relief of itching associated with minor skin irritations and rashes due to eczema, insect bites, poison ivy, poison oak, poison sumac, soaps, detergents, cosmetics, jewelry, seborrheic dermatitis, or psoriarsis. Other uses of this product should be only under the advice and supervision of a physician.

Directions: Adults: When practical, cleanse the affected area with mild soap and warm water and rinse thoroughly. Gently dry by patting or blotting with toilet tissue or a soft cloth before application of this product. Apply to affected area not more than 3 to 4 times daily. **Children under 12 years of age:** Consult a physician.

Warnings: For external use only. Avoid contact with the eyes. If condition worsens, or if symptoms persist for more than 7 days or clear up and occur again within a few days, stop use of this product and do not begin use of any other hydrocortisone product unless you have consulted a physician. Do not use for the treatment of diaper rash; consult a physician. Do not exceed the recommended daily dosage unless directed by a physician. In case of bleeding, consult a physician promptly. Do not put this product into the rectum by using fingers or any mechanical device or applicator. KEEP THIS AND ALL MEDICATION OUT OF REACH OF CHILDREN. In case of accidental ingestion, seek professional assistance or contact a poison control center immediately.

Active Ingredient: Hydrocortisone Acetate USP (equivalent to Hydrocortisone Free Base 1%).

Inactive Ingredients: Cetostearyl Alcohol, Sodium Lauryl Sulfate, White Petrolatum, Propylene Glycol, Purified Water.

How Supplied: Nupercainal Hydrocortisone Cream is available in a 1 ounce tube. See crimp of tube for lot number and expiration date.
Store at controlled room temperature 15–30°C (59°–86°F).
NDC 0083-5700-96
Nupercainal is a registered trademark of Ciba Self-Medication, Inc.
Distributed by: Ciba Self-Medication, Inc., 581 Main Street, Woodbridge, NJ 07095

Made in Canada
Shown in Product Identification Guide, page 509

NUPERCAINAL®
Pain-Relief Cream

Active Ingredient: 0.5% dibucaine USP.

Inactive Ingredients: acetone sodium bisulfite, fragrance, glycerin, potassium hydroxide, purified water, stearic acid, and trolamine.

Indications: For prompt, temporary relief of pain and itching due to sunburn, minor burns, cuts, scrapes, scratches, and nonpoisonous insect bites.

Directions: Puncture tube seal with cap or sharp object. Apply to affected area, rub in gently. **Do not use in or near eyes.**

Caution: IF SWALLOWED, CONSULT A PHYSICIAN OR POISON CONTROL CENTER IMMEDIATELY. Not for prolonged use. Not more than ⅔ tube should be applied in 24 hours for adults or ⅙ tube to a child. If the symptom being treated does not subside or rash, irritation, swelling, pain, or other symptoms develop or increase, discontinue use and consult a physician.

How Supplied: Nupercainal Pain-Relief Cream is available in tubes of 1½ ounces. See crimp of tube for lot number and expiration date. Store between 15°–30°C (59°–86°F).
NDC 0083-5830-91.
Nupercainal is a registered trademark of Ciba Self-Medication, Inc.
Distributed by: Ciba Self-Medication, Inc., 581 Main Street, Woodbridge, NJ 07095
Shown in Product Identification Guide, page 509

NUPERCAINAL®
Suppositories

Indications: Nupercainal Rectal Suppositories give temporary relief of itching, burning, and discomfort associated with hemorrhoids or other anorectal disorders.

Ingredients: 2.1 grams cocoa butter, NF and .25 gram zinc oxide. Also contains acetone sodium bisulfite and bismuth subgallate.

Directions: ADULTS—When practical, cleanse the affected area. Tear one suppository at the "V" cut, peel foil downward and remove foil wrapper before inserting into the rectum. Gently

Continued on next page

The full prescribing information for each Ciba Self-Medication, Inc., product is contained herein and is that in effect as of December 15, 1995

Ciba Self-Medication, Inc.—Cont.

insert the suppository rectally, rounded end first. Use one suppository up to 6 times daily or after each bowel movement. CHILDREN UNDER 12 YEARS OF AGE—Consult a physician.

WARNING: IF ACCIDENTALLY SWALLOWED, CONSULT A PHYSICIAN OR POISON CONTROL CENTER IMMEDIATELY.

If condition worsens or does not improve within 7 days, consult a physician. Do not exceed the recommended daily dosage unless directed by a physician. In case of bleeding consult a physician promptly. As with any drug, if you are pregnant or nursing a baby, seek the advice of a health professional before using this product.
Keep this and all medications out of reach of children.

How Supplied: Nupercainal Suppositories are available in tamper-evident packages of 12 and 24.
Do not store above 30℃ (86°F).
NDC 0083-5841-25 24 count.
NDC 0083-5841-12 12 count.
Nupercainal is a registered trademark of Ciba Self-Medication, Inc.
Distributed by:
Ciba Self-Medication, Inc.
581 Main St.
Woodbridge NJ 07095
C86-42 (Rev. 9/86)

OTRIVIN®
Nasal Decongestant

Active Ingredient: xylometazoline hydrochloride USP (Nasal Spray and Nasal Drops 0.1%, Pediatric Nasal Drops 0.05%).

Inactive Ingredients: Otrivin Nasal Spray/Nasal Drops—benzalkonium chloride, dibasic sodium phosphate, disodium edetate, monobasic sodium phosphate, purified water and sodium chloride. They are available in an unbreakable plastic spray package of 0.66 fl oz (20 ml) and in a plastic dropper bottle of 0.83 fl oz (25 ml).
Otrivin Pediatric Nasal Drops—benzalkonium chloride, dibasic sodium phosphate, disodium edetate, monobasic sodium phosphate, purified water and sodium chloride. It is available in a plastic dropper bottle of 0.83 fl oz (25 ml).

One application provides long-lasting relief.
Otrivin has been prescribed by doctors for many years. Here is how you use it:

Directions: Nasal Spray 0.1%—for adults and children 12 years and older. Spray 2 or 3 times into each nostril every 8–10 hours. **Do not give Nasal Spray 0.1% to children under 12 years of age unless directed by a doctor.**
Nasal Drops 0.1%—for adults and children 12 years and older. Put 2 or 3 drops into each nostril every 8 to 10 hours. **Do not give Nasal Drops 0.1% to children**

under 12 years except under the advice and supervision of a physician.
Pediatric Nasal Drops 0.05%—children 6 to 12 years of age (with adult supervision): 2 or 3 drops in each nostril not more often than every 8 to 10 hours. Children 2 to 6 years of age (with adult supervision): 2 to 3 drops in each nostril not more often than every 8 to 10 hours. Use dropper provided. Use only recommended amount. Do not exceed 3 doses in any 24 hour period. Children under 2 years of age: consult a doctor.

Warning: Do not exceed recommended dosage. This product may cause temporary discomfort such as burning, stinging, sneezing, or an increase in nasal discharge. Do not use this product for more than 3 days. Use only as directed. Frequent or prolonged use may cause nasal congestion to recur or worsen. If symptoms persist, consult a doctor. Do not use this product if you have heart disease, high blood pressure, thyroid disease, diabetes, or difficulty in urination due to enlargement of the prostate gland unless directed by a doctor. The use of this container by more than one person may spread infection.
KEEP THIS AND ALL DRUGS OUT OF THE REACH OF CHILDREN. In case of accidental ingestion, seek professional assistance or contact a poison control center immediately.
Overdosage in young children may cause marked sedation.

Caution: Do not use if the clear overwrap with the name Otrivin® or the printed band on the bottle is missing or damaged.

Shown in Product Identification Guide, page 509

PERDIEM®
[pĕr "dē 'ŭm]
Bulk-Forming/Stimulant Laxative

Description: Perdiem®, with its 100% natural, gentle action provides relief from occasional constipation. Perdiem® is a unique combination of bulk-forming fiber and natural stimulant. Each rounded teaspoonful (6.0 g) contains approximately 3.25 g psyllium. 0.02 g sennosides, 1.8 mg of sodium, and 35.5 mg of potassium. Perdiem® is dye free and contains no artificial sweeteners.

Indications: For relief of occasional constipation. This product generally produces bowel movement in 12 to 72 hours.

Active Ingredients: Psyllium and Sennosides.

Inactive Ingredients: Acacia, iron oxides, natural flavors, paraffin, sucrose, talc.

Directions for Use: TAKE THIS PRODUCT (CHILD OR ADULT DOSE) WITH AT LEAST 8 OUNCES (A FULL GLASS) OF COOL WATER OR OTHER FLUID. TAKING THIS PRODUCT WITHOUT ENOUGH LIQUID

MAY CAUSE CHOKING. SEE WARNINGS.
Adults and Children 12 years and older: In the evening and/or before breakfast, 1 to 2 rounded teaspoonfuls of Perdiem® (in full or partial doses) should be placed in the mouth and swallowed with at least 8 ounces of cool liquid. Perdiem® should not be chewed.
Children 7 to 11 years: One (1) rounded teaspoon one to two times daily with at least 8 ounces of cool liquid.
For Severe Cases of Constipation: Perdiem® may be taken more frequently, up to 2 rounded teaspoonfuls every 6 hours not to exceed 5 teaspoonfuls in a 24-hour period. Perdiem® generally takes effect within 12 hours; in severe cases, 24 to 72 hours may be required for optimal relief.

Warnings: TAKING THIS PRODUCT WITHOUT ADEQUATE FLUID MAY CAUSE IT TO SWELL AND BLOCK YOUR THROAT OR ESOPHAGUS AND MAY CAUSE CHOKING. DO NOT TAKE THIS PRODUCT IF YOU HAVE DIFFICULTY IN SWALLOWING. IF YOU EXPERIENCE CHEST PAIN, VOMITING OR DIFFICULTY IN SWALLOWING OR BREATHING AFTER TAKING THIS PRODUCT, SEEK IMMEDIATE MEDICAL ATTENTION.
Patients with esophageal narrowing should not use bulk-forming agents.
Do not use laxative products when abdominal pain, nausea, or vomiting are present unless directed by a doctor. If you have noticed a sudden change in bowel habits that persists over a period of 2 weeks, consult a doctor before using a laxative. Laxative products should not be used for a period longer than 1 week unless directed by a doctor. Rectal bleeding or failure to have a bowel movement after use of a laxative may indicate a serious condition. Discontinue use and consult your doctor. Do not use if you have a history of psyllium allergy.
If you are pregnant or nursing a baby, seek the advice of a health professional before using this product. In case of accidental overdose, seek professional assistance or contact a poison control center immediately. Keep this and all drugs out of the reach of children.
Suggested Use—Clinical Regulation: For patients confined to bed that experience occasional constipation. Up to 2 rounded teaspoonfuls every 6 hours not to exceed 5 teaspoonfuls in a 24-hour period.

How Supplied: Granules: 250-gram (8.8 oz) (0067-0690-70) plastic container and 6 single serving packets 6 g (0067-0690-16).

Shown in Product Identification Guide, page 509

PERDIEM® FIBER
[pĕr "dē 'ŭm]
Bulk-Forming Laxative

Description: Perdiem® Fiber is a 100% natural, bulk-forming fiber for the relief of occasional constipation (irregularity). Perdiem Fiber's unique form is easy to swallow and requires no mixing but must be followed by at least 8 ounces of cool liquid. Perdiem® Fiber contains no chemical stimulants. Each rounded teaspoonful (6.0 g) contains 4.03 g psyllium, 1.8 mg sodium, and 36.1 mg of potassium. Perdiem® is dye free and contains no artificial sweeteners.

Indications: For relief of occasional constipation. This product generally produces bowel movement in 12 to 72 hours.

Active Ingredients: Psyllium

Inactive Ingredients: Acacia, iron oxides, natural flavors, paraffin, sucrose, talc, titanium dioxide.

Directions for Use: TAKE THIS PRODUCT (CHILD OR ADULT DOSE) WITH AT LEAST 8 OUNCES (A FULL GLASS) OF COOL WATER OR OTHER FLUID. TAKING THIS PRODUCT WITHOUT ENOUGH LIQUID MAY CAUSE CHOKING. SEE WARNINGS.
Adults and Children 12 years of age and older: In the evening and/or before breakfast, 1 to 2 rounded teaspoonfuls of Perdiem® Fiber (in full or partial doses) should be placed in the mouth and swallowed with at least 8 ounces (a full glass) of cool liquid. Perdiem® Fiber should not be chewed.
Children 7 to under 11 years: One (1) rounded teaspoonful with at least 8 ounces (a full glass) of cool liquid.
For Severe Cases of Constipation: Perdiem Fiber may be taken more frequently, up to 2 rounded teaspoonfuls every 6 hours not to exceed 5 teaspoonfuls in a 24-hour period. Perdiem Fiber generally takes effect after 12 hours; in severe cases, 48 to 72 hours may be required for optimal relief.

Warnings: TAKING THIS PRODUCT WITHOUT ADEQUATE FLUID MAY CAUSE IT TO SWELL AND BLOCK YOUR THROAT OR ESOPHAGUS AND MAY CAUSE CHOKING. DO NOT TAKE THIS PRODUCT IF YOU HAVE DIFFICULTY IN SWALLOWING. IF YOU EXPERIENCE CHEST PAIN, VOMITING, OR DIFFICULTY IN SWALLOWING OR BREATHING AFTER TAKING THIS PRODUCT, SEEK IMMEDIATE MEDICAL ATTENTION.
Patients with esophageal narrowing should not use bulk-forming agents. Do not use laxative products when abdominal pain, nausea, or vomiting are present unless directed by a doctor. If you have noticed a sudden change in bowel habits that persists over a period of 2 weeks, consult a doctor before using a laxative. Laxative products should not be used for a period longer than 1 week unless directed by a doctor. Rectal bleeding or failure to have a bowel movement after use of a laxative may indicate a serious condition. Discontinue use and consult your doctor. Do not use if you have a history of psyllium allergy.

In case of accidental overdose, seek professional assistance or contact a poison control center immediately. Keep this and all drugs out of the reach of children.

How Supplied: Granules: 250-gram (8.8 oz) (0067-0795-70) plastic container.
Shown in Product Identification Guide, page 509

PRIVINE®
Naphazoline Hydrochloride, USP
Nasal Decongestant

Active Ingredient: Naphazoline Hydrochloride, USP.

Other Ingredients: Benzalkonium chloride, dibasic sodium phosphate, disodium edetate, monobasic sodium phosphate, purified water, and sodium chloride. It is available in plastic squeeze bottles of 0.66 fl oz (20 ml).

Privine is a nasal decongestant that comes in two forms: Nasal Drops (in a bottle with a dropper) and Nasal Spray (in a plastic squeeze bottle). Both are for prompt and prolonged relief of nasal congestion due to common colds, sinusitis, hay fever, etc.

Indications: For the temporary relief of nasal congestion due to the common cold, hay fever or other respiratory allergies, or associated with sinusitis.

Warnings: Do not exceed recommended dosage. This product may cause temporary discomfort such as burning, stinging, sneezing, or an increase in nasal discharge. Do not use this product for more than 3 days. Use only as directed. Frequent or prolonged use may cause nasal congestion to recur or worsen. If symptoms persist, consult a doctor. Do not use this product if you have heart disease, high blood pressure, thyroid disease, diabetes, or difficulty in urination due to enlargement of the prostate gland unless directed by a doctor. Do not use this product in children under 12 years of age because it may cause sedation if swallowed. The use of this container by more than one person may spread infection. Keep this and all drugs out of the reach of children. In case of accidental ingestion, seek professional assistance or contact a poison control center immediately.

Directions: Nasal Drops: Adults and children 12 years of age and over: 1 or 2 drops in each nostril not more often than every 6 hours. Do not give to children under 12 years of age unless directed by a doctor.

Nasal Spray: Adults and children 12 years of age and over: 1 or 2 sprays in each nostril not more often than every 6 hours. Do not give to children under 12 years of age unless directed by a doctor.
Shown in Product Identification Guide, page 509

SINAREST® TABLETS, EXTRA STRENGTH CAPLETS, AND NO DROWSINESS CAPLETS

Active Ingredients: *Tablets*—Acetaminophen 325 mg, chlorpheniramine maleate 2 mg, pseudoephedrine HCl 30 mg.
No Drowsiness Caplets—Acetaminophen 325 mg, pseudoephedrine HCl 30 mg.
Extra Strength Caplets—Acetaminophen 500 mg, chlorpheniramine maleate 2 mg, pseudoephedrine HCl 30 mg.

Other Ingredients: *Tablets*—Corn starch, D & C Yellow No. 10, FD & C Yellow No. 6, hydroxypropyl methylcellulose, microcrystalline cellulose, polyethylene glycol, polysorbate 80, polyvinylpyrrolidone, stearic acid, titanium dioxide.
No Drowsiness Caplets—Corn starch, hydroxypropyl methylcellulose, microcrystalline cellulose, polyethylene glycol, polysorbate 80, stearic acid, titanium dioxide.
Extra Strength Caplets—Corn starch, hydroxypropyl methylcellulose, microcrystalline cellulose, polyethylene glycol, polysorbate 80, polyvinylpyrrolidone, stearic acid, titanium dioxide.

Indications: *Tablets and Extra Strength*—Temporarily relieves nasal congestion, runny nose, sneezing, itching of the nose or throat, and itchy, watery eyes due to hay fever or other upper respiratory allergies, or associated with sinusitis. For temporary relief of minor aches, pains, and headache.
No Drowsiness—Temporarily relieves nasal congestion due to hay fever or other upper respiratory allergies, or associated with sinusitis. For temporary relief of minor aches, pains and headache.

Warnings: *All Products*—**Do not exceed recommended dosage.** If nervousness, dizziness, or sleeplessness occur, discontinue use and consult a physician. Do not take this product for more than 10 days (for adults) or 5 days (for children). If symptoms do not improve or are accompanied by fever that lasts for more than 3 days, or if new symptoms occur, consult a physician. Do not take this product, unless directed by a physician, if you have heart disease, high blood pressure, thyroid disease, diabetes, or difficulty in urination due to enlargement of the prostate gland. As with any drug, if you are pregnant or nursing a baby, seek the advice of a health professional before using this product. Keep this and all drugs out of the reach of children. In case of accidental overdose, seek professional assistance or contact a Poison Control Center immediately. Prompt medical

Continued on next page

The full prescribing information for each Ciba Self-Medication, Inc., product is contained herein and is that in effect as of December 15, 1995

Ciba Self-Medication, Inc.—Cont.

attention is critical for adults as well as for children even if you do not notice any signs or symptoms.

Tablets and Extra Strength Caplets—Do not take this product, unless directed by a physician, if you have a breathing problem such as emphysema or chronic bronchitis, or glaucoma. May cause excitability, especially in children. May cause drowsiness; alcohol, sedatives, and tranquilizers may increase the drowsiness effect. Avoid alcoholic beverages while taking this product. Do not take this product if you are taking sedatives or tranquilizers, without first consulting your physician. Use caution when driving a motor vehicle, or operating machinery.

Drug Interaction Precaution: *All Products*—Do not use this product if you are now taking a prescription monoamine oxidase inhibitor (MAOI) (certain drugs for depression, psychiatric or emotional conditions, or Parkinson's disease), or for 2 weeks after stopping the MAOI drug. If you are uncertain whether your prescription drug contains an MAOI, consult a health professional before taking this product.

Directions: *Tablets*—Dose as follows while symptoms persist, or as directed by a physician. Adults and children 12 years of age and over: 2 tablets every 4 to 6 hours, not to exceed 8 tablets in 24 hours. Children 6 to under 12 years of age: 1 tablet every 4 to 6 hours, not to exceed 4 tablets in 24 hours. Children under 6 years of age: Consult a physician.
No Drowsiness—Dose as follows while symptoms persist, or as directed by a physician. Adults and children 12 years of age and over: 2 caplets every 4 to 6 hours, not to exceed 8 caplets in 24 hours. Children 6 to under 12 years of age: 1 caplet every 4 to 6 hours, not to exceed 4 caplets in 24 hours. Children under 6 years of age: Consult a physician.
Extra Strength Caplets—Dose as follows while symptoms persist, or as directed by a physician. Adults and children 12 years of age and older: 2 caplets every 6 hours, not to exceed 8 caplets in 24 hours. Children under 12 years of age: Consult a physician.

How Supplied:
Tablets—Boxes of 20 and 40 tablets.
No Drowsiness—Boxes of 20 caplets.
Extra Strength Caplets—Boxes of 24 caplets.
Sinarest is a registered trademark of Ciba Self-Medication, Inc.

SLOW FE®
Slow Release Iron Tablets

Description: SLOW FE supplies ferrous sulfate for the treatment of iron deficiency and iron deficiency anemia with a significant reduction in the incidence of the common side effects of oral iron preparations. The wax matrix delivery system of SLOW FE is designed to maximize the release of ferrous sulfate in the duodenum and the jejunum where it is best tolerated and absorbed. SLOW FE has been clinically shown to be associated with a lower incidence of constipation, diarrhea and abdominal discomfort when compared to regular iron tablets and the leading capsule.

Formula: Each tablet contains 160 mg. dried ferrous sulfate USP, equivalent to 50 mg. elemental iron. Also contains cetostearyl alcohol, FD&C Blue No. 2, hydroxypropyl methylcellulose, lactose, magnesium stearate, polysorbate, talc, titanium dioxide, yellow iron oxide.

Dosage: ADULTS—one or two tablets daily or as recommended by a physician. A maximum of four tablets daily may be taken. CHILDREN—one tablet daily. Tablets must be swallowed whole.

Warning: Close tightly and keep out of reach of children. Contains iron, which can be harmful or fatal to children in large doses. In case of accidental overdose, seek professional assistance or contact a Poison Control Center immediately. The treatment of any anemic condition should be under the advice and supervision of a physician. As oral iron products interfere with absorption of oral tetracycline antibiotics, these products should not be taken within two hours of each other. As with any drug, if you are pregnant or nursing a baby, seek the advice of a health professional before using this product.
Keep this and all medications out of the reach of children.
Tamper-Evident Packaging.

How Supplied: Child-resistant blister packages of 30, 60, and child-resistant bottles of 100. Do Not Store Above 86°F. Protect From Moisture.
Shown in Product Identification Guide, page 509

SLOW FE WITH FOLIC ACID
(Slow Release Iron, Folic Acid)

Description: Slow Fe + Folic Acid delivers 50 mg. elemental iron (160 mg. dried ferrous sulfate) plus 400 mcg. folic acid using the unique wax matrix delivery system described above (for SLOW FE® Slow Release Iron Tablets).
Provides women of childbearing potential with the daily target level of folic acid to reduce the risk of neural tube birth defects. These birth defects are rare, but serious, and occur within 28 days of conception, often before a woman knows she's pregnant.

Formula: Each tablet contains: Active Ingredients: 160 mg. dried ferrous sulfate, USP (equivalent to 50 mg. elemental iron) and 400 mcg. folic acid. Inactive Ingredients: cetostearyl alcohol, hydroxypropyl methylcellulose, lactose, magnesium stearate, polysorbate 80, talc, titanium dioxide, yellow iron oxide 17628.

Dosage: ADULTS—One or two tablets once a day or as recommended by a physician. A maximum of two tablets daily may be taken. CHILDREN UNDER 12—Consult a physician. Tablets must be swallowed whole.

Warning: The treatment of any anemic condition should be under the advice and supervision of a physician. As oral iron products interfere with absorption of oral tetracycline antibiotics, these products should not be taken within two hours of each other. Intake of folic acid from all sources should be limited to 1000 mcg. per day to prevent the masking of Vitamin B12 deficiencies. Should you become pregnant while using this product, consult a physician as soon as possible about good prenatal care and the continued use of this product. If you are already pregnant or nursing a baby, seek the advice of a health care professional before using this product. KEEP THIS PRODUCT AND ALL MEDICATIONS OUT OF THE REACH OF CHILDREN: Contains iron, which can be harmful or fatal to children in large doses. In case of accidental overdose, contact a physician or a poison control center immediately.

How Supplied: Blister packages of 20 supplied in Child-Resistant packaging. Do not store above 86°F. Protect from moisture.
Distributed by: Ciba Self-Medication, Inc.
Woodbridge, NJ 07095
Tablets made in Great Britain
©1994 Ciba Self-Medication, Inc.
Shown in Product Identification Guide, page 509

SUNKIST® CHILDREN'S CHEWABLE MULTIVITAMINS— REGULAR

Nutrition Facts
Serving Size   1 Tablet
Amount Per Tablet
Total Carbohydrate less than 1 g
[See table at top of next page.]

Ingredients: Sorbitol, Sodium Ascorbate, Ascorbic Acid, Natural Flavors, Mono & Diglycerides, Starch, Stearic Acid, Hydrolyzed Protein, Vitamin E Acetate, Niacinamide, Carrageenan, Hydrogenated Vegetable Oils, Magnesium Stearate, Citric Acid, Aspartame, Calcium Silicate, Silica, FD&C Yellow #6, FD&C Red #40, Vitamin A Palmitate, Cellulose, FD&C Yellow #5, Gelatin, Riboflavin, Thiamin, Vitamin B6, Folic Acid, Beta Carotene, Vitamin D, Vitamin K, Vitamin B12.

Directions: Adults and children 2 years and older—Chew one tablet daily. PHENYLKETONURICS: CONTAINS PHENYLALANINE
Store at controlled room temperature, 15°–30°C (59°–86°F) Protect from moisture.

SUNKIST® CHILDREN'S CHEWABLE MULTIVITAMINS-REGULAR

Amount Per Tablet	% Daily Value for Children 2–4 Years of Age	% Daily Value for Adults and Children 4 or More Years of Age
Vitamin A 2500 I.U.	100%	50%
Vitamin C 60 mg	150%	100%
Vitamin D 400 I.U.	100%	100%
Vitamin E 15 I.U.	150%	50%
Vitamin K 5 mcg	*	*
Thiamin 1.1 mg	160%	70%
Riboflavin 1.2 mg	150%	70%
Niacin 14 mg	160%	70%
Vitamin B_6 1 mg	140%	50%
Folate 0.3 mg	150%	80%
Vitamin B_{12} 5 mcg	170%	80%

*Daily Value not established.

How Supplied: 60 TABLETS
Manufactured for and distributed by Ciba Self-Medication, Inc., Woodbridge, NJ 07095 under a trademark license from Sunkist Growers, Inc. Sunkist® is a registered trademark of Sunkist Growers, Inc., Sherman Oaks, CA 91423.©
Shown in Product Identification Guide, page 509

**CHILDREN'S CHEWABLE SUNKIST VITAMINS + EXTRA C
60 TABLETS**

Nutrition Facts
Serving Size 1 Tablet

Amount Per Tablet
Calories 5
Total Carbohydrate 1 g

Amount Per Tablet	% Daily Value for Children 2–4 Years of Age	% Daily Value for Adults and Children 4 or more Years of Age
Vitamin A 2500 I.U.	100%	50%
Vitamin C 250 mg	630%	420%
Vitamin D 400 I.U.	100%	100%
Vitamin E 15 I.U.	150%	50%
Vitamin K 5 mcg	*	*
Thiamin 1.1 mg	160%	70%
Riboflavin 1.2 mg	150%	70%
Niacin 14 mg	160%	70%
Vitamin B_6 1 mg	140%	50%
Foiate 0.3 mg	150%	80%
Vitamin B_{12} 5 mcg	170%	80%

*Daily Value not established.

Ingredients: Sorbitol, Sodium Ascorbate, Ascorbic Acid, Natural Flavors, Mono & Diglycerides, Starch, Stearic Acid, Hydrolyzed Protein, Vitamin E Acetate, Niacinamide, Aspartame Hydrogenated Vegetable Oils, *Magnesium Stearate, FD&C Yellow #6, Calicum Silicate, Silica, FD&C Red #40, Vitamin A Palmitate Cellulose, FD&C Yellow #5, Gelatin, Riboflavin, Thiamin, Vitamin B_6, Folic Acid, Beta Carotene, Vitamin D, Vitamin K, Vitamin B_{12}.

Directions: Adults and children 2 years and older—Chew one tablet daily. PHENYLKETONURICS CONTAINS PHENYLALANINE
Store at controlled room temperature, 15°–30°C (59°–86°F). Protect from moisture.
Manufactured for and distributed by Ciba Self-Medication, Inc., Woodbridge, NJ 07095 under a trademark license from Sunkist Growers, Inc. Sunkist® is a registered trademark of Sunkist Growers, Inc., Sherman Oaks, CA 91423
Shown in Product Identification Guide, page 509

**CHILDREN'S CHEWABLE SUNKIST VITAMINS +IRON
60 TABLETS**

Nutrition Facts
Serving Size 1 Tablet

Amount Per Tablet
Sodium 5mg
Total Carbohydrate less than 1g

Amount Per Tablet	% Daily Value for Children 2–4 Years of Age	% Daily Value for Adults and Children 4 or more Years of Age
Vitamin A 2500 I.U.	100%	50%
Vitamin C 60 mg	150%	100%
Vitamin D 400 I.U.	100%	100%
Vitamin E 15 I.U.	150%	50%
Vitamin K 5 mcg	*	*
Thiamin 1.1 mg	160%	70%
Riboflavin 1.2 mg	150%	70%
Niacin 14 mg	160%	70%
Vitamin B_6 1 mg	140%	50%
Foiate 0.3 mg	150%	80%
Vitamin B_{12} 5 mcg	170%	80%
Iron 15 mg	150%	80%

*Daily Value not established.

Ingredients: Sorbitol, Sodium Ascorbate, Ascorbic Acid, Natural Flavors, Mono & Diglycerides, Starch, Stearic Acid, Carrageenan, Hydrolyzed Protein, Vitamin E Acetate, Ferrous Fumarate, Niacinamide, Aspartame, Magnesium Stearate, Hydrogenated Vegetable Oils, FD&C Red #40, Calcium Silicate, Silica, FD&C Yellow #5, FD&C Yellow #6, Vitamin A Palmitate, Cellulose, Gelatin, Riboflavin, Thiamin, Vitamin B_6, Folic Acid, Beta Carotene, Vitamin D, Vitamin K, Vitamin B_{12}.

Directions: Adults and children 2 years and older—Chew one tablet daily. PHENYLKETONURICS CONTAINS PHENYLALANINE

Warning: Close tightly and keep out of reach of children. Contains iron, which can be harmful or fatal in children in large doses. In case of accidental overdose, seek professional assistance or contact a poison control center immediately. Store at controlled room temperature 15°–30°C (59°–86°F). Protect from moisture.
Manufactured for and distributed by Ciba Self-Medication, Inc., Woodbridge, NJ 07095 under a trademark license from Sunkist Growers, Inc. Sunkist® is a registered trademark of Sunkist Growers, Inc., Sherman Oaks, CA 91423.
Shown in Product Identification Guide, page 509

**SUNKIST® CHILDREN'S CHEWABLE MULTIVITAMINS— COMPLETE
WITH CALCIUM, IRON & MINERALS**

Nutrition Facts
Serving Size ½ Tablet or 1 Tablet, depending on age (see Directions)
Servings Per Container 120 ½-tablet servings or 60 single-tablets servings
Amount Per Tablet
Sodium 8g
Total Carbohydrate less than 1g
[See table at top of next page.]

Directions: Ages 2 to 4 years—Chew one-half tablet daily. Ages 4 years and older—Chew one tablet daily.

Ingredients: Sorbitol, Dicalcium Phosphate, Mono & Diglycerides, Ferrous Fumarate, Stearic Acid, Carrageenan, Starch, Sodium Ascorbate, Vitamin E, Magnesium Oxide, Hydrolyzed Protein, Ascorbic Acid, Niacinamide, Citric Acid, FD&C Yellow #6, Zinc Oxide, Gelatin, Magnesium Stearate, FD&C Red #40, Calcium Pantothenate, FD&C Yellow #5, Aspartame, Silica, Calcium Silicate, Vitamin A Palmitate, Cellulose, Manganese Sulfate, Vitamin B_6, Cupric Oxide, Riboflavin, Hydrogenated Vegetable Oils, Thiamin, Folic Acid, Beta Carotene, Potassium Iodide, Biotin, Calcium

Continued on next page

The full prescribing information for each Ciba Self-Medication, Inc., product is contained herein and is that in effect as of December 15, 1995

Ciba Self-Medication, Inc.—Cont.

SUNKIST® CHILDREN'S CHEWABLE MULTIVITAMINS-COMPLETE

Amount Per Tablet	% Daily Value for Children 2–4 Years of Age	% Daily Value for Adults and Children 4 or More Years of Age
Vitamin A 5000 I.U.	100%	100%
Vitamin C 60 mg	80%	100%
Vitamin D 400 I.U.	50%	100%
Vitamin E 30 I.U.	150%	100%
Vitamin K 10 mcg	*	*
Thiamin 1.5 mg	110%	100%
Riboflavin 1.7 mg	110%	100%
Niacin 20 mg	110%	100%
Vitamin B$_6$ 2 mg	140%	100%
Folate 0.4 mg	100%	100%
Vitamin B$_{12}$ 6 mcg	100%	100%
Biotin 40 mcg	15%	15%
Pantothenic Acid 10 mg	100%	100%
Calcium 100 mg	6%	10%
Iron 18 mg	90%	100%
Phosphorus 78 mg	4%	8%
Iodine 150 mcg	110%	100%
Magnesium 20 mg	5%	6%
Zinc 10 mg	60%	60%
Copper 2.0 mg	100%	100%
Manganese 1 mg	*	30%

*Daily Value not established.

Stearate, Vitamin K, Vitamin D, Vitamin B$_{12}$.
PHENYLKETONURICS: CONTAINS PHENYLALANINE

Warning: Close tightly and keep out of reach of children. Contains iron, which can be harmful or fatal to children in large doses. In case of accidental overdose, seek professional assistance or contact a poison control center immediately.
Store at controlled room temperature, 15°–30°C (59°–86°F). Protect from moisture.

How Supplied: 60 TABLETS
Mfd. for and dist. by Ciba Self-Medication, Inc., Woodbridge, NJ 07095 under a trademark license from Sunkist Growers, Inc. Sunkist® is a registered trademark of Sunkist Growers, Inc. Sherman Oaks, CA 91423.©

Shown in Product Identification Guide, page 509

SUNKIST® VITAMIN C
Citrus Complex
Chewable Tablets
Easy to Swallow Caplets

Description: All Sunkist Vitamin C chewable tablets have a delicious orange flavor unlike any other Vitamin C tablet. Each 60 mg chewable tablet contains 100% of the U.S. RDA* of Vitamin C. Each 250 mg chewable tablet contains 417% of the U.S. RDA* of Vitamin C. Each 500 mg chewable tablet contains 833% of the U.S. RDA* of Vitamin C.

Each 500 mg easy to swallow caplet contains 833% of the U.S. RDA* of Vitamin C.

Sunkist Vitamin C chewable tablets and easy to swallow caplets do not contain artificial flavors or colors.

*U.S. Recommended Daily Allowance for adults and children over 4 years of age.

Indication: Dietary supplementation.

How Supplied: 60 mg Chewable Tablets—Rolls of 11.
250 mg and 500 mg Chewable Tablets—Bottles of 60.
500 mg Easy to Swallow Caplets—Bottles of 60.

Manufactured & Distributed by
Ciba Self-Medication, Inc.
581 Main St.
Woodbridge, NJ 07095
Sunkist® is a registered trademark of Sunkist Growers, Inc., Sherman Oaks, CA 91423.©

Shown in Product Identification Guide, page 509

TING® ANTIFUNGAL CREAM, SPRAY LIQUID

Active Ingredient: Tolnaftate, 1%.

Other Ingredients: *Cream* —BHT, fragrance, polyethylene glycol 400, polyethylene glycol 3350, titanium dioxide, white petrolatum. *Spray Liquid* —BHT, fragrance, isobutane (propellant), polyethylene glycol 400, SD alcohol 40-B (41% w/w).

Indications: Cures athlete's foot and jock itch with a clinically proven ingredient. Relieves itching and burning. Prevents the recurrence of athlete's foot with daily use.

Warnings: Do not use on children under 2 years of age unless directed by a doctor. For external use only. Avoid contact with the eyes. If irritation occurs or

if there is no improvement within 4 weeks for athlete's foot or within 2 weeks for jock itch, discontinue use and consult a doctor. **Keep this and all drugs out of the reach of children.** In case of accidental ingestion, seek professional assistance or contact a Poison Control Center immediately. *For Spray Liquid only* —Avoid inhaling. Avoid contact with the eyes or other mucous membranes. Contents under pressure; do not puncture or incinerate. Flammable mixture, do not use near fire or flame. Do not expose to heat or temperatures above 49°C (120°F). Use only as directed. Intentional misuse by deliberately concentrating and inhaling contents can be harmful or fatal.

Directions: Clean the affected area and dry thoroughly. Apply a thin layer of the product over affected area twice daily (morning and night) or as directed by a doctor. Supervise children in the use of this product. For athlete's foot: pay special attention to the spaces between the toes, wear well-fitting, ventilated shoes, and change shoes and socks at least once daily. For athlete's foot, use daily for 4 weeks; for jock itch, use daily for 2 weeks. If condition persists longer, consult a doctor. This product is not effective on the scalp or nails. To prevent athlete's foot, apply a thin layer of the product to the feet once or twice daily (morning and/or night) following the above directions.

How Supplied: *Cream* —½ oz (14 g) tube, *Spray Liquid* —3 oz (85 g) aerosol container.
TING is a registered trademark of Ciba Self-Medication, Inc.
581 Main St
Woodbridge NJ 07095
Shown in Product Identification Guide, page 509

TING® ANTIFUNGAL SPRAY POWDER

Active Ingredient: Miconazole Nitrate, 2%.

Other Ingredients: Aloe vera gel, aluminum starch octenylsuccinate, Isopropyl myristate, propylene carbonate, SD alcohol 40-B (10% w/w), sorbitan monooleate, stearalkonium hectorite.

Propellant: Isobutane/propane.

Indications: Proven clinically effective in the treatment of athlete's foot and ring worm. Relieves the itching, scaling, burning, and discomfort that can accompany athlete's foot. Specially formulated to aid the drying of moist areas of the feet.

Warnings: Do not use on children under 2 years of age, unless directed by a doctor. For external use only. Avoid inhaling. Avoid contact with the eyes or other mucous membranes. If irritation occurs or if there is no improvement within 4 weeks, discontinue use and consult a physician. Contents under pressure. Do not puncture or incinerate.

Flammable mixture, do not use near fire or flame. Do not expose to heat or temperatures above 49℃ (120°F). Use only as directed. Intentional misuse by deliberately concentrating and inhaling contents can be harmful or fatal. **Keep this and all drugs out of the reach of children**. In case of accidental ingestion, seek professional assistance or contact a Poison Control Center immediately.

Directions: Clean the affected area and dry thoroughly. Shake can well, hold 4″ to 6″ from skin. Spray a thin layer of the product over affected area twice daily (morning and night) or as directed by a doctor. Supervise children in the use of this product. Pay special attention to the spaces between the toes. Wear well-fitting, ventilated shoes, and change shoes and socks at least once daily. Use daily for 4 weeks. If condition persists longer, consult a doctor. This product is not effective on the scalp or nails.

How Supplied: Spray Powder 3 oz (85g) aerosol container.
Shown in Product Identification Guide, page 509

VITRON–C® TABLETS
[vī'tron c]

Active Ingredients: Each tablet contains
Ferrous fumarate, USP .... 200 mg
equivalent to 66 mg elemental iron (365% U.S. RDA)
Ascorbic acid .... 125 mg (200% U.S. RDA)
Present in part as sodium ascorbate, USP

Other Ingredients: Colloidal silicon dioxide, flavor, glycine, hydroxypropyl methylcellulose, iron oxides, magnesium stearate, microcrystalline cellulose, polyethylene glycol, polysorbate 80, povidone, saccharin sodium, talc, titanium dioxide.

Indications: For iron deficiency anemia.

Actions: Ascorbic acid only enhances iron absorption at doses ≤ 200 mg. Vitron-C, a well-tolerated formula, is especially useful when pregnancy, menstruation, or chronic blood loss increases iron needs.

Warning: Close tightly and keep out of reach of children. Contains iron, which can be harmful or fatal to children in large doses. In case of accidental overdose, seek professional assistance or contact a Poison Control Center immediately.
The treatment of any anemic condition should be under the advice and supervision of a physician. As oral iron products interfere with absorption of oral tetracycline antibiotics, these products should not be taken within two hours of each other. As with any drug, if you are pregnant or nursing a baby, seek the advice of a health professional before using this product.

Directions: Adults—one or two tablets daily or as directed by a physician. Tablet may be swallowed whole, chewed or sucked like a lozenge.

How Supplied: Bottles of 100 tablets with child-resistant safety closure.
Distributed By:
CIBA Self-Medication, Inc.
581 Main St
Woodbridge, NJ 07095

Del Pharmaceuticals, Inc.
A Subsidiary of Del Laboratories, Inc.
**163 E. BETHPAGE ROAD
PLAINVIEW, NY 11803**

Direct Inquiries to:
Charles J. Hinkaty, President
(516) 844-2020
FAX: (516) 293-9018

For Medical Emergencies Contact:
Serap Ozelkan, Director
Pharmaceutical Product Development
(516) 844-2020

ARTHRICARE®
**Extra Strength
Pain Relieving Rubs**

Description: ArthriCare Odor Free is perfect for daytime use anywhere. Its unique greaseless and stainless formula provides the warming pain relief of medicinal rubs without the embarrassing medicinal odor. This special formula provides temporary relief of minor aches and pains of muscles and joints associated with arthritis, simple back pain, sprains and strains. This unique formulation contains Capsicum Oleoresin (containing Capsaicin 0.025%), a strong, penetrating pain blocker not commonly found in other rubs. In addition, it has two added fast-acting pain relievers to ease stiffness of muscles and joints.
ArthriCare Triple Medicated is specially formulated with three fast acting pain relievers. It's strong medicine that penetrates deep. You don't have to rub it in; just apply gently. ArthriCare Triple-Medicated provides temporary relief of minor aches and pains of muscles and joints associated with arthritis, simple backache, sprains and strains. Perfect for nightime use to help one sleep.
Active Ingredients: ArthriCare Odor Free Menthol 1.25%, Methyl Nicotinate 0.25%, Capsicum Oleoresin (containing Capsaicin 0.025%).
ArthriCare Triple Medicated Methyl Salicylate 30%, Menthol 1.25%, Methyl Nicotinate 0.25%.
Inactive Ingredients: ArthriCare Odor Free Aloe Vera Gel, Carbomer 940, Cetyl Alcohol, DMDM Hydantoin, Emulsifying Wax, Glyceryl Stearate SE, Isocatyl Alcohol, Myristyl Propionate, Propylparaben, Purified Water, Stearyl Alcohol, Triethanolamine.
ArthriCare Triple Medicated Carbomer 940, Dioctyl Sodium Sulfosucci-

nate, FD&C Blue No. 1, Glycerin, Isopropyl Alcohol, Polysorbate 60, Propylene Gycol, Purified Water.

Directions: Adults and children 2 years of age and older: Apply to affected area not more than 3 to 4 times daily. Children under 2 years of age: Consult a physician.

Warnings: For external use only. Avoid contact with the eyes. If condition worsens, or if symptoms persist for more than 7 days or clear up and occur again within a few days, discontinue use of this product and consult a physician. Do not apply to wounds or damaged skin. Do not bandage tightly. Avoid contact with mucous membranes, broken or irritated skin. Do not use with a heating pad, or immediately before or after taking a shower or bath. As part of its warming action, temporary redness may occur Keep this and all drugs out of the reach of children. In case of accidental ingestion, seek professional assistance or contact a Poison Control Center immediately. Store at room temperature 15–30 C (59–86 F).
Shown in Product Identification Guide, page 509

BABY ORAJEL®
Teething Pain Medicine

Description: Baby Orajel with fast-acting benzocaine (7.5%) relieves teething pain within one minute. It's pleasant tasting and contains no alcohol.

Active Ingredient: Benzocaine 7.5%.

Inactive Ingredients: FD&C Red No. 40, Flavor, Glycerin, Polyethylene Glycols, Purified Water, Sodium Saccharin, Sorbic Acid, Sorbitol.

Indications: For the temporary relief of sore gums due to teething in infants and children 4 months of age and older. Baby Orajel is a safe, soothing, pleasantly flavored product which helps to immediately relieve teething pain by its topical anesthetic effect on the gums.

Actions: Benzocaine is a topical, local anesthetic commonly used for pain, discomfort, or pruritis associated with wounds, mucous membranes and skin irritations.

Warnings: Do not use this product for more than 7 days unless directed by a dentist or physician. If sore mouth symptoms do not improve in 7 days; if irritation, pain or redness persists or worsens; or if swelling, rash or fever develops, see your dentist or physician promptly. Do not exceed recommended dosage. Do not use this product if you have a history of allergy to local anesthetics such as procaine, butacaine, benzocaine, or other "caine" anesthetics. Fever and nasal congestion are not symptoms of teething and may indicate the presence of infection. If these symptoms persist, consult your physician. Keep this and all drugs out of

Continued on next page

Del—Cont.

the reach of children. In case of accidental overdose, seek professional assistance or contact a Poison Control Center immediately. Do not use if tube tip is cut prior to opening.

Precaution: For persistent or excessive teething pain, consult your physician.

Directions: Wash hands. Cut open tip of tube on score mark. Use your fingertip or cotton applicator to apply a small pea-size amount of Baby Orajel. Apply to affected area not more than four times daily or as directed by a dentist or physician. For infants under 4 months of age, there is no recommended dosage or treatment except under the advice and supervision of a dentist or physician.

How Supplied: Baby Orajel: Gel in ⅓ oz (9.45 g) tube.
Shown in Product Identification Guide, page 510

BABY ORAJEL® TOOTH & GUM CLEANSER

Description: Baby Orajel Tooth & Gum Cleanser is specifically designed for children under four. Safe to swallow, non-foaming, fluoride- and abrasive-free, it contains Microdent®, which helps remove plaque and fight its build-up. Available in Fruit and Peaches 'n Cream flavors.

Active Ingredients: Microdent® (Poloxamer 407 2.0%, Simethicone 0.12%).

Inactive Ingredients: Carboxymethylcellulose Sodium, Citric Acid, Flavor, Glycerin, Methylparaben, Potassium Sorbate, Propylene Glycol, Propylparaben, Purified Water, Sodium Saccharin, Sorbitol.

Indications and Actions: Baby Orajel Tooth & Gum Cleanser is the first oral cleanser specially formulated to remove the plaque-like film on babies' teeth and gums. It's fluoride-free, non-abrasive and does not foam so it's safe to swallow. It's sugar-free and has a flavor babies love. Only Baby Orajel Tooth & Gum Cleanser contains patented Microdent® to help remove plaque and fight its buildup.

Warnings: Keep out of the reach of children. Do not use if tube tip is cut prior to opening.

Dosage and Administration: Wash hands. Cut open tip of tube on score mark. Apply a small amount to baby's gums and teeth with your finger, a gauze pad or a toothbrush. Gently rub or brush the gums and teeth to remove food and plaque-like film. For best results, use in the morning and at bedtime.

How Supplied: Gel in ½ oz. (14.2g) tube. Available in assorted flavors.
Shown in Product Identification Guide, page 510

Maximum Strength ORAJEL®
[ōr 'ah-jel]
Toothache Medicine

Description: Maximum Strength Orajel with 20% benzocaine provides immediate, long lasting toothache pain relief.

Active Ingredient: Benzocaine 20%.

Inactive Ingredients: Flavor, Polyethylene Glycols, Sodium Saccharin, Sorbic Acid.

Indications: Maximum Strength Orajel is formulated to provide fast, long lasting relief from toothache pain for hours.

Actions: Benzocaine is a topical, local anesthetic commonly used for pain, discomfort, or pruritis associated with wounds, mucous membranes and skin irritation.

Warning: Keep this and all drugs out of the reach of children. Do not use if tube tip is cut prior to opening. Do not use this product if you have a history of allergy to local anesthetics such as procaine, butacaine, benzocaine or other "caine" anesthetics. In case of accidental overdose, seek professional assistance or contact a Poison Control Center immediately.

Precaution: This preparation is intended for use in cases of toothache only as a temporary expedient until a dentist can be consulted. Do not use continuously.

Directions: Remove cap. Cut open tip of tube on score mark. Squeeze a small quantity of Maximum Strength Orajel directly into cavity and around gum surrounding the teeth.

How Supplied: Gel in two sizes— ³⁄₁₆ oz (5.3 g) and ⅓ oz (9.45 g) tubes.
Shown in Product Identification Guide, page 510

ORAJEL® COVERMED™
Fever Blister/Cold Sore Treatment

Description: Orajel CoverMed conceals unsightly cold sores or fever blisters for hours as it protects and relieves pain.

Active Ingredients: Dyclonine Hydrochloride 1.0%, Allantoin 0.5%.

Inactive Ingredients: Beeswax, Citric Acid, Colloidal Silicone Dioxide, Flavor, Iron Oxides, Lanolin, Petrolatum, Propylene Glycol, Purified Water, PVP/Hexadecene Copolymer, Titanium Dioxide.

Warnings: For external use only. Avoid contact with the eyes. If condition worsens, or if symptoms persist for more than 7 days or clear up and occur again within a few days, discontinue use of this product and consult a physician. Keep this and all drugs out of the reach of children. In case of accidental overdose, seek professional assistance or contact a Poi-

son Control Center immediately. Do not use if tube tip is cut prior to opening.

Dosage and Administration: Remove cap and cut open tip of tube on score mark. Adults and children 2 years of age and older: Apply to fever blisters/cold sores not more than 3 to 4 times daily. Children under 2 years of age: consult a physician.

How Supplied: Available in ³⁄₁₆ oz. (5.3g) tube.
Shown in Product Identification Guide, page 510

ORAJEL® Mouth-Aid®
[ōr 'ah-jel]
Cold/Canker Sore Medicine

Description: Orajel Mouth-Aid is a unique triple-acting medication which provides fast relief from painful minor mouth and lip sores. It has a protective formula that stays on the sore.

Active Ingredients: Benzocaine 20%, Benzalkonium Chloride 0.02%, Zinc Chloride 0.1%.

Inactive Ingredients: Allantoin, Carbomer, Edetate Disodium, Peppermint Oil, Polyethylene Glycol, Polysorbate 60, Propyl Gallate, Propylene Glycol, Purified Water, Povidone, Sodium Saccharin, Sorbic Acid, Stearyl Alcohol.

Indications: For the temporary relief of pain associated with canker sores, cold sores, fever blisters and minor irritation or injury of the mouth and gums.

Actions: Benzocaine is a topical, local anesthetic commonly used for pain, discomfort, or pruritis associated with wounds, mucous membranes and skin irritations. Benzalkonium chloride is a rapidly acting surface disinfectant and detergent. Zinc chloride provides an astringent effect.

Warnings: Do not use this product for more than 7 days unless directed by a dentist or physician. If sore mouth symptoms do not improve in 7 days; if irritation, pain, or redness persists or worsens; or if swelling, rash or fever develops, see your dentist or physician promptly. Do not exceed recommended dosage. Do not use this product if you have a history of allergy to local anesthetics such as procaine, butacaine, benzocaine or other "caine" anesthetics. Keep this and all drugs out of the reach of children. In case of accidental overdose, seek professional assistance or contact a Poison Control Center immediately. Do not use if tube tip is cut prior to opening.

Precaution: If condition persists, discontinue use and consult your physician or dentist. Not for prolonged use.

Directions: Cut open tip of tube on score mark. Adults and children 2 years and older: Apply to the affected area. Use up to 4 times daily or as directed by a dentist or physician. Children under 12 years of age should be supervised in the use of the product. Children under 2 years of age: Consult a dentist or physician.

How Supplied: Gel in 2 sizes—a 1/3 oz (9.45 g) tube and a 3/16 oz (5.3 g) tube.
Shown in Product Identification Guide, page 510

ORAJEL®PERIOSEPTIC®

Description: Orajel Perioseptic is an oxygenating saline cleanser for sore and irritated gums. A pleasant tasting alternative to plain salt water rinses, it contains the maximum amount of the active ingredient carbamide peroxide. Developed by a dentist, Orajel Perioseptic is a safe and effective oral antiseptic wound cleanser that can help decrease the number of micro-organisms populating a wound by its oxygenating action.

Active Ingredient: Carbamide Peroxide 15% in anhydrous glycerin.

Inactive Ingredients: Citric Acid, Edetate Disodium, Flavor, Methylparaben, Propylene Glycol, Purified Water, Sodium Chloride, Sodium Saccharin.

Indications: For temporary use in cleansing minor wounds or minor gum inflammation resulting from minor dental procedures, dentures, orthodontic appliances, accidental injury, or other irritations of the mouth or gums. For temporary use to cleanse canker sores.

Warning: Do not use this product for more than 7 days unless directed by a dentist or doctor. If sore mouth symptoms do not improve in 7 days; if irritation, pain, or redness persists or worsens, or if swelling, rash, or fever develops, see your dentist or doctor promptly. Cap bottle tightly. Keep away from heat and direct sunlight.

Dosage and Administration: Adults and children 2 years of age and older: Apply several drops directly to the affected area of the mouth with cotton swab or applicator. Allow the medication to remain in place at least 1 minute and then spit out. Use up to 4 times daily after meals and at bedtime or as directed by a dentist or doctor. Children under 12 years of age should be supervised in the use of this product. Children under 2 years of age: Consult a dentist or doctor.

How Supplied: 0.45 fl. oz. (13.3 ml) bottle
Shown in Product Identification Guide, page 510

PRONTO® Lice Killing Shampoo & Conditioner in One Kit

Description: Pronto Concentrate Lice Killing Shampoo & Conditioner in One contains the maximum strength of pyrethrum extract and piperonyl butoxide. In laboratory testing it has been shown to be effective in killing 100% of lice and their eggs. In addition, a conditioner is included in the formulation to reduce tangles, for easy, effective comb-out of lice and eggs.

Active Ingredients: Piperonyl Butoxide 4%, Pyrethrum Extract 0.33%

Inactive Ingredients: Ammonium Laureth Sulfate, Benzyl Alcohol, BHT, Decyl Alcohol, Disodium EDTA, Fragrance, Isopropyl Alcohol, Glycerin, PEG-14M, Poloxamer 183, Purified Water

Indications: For the treatment of head, pubic (crab), and body lice.

Actions: Pronto contains the maximum strength of pyrethrum extract and piperonyl butoxide. Pyrethrum extract acts directly on the nervous system of insects and piperonyl butoxide enhances the neurotoxic effect of pyrethrum extract by inhibiting the oxidative breakdown of pyrethrum extract by the insect's detoxification system. This results in a longer amount of time which the pyrethrum extract may exert its toxic effect on the insect.

Warning: Use with caution on persons allergic to ragweed. For external use only. Do not use near the eyes or permit contact with mucous membranes, such as inside the nose, mouth, or vagina, as irritation may occur. Keep out of eyes when rinsing hair. Adults and children: Close eyes tightly and do not open eyes until product is rinsed out. Also, protect children's eyes with washcloth, towel or other suitable material, or by similar method. If product gets into the eyes, immediately flush with water. If skin irritation or infection is present or develops, discontinue use and consult a doctor. Consult a doctor if infestation of eyebrows or eyelashes occurs. Wash thoroughly with soap and water after handling. Do not exceed two applications within 24 hours.

Directions: Shake well. Apply to affected area until all the hair is thoroughly wet with product. Allow product to remain on area for 10 minutes but no longer. Add sufficient warm water to form a lather and shampoo as usual. Rinse thoroughly. A fine-toothed comb or a special lice/nit-removing comb may be used to help remove dead lice or their eggs (nits) from hair. A second treatment must be done in 7 to 10 days to kill any newly hatched lice. Handy applicator gloves are provided for your convenience in applying the shampoo to avoid contact with lice.

How Supplied: 2 fl. oz. (59 ml) and 4 fl. oz. (118 ml) plastic bottles.
Shown in Product Identification Guide, page 510

TANAC® Medicated Gel
Fever Blister/Cold Sore Treatment

Description: Tanac Medicated Gel treats cold sores with a unique, long lasting maximum strength pain reliever, Dyclonine Hydrochloride (1.0%). It also protects lip sores while it treats them.

Active Ingredients: Dyclonine Hydrochloride 1.0%, Allantoin 0.5%.

Inactive Ingredients: Citric Acid, Flavor, Hydroxylated Lanolin, Petrolatum, Propylene Glycol, Purified Water, PVP/Hexadecene Copolymer, Yellow Wax.

Indications: For the temporary relief of pain and itching associated with fever blisters and cold sores. Relieves dryness and softens cold sores and fever blisters.

Warnings: DO NOT USE IF TIP IS CUT PRIOR TO OPENING. For external use only. Avoid contact with the eyes. If condition worsens, or if symptoms persist for more than 7 days or clear up and occur again within a few days, discontinue use of this product and consult a physician. Keep this and all other drugs out of reach of children. In case of accidental ingestion, seek professional assistance, or contact a Poison Control Center immediately.

Dosage and Administration: Cut open tip of tube on score mark. Adults and children 2 years of age and older: Apply to fever blisters/cold sores not more than 3 to 4 times daily. Children under 2 years of age: consult a physician.

How Supplied: Available in 1/3 oz. (9.45g) plastic tube.
Shown in Product Identification Guide, page 510

TANAC® No Sting Liquid
Canker Sore Medicine

Description: Tanac Liquid provides fast, soothing relief from painful canker sores and other gum irritations because it contains an effective anesthetic plus an antiseptic. It's alcohol-free so it doesn't sting.

Active Ingredients: Benzocaine 10%, Benzalkonium Chloride 0.12%.

Inactive Ingredients: Flavor, Polyethylene Glycol 400, Propylene Glycol, Sodium Saccharin, Tannic Acid.

Indications: For temporary relief of pain from mouth sores, canker sores, fever blisters and gum irritations.

Warnings: If the condition for which this preparation is used persists or if a rash or irritation develops, discontinue use and consult a physician. Use as indicated but not for more than 5 consecutive days. Not for prolonged use. Avoid getting into eyes. Do not use if you have a history of allergy to local anesthetics such as procaine, butacaine, benzocaine, or other "caine" anesthetics. KEEP THIS AND ALL DRUGS OUT OF THE REACH OF CHILDREN. In case of accidental ingestion, seek professional assistance or contact a Poison Control Center immediately. Do not use if imprinted bottle cap safety seal is broken or missing prior to opening.

Continued on next page

Del—Cont.

Dosage and Administration: Apply with cotton or cotton swab to affected area not more than 3 to 4 times daily.

How Supplied: Available in 0.45 fl. oz. (13 ml) glass bottle.
Shown in Product Identification Guide, page 510

Effcon Laboratories, Inc.
P.O. BOX 7499
MARIETTA, GA 30065-1499

Address inquiries to:
Jan Sugrue
(800-722-2428)
Fax: (770-428-6811)

For Medical Emergency Contact:
J. Kent Burklow,
(800-722-2428)
Fax: (770-428-6811)

PIN-X®
Pinworm Treatment

Description: Each 1 mL of liquid for oral administration contains:
Pyrantel base .... 50 mg
(as Pyrantel Pamoate)

Indication: For the treatment of pinworms.

Warnings: Keep this and all drugs out of the reach of children. In case of accidental overdose, seek professional assistance or contact a poison control center immediately.
If you are pregnant or have liver disease, do not take this product unless directed by a doctor.

Directions for Use: Adults and children 2 years to under 12 years of age: oral dosage is a single dose of 5 milligrams of pyrantel base per pound, or 11 milligrams per kilogram, of body weight not to exceed 1 gram. Dosage information is summarized on the following dosing schedule:

Weight	Dosage
	(taken as a single dose)
25 to 37 lbs.	= ½ tsp.
38 to 62 lbs.	= 1 tsp.
63 to 87 lbs.	= 1½ tsp.
88 to 112 lbs.	= 2 tsp.
113 to 137 lbs.	= 2½ tsp.
138 to 162 lbs.	= 3 tsp. (1 tbsp.)
163 to 187 lbs.	= 3½ tsp.
188 lbs. & over	= 4 tsp.

SHAKE WELL BEFORE USING

How Supplied: Pin-X is supplied as a tan to yellowish, caramel-flavored suspension which contains 50 mg of pyrantel base (as pyrantel pamoate) per mL, in bottles of 30 mL (1 fl oz). NDC 55806-024-10

Store at controlled room temperature 15°–30°C (59°–86°F).
Manufactured for:
Effcon Laboratories Inc.
Marietta, GA 30065-1499
Manufactured by:
MIKART, INC.
Atlanta, GA 30318
Rev. 1/89
Code 587A00
Shown in Product Identification Guide, page 510

Fisons Corporation
P.O. BOX 1766
ROCHESTER, NY 14603

Mailing Address:
P.O. Box 1766
Rochester, NY 14603

Direct Inquiries to:
Medical Information Dept.
P.O. Box 1766
Rochester, NY 14603
(716) 475-9000

DELSYM® Cough Formula
[*del'sĭm*]
(dextromethorphan polistirex)
Extended-Release Suspension
12-Hour Cough Relief

Active Ingredient: Each teaspoonful (5 mL) contains dextromethorphan polistirex equivalent to 30 mg dextromethorphan hydrobromide.

Inactive Ingredients: Citric acid, ethylcellulose, FD&C Yellow No. 6, flavor, high fructose corn syrup, methylparaben, polyethylene glycol 3350, polysorbate 80, propylene glycol, propylparaben, purified water, sucrose, tragacanth, vegetable oil, xanthan gum.

Indications: Temporarily relieves cough due to minor throat and bronchial irritation as may occur with the common cold or inhaled irritants.

Warnings: Do not take this product for persistent or chronic cough such as occurs with smoking, asthma, or emphysema, or if cough is accompanied by excessive phlegm (mucus) unless directed by a physician. A persistent cough may be a sign of a serious condition. If cough persists for more than 1 week, tends to recur, or is accompanied by fever, rash, or persistent headache, consult a physician. As with any drug, if you are pregnant or nursing a baby, seek the advice of a health professional before using this product. **Keep this and all drugs out of the reach of children.** In case of accidental overdose, seek professional assistance or contact a Poison Control Center immediately.

Drug Interaction Precaution: Do not use this product if you are now taking a prescription monoamine oxidase inhibitor (MAOI) (certain drugs for depression, psychiatric or emotional conditions, or Parkinson's disease), or for 2 weeks after

stopping the MAOI drug. If you are uncertain whether your prescription drug contains an MAOI, consult a health professional before taking this product.

Directions: **Shake Bottle Well Before Using.** Dose as follows or as directed by a physician.
Adults and Children 12 years of age and over: 2 teaspoonfuls every 12 hours, not to exceed 4 teaspoonfuls in 24 hours.
Children 6 to under 12 years of age: 1 teaspoonful every 12 hours, not to exceed 2 teaspoonfuls in 24 hours.
Children 2 to under 6 years of age: ½ teaspoonful every 12 hours, not to exceed 1 teaspoonful in 24 hours.
Children under 2 years of age: Consult a physician.

How Supplied: 89 mL (3 fl oz) bottles NDC 0585-0842-61
Store at 15°–30°C (59°–86°F).
FISONS Pharmaceuticals
Fisons Corporation
Rochester, NY 14623 U.S.A.
DELSYM is a registered trademark of Fisons Corporation.

Fleming & Company
1600 FENPARK DR.
FENTON, MO 63026

Direct Inquiries to:
John J. Roth, M.D.
(314) 343-8200

For Medical Emergencies Contact:
John R. Roth, M.D.
(314) 343-8200

CHLOR-3
Medicinal Condiment

Active Ingredients: A troika of sodium chloride (50% 24.3 mEq/half tsp. iodized); potassium chloride (30% 11.5 mEq/half tsp.); magnesium chloride (20% 5.6 mEq/half tsp.).

Indications: The first medicinal condiment to restore needed K^+ & Mg^{++} lost during diuresis, at the expense of Na^+. To restore electrolytes lost by overcooking foods, or to add to diets that lack green vegetables, bananas, etc. And to replace conventional salting of foods in culinary and gourmet arts.

Symptoms and Treatment of Oral Overdosage: Hyperkalemia and hypermagnesemia are not end-stage results of usage.

How Supplied: In 8-oz plastic shaker, tamper-evident bottles.

IMPREGON Concentrate

Active Ingredient: Tetrachlorosalicylanilide 2%

Indications: Diaper Rash Relief, 'Staph' control, Mold inhibitor.

Actions: This is a bacteriostatic/fungistatic agent for home usage and hospital usage.

Warnings: Impregon should not be exposed to direct sunlight for long periods after applications.

Precaution: Addition of bleach prior to diaper treatment negates application effects.

Dosage and Administration: One capful (5ml) per gallon of water to impregnate diapers in the diaper pail. Dilutions for many home areas accompany the full package.

Note: For disposable-type diapers, add one teaspoonful to 8 oz of water to a 'Windex-type' sprayer. Spray middle half area of diapers until damp, and allow to dry before using, to prevent rashes.

How Supplied: Four ounce amber plastic bottles.

MAGONATE TABLETS
MAGONATE LIQUID
Magnesium Gluconate (Dihydrate)

Active Ingredients: Each tablet contains magnesium gluconate (dihydrate) 500mg (27mg of Mg^{++}). Each 5cc of Magonate Liquid contains magnesium gluconate (dihydrate) 1000mg (54mg of Mg^{++}).

Indications: For all patients in negative magnesium balance.

Precaution: Excessive dosage may cause loose stools.

Dosage and Administration: Magonate is recommended during and for three weeks after a course in chemotherapy, then monitored regularly.
Adults and children over 12 yrs.—one or two tablets or ½ to 1 teaspoon of liquid t.i.d. Under 12 yrs.—one tablet or ½ teaspoon of liquid t.i.d. Dosage may be increased in severe cases.

How Supplied: Magonate Tablets are supplied in bottles of 100 and 1000 tablets. Magonate Liquid is supplied in pints and gallons.

MARBLEN Suspension and Tablet

Composition: A modified 'Sippy Powder' antacid containing magnesium and calcium carbonates.

Action and Uses: The peach/apricot (pink) antacid suspension is sugar-free and neutralizes 18 mEq acid per teaspoonful with a low sodium content of 18mg per fl. oz. Each pink tablet consumes 18.0 mEq acid.

Administration and Dosage: One teaspoonful rather than a tablespoonful or one tablet to reduce patient cost by ⅔.

How Supplied: Plastic pints and bottles of 100 and 1000.

NEPHROX SUSPENSION
(aluminum hydroxide)
Antacid Suspension

Composition: A watermelon flavored aluminum hydroxide (320mg as gel)/mineral oil (10% by volume) antacid per teaspoonful.

Action and Uses: A sugar-free/saccharin-free pink suspension containing no magnesium and low sodium (19mg/oz). Extremely palatable and especially indicated in renal patients. Each teaspoon consumes 9 mEq acid.

Administration and Dosage: Two teaspoonfuls or as directed by a physician.

Caution: To be taken only at bedtime. Do not use at any other time or administer to infants, expectant women, and nursing mothers except upon the advice of a physician as this product contains mineral oil.

How Supplied: Plastic pints and gallons.

NICOTINEX Elixir
nicotinic acid

Composition: Contains niacin 50 mg./tsp. in a sherry wine base (amber color).

Action and Uses: Produces flushing when tablets fail. To increase micro-circulation of inner-ear in Meniere's, tinnitus and labyrinthine syndromes. For 'cold hands & feet', and as a vehicle for additives.

Administration and Dosage: One or two teaspoonsful on fasting stomach.

Side Effects: Patients should be warned of dermal flush. Ulcer and gout patients may be affected by 14% alcoholic content.

Contraindications: Severe hypotension and hemorrhage.

How Supplied: Plastic pints and gallons.

OCEAN MIST
(buffered saline)

Composition: A 0.65% special saline made isotonic by a dual preservative system and buffering excipients prevent nasal irritation.

Action and Uses: Rhinitis medicamentosa, rhinitis sicca and atrophic rhinitis. For patients 'hooked on nose drops' and glaucoma patients on diuretics having dry nasal capillaries. OCEAN may also be used as a mist or drop.

Administration and Dosage: One or two squeezes in each nostril P.R.N.

Supplied: Plastic 45cc spray bottles and pints.

PURGE
(flavored castor oil)

Composition: Contains 95% castor oil (USP) in a sweetened lemon flavored base that completely masks the odor and taste of the oil.

Indications: Preparation of the bowel for x-ray, surgery and proctological procedures, IVPs, and constipation.

Dosage: Infants—1-2 teaspoonfuls. Children—adjust between infant and adult dose. Adult—2-4 tablespoonfuls.

Precaution: Not indicated when nausea, vomiting, abdominal pain or symptoms of appendicitis occur. Pregnancy, use only on advice of physician.

Supplied: Plastic 1 oz. & 2 oz. bottles.

A.C. Grace Co.
**1100 QUITMAN ROAD
P.O. BOX 570
BIG SANDY, TX 75755**

Direct Inquiries to:
Roy Erickson
(903) 636-4368
FAX: (903) 636-4051

For Medical Emergencies Contact:
Roy Erickson
(903) 636-4368
FAX: (903) 636-4051

UNIQUE E™ Vitamin E

Description: Each beef gelatin 400 I.U. Softgel Capsule contains All-Natural *Un*esterified Extra-High Antioxidant Concentrated Mixed Tocopherols. Not esterified acetate, succinate, *ordinary* Mixed Tocopherols nor d*l* synthetic. Contains *NO* SOY OIL, WHEAT GERM OIL or *ANY* OTHER OIL *DILUENT* which will turn rancid causing harmful free radical pathology. NO ALLERGENS, PRESERVATIVES, COLORS OR FLAVORS. Minimum shelf life FIVE YEARS.
All known natural related tocopherols for extra-high antioxidant function *PLUS* full biological activity and synergistic benefits of the complete all-natural Vitamin E Complex. The *ONLY* form providing all known vital functions of Vitamin E.
Unlike *ordinary* Mixed Tocopherols which can vary in the important d-alpha tocopherol potency, UNIQUE E Softgel capsules are stabilized and Certified by Assay to provide 400 I.U. (International Units) of d-alpha tocopherol *PLUS* all vital antioxidant factors.

Dosage: One or more capsules as directed by physician. Take *ENTIRE* daily dosage just before or with morning meal.

How Supplied: Bottles of 180 and 90 Softgel Capsules in safety-sealed, light protected plastic bottles.

Hogil Pharmaceutical Corp.
**TWO MANHATTANVILLE RD.
PURCHASE, NY 10577**

Direct Inquiries to:
Tanya Costagna
(914) 696-7600
FAX: (914) 696-4600

For Medical Information Contact:
Dr. Gilbert Spector
(914) 696-7600
FAX: (914) 696-4600

A•200®
GEL CONCENTRATE

Description:

Active Ingredients:
Pyrethrum Extract 0.33%
Piperonyl Butoxide 4.0%

Other Ingredients: Benzyl Alcohol, Carbomer-934, D&C Red # 33, FD&C Blue # 1, Fragrance, Isopropyl Alcohol, Octoxynol-9, Trolamine, Water.

Indications: A•200 Gel is indicated for the treatment of head, pubic(crab) and body lice.

Actions: Pyrethrum extract disrupts nervous transmission in lice resulting in paralysis and death. Piperonyl Butoxide is a synergist that potentiates the lethal actions of pyrethum extract by blocking detoxification of the drug by the lice. Pyrethrum extract is poorly absorbed through the skin.

Warning: Should be used with caution on persons allergic to ragweed.

Precautions: For external use only. Do not use near the eyes or permit contact with mucous membranes, such as inside the nose, mouth or vagina, as irritation may occur. Keep out of eyes when rinsing hair. Adults and children: Close eyes tightly and do not open until product is rinsed out. Also protect children's eyes with washcloth, towel or other suitable material, or by a similar method. If product gets in the eyes: immediately flush with water. If skin irritation or infection is present or develops, discontinue use and consult a physician. Consult a physician if infestation of eyebrows or eye-lashes occurs. In case of accidental ingestion, seek professional assistance or call a poison control center. If pregnant or nursing a baby, seek advice from a health professional before using this product.

Directions for Use: Apply to affected area until all hair is thoroughly covered with product. Allow product to remain on the area for 10 minutes but no longer. Wash area thoroughly with warm water and soap or shampoo. Use the special A•200 Lice/Nit Comb supplied to remove dead lice and their eggs(nits) from the hair. A second treatment must be done in 7 to 10 days to kill any newly hatched lice. In case of accidental ingestion, seek professional assistance or call a poison control center. As with any drug, if you are pregnant or nursing a baby, seek the advice of a health care professional before using this product.

How Supplied: Consumer package containing ¾ oz. tube, a special patented A•200 Lice/Nit Comb for lice and egg(nit) removal and a patient insert in both English and Spanish.
Shown in Product Identification Guide, page 510

A•200®
Lice Control Spray

Description: A•200 Lice Control Spray contains the synthetic pyrethroid permithrin.

Active Ingredients:
*Permethrin 0.50%
Inert Ingredients 99.50%
100.00%
*(3-phenoxyphenyl) methyl (+/−) cis/trans 3-(2,2-dichloroethenyl) 2,2- dimethylcyclopropanecarboxylate. Cis/ trans ratio: Min. 35% (+/−) cis and max. 65% (+/−) trans.

Indications: A•200 Lice control Spray is indicated for use only on garments, bedding, furniture, carpeting, upholstery and other inanimate objects infested with lice. Also for control of fleas and ticks on dogs.

Actions: Permethrin, a highly active synthetic pyrethroid, acts on nerve cell membranes to disrupt polarization creating paralysis of the insect.

Warnings: PRECAUTIONARY STATEMENTS: HAZARDS TO HUMANS AND DOMESTIC ANIMALS-CAUTION: Harmful if swallowed. May be absorbed through the skin. Avoid inhalation of spray mist. Avoid contact with skin, eyes or clothing. Wash thoroughly after handling and before smoking or eating. Avoid contamination of feed and food-stuffs. Remove pets and birds and cover fish aquaria before space spraying or surface applications. **THIS PRODUCTS IS NOT FOR USE ON HUMANS. ANIMALS:** Do not spray directly in/on eyes, mouth or genitalia. Do not cause exposure to puppies less than four weeks old.
Environmental Hazards: This product is toxic to fish. Do not apply directly to water.
STATEMENT OF PRACTICAL TREATMENT: IF INHALED: Remove affected person to fresh air. Apply artificial respiration if indicated.
IF IN EYES: Flush with plenty of water. Contact a physician if irritation persists.
IF ON SKIN: Wash affected areas immediately with soap and water. Get medical attention if irritation persists.
Physical or Chemical Hazards: Contents under pressure. Do not use or store near heat or open flame. Do not puncture or incinerate container. Exposure to temperatures above 130°F may cause bursting.

Directions For Use: It is a violation of Federal law to use this product in a manner inconsistent with its labeling. Do not use in food areas of food handling establishments, restaurants or other areas where food is commercially prepared or processed. Do not use in serving areas while food is exposed or facility is in operation. Serving areas are areas where prepared foods are served such as dining rooms but excluding areas where foods may be preapred or held. In the home, all food processing surfaces and utensils should be covered during treatment or thoroughly washed before use. Exposed food should be covered or removed. Do not use this product in or on electrical equipment due to the possibility of shock hazards.
SHAKE WELL BEFORE USING. Remove protective cap, hold container upright and spray from a distance of 12 to 15 inches. Remove birds and cover fish aquariums before spraying.
To Kill Lice and Louse Eggs: Spray in an inconspicuous area to test for possible staining or discoloration. Inspect again after drying, then proceed to spray entire area to be treated. Hold container upright with nozzle away from you. Depress valve and spray from a distance of 8 to 10 inches. Spray each square foot for three seconds.
Spray only those garments and parts of bedding, including mattresses and furniture that can not be either laundered or dry cleaned. Allow all sprayed articles to dry thoroughly before use.

Storage and Disposal: Store in a cool dry area. Do not transport or store below 32°F. Storage. Wrap container in several layers of newspaper and dispose of in trash. Do not incinerate or puncture.

How Supplied: 6 Oz. aerosol can. Also available in combination with A•200 Lice Treatment Kit.
Shown in Product Identification Guide, page 510

A•200®
LICE KILLING SHAMPOO

Description: A•200 Pediculicide, a synergized pyrethrum extract contains:

Active Ingredients:
Pyrethrum Extract 0.33%
Piperonyl Butoxide 4.0%

Other Ingredients: Benzyl Alcohol, $C_{13}C_{14}$Isoparaffin, Isopropyl Alcohol, Fragrance, Octoxynol-9, Water.

Indications: A•200 is indicated for the treatment of head and body lice.

Actions: Pyrethrum Extract disrupts nervous transmission in lice resulting in paralysis and death. Piperonyl Butoxide is a synergist that potentiates the lethal actions of pyrethrum extract by blocking detoxification of the drug by the lice. Pyrethrum extract is poorly absorbed through the skin.

Warning: Should be used with caution on persons allergic to ragweed.

Precautions: For external use only. Do not use near the eyes or permit contact with mucous membranes, such as inside the nose, mouth or vagina, as irritation may occur. Keep out of eyes when rinsing hair. Adults and children: Close eyes tightly and do not open until product is rinsed out. Also protect children's eyes with washcloth, towel or other suitable material, or by a similar method. If product gets in the eyes: immediately flush with water. If skin irritation or infection is present or develops, discontinue use and consult a physician. Consult a physician if infestation of eyebrows or eye-lashes occurs. In case of accidental ingestion, seek professional assistance or call a poison control center. If pregnant or nursing a baby, seek advice from a health professional before using this product.

Storage and Disposal: Do not contaminate water, food or feed by storage or disposal. Do not reuse container. Wrap and put in trash collection. Do not transport or store below 32°F (0°C).

Directions for Use: Important—Read Warnings Before Using. Shake well before using. Apply to the affected area until all the hair is thoroughly wet with product. Allow product to remain on the area for 10 minutes but no longer. Then add sufficient warm water to form a lather and shampoo as usual. Rinse thoroughly, Use the special A•200 Lice/Nit comb supplied to help remove the dead lice and their eggs(nits) from the hair. A second treatment must be done in 7 to 10 days to kill any newly hatched lice.

How Supplied: In 2 and 4 oz. unbreakable plastic bottles. A special patented A•200 Lice/Nit Comb for lice and egg (nit) removal and a patient insert in both English and Spanish are included.
Shown in Product Identification Guide, page 510

INNOGel PLUS®
Pubic(Crab) Lice Treatment Gel

Description: Active Ingredients: Pyrethrum Extract 0.30% Piperonyl Butoxide 3.0%

Other Ingredients: Benzyl Alcohol, Carbomer 934, D&C Red #33, FD&C Blue #1, Isopropyl Alcohol, Octoxynol-9, Trolamine, Water.

Indications: InnoGel Plus is indicated for the treatment of pubic(crab) and body lice.

Actions: Pyrethrum extract disrupts nervous transmission in lice resulting in paralysis and death. Piperonyl Butoxide is a synergist that potentiates the lethal actions of pyrethum extract by blocking detoxification of the drug by the lice. Pyrethrum extract is poorly absorbed through the skin.

Warning: Should be used with caution on persons allergic to ragweed.

Precautions: For external use only. Do not use near the eyes or permit contact with mucous membranes, such as inside the nose, mouth or vagina, as irritation may occur. Keep out of eyes when rinsing hair. Adults and children: Close eyes tightly and do not open until product is rinsed out. Also protect children's eyes with washcloth, towel or other suitable material, or by a similar method. If product gets in the eyes: immediately flush with water. If skin irritation or infection is present or develops, discontinue use and consult a physician. Consult a physician if infestation of eyebrows or eyelashes occurs. In case of accidental ingestion, seek professional assistance or call a poison control center. If pregnant or nursing a baby, seek advice from a health professional before using this product.

Directions for Use: Apply InnoGel Plus to affected area until hair is thoroughly covered with product. Allow product to remain on the area for 10 minutes but no longer. Wash area thoroughly with warm water and soap or shampoo. Use the special InnoGel Plus Lice/Nit Comb supplied to remove dead lice and their eggs(nits) from the hair. A second treatment must be done in 7 to 10 days to kill any newly hatched lice.

How Supplied: Consumer package containing 3-4 gram pre-dosed gel packettes and a special InnoGel Lice/Nit Comb.
Shown in Product Identification Guide, page 510

SINE–OFF®
No Drowsiness Formula Caplets

Relieves sinus headache, pain, pressure and congestion.

Active Ingredients: Each caplet contains: Pseudoephedrine Hydrochloride 30 mg., Acetaminophen 500 mg.

Inactive Ingredients: Crospovidone, FD & C Red 40, Hydroxypropyl Methylcellulose, Magnesium Stearate, Microcrystalline Cellulose, Polyethylene Glycol, Polysorbate 80, Povidone, Starch, and Titanium Dioxide.
For full prescribing information on Sine-Off No Drowsiness Formula Caplets, see Smithkline Beecham.

SINE–OFF® Sinus Medicine Caplets
Relieves sinus headache, pain, pressure, congestion, runny nose, sneezing & itchy, watery eyes.

Active Ingredients: Each caplet contains: Chlorpheniramine 2 mg, Pseudoephedrine Hydrochloride 30 mg., Acetaminophen 500 mg.

Inactive Ingredients: Carnauba Wax, Hydroxypropyl Methylcellulose, Magnesium Stearate, Microcrystalline Cellulose, Polydextrose, Polyethylene Glycol, Povidone, Sodium Starch Glycolate, Starch, Stearic Acid, Titanium Dioxide, Triacetin, FD & C Yellow #6, D & C Yellow 10.
For full prescribing information on Sine-Off Sinus Medicine caplets, see Smithkline Beecham.

TELDRIN®
Chlorpheniramine Maleate/ Phenylpropanolamine Hydrochloride Timed-Release 12 hour Allergy Relief Capsules
IMPROVED!
Now relieves congestion too!
PLEASE NOTE: This description replaces the previous formulation of TELDRIN—Timed Release Allergy Capsules which contained Chlorpheniramine 12 mg. per capsule.

Active Ingredients: Each capsule contains Chlorpheniramine Maleate 8 mg. and Phenylpropanolamine Hydrochloride 75 mg.

Inactive Ingredients: Benzyl Alcohol, Butylparaben, D & C Red No. 33, Edetate Calcium Disodium, FD & C Red No. 3, FD & C Yellow No. 6, Gelatin, Methylparaben, Pharmaceutical Glaze, Propylparaben, Sodium Lauryl Sulfate, Sodium Propionate, Starch, Sucrose, and other ingredients. May also contain Polysorbate 80.
For full prescribing information on Teldrin, see Smithkline Beecham.

EDUCATIONAL MATERIAL

The Contemporary Approach to the Control of Head Lice in Schools and communities. (A comprehensive training Manual for health Professionals)
Head Lice: Differential Diagnosis Cards

Inter-Cal Corporation
533 MADISON AVENUE
PRESCOTT, AZ 86301

Direct Inquiries to:
Dr. Jack Hegenauer: (520) 445-8063
FAX: (520) 778-7986

For Medical Emergency Contact:
Dr. Jack Hegenauer: (520) 445-8063
FAX: (520) 778-7986

ESTER–C®
(Calcium Ascorbate with C Metabolites)

Description: Each Ester-C® tablet, caplet, or capsule contains 500 mg Vita-

Continued on next page

Inter-Cal—Cont.

min C in the form of calcium ascorbate, 650 mg. Tablets and caplets may also contain vegetable-derived cellulose and lecithin as excipients. Ester-C® contains no preservatives, sugars, artificial colorings, or flavorings. As the calcium salt of L-ascorbic acid, calcium ascorbate, the primary constituent of Ester-C®, has an empirical formula of $CaC_{12}H_{14}O_{12}$ and a formula weight of 390.3. The water-based neutralization process yields natural C metabolites, including dehydroascorbic acid and the calcium salt of threonic acid, which are also present in the patented Ester-C® complex.

Actions: Vitamin C is essential for the prevention of scurvy. In humans, an exogenous source of the vitamin is required for collagen formation and tissue repair. Ascorbate is reversibly oxidized to dehydroascorbic acid in the body. Both of these are active forms of the vitamin and are considered to play important roles in biochemical reduction and oxidation reactions. The C metabolites (e.g., threonic acid) present in Ester-C® have been shown in cell culture and clinical studies to enhance cellular uptake of the vitamin. Biochemically, Vitamin C serves as a reducing agent in many important hydroxylation reactions in the body. The vitamin participates in collagen cross-linking and synthesis; synthesis of adrenal hormones and vasoactive amines; microsomal drug metabolism; carnitine synthesis; iron metabolism; folate metabolism; leukocyte activity and resistance to infection; and wound healing.

Indications and Usage: Vitamin C and its salts, such as calcium ascorbate, are recommended as nutritional supplements in the prevention of scurvy. In scurvy, a deficiency of ascorbate results in impaired collagen formation. These defects result in impaired bone formation, poor wound healing, and rupture of capillaries. Symptoms of mild deficiency may include faulty development of bones, bleeding gums, gingivitis, and loose teeth. An increased need for the vitamin exists in febrile states, chronic illness, and infection, e.g., rheumatic fever, pneumonia, tuberculosis, whooping cough, diphtheria, sinusitis, etc. Additional increases in the daily intake of ascorbate are indicated in trauma, burns, physical stress, delayed healing of bone fractures and wounds, and hemovascular disorders. Requirements of Vitamin C are increased for smokers.

Contraindications: Because of its calcium content, Ester-C® is contraindicated in hypercalcemic states, e.g., from dosing with parathyroid hormone, overdosage of Vitamin D, or dysfunctional calcium metabolism.

Adverse Reactions: There are no known adverse reactions following ingestion of Ester-C® tablets, caplets, capsules, or powder. The gastric disturbances characteristic of large doses of ascorbic acid are absent or greatly diminished when the pH-neutral form of calcium ascorbate present in Ester-C® tablets, caplets, capsules, or powder is utilized as the source of Vitamin C supplementation.

Dosage and Administration: The minimum U.S. Recommended Dietary Allowance (RDA) for Vitamin C to prevent diseases such as scurvy is 60 mg per day. The RDA for smokers is 100 mg per day. Optimum daily allowances, e.g., for the maintenance of increased cellular and body reserves, are significantly greater. For adults, the recommended average preventive dose of the vitamin is 70 to 150 mg daily. The recommended average optimum dose of Ester-C® calcium ascorbate is 650 to 1950 mg (1 to 3 tablets, caplets, or capsules) daily.

For frank scurvy, doses of 300 mg to one gram of Vitamin C daily have been recommended. Normal adults, however, have received as much as 12 grams of the vitamin daily without evidence of adverse reactions. For enhancement of wound healing, doses of the vitamin provided by two Ester-C® tablets, caplets, or capsules (one gram of Vitamin C) daily for 7–10 days both preoperatively and postoperatively are generally adequate; considerably larger amounts may be recommended in some cases. In the treatment of burns, the recommended daily dosage of Ester-C® calcium ascorbate is governed by the extent of tissue injury. For severe burns, daily doses of 2 to 4 tablets, caplets, or capsules (approximately 1–2 grams of Vitamin C) are recommended.

How Supplied: 650-mg tablets, caplets, or capsules of Ester-C® (equal to 500 mg of Vitamin C) in 100- or 250-count bottles. The Inter-Cal Corporation manufactures Ester-C® ascorbates as powdered raw materials. Tablets, caplets, capsules, and powders are available from many distributors in varying potencies, formulations, and packages. Used in food fortification and preservation, as a cosmetic ingredient, and in oral health applications. Also available as magnesium, potassium, sodium and zinc salts. Store at room temperature.

U.S. Patent No. 4,822,816, granted April 18, 1989.
Literature revised: July 1995.
Mfd. by Inter-Cal Corp.
Prescott, AZ 86301

**IF YOU SUSPECT
AN INTERACTION...**
The 1,500-page
PDR Guide to Drug Interactions •
Side Effects • Indications
can help.
Use the order form
in the front of this book.

IYATA Pharmaceutical, Inc.

735 NORTH WATER STREET
SUITE 612
MILWAUKEE, WI 53202

Direct Inquiries to:
Michael B. Adekunle, M.D.:
(414) 272-1982
FAX: (414) 272-2919

For Medical Emergency Contact:
(414) 272-1982
(800) 809-7918
FAX: (414) 272-1982

CAPSAGEL®

Product Information: Capsagel® contains natural purified capsaicin in a patented gel formulation developed by doctors.

Indications: For the temporary relief of minor aches and pains associated with Arthritis, Joint aches, Backaches, Sprains, Strains, Bruises, Bursitis, Tendinitis, Athralgias and Neuralgia.

Warnings: For external use only. Keep this and all medicines out of the reach of children. Avoid contact with eyes and mucous membranes. Do not apply to open or damaged skin. Do not bandage tightly. If condition worsens or if symptoms persist for more than seven days, or clear up and occur again within a few days, discontinue use and consult a doctor. If pregnant, consult your physician before using this product.

Directions: For adults and children over the age of two years. Apply a 1/8 inch dab (about the size of a pea) to the affeected area and massage until the gel is completely absorbed into the skin. Wash hands thoroughly with soap and water after each application. Capsagel® may be applied three to four times daily, as needed.

Inactive Ingredients: Carbopol 1382, Neutrol TE, Polysorbate 20, Uvinol MS 40, Germall II, Disodium EDTA USP, Ethyl alcohol SDA 40, Ion exchanged or Distilled water q. ed.

How Supplied: Capsagel is available in 3 strengths: .025%, .05% and .075% natural purified capsaicin in a unique patented gel formula.
U.S. patents: 6,178,879; 5,296,225 and 5,431,914
Distributed by IYATA Pharmaceutical Inc. Capsagel® is a registered trademark of IYATA Pharmaceutical Inc., Milwaukee, WI 53202 Made in U.S.A.

Johnson & Johnson •
MERCK
Consumer Pharmaceuticals Co.
CAMP HILL ROAD
FORT WASHINGTON, PA 19034

Direct Inquiries to:
Consumer Affairs Department
(215) 233-7000

For Medical Emergencies Contact:
(215) 233-7000

ALternaGEL™
[al-tern 'a-jel]
Liquid
High-Potency Aluminum Hydroxide Antacid

Description: ALternaGEL is available as a white, pleasant-tasting, high-potency aluminum hydroxide liquid antacid.

Ingredients: Each 5 mL teaspoonful contains: Active: 600 mg aluminum hydroxide (equivalent to dried gel, USP) providing 16 milliequivalents (mEq) of acid-neutralizing capacity (ANC), and less than 2.5 mg (0.109 mEq) of sodium and no sugar. Inactive: butylparaben, flavors, propylparaben, purified water, simethicone, and other ingredients.

Indications: ALternaGEL is indicated for the symptomatic relief of hyperacidity associated with peptic ulcer, gastritis, peptic esophagitis, gastric hyperacidity, hiatal hernia, and heartburn.
ALternaGEL will be of special value to those patients for whom magnesium-containing antacids are undesirable, such as patients with renal insufficiency, patients requiring control of attendant GI complications resulting from steroid or other drug therapy, and patients experiencing the laxation which may result from magnesium or combination antacid regimens.

Directions: One to two teaspoonfuls, as needed, between meals and at bedtime, or as directed by a physician: May be followed by a sip of water if desired. Concentrated product. Shake well before using. Keep tightly closed.

Warnings: Keep this and all drugs out of the reach of children. ALternaGEL may cause constipation.
Except under the advice and supervision of a physician: do not take more than 18 teaspoonfuls in a 24-hour period, or use the maximum dose of ALternaGEL for more than two weeks. ALternaGEL may cause constipation.
Prolonged use of aluminum-containing antacids in patients with renal failure may result in or worsen dialysis osteomalacia. Elevated tissue aluminum levels contribute to the development of the dialysis encephalopathy and osteomalacia syndromes. Small amounts of aluminum are absorbed from the gastrointestinal tract and renal excretion of aluminum is impaired in renal failure. Aluminum is not well removed by dialysis because it is bound to albumin and transferrin, which do not cross dialysis membranes. As a result, aluminum is deposited in bone, and dialysis osteomalacia may develop when large amounts of aluminum are ingested orally by patients with imparied renal function.
Aluminum forms insoluble complexes with phosphate in the gastrointestinal tract, thus decreasing phosphate absorption. Prolonged use of aluminum-containing antacids by normophosphatemic patients may result in hypophosphatemia if phosphate intake is not adequate. In its more severe forms, hypophosphatemia can lead to anorexia, malaise, muscle weakness, and osteomalacia.

Drug Interaction Precaution: Antacids may interact with certain prescription drugs. If you are presently taking a prescription drug, do not take this product without checking with your physician or other health professional.

How Supplied: ALternaGEL is available in bottles of 12 fluid ounces and 1 fluid ounce hospital unit doses. NDC 16837-860.
Shown in Product Identification Guide, page 510

DIALOSE® Tablets
[di 'a-lose]
Stool Softener Laxative

Description: DIALOSE is a very low sodium, nonhabit forming, stool softener containing 100 mg docusate sodium per tablet.
The docusate in DIALOSE is a highly efficient surfactant which facilitates absorption of water by the stool to form a soft, easily evacuated mass. Unlike stimulant laxatives, DIALOSE does not interfere with normal peristalsis, neither does it cause griping nor sensations of urgency.

Ingredients: Active: Docusate Sodium, 100 mg per tablet
Inactive: Colloidal Silicone Dioxide, Dextrates, Flavors, Hydroxypropyl Methylcellulose, Magnesium Stearate, Microcrystalline Cellulose, Polyethylene Glycol, Polysorbate 80, Pregelatinized Starch, Propylene Glycol, Sodium Starch Glycolate, Titanium Dioxide, D&C Red No. 28, D&C Red No. 27 Aluminum Lake, FD&C Blue No. 1, FD&C Blue No. 1 Aluminum Lake, FD&C Red No. 40.

Indications: DIALOSE is indicated for the relief of occasional constipation (irregularity).
DIALOSE is an effective aid to soften or prevent formation of hard stools in a wide range of conditions that may lead to constipation. DIALOSE helps to eliminate straining associated with obstetric, geriatric, cardiac, surgical, anorectal, or proctologic conditions. In cases of mild constipation, the fecal softening action of DIALOSE can prevent constipation from progressing and relieve painful defecation.

Directions: *Adults:* One tablet, one to three times daily; adjust dosage as needed.
Children 6 to under 12 years: One tablet daily as needed.
Children under 6 years: As directed by physician.
It is helpful to increase the daily intake of fluids by taking a glass of water with each dose.

Warnings: Unless directed by a physician: Do not use when abdominal pain, nausea, or vomiting are present. Do not use for a period longer than one week. Do not take this product if you are presently taking a prescription drug or mineral oil. As with any drug, if you are pregnant or nursing a baby, seek the advice of a health professional before using this product. Keep out of the reach of children.

How Supplied: Bottles of 100 pink tablets. Also available in 100 tablet unit dose boxes (10 strips of 10 tablets each). NDC-16837-870.
Shown in Product Identification Guide, page 510

DIALOSE® PLUS Tablets
[di 'a-lose Plus]
Stool Softener/Stimulant Laxative

Description: DIALOSE PLUS provides a very low sodium tablet formulation of 100 mg docusate sodium and 65 mg yellow phenolphthalein.

Ingredients: Each tablet contains: Actives: Docusate Sodium, 100 mg., yellow phenolphthalein, 65 mg.
Inactive: Dextrates, Dibasic Calcium Phosphate Dihydrate, Flavors, Hydroxypropyl Methylcellulose, Magnesium Stearate, Microcrystalline Cellulose, Polydextrose, Polythylene Glycol, Polysorbate 80, Propylene Glycol, Sodium Starch Glycolate, Titanium Dioxide, Triacetin, D&C Yellow NO. 10 Aluminum Lake, D&C Red NO. 28, FD&C Blue NO. 1, FD&C Red NO. 40, FD&C Red NO. 40 Aluminum Lake.

Indications: DIALOSE PLUS is indicated for the treatment of constipation characterized by lack of moisture in the intestinal contents, resulting in hardness of stool and decreased intestinal motility. DIALOSE PLUS combines the advantages of the stool softener, docusate sodium, with the peristaltic activating effect of yellow phenolphthalein.

Directions: *Adults:* One or two tablets daily as needed, at bedtime or on arising
Children 6 to under 12 years: One tablet daily as needed
Children under 6 years: As directed by physician.
It is helpful to increase the daily intake of fluids by taking a glass of water with each dose.

Continued on next page

J&J • Merck—Cont.

Warnings: Unless directed by a physician: Do not use when abdominal pain, nausea, or vomiting are present. Do not use for a period longer than one week. If skin rash appears do not use this product or any other preparation containing phenolphthalein. Frequent or prolonged use may result in dependence on laxatives. Do not take this product if you are presently taking a prescription drug or mineral oil.

As with any drug, if you are pregnant or nursing a baby, seek the advice of a health professional before using this Keep out of the reach of children.

How Supplied: Bottles of 100 yellow tablets. Also available in 100 tablet unit dose boxes (10 strips of 10 tablets each). NDC 16837-871.

Shown in Product Identification Guide, page 510

INFANTS' MYLICON® Drops
[*my'li-con*]
Antiflatulent

Ingredients: Each 0.6 mL of drops contains: Active: simethicone, 40 mg. Inactive: carbomer 934P, citric acid, flavors, hydroxypropyl methylcellulose, purified water, Red 3, saccharin calcium, sodium benzoate, sodium citrate.

Indications: For relief of the painful symptoms of excess gas in the digestive tract. Such gas is frequently caused by excessive swallowing of air or by eating foods that disagree. The defoaming action of INFANTS' MYLICON® Drops relieves flatulence by dispersing and preventing the formation of mucus-surrounded gas pockets in the gastrointestinal tract. INFANTS' MYLICON® Drops act in the stomach and intestines to change the surface tension of gas bubbles enabling them to coalesce, thereby freeing and eliminating the gas more easily by belching or passing flatus.

Directions: Infants (under 2 years): 0.3 ml four times daily after meals and at bedtime, or as directed by a physician. The dosage can also be mixed with 1 oz of cool water, infant formula or other suitable liquids to ease administration. Adults and children: 0.6 ml four times daily, after meals and at bedtime, or as directed by a physician.

Warnings: Do not exceed 12 doses per day except under the advice and supervision of a physician. Keep this and all drugs out of the reach of chldren.

How Supplied: INFANTS' MYLICON® Drops are available in bottles of 15 ml (0.5 fl oz) and 30 ml (1.0 fl oz) pink, pleasant tasting liquid. NDC 16837-630.

Shown in Product Identification Guide, page 511

MYLANTA® AND MYLANTA® DOUBLE STRENGTH
[*my-lan'ta*]
Aluminum, Magnesium and Simethicone Liquid Antacid/Anti-Gas

Description: MYLANTA® and MYLANTA® Double Strength are well-balanced, pleasant-tasting, antacid/anti-gas medications that provide consistent, effective relief of symptoms associated with gastric hyperacidity and excess gas. Non-constipating and considered dietetically low sodium or sodium free, MYLANTA® and MYLANTA® Double Strength contain two proven antacids, aluminum hydroxide and magnesium hydroxide, plus simethicone for gas relief.

Active Ingredients: Each 5 mL teaspoon contains:

	MYLANTA®	MYLANTA® Double Strength
Aluminum Hydroxide	200 mg	400 mg
Magnesium Hydroxide	200 mg	400 mg
Simethicone	20 mg	40 mg

Inactive Ingredients:
LIQUIDS:
Butylparaben, carboxymethylcellulose sodium, flavors, hydroxypropyl methylcellulose, microcrystalline cellulose, propylparaben, purified water, saccharin sodium, and sorbitol.

Sodium Content: Each 5 mL teaspoon contains the following amount of sodium:

	MYLANTA®	MYLANTA® Double Strength
Liquid	0.68 mg (0.03 mEq)*	1.14 mg (0.05 mEq)*

* considered dietetically sodium free

Acid Neutralizing Capacity: Two teaspoonfuls have the following acid neutralizing capacity:

	MYLANTA®	MYLANTA® Double Strength
Liquid	25.4 mEq	50.8 mEq

Indications: MYLANTA® and MYLANTA® Double Strength are indicated for the relief of acid indigestion, heartburn, sour stomach, and symptoms of gas and upset stomach associated with those conditions. MYLANTA® and MYLANTA® Double Strength are also indicated as antacids for the symptomatic relief of hyperacidity associated with the diagnosis of peptic ulcer, gastritis, peptic esophagitis, heartburn and hiatal hernia and as antiflatulents to alleviate the symptoms of mucus-entrapped gas, including postoperative gas pain.

Advantages: MYLANTA® and MYLANTA® Double Strength are homogenized for a smooth, creamy taste. The choice of three pleasant-tasting liquid flavors and the non-constipating formula encourage patient acceptance, thereby minimizing the skipping of prescribed doses. MYLANTA® and MYLANTA® Double Strength are also available in tablets, and both the liquid and tablet forms are considered dietetically low sodium or sodium free. MYLANTA® and MYLANTA® Double Strength Liquids provide consistent relief in patients suffering from distress associated with hyperacidity, mucus-entrapped gas, or swallowed air.

Directions:
Liquid:
Shake well. 2-4 teaspoonfuls between meals and at bedtime, or as directed by a physician.

Warnings: Keep this and all drugs out of the reach of children. Do not take more than 24 tsps of MYLANTA® or 12 tsps of MYLANTA® Double Strength in a 24-hour period or use the maximum dose of this product for more than two weeks, except under the advice and supervison of a physician. Do not use this product if you have kidney disease.

Prolonged use of aluminum-containing antacids in patients with renal failure may result in or worsen dialysis osteomalacia. Elevated tissue aluminum levels contribute to the development of the dialysis encephalopathy and osteomalacia syndromes. Small amounts of aluminum are absorbed from the gastrointestinal tract and renal excretion of aluminum is impaired in renal failure. Aluminum is not well removed by dialysis because it is bound to albumin and transferrin, which do not cross dialysis membranes. As a result, aluminum is deposited in bone, and dialysis osteomalacia may develop when large amounts of aluminum are ingested orally by patients with impaired renal function.

Aluminum forms insoluble complexes with phosphate in the gastrointestinal tract, thus decreasing phosphate absorption. Prolonged use of aluminum-containing antacids by normophosphatemic patients may result in hypophosphatemia if phosphate intake is not adequate. In its more severe forms, hypophosphatemia can lead to anorexia, malaise, muscle weakness, and osteomalacia.

Drug Interaction Precaution: Antacids may interact with certain prescription drugs. If you are presently taking a prescription drug, do not take this product without checking with your physician or other health professional.

How Supplied: MYLANTA® and MYLANTA® Double Strength are available as white liquid suspensions in pleasant-tasting flavors, Original, Cherry Creme and Cool Mint Creme. Liquids are supplied in bottles of 5 oz, 12 oz, and 24 oz. Also available for hospital use in liquid unit dose bottles of 1 oz and bottles of 5 oz.

MYLANTA®
NDC 16837-610 ORIGINAL LIQUID
NDC 16837-629 COOL MINT CREME LIQUID

NDC 16837-621 CHERRY CREME LIQUID

MYLANTA® Double Strength
NDC 16837-652 ORIGINAL LIQUID
NDC 16837-624 COOL MINT CREME LIQUID
NDC 16837-622 CHERRY CREME LIQUID

Professional Labeling

Indications: Stress-induced upper gastrointestinal hemorrhage: MYLANTA DOUBLE STRENGTH is indicated for the prevention of stress-induced upper gastrointestinal hemorrhage. Hyperacidic conditions: As an antacid, for the symptomatic relief of hyperacidity associated with the diagnosis of peptic ulcer and other gastrointestinal conditions where a high degree of acid neutralization is desired.

Directions: Prevention of stress-induced upper gastrointestinal hemorrhage: 1) Aspirate stomach via nasogastric tube* and record pH. 2) Instill 10 mL of MYLANTA DOUBLE STRENGTH followed by 30 mL of water via nasogastric tube. Clamp tube. 3) Wait one hour. Aspirate stomach and record pH. 4a) If pH equals or exceeds 4.0, apply drainage or intermittent suction for one hour, then repeat the cycle. 4b) If pH is less than 4.0, instill double (20 mL) MYLANTA DOUBLE STRENGTH followed by 30 mL of water. Clamp tube. 5) Wait one hour. If pH equals or exceeds 4.0, see number 7, if pH is still less than 4.0, instill double (40 mL) MYLANTA DOUBLE STRENGTH followed by 30 mL of water. Clamp tube. 6) Wait one hour. If pH equals or exceeds 4.0, see number 7. If pH is still less than 4.0, instill double (80 mL)† MYLANTA DOUBLE STRENGTH followed by 30 mL of water. 7) Drain for one hour and repeat cycle with the effective dosage of MYLANTA DOUBLE STRENGTH.
*If nasogastric tube is not in place, administer 20 mL of MYLANTA DOUBLE STRENGTH orally q2h.
†In a recent clinical study[1] 20 mL of MYLANTA DOUBLE STRENGTH, q2h, was sufficient in more than 85 percent of the patients. No patient studied required more than 80 mL of MYLANTA DOUBLE STRENGTH q2h.
In hyperacid states for symptomatic relief: One or two teaspoonfuls as needed between meals and at bedtime or as directed by a physician. Higher dosage regimens may be employed under the direct supervision of a physician in the treatment of active peptic ulcer disease.

Precaution: Aluminum-magnesium hydroxide containing antacids should be used with caution in patients with renal impairment.

Adverse Effects: Occasional regurgitation and mild diarrhea have been reported with the dosage recommended for the prevention of stress-induced upper gastrointestinal hemorrhage.

References: 1. Zinner MJ, Zuidema GD, Smigh PL, Mignosa M: The prevention of upper gastrointestinal tract bleeding in patients in an intensive care unit. *Surg Gynecol Obster* 153:214–220, 1981. 2. Lucas CE, Sugawa C, Riddle J, et al.: Natural history and surgical dilemma of "stress" gastric bleeding. *Arch Surg* 102:266–273, 1971. 3. Hastings PR, Skillman JJ, Bushnell LS, Silen W: Antacid titration in the prevention of acute gastrointestinal bleeding: a controlled, randomized trial in 100 critically ill patients. *N Engl J Med* 298:1042–1045, 1978. 4. Day SB, MacMillan BG, Altemeier WA: *Curling 's Ulcer, An Experience of Nature.* Springfield, IL, Charles C Thomas Co., 1972, p. 205. 5. Skillman JJ, Bushnell LS, Goldman H, Silen W: Respiratory failure, hypotension, sepsis, and jaundice. A clinical syndrome associated with lethal hemorrhage from acute stress ulceration of the stomach. *Am J Surg* 117:523–530, 1969. 6. Priebe HJ, Skillman J, Bushnell LS, et al. Antacid versus cimetidine in preventing acute gastrointestinal bleeding. *N Engl J Med* 302:426–430, 1980. 7. Silen W: The prevention and management of stress ulcers. *Hosp Pract* 15:93–97, 1980. 8. Herrmann V, Kaminski DL: Evaluation of intragastric pH in acutely ill patients. *Arch Surg* 114:511–514, 1979. 9. Martin LF, Staloch DK, Simonowitz DA, et al.: Failure of cimetidine prophylaxis in the critically ill. *Arch Surg* 114:492–496, 1979. 10. Zinner MJ, Turtinen L, Gurll NJ, Reynolds DG: The effect of metiamide on gastric mucosal injury in rat restraint. *Clin Res* 23:484A, 1975. 11. Zinner M, Turtinen BA, Gurll NJ: The role of acid and ischemia in production of stress ulcers during canine hemorrhagic shock. *Surgery* 77:807–816, 1975. 12. Winans CS: Prevention and treatment of stress ulcer bleeding: Antacids or cimetidine? *Drug Ther Bull* (hospital) 12:37–45, 1981.

Shown in Product Identification Guide, page 510

MYLANTA AND MYLANTA DOUBLE STRENGTH

[mylan 'ta]
Calcium Carbonate and Magnesium Hydroxide Tablets Antacid

Description: Mylanta and Mylanta Double Strength are well balanced, pleasant tasting antacid medications that provide consistent, effective relief of symptoms associated with gastric hyperacidity. Non-constipating and considered dietetically sodium free, Mylanta and Mylanta Double Strength contain two proven antacids, calcium carbonate and magnesium hydroxide.

Active Ingredients: Each tablet contains:

	Mylanta	Mylanta Double Strength
Calcium Carbonate	350mg	700mg
Magnesium Hydroxide	150mg	300mg

Inactive Ingredients: Citric acid, confectioner's sugar, flavors, magnesium stearate, sorbitol, FD&C Blue 1 or D&C Yellow 10 or D&C Red 27

Sodium Content
Each chewable tablet contains the following amount of sodium:

Mylanta	Mylanta Double Strength
0.3mg *	0.6mg *

* considered dietetically sodium free

Acid Neutralizing Capacity
Two chewable tablets have the following acid neutralizing capacity:

Mylanta	Mylanta Double Strength
24.0mEq	48.0mEq

Indications: Mylanta and Mylanta Double Strength are indicated for the relief of heartburn, acid indigestion, sour stomach and upset stomach associated with these conditions. Mylanta and Mylanta Double Strength are also indicated as antacids for the symptomatic relief of hyperacidity associated with the diagnosis of peptic ulcer, gastritis, peptic esophagitis, heartburn and hiatal hernia.

Directions: Thoroughly chew 2–4 tablets between meals, at bedtime or as directed by a physician.

Warnings: Keep this and all drugs out of the reach of children. Do not take more than 10 tablets of Mylanta or 20 tablets of Mylanta Double Strength in a 24-hour period, or use the maximum dosage for more than two weeks. Do not use this product if you have kidney disease, except under the advise and supervision of a physician.

Drug Interaction Precaution: Antacids may interact with certain prescription drugs. If you are presently taking a prescription drug, do not take this product without checking with your physician or other health professional.

How Supplied: Mylanta is available as a green Cool Mint Creme chewable tablet. Mylanta Double Strength is available as a green Cool Mint Creme Chewable tablet and pink Cherry Creme chewable tablet.
Mylanta
NDC 16837-848 Cool Mint Creme
Mylanta Double Strength
NDC 16837-869 Cherry Creme
NDC 16837-849 Cool Mint Creme
Shown in Product Identification Guide, page 511

MYLANTA® GAS Relief Tablets
Maximum Strength MYLANTA®
GAS Relief Tablets
MYLANTA® GAS Relief Gelcaps
[My-lan '-ta]
Antiflatulent

Active Ingredients:
Each chewable tablet contains:

Continued on next page

J&J • Merck—Cont.

	Simethicone
MYLANTA® GAS Relief Maximum Strength	80 mg
MYLANTA® GAS Relief	125 mg
MYLANTA® GAS Relief Gelcaps	62.5 mg

Inactive Ingredients: Tablets: Dextrates, flavor, sorbitol, stearic acid, tricalcium phosphate. Cherry: Red 7.
Gelcaps: Benzyl alcohol, butylparaben, castor oil, croscarmellose sodium, D&C Red 28, D&C Yellow 10, dextrose, dibasic calcium phosphate dihydrate, edetate calcium disodium, FD&C Blue 1, FD&C Red 28, gelatin, hydroxypropyl methylcellulose, maltodextrin, methylparaben, microcrystalline cellulose, propylene glycol, propylparaben, silicon dioxide, sodium lauryl sulfate, sodium propionate, sorbitol, stearic acid, titanium dioxide, tribasic calcium phosphate.

Indications: For relief of the painful symptoms of excess gas in the digestive tract. Such gas is frequently caused by excessive swallowing of air or by eating foods that disagree. MYLANTA® GAS Relief Gelcaps, MYLANTA® GAS Relief Tablets, and Maximum Strength MYLANTA® GAS Relief Tablets are high capacity antiflatulents for adjunctive treatment of many conditions in which the retention of gas may be a problem, such as the following: air swallowing, postoperative gaseous distention, peptic ulcer, spastic or irritable colon, diverticulosis. If condition persists, consult your physician.
MYLANTA® GAS Relief Gelcaps, MYLANTA® GAS Relief Tablets and Maximum Strength MYLANTA®GAS Relief Tablets have a defoaming action that relieves flatulence by dispersing and preventing the formation of mucus-surrounded gas pockets in the gastrointestinal tract. MYLANTA® GAS Relief Gelcaps, MYLANTA® GAS Relief Tablets, and Maximum Strength MYLANTA® GAS Relief Tablets act in the stomach and intestines to change the surface tension of gas bubbles enabling them to coalesce, thereby freeing and eliminating the gas more easily by belching or passing flatus.

Directions:
MYLANTA® GAS Relief Tablets
One tablet four times daily after meals and at bedtime. May also be taken as needed up to six tablets daily or as directed by a physician.
Maximum Strength MYLANTA® GAS Relief Tablets
One tablet four times daily after meals and at bedtime or as directed by a physician.
TABLETS SHOULD BE CHEWED THOROUGHLY
MYLANTA® Gas Relief Gelcaps
Swallow 2–4 gelcaps as needed after meals and at bedtime. Do not exceed 8 gelcaps per day unless directed by a physician.

Warnings: Keep this and all drugs out of the reach of children.

How Supplied: MYLANTA® GAS Relief Tablets are available as white (mint) or pink (cherry) scored, chewable tablets identified "MYL GAS 80." Mint flavor is available in bottles of 60 and 100 tablets and individually wrapped 12 and 30 tablet packages. Cherry flavor is available in packages of 12 individually wrapped tablets. Mint NDC 16837-858. Cherry NDC 16837-859.
Maximum Strength MYLANTA® GAS Relief Tablets are available as white, scored, chewable tablets identified "MYL GAS 125" in individually wrapped 12 and 24 tablet packages and economical 48 tablet bottles. NDC 16837-455.
Mylanta® Gas Relief Gelcaps are available as blue and yellow gelcaps identified as "Mylanta Gas," in individually wrapped 24 tablet packages.
Shown in Product Identification Guide, page 510

MYLANTA® GELCAPS
[my-lan'ta]
Antacid

Description: MYLANTA® GELCAPS are an easy-to-swallow, non-chalky alternative to liquid and tablet antacids. The gelcaps contain two antacid ingredients, calcium carbonate and magnesium hydroxide, have no chalky taste, are low in sodium and provide fast, effective acid pain relief.

Ingredients: Each gelcap contains:
Active: Calcium Carbonate 550 mg and Magnesium Hydroxide 125 mg.
Inactive: Benzyl Alcohol, Butylparaben, Castor Oil, D&C Yellow 10, Disodium Calcium Edetate, FD&C Blue 1, Gelatin, Hydroxypropyl Cellulose, Magnesium Stearate, Methylparaben, Microcrystalline Cellulose, Propylparaben, Sodium Croscarmellose, Sodium Lauryl Sulfate, Sodium Propionate, Titanium Dioxide.
Sodium Content: MYLANTA® GELCAPS contain a very low amount of sodium per daily dose. Typical value is 2.5 mg (.1087 mEq) sodium per gelcap.
Acid Neutralizing Capacity: Two MYLANTA® GELCAPS have an acid neutralizing capacity of 23.0 mEq.

Indications: For the relief of acid indigestion, heartburn, sour stomach and upset stomach associated with these symptoms.

Advantages: MYLANTA® GELCAPS are easy to swallow, provide fast, effective relief, eliminate antacid taste and are low in sodium. Convenience of dosage in the unique gelcap form can promote patient compliance.

Directions: 2–4 gelcaps as needed or as directed by a physician.

Warnings: Keep this and all other drugs out of the reach of children. Do not take more than 24 gelcaps in a 24-hour period or use the maximum dosage for more than two weeks or use if you have kidney disease, except under the advice and supervision of a physician.

Drug Interaction Precaution: Antacids may interact with certain prescription drugs. If you are presently taking a prescription drug, do not take this product without checking with your physician or other health professional.

How Supplied: MYLANTA® GELCAPS are available as a blue and white gelcap in convenient blister packs in boxes of 24 solid gelcaps or in bottles of 50 and 100 solid gelcaps.
NDC 16837-850   1/93
Shown in Product Identification Guide, page 510

MYLANTA® SOOTHING LOZENGES
[mi-lan'ta]
ANTACID

Description: MYLANTA® SOOTHING LOZENGES are a dietically sodium free calcium rich antacid which dissolve in your mouth to quickly soothe your heartburn pain or acid indigestion.

Ingredients: Each MYLANTA® SOOTHING LOZENGE contains:

Active: Calcium Carbonate, 600 mg

Inactive: Citric Acid, Corn Syrup, FD&C Red 40, Flavor, Propylene Glycol, Soybean Oil, Sucrose, Titanium Dioxide

Indications: For the relief of heartburn, acid indigestion, sour stomach and upset stomach associated with these symptoms.

Acid Neutralizing Capacity: Each MYLANTA® SOOTHING LOZENGE has an acid neutralizing capacity of 11.4 mEq.

Directions: Allow 1 lozenge to dissolve in your mouth and if necessary, follow with a second. Repeat as needed or as directed by a physician.

Warnings: Keep this and all other drugs out of the reach of children. Do not take more than 12 lozenges in a 24-hour period or use the maximum dosage for more than two weeks, except under the advice and supervision of a physician.

Drug Interaction Precaution: Antacids may interact with certain prescription drugs. If you are presently taking a prescription drug, do not take this product without checking with your physician or other health professional.

How Supplied: MYLANTA® SOOTHING LOZENGES are available as green Cool Mint Creme flavored lozenges, and as pink Cherry Creme flavored lozenges identified as "M". Lozenges supplied in 18 count boxes and 50 count bottles.
NDC 16837-876 (Cherry Creme)
NDC 16837-875 (Cool Mint Creme)
Shown in Product Identification Guide, page 511

PEPCID AC

Description:
Active Ingredient: Famotidine 10 mg per tablet.
Inactive Ingredients: Hydroxypropyl cellulose, hydroxypropyl methylcellulose, red iron oxide, magnesium stearate, microcrystalline cellulose, starch, talc, titanium dioxide.

Product Benefits:
1 tablet relieves heartburn and acid indigestion.
Pepcid AC Acid Controller prevents heartburn and acid indigestion brought on by consuming food and beverages.
It contains famotidine, a prescription-proven medicine.
The ingredient in PEPCID AC Acid Controller, famotidine, has been prescribed by doctors for years to treat millions of patients safely and effectively. The active ingredient in PEPCID AC Acid Controller has been taken safely with many frequently prescribed medications.

Action: It is normal for the stomach to produce acid, especially after consuming food and beverages. However, acid in the wrong place (the esophagus), or too much acid, can cause burning pain and discomfort that interfere with everyday activities.

Heartburn—Caused by acid in the esophagus

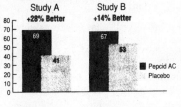

A valve-like muscle called the lower esophageal sphincter (LES) is relaxed in an open position — Burning pain/discomfort — Excess acid moves up into esophagus

In clinical studies, PEPCID AC Acid Controller was significantly better than placebo pills in relieving and preventing heartburn.

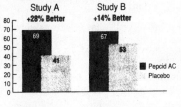

Study A +28% Better — 69 / 41
Study B +14% Better — 67 / 53
Pepcid AC / Placebo

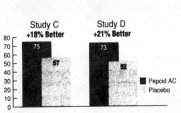

Study C +18% Better — 75 / 57
Study D +21% Better — 73 / 52
Pepcid AC / Placebo

Uses:
For Relief of heartburn, acid indigestion, and sour stomach;
For Prevention of these symptoms brought on by consuming food and beverages.

How to help avoid symptoms
Do not lie down soon after eating.
If your are overweight, lose weight.
If you smoke, stop or cut down.
Avoid or limit foods such as caffeine, chocolate, fatty foods and alcohol.
Do not eat just before bedtime.

Warnings: Do not take the maximum daily dosage for more than 2 weeks continuously except under the advice and supervision of a doctor.
As with any drug, if you are pregnant or nursing a baby, seek the advice of a health professional before using this product.
If you have trouble swallowing, or persistent abdominal pain, see your doctor promptly. You may have a serious condition that may need different treatment.
Keep this and all drugs out of the reach of children.
In case of accidental overdose, seek professional assistance or contact a poison control center immediately.

Caution: Heartburn and acid indigestion are common, but you should see your doctor promptly if:
You have trouble swallowing or persistent abdominal pain. You may have a serious condition that may need different treatment.
You have used the maximum dosage every day for two weeks continously.
Important: As with any drug, if you are pregnant or nursing a baby, seek the advice of a health professional before using this product. This product should not be given to children under 12 years old, unless directed by a doctor. Keep this and all drugs out of the reach of children. In case of accidental overdose, seek professional assistance or contact a poison control center immediately.

Directions: For **Relief** of symptoms **swallow 1 tablet with water.**
For **Prevention** of symptoms brought on by consuming food and beverages **swallow 1 tablet 1 hour before eating a meal you expect to cause symptoms.**
Can be used up to twice daily (up to 2 tablets in 24 hours).
This product should not be given to children under 12 years old unless directed by a doctor.

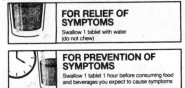

FOR RELIEF OF SYMPTOMS
Swallow 1 tablet with water (do not chew)

FOR PREVENTION OF SYMPTOMS
Swallow 1 tablet 1 hour before consuming food and beverages you expect to cause symptoms

How Supplied: PEPCID AC Acid Controller is available as a rose-tablet identified as PEPCID AC. PEPCID AC Acid Controller is available in blister packs in boxes of 6, 12, 18, and 30 tablets. NDC 16837-872. Read the directions and warnings before use.
Keep the carton. It contains important information.

Store at temperatures up to 30°C (86°F).
Protect from moisture.
DO NOT USE IF THE INDIVIDUAL BLISTER UNIT IS OPEN OR BROKEN.
Shown in Product Identification Guide, page 511

Konsyl Pharmaceuticals, Inc.
4200 S. HULEN
FORT WORTH, TX 76109

Direct Inquiries to:
Bill Steiber
(817) 763-8011, Ext. 23
FAX: (817) 731-9389

KONSYL® Fiber Tablets
(Calcium Polycarbophil 625mg)

Description: KONSYL Fiber Tablets is a bulk forming fiber laxative for restoring and maintaining regularity. Promotes normal function of the bowel by increasing bulk volume and water content of stool. KONSYL Fiber Tablets contain 625 mg calcium polycarbophil equivalent to 500 mg polycarbophil.

Inactive Ingredients: Caramel, Crospovidone, Ethycellulose, Hydroxypropyl Methylcellulose, Magnesium Stearate, Microcrystalline Cellulose, Polyethylene Glycol, Povidone, Silicon Dioxide.

Actions: KONSYL Fiber Tablets provide bulk that promotes normal elimination. KONSYL Fiber Tablets provide convenience of a bulk forming laxative in a tablet form. The product is easy-to-swallow and non-irritative in the gastrointestinal tract.

Indications: KONSYL Fiber Tablets are indicated in the management of chronic constipation, irritable bowel syndrome, as adjunctive therapy in the constipation of diverticular disease, bowel management of patients with hemorrhoids, and for constipation during pregnancy, convalescence, and senility. KONSYL Fiber Tablets are also used for other indications as prescribed by physician.

Contraindications: Intestinal obstruction, fecal impaction.

Warnings: KEEP THIS AND ALL DRUGS OUT OF THE REACH OF CHILDREN. TAKING THIS PRODUCT WITHOUT ADEQUATE FLUID MAY CAUSE IT TO SWELL AND BLOCK YOUR THROAT OR ESOPHAGUS AND MAY CAUSE CHOKING. DO NOT TAKE THIS PRODUCT IF YOU HAVE DIFFICULTY IN SWALLOWING. IF YOU EXPERIENCE CHEST PAIN, VOMITING, OR DIFFICULTY IN SWALLOWING OR BREATHING AFTER TAKING THIS PRODUCT, SEEK IMMEDIATE MEDICAL ATTENTION.

Continued on next page

Konsyl—Cont.

Interaction Precaution: Contains calcium. If you are taking any form of tetracycline antibiotic, this product should be taken at least 1 hour before or 2 hours after you have taken the antibiotic. Store at controlled room temperature 59°–86°F (15°–30°C). Protect from moisture.

Dosage and Administration: TAKE THIS PRODUCT (CHILD OR ADULT DOSE) WITH AT LEAST 8 OUNCES (A FULL GLASS) OF WATER OR OTHER FLUID. TAKING THIS PRODUCT WITHOUT ENOUGH LIQUID MAY CAUSE CHOKING. SEE WARNINGS. **ADULTS:** 2 TABLETS 1 TO 4 TIMES A DAY. **CHILDREN** (6 TO 12 YEARS OLD): 1 TABLET 1 TO 3 TIMES A DAY. CHILDREN UNDER 6 YEARS CONSULT A PHYSICIAN. DOSAGE WILL VARY ACCORDING TO DIET, EXERCISE, PREVIOUS LAXATIVE USE OR SEVERITY OF CONSTIPATION. THE RECOMMENDED ADULT STARTING DOSE IS 2 TO 4 TABLETS DAILY. MAY BE INCREASED UP TO 8 TABLETS DAILY.

How Supplied: Tablets, containers of 90 tablets.
Is this product OTC? Yes

KONSYL® POWDER
(psyllium hydrophilic mucilloid)
Sugar Free, Sugar Substitute Free.
6.0 grams of psyllium per
TEASPOON

Description: Konsyl is a bulk-forming natural therapeutic fiber for restoring and maintaining regularity. Konsyl contains 100% psyllium hydrophilic mucilloid, a highly efficient dietary fiber derived from the husk of the psyllium seed. Konsyl contains no chemical stimulants and is non-addictive. Each dose contains 6.0 grams of psyllium compared to 3.4 grams of psyllium in most other products.

Inactive Ingredients: None. Each 6 gram dose provides 3 calories. Konsyl is sodium free. Since Konsyl is sugar free, it is excellent for diabetics who require a bowel normalizer.

Actions: Konsyl provides bulk that promotes normal elimination. The product is uniform, instantly miscible, palatable, and non-irritative in the gastrointestinal tract.

Indications: Konsyl is indicated in the management of chronic constipation, irritable bowel syndrome, as adjunctive therapy in the constipation of diverticular disease, bowel management of patients with hemorrhoids, and for constipation during pregnancy, convalescence, and senility. Konsyl is also indicated for other indications as prescribed by physician.

Contraindications: Intestinal obstruction, fecal impaction.

Warnings: KEEP THIS AND ALL DRUGS OUT OF THE REACH OF CHILDREN. TAKING THIS PRODUCT WITHOUT ADEQUATE FLUID MAY CAUSE IT TO SWELL AND BLOCK YOUR THROAT OR ESOPHAGUS AND MAY CAUSE CHOKING. DO NOT TAKE THIS PRODUCT IF YOU HAVE DIFFICULTY IN SWALLOWING. IF YOU EXPERIENCE CHEST PAIN, VOMITING OR DIFFICULTY IN SWALLOWING OR BREATHING AFTER TAKING THIS PRODUCT, SEEK IMMEDIATE MEDICAL ATTENTION.

Precautions: May cause allergic reaction in people sensitive to inhaled or ingested psyllium powder.

Dosage and Administration:
MIX THIS PRODUCT (CHILD OR ADULT DOSE) WITH AT LEAST 8 OUNCES OF WATER OR OTHER FLUID. TAKING THIS PRODUCT WITHOUT ENOUGH LIQUID MAY CAUSE CHOKING. SEE WARNINGS. **ADULTS:** Place one rounded teaspoon (6.0 grams) into a dry shaker cup or container that can be closed. Add 8 oz. of juice, cold water or your favorite beverage. Shake, don't stir, for 3–5 seconds. Drink promptly. If mixture thickens, add more liquid and shake. Follow with an 8 oz. glass of juice or water to aid product action. Konsyl can be taken one to three times daily, depending on need and response. Konsyl generally produces results within 12–72 hours. Take Konsyl at any convenient time, morning or evening; before or after meals. When taking Konsyl, one should drink several 8 oz. glasses of water a day to aid product action. **CHILDREN:** (6–12 years old) Use ½ adult dose in 8 oz. of liquid, 1–3 times daily.

New Users: Easy Does It. Medical research shows that higher fiber intake is important for good digestive health. To help the body adjust and avoid minor gas and bloating sometimes associated with high fiber intake, it may be necessary to take one half dose over several days and then slowly increase the dosage over several days. Always follow with 8 oz. of liquid.

How Supplied: Powder, containers of 10.6 oz. (300 g), 15.9 oz. (450 g) and 30 single dose (6.0 g) packets.
Is this product OTC? Yes.

Kyolic Ltd.
Division of Wakunaga
of America Co., Ltd.
23501 MADERO
MISSION VIEJO, CA 92691

Direct Inquiries to:
(800) 421-2998

BE SURE®

Prevents flatulence
Digestive enzymes: 1–2 capsules to be taken with offending foods. Comes in boxes of 30 and bottles of 60 capsules.

GINKGO BILOBA PLUS™
Dietary Supplement

Active Ingredients: Each capsule contains Ginkgo Biloba Extract 50:1 (40 mg), Aged Garlic Extract (200 mg) and Siberian Ginseng Extract 5:1 (80 mg).

Suggested Use: As a dietary supplement, take 3 capsules daily with food.

How Supplied: Bottles of 45 and 90 Capsules.

KYOLIC®
Odor Modified Garlic Supplement

Active Ingredient: Each caplet contains 600 mg Aged Garlic Extract™.

Suggested Use: As a dietary supplement, take 1 or more caplets daily with food.

How Supplied: Boxes of 30 Caplets.
Shown in Product Identification Guide, page 523

KYO-CHROME™
Odor Modified Garlic-Containing Supplement

Active Ingredients: Each caplet contains Aged Garlic Extract Powder (500 mg), Niacin (20 mg) and Chromium Picolinante (200 µg).

Suggested Use: As a dietary supplement, take 1 caplet daily with food.

How Supplied: Boxes of 30 Caplets.

KYO-DOPHILUS®
Probiotic Dietary Supplements

Suggested Use: 1 capsule/tablet, twice daily with meals to replace beneficial bacteria.

How Supplied:
Kyo-Dophilus® *Capsules:* 1.5 billion cells of *L. acidophilus, B. bifidum,* and *B. longum;* Bottles of 45 and 90.
Kyo-Dophilus® *Tablets:* 1 billion live cells of *L. acidophilus;* Bottles of 90.
Acidophilase® *Capsules:* 1 billion live cells of *L. acidophilus* and *B. bifidum,*

Amylase, Protease and Lipase; Bottles of 60.

Other Products Available: Kyo-Green®, **PREMIUM KYOLIC®-EPA,** Professional label **A.G.E.™/SGP®** Formula. *Please see Manufacturer's Index.*

Lavoptik Company, Inc.
661 WESTERN AVENUE N.
ST. PAUL, MN 55103

Direct Inquiries to:
661 Western Avenue North
St. Paul, MN 55103-1694
(612) 489-1351

For Medical Emergencies Contact:
B. C. Brainard
(612) 489-1351
FAX: (612) 489-0760

LAVOPTIK® Eye Cups

Description: Device—Sterile disposable eye cups.

How Supplied: Individually bagged eye cups are packed 12 per box, NDC 10651-01004.

LAVOPTIK® Eye Wash

Description: Isotonic LAVOPTIK Eye Wash is a buffered solution designed to help physically remove contaminants from the surface of the eye and lids. Formulated to buffer contaminants toward the safe range and help restore normal salts and water ratios in the tears.

Contents: Each 100 ml
Sodium Chloride	0.49	gram
Sodium Biphosphate	0.40	gram
Sodium Phosphate	0.45	gram
Preservative Agent		
Benzalkonium Chloride	0.005	gram

Precautions: If you experience severe eye pain, headache, rapid change in vision (side or straight ahead); sudden appearance of floating objects, acute redness of the eyes, pain on exposure to light or double vision consult a physician at once. If symptoms persist or worsen after use of this product, consult a physician. If solution changes color or becomes cloudy do not use. Keep this and all medicines out of reach of children. Keep container tightly closed. Do not use if safety seal is broken at time of purchase.

Administration: 6 ounce size with Eye Cup.
Rinse cup with clean water immediately before and after each use, avoid contamination of rim and inside surfaces of cup. Apply cup, half-filled with LAVOPTIK Eye Wash tightly to the eye. Tilt head backward. Open eyelids wide, rotate eyeball and blink several times to insure thorough washing. Discard washings. Repeat other eye. Tightly cap bottle.

32 ounce size.
Break seal as you remove cap and pour directly on contaminated area.

How Supplied: 6 ounce bottle with eyecup, NDC 10651-01040.
32 ounce bottle, NDC 10651-01019.

Lederle Consumer Health
A Division of Whitehall-Robins Healthcare
FIVE GIRALDA FARMS
MADISON, NJ 07940

Direct Inquiries to:
Lederle Consumer Product Information
(800) 282-8805

CALTRATE® 600
[căl-trāte]
High Potency Calcium Supplement
Nature's Most Concentrated Form of Calcium®
No Sugar, No Salt, No Lactose, No Preservatives, Tablet Shape Specially Designed for Easier Swallowing

Caltrate 600 is a dietary supplement that meets USP standards for purity, potency and dissolution.

Nutrition Facts
Serving Size 1 Tablet

Each Tablet Contains	% Daily Value
Calcium 600 mg	60%

Recommended Intake: One or two tablets daily or as directed by your physician.

Warning: Keep out of reach of children.

Ingredients: Calcium Carbonate, Maltodextrin, Cellulose, Mineral Oil, Hydroxypropyl Methylcellulose, Titanium Dioxide, Sodium Lauryl Sulfate, Gelatin, Crospovidone, Stearic Acid and Magnesium Stearate.

How Supplied: Bottle of 60
Store at Room Temperature.

CALTRATE® 600 + D
[căl-trāte]
High Potency Calcium Supplement
With Vitamin D
Nature's Most Concentrated Form of Calcium®
No Sugar, No Salt, No Lactose, No Preservatives, Tablet Shape Specially Designed for Easier Swallowing

CALTRATE® 600 + D is a dietary supplement that meets USP standards for purity, potency and dissolution.

Nutrition Facts
Serving Size 1 Tablet

Each Tablet Contains	% Daily Value
Vitamin D 200 IU	50%
Calcium 600 mg	60%

Recommended Intake: One or two tablets daily or as directed by your physician.

Warning: Keep out of reach of children.

Ingredients: Calcium Carbonate, Maltodextrin, Cellulose, Mineral Oil, Hydroxypropyl Methylcellulose, Titanium Dioxide, Vitamin D, Sodium Lauryl Sulfate, FD&C Yellow No. 6, Gelatin, Crospovidone, Stearic Acid and Magnesium Stearate.

How Supplied: Bottle of 60
Store at Room Temperature.
© 1994

CALTRATE® PLUS™
[căl-trāte]
High Potency Calcium Supplement
With Vitamin D & Minerals
Nature's Most Concentrated Form of Calcium®
No Sugar, No Salt, No Lactose, No Preservatives, Tablet Shape Specially Designed for Easier Swallowing

Nutrition Facts
Serving Size 1 Tablet

Each Tablet Contains	% Daily Value
Vitamin D 200 IU	50%
Calcium 600 mg	60%
Magnesium 40 mg	10%
Zinc 7.5 mg	50%
Copper 1 mg	50%
Manganese 1.8 mg	*
Boron 250 mcg	*
*Daily Value Not Established	

Recommended Intake: One or two tablets daily or as directed by your physician.

Warning: Keep out of reach of children.

Ingredients: Calcium Carbonate, Maltodextrin, Magnesium Oxide, Cellulose, Mineral Oil, Hydroxypropyl Methylcellulose, Zinc Oxide, Titanium Dioxide, Manganese Sulfate, Vitamin D, Sodium Lauryl Sulfate, Sodium Borate, Cupric Oxide, FD&C Red No. 40, FD&C Yellow No. 6, FD&C Blue No. 1, Gelatin, Crospovidone, Stearic Acid and Magnesium Stearate.

Continued on next page

Lederle Consumer Health—Cont.

How Supplied: Bottle of 60
Store at Room Temperature.
*Shown in Product Identification
Guide, page 511*

CENTRUM®
[sĕn-trŭm]
**High Potency
Multivitamin-Multimineral Formula,
Advanced Formula
From A to Zinc®**

**Nutrition Facts
Serving Size 1 Tablet**

Each Tablet Contains	%DV
Vitamin A 5000 IU	100%
(40% as Beta Carotene)	
Vitamin C 60 mg	100%
Vitamin D 400 IU	100%
Vitamin E 30 IU	100%
Thiamin 1.5 mg	100%
Riboflavin 1.7 mg	100%
Niacinamide 20 mg	100%
Vitamin B₆ 2 mg	100%
Folic Acid 400 mcg	100%
Vitamin B₁₂ 6 mcg	100%
Biotin 30 mcg	10%
Pantothenic Acid 10 mg	100%
Calcium 162 mg	16%
Iron 18 mg	100%
Phosphorus 109 mg	11%
Iodine 150 mcg	100%
Magnesium 100 mg	25%
Zinc 15 mg	100%
Copper 2 mg	100%
Potassium 80 mg	2%
Vitamin K 25 mcg	*
Selenium 20 mcg	*
Manganese 3.5 mg	*
Chromium 65 mcg	*
Molybdenum 160 mcg	*
Chloride 72 mg	*
Nickel 5 mcg	*
Tin 10 mcg	*
Silicon 2 mg	*
Vanadium 10 mcg	*
Boron 150 mcg	*

*Daily Value (%DV) not established.

Recommended Intake: Adults, 1 tablet daily.

Warning: Close tightly and keep out of reach of children. Contains iron, which can be harmful or fatal to children in large doses. In case of accidental overdose, seek professional assistance or contact a Poison Control Center immediately.

Ingredients: Calcium Phosphate, Magnesium Oxide, Calcium Carbonate, Potassium Chloride, Ascorbic Acid (Vit. C), Ferrous Fumarate, Microcrystalline Cellulose, dl-alpha Tocopheryl Acetate (Vit. E), Gelatin, Crospovidone, Niacinamide, Zinc Oxide, Hydroxypropyl Methylcellulose, Calcium Pantothenate, Vitamin A Acetate/Vitamin D, Titanium Di-

CENTRUM, JR.® + EXTRA C Children's Chewable Vitamin/Mineral Formula Each Tablet Contains	Children 2–4 Years Old (½ tablet)	% Daily Value	Children Over 4 Years Old (1 tablet)	% Daily Value
Vitamin A (20% as Beta Carotene)	2500 IU	100%	5000 IU	100%
Vitamin C	150 mg	375%	300 mg	500%
Vitamin D	200 IU	50%	400 IU	100%
Vitamin E	15 IU	150%	30 IU	100%
Thiamin	0.75 mg	107%	1.5 mg	100%
Riboflavin	0.85 mg	106%	1.7 mg	100%
Niacinamide	10 mg	111%	20 mg	100%
Vitamin B₆	1 mg	143%	2 mg	100%
Folic Acid	200 mcg	100%	400 mcg	100%
Vitamin B₁₂	3 mcg	100%	6 mcg	100%
Biotin	22.5 mcg	15%	45 mcg	15%
Pantothenic Acid	5 mg	100%	10 mg	100%
Calcium	54 mg	7%	108 mg	11%
Iron	9 mg	90%	18 mg	100%
Phosphorous	25 mg	3%	50 mg	5%
Iodine	75 mcg	107%	150 mcg	100%
Magnesium	20 mg	10%	40 mg	10%
Zinc	7.5 mg	94%	15 mg	100%
Copper	1 mg	100%	2 mg	100%
Vitamin K	5 mcg	*	10 mcg	*
Manganese	0.5 mg	*	1 mg	*
Chromium	10 mcg	*	20 mcg	*
Molybdenum	10 mcg	*	20 mcg	*

*Daily Value not established.

oxide, Manganese Sulfate, Magnesium Stearate, Stearic Acid, Silicon Dioxide, Pyridoxine Hydrochloride (Vit. B₆), Cupric Oxide, Riboflavin (Vit. B₂), Triethyl Citrate, Thiamin Mononitrate (Vit. B₁), Polysorbate 80, Beta Carotene, FD&C Yellow #6, Folic Acid, Sodium Selenate, Potassium Iodide, Chromium Chloride, Sodium Metasilicate, Sodium Molybdate, Borates, Phytonadione (Vit. K), Biotin, Sodium Metavanadate, Stannous Chloride, Nickelous Sulfate and Cyanocobalamin (Vit. B₁₂).

How Supplied: Light peach, engraved CENTRUM C1.
Bottle of 60
Combopack†
†Bottles of 100 plus 30
Store at Room Temperature.
Shown in Product Identification Guide, page 511

CENTRUM, JR.®
[sĕn-trŭm]
**Shamu and his Crew™
+ EXTRA C
Children's Chewable
Vitamin/Mineral Formula**

[See table above.]

Inactive Ingredients: Artificial Flavorings, Aspartame,† Blue 2, Citric Acid, FD&C Yellow No. 6, Lactose, Magnesium Stearate, Microcrystalline Cellulose, Pregelatinized Starch, Red 40, Silica Gel, Sorbitol, Stearic Acid, and Sucrose.

Phenylketonurics: Contains Phenylalanine.

Warnings: CONTAINS IRON, WHICH CAN BE HARMFUL OR FATAL TO CHILDREN IN LARGE DOSES. CLOSE TIGHTLY AND KEEP OUT OF THE REACH OF CHILDREN. IN CASE OF ACCIDENTAL OVERDOSE, SEEK PROFESSIONAL ASSISTANCE OR CONTACT A POISON CONTROL CENTER IMMEDIATELY. CONTAINS ASPARTAME.

Recommended Intake: Children 2 to 4 years of age: Chew approximately one-half tablet daily. Children over 4 years of age: Chew one tablet daily.

How Supplied: Bottle of 60

Tamper-evident feature: Bottle sealed with printed foil under cap. If foil is torn, do not accept.
Store at Room Temperature.
© 1995
Sea World Characters ©1993 Sea World, Inc. All Rights Reserved.
Shamu and his Crew™ are trademarks and copyrights of Sea World, Inc. CENTRUM, JR.®, The Spectrum Design and all other marks and indicia are trademarks and copyrights of Lederle.
Shown in Product Identification Guide, page 511

CENTRUM, JR.®
[sĕn-trŭm]
**Shamu and his Crew™
+EXTRA CALCIUM
Children's Chewable
Vitamin/Mineral Formula**

[See table at top of next page.]

Inactive Ingredients: Artificial Flavorings, Aspartame,† Blue 2, Citric Acid, FD&C Yellow No. 6, Lactose, Magnesium Stearate, Microcrystalline Cellulose, Pregelatinized Starch, Red 40, Silica Gel, Sorbitol, Stearic Acid, and Sucrose.

Phenylketonurics: Contains Phenylalanine.

Recommended Intake: Children 2 to 4 years of age: chew approximately one-half tablet daily. Children over 4 years of age: chew one tablet daily.

How Supplied: Bottle of 60

Tamper-evident feature: Bottle sealed with printed foil under cap. If foil is torn, do not accept.

Store at Room Temperature.
© 1995
Sea World Characters ©1993 Sea World, Inc. All Rights Reserved.

Shamu and his Crew™ are trademarks and copyrights of Sea World, Inc. CENTRUM, JR.®, The Spectrum Design and all other marks and indicia are trademarks and copyrights of Lederle.

CENTRUM, JR.®
[sĕn-trŭm]
Shamu and his Crew™ + IRON
Children's Chewable Vitamin/Mineral Formula

[See second table from top of page.]

Inactive Ingredients: Artificial Flavorings, Aspartame,† Blue 2, Citric Acid, FD&C Yellow No. 6, Lactose, Magnesium Stearate, Microcrystalline Cellulose, Pregelatinized Starch, Red 40, Silica Gel, Sorbitol, Stearic Acid, and Sucrose.

Phenylketonurics: Contains Phenylalanine.

Recommended Intake: Children 2 to 4 years of age: Chew approximately one-half tablet daily. Children over 4 years of age: Chew one tablet daily.

How Supplied: Assorted Flavors—Uncoated Tablet—Partially Scored—Engraved Lederle C2 and CENTRUM, JR. Bottle of 60

Tamper-evident feature: Bottle sealed with printed foil under cap. If foil is torn, do not accept.

CENTRUM, JR.® + EXTRA CALCIUM
Children's Chewable Vitamin/Mineral Formula

Each Tablet Contains	Children 2–4 Years Old (½ tablet)	% Daily Value	Children Over 4 Years Old (1 tablet)	% Daily Value
Vitamin A (20% as Beta Carotene)	2500 IU	100%	5000 IU	100%
Vitamin C	30 mg	75%	60 mg	100%
Vitamin D	200 IU	50%	400 IU	100%
Vitamin E	15 IU	150%	30 IU	100%
Thiamin	0.75 mg	107%	1.5 mg	100%
Riboflavin	0.85 mg	106%	1.7 mg	100%
Niacinamide	10 mg	111%	20 mg	100%
Vitamin B$_6$	1 mg	143%	2 mg	100%
Folic Acid	200 mcg	100%	400 mcg	100%
Vitamin B$_{12}$	3 mcg	100%	6 mcg	100%
Biotin	22.5 mcg	15%	45 mcg	15%
Pantothenic Acid	5 mg	100%	10 mg	100%
Calcium	80 mg	10%	160 mg	16%
Iron	9 mg	90%	18 mg	100%
Phosphorous	25 mg	3%	50 mg	5%
Iodine	75 mcg	107%	150 mcg	100%
Magnesium	20 mg	10%	40 mg	10%
Zinc	7.5 mg	94%	15 mg	100%
Copper	1 mg	100%	2 mg	100%
Vitamin K	5 mcg	*	10 mcg	*
Manganese	0.5 mg	*	1 mg	*
Chromium	10 mcg	*	20 mcg	*
Molybdenum	10 mcg	*	20 mcg	*

*Daily Value not established.

CENTRUM, JR.® + IRON
Children's Chewable Vitamin/Mineral Formula

Each Tablet Contains	Children 2–4 Years Old (½ tablet)	% Daily Value	Children Over 4 Years Old (1 tablet)	% Daily Value
Vitamin A (20% as Beta Carotene)	2500 IU	100%	5000 IU	100%
Vitamin C	30 mg	75%	60 mg	100%
Vitamin D	200 IU	50%	400 IU	100%
Vitamin E	15 IU	150%	30 IU	100%
Thiamin	0.75 mg	107%	1.5 mg	100%
Riboflavin	0.85 mg	106%	1.7 mg	100%
Niacinamide	10 mg	111%	20 mg	100%
Vitamin B$_6$	1 mg	143%	2 mg	100%
Folic Acid	200 mcg	100%	400 mcg	100%
Vitamin B$_{12}$	3 mcg	100%	6 mcg	100%
Biotin	22.5 mcg	15%	45 mcg	15%
Pantothenic Acid	5 mg	100%	10 mg	100%
Calcium	54 mg	7%	108 mg	11%
Iron	9 mg	90%	18 mg	100%
Phosphorous	25 mg	3%	50 mg	5%
Iodine	75 mcg	107%	150 mcg	100%
Magnesium	20 mg	10%	40 mg	10%
Zinc	7.5 mg	94%	15 mg	100%
Copper	1 mg	100%	2 mg	100%
Vitamin K	5 mcg	*	10 mcg	*
Manganese	0.5 mg	*	1 mg	*
Chromium	10 mcg	*	20 mcg	*
Molybdenum	10 mcg	*	20 mcg	*

*Daily Value not established.

Store at Room Temperature.
© 1995

Sea World Characters ©1993 Sea World, Inc. All Rights Reserved.

Shamu and his Crew™ are trademarks and copyrights of Sea World, Inc.

CENTRUM, JR.®, The Spectrum Design and all other marks and indicia are trademarks and copyrights of Lederle.

CENTRUM® SILVER®
Specially Formulated Multivitamin-Multimineral for Adults 50+
Complete From A to Zinc®

Nutrition Facts
Serving Size 1 Tablet

Continued on next page

Lederle Consumer Health—Cont.

Each Tablet Contains	%DV
Vitamin A 5000 IU	100%
(50% as Beta Carotene)	
Vitamin C 60 mg	100%
Vitamin D 400 IU	100%
Vitamin E 45 IU	150%
Thiamin 1.5 mg	100%
Riboflavin 1.7 mg	100%
Niacinamide 20 mg	100%
Vitamin B$_6$ 3 mg	150%
Folic Acid 400 mcg	100%
Vitamin B$_{12}$ 25 mcg	416%
Biotin 30 mcg	10%
Pantothenic Acid 10 mg	100%
Calcium 200 mg	20%
Iron 4 mg	22%
Phosphorus 48 mg	5%
Iodine 150 mcg	100%
Magnesium 100 mg	25%
Zinc 15 mg	100%
Copper 2 mg	100%
Potassium 80 mg	2%
Vitamin K 10 mcg	*
Selenium 20 mcg	*
Manganese 3.5 mg	*
Chromium 130 mcg	*
Molybdenum 160 mcg	*
Chloride 72 mg	*
Nickel 5 mcg	*
Silicon 2 mg	*
Vanadium 10 mcg	*
Boron 150 mcg	*

*Daily Value (% DV) not established.

Recommended Intake:
Adults, 1 tablet daily.

Warning: Close tightly and keep out of reach of children. Contains iron, which can be harmful or fatal to children in large doses. In case of accidental overdose, seek professional assistance or contact a Poison Control Center immediately.

Ingredients: Calcium Carbonate, Calcium Phosphate, Magnesium Oxide, Potassium Chloride, Microcrystalline Cellulose, Ascorbic Acid (Vit. C), Gelatin, d*l*-alpha Tocopheryl Acetate (Vit. E), Modified Food Starch, Maltodextrin, Crospovidone, Ferrous Fumarate, Hydroxypropyl Methylcellulose, Niacinamide, Zinc Oxide, Calcium Pantothenate, Manganese Sulfate, Vitamin D, Titanium Dioxide, Vitamin A, Magnesium Stearate, Stearic Acid, Pyridoxine Hydrochloride (Vit. B$_6$), Riboflavin (Vit. B$_2$), Silicon Dioxide, Cupric Oxide, Beta Carotene, Dextrose, Thiamin Mononitrate (Vit. B$_1$), Triethyl Citrate, Polysorbate 80, Chromium Chloride, FD&C Blue #2, FD&C Yellow #6, Folic Acid, Potassium Iodide, FD&C Red #40, Sodium Metasilicate, Sodium Molybdate, Borates, Sodium Selenate, Biotin, Sodium Metavanadate, Cyanocobalamin (Vit. B$_{12}$), Nickelous Sulfate and Phytonadione (Vit. K).

How Supplied: Bottle of 60
Bottle of 100
Store at Room Temperature.
© 1995
Shown in Product Identification Guide, page 511

FERRO-SEQUELS®
[fer″rō-sē′quls]
High potency, time-release iron supplement.
Specially designed to optimize iron absorption, yet minimize digestive upset. Easy to swallow tablets.
Low sodium, no sugar.

The Ferro-Sequels timed-release system delivers iron slowly and gently to maximize absorption while reducing gastric upset common with regular iron tablets. Ferro-Sequels is the effective and gentle way to treat simple iron deficiency and iron deficiency anemia.

Nutrition Facts
Serving Size 1 Tablet

Each Tablet Contains	% Daily Value
Iron 50 mg	277%

Recommended Intake: One tablet daily or as directed by a health care professional.

Warning: Keep out of reach of children. Contains iron, which can be harmful or fatal to children in large doses. In case of accidental overdose, seek professional assistance or contact a Poison Control Center immediately. As with any supplement, if you are pregnant or nursing a baby, seek the advice of a health care professional before using this product.

Ingredients: Lactose, Ferrous Fumarate, Microcrystalline Cellulose, Hydroxypropyl Methylcellulose, Docusate Sodium, Magnesium Stearate, Sodium Benzoate, Silicon Dioxide, Mineral Oil, Titanium Dioxide, Yellow #10, Blue #1 and Sodium Lauryl Sulfate.
Store at Room Temperature.

How Supplied: Box of 30 tablets
Bottle of 30 tablets
Bottle of 100 tablets
Blister pack of 30 tablets
Store at Room Temperature
LEDERLE CONSUMER HEALTH
DIVISION
MADE IN USA
©1994

FIBERCON®
[fĭ-bĕr-cŏn]
Calcium Polycarbophil
Bulk-Forming Fiber Laxative

Indications: To help restore and maintain regularity, to relieve constipation, and to promote normal function of the bowel.

Directions: FIBERCON dosage will vary according to diet, exercise, previous laxative use or severity of constipation. FIBERCON works naturally so continued use for one to three days is normally required to provide full benefit. Recommended Adult Starting Dose: 2 or 4 caplets daily. May be increased up to 8 caplets daily.

Dosage Recommendations
Adults: 2 caplets 1 to 4 times a day.
Children (6 to 12 Years): 1 caplet 1 to 3 times a day.
Under 6 years: consult a physician.

TAKE THIS PRODUCT (CHILD OR ADULT DOSE) WITH AT LEAST 8 OUNCES (A FULL GLASS) OF WATER OR OTHER FLUID. TAKING THIS PRODUCT WITHOUT ENOUGH LIQUID MAY CAUSE CHOKING. SEE WARNINGS.

Warnings: Any sudden change in bowel habits may indicate a more serious condition than constipation. Consult your physician if symptoms such as nausea, vomiting, abdominal pain, or rectal bleeding occur or if this product has no effect within one week. For chronic or continued constipation consult your physician. TAKING THIS PRODUCT WITHOUT ADEQUATE FLUID MAY CAUSE IT TO SWELL AND BLOCK YOUR THROAT OR ESOPHAGUS AND MAY CAUSE CHOKING. DO NOT TAKE THIS PRODUCT IF YOU HAVE DIFFICULTY IN SWALLOWING. IF YOU EXPERIENCE CHEST PAIN, VOMITING, OR DIFFICULTY IN SWALLOWING OR BREATHING AFTER TAKING THIS PRODUCT, SEEK IMMEDIATE MEDICAL ATTENTION.

Interaction Precaution: Contains calcium. If you are taking any form of tetracycline antibiotic, FIBERCON should be taken at least 1 hour before or 2 hours after you have taken the antibiotic.
Keep this and all medicines out of the reach of children.

Ingredients: Each caplet contains 625 mg calcium polycarbophil equivalent to 500 mg polycarbophil.

Inactive Ingredients: Calcium Carbonate, Caramel, Crospovidone, Hydroxypropyl Methylcellulose, Magnesium Stearate, Microcrystalline Cellulose, Mineral Oil, Povidone, Silica Gel and Sodium Lauryl Sulfate.
Store At Controlled Room Temperature 15–30° C (59–86°F).
Protect Contents From Moisture.

TAMPER RESISTANT FEATURE:
Bottle sealed in clear plastic overwrap. Do not accept if plastic overwrap is torn.

If you have any questions or comments about **FIBERCON**, please call us **TOLL-FREE 1-800-282-8805.**
(Monday–Friday, 9:00 a.m. to 4.00 p.m. Eastern Time)

How Supplied: Film-coated caplets, scored, engraved LL and F66.
Package of 36 caplets, NDC 0005-2500-02
Package of 60 caplets, NDC 0005-2500-86
Bottle of 90 caplets, NDC 0005-2500-33
LEDERLE CONSUMER HEALTH DIVISION
Shown in Product Identification Guide, page 511

PROTEGRA®
[prō-tĕg-rǎ]
Antioxidant Vitamin & Mineral Supplement
Each softgel contains:

	For Adults—Percentage of US Recommended Daily Allowance (US RDA)	
Vitamin E	200 IU	667%
Vitamin C	250 mg	417%
Beta Carotene	3 mg	100%*
Zinc	7.5 mg	50%
Copper	1 mg	50%
Selenium	15 mcg	**
Manganese	1.5 mg	**

*US RDA for Vitamin A.
**No US RDA established but essential.

Inactive Ingredients: Gelatin, Cottonseed Oil, Glycerin, Dibasic Calcium Phosphate, Lecithin, Partially Hydrogenated Cottonseed and Soybean Oils, Beeswax, Titanium Dioxide, FD&C Yellow #6, and FD&C Red #40.

Recommended Intake: Adults: One softgel daily or as directed by your physician. PROTEGRA® can be taken by itself or with a multiple vitamin.

How Supplied: Bottle of 50
Store at Controlled Room Temperature 15°–30°C (59°–86°F)
Protect Contents From Moisture
Natural color variations in the softgels may occur.

Warning: Keep out of the reach of children.
Shown in Product Identification Guide, page 511

STRESSTABS®
[strĕss-tăbs]
High Potency
Stress Formula Vitamins

Nutrition Facts
Serving Size 1 Tablet

Each Tablet Contains	% Daily Value
Vitamin C 500 mg	833%
Vitamin E 30 IU	100%
Thiamin 10 mg	667%
Riboflavin 10 mg	588%
Niacinamide 100 mg	500%
Vitamin B_6 5 mg	250%
Folic Acid 400 mcg	100%
Vitamin B_{12} 12 mcg	200%
Biotin 45 mcg	15%
Pantothenic Acid 20 mg	200%

Recommended Intake: Adults, 1 tablet daily or as directed by physician.

Warning: Keep out of reach of children

Ingredients: Ascorbic Acid (Vit. C), Calcium Carbonate, Niacinamide, Microcrystalline Cellulose, dl-Tocopheryl Acetate (Vit. E), Modified Food Starch, Calcium Pantothenate, Thiamin Mononitrate (Vit. B_1), Riboflavin (Vit. B_2), Magnesium Stearate, Mineral Oil, Pyridoxine Hydrochloride (Vit. B_6), Silicon Dioxide, FD&C Yellow #6, Biotin, Stearic Acid, Cyanocobalamin (Vit. B_{12}) and Folic Acid.

How Supplied: Capsule-shaped tablet (film coated, orange, scored). Engraved LL and S1.
Bottle of 60
Store at Room Temperature.
LEDERLE CONSUMER HEALTH DIVISION

STRESSTABS® + IRON
[strĕss-tăbs]
High Potency
Stress Formula Vitamins

Nutrition Facts
Serving Size 1 Tablet

Each Tablet Contains	% Daily Value
Vitamin C 500 mg	833%
Vitamin E 30 IU	100%
Thiamin 10 mg	667%
Riboflavin 10 mg	588%
Niacinamide 100 mg	500%
Vitamin B_6 5 mg	250%
Folic Acid 400 mcg	100%
Vitamin B_{12} 12 mcg	200%
Biotin 45 mcg	15%
Pantothenic Acid 20 mg	200%
Iron 18 mg	100%

Recommended Intake: Adults, 1 tablet daily or as directed by the physician.

Warning: Always replace pop-lock top, close tightly, and keep out of reach of children. Contains iron, which can be harmful or fatal to children in large doses. In case of accidental overdose, seek professional assistance or contact a Poison Control Center immediately.

Ingredients: Ascorbic Acid (Vit. C), Calcium Carbonate, Niacinamide, Microcrystalline Cellulose, dl-Tocopheryl Acetate (Vit. E), Ferrous Fumarate, Modified Food Starch, Calcium Pantothenate, Thiamin Mononitrate (Vit. B_1), Stearic Acid, Riboflavin (Vit. B_2), Magnesium Stearate, Mineral Oil, Silicon Dioxide, Pyridoxine Hydrochloride (Vit. B_6), Biotin, FD&C Yellow #6, FD&C Red #40, Cyanocobalamin (Vit. B_{12}) and Folic Acid.

How Supplied: Capsule-shaped tablets (film coated, orange red, scored). Engraved LL and S2.
Bottle of 60
Store at Room Temperature.
LEDERLE CONSUMER HEALTH DIVISION
Shown in Product Identification Guide, page 511

STRESSTABS® + ZINC
[strĕss-tăbs]
High Potency
Stress Formula Vitamins

Nutrition Facts
Serving Size 1 Tablet

Each Tablet Contains	% Daily Value
Vitamin C 500 mg	833%
Vitamin E 30 IU	100%
Thiamin 10 mg	667%
Riboflavin 10 mg	588%
Niacinamide 100 mg	500%
Vitamin B_6 5 mg	250%
Folic Acid 400 mcg	100%
Vitamin B_{12} 12 mcg	200%
Biotin 45 mcg	15%
Pantothenic Acid 20 mg	200%
Zinc 23.9 mg	159%
Copper 3 mg	150%

Recommended Intake: Adults, 1 tablet daily or as directed by the physician.

Warning: Keep out of reach of children.

Ingredients: Ascorbic Acid (Vit. C), Calcium Carbonate, Niacinamide, Microcrystalline Cellulose, dl-Tocopheryl Acetate (Vit. E), Modified Food Starch, Calcium Pantothenate, Zinc Oxide, Thiamin Mononitrate (Vit. B_1), Riboflavin (Vit. B_2), Mineral Oil, Pyridoxine Hydrochloride (Vit. B_6), Silicon Dioxide, Biotin, Stearic Acid, Magnesium Stearate, Cupric Oxide, Cyanocobalamin (Vit. B_{12}), FD&C Yellow #6 and Folic Acid.

How Supplied: Capsule-shaped tablet (film coated, peach color, scored). Engraved LL and S3.
Bottle of 60
Store at Room Temperature.
LEDERLE CONSUMER HEALTH DIVISION

EDUCATIONAL MATERIAL

Everyone Needs to Know About Antioxidant Nutrients
6-page pamphlet explaining the importance of antioxidants in a healthy diet and good sources of antioxidants in food and vitamin supplements.

Continued on next page

Lederle Consumer Health—Cont.

Write to: Lederle Promotional Center
2200 Bradley Hill Road
Blauvelt, NY 10913

Lenes Pharmacal, Inc.
**1990 S.W. 27TH AVENUE
3RD FLOOR
MIAMI, FL 33145**

Direct Inquiries to:
P.O. Box 45-1350
(305) 858-8111

For Medical Emergency Contact:
Abdon S. Borges, Jr., M.D.
(305) 858-8111

VENOLAX
[vənōlax]
Ascorbic Acid & Pyridoxine HCl

DIETARY SUPPLEMENT
Each red coated tablet for oral administration contains:

		% U.S. RDA*
Ascorbic Acid	200mg	333.3
Pyridoxine HCL	7.5 mg	375.0

Manufactured in special base containing. Hamamelis Virginiana Leaves, Hydratis Canadensis, Aesculus Hippocastanum and Rutin for which no known need in human nutrition is established.

Indications: For use as Dietary Supplement, to relieve symptoms such as pain, cramps and heat sensation associated with faulty peripheral vascular circulation.

Usual Adult Dosage: Take 1 tablet 3 times daily or as directed by a physician.

Warning: Keep this and all drugs out of the reach of children. DO NOT USE IF IMPRINTED SAFETY SEAL IS BROKEN.
*U.S.A. Recommended Daily Allowance for adults and children 4 or more years of age.
In case of pregnancy or nursing consult your physician before using.
Store at controlled room temperature 15–30°C (59–80°).
Lot. No. 951128
Exp. 12–98.
NDC 495-23-20706
Manufactured by:
LEX INCORPORATED
Medley, Fl 33166
MANUFACTURED FOR
LENES PHARMACAL INC.
P.O. BOX 45-1350 • MIAMI, FL 33245-1350
Shown in Product Identification Guide, page 511

Lever Brothers Company
**390 PARK AVENUE
NEW YORK, NY 10022**

Direct Inquiries to:
(212) 688-6000

DOVE®

Active Ingredients: Sodium Cocoyl Isethionate, Stearic Acid, Sodium Tallowate, Water, Sodium Isethionate, Coconut Acid, Sodium Stearate, Sodium Dodecylbenzenesulfonate, Sodium Cocoate, Fragrance, Sodium Chloride, Titanium Dioxide.

Actions and Uses: Dove is specially formulated to be predictably gentle to all kinds of skin including those with common dermatoses. The mildness of Dove is suitable for Acne and Rosacea patients on drying topical medications and Dove is non-acnegenic, non-comedogenic and oil-free.
Dove is also available in Sensitive Skin Formula that provides clinically proven superior mildness in a nonsensitizing 100% fragrance-free formula.
A new addition to the Dove product line is also available: Dove® Moisturizing Body Wash, a cleanser with special moisturizers that replenish and protect skin's natural moisture for up to 8 hours.

Directions: Instruct patients to use Dove as they would any other cleanser.

How Supplied: Original Dove 3.5 oz. and 4.75 bars; Unscented Dove 4.75 oz.; Sensitive Skin Formula Dove 4.25 oz. bars. Liquid Dove Beauty Wash 6 oz. pump dispenser; Dove Moisturizing Body Wash 6 oz. starter kit, 10 oz. bottle.
Shown in Product Identification Guide, page 512

LEVER 2000®
Antibacterial Bar and Liquid

Active Ingredients: Triclosan. Other ingredients: Sodium tallowate, sodium cocoyl isethionate, sodium cocoate, water, sodium isethionate, stearic acid, coconut fatty acid, fragrance, titanium dioxide, sodium chloride, tetrasodium EDTA, disodium phosphate, trisodium etidronate, BHT.

Actions and Uses: Lever 2000® is the mildest antibacterial bar soap available. Lever 2000® offers broad spectrum antibacterial activity against both gram-negative and gram-positive pathogens. It is a useful adjunct to any therapeutic regimen that fights topical bacterial infection. It is also milder to the skin than any other antibacterial or deodorant bar soap. Lever 2000® has been proven mild enough for children's tender skin as young as 18 months and can also be used by adolescents and adults.

Directions: Instruct patients to use Lever 2000® as they would any other mild antibacterial or deodorant soap.

How Supplied: Antibacterial Lever 2000 5.0 oz bar, Liquid Lever 2000 7 oz pump, 14 oz refill; 28 oz Wall Dispenser.
Shown in Product Identification Guide, page 512

3M
**BUILDING 275-5W-05
ST PAUL, MN 55144-1000**

Direct Inquiries to:
Customer Service
(800) 537-2191

For Medical Emergencies Contact:
(612) 733-2882 (answered 24 hrs.)

Sales and Ordering or Returns:
(800) 832-2189

TITRALAC™ REGULAR AND EXTRA STRENGTH
[T ĭ' tră lăc]

Active Ingredients: Calcium Carbonate: *Regular:* 420mg./tablet (168 mg. elemental calcium). *Extra Strength:* 750mg/tablet (300 mg. elemental calcium).

Inactive Ingredients: Glycine, Magnesium Stearate, Saccharin, Spearmint Oil, Starch.

Indications: A spearmint flavored non-chalky antacid tablet which quickly relieves heartburn, sour stomach, acid indigestion and upset stomach associated with these symptoms.

Dosage and Administration: *Regular:* Two tablets every two or three hours as symptoms occur or as directed by a physician. Tablets can be chewed, swallowed or allowed to melt in the mouth. *Extra Strength:* One or two tablets every two or three hours as symptoms occur or as directed by a physician. Tablets can be chewed or allowed to melt in the mouth.

Warnings: *Regular:* Do not take more than 19 tablets in a 24-hour period or use maximum dosage for more than two weeks, except under the advise and supervision of a physician. *Extra Strength:* Do not take more than ten tablets in a 24-hour period or use maximum dosage for more than two weeks, except under the advice and supervision of a physician. **Keep this and all medication out of the reach of children**

Drug Interaction Precaution: Antacids may interact with certain prescription drugs. If you are presently taking a prescription drug, do not take this product without checking with your physician or other health professional.

Dietary Guidelines: Titralac™ Antacid is sodium free and sugar free. Also aluminum free.

How Supplied: *Regular:* Available in bottles of 40, 100, 1000 tablets. *Extra Strength:* Available in bottles of 100 tablets.
Shown in Product Identification Guide, page 512

PRODUCT INFORMATION/687

TITRALAC PLUS ANTACID
[T ĭ 'tră lăc]
TITRALAC PLUS™ LIQUID AND TABLETS

Active Ingredients: *Tablets:* Calcium Carbonate: 420 mg/tablet (168 mg elemental calcium), Simethicone: 21 mg/tablet. *Liquid:* Calcium Carbonate: 1000 mg/2 teaspoons (10 ml.) (400 mg elemental calcium), Simethicone: 40 mg/2 teaspoons (10 ml.)

Inactive Ingredients: *Tablets:* Glycine, Magnesium Stearate, Saccharin, Spearmint Oil, Starch. May also contain Croscarmellose Sodium. *Liquid:* Benzyl Alcohol, Colloidal Silicon Dioxide, Glyceryl Laurate, Methylparaben, Potassium Benzoate, Propylparaben, Saccharin, Sorbitol, Spearmint Flavor, Water, Xanthan Gum.

Indications: A spearmint flavored non-chalky antacid which quickly relieves heartburn, sour stomach, acid indigestion, and accompanying gas often associated with these symptoms.

Dosage and Administration: *Tablets:* Two tablets every two or three hours as symptoms occur or as directed by a physician. Tablets can be chewed, swallowed or allowed to melt in the mouth. *Liquid:* Two teaspoons, between meals and at bedtime or as directed by a physician. Shake well before using.

Warnings: *Tablets:* Do not take more than 19 tablets in a 24-hour period or use maximum dosage for more than two weeks, except under the advice and supervision of a physician. *Liquid:* do not take more than 16 teaspoons in a 24-hour period, or use maximum dosage for more than two weeks, except under the advice and supervision of a physician. Keep this and all medication out of the reach of children.

Drug Interaction Precaution: Antacids may interact with certain prescription drugs. If you are presently taking a prescription drug, do not take this product without checking with your physician or other health professional.

Dietary Guidelines: Tablets and liquid are sodium free, sugar free, and aluminum free.

How Supplied: *Tablets:* Available in bottles of 100 tablets. *Liquid:* Available in 12 fl. oz. bottles.

Shown in Product Identification Guide, page 512

Marlyn Nutraceuticals
14851 N. SCOTTSDALE RD
SCOTTSDALE, AZ 85254

Direct Inquiries to:
Kelly Easton
(602) 991-0200
FAX: (602) 991-0551

MARLYN FORMULA 50®

PRODUCT OVERVIEW

Key Facts: MARLYN FORMULA 50 is a combination of amino acids and B6 in a gelatin capsule which provides protein "building blocks" important to growth and development of all protein containing tissue including nails, hair and skin.

Major Uses: Dermatologists recommend Formula 50 not only for splitting, peeling nails but also prescribe it in conjunction with their favorite topical cream for control of nail fungus. OB-Gyn's recommend it for help in controlling excessive hair fall-out after child birth.
The recommended daily dose is six capsules daily.

Safety Information: There are no known contraindications or adverse reactions.

PRESCRIBING INFORMATION
MARLYN FORMULA 50®

Composition: Each capsule contains:
Amino Acids..............................0.3 Gm*
Vitamin B6 (pyridoxine HCl)......1.0 mg.
*Approximate analysis of the amino acids: indispensable amino acids (lysine, tryptophan, phenylalanine, methionine, threonine, leucine, isoleucine, valine), 35.30%; semi-dispensable amino acids (arginine, histidine, tyrosine, cystine, glycine), 19.18%; dispensable amino acids (glutamic acid, alanine, aspartic acid, serine, proline), 45.56%.
Amino acids: Protein "building blocks" important to growth and development of all protein containing tissue including nails, hair, and skin.

Dosage and Administration: The recommended daily dose is 6 capsules daily.

Supply: Bottles of 100, 250.

UNKNOWN DRUG?
Consult the
Product Identification Guide
(Gray Pages)
for full-color photos of
leading over-the-counter
medications

McNeil Consumer Products Company
Division of McNeil-PPC, Inc.
FORT WASHINGTON, PA 19034

Direct Inquiries to:
Consumer Affairs Department
Fort Washington, PA 19034
(215) 233-7000

Children's MOTRIN®
Ibuprofen Oral Suspension

Description: Children's MOTRIN Ibuprofen Oral Suspension is an alcohol-free, berry-flavored liquid specially developed for children. Each 5 ml (teaspoon) contains ibuprofen 100 mg.

Indications: Children's MOTRIN Ibuprofen Oral Suspension is indicated for temporary relief of fever, and minor aches and pains due to colds, flu, sore throat, headaches and toothaches. One dose lasts 6–8 hours.

Directions: Shake well before using. A calibrated dosage cup is provided for accurate dosing of Children's MOTRIN Suspension. If possible, use weight to dose; otherwise use age. 2–3 years (24–35 lbs): 1 tsp, 4–5 years (36–47 lbs): 1.5 tsp, 6–8 years (48–59 lbs): 2 tsp, 9–10 years (60–71 lbs): 2.5 tsp, 11 years (72–95 lbs): 3 tsp. Administer to children under 2 years only on advise of a physician. Repeat dose every 6–8 hours, if needed. Do not use more than 4 times a day.

Warnings: ASPIRIN SENSITIVE CHILDREN:
- **This product contains no aspirin, but may cause a severe reaction in people allergic to aspirin.**
- **Do not use this product if your child has had an allergic reaction to aspirin such as asthma, swelling, shock or hives.**

CALL YOUR DOCTOR IF:
- Your child is under a doctor's care for any serious condition or is taking any other drug.
- Your child has problems or serious side effects from taking fever reducers or pain relievers.
- Your child does not get any relief within first day (24 hours) of treatment, or pain or fever gets worse.
- Redness or swelling is present in the painful area.
- Sore throat is severe, lasts for more than 2 days or occurs with fever, headache, rash, nausea or vomiting.
- Any new symptoms appear.

DO NOT USE:
- With any other product that contains ibuprofen, aspirin, naproxen sodium, or acetaminophen.
- For more than **3 days** for fever or pain unless directed by a doctor.
- For stomach pain unless directed by a doctor.

Continued on next page

McNeil Consumer—Cont.

- If your child is dehydrated (significant fluid loss) due to continued vomiting, diarrhea or lack of fluid intake.
- If imprinted plastic bottle wrap or imprinted foil seal is broken.

IMPORTANT:
- **Keep this and all drugs out of the reach of children. In case of accidental overdose, seek professional assistance or contact a poison control center immediately.**
- If stomach upset occurs while taking this product, give with food or milk. If stomach upset gets worse or lasts, call your doctor.

Inactive Ingredients: Citric acid, corn starch, artificial flavors, glycerin, polysorbate 80, purified water, sodium benzoate, sucrose, xanthan gum, FD&C Red #40, D&C Yellow #10.

How Supplied: Orange colored liquid in tamper-resistant bottles of 2 and 4 fl. oz.
Shown in Product Identification Guide, page 512

CHILDREN'S TYLENOL®
acetaminophen
Chewable Tablets, Elixir, Drops
Suspension Liquid and Drops

Description: Infants' TYLENOL acetaminophen Drops are stable, alcohol-free, fruit-flavored and orange in color. Infants' TYLENOL Suspension Drops are alcohol-free, grape-flavored and purple in color. Each 0.8 ml (one calibrated dropperful) contains 80 mg acetaminophen. Children's TYLENOL Elixir is stable and alcohol-free, cherry-flavored, and red in color or grape-flavored, and purple in color. Children's TYLENOL Suspension Liquid is alcohol-free, cherry-flavored, and red in color or bubble gum flavored, and pink in color. Each 5 ml contains 160 mg acetaminophen. Each Children's TYLENOL Chewable Tablet contains 80 mg acetaminophen in a grape, fruit, or bubble gum flavor.

Actions: Acetaminophen is a clinically proven analgesic/antipyretic. Acetaminophen produces analgesia by elevation of the pain threshold and antipyresis through action on the hypothalamic heat regulating center. Acetaminophen is equal to aspirin in analgesic and antipyretic effectiveness and it is unlikely to produce many of the side effects associated with aspirin and aspirin containing products.

Indications: Children's TYLENOL Chewable Tablets, Elixir, Drops, Suspension Liquid and Suspension Drops are designed for treatment of infants and children with conditions requiring temporary relief of fever and discomfort due to colds and "flu," and of simple pain and discomfort due to teething, immunizations and tonsillectomy.

Precautions: If a rare sensitivity reaction occurs, the drug should be stopped.

Usual Dosage: All dosages may be repeated every 4 hours, but not more than 5 times daily. Administer to children under 2 years only on the advice of a physician. Children's TYLENOL Chewable Tablets: 2–3 years: two tablets. 4–5 years: three tablets, 6–8 years: four tablets. 9–10 years: five tablets. 11–12 years: six tablets.
Children's TYLENOL Elixir and Suspension Liquid: (special cup for measuring dosage is provided) 4–11 months: one-half teaspoon. 12–23 months: three-quarters teaspoon, 2–3 years: one teaspoon. 4–5 years: one and one-half teaspoons. 6–8 years: 2 teaspoons. 9–10 years: two and one-half teaspoons. 11–12 years: three teaspoons.
Infants' TYLENOL Drops and Suspension Drops: 0–3 months: 0.4 ml. 4–11 months: 0.8 ml. 12–23 months: 1.2 ml. 2–3 years: 1.6 ml. 4–5 years: 2.4 ml.

Warnings: Do not take for pain more than 5 days or for fever for more than 3 days unless directed by a physician. If pain or fever persists or gets worse, if new symptoms occur, or if redness or swelling is present, consult a physician because these could be signs of a serious condition. Keep this and all drugs out of the reach of children. In case of accidental overdose, contact a physician or poison control center immediately. Prompt medical attention is critical even if you do not notice any signs or symptoms. Do not use with other products containing acetaminophen.
NOTE: In addition to the above:
Infants' TYLENOL® Drops and Suspension Drops—Do not use if printed carton overwrap or printed plastic bottle wrap is broken or missing or if carton is opened.
Children's TYLENOL Elixir and Suspension Liquid—Do not use if printed carton overwrap is broken or missing or if carton is opened. Do not use if printed plastic bottle wrap or printed foil inner seal is broken. Not a USP elixir.
Children's TYLENOL Chewables—Do not use if carton is opened or if printed plastic bottle wrap or printed foil inner seal is broken. Phenylketonurics: contains phenylalanine 3 mg per tablet, bubble gum contains 3 mg per tablet.

Overdosage: Acetaminophen in massive overdosage may cause hepatic toxicity in some patients. In adults and adolescents, hepatic toxicity has rarely been reported following ingestion of acute overdoses of less than 10 grams. Fatalities are infrequent (less than 3–4% of untreated cases) and have rarely been reported with overdoses of less than 15 grams. In children, an acute overdosage of less than 150 mg/kg has not been associated with hepatic toxicity.
Early symptoms following a potentially hepatotoxic overdose may include: nausea, vomiting, diaphoresis and general malaise. Clinical and laboratory evidence of hepatic toxicity may not be apparent until 48 to 72 hours postingestion.

In adults and adolescents, regardless of the quantity of acetaminophen reported to have been ingested, administer MUCOMYST® acetylcysteine immediately if 24 hours or less have elapsed from the reported time of ingestion. For full prescribing information, refer to the MUCOMYST package insert. Do not await results of assays for acetaminophen level before initiating treatment with MUCOMYST acetylcysteine. The following additional procedures are recommended: The stomach should be emptied promptly by lavage or by induction of emesis with syrup of ipecac. A serum acetaminophen assay should be obtained as early as possible, but no sooner than four hours following ingestion. Liver function studies should be obtained initially and repeated at 24-hour intervals.
Serious toxicity or fatalities are extremely infrequent in children, possibly due to differences in the way they metabolize acetaminophen. In children, the maximum potential amount ingested can be more easily estimated. If more than 150 mg/kg or an unknown amount was ingested, obtain an acetaminophen plasma level. The acetaminophen plasma level should be obtained as soon as possible, but no sooner than 4 hours following the ingestion. Induce emesis using syrup of ipecac. If the plasma level is obtained and falls above the broken line on the acetaminophen overdose nomogram, the MUCOMYST acetylcysteine therapy should be initiated and continued for a full course of therapy. If acetaminophen plasma assay capability is not available, and the estimated acetaminophen ingestion exceeds 150 mg/kg, MUCOMYST acetylcysteine therapy should be initiated and continued for a full course of therapy.
For additional emergency information, call your regional poison center or call the Rocky Mountain Poison Center toll free, (1-800-525-6115).

Inactive Ingredients: Children's TYLENOL Fruit Flavored Chewable Tablets—Aspartame, Cellulose, Citric Acid, Cornstarch, Ethylcellulose, Flavors, Magnesium Stearate, Mannitol, and Red #7.
Children's TYLENOL Grape Flavored Chewable Tablets—Aspartame, Cellulose, Cellulose Acetate, Citric Acid, Cornstarch, Flavors, Magnesium Stearate, Mannitol, Povidone. Blue #1, Red #7, and Red #30.
Children's TYLENOL Bubble Gum Flavored Chewable Tablets—Aspartame, Cellulose, Cellulose Acetate, Cornstarch, Flavors, Magnesium Stearate, Mannitol, Povidone and Red #7.
Children's TYLENOL Elixir—Benzoic Acid, Citric Acid, Flavors, Glycerin, Polyethylene Glycol, Propylene Glycol, Sodium Benzoate, Sorbitol, Sucrose, Purified Water, Red #40. In addition to the above ingredients cherry flavored elixir contains Red #33 and grape flavored elixir contains Malic Acid and Blue #1.

Children's TYLENOL Suspension Liquid—Butylparaben, Cellulose, Citric Acid, Corn Syrup, Flavors, Glycerin, Propylene Glycol, Purified Water, Sodium Benzoate, Sorbitol, Xanthan Gum, FD&C Red #40. In addition to the above ingredients bubble gum flavored suspension contains D&C Red #33.

Infant's TYLENOL Drops—Butylparaben, Citric Acid, Flavors, Glycerin, Polyethylene Glycol, Propylene Glycol, Saccharin, Sodium Citrate, Purified Water and Yellow #6.

Infant's TYLENOL Suspension Drops—Butylparaben, Cellulose, Citric Acid, Corn Syrup, Flavors, Glycerin, Propylene Glycol, Purified Water, Sodium Benzoate, Sorbitol, Xanthan Gum, D&C Red #33 and D&C Blue #1.

How Supplied: Chewable Tablets (pink colored fruit, purple colored grape, pink colored bubble gum, scored, imprinted "TYLENOL")—Bottles of 30 and child resistant blister packs of 48 (fruit only). Elixir (cherry colored red and grape colored purple), Suspension liquid (cherry colored red)—bottles of 2 and 4 fl. oz. (bubble gum flavored colored pink)—bottle of 4 fl. oz. Drops (colored orange)—bottle of ½ oz. (15 ml.) and 1 oz. (30 ml.) with calibrated plastic dropper. Suspension drops (grape colored purple)—bottles of ½ oz (15 ml) with calibrated plastic dropper.
All packages listed above have child-resistant safety caps.

Shown in Product Identification Guide, page 512 & 513

CHILDREN'S TYLENOL COLD®
Multi Symptom Chewable Tablets and Liquid

Description: Each CHILDREN'S TYLENOL COLD Multi Symptom Chewable Grape-Flavored Tablet contains acetaminophen 80 mg, chlorpheniramine maleate 0.5 mg and pseudoephedrine hydrochloride 7.5 mg. CHILDREN'S TYLENOL COLD Multi Symptom Liquid is grape flavored and contains no alcohol. Each teaspoon (5 ml) contains acetaminophen 160 mg, chlorpheniramine maleate 1 mg, and pseudoephedrine hydrochloride 15 mg.

Actions: CHILDREN'S TYLENOL COLD Multi Symptom Chewable Tablets and Liquid combine the analgesic-antipyretic acetaminophen with the decongestant pseudoephedrine hydrochloride and the antihistamine chlorpheniramine maleate to help relieve nasal congestion, dry runny noses and prevent sneezing as well as to relieve the fever, aches, pains and general discomfort associated with colds and upper respiratory infections. Acetaminophen is equal to aspirin in analgesic and antipyretic effectiveness and it is unlikely to produce the side effects often associated with aspirin or aspirin-containing products.

Indications: Provides fast, effective temporary relief of nasal congestion, runny nose, sore throat, sneezing, minor aches and pains, headaches and fever due to the common cold, hay fever or other upper respiratory allergies.

Precautions: If a rare sensitivity reaction occurs, the drug should be stopped.

Usual Dosage: All doses may be repeated every 4–6 hours, not to exceed 4 doses in 24 hours.
Administer to children under 6 years only on the advice of a physician. Children's Tylenol Cold Chewable Tablets: 2–5 years—2 tablets: 6–11 years—4 tablets.
Children's Tylenol Cold Liquid Formula: 2–5 years—1 teaspoonful; 6–11 years—2 teaspoonsful. Measuring cup is provided and marked for accurate dosing.

Warning: KEEP THIS AND ALL MEDICATION OUT OF THE REACH OF CHILDREN. IN CASE OF ACCIDENTAL OVERDOSAGE, CONTACT A PHYSICIAN OR POISON CONTROL CENTER IMMEDIATELY. PROMPT MEDICAL ATTENTION IS CRITICAL EVEN IF YOU DO NOT NOTICE ANY SIGNS OR SYMPTOMS. DO NOT USE WITH OTHER PRODUCTS CONTAINING ACETAMINOPHEN. DO NOT EXCEED RECOMMENDED DOSAGE. Do not take for pain for more than 5 days or for fever for more than 3 days unless directed by a doctor, if pain or fever persists or get worse. If new symptoms occur, or if redness or swellin gis present, consult a doctor because these could be signs of a serious condition. If sore throat is severe, persists for more than 2 days, is accompanied or followed by fever, headache, rash, nausea, or vomiting, consult a doctor promptly. If nervousness, dizziness, or sleeplessness occur discontinue use and consult a doctor. May cause excitability especially in children. Do not give this product to children who have a breathing problem such as chronic bronchitis, or who have glaucoma, heart disease, high blood pressure, thyroid disease, or diabetes without first consulting the child's physician. May cause drowsiness. Sedatives and tranquilizers may increase the drowsiness effect. Do not give this product to children who are taking sedatives or tranquilizers, without first consulting the child's doctor.
NOTE: In addition to the above:
Children's TYLENOL COLD Chewables—DO NOT USE IF CARTON IS OPENED, OR IF PRINTED NECK WRAP OR PRINTED FOIL INNER SEAL IS BROKEN. PHENYLKETONURICS: CONTAINS PHENYLALANINE 6 MG PER TABLET.
Children's TYLENOL COLD Liquid—DO NOT USE IF CARTON IS OPENED, OR IF PRINTED PLASTIC BOTTLE WRAP OR PRINTED FOIL INNER SEAL IS BROKEN.

Drug Interaction Precaution: Do not give this product to a child who is taking a prescription monamine omidase inhibitor (MAOI) (certain drugs for depression, psychiatric or emotional conditions), or for 2 weeks after stopping the MAOI drug. If you are uncertain whether your child's prescription drug contains an MAOI, consult a health professional before giving this product.

Overdosage: Acetaminophen in massive overdosage may cause hepatic toxicity in some patients. In adults and adolescents, hepatic toxicity has rarely been reported following ingestion of acute overdosage of less than 10 grams. Fatalities are infrequent (less than 3–4% of untreated cases) and have rarely been reported with overdoses of less than 15 grams. In children, an acute overdosage of less than 150 mg/kg has not been associated with hepatic toxicity.
Early symptoms following a potentially hepatotoxic overdose may include: nausea, vomiting, diaphoresis and general malaise. Clinical and laboratory evidence of hepatic toxicity may not be apparent until 48 to 72 hours postingestion. In adults and adolescents, regardless of the quantity of acetaminophen reported to have been ingested, administer MUCOMYST® acetylcysteine immediately if 24 hours or less have elapsed from the reported time of ingestion. For full prescribing information, refer to the MUCOMYST package insert. Do not await the results of assays for acetaminophen level before initiating treatment with MUCOMYST acetylcysteine. The following additional procedures are recommended: The stomach should be emptied promptly by lavage or by induction of emesis with syrup of ipecac. A plasma acetaminophen assay should be obtained as early as possible, but no sooner than four hours following ingestion. Liver function studies should be obtained initially and repeated at 24-hour intervals.
Serious toxicity or fatalities are extremely infrequent in children, possibly due to differences in the way they metabolize acetaminophen. In children, the maximum potential amount ingested can be more easily estimated. If more than 150 mg/kg or an unknown amount was ingested, obtain an plasma acetaminophen level. The acetaminophen plasma level should be obtained as soon as possible, but no sooner than 4 hours following the ingestion. Induce emesis using syrup of ipecac. If the plasma level is obtained and falls above the broken line on the acetaminophen overdose nomogram, the MUCOMYST acetylcysteine therapy should be initiated and continued for a full course of therapy. If acetaminophen plasma assay capability is not available, and the estimated acetaminophen ingestion exceeds 150 mg/kg, MUCOMYST acetylcysteine therapy should be initiated and continued for a full course of therapy.
For additional emergency information, call your regional poison center or call the Rocky Mountain Poison Center toll-free, (1-800-525-6115).

Continued on next page

McNeil Consumer—Cont.

Chlorpheniramine toxicity should be treated as you would an antihistamine/anticholinergic overdose and is likely to be present within a few hours after acute ingestion.

Symptoms from pseudoephedrine overdose consist most often of mild anxiety, tachycardia and/or mild hypertension. Symptoms usually appear within 4 to 8 hours of ingestion and are transient, usually requiring no treatment.

Inactive Ingredients: Chewable Tablets—Aspartame, Basic Polymuth acrylate, cellulose acetate, citric acid, flavors, hydroxypropyl methylcellulose, magnesium stearate, mannitol, microcrystalline cellulose, Blue #1, Red #7. Liquid—Benzoic acid, citric acid, flavors, glycerin, malic acid, polyethylene glycol, propylene glycol, sodium benzoate, sorbitol, sucrose, purified water, Blue #1 and Red #40.

How Supplied: Chewable Tablets (colored purple, scored, imprinted "Tylenol Cold") on one side and "TC" on opposite side—bottles of 24. Cold Formula—bottles (colored purple) of 4 fl. oz.
Shown in Product Identification Guide, page 513

CHILDREN'S TYLENOL® COLD Multi Symptom PLUS COUGH
Chewable Tablets and Liquid

Description: Each CHILDREN'S TYLENOL COLD Multi Symptom PLUS COUGH Chewable Cherry-Flavored Tablet contains:
  acetaminophen 80 mg
  chlorpheniramine maleate 0.5 mg
  dextromethorphan hydrobromide 2.5 mg
  pseudoephedrine hydrochloride 7.5 mg
CHILDREN'S TYLENOL COLD Multi Symptom PLUS COUGH Liquid is cherry flavored and contains no alcohol. Each teaspoon (5 ml) contains acetaminophen 160 mg, chlorpheniramine maleate 1 mg, dextromethorphan hydrobromide 5 mg and pseudoephedrine hydrochloride 15 mg.

Actions: CHILDREN'S TYLENOL COLD Multi Symptom PLUS COUGH Chewable Tablets and Liquid combines the analgesic-antipyretic acetaminophen with the decongestant pseudoephedrine hydrochloride, the cough suppressant dextromethorphan hydrobromide, and the antihistamine chlorpheniramine maleate to help relieve coughs, nasal congestion, and sore throat, dry runny noses, and prevent sneezing as well as to relieve the fever, aches, pains and general discomfort associated with colds and upper respiratory infections.
Acetaminophen is equal to aspirin in analgesic and antipyretic effectiveness and it is unlikely to produce the side effects often associated with aspirin or aspirin-containing products.

Indications: For temporary relief of coughs, nasal congestion, runny nose, sore throat, sneezing, minor aches and pains, headaches and fever due to the common cold, hay fever or other upper respiratory allergies.

Precaution: If a rare sensitivity reaction occurs, the drug should be stopped.

Directions: All doses may be repeated every 4–6 hours, not to exceed 4 doses in 24 hours.
Administer to children under 6 years only on the advice of a physician.
Children's Tylenol Cold Plus Cough Chewable Tablets: 2–5 years—2 tablets, 6–11 years—4 tablets.
Children's Tylenol Cold Plus Cough Liquid Formula: 2–5 years—1 teaspoonful, 6–11 years—2 teaspoonfuls. Measuring cup is provided and marked for accurate dosing.

Warning: KEEP THIS AND ALL MEDICATION OUT OF THE REACH OF CHILDREN. IN CASE OF ACCIDENTAL OVERDOSE, CONTACT A DOCTOR OR POISON CONTROL CENTER IMMEDIATELY. PROMPT MEDICAL ATTENTION IS CRITICAL EVEN IF YOU DO NOT NOTICE ANY SIGNS OR SYMPTOMS. DO NOT USE WITH OTHER PRODUCTS CONTAINING ACETAMINOPHEN. DO NOT EXCEED RECOMMENDED DOSAGE. Do not take for pain for more than 5 days or for fever for more than 3 days unless directed by a doctor. If pain or fever persists for gets worse, if new symptoms occur, or if redness or swelling is present, consult a doctor because these could be signs of a serious condition. If sore throat is severe, persists for more than 2 days, is accompanied or followed by fever, headache, rash, nausea or vomiting, consult a doctor promptly. If nervousness, dizziness, or sleeplessness occur, discontinue use and consult a doctor. May cause excitability especially in children. Do not give this product to children who have a breathing problem such as chronic bronchitis, or who have glaucoma, heart disease, high blood pressure, thyroid disease, or diabetes, without first consulting the child's doctor. May cause drowsiness. Sedatives and tranquilizers may increase the drowsiness effect. Do not give this product to children who are taking sedatives or tranquilizers, without first consulting the child's doctor. A persistent cough may be a sign of a serious condition. If cough persists for more than 1 week, tends to recur, or is accompanied by fever, rash or persistent headache, consult a doctor. Do not give this product for persistent or chronic cough such as occurs with asthma or if cough is accompanied by excessive phlegm (mucus) unless directed by a doctor.
NOTE: In addition to the above:
Chewable Tablets—DO NOT USE IF CARTON IS OPENED, OR IF PRINTED NECK WRAP OR PRINTED FOIL INNER SEAL IS BROKEN. PHENYLKETONURICS: CONTAINS PHENYLALANINE 4 MG PER TABLET.

Liquid—DO NOT USE IF CARTON IS OPENED, OR IF PRINTED PLASTIC BOTTLE WRAP OR PRINTED FOIL INNER SEAL IS BROKEN.

Drug Interaction Precaution: Do not give this product to a child who is taking a prescription monoamine oxidase inhibitor (MAOI) (certain drugs for depression, psychiatric or emotional conditions), or for 2 weeks after stopping the MAOI drug. If you are uncertain whether your child's prescription drug contains an MAOI, consult a health professional before giving this product.

Overdosage Information: Acetaminophen in massive overdosage may cause hepatic toxicity in some patients. In adults and adolescents, hepatic toxicity has rarely been reported following ingestion of acute overdoses of less than 10 grams. Fatalities are infrequent (less than 3–4% of untreated cases) and have rarely been reported with overdoses of less than 15 grams. In children, an acute overdosage of less than 150 mg/kg has not been associated with hepatic toxicity. Early symptoms following a potentially hepatotoxic overdose may include: nausea, vomiting, diaphoresis and general malaise. Clinical and laboratory evidence of hepatic toxicity may not be apparent until 48 to 72 hours postingestion. In adults and adolescents, regardless of the quantity of acetaminophen reported to have been ingested, administer acetylcysteine immediately if 24 hours or less have elapsed from the reported time of ingestion. For full prescribing information, refer to the acetylcysteine package insert. Do not await the results of assays for plasma acetaminophen level before initiating treatment with acetylcysteine. The following additional procedures are recommended: The stomach should be emptied promptly by lavage or by induction of emesis with syrup of ipecac. A plasma acetaminophen assay should be obtained as early as possible, but no sooner than four hours following ingestion. If plasma level falls above the lower treatment line on the acetaminophen overdose nomogram, acetylcysteine therapy should be continued. Liver function studies should be obtained initially and repeated at 24-hour intervals.
Serious toxicity or fatalities are extremely infrequent in children, possibly due to differences in the way they metabolize acetaminophen. In children, the maximum potential amount ingested can be more easily estimated. If more than 150 mg/kg or an unknown amount was ingested, obtain an plasma acetaminophen level. The plasma acetaminophen level should be obtained as soon as possible, but no sooner than 4 hours following the ingestion. If plasma level falls above the lower treatment line on the acetaminophen overdose nomogram, the acetylcysteine therapy should be initiated and continued for a full course of therapy. If plasma acetaminophen assay capability is not available, and the estimated acetaminophen ingestion exceeds 150 mg/kg, acetylcysteine therapy

should be initiated and continued for a full course of therapy.

For additional emergency information, call your regional poison center or call the Rocky Mountain Poison Center toll-free, (1-800-525-6115).

Chlorpheniramine toxicity should be treated as you would an antihistamine/anticholinergic overdose and is likely to be present within a few hours after acute ingestion.

Symptoms from pseudoephedrine overdose consist most often of mild anxiety, tachycardia and/or mild hypertension. Symptoms usually appear within 4 to 8 hours of ingestion and are transient, usually requiring no treatment.

Acute dextromethorphan overdose usually does not result in serious signs and symptoms unless massive amounts have been ingested. Signs and symptoms of a substantial overdose may include nausea and vomiting, visual disturbances, CNS disturbances, and urinary retention.

Inactive Ingredients: Chewable Tablets—Aspartame, Basic Polymethacrylate, Cellulose Acetate, Colloidal Silicon Dioxide, Flavors, Hydroxypropyl Methylcellulose, Mannitol, Microcrystalline Cellulose, Stearic Acid and Red #7. Liquid—Citric Acid, Corn Syrup, Flavors, Polyethylene Glycol, Propylene Glycol, Sodium Benzoate, Sodium Carboxymethylcellulose, Sorbitol, Purified Water, Red #33 and Red #40.

How Supplied: Chewable Tablets (colored pink, imprinted "TYLENOL C/C" on one side and "TC/C" on the opposite side)—bottles of 24.
Liquid Formula—(red colored) bottles of 4 fl. oz.

Shown in Product Identification Guide, page 513

INFANTS' TYLENOL® COLD
Decongestant & Fever Reducer Drops

Description: INFANTS' TYLENOL COLD Decongestant & Fever Reducer Drops are alcohol-free, bubble gum flavored and red in color. Each 0.8 ml (dropperful) contains acetaminophen 80 mg and pseudoephedrine HCl 7.5 mg.

Actions: Acetaminophen is a clinically proven analgesic/antipyretic. Acetaminophen produces analgesia by elevation of the pain threshold and antipyresis through action on the hypothalamic heat regulating center. Acetaminophen is equal to aspirin in analgesic and antipyretic effectiveness and it is unlikely to product many of the side effects associated with aspirin and aspirin containing products. Pseudoephedrine hydrochloride is a sympathomimetic amine which provides temporary relief of nasal congestion.

Indications: INFANTS' TYLENOL COLD Decongestant & Fever Reducer Drops are indicated for the temporary relief of nasal congestion, minor aches and pains, headaches and fever due to

the common cold, hay fever or other upper respiratory allergies.

Precautions: If a rare sensitivity reaction occurs, the drug should be stopped.

Usual Dosage: All dosages may be repeated every 4–6 hours, but not more than 4 times daily. Administer to children under 2 years only on the advice of a physician. 0–3 months: 0.4 ml, 4–11 months: 0.8 ml, 12–23 months: 1.2 ml, 2–3 years: 1.6 ml, 4–5 years: 2.4 ml.

Warnings: Do not use if printed carton overwrap or printed plastic bottle wrap is broken or missing or if carton is opened. Keep this and all medication out of the reach of children. In case of accidental overdose, contact a doctor or poison control center immediately. Prompt medical attention is critical even if you do not notice any signs or symptoms. Do not exceed recommended dosage. Do not take for pain for more than 5 days or for fever for more than 3 days unless directed by a doctor. If pain or fever persists or get worse, if new symptoms occur, or if redness or swelling is present, consult a doctor because these could be signs of a serious condition. If nervousness, dizziness or sleeplessness occur, discontinue use and consult a doctor. Do not give this product to a child who has heart disease, high blood pressure, thyroid disease, or diabetes unless directed by a doctor. Do not use with other products containing acetaminophen.

Drug Interaction Precaution: Do not give this product to a child who is taking a prescription monoamine oxidase inhibitor (MAOI) (certain drugs for depression, psychiatric or emotional conditions), or for 2 weeks after stopping the MAOI drug. If you are uncertain whether your child's prescription drug contains an MAOI, consult a health professional before giving this product.

Overdosage Information: Acetaminophen in massive overdosage may cause hepatic toxicity in some patients. In adults and adolescents, hepatic toxicity has rarely been reported following ingestion of acute overdoses of less than 10 grams. Fatalities are infrequent (less than 3–4% of untreated cases) and have rarely been reported with overdoses of less than 15 grams. In children, an acute overdosage of less than 150 mg/kg has not been associated with hepatic toxicity. Early symptoms following a potentially hepatotoxic overdose may include: nausea, vomiting, diaphoresis and general malaise. Clinical and laboratory evidence of hepatic toxicity may not be apparent until 48 to 72 hours postingestion. In adults and adolescents, regardless of the quantity of acetaminophen reported to have been ingested, administer acetylcysteine immediately if 24 hours or less have elapsed from the reported time of ingestion. For full prescribing information, refer to the acetylcysteine package insert. Do not await results of assays for plasma acetaminophen level before initi-

ating treatment with acetylcysteine. The following additional procedures are recommended. The stomach should be emptied promptly by lavage or by induction of emesis with syrup of ipecac. A plasma acetaminophen assay should be obtained as early as possible, but no sooner than four hours following ingestion. If plasma level falls above the lower treatment line on the acetaminophen overdose nomogram, acetylcysteine therapy should be continued. Liver function studies should be obtained initially and repeated at 24-hour intervals.

Serious toxicity or fatalities are extremely infrequent in children, possibly due to differences in the way they metabolize acetaminophen. In children, the maximum potential amount ingested can be more easily estimated. If more than 150 mg/kg or an unknown amount was ingested, obtain a plasma acetaminophen level. The plasma acetaminophen level should be obtained as soon as possible, but no sooner than 4 hours following the ingestion. If plasma level falls above the lower treatment line on the acetaminophen overdose nomogram, the acetylcysteine therapy should be initiated and continued for a full course of therapy. If plasma acetaminophen assay capability is not available, and the estimated acetaminophen ingestion exceeds 150 mg/kg, acetylcysteine therapy should be initiated and continued for a full course of therapy.

For additional emergency information, call your regional poison center or call the Rocky Mountain Poison Center toll-free (1-800-525-6115).

Symptoms from pseudoephedrine overdose consist most often of mild anxiety, tachycardia and/or mild hypertension. Symptoms usually appear within 4 to 8 hours of ingestion and are transient, usually requiring no treatment.

Inactive Ingredients: Citric acid, corn syrup, flavors, polyethylene glycol, propylene glycol, purified water, sodium benzoate, saccharin, FD&C red #40.

How Supplied: Drops (colored red)—bottles of ½ fl. oz.

Shown in Product Identification Guide, page 513

IMODIUM® A-D
(loperamide hydrochloride)

Description: Each 5 ml (teaspoon) of Imodium A-D liquid contains loperamide hydrochloride 1 mg. Imodium A-D liquid is stable, cherry flavored, and clear in color.
Each caplet of Imodium AD contains 2 mg of loperamide and is scored and colored green.

Actions: Imodium A-D contains a clinically proven antidiarrheal medication. Loperamide HCl acts by slowing intestinal motility and by affecting water and electrolyte movement through the bowel.

Continued on next page

McNeil Consumer—Cont.

Indication: Imodium A-D is indicated for the control and symptomatic relief of acute nonspecific diarrhea, including travelers' diarrhea.

Usual Dosage: Adults: Take four teaspoonfuls or two caplets after first loose bowel movement. If needed, take two teaspoonfuls or one caplet after each subsequent loose bowel movement. Do not exceed eight teaspoonfuls or four caplets in any 24 hour period, unless directed by a physician.

9–11 years old (60–95 lbs.): Two teaspoonfuls or one caplet after first loose bowel movement, followed by one teaspoonful or one-half caplet after each subsequent loose bowel movement. Do not exceed six teaspoonfuls or three caplets a day.

6–8 years old (48–59 lbs.): Two teaspoonfuls or one caplet after first loose bowel movement, followed by one teaspoonful or one-half caplet after each subsequent loose bowel movement. Do not exceed four teaspoonfuls or two caplets a day. Professional Dosage Schedule for children two-five years old (24–47 lbs): one teaspoon after first loose bowel movement, followed by one after each subsequent loose bowel movement. Do not exceed three teaspoonfuls a day.

Warnings: KEEP THIS AND ALL DRUGS OUT OF THE REACH OF CHILDREN. Do not use for more than two days unless directed by a physician. DO NOT USE IF DIARRHEA IS ACCOMPANIED BY HIGH FEVER (GREATER THAN 101°F), OR IF BLOOD OR MUCUS IS PRESENT IN THE STOOL, OR IF YOU HAVE HAD A RASH OR OTHER ALLERGIC REACTION TO LOPERAMIDE HCl. If you are taking antibiotics or have a history of liver disease, consult a physician before using this product. As with any drug, if you are pregnant or nursing a baby, seek the advice of a health professional before using this product. In case of accidental overdose, seek professional assistance or contact a poison control center immediately.

Overdosage: Overdosage of loperamide HCl in man may result in constipation, CNS depression and nausea. A slurry of activated charcoal administered promptly after ingestion of loperamide hydrochloride can reduce the amount of drug which is absorbed. If vomiting occurs spontaneously upon ingestion, a slurry of 100 grams of activated charcoal should be administered orally as soon as fluids can be retained. If vomiting has not occurred, and CNS depression is evident, gastric lavage should be performed followed by administration of 100 gms of the activated charcoal slurry through the gastric tube. In the event of overdosage, patients should be monitored for signs of CNS depression for at least 24 hours. Children may be more sensitive to central nervous system effects than adults. If CNS depression is

observed, naloxone may be administered. If responsive to naloxone, vital signs must be monitored carefully for recurrence of symptoms of drug overdose for at least 24 hours after the last dose of naloxone.

Inactive Ingredients: Liquid: Alcohol (5.25%), citric acid, flavors, glycerin, methylparaben, propylparaben and purified water.
Caplets: Dibasic calcium phosphate, magnesium stearate, microcrystalline cellulose, colloidal silicon dioxide, FD&C Blue #1 and D&C Yellow #10.

How Supplied: Cherry flavored liquid (clear) 2 fl. oz., and 4 fl. oz. tamper resistant bottles with child resistant safety caps and special dosage cups.
Green Scored caplets in 6's and 12's and 18's blister packaging which is tamper resistant and child resistant.

Shown in Product Identification Guide, page 512

JUNIOR STRENGTH TYLENOL®
acetaminophen
Coated Caplets and Chewable Tablets

Description: Each Junior Strength TYLENOL Coated Caplet or Chewable Tablet contains 160 mg acetaminophen in a small, coated, capsule shaped tablet or grape or fruit flavored chewable tablet.

Actions: Acetaminophen is a clinically proven analgesic/antipyretic. Acetaminophen produces analgesia by elevation of the pain threshold and antipyresis through action on the hypothalamic heat-regulating center. Acetaminophen is equal to aspirin in analgesic and antipyretic effectiveness and it is unlikely to produce many of the side effects associated with aspirin and aspirin-containing products.

Indications: Junior Strength TYLENOL Caplets are designed for easy swallowability in older children and young adults. Both Junior Strength TYLENOL Caplets and Junior Strength Chewable Tablets provide fast, effective temporary relief of fever and discomfort due to colds and "flu," and pain and discomfort due to simple headaches, minor muscle aches, sprains and overexertion.

Precautions: If a rare sensitivity reaction occurs, the drug should be stopped.

Usual Dosage: Caplets should be taken with liquid. Chewable tablets should be well chewed. All dosages may be repeated every 4 hours, but not more than 5 times daily. For ages: 6–8 years: two caplets or tablets, 9–10 years: two and one-half caplets or tablets, 11 years: three caplets or tablets, 12 years: four caplets or tablets.

Warning: Do not use if carton is opened or if a blister unit is broken. Do not take for pain for more than 5 days or for fever for more than 3 days unless directed by a physician. If pain or fever persists or gets worse, if new symptoms oc-

cur, or if redness or swelling is present consult a physician because these could be signs of a serious condition. Keep this and all drugs out of reach of children. In case of accidental overdose, contact a physican or poison control center immediately. Prompt medical attention is critical even if you do not notice any signs or symptoms. Do not use with other products containing acetaminophen. As with any drug, if you are pregnant or nursing a baby, seek the advice of a health professional before using this product. In addition the caplet package states: Not for children who have difficulty swallowing tablets. In addition the Chewable Tablet package states: Phenylketonurics: contains phenylalanine 6 mg per tablet.

Overdosage: Acetaminophen in massive overdosage may cause hepatic toxicity in some patients. In adults and adolescents, hepatic toxicity has rarely been reported following ingestion of acute overdosage of less than 10 grams. Fatalities are infrequent (less than 3–4% of untreated cases) and have rarely been reported with overdoses of less than 15 grams. In children, an acute overdosage of less than 150 mg/kg has not been associated with hepatic toxicity.
Early symptoms following a potentially hepatotoxic overdose may include: nausea, vomiting, diaphoresis and general malaise. Clinical and laboratory evidence of hepatic toxicity may not be apparent until 48 to 72 hours postingestion. In adults and adolescents, regardless of the quantity of acetaminophen reported to have been ingested, administer MUCOMYST® acetylcysteine immediately if 24 hours or less have elapsed from the reported time of ingestion. For full prescribing information, refer to the MUCOMYST package insert. Do not await the results of assays for acetaminophen level before initiating treatment with MUCOMYST acetylcysteine. The following additional procedures are recommended: The stomach should be emptied promptly by lavage or by induction of emesis with syrup of ipecac. A serum acetaminophen assay should be obtained as early as possible, but no sooner than four hours following ingestion. Liver function studies should be obtained initially and repeated at 24-hour intervals.
Serious toxicity or fatalities are extremely infrequent in children, possibly due to differences in the way they metabolize acetaminophen. In children, the maximum potential amount ingested can be more easily estimated. If more than 150 mg/kg or an unknown amount was ingested, obtain an acetaminophen plasma level. The acetaminophen plasma level should be obtained as soon as possible, but no sooner than 4 hours following the ingestion. Induce emesis using syrup of ipecac. If the plasma level is obtained and falls above the broken line on the acetaminophen overdose nomogram, the MUCOMYST acetylcysteine therapy should be initiated and continued for a full course of therapy. If acet-

aminophen plasma assay capability is not available, and the estimated acetaminophen ingestion exceeds 150 mg/kg, MUCOMYST acetylcysteine therapy should be initiated and continued for a full course of therapy.

For additional emergency information, call your regional poison center or call the Rocky Mountain Poison Center toll-free (1-800-525-6115).

Inactive Ingredients: Junior Strength Caplets: Cellulose, Cornstarch, Ethylcellulose, Magnesium Stearate, Sodium Lauryl Sulfate, Sodium Starch Glycolate.

Junior Strength Fruit Chewable Tablets: Aspartame, Cellulose, Citric acid, Cornstarch, Ethylcellulose, Flavors, Magnesium Stearate, Mannitol, and Red #7.

Junior Strength Grape Flavored Chewable Tablets: Aspartame, Cellulose, Cellulose Acetate, Citric Acid, Cornstarch, Flavors, Magnesium Stearate, Mannitol, Povidone, Blue #1, Red #7 and Red #30.

How Supplied: Coated Caplets, (colored white, coated, scored, imprinted "TYLENOL 160") Package of 30.

Chewable Tablets (colored purple or pink, imprinted "TYLENOL 160") Package of 24. All packages are safety sealed and use child resistant blister packaging.
Shown in Product Identification Guide, page 513

LACTAID® Original Strength Caplets
(lactase enzyme)

LACTAID® Extra Strength Caplets
(lactase enzyme)

PRODUCT OVERVIEW

Key Facts: Lactaid® is the original dairy digestive lactose dietary supplement that makes milk and dairy foods more digestible. Lactaid® lactase enzyme hydrolyzes lactose into two digestible simple sugars: glucose and galactose. Lactaid Caplets are taken orally for *in vivo* hydrolysis of lactose.

Major Uses: Lactose intolerance, suspected from gastrointestinal discomfort (ie, gas, bloating, cramps, and diarrhea) after drinking milk or ingesting other dairy foods such as cheese and ice cream.

PRESCRIBING INFORMATION

Description: Each Lactaid Original Strength Caplet contains 3000 FCC (Food Chemical Codex) units of lactase enzyme (derived from *Aspergillus oryzae*).

Each Lactaid Extra Strength Caplet contains 4500 FCC units of lactase enzyme (derived from *Aspergillus oryzae*).

Action: Lactaid Caplets work to naturally replenish lactase enzyme that aids in dairy food digestion. Lactase enzyme hydrolyzes lactose sugar (a double sugar) into its simple sugar components, glucose and galactose.

Indications: Lactose intolerance, suspected from gastrointestinal discomfort (ie, gas, bloating, flatulence, cramps, and diarrhea) after drinking milk or ingesting other dairy foods such as cheese and ice cream.

Usual Dosage: These convenient, portable caplets are easy to swallow or chew and can be used with milk or any dairy food. Original Strength: swallow or chew 3 caplets with the first bite of dairy food. Take no more than 6 caplets at a time. Extra Strength: swallow or chew 2 caplets with first bite of dairy food. Don't be discouraged if at first Lactaid does not work to your satisfaction. Because the degree of enzyme deficiency naturally varies from person to person and from food to food, you may have to adjust the number of caplets up or down to find your own level of comfort. Since Lactaid Caplets work only on the food as you eat it, use them every time you enjoy dairy foods.

Warning: If you experience any symptoms which are unusual or seem unrelated to the condition for which you took this product, consult a doctor before taking any more of it. Do not use if carton is opened or if printed plastic neckwrap is broken.

Ingredients: Mannitol, Cellulose, Lactase Enzyme, Dextrose, and Sodium Citrate Magnesium Stearate.

How Supplied: Lactaid Original Strength Caplets are available in bottles of 60, and 120 counts. Lactaid Extra Strength Caplets are available in bottles of 24, and 50 counts. Store at or below room temperature (below 77°F) but do not refrigerate. Keep away from heat. Lactaid Caplets are certified kosher from the Orthodox Union.

Also available: 70% lactose reduced Lactaid Milk and 100% lactose-free Lactaid Milk.
Shown in Product Identification Guide, page 512

LACTAID® Drops
(lactase enzyme)

PRODUCT OVERVIEW

Key Facts: Lactaid® is the original dairy digestive supplement that makes milk more digestible. Lactaid® lactase enzyme hydrolyzes lactose into two digestible simple sugars: glucose and galactose. Lactaid Drops are added to milk for *in vitro* hydrolysis of lactose.

Major Uses: Lactose intolerance, suspected from gastrointestinal discomfort (ie, gas, bloating, cramps, and diarrhea) after drinking milk.

PRESCRIBING INFORMATION

Description: Lactaid drops contain sufficient lactase enzyme (derived from *Kluyveromyces lactis*) to hydrolyze lactose in milk.

Action: Lactaid Drops are a liquid form of the natural lactase enzyme that makes milk more digestible. The lactase enzyme hydrolyzes the lactose sugar (a double sugar) into its simple sugar components, glucose and galactose.

Indications: Lactose intolerance, suspected from gastrointestinal discomfort (ie, gas, bloating, cramps, and diarrhea) after drinking milk.

Usual Dosage: Lactaid drops are a liquid form of the natural lactase enzyme that makes milk more digestible. To use, add Lactaid drops to a quart of milk, shake gently and refrigerate for 24 hours. We recommend starting with 5–7 drops per quart of milk but because sensitivity to lactose can vary you may have to adjust the number of drops you use. If you are still experiencing discomfort after consuming milk with 5–7 Lactaid drops per quart, you may want to add 10 drops per quart or even 15 drops per quart. 15 drops per quart should remove nearly all of the lactose in the milk. Lactaid can be used with any kind of milk: whole, 1%, 2%, non-fat, skim, powdered and chocolate milk.

Warning: If you experience any symptoms which are unusual or seem unrelated to the condition for which you took this product, consult a doctor before taking any more of it. Do not use if carton is opened or if printed plastic bodywrap is broken.

Inactive Ingredients: Glycerin, Water

How Supplied: Lactaid Drops are available in .22 fl. oz. (7 mL), (30 quart supply). Store at or below room temperature (below 77°F). Refrigerate after opening.

Lactaid Drops are certified kosher from the Orthodox Union.

Also available: 70% lactose reduced Lactaid Milk and 100% lactose-free Lactaid Milk.
Shown in Product Identification Guide, page 512

PEDIACARE® Cough-Cold Liquid and Chewable Tablets
PEDIACARE® NightRest Cough-Cold Liquid
PEDIACARE® Infants' Drops Decongestant
PEDIACARE® Infants' Drops Decongestant Plus Cough

Description: Each 5 ml of PEDIACARE Cough-Cold Liquid contains pseudoephedrine hydrochloride 15 mg, chlorpheniramine maleate 1 mg and dextromethorphan hydrobromide 5 mg. Each PEDIACARE Cough-Cold Formula Chewable Tablet contains pseudoephedrine hydrochloride 15 mg, chlorpheniramine maleate 1 mg and dextromethorphan hydrobromide 5 mg. Each 0.8 ml oral dropper of PEDIACARE Infants' Drops Decongestant contains pseudoephedrine hydrochloride 7.5 mg. Each 0.8 oral dropper of PEDIACARE Infants' Drops Decongestant Plus Cough contains pseudoephedrine hydrochloride 7.5 mg and dextromethorphan hydrobromide

Continued on next page

McNeil Consumer—Cont.

2.5 mg. PEDIACARE NightRest Cough-Cold Liquid contains pseudoephedrine hydrochloride 15 mg, chlorpheniramine maleate 1 mg and dextromethorphan hydrobromide 7.5 mg per 5 ml. PEDIACARE Cough-Cold Liquid and NightRest Cough-Cold Liquid are stable, cherry flavored and red in color. PEDIACARE Infants' Drops are fruit flavored alcohol free and red in color. PEDIACARE Infants' Drops Decongestant Plus Cough are cherry flavored, alcohol free and clear, non-staining in color. PEDIACARE Cough-Cold Chewable Tablets are fruit flavored and pink in color.

Actions: PEDIACARE Products are available in four different formulas, allowing you to select the ideal product to temporarily relieve the patient's symptoms. PEDIACARE Cough-Cold Liquid and Chewable Tablets contain an antihistamine, chlorphiniramine maleate, a nasal decongestant, pseudoephedrine HCl and a cough suppressant, dextromethorphan hydrobromide, to provide temporary relief of nasal congestion, runny nose, sneezing and coughing due to the common cold, hay fever or other upper respiratory allergies. PEDIACARE NightRest Cough-Cold Liquid contains a decongestant, pseudoephedrine hydrochloride, an antihistamine, chlorpheniramine maleate, and a cough suppressant, dextromethorphan hydrobromide, to provide temporary relief of coughs, nasal congestion, runny nose and sneezing due to the common cold hayfever or other upper respiratory allergies. PEDIACARE NightRest may be used day or night to relieve cough and cold symptoms. PEDIACARE Infants' Drops Decongestant contain a decongestant, pseudoephedrine hydrochloride, to provide temporary relief of nasal congestion due to the common cold, hay fever or other upper respiratory allergies. PEDIACARE Infants' Drops Decongestant Plus Cough contain a decongestant, pseudoephedrine hydrochloride, and a cough suppressant, dextromethorphan hydrobromide to provide temporary relief of nasal congestion and coughing due to common cold, hay fever or other upper respiratory allergies.

Professional Dosage: A calibrated dosage cup is provided for accurate dosing of the PEDIACARE Liquid formulas. A calibrated oral dropper is provided for accurate dosing of PEDIACARE Infants' Drops. All doses of PEDIACARE Cough-Cold Liquid and Chewable Tablets, as well as PEDIACARE Infants' Drops may be repeated every 4–6 hours, not to exceed 4 doses in 24 hours. PEDIACARE NightRest Liquid may be repeated every 6–8 hrs, not to exceed 4 doses in 24 hours. [See table below.]

Warnings: DO NOT USE IF CARTON IS OPENED, OR IF PRINTED PLASTIC BOTTLE WRAP OR FOIL INNER SEAL IS BROKEN. KEEP THIS AND ALL MEDICATION OUT OF THE REACH OF CHILDREN. IN CASE OF ACCIDENTAL OVERDOSAGE, CONTACT A PHYSICIAN OR POISON CONTROL CENTER IMMEDIATELY.

The following information appears on the appropriate package labels:

PEDIACARE Cough-Cold Chewable Tablets:
PHENYLKETONURICS: CONTAINS PHENYLALANINE 6MG PER TABLET.

PEDIACARE Cough-Cold Liquid and Chewable Tablets, Night Rest Cough-Cold Liquid: Do not exceed recommended dosage. If nervousness, dizziness or sleeplessness occur, discontinue use and consult a doctor. If symptoms do not improve within 7 days or are accompanied by fever, consult a doctor. A persistent cough may be a sign of a serious condition. If cough persists for more than one week, tends to recur or is accompanied by fever, rash, or persistent headache, consult a doctor. Do not give this product for persistent or chronic cough such as occurs with asthma or if cough is accompanied by excessive phlegm (mucus) unless directed by a doctor. May cause excitability especially in children. May cause drowsiness. Sedatives and tranquilizers may increase the drowsiness effect. Do not give this product to children who are taking sedatives or tranquilizers without first consulting the child's doctor. Do not give this product to children who have a breathing problem such as chronic bronchitis, or who have glaucoma, heart disease, high blood pressure, thyroid disease or diabetes, without first consulting the child's doctor.

PEDIACARE Infants' Drops Decongestant: Do not exceed the recommended dosage. If nervousness, dizziness or sleeplessness occur discontinue use and consult a doctor. If symptoms do not improve within 7 days or are accompanied by fever, consult a physician. Do not give this product to a child who has heart disease, high blood pressure, thyroid disease or diabetes unless directed by a doctor. Take by mouth only. Not for nasal use.

PEDIACARE Infants' Drops Decongestant Plus
Cough: Do not exceed recommended dosage. If nervousness, dizziness, or sleeplessness occur, discontinue use and consult a doctor. If symptoms do not improve within 7 days or are accompanied by fever, consult a doctor. A persistent cough may be a sign of a serious condition. If cough persists for more than one week, tends to recur or is accompanied by fever, rash, or persistent headache, consult a doctor. Do not give this product for persistent or chronic cough such as occurs with asthma or if cough is accompanied by excessive phlegm (mucus) unless directed by a doctor. Do not give this product to a child who has heart disease, high blood pressure, thyroid disease or diabetes unless directed by a doctor. Take by mouth only. Not for nasal use.

Drug Interaction Precaution: Do not give this product to a child who is taking a prescription monoamine oxidase inhibitor (MAOI) (certain drugs for depression, psychiatric or emotional conditions), or for 2 weeks after stopping the MAOI drug. If you are uncertain whether your child's prescription drug contains an MAOI, consult a health professional before giving this product.

Inactive Ingredients: PEDIACARE Cough-Cold Liquid: Citric acid, corn syrup, flavors, glycerin, propylene glycol, sodium benzoate, sodium carboxymethylcellulose, sorbitol, purified water and Red #40.
PEDIACARE NightRest Cough-Cold Liquid: Citric acid, corn syrup, flavors, glycerin, propylene glycol, sodium benzoate, sodium carboxymethylcellulose, sorbitol, purified water and Red #40.

Age Group	0–3 mos	4–11 mos	12–23 mos	2–3 yrs	4–5 yrs	6–8 yrs	9–10 yrs	11 yrs	Dosage
Weight (lbs)	6–11 lb	12–17 lb	18–23 lb	24–35 lb	36–47 lb	48–59 lb	60–71 lb	72–95 lb	
PEDIACARE Infants' Drops Decongestant*	½ dropper (0.4 ml)	1 dropper (0.8 ml)	1½ droppers (1.2 ml)	2 droppers (1.6 ml)					q4–6h
PEDIACARE Infants' Drops Decongestant Plus Cough*	½ dropper (0.4 ml)	1 dropper (0.8 ml)	1½ droppers (1.2 ml)	2 droppers (1.6 ml)					q4–6h
PEDIACARE Cough-Cold Liquid** and Chewable Tablets**				1 tsp / 1 tab	1½ tsp / 1½ tabs	2 tsp / 2 tabs	2½ tsp / 2½ tabs	3 tsp / 3 tabs	q4–6h
PEDIACARE NightRest Liquid**				1 tsp	1½ tsp	2 tsp	2½ tsp	3 tsp	q6–8h

*Administer to children under 2 years only on the advice of a physician.
**Administer to children under 6 years only on the advice of a physician.

PEDIACARE Cough-Cold Chewable Tablets: Aspartame, cellulose, citric acid, flavors, magnesium stearate, magnesium trisilicate, mannitol, corn starch and Red #7.
PEDIACARE Infants' Drops Decongestant: Benzoic acid, citric acid, flavors, glycerin, polyethylene glycol, propylene glycol, purified water, sodium benzoate, sorbitol, sucrose and Red #40.
PEDIACARE Infants's Drops Decongestant Plus Cough: Citric acid, flavors, glycerin, purified water, sodium benzoate, and sorbitol.

Overdosage: Acute dextromethorphan overdose usually does not result in serious signs and symptoms unless massive amounts have been ingested. Signs and symptoms of a substantial overdose may include nausea and vomiting, visual disturbances, CNS disturbances, and urinary retention. Symptoms from pseudoephedrine overdose consist most often of mild anxiety, tachycardia and/or mild hypertension. Symptoms usually appear within 4 to 8 hours of ingestion and are transient, usually requiring no treatment. Chlorpheniramine toxicity should be treated as you would an antihistamine/anticholinergic overdose and is likely to be present within a few hours after acute ingestion. Symptoms from pseudoephedrine overdose consist often of mild anxiety, tachycardia and/or mild hypertension. Symptoms usually appear within 4 to 8 hours of ingestion and are transient, usually requiring no treatment.

How Supplied: PEDIACARE Cough-Cold Liquid and NightRest Cough-Cold Liquid (colored red)—bottles of 4 fl. oz. (120 ml) with child-resistant safety cap and calibrated dosage cup. PEDIACARE Cough-Cold Chewable Tablets (pink, scored)—blister packs of 16. PEDIACARE Infants' Drops Decongestant (colored red) and PEDIACARE Infants' Drops Decongestant Plus Cough (clear)—bottles of ½ fl. oz (15 ml) with calibrated dropper.
Shown in Product Identification Guide, page 512

**Maximum Strength
SINE-AID®
Sinus Medication Gelcaps, Caplets and Tablets**

Description: Each Maximum Strength SINE-AID® Gelcap, Caplet or Tablet contains acetaminophen 500 mg and pseudoephedrine hydrochloride 30 mg.

Actions: Maximum Strength SINE-AID® Gelcaps, Caplets and Tablets contain a clinically proven analgesic-antipyretic and a decongestant. Maximum allowable non-prescription levels of acetaminophen and pseudoephedrine provide temporary relief of sinus congestion and pain. Acetaminophen is equal to aspirin in analgesic and antipyretic effectiveness and it is unlikely to produce many of the side effects associated with aspirin and aspirin-containing products.

Acetaminophen produces analgesia by elevation of the pain threshold and antipyresis through action on the hypothalamic heat-regulating center. Pseudoephedrine hydrochloride is a sympathomimetic amine that promotes sinus cavity drainage by reducing nasopharyngeal mucosal congestion.

Indications: Maximum Strength SINE-AID® Gelcaps, Caplets and Tablets provide effective symptomatic relief from sinus headache pain and congestion. SINE-AID® is particularly well-suited in patients with aspirin allergy, hemostatic disturbances (including anticoagulant therapy), and bleeding diatheses (e.g. hemophilia) and upper gastrointestinal disease (e.g. ulcer, gastritis, hiatus hernia).

Precautions: If a rare sensitivity occurs, the drug should be discontinued. Although pseudoephedrine is virtually without pressor effect in normotensive patients, it should be used with caution in hypertensives.

Directions: Adults & children 12 years of age and older: Two gelcaps, caplets or tablets every four to six hours. Do not exceed eight gelcaps, caplets or tablets in any 24 hour period. Not for use in children under 12 years of age.

Warnings: Do not use if carton is open or if blister unit is broken.
Do not take for pain for more than 7 days or for fever for more than 3 days unless directed by a doctor. If pain or fever persists, or gets worse, if new symptoms occur, or if redness or swelling is present, consult a doctor because these could be signs of a serious condition. **Do not exceed recommended dosage.** If nervousness, dizziness or sleeplessness occur, discontinue use and consult a doctor. Do not take this product if you have heart disease, high blood pressure, thyroid disease, diabetes or difficulty in urination due to enlargement of the prostate gland unless directed by a doctor.
As with any drug, if you are pregnant or nursing a baby, seek the advice of a health professional before using this product. Keep this and all drugs out of the reach of children. In case of accidental overdose, contact a doctor or poison control center immediately. Prompt medical attention is critical for adults as well as for children even if you do not notice any signs or symptoms. Do not use with other products containing acetaminophen.

Alcohol Warning: If you generally consume 3 or more alcohol-containing drinks per day, you should consult your physician for advice on when and how you should take Maximum Strength SINE-AID and other pain relievers.

Drug Interaction Precaution: Do not use this product if you are now taking a prescription monoamine oxidase inhibitor (MAOI) (certain drugs for depression, psychiatric or emotional conditions, or Parkinson's disease), or for 2 weeks after stopping the MAOI drug. If you are un-

certain whether your prescription drug contains an MAOI, consult a health professional before taking this product.

PROFESSIONAL INFORMATION

Overdosage Information: Acetaminophen in massive overdosage may cause hepatic toxicity in some patients. In adults and adolescents, hepatic toxicity has rarely been reported following ingestion of acute overdoses of less than 10 grams. Fatalities are infrequent (less than 3–4% of untreated cases) and have rarely been reported with overdoses of less than 15 grams. In children, an acute overdosage of less than 150 mg/kg has not been associated with hepatic toxicity. Early symptoms following a potentially hepatotoxic overdose may include: nausea, vomiting, diaphoresis and general malaise. Clinical and laboratory evidence of hepatic toxicity may not be apparent until 48 to 72 hours postingestion. In adults and adolescents, regardless of the quantity of acetaminophen reported to have been ingested, administer acetylcysteine immediately if 24 hours or less have elapsed from the reported time of ingestion. For full prescribing information, refer to the acetylcysteine package insert. Do not await results of assays for plasma acetaminophen level before initiating treatment with acetylcysteine. The following additional procedures are recommended: The stomach should be emptied promptly by lavage or by induction of emesis with syrup of ipecac. A plasma acetaminophen assay should be obtained as early as possible, but no sooner than four hours following ingestion. If plasma level falls above the lower treatment line on the acetaminophen overdose nomogram, acetylcysteine therapy should be continued. Liver function studies should be obtained initially and repeated at 24-hour intervals.
Serious toxicity or fatalities are extremely infrequent in children, possibly due to differences in the way they metabolize acetaminophen. In children, the maximum potential amount ingested can be more easily estimated. If more than 150 mg/kg or an unknown amount was ingested, obtain a plasma acetaminophen level. The plasma acetaminophen level should be obtained as soon as possible, but no sooner than 4 hours following the ingestion. If plasma level falls above the lower treatment line on the acetaminophen overdose nomogram, the acetylcysteine therapy should be initiated and continued for a full course of therapy. If plasma acetaminophen assay capability is not available, and the estimated acetaminophen ingestion exceeds 150 mg/kg, acetylcysteine therapy should be initiated and continued for a full course of therapy.
For additional emergency information, call your regional poison center or call the Rocky Mountain Poison Center toll-free, (1-800-525-6115).
Symptoms from pseudoephedrine overdose consist most often of mild anxiety,

Continued on next page

McNeil Consumer—Cont.

tachycardia and/or mild hypertension. Symptoms usually appear within 4 to 8 hours of ingestion and are transient, usually requiring no treatment.

Alcohol Information: Chronic heavy alcohol abusers may be at increased risk of liver toxicity from excessive acetaminophen use, although reports of this event are rare. Reports almost invariably involve cases of severe chronic alcoholics and the dosages of acetaminophen most often exceed recommended doses and often involve substantial overdose. Professionals should alert their patients who regularly consume large amounts of alcohol not to exceed recommended doses of acetaminophen.

Inactive Ingredients: Gelcaps: Benzyl Alcohol, Butylparaben, Castor Oil, Cellulose, Corn Starch, Edetate Calcium Disodium, Gelatin, Hydroxypropyl Methylcellulose, Iron Oxide Black, Magnesium Stearate, Methylparaben, Propylparaben, Sodium Lauryl Sulfate, Sodium Propionate, Sodium Starch Glycolate, Titanium Dioxide, FD&C Red #40. Caplets: Cellulose, Corn Starch, Hydroxypropyl Methylcellulose, Magnesium Stearate, Polyethylene Glycol, Sodium Starch Glycolate, Titanium Dioxide, Blue #1 and Red #40. Tablets: Cellulose, Corn Starch, Magnesium Stearate and Sodium Starch Glycolate.

How Supplied: Gelcaps (colored red and white imprinted "SINE-AID")—blister package of 20 and tamper resistant bottle of 40. Caplets (colored white imprinted "Maximum SINE-AID")—blister package of 24 and tamper resistant bottle of 50. Tablets (colored white embossed "SINE-AID")—blister package of 24 and tamper resistant bottle of 50.

Shown in Product Identification Guide, page 512

**Extra Strength
TYLENOL® acetaminophen
Gelcaps, Geltabs, Caplets, Tablets
Extra Strength
TYLENOL® acetaminophen
Adult Liquid Pain Reliever
Regular Strength
TYLENOL® acetaminophen
Caplets and Tablets
TYLENOL® Extended Relief
acetaminophen extended release
Caplets**

Product information for all dosage forms of Adult TYLENOL acetaminophen have been combined under this heading.

Description: Each *Extra Strength TYLENOL Gelcap, Geltab, Caplet, or Tablet* contains acetaminophen 500 mg. Each 15 ml (½ fl oz or one tablespoonful) of *Extra Strength TYLENOL acetaminophen Adult Liquid Pain Reliever* contains 500 mg acetaminophen (alcohol 7%).
Each *Regular Strength TYLENOL Caplet or Tablet* contains acetaminophen 325 mg.
Each *TYLENOL Extended Relief Caplet* contains acetaminophen 650 mg.

Actions: Acetaminophen is a clinically proven analgesic and antipyretic. Acetaminophen produces analgesia by elevation of the pain threshold and antipyresis through action on the hypothalamic heat-regulating center. Acetaminophen is equal to aspirin in analgesic and antipyretic effectiveness and it is unlikely to produce many of the side effects associated with aspirin and aspirin-containing products.
Tylenol Extended Relief uses a unique, patented bilayer caplet. The first layer dissolves quickly to provide prompt relief while the second layer is time released to provide up to 8 hours of relief.

Indications: For the temporary relief of minor aches and pains associated with the common cold, headache, toothache, muscular aches, back ache, for the minor pain of arthritis, for the pain of menstrual cramps and for the reduction of fever.

Directions: *Extra Strength TYLENOL Gelcaps, Geltabs, Caplets, or Tablets:* Adults and Children 12 years of Age and Older: Take two gelcaps, geltabs, caplets, or tablets every 4 to 6 hours. Not to exceed 8 gelcaps, geltabs, caplets, or tablets in any 24-hour period. Not for use in children under 12 years of age.
Extra Strength TYLENOL Adult Liquid Pain Reliever: Adults and Children 12 years of Age and Older: Fill measuring cup once to 2-tablespoon line (1,000 mg) which is equivalent to two 500 mg Extra Strength TYLENOL® Gelcaps, Geltabs, Caplets or Tablets. Take every 4–6 hours. No more than 4 doses in any 24-hour period, or as directed by a doctor. Not for use in children under 12 years of age.
Regular Strength TYLENOL Caplets or Tablets: Adults and Children 12 years of Age and Older: Take two caplets or tablets every 4 to 6 hours. No more than a total of 12 caplets or tablets in any 24-hour period, or as directed by a doctor. Children (6–11): ½ to 1 caplet or tablet every 4 to 6 hours, not to exceed 5 doses in 24 hours. Consult a physician for use by children under 6 years of age.
TYLENOL Extended Relief Caplets: Adults and Children 12 years of Age and Older: Take two caplets every 8 hours, not to exceed 6 caplets in any 24-hour period. TAKE TWO CAPLETS WITH WATER, SWALLOW EACH CAPLET WHOLE. DO NOT CRUSH, CHEW, OR DISSOLVE THE CAPLET. Not for use in children under 12 years of age.

Precautions: If a rare sensitivity reaction occurs, the drug should be discontinued.

Warnings: Do not use if carton is opened or printed red neck wrap or printed full inner seal is broken. Do not take for pain for more than 10 days or for fever for more than 3 days unless directed by a physician. If pain or fever persists, or gets worse, if new symptoms occur, or if redness or swelling is present, consult a physician because these could be signs of a serious condition. As with any drug, if you are pregnant or nursing a baby, seek the advice of a health professional before using this product. Keep this and all drugs out of the reach of children. In case of accidental overdose, contact a physician or poison control center immediately. Prompt medical attention is critical for adults as well as for children even if you do not notice any signs or symptoms. Do not use with other products containing acetaminophen.

Alcohol Warning: If you generally consume 3 or more alcohol-containing drinks per day, you should consult your physician for advice on when and how you should take [product] and other pain relievers.

PROFESSIONAL INFORMATION

Overdosage Information: Acetaminophen in massive overdosage may cause hepatic toxicity in some patients. In adults and adolescents, hepatic toxicity has rarely been reported following ingestion of acute overdoses of less than 10 grams. Fatalities are infrequent (less than 3–4% of untreated cases) and have rarely been reported with overdoses of less than 15 grams. In children, an acute overdosage of less than 150 mg/kg has not been associated with hepatic toxicity. Early symptoms following a potentially hepatotoxic overdose may include: nausea, vomiting, diaphoresis and general malaise. Clinical and laboratory evidence of hepatic toxicity may not be apparent until 48 to 72 hours postingestion. In adults and adolescents, regardless of the quantity of acetaminophen reported to have been ingested, administer acetylcysteine immediately if 24 hours or less have elapsed from the reported time of ingestion. For full prescribing information, refer to the acetylcysteine package insert. Do not await results of assays for plasma acetaminophen level before initiating treatment with acetylcysteine. The following additional procedures are recommended: The stomach should be emptied promptly by lavage or by induction of emesis with syrup of ipecac. A plasma acetaminophen assay should be obtained as early as possible, but no sooner than four hours following ingestion. If an acetaminophen extended release product is involved, it may be appropriate to obtain an additional plasma acetaminophen level 4–6 hours following the initial plasma acetaminophen level. If either plasma level falls above the lower treatment line on the acetaminophen overdose nomogram, acetylcysteine therapy should be continued. Liver function studies should be obtained initially and repeated at 24-hour intervals.

Serious toxicity or fatalities are extremely infrequent in children, possibly due to differences in the way they metabolize acetaminophen. In children, the maximum potential amount ingested can be more easily estimated. If more than 150 mg/kg or an unknown amount was ingested, obtain a plasma acetaminophen level. The plasma level should be obtained as soon as possible, but no sooner than 4 hours following the ingestion. If an acetaminophen *extended release* product is involved, it may be appropriate to obtain an additional plasma acetaminophen level 4–6 hours following the initial plasma acetaminophen level. If either plasma level falls above the lower treatment line on the acetaminophen overdose nomogram, the acetylcysteine therapy should be initiated and continued for a full course of therapy. If plasma acetaminophen assay capability is not available, and the estimated acetaminophen ingestion exceeds 150 mg/kg, acetylcysteine therapy should be initiated and continued for a full course of therapy.

For additional emergency information, call your regional poison center or call the Rocky Mountain Poison Center toll-free, (1-800-525-6115).

Alcohol Information: Chronic heavy alcohol abusers may be at increased risk of liver toxicity from excessive acetaminophen use, although reports of this event are rare. Reports almost invariably involve cases of severe chronic alcoholics and the dosages of acetaminophen most often exceed recommended doses and often involve substantial overdose. Professionals should alert their patients who regularly consume large amounts of alcohol not to exceed recommended doses of acetaminophen.

Inactive Ingredients: *Extra Strength TYLENOL:* **Tablets**—Magnesium Stearate, Cellulose, Sodium Starch Glycolate and Starch. **Caplets**—Cellulose, Cornstarch, Hydroxypropyl Methylcellulose, Magnesium Stearate, Polyethylene Glycol, Sodium Starch Glycolate, and Red #40. **Gelcaps**—Benzyl Alcohol, Butylparaben, Castor Oil, Cellulose, Edetate Calcium Disodium, Gelatin, Hydroxypropyl Methylcellulose, Magnesium Stearate, Methylparaben, Propylparaben, Sodium Lauryl Sulfate, Sodium Propionate, Sodium Starch Glycolate, Starch, Titanium Dioxide, Blue #1 and #2, Red #40, and Yellow #10. **Geltabs**—Benzyl Alcohol, Butylparaben, Castor Oil, Cellulose, Corn Starch, Edetate Calcium Disodium, Gelatin, Hydroxypropyl Methylcellulose, Magnesium Stearate, Methylparaben, Propylparaben, Sodium Lauryl Sulfate, Sodium Propionate, Sodium Starch Glycolate, Titanium Dioxide, Blue #1 and #2, Red #40, and Yellow #10.
Extra Strength TYLENOL Adult Liquid Pain Reliever: Alcohol (7%), Citric Acid, Flavors, Glycerin, Polyethylene Glycol, Purified Water, Sodium Benzoate, Sorbitol, Sucrose, Yellow #6 (Sunset Yellow), Yellow #10 and Blue #1.

Regular Strength TYLENOL: **Tablets**—Magnesium Stearate, Cellulose, Sodium Starch Glycolate and Starch. **Caplets**—Cellulose, Hydroxypropyl Methylcellulose, Magnesium Stearate, Polyethylene Glycol, Sodium Starch Glycolate, Starch and Red #40.
TYLENOL Extended Relief Caplets: Corn Starch, Hydroxyethyl Cellulose, Hydroxypropyl Methylcellulose, Magnesium Stearate, Microcrystalline Cellulose, Povidone, Powdered Cellulose, Pregelatinized Starch, Sodium Starch Glycolate, Titanium Dioxide, Triacetin.

How Supplied: *Extra Strength TYLENOL:* **Tablets** (colored white, imprinted "TYLENOL" and "500")—vials of 10, and tamper-resistant bottles of 30, 60, 100, and 200. **Caplets** (colored white, imprinted "TYLENOL 500 mg")—vials of 10, 10 blister packs, and tamper-resistant bottles of 24, 50, 100, 175, and 250 and FastCap package of 72. **Gelcaps** (colored yellow and red, imprinted "Tylenol 500") vials of 10 and tamper-resistant bottles of 24, 50, 100, and 225 and FastCap package of 72. **Geltabs** (colored yellow and red, imprinted "Tylenol 500") tamper-resistant bottles of 24, 50, and 100.
Extra Strength TYLENOL Adult Liquid Pain Reliever: Mint-flavored liquid (colored green) 8 fl. oz. tamper-resistant bottle with child resistant safety cap and special dosage cup.
Regular Strength TYLENOL: **Tablets** (colored white, scored, imprinted "TYLENOL")—tamper-resistant bottles of 24, 50, 100 and 200. **Caplets** (colored white, "TYLENOL")—tamper-resistant bottles of 24, 50, 100.
TYLENOL Extended Relief Caplets: (colored white, engraved "TYLENOL ER") tamper-resistant bottles of 24, 50, and 100's.

Shown in Product Identification Guide, page 514

**Maximum Strength
TYLENOL® ALLERGY SINUS
Medication
Caplets, Gelcaps, Geltabs**

Description: Each Maximum Strength TYLENOL® ALLERGY SINUS Caplet, Gelcap or Geltab contains acetaminophen 500 mg, chlorpheniramine maleate 2 mg, and pseudoephedrine hydrochloride 30 mg.

Actions: Maximum Strength TYLENOL® ALLERGY SINUS Caplets or Gelcaps contain a clinically proven analgesic-antipyretic, decongestant, and antihistamine. Acetaminophen produces analgesia by elevation of the pain threshold and antipyresis through action on the hypothalamic heat-regulating center. Acetaminophen is equal to aspirin in analgesic and antipyretic effectiveness, and it is unlikely to produce many of the side effects associated with aspirin and aspirin-containing products. Pseudoephedrine hydrochloride is a sympathomimetic amine which provides temporary

relief of nasal congestion. Chlorpheniramine is an antihistamine which helps provide temporary relief of runny nose, sneezing and watery and itchy eyes.

Indications: TYLENOL® ALLERGY SINUS provides effective temporary relief of these upper respiratory allergy, hay fever and sinusitis symptoms: sneezing, itchy, watery eyes, runny nose, itching of the nose or throat, nasal and sinus congestion and sinus pain and headaches.

Precautions: If a rare sensitivity reaction occurs, the drug should be stopped. Although pseudoephedrine is virtually without pressor effect in normotensive patients, it should be used with caution in hypertensives.

Directions: Adults and children 12 years of age and older: Two caplets, gelcaps or geltabs every 6 hours, not to exceed 8 caplets, gelcaps or geltabs in 24 hours. Not for use in children under 12 years of age.

Warnings: Do not use if carton is open or if green neck wrap or printed foil inner seal is broken.
Do not take for pain for more than 7 days or for fever for more than 3 days unless directed by a doctor. If pain or fever persists, or get worse, if new symptoms occur, or if redness or swelling is present, consult a doctor because these could be signs of a serious condition. **Do not exceed recommended dosage.** If nervousness, dizziness or sleeplessness occur, discontinue use and consult a doctor. May cause excitability, especially in children. Do not take this product, unless directed by a doctor, if you have a breathing problem such as emphysema or chronic bronchitis, or if you have glaucoma or difficulty in urination due to enlargement of the prostate gland. Do not take this product if you have heart disease, high blood pressure, thyroid disease or diabetes unless directed by a doctor. May cause drowsiness; alcohol, sedatives and tranquilizers may increase the drowsiness effect. Avoid alcoholic beverages while taking this product. Do not take this product if you are taking sedatives or tranquilizers without first consulting your doctor. Use caution when driving a motor vehicle or operating machinery. As with any drug, if you are pregnant or nursing a baby, seek the advice of a health professional before using this product. Keep this and all drugs out of the reach of children. In case of accidental overdose, contact a doctor or poison control center immediately. Prompt medical attention is critical for adults as well as for children even if you do not notice any signs or symptoms. Do not use with other products containing acetaminophen.

Alcohol Warning: If you generally consume 3 or more alcohol-containing drinks per day, you should consult your physician for advice on when and how you should take Maximum Strength

Continued on next page

McNeil Consumer—Cont.

TYLENOL ALLERGY SINUS Medication and other pain relievers.

Drug Interaction Precaution: Do not use this product if you are now taking a prescription monoamine oxidase inhibitor (MAOI) (certain drugs for depression, psychiatric or emotional conditions, or Parkinson's disease), or for 2 weeks after stopping the MAOI drug. If you are uncertain whether your prescription drug contains an MAOI, consult a health care professional before taking this product.

PROFESSIONAL INFORMATION

Overdosage Information: Acetaminophen in massive overdosage may cause hepatic toxicity in some patients. In adults and adolescents, hepatic toxicity has rarely been reported following ingestion of acute overdoses of less than 10 grams. Fatalities are infrequent (less than 3–4% of untreated cases) and have rarely been reported with overdoses of less than 15 grams. In children, an acute overdosage of less than 150 mg/kg has not been associated with hepatic toxicity. Early symptoms following a potentially hepatotoxic overdose may include: nausea, vomiting, diaphoresis and general malaise. Clinical and laboratory evidence of hepatic toxicity may not be apparent until 48 to 72 hours postingestion. In adults and adolescents, regardless of the quantity of acetaminophen reported to have been ingested, administer acetylcysteine immediately if 24 hours or less have elapsed from the reported time of ingestion. For full prescribing information, refer to the acetylcysteine package insert. Do not await results of assays for plasma acetaminophen level before initiating treatment with acetylcysteine. The following additional procedures are recommended: The stomach should be emptied promptly by lavage or by induction of emesis with syrup of ipecac. A plasma acetaminophen assay should be obtained as early as possible, but no sooner than four hours following ingestion. If plasma level falls above the lower treatment line on the acetaminophen overdose nomogram, acetylcysteine therapy should be continued. Liver function studies should be obtained initially and repeated at 24-hour intervals.

Several toxicity or fatalities are extremely infrequent in children, possibly due to differences in the way they metabolize acetaminophen. In children, the maximum potential amount ingested can be easily estimated. If more than 150 mg/kg or an unknown amount was ingested, obtain a plasma acetaminophen level. The plasma acetaminophen level should be obtained as soon as possible, but no sooner than 4 hours following ingestion. If plasma level falls above the lower treatment line on the acetaminophen overdose nomogram, the acetylcysteine therapy should be initiated and continued for a full course of therapy. If plasma acetaminophen assay

capability is not available, and the estimated acetaminophen ingestion exceeds 150 mg/kg, acetylcysteine therapy should be initiated and continued for a full course of therapy.

For additional emergency information, call your regional poison center or call the Rocky Mountain Poison Control Center toll-free, (1-800-525-6115).

Chlorpheniramine toxicity should be treated as you would an antihistamine/anticholinergic overdose and is likely to be present within a few hours after acute ingestion.

Symptoms from pseudophedrine overdose consist most often of mild anxiety, tachycardia and/or hypertension. Symptoms usually appear within 4 to 8 hours of ingestion and are transient, usually requiring no treatment.

Alcohol Information: Chronic heavy alcohol abusers may be at increased risk of liver toxicity from excessive acetaminophen use, although reports of this event are rare. Reports almost invariably involve cases of severe chronic alcoholics and the dosages of acetaminophen most often exceed recommended doses and often involve substantial overdose. Professionals should alert their patients who regularly consume large amounts of alcohol not to exceed recommended doses of acetaminophen.

Inactive Ingredients: Caplets: Cannuba Wax, Cellulose, Cornstarch, Hydroxypropyl Cellulose, Hydroxypropyl Methylcellulose, Iron Oxide Black, Magnesium Stearate, Polyethylene Glycol, Sodium Starch Glycolate, Titanium Dioxide, Blue #1, Yellow #6, Yellow #10. Gelcaps: Benzyl Alcohol, Butylparaben, Castor oil, Cellulose, Cornstarch, Edetate Calcium Disodium, Gelatin, Hydroxypropyl Methylcellulose, Magnesium Stearate, Methylparaben, Propylparaben, Sodium Lauryl Sulfate, Sodium Propionate, Sodium Starch Glycolate, Titanium Dioxide, Blue #1 and #2 and Yellow #10. Geltabs: Benzyl Alcohol, Butylparaben, Castor oil, Cellulose, Cornstarch, Edetate Calcium Disodium, Gelatin, Hydroxypropyl Methylcellulose, Magnesium Stearate, Methylparaben, Propylparaben, Sodium Lauryl Sulfate, Sodium Propionate, Sodium Starch Glycolate, Titanium Dioxide, Blue #1, Blue #2 and Yellow #10.

How Supplied: Caplets: (dark yellow, imprinted "TYLENOL Allergy Sinus")—Blister packs of 24 and tamper-resistant bottles of 60. Gelcaps: (dark green and dark yellow, imprinted "TYLENOL A/S")—Blister packs of 24 and tamper-resistant bottles of 60. Geltabs: (dark green and dark yellow, imprinted "Tylenol A/S")—Blister packs of 24 and tamper-resistant bottles of 60.

Shown in Product Identification Guide, page 513

**Maximum Strength
TYLENOL® ALLERGY SINUS
NIGHTTIME Medication
Caplets**

Description: Each Maximum Strength TYLENOL® ALLERGY SINUS NIGHTTIME Caplet contains Acetaminophen 500mg, Pseudoephedrine Hydrochloride 30mg, and Diphenhydramine Hydrochloride 25mg.

Actions: Maximum Strength TYLENOL® ALLERGY SINUS NIGHTTIME Medication contains a clinically proven analgesic-antipyretic, decongestant, and antihistamine. Acetaminophen produces analgesia by elevation of the pain threshold and antipyresis through action on the hypothalamic heat-regulating center. Acetaminophen is equal to aspirin in analgesic and antipyretic effectiveness, and it is unlikely to produce many of the side effects associated with aspirin and aspirin-containing products. Pseudoephedrine Hydrochloride is a sympathomimetic amine which provides temporary relief of nasal congestion. Diphenhydramine Hydrochloride is an antihistamine with sedative properties which helps provide temporary relief of runny nose, sneezing and watery and itchy eyes.

Indications: TYLENOL® ALLERGY SINUS NIGHTTIME provides effective temporary relief of these upper respiratory allergy, hay fever and sinusitis symptoms: sneezing, itchy, watery eyes, runny nose, itching of the nose or throat, nasal and sinus congestion, and sinus pain and headaches.

Precautions: If a rare sensitivity reaction occurs, the drug should be stopped. Although psuedoephedrine is virtually without pressor effect in normotensive patients, it should be used with caution in hypertensives.

Directions: Adults and children 12 years of age and older: Two caplets at bedtime. Not for use in children under 12 years of age.

Warnings: Do not use if carton is open or if blister unit is broken.

Do not take for pain for more than 7 days or for fever for more than 3 days unless directed by a doctor. If pain or fever persists, or get worse, if new symptoms occur, or if redness or swelling is present, consult a doctor because these could be signs of a serious condition. **Do not exceed recommended dosage.** If nervousness, dizziness or sleeplessness occur, discontinue use and consult a doctor. May cause excitability, especially in children. Do not take this product, unless directed by a doctor, if you have a breathing problem such as emphysema or chronic bronchitis, or if you have glaucoma or difficulty in urination due to enlargement of the prostate gland. Do not take this product if you have heart disease, high blood pressure, thyroid disease or diabetes unless directed by a doctor. May cause marked drowsiness; alcohol, sedatives and tranquilizers may increase the drowsiness effect. Avoid alcoholic beverages while taking this product. Do not take this product if you are taking sedatives or tranquilizers, without first consulting your doctor. Use caution when driving a motor vehicle or operating machinery.

As with any drug, if you are pregnant or nursing a baby, seek the advice of a health professional before using this product. Keep this and all drugs out of the reach of children. In case of accidental overdose, contact a doctor or poison control center immediately. Prompt medical attention is critical for adults as well as for children even if you do not notice any signs or symptoms. Do not use with other products containing acetaminophen.

Alcohol Warning: If you generally consume 3 or more alcohol-containing drinks per day, you should consult your physician for advice on when and how you should take Maximum Strength TYLENOL® ALLERGY SINUS NIGHTTIME and other pain relievers.

Drug Interaction Precaution: Do not use this product if you are now taking a prescription monomaine oxidase inhibitor (MAOI) (certain drugs for depression, psychiatric or emotional conditions, or Parkinson's disease), or for 2 weeks after stopping the MAOI drug. If you are uncertain whether your prescription drug contains an MAOI, consult a health professional before taking this product.

PROFESSIONAL INFORMATION

Overdosage Information: Acetaminophen in massive overdosage may cause hepatic toxicity in some patients. In adults and adolescents, hepatic toxicity has rarely been reported following ingestion of acute overdose of less than 10 grams. Fatalities are infrequent (less than 3–4% of untreated cases) and have rarely been reported with overdoses of less than 15 grams. In children, an acute overdoses of less than 150 mg/kg has not been associated with hepatic toxicity. Early symptoms following a potentially hepatotoxic overdose may include: nausea, vomiting, diaphoresis and general malaise. Clinical and laboratory evidence of hepatic toxicity may not be apparent until 48 to 72 hours postingestion. In adults and adolescents, regardless of the quantity of acetaminophen reported to have been ingested, administer acetylcysteine immediately if 24 hours or less have elapsed from the reported time of ingestion. For full prescribing information, refer to the acetylcysteine package insert. Do not await results of assays for plasma acetaminophen level before initiating treatment with acetylcysteine. The following additional procedures are recommended: The stomach should be emptied promptly by lavage or by induction of emesis with syrup of ipecac. A plasma acetaminophen assay should be obtained as early as possible, but no sooner than four hours following ingestion. If plasma level falls above the lower treatment line on the acetaminophen overdose nomogram, acetylcysteine ther-

apy should be continued. Liver function studies should be obtained initially and repeated at 24-hour intervals.

Serious toxicity or fatalities are extremely infrequent in children, possibly due to differences in the way they metabolize acetaminophen. In children, the maximum potential amount ingested can be more easily estimated. If more than 150 mg/kg or an unknown amount was ingested, obtain an plasma acetaminophen level. The plasma acetaminophen level should be obtained as soon as possible, but no sooner than 4 hours following ingestion. If plasma level falls above the lower treatment line on the acetaminophen overdose nomogram, the acetylcysteine therapy should be initiated and continued for a full course of therapy. If plasma acetaminophen assay capability is not available, and the estimated acetaminophen ingestion exceeds 150 mg/kg, acetylcysteine therapy should be initiated and continued for a full course of therapy.

For additional emergency information, call your regional poison control center or call the Rocky Mountain Poison Control Center toll-free, at (1-800-525-6115). Symptoms for pseudoephedrine overdose consist most often of mild anxiety, tachycardia and/or hypertension. Symptoms usually appear within 4 to 8 hours of ingestion and are transient, usually requiring no treatment.

Diphenhydramine toxicity should be treated as you would an antihistamine/anticholinergic overdose and is likely to be present within a few hours after acute ingestion.

Alcohol Information: Chronic heavy alcohol abusers may be at increased risk of liver toxicity from excessive acetaminophen use, although reports of this event are rare. Reports almost invariably involve cases of severe chronic alcoholics and the dosages of acetaminophen most often exceed recommended doses and often involve substantial overdose. Professionals should alert their patients who regularly consume large amounts of alcohol not to exceed recommended doses of acetaminophen.

Inactive Ingredients: Caplet: Cellulose, Corn Starch, Hydroxypropyl Methylcellulose, Iron Oxide Black, Magnesium Stearate, Polyethylene Glycol, Polysorbate 80, Sodium Citrate, Sodium Starch Glycolate, Titanium Dioxide, Blue #1, Yellow #10.

How Supplied: Caplets (light blue, imprinted "TYLENOL A/S Night Time") —Child-resistant blister packs of 24.

Shown in Product Identification Guide, page 513

TYLENOL® COLD Medication No Drowsiness Formula Caplets and Gelcaps

Multi-Symptom Formula TYLENOL® COLD Medication Tablets and Caplets

TYLENOL® COLD Multi-Symptom Hot Medication Liquid Packets

Product information for all dosage forms of TYLENOL COLD have been combined under this heading.

Description: Each *TYLENOL COLD Medication No Drowsiness Formula Caplet and Gelcap* contains acetaminophen 325 mg, pseudoephedrine hydrochloride 30 mg, and dextromethorphan hydrobromide 15 mg.

Each *Multi-Symptom Formula TYLENOL COLD Tablet or Caplet* contains acetaminophen 325 mg, chlorpheniramine maleate 2 mg, pseudoephedrine hydrochloride 30 mg, and dextromethorphan hydrobromide 15 mg.

Each packet of *TYLENOL COLD Multi-Symptom Hot Medication* contains acetaminophen 650 mg, chlorpheniramine maleate 4 mg, pseudoephedrine hydrochloride 60 mg, and dextromethorphan hydrobromide 30 mg.

Actions: *TYLENOL COLD Medication No Drowsiness Formula* contains a clinically proven analgesic-antipyretic, decongestant and cough suppressant. Acetaminophen produces analgesia by elevation of the pain threshold and antipyresis through action on the hypothalamic heat-regulating center. Acetaminophen is equal to aspirin in analgesic and antipyretic effectiveness and it is unlikely to produce many of the side effects associated with aspirin and aspirin-containing products. Pseudoephedrine is a sympathomimetic amine which provides temporary relief of nasal congestion. Dextromethorphan is a cough suppressant which provides temporary relief of coughs due to minor throat irritations that may occur with the common cold. *Multi-Symptom Formula TYLENOL COLD Medication* and *TYLENOL COLD Multi-Symptom Hot Medication* contain, in addition to the above ingredients, an antihistamine. Chlorpheniramine is an antihistamine which helps provide temporary relief of runny nose, sneezing and watery and itchy eyes.

Indications: *TYLENOL COLD Medication No Drowsiness Formula* provides effective temporary relief of nasal congestion, coughing, and body aches, pains, headache, sore throat and fever due to a cold or "flu."

Multi-Symptom Formula TYLENOL COLD Medication and *TYLENOL COLD Multi-Symptom Hot Medication* provide effective temporary relief of runny nose, sneezing, watery and itchy eyes, nasal congestion, coughing and body aches, pains, headache, sore throat and fever due to a cold or "flu."

Continued on next page

McNeil Consumer—Cont.

Directions: *TYLENOL COLD No Drowsiness Formula and Multi-Symptom Formula TYLENOL COLD Medication:* Adults (12 years and older): Two every 6 hours, not to exceed 8 in 24 hours. Children (6–11 years): One every 6 hours, not to exceed 4 in 24 hours. Not for use in children under 6 years of age.
TYLENOL COLD Multi-Symptom Hot Medication: Adults (12 years and older): dissolve one packet in 6 oz. cup of hot water. Sip while hot. Sweeten to taste, if desired. May repeat every 6 hours, not to exceed 4 doses in 24 hours. Not for use in children under 12 years of age.

Precautions: *TYLENOL COLD Medication No Drowsiness Formula, Multi-Symptom Formula TYLENOL COLD Medication* and *TYLENOL COLD Multi-Symptom Hot Medication:* If a rare sensitivity reaction occurs, the drug should be stopped. Although pseudoephedrine is virtually without pressor effect in normotensive patients, it should be used with caution in hypertensives.
TYLENOL COLD Medication No Drowsiness Formula: Do not take this product for more than 7 days or for fever for more than 3 days unless directed by a doctor. If symptoms do not improve or are accompanied by fever, consult a doctor. If sore throat is severe, persists for more than 2 days, is accompanied or followed by fever, headache, rash, nausea or vomiting, consult a doctor promptly. A persistent cough may be a sign of a serious condition. If cough persists for more than 1 week, tends to recur or is accompanied by fever, rash or persistent headache, consult a doctor. Do not take this product for persistent or chronic cough such as occurs with smoking, asthma, emphysema or if cough is accompanied by excessive phlegm (mucus) unless directed by a doctor. Do not exceed recommended dosage because at higher doses, nervousness, dizziness or sleeplessness may occur. Do not take this product if you have heart disease, high blood pressure, thyroid disease, diabetes or difficulty in urination due to enlargement of the prostate gland unless directed by a doctor. Do not use with other products containing acetaminophen.
DO NOT USE IF CARTON IS OPENED OR IF A BLISTER UNIT IS BROKEN. KEEP THIS AND ALL MEDICATION OUT OF THE REACH OF CHILDREN. AS WITH ANY DRUG, IF YOU ARE PREGNANT OR NURSING A BABY, SEEK THE ADVICE OF A HEALTH PROFESSIONAL BEFORE USING THIS PRODUCT. IN CASE OF ACCIDENTAL OVERDOSE, CONTACT A DOCTOR OR POISON CONTROL CENTER IMMEDIATELY. PROMPT MEDICAL ATTENTION IS CRITICAL FOR ADULTS AS WELL AS FOR CHILDREN EVEN IF YOU DO NOT NOTICE ANY SIGNS OR SYMPTOMS.

Multi-Symptom Formula TYLENOL COLD Medication: Do not take this product for more than 7 days or for fever for more than 3 days unless directed by a doctor. If symptoms do not improve or are accompanied by fever, consult a doctor. If sore throat is severe, persists for more than 2 days, is accompanied or followed by fever, headache, rash, nausea or vomiting, consult a doctor promptly. A persistent cough may be a sign of a serious condition. If cough persists for more than 1 week, tends to recur or is accompanied by fever, rash or persistent headache, consult a doctor. Do not take this product for persistent or chronic cough such as occurs with smoking, asthma, emphysema or if cough is accompanied by excessive phlegm (mucus) unless directed by a doctor. Do not exceed recommended dosage because at higher doses, nervousness, dizziness or sleeplessness may occur. May cause excitability in children. Do not take this product unless directed by a doctor, if you have a breathing problem such as emphysema or chronic bronchitis, or if you have glaucoma or difficulty in urination due to enlargement of the prostate gland. Do not take this product if you have heart disease, high blood pressure, thyroid disease or diabetes unless directed by a doctor. May cause drowsiness; alcohol, sedatives and tranquilizers may increase the drowsiness effect. Avoid alcoholic beverages while taking this product. Do not take this product if you are taking sedatives or tranquilizers without first consulting your doctor. Use caution when driving a motor vehicle or operating machinery. Do not use with other products containing acetaminophen.
DO NOT USE IF CARTON IS OPENED OR IF A BLISTER UNIT IS BROKEN. KEEP THIS AND ALL MEDICATION OUT OF THE REACH OF CHILDREN. AS WITH ANY DRUG, IF YOU ARE PREGNANT OR NURSING A BABY, SEEK THE ADVICE OF A HEALTH PROFESSIONAL BEFORE USING THIS PRODUCT. IN CASE OF ACCIDENTAL OVERDOSE, CONTACT A DOCTOR OR POISON CONTROL CENTER IMMEDIATELY. PROMPT MEDICAL ATTENTION IS CRITICAL FOR ADULTS AS WELL AS FOR CHILDREN EVEN IF YOU DO NOT NOTICE ANY SIGNS OR SYMPTOMS.

Warning: *TYLENOL COLD Multi-Symptom Hot Medication:* Do not take this product for more than 7 days or for fever for more than 3 days unless directed by a doctor. If symptoms do not improve or are accompanied by fever, consult a doctor. If sore throat is severe, persists for more than 2 days, is accompanied or followed by fever, headache, rash, nausea or vomiting, consult a doctor promptly. A persistent cough may be a sign of a serious condition. If cough persists for more than 1 week, tends to recur or is accompanied by fever, rash or persistent headache, consult a doctor. Do not take this product for persistent or

chronic cough such as occurs with smoking, asthma, emphysema or if cough is accompanied by excessive phlegm (mucus) unless directed by a doctor. Do not exceed recommended dosage because at higher doses, nervousness, dizziness or sleeplessness may occur. May cause excitability especially in children. Do not take this product, unless directed by a doctor, if you have a breathing problem such as emphysema or chronic bronchitis, or if you have glaucoma or difficulty in urination due to enlargement of the prostate gland. Do not take this product if you have heart disease, high blood pressure, thyroid disease or diabetes unless directed by a doctor. May cause drowsiness; alcohol, sedatives and tranquilizers may increase the drowsiness effect. Avoid alcoholic beverages while taking this product. Do not take this product if you are taking sedatives or tranquilizers without first consulting your doctor. Use caution when driving a motor vehicle or operating machinery. Do not use with other products containing acetaminophen.

DO NOT USE IF PRINTED CARTON OVERWRAP IS BROKEN OR MISSING OR IF FOIL PACKET IS TORN OR BROKEN. KEEP THIS AND ALL MEDICATION OUT OF THE REACH OF CHILDREN. AS WITH ANY DRUG, IF YOU ARE PREGNANT OR NURSING A BABY, SEEK THE ADVICE OF A HEALTH PROFESSIONAL BEFORE USING THIS PRODUCT. IN CASE OF ACCIDENTAL OVERDOSE, CONTACT A DOCTOR OR POISON CONTROL CENTER IMMEDIATELY. PROMPT MEDICAL ATTENTION IS CRITICAL FOR ADULTS AS WELL AS FOR CHILDREN EVEN IF YOU DO NOT NOTICE ANY SIGNS OR SYMPTOMS.
PHENYLKETONURICS: CONTAINS PHENYLALANINE 11 MG PER PACKET.

Alcohol Warning: If you generally consume 3 or more alcohol-containing drinks per day, you should consult your physician for advice on when and how you should take [product] or other pain relievers.

Drug Interaction Precaution: *TYLENOL COLD Medication No Drowsiness Formula, Multi-Symptom Formula TYLENOL COLD Medication* and *TYLENOL COLD Multi-Symptom Hot Medication:* Do not take this product if you are presently taking a prescription drug for high blood pressure or you are now taking a prescription monoamine oxidase inhibitor (MAOI) (certain drugs for depression, psychiatric or emotional conditions, or Parkinson's disease), or for 2 weeks after stopping the MAOI drug. If you are uncertain whether your prescription drug contains an MAOI, consult a health professional before taking this product.

PROFESSIONAL INFORMATION

Overdosage Information: *TYLENOL COLD Medication No Drowsiness Formula, Multi-Symptom Formula TYLENOL COLD Medication and TYLENOL COLD Multi-Symptom Hot Medication:* Acetaminophen in massive overdosage may cause hepatic toxicity in some patients. In adults and adolescents, hepatic toxicity has rarely been reported following ingestion of acute overdoses of less than 10 grams. Fatalities are infrequent (less than 3–4% of untreated cases) and have rarely been reported with overdoses of less than 15 grams. In children, an acute overdosage of less than 150 mg/kg has not been associated with hepatic toxicity.

Early symptoms following a potentially hepatotoxic overdose may include: nausea, vomiting, diaphoresis and general malaise. Clinical and laboratory evidence of hepatic toxicity may not be apparent until 48 to 72 hours postingestion. In adults and adolescents, regardless of the quantity of acetaminophen reported to have been ingested, administer acetylcysteine immediately if 24 hours or less have elapsed from the reported time of ingestion. For full prescribing information, refer to the acetylcysteine package insert. Do not await results of assays for plasma acetaminophen level before initiating treatment with acetylcysteine. The following additional procedures are recommended. The stomach should be emptied promptly by lavage or by induction of emesis with syrup of ipecac. A plasma acetaminophen assay should be obtained as early as possible, but no sooner than four hours following ingestion. If plasma level falls above the lower treatment line on the acetaminophen overdose nomogram, acetylcysteine therapy should be continued. Liver function studies should be obtained initially and repeated at 24-hour intervals.

Serious toxicity or fatalities are extremely infrequent in children, possibly due to differences in the way they metabolize acetaminophen. In children, the maximum potential amount ingested can be more easily estimated. If more than 150 mg/kg or an unknown amount was ingested, obtain a plasma acetaminophen level. The plasma acetaminophen level should be obtained as soon as possible, but no sooner than 4 hours following the ingestion. If plasma level falls above the lower treatment line on the acetaminophen overdose nomogram, the acetylcysteine therapy should be initiated and continued for a full course of therapy. If plasma acetaminophen assay capability is not available, and the estimated acetaminophen ingestion exceeds 150 mg/kg, acetylcysteine therapy should be initiated and continued for a full course of therapy.

For additional emergency information, call your regional poison center or call the Rocky Mountain Poison Center toll-free, (1-800-525-6115).

Symptoms from pseudoephedrine overdose consist most often of mild anxiety, tachycardia and/or mild hypertension. Symptoms usually appear within 4 to 8 hours of ingestion and are transient, usually requiring no treatment.

Acute dextromethorphan overdose usually does not result in serious signs and symptoms unless massive amounts have been ingested. Signs and symptoms of a substantial overdose may include nausea and vomiting, visual disturbances, CNS disturbances, and urinary retention. Chlorpheniramine toxicity should be treated as you would an antihistamine/anticholinergic overdose and is likely to be present within a few hours after acute ingestion.

Alcohol Information: *TYLENOL COLD Medication No Drowsiness Formula, Multi-symptom Formula TYLENOL COLD Medication and TYLENOL COLD Multi-Symptom Hot Medication:* Chronic heavy alcohol abusers may be at increased risk of liver toxicity from excessive acetaminophen use, although reports of this event are rare. Reports almost invariably involve cases of severe chronic alcoholics and the dosages of acetaminophen most often exceed recommended doses and often involve substantial overdose. Professionals should alert their patients who regularly consume large amounts of alcohol not to exceed recommended doses of acetaminophen.

Inactive Ingredients: *TYLENOL COLD No Drowsiness Formula:* Caplet: cellulose, corn starch, glyceryl triacetate, hydroxypropyl methylcellulose, iron oxide black, magnesium stearate, sodium starch glycolate, titanium dioxide, Blue #1 and Yellow #10. Gelcap: benzyl alcohol, butylparaben, castor oil, cellulose, corn starch, edetate calcium disodium, gelatin, hydroxypropyl methylcellulose, magnesium stearate, methylparaben, propylparaben, sodium propionate, sodium lauryl sulfate, sodium starch glycolate, titanium dioxide, Red #40 and Yellow #10.

Multi-Symptom Formula TYLENOL COLD Medication: Tablets: cellulose, cornstarch, magnesium stearate, Yellow #6 and Yellow #10. Caplets: cellulose, cornstarch, glyceryl triacetate, hydroxypropyl methylcellulose, iron oxide black, magnesium stearate, sodium starch glycolate, titanium dioxide, Blue #1 and Yellow #6 and #10.

TYLENOL COLD Multi-Symptom Hot Medication: Aspartame, citric acid, corn starch, sodium citrate, sucrose, Red #40 and Yellow #10.

How Supplied: *TYLENOL COLD No Drowsiness Formula:* Caplets (colored white, imprinted "TYLENOL COLD") blister packs of 24 and tamper-resistant bottles of 50. Gelcaps (colored red and tan, imprinted "TYLENOL COLD") blister packs of 20 and tamper-resistant bottles of 40.

Multi-Symptom Formula TYLENOL COLD Medication: Tablets (colored yellow, imprinted "TYLENOL Cold") blister packs of 24 and tamper-resistant bottles of 50. Caplets (light yellow, imprinted "TYLENOL Cold") blister packs of 24 and tamper-resistant bottles of 50.

TYLENOL COLD Multi-Symptom Hot Medication: Packets of powder (yellow colored) in cartons of 6 tamper-resistant foil packets.

Shown in Product Identification Guide, page 514

Multi-Symptom
TYLENOL® COUGH Medication

Multi-Symptom
TYLENOL® COUGH Medication
with Decongestant

Product information for all dosage forms of TYLENOL COUGH have been combined under this heading.

Description: Each 15 ml (3 tsp.) adult dose of *Multi-Symptom TYLENOL COUGH Medication* contains dextromethorphan HBr 30 mg, and acetaminophen 650 mg.

Each 15 ml (3 tsp.) adult dose of *Multi-Symptom TYLENOL COUGH Medication with Decongestant* contains dextromethorphan HBr 30 mg, acetaminophen 650 mg, and pseudoephedrine HCl 60 mg.

Actions: *Multi-Symptom TYLENOL® COUGH Medication* contains a clinically proven cough suppressant, and an analgesic-antipyretic. Acetaminophen produces analgesia by elevation of the pain threshold and antipyresis through action on the hypothalamic heat-regulating center. Dextromethorphan is a cough suppressant which provides temporary relief of coughs due to minor throat irritations that may occur with the common cold.

Multi-Symptom TYLENOL COUGH Medication with Decongestant contains, in addition to the above ingredients, a sympathomimetic amine, pseudoephedrine HCl, which provides temporary relief of nasal congestion.

Indications: *Multi-Symptom TYLENOL® COUGH Medication* provides effective, temporary relief of coughing, and the aches, pains and sore throat that may accompany a cough due to a cold.

Multi-Symptom TYLENOL COUGH Medication with Decongestant provides effective, temporary relief of coughing, nasal congestion and the aches, pains and sore throat that may accompany a cough due to a cold.

Directions: *Multi-Symptom TYLENOL COUGH Medication and Multi-Symptom TYLENOL COUGH Medication with Decongestant:* Adults (12 years and older): 1 tablespoon or 3 teaspoons every 6–8 hours, not to exceed 4 doses in 24 hours. Children: (ages 6–11) 1½ teaspoons every 6–8 hours, not to exceed 4 doses in 24 hours. Not for use in children under 6 years of age.

Precautions: *Multi-Symptom TYLENOL COUGH Medication:* If a rare sen-

Continued on next page

McNeil Consumer—Cont.

sitivity reaction occurs, the drug should be discontinued.

Multi-Symptom TYLENOL COUGH Medication with Decongestant: If a rare sensitivity reaction occurs, the drug should be discontinued. Although pseudoephedrine is virtually without pressor effect in normotensive patients, it should be used with caution in hypertensives.

Warning: ***Multi-Symptom TYLENOL COUGH Medication:*** Do not take this product for more than 10 days or for fever for more than 3 days unless directed by a physician. Severe or recurrent pain or high or continued fever may be indicative of serious illness. Under these conditions, consult a doctor. A persistent cough may be a sign of a serious condition. If cough persists for more than 1 week, tends to recur or is accompanied by fever, rash or persistent headache, consult a doctor. Do not take this product for persistent or chronic cough such as occurs with smoking, asthma, emphysema, or if cough is accompanied by excessive phlegm (mucus) unless directed by a doctor. If sore throat is severe, persists for more than 2 days, is accompanied or followed by fever, headache, rash, nausea or vomiting, consult a doctor promptly. Do not use with other products containing acetaminophen.

DO NOT USE IF PRINTED PLASTIC BOTTLE WRAP OR PRINTED FOIL INNER SEAL IS BROKEN. **As with any drug, if you are pregnant or nursing a baby, seek the advice of a health professional before using this product. Keep this and all medication out of the reach of children. In case of accidental overdosage, contact a doctor or poison control center immediately. Prompt medical attention is critical for adults as well as children even if you do not notice any signs or symptoms.**

Multi-Symptom TYLENOL COUGH Medication with Decongestant: Do not take this product for more than 7 days or for fever for more than 3 days unless directed by a doctor. If symptoms do not improve or are accompanied by fever, consult a doctor. A persistent cough may be a sign of a serious condition. If cough persists for more than 1 week, tends to recur or is accompanied by fever, rash or persistent headache, consult a doctor. Do not take this product for persistent or chronic cough such as occurs with smoking, asthma, emphysema, or if cough is accompanied by excessive phlegm (mucus) unless directed by a doctor. Do not exceed the recommended dosage because at higher doses nervousness, dizziness or sleeplessness may occur. Do not take this product if you have heart disease, high blood pressure, thyroid disease, diabetes or difficulty in urination due to enlargement of the prostate gland unless directed by a doctor. If sore throat is severe, persists for more than 2 days, is accompanied or followed by fever, headache, rash, nausea or vomiting, consult a

doctor promptly. Do not use with other products containing acetaminophen.

DO NOT USE IF PRINTED PLASTIC BOTTLE WRAP OR PRINTED FOIL INNER SEAL IS BROKEN. **As with any drug, if you are pregnant or nursing a baby, seek the advice of a health professional before using this product. Keep this and all medication out of the reach of children. In case of accidental overdosage, contact a doctor or poison control center immediately. Prompt medical attention is critical for adults as well as children even if you do not notice any signs or symptoms.**

Alcohol Warning: ***Multi-Symptom TYLENOL COUGH Medication and Multi-Symptom TYLENOL COUGH Medication with Decongestant:*** If you generally consume 3 or more alcohol-containing drinks per day, you should consult your physician for advice on when and how you should take [product] and other pain relievers.

Drug Interaction Precaution: ***Multi-Symptom TYLENOL COUGH Medication:*** Do not use this product if you are presently taking a prescription monoamine oxidase inhibitor (MAOI) (certain drugs for depression, psychiatric or emotional conditions, or Parkinson's Disease), or for 2 weeks after stopping the MAOI drug. If you are uncertain whether your prescription drug contains an MAOI, consult a health professional before taking this product.

Multi-Symptom TYLENOL COUGH Medication with Decongestant: Do not use this product if you are presently taking a prescription drug for high blood pressure or you are now taking a prescription monoamine oxidase inhibitor (MAOI) (certain drugs for depression or psychiatric or emotional conditions, or Parkinson's Disease), or for 2 weeks after stopping the MAOI drug. If you are uncertain whether your prescription drug contains an MAOI, consult a health professional before taking this product.

PROFESSIONAL INFORMATION

Overdosage Information: ***Multi-Symptom TYLENOL COUGH Medication and Multi-Symptom TYLENOL COUGH Medication with Decongestant:*** Acetaminophen in massive overdosage may cause hepatic toxicity in some patients. In adults and adolescents, hepatic toxicity has rarely been reported following ingestion of acute overdoses of less than 10 grams. Fatalities are infrequent (less than 3–4% of untreated cases) and have rarely been reported with overdoses of less than 15 grams. In children, an acute overdosage of less than 150 mg/kg has not been associated with hepatic toxicity.

Early symptoms following a potentially hepatotoxic overdose may include: nausea, vomiting, diaphoresis and general malaise. Clinical and laboratory evidence of hepatic toxicity may not be apparent until 48 to 72 hours postingestion. In adults and adolescents, regardless of

the quantity of acetaminophen reported to have been ingested, administer acetylcysteine immediately if 24 hours or less have elapsed from the reported time of ingestion. For full prescribing information, refer to the acetylcysteine package insert. Do not await results of assays for plasma acetaminophen level before initiating treatment with acetylcysteine. The following additional procedures are recommended. The stomach should be emptied promptly by lavage or by induction of emesis with syrup of ipecac. A plasma acetaminophen assay should be obtained as early as possible, but no sooner than four hours following ingestion. If plasma level falls above the lower treatment line on the acetaminophen overdose nomogram, acetylcysteine therapy should be continued. Liver function studies should be obtained initially and repeated at 24-hour intervals.

Serious toxicity or fatalities are extremely infrequent in children, possibly due to differences in the way they metabolize acetaminophen. In children, the maximum potential amount ingested can be more easily estimated. If more than 150 mg/kg or an unknown amount was ingested, obtain a plasma acetaminophen level. The plasma acetaminophen level should be obtained as soon as possible, but no sooner than 4 hours following the ingestion. If the plasma level falls above the lower treatment line on the acetaminophen overdose nomogram, the acetylcysteine therapy should be initiated and continued for a full course of therapy. If plasma acetaminophen assay capability is not available, and the estimated acetaminophen ingestion exceeds 150 mg/kg, acetycysteine therapy should be initiated and continued for a full course of therapy.

For additional emergency information, call your regional poison center or call the Rocky Mountain Poison Center toll-free (1-800-525-6115).

Acute dextromethorphan overdose usually does not result in serious signs and symptoms unless massive amounts have been ingested. Signs and symptoms of a substantial overdose may include nausea and vomiting, visual disturbances, CNS disturbances, and urinary retention.

Symptoms from pseudoephedrine overdose consist most often of mild anxiety, tachycardia and/or mild hypertension. Symptoms usually appear within 4 to 8 hours of ingestion and are transient, usually requiring no treatment.

Alcohol Information: ***Multi-Symptom TYLENOL COUGH Medication and Multi-Symptom TYLENOL COUGH Medication with Decongestant:*** Chronic heavy alcohol abusers may be at increased risk of liver toxicity from excessive acetaminophen use, although reports of this event are rare. Reports almost invariably involve cases of severe chronic alcoholics and the dosages of acetaminophen most often exceed recommended doses and often involve substantial overdose. Professionals should alert their patients who regularly consume large amounts of alcohol not to exceed recommended doses of acetaminophen.

Inactive Ingredients: *Multi-Symptom TYLENOL COUGH Medication:* Alcohol (5%), citric acid, flavors, high fructose corn syrup, polyethylene glycol, propylene glycol, purified water, sodium benzoate, sodium carboxymethylcellulose, sodium saccharin, sorbitol, Red #40.

Multi-Symptom TYLENOL COUGH Medication with Decongestant: Alcohol (5%), citric acid, flavors, high fructose corn syrup. polyethylene glycol, propylene glycol, purified water, sodium benzoate, sodium carboxymethylcellulose, sodium saccharin, sorbitol, Blue #1, and Red #40.

How Supplied: *Multi-Symptom TYLENOL® COUGH Medication* is available in a 4 oz. bottle with child resistant safety cap and tamper resistant packaging.

Multi-Symptom TYLENOL COUGH Medication with Decongestant is available in a 4 oz. bottle with child resistant safety cap, and tamper resistant packaging.

Shown in Product Identification Guide, page 514

**Maximum Strength
TYLENOL® FLU Medication
No Drowsiness Formula Gelcaps**

**Maximum Strength
TYLENOL® FLU NightTime
Medication Gelcaps**

**Maximum Strength
TYLENOL® FLU NightTime
Hot Medication Packets**

Product information for all dosage forms of TYLENOL FLU have been combined under this heading.

Description: Each *Maximum Strength TYLENOL FLU Medication No Drowsiness Formula Gelcap* contains acetaminophen 500 mg, pseudoephedrine hydrochloride 30 mg, and dextromethorphan hydrobromide 15 mg.

Each *Maximum Strength TYLENOL FLU NightTime Medication Gelcap* contains acetaminophen 500 mg, pseudoephedrine hydrochloride 30 mg, and diphenhydramine hydrochloride 25 mg.

Each packet of *Maximum Strength TYLENOL FLU NightTime Hot Medication* contains acetaminophen 1000 mg, pseudoephedrine hydrochloride 60 mg and diphenhydramine hydrochloride 50 mg.

Actions: *Maximum Strength TYLENOL FLU Medication No Drowsiness Formula* contains a clinically proven analgesic-antipyretic, decongestant and cough suppressant. Acetaminophen produces analgesia by elevation of the pain threshold and antipyresis through action on the hypothalamic heat-regulating center. Acetaminophen is equal to aspirin in analgesic and antipyretic effectiveness and it is unlikely to produce many of

the side effects associated with aspirin and aspirin-containing products. Pseudoephedrine hydrochloride is a sympathomimetic amine which provides temporary relief of nasal congestion. Dextromethorphan is a cough suppressant which provides temporary relief of coughs due to minor throat irritations that may occur with the common cold.

Maximum Strength TYLENOL FLU NightTime Medication and *Maximum Strength TYLENOL FLU NightTime Hot Medication* contains the same clinically proven analgesic-antipyretic and decongestant as Maximum Strength TYLENOL FLU Medication No Drowsiness Formula along with an antihistamine. Diphenhydramine is an antihistamine which helps provide temporary relief of runny nose and sneezing.

Indications: *Maximum Strength TYLENOL FLU Medication No Drowsiness Formula* provides effective temporary relief of body aches, headaches, fever, sore throat, coughing and nasal congestion due to a cold or "flu."

Maximum Strength TYLENOL FLU NightTime Medication and *Maximum Strength TYLENOL FLU NightTime Hot Medication* provides effective temporary relief of body aches, headaches, fever, sore throat, nasal congestion, and runny nose/sneezing due to a cold or "flu" so you can rest.

Directions: *Maximum Strength TYLENOL FLU Medication No Drowsiness Formula:* Adults (12 years and older): Two gelcaps every 6 hours, not to exceed 8 gelcaps in 24 hours. Not for use in children under 12 years of age.

Maximum Strength TYLENOL FLU NightTime Medication: Adults (12 years and older): Two gelcaps at bedtime. May repeat every 6 hours, not to exceed 8 gelcaps in 24 hours. Not for use in children under 12 years of age.

Maximum Strength TYLENOL FLU NightTime Hot Medication: Adults (12 years and older): Dissolve one packet in 6 oz. cup of hot water. Sip while hot. Sweeten to taste, if desired. May repeat every 6 hours, not to exceed 4 doses in 24 hours. Not for use in children under 12 years of age.

Precautions: *Maximum Strength TYLENOL FLU Medication No Drowsiness Formula, Maximum Strength TYLENOL FLU NightTime Medication, and Maximum Strength TYLENOL FLU NightTime Hot Medication:* If a rare sensitivity reaction occurs, the drug should be stopped. Although pseudoephedrine is virtually without pressor effect in normotensive patients, it should be used with caution in hypertensives.

Warnings: *Maximum Strength TYLENOL FLU Medication No Drowsiness Formula:* Do not take this product for more than 7 days or for fever for more than 3 days unless directed by a doctor. If symptoms do not improve or are accompanied by fever, consult a doctor. A persistent cough may be a sign of a serious condition. If cough persists for

more than 1 week, tends to recur or is accompanied by fever, rash or persistent headache, consult a doctor. Do not take this product for persistent or chronic cough such as occurs with smoking, asthma, emphysema or if cough is accompanied by excessive phlegm (mucus) unless directed by a doctor. If sore throat is severe, persists for more than 2 days, is accompanied or followed by fever, headache, rash, nausea or vomiting, consult a doctor promptly. Do not exceed recommended dosage because at higher doses, nervousness, dizziness or sleeplessness may occur. Do not take this product if you have heart disease, high blood pressure, thyroid disease, diabetes or difficulty in urination due to enlargement of the prostate gland unless directed by a doctor. Do not use with other products containing acetaminophen.
DO NOT USE IF CARTON IS OPENED OR IF A BLISTER UNIT IS BROKEN. KEEP THIS AND ALL MEDICATION OUT OF THE REACH OF CHILDREN. AS WITH ANY DRUG, IF YOU ARE PREGNANT OR NURSING A BABY, SEEK THE ADVICE OF A HEALTH PROFESSIONAL BEFORE USING THIS PRODUCT. IN CASE OF ACCIDENTAL OVERDOSE, CONTACT A DOCTOR OR POISON CONTROL CENTER IMMEDIATELY. PROMPT MEDICAL ATTENTION IS CRITICAL FOR ADULTS AS WELL AS CHILDREN EVEN IF YOU DO NOT NOTICE ANY SIGNS OR SYMPTOMS.
Maximum StrengthTYLENOL FLU NightTime Medication Gelcaps: Do not exceed the recommended dosage, because at higher doses, nervousness, dizziness or sleeplessness may occur. Do not take this product for more than 7 days or for fever for more than 3 days unless directed by a doctor. If symptoms do not improve or are accompanied by fever, consult a doctor. If sore throat is severe, persists for more than 2 days, is accompanied by fever, headache, rash nausea or vomiting, consult a doctor promptly. May cause excitability, especially in children. Do not take this product, unless directed by a doctor, if you have a breathing problem such as emphysema or chronic bronchitis, or if you have glaucoma or difficulty in urination due to enlargement of the prostate gland. Do not take this product if you have heart disease, high blood pressure, thyroid disease, or diabetes unless directed by a doctor. May cause marked drowsiness: alcohol, sedatives and tranquilizers may increase the drowsiness effect. Avoid alcoholic beverages while taking this product. Do not take this product if you are taking sedatives or tranquilizers without first consulting your doctor. Use caution when driving a motor vehicle or operating machinery. Do not use with other products containing acetaminophen.
DO NOT USE IF CARTON IS OPENED OR IF A BLISTER UNIT IS BROKEN. KEEP THIS AND ALL MEDICATION OUT OF THE REACH OF CHILDREN.

Continued on next page

McNeil Consumer—Cont.

AS WITH ANY DRUG, IF YOU ARE PREGNANT OR NURSING A BABY, SEEK THE ADVICE OF A HEALTH PROFESSIONAL BEFORE USING THIS PRODUCT. IN CASE OF ACCIDENTAL OVERDOSE, CONTACT A DOCTOR OR POISON CONTROL CENTER IMMEDIATELY. PROMPT MEDICAL ATTENTION IS CRITICAL FOR ADULTS AS WELL AS CHILDREN EVEN IF YOU DO NOT NOTICE ANY SIGNS OR SYMPTOMS.

Maximum Strength TYLENOL FLU NightTime Hot Medication: Do not exceed the recommended dosage, because at higher doses, nervousness, dizziness or sleeplessness may occur. Do not take this product for more than 7 days or for fever for more than 3 days unless directed by a doctor. If symptoms do not improve or are accompanied by fever, consult a doctor. If sore throat is severe, persists for more than 2 days, is accompanied or followed by fever, headache, rash, nausea or vomiting, consult a doctor promptly. May cause excitability especially in children. Do not take this product, unless directed by a doctor, if you have a breathing problem such as emphysema or chronic bronchitis, or if you have glaucoma or difficulty in urination due to enlargement of the prostate gland. Do not take this product if you have heart disease, high blood pressure, thyroid disease or diabetes unless directed by a doctor. May cause marked drowsiness: alcohol, sedatives and tranquilizers may increase the drowsiness effect. Avoid alcoholic beverages while taking this product. Do not take this product if you are taking sedatives or tranquilizers without first consulting your doctor. Use caution when driving a motor vehicle or operating machinery. Do not use with other products containing acetaminophen.

DO NOT USE IF PRINTED CARTON OVERWRAP IS BROKEN OR MISSING OR IF CARTON IS OPENED OR FOIL PACKET IS TORN OR BROKEN. KEEP THIS AND ALL MEDICATION OUT OF THE REACH OF CHILDREN. AS WITH ANY DRUG, IF YOU ARE PREGNANT OR NURSING A BABY, SEEK THE ADVICE OF A HEALTH PROFESSIONAL BEFORE USING THIS PRODUCT. IN CASE OF ACCIDENTAL OVERDOSE, CONTACT A DOCTOR OR POISON CONTROL CENTER IMMEDIATELY. PROMPT MEDICAL ATTENTION IS CRITICAL FOR ADULTS AS WELL AS CHILDREN EVEN IF YOU DO NOT NOTICE ANY SIGNS OR SYMPTOMS.

PHENYLKETONURICS: CONTAINS PHENYLALANINE 67 MG PER PACKET.

Alcohol Warning: *Maximum Strength TYLENOL FLU Medication No Drowsiness Formula, Maximum Strength TYLENOL FLU NightTime Medication, and Maximum Strength TYLENOL FLU NightTime Hot Medication:* If you generally consume 3 or more alcohol-containing drinks per day, you should consult your physician for advice on when and how you should take [product] and other pain relievers.

Drug Interaction Precaution: *Maximum Strength TYLENOL FLU Medication No Drowsiness Formula, Maximum Strength TYLENOL FLU NightTime Medication, and Maximum Strength TYLENOL FLU NightTime Hot Medication:* Do not take this product if you are presently taking a prescription drug for high blood pressure or you are now taking a prescription monoamine oxidase inhibitor (MAOI) (certain drugs for depression, psychiatric or emotional conditions, or Parkinson's disease), or for 2 weeks after stopping the MAOI drug. If you are uncertain whether your prescription drug contains an MAOI, consult a health professional before taking this product.

PRODUCT INFORMATION

Overdosage Information: *Maximum Strength TYLENOL FLU Medication No Drowsiness Formula, Maximum Strength TYLENOL FLU NightTime Medication, and Maximum Strength TYLENOL FLU NightTime Hot Medication:* Acetaminophen in massive overdosage may cause hepatic toxicity in some patients. In adults and adolescents, hepatic toxicity has rarely been reported following ingestion of acute overdoses of less than 10 grams. Fatalities are infrequent (less than 3–4% of untreated cases) and have rarely been reported with overdosage of less than 15 grams. In children, an acute overdosage of less than 150 mg/kg has not been associated with hepatic toxicity.

Early symptoms following a potentially hepatotoxic overdose may include: nausea, vomiting, diaphoresis and general malaise. Clinical and laboratory evidence of hepatic toxicity may not be apparent until 48 to 72 hours postingestion. In adults and adolescents, regardless of the quantity of acetaminophen reported to have been ingested, administer acetylcysteine immediately if 24 hours or less have elapsed from the reported time of ingestion. For full prescribing information, refer to the acetylcysteine package insert. Do not await results of assays for plasma acetaminophen level before initiating treatment with acetylcysteine. The following additional procedures are recommended: The stomach should be emptied promptly by lavage or by induction of emesis with syrup of ipecac. A plasma acetaminophen assay should be obtained as early as possible, but not sooner than four hours following ingestion. If plasma level falls above the lower treatment line on the acetaminophen overdose nomogram, acetylcysteine therapy should be continued. Liver function studies should be obtained initially and repeated at 24-hour intervals.

Serious toxicity or fatalities are extremely infrequent in children, possibly due to differences in the way they metabolize acetaminophen. In children, the maximum potential amount ingested can be more easily estimated. If more than 150 mg/kg or an unknown amount was ingested, obtain an plasma acetaminophen level. The plasma acetaminophen level should be obtained as soon as possible, but no sooner than 4 hours following the ingestion. If plasma level falls above the lower treatment line on the acetaminophen overdose nomogram, the acetylcysteine therapy should be initiated and continued for a full course of therapy. If plasma acetaminophen assay capability is not available, and the estimated acetaminophen ingestion exceeds 150 mg/kg, acetylcysteine therapy should be initiated and continued for a full course of therapy.

For additional emergency information, call your regional poison center or call the Rocky Mountain Poison Center toll-free, (1-800-525-6115).

Symptoms from pseudoephedrine overdose consist most often of mild anxiety, tachycardia and/or mild hypertension. Symptoms usually appear within 4 to 8 hours of ingestion and are transient, usually requiring no treatment.

Acute dextromethorphan overdose usually does not result in serious signs and symptoms unless massive amounts have been ingested. Signs and symptoms of a substantial overdose may include nausea and vomiting, visual disturbances, CNS disturbances, and urinary retention.

Diphenhydramine toxicity should be treated as you would an antihistamine/anticholinergic overdose and is likely to be present within a few hours after acute ingestion.

Alcohol Information: *Maximum Strength TYLENOL FLU Medication No Drowsiness Formula, Maximum Strength TYLENOL FLU NightTime Medication, and Maximum Strength TYLENOL FLU NightTime Hot Medication:* Chronic heavy alcohol abusers may be at increased risk of liver toxicity from excessive acetaminophen use, although reports of this event are rare. Reports almost invariably involve cases of severe chronic alcoholics and the dosages of acetaminophen most often exceed recommended doses and often involve substantial overdose. Professionals should alert their patients who regularly consume large amounts of alcohol not to exceed recommended doses of acetaminophen.

Inactive Ingredients: *Maximum Strength TYLENOL FLU Medication No Drowsiness Formula:* Benzyl alcohol, butylparaben, castor oil, cellulose, corn starch edetate calcium disodium, gelatin, hydroxypropyl methylcellulose, iron oxide black, magnesium stearate, methylparaben, propylparaben, sodium lauryl sulfate, sodium propionate, sodium starch glycolate, titanium dioxide, Red #40 and Blue #1.

Maximum Strength TYLENOL FLU NightTime Medication: Benzyl alcohol, butylparaben, castor oil, cellulose, corn starch, edetate calcium disodium, gelatin, hydroxypropyl methylcellulose, iron oxide black, magnesium stearate, methylparaben, propylparaben, sodium citrate, sodium laurel sulfate, sodium propionate, sodium citrate, sucrose, sodium starch glycolate, titanium dioxide, Red #28 and Blue #1.

Maximum Strength TYLENOL FLU Hot Medication Packets: Ascorbic acid (vitamin C), aspartame, citric acid, flavors, sodium citrate, sucrose, Yellow #10, Blue #1, Red #40, and Yellow #6. May also contain: silicon dioxide.

How Supplied: *Maximum Strength TYLENOL FLU Medication No Drowsiness Formula:* Gelcaps (colored burgundy and white, imprinted "TYLENOL FLU") in blister packs of 10 and 20.

Maximum Strength TYLENOL FLU NightTime Medication: Gelcaps (colored blue and white, imprinted "TYLENOL FLU NT") in blister packs of 10 and 20.

Maximum Strength TYLENOL FLU Hot Medication Packets: Packets of powder (yellow colored) in cartons of 6 tamper-resistant foil packets.

Shown in Product Identification Guide, page 514

**Extra Strength
TYLENOL® HEADACHE PLUS
Pain Reliever with Antacid Caplets**

Description: Each Extra Strength TYLENOL® HEADACHE PLUS Pain Reliever with Antacid Caplet contains acetaminophen 500 mg. and calcium carbonate 250 mg.

Actions: TYLENOL® HEADACHE PLUS contains a clinically proven analgesic and antacid. Acetaminophen produces analgesia by elevation of the pain threshold. Acetaminophen is equal to aspirin in analgesic effectiveness, and it is unlikely to produce many of the side effects associated with aspirin and aspirin-containing products. The antacid, calcium carbonate, provides fast relief of heartburn or acid indigestion and upset stomach associated with these symptoms.

Indications: TYLENOL® HEADACHE PLUS provides temporary relief of minor aches and pains with heartburn or acid indigestion and upset stomach associated with these symptoms.

Directions: Adults and children 12 years of age and older: Two caplets every 6 hours. No more than a total of 8 caplets in any 24 hour period or as directed by a physician. Not for use in children under 12 years of age.

Precautions: If a rare sensitivity reaction occurs, the drug should be stopped.

Warnings: Do not use the maximum dosage of this product for more than 10 days except under the advice and supervision of a physician. Do not take the product for pain for more than 10 days, or for fever for more than 3 days unless directed by a physician. If pain or fever persists or gets worse, if new symptoms

occur, or if redness or swelling is present, consult a physician because these could be signs of a serious condition. Do not use with other products containing acetaminophen.

DO NOT USE IF CARTON IS OPENED, OR IF PRINTED NECK WRAP OR PRINTED FOIL SEAL IS BROKEN. KEEP THIS AND ALL MEDICATION OUT OF THE REACH OF CHILDREN. AS WITH ANY DRUG, IF YOU ARE PREGNANT OR NURSING A BABY, SEEK THE ADVICE OF A HEALTH PROFESSIONAL BEFORE USING THIS PRODUCT. IN THE CASE OF ACCIDENTAL OVERDOSE, CONTACT A DOCTOR OR A POISON CONTROL CENTER IMMEDIATELY. PROMPT MEDICAL ATTENTION IS CRITICAL FOR ADULTS AS WELL AS FOR CHILDREN EVEN IF YOU DO NOT NOTICE ANY SIGNS OR SYMPTOMS.

Alcohol Warning: If you generally consume 3 or more alcohol-containing drinks per day, you should consult your physician for advice on when and how you should take Extra Strength TYLENOL® HEADACHE PLUS and other pain relievers.

Drug Interaction Precaution: Antacids may interact with certain prescription drugs. If you are presently taking a prescription drug, do not take this product without checking with your physician or other health professional.

PROFESSIONAL INFORMATION

Overdosage Information: Acetaminophen in massive overdosage may cause hepatic toxicity in some patients. In adults and adolescents, hepatic toxicity has rarely been reported following ingestion of acute overdosage of less than 10 grams. Fatalities are infrequent (less than 3–4% of untreated cases) and have rarely been reported with overdoses of less than 15 grams. In children, an acute overdosage of less than 150 mg/kg has not been associated with hepatic toxicity. Early symptoms following a potentially hepatotoxic overdose may include: nausea, vomiting, diaphoresis and general malaise. Clinical and laboratory evidence of hepatic toxicity may not be apparent until 48 to 72 hours postingestion. In adults and adolescents, regardless of the quantity of acetaminophen reported to have been ingested, administer acetylcysteine immediately if 24 hours or less have elapsed from the reported time of ingestion. For full prescribing information, refer to the acetylcysteine package insert. Do not await results of assays for plasma acetaminophen level before initiating treatment with acetylcysteine. The following additional procedures are recommended. The stomach should be emptied promptly by lavage or by induction of emesis with syrup of ipecac. A plasma acetaminophen assay should be obtained as early as possible, but no sooner than four hours following ingestion. If plasma level falls above the lower treatment line on the acetaminophen

overdose nomogram, acetylcysteine therapy should be continued. Liver function studies should be obtained initially and repeated at 24-hour intervals.

Serious toxicity or fatalities are extremely infrequent in children, possibly due to differences in the way they metabolize acetaminophen. In children, the maximum potential amount ingested can be more easily estimated. If more than 150 mg/kg or an unknown amount was ingested, obtain a plasma acetaminophen level. The plasma acetaminophen level should be obtained as soon as possible, but no sooner than 4 hours following the ingestion. If the plasma level falls above the lower treatment line on the acetaminophen overdose nomogram, the acetylcysteine therapy should be initiated and continued for a full course of therapy. If plasma acetaminophen, assay capability is not available, and the estimated acetaminophen ingestion exceeds 150 mg/kg, acetylcysteine therapy should be initiated and continued for a full course of therapy.

For additional emergency information, call your regional poison center or call the Rocky Mountain Poison Center toll-free (1-800-525-6115).

Alcohol Information: Chronic heavy alcohol abusers may be at increased risk of liver toxicity from excessive acetaminophen use, although reports of this event are rare. Reports almost invariably involve cases of severe chronic alcoholics and the dosages of acetaminophen most often exceed recommended doses and often involve substantial overdose. Professionals should alert their patients who regularly consume large amounts of alcohol not to exceed recommended doses of acetaminophen.

Inactive Ingredients: Acacia, Cellulose, Corn Starch, Croscarmellose Sodium, Hydroxypropyl Methylcellulose, Magnesium Stearate, Maltodextrin, Propylene Glycol, Sodium Starch Glycolate, Titanium Dioxide, Triacetin, Blue #1 and Blue #2.

How Supplied: Caplets (white with royal blue imprinted "TYLENOL Headache Plus"). Tamper resistant bottles of 24 and 50.

Shown in Product Identification Guide, page 514

**Extra Strength
TYLENOL® PM
Pain Reliever/Sleep Aid Caplets,
Geltabs and Gelcaps**

Description: Each Extra Strength TYLENOL® PM Caplet, Geltab or Gelcap contains acetaminophen 500 mg and diphenhydramine HCl 25 mg.

Actions: Extra Strength TYLENOL® PM Caplets, Geltabs and Gelcaps contain a clinically proven analgesic-antipyretic and an antihistamine. Maximum allowable non-prescription levels of acetami-

Continued on next page

McNeil Consumer—Cont.

nophen and diphenhydramine provide temporary relief of occasional headaches and minor aches and pains accompanying sleeplessness. Acetaminophen is equal to aspirin in analgesic and antipyretic effectiveness and it is unlikely to produce many of the side effects associated with aspirin containing products. Acetaminophen produces analgesia by elevation of the pain threshold. Diphenhydramine HCl is an antihistamine with sedative properties.

Indications: Extra Strength TYLENOL® PM Caplets, Geltabs and Gelcaps provide temporary relief of occasional headaches and minor aches and pains with accompanying sleeplessness.

Precautions: If a rare sensitivity reaction occurs, the drug should be discontinued.

Directions: Adults and Children 12 years of Age and Older: Two caplets, geltabs or gelcaps at bedtime or as directed by physician. Do not exceed recommended dosage. Not for use in children under 12 years of age.

Warnings: Do not use if carton is opened or printed neck wrap or printed foil inner seal is broken. Do not give to children under 12 years of age. If sleeplessness persists continuously for more than 2 weeks, consult your doctor. Insomnia may be a symptom of serious underlying medical illness. Do not take for pain for more than 10 days or for fever for more than 3 days unless directed by a doctor. If pain or fever persists, or gets worse, if new symptoms occur, or if redness or swelling is present, consul a doctor because these could be signs of a serious condition. Do not take this product, unless directed by a doctor, if you have a breathing problem such as emphysema or chronic bronchitis, or if you have glaucoma or difficulty in urination due to enlargement of the prostate gland. Avoid alcoholic beverages while taking this product. Do not take this product if your are taking sedatives or tranquilizers without first consulting your doctor.
As with any drug, if you are pregnant or nursing a baby, seek the advice of a health professional beffore using this product. Keep this and all drugs out of the reach of children. In case of accidental overdose, contact a doctor or poison control center immediately. Prompt medical attention is critical for adults as well as for children even if you do not notice any signs or symptoms. Do not use with other products containing acetaminophen.

Alcohol Warning: If you generally consume 3 or more alcohol-containing drinks per day, you should consult your physician for advice on when and how you should take Extra Strength TYLENOL® PM and other pain relievers.

Caution: This product will cause drowsiness. Do not drive a motor vehicle or operate machinery after use.

PROFESSIONAL INFORMATION

Overdosage Information: Acetaminophen in massive overdosage may cause hepatic toxicity in some patients. In adults and adolescents, hepatic toxicity has rarely been reported following ingestion of acute overdoses of less than 10 grams. Fatalities are infrequent (less than 3–4% of untreated cases) and have rarely been reported with overdoses of less than 15 grams. In children, an acute overdosage of less than 150 mg/kg has not been associated with hepatic toxicity. Early symptoms following a potentially hepatotoxic overdose may include: nausea, vomiting, diaphoresis and general malaise. Clinical and laboratory evidence of hepatic toxicity may not be apparent until 48 to 72 hours postingestion. In adults and adolescents, regardless of the quantity of acetaminophen reported to have been ingested, administer acetylcysteine immediately if 24 hours or less have elapsed from the reported time of ingestion. For full prescribing information, refer to the acetylcysteine package insert. Do not await results of assays for plasma acetaminophen level before initiating treatment with acetylcysteine. The following additional procedures are recommended. The stomach should be emptied promptly by lavage or by induction of emesis with syrup of ipecac. A plasma acetaminophen assay should be obtained as early as possible, but no sooner than four hours following ingestion. If plasma level falls above the lower treatment line on the acetaminophen overdose nomogram, acetylcysteine therapy should be continued. Liver function studies should be obtained initially and repeated at 24-hour intervals.
Serious toxicity or fatalities are extremely infrequent in children, possibly due to differences in the way they metabolize acetaminophen. In children, the maximum potential amount ingested can be more easily estimated. If more than 150 mg/kg or an unknown amount was ingested, obtain a plasma acetaminophen level. The plasma acetaminophen level should be obtained as soon as possible, but no sooner than 4 hours following the ingestion. If the plasma level falls above the lower treatment line on the acetaminophen overdose nomogram, the acetylcysteine therapy should be initiated and continued for a full course of therapy. If plasma acetaminophen assay capability is not available, and the estimated acetaminophen ingestion exceeds 150 mg/kg, acetylcysteine therapy should be initiated and continued for a full course of therapy.
For additional emergency information, call your regional poison center or call the Rocky Mountain Poison Center toll-free, (1-800-525-6115).
Diphenhydramine toxicity should be treated as you would an antihistamine/anticholinergic overdose and is likely to

be present within a few hours after acute ingestion.

Alcohol Information: Chronic heavy alcohol abusers may be at increased risk of liver toxicity from excessive acetaminophen use, although reports of this event are rare. Reports almost invariably involve cases of severe chronic alcoholics and the dosages of acetaminophen most often exceed recommended doses and often involve substantial overdose. Professionals should alert their patients who regularly consume large amounts of alcohol not to exceed recommended doses of acetaminophen.

Inactive Ingredients: Caplets: Cellulose, Cornstarch, Hydroxypropyl Methylcellulose, Magnesium Stearate or Stearic Acid and Colloidal Silicon Dioxide, Polyethylene Glycol, Polysorbate 80, Sodium Citrate, Sodium Starch Glycolate, Titanium Dioxide, Blue #1 and Blue #2.
Geltabs/Gelcaps: Benzyl Alcohol, Butylparaben, Castor Oil, Cellulose, Cornstarch, Edetate Calcium Disodium, Gelatin, Hydroxypropyl Methylcellulose, Magnesium Stearate, Propylparaben, Sodium Lauryl Sulfate, Sodium Citrate, Sodium Propionate, Sodium Starch Glycolate, Titanium Dioxide, Blue #1 and Red #28.

How Supplied: Caplets (colored light blue imprinted "Tylenol PM") tamper-resistant bottles of 24, 50, and 100.
Geltabs/Gelcaps (colored blue and white imprinted "TYLENOL PM") tamper-resistant bottles of 24 and 50.
Shown in Product Identification Guide, page 514

TYLENOL® SEVERE ALLERGY
Medication Caplets

Description: Each TYLENOL® SEVERE ALLERGY Caplet contains acetaminophen 500 mg. and Diphenhydramine hydrochloride 12.5 mg.

Actions: TYLENOL® SEVERE ALLERGY Caplets contain a clinically proven analgesic-antipyretic, and antihistamine. Acetaminophen produces analgesia by elevation of the pain threshold and antipyresis through action on the hypothalamic heat-regulating center. Acetaminophen is equal to aspirin in analgesic and antipyretic effectiveness, and it is unlikely to produce many of the side effects associated with aspirin and aspirin-containing products. Diphenhydramine is an antihistamine which helps provide temporary relief of itchy, watery eyes, runny nose, sneezing, itching of the nose or throat due to hay fever or other respiratory allergies.

Indications: TYLENOL® SEVERE ALLERGY provides effective temporary relief of itchy, watery eyes, runny nose, sneezing, sore or scratchy throat and itching of the nose or throat due to hay fever or other upper respiratory allergies.

Precautions: If a rare sensitivity reaction occurs, the drug should be stopped.

Directions: Adults and children 12 years of age and older: Two caplets every 4 to 6 hours, do not exceed 8 caplets in any 24 hours period. Not for use in children under 12 years of age.

Warnings: DO NOT USE IF CARTON IS OPEN OR IF A BLISTER UNIT IS BROKEN. Do not take for pain for more than 10 days or for fever for more than 3 days unless directed by a doctor if pain or fever persists, or gets worse, if new symptoms occur, or if redness or swelling is present, consult a doctor because these could be signs of a serious condition. If sore throat is severe, persists for more than 2 days, is accompanied or followed by fever, headache, rash, nausea or vomiting, consult a doctor promptly. May cause excitability especially in children. Do not take this product, unless directed by a doctor if you have a breathing problem such as emphysema or chronic bronchitis or if you have glaucoma or difficulty in urination due to enlargement of the prostate gland. May cause marked drowsiness; alcohol, sedatives and tranquilizers may increase the drowsiness effect. Avoid alcoholic beverages while taking this product. Do not take this product if you are taking sedatives or tranquilizers without first consulting your doctor. Use caution when driving a motor vehicle or operating machinery. As with any drug, if you are pregnant or nursing a baby, seek the advice of a health professional before using this product. Keep this and all drugs out of reach of children. In case of accidental overdose, contact a doctor or poison control center immediately. Prompt medical attention is critical for adults as well as for children even if you do not notice any signs or symptoms. Do not use with other products containing acetaminophen.

Alcohol Warning: If you generally consume 3 or more alcohol-containing drinks per day, you should consult your physician for advice on when and how you should take Tylenol® SEVERE ALLERGY Caplets and other pain relievers.

PROFESSIONAL INFORMATION

Overdosage Information: Acetaminophen in massive overdosage may cause hepatic toxicity in some patients. In adults and adolescents, hepatic toxicity has rarely been reported following ingestion of acute overdoses of less than 10 grams. Fatalities are infrequent (less than 3-4% of untreated cases) and have rarely been reported with overdoses of less than 15 grams. In children, an acute overdosage of less than 150 mg/kg has not been associated with hepatic toxicity. Early symptoms following a potentially hepatotoxic overdose may include: nausea, vomiting, diaphoresis and general malaise. Clinical and laboratory evidence of hepatic toxicity may not be apparent until 48 to 72 hours postingestion. In adults and adolescents, regardless of

the quantity of acetaminophen reported to have been ingested, administer acetylcysteine immediately if 24 hours or less have elapsed from the reported time of ingestion. For full prescribing information, refer to the acetylcysteine package insert. Do not await results of assays for plasma acetaminophen level before initiating treatment with acetylcysteine. The following additional procedures are recommended. The stomach should be emptied promptly by lavage or by induction of emesis with syrup of ipecac. A plasma acetaminophen assay should be obtained as early as possible, but no sooner than four hours following ingestion. If plasma level falls above the lower treatment line on the acetaminophen overdose nomogram, acetylcysteine therapy should be continued. Liver function studies should be obtained initially and repeated at 24-hour intervals.

Serious toxicity or fatalities are extremely infrequent in children, possibly due to differences in the way they metabolize acetaminophen. In children, the maximum potential amount ingested can be more easily estimated. If more than 150 mg/kg or an unknown amount was ingested, obtain a plasma acetaminophen level. The plasma acetaminophen level should be obtained as soon as possible, but no sooner than 4 hours following the ingestion. If plasma level falls above the lower treatment line on the acetaminophen overdose nomogram, the acetylcysteine therapy should be initiated and continued for a full course of therapy. If plasma acetaminophen assay capability is not available, and the estimated acetaminophen ingestion exceeds 150 mg/kg, acetylcysteine therapy should be initiated and continued for a full course of therapy.

For additional emergency information, call your regional poison center or call the Rocky Mountain Poison Center toll-free (1-800-525-6115).

Diphenhydramine toxicity should be treated as you would an antihistamine/anticholinergic overdose and is likely to be present within a few hours after acute ingestion.

Alcohol Information Chronic heavy alcohol abusers may be at increased risk of liver toxicity from excessive acetaminophen use, although reports of this event are rare. Reports almost invariably involve cases of severe chronic alcoholics and the dosages of acetaminophen most often exceed recommended doses and often involve substantial overdose. Professionals should alert their patients who regularly consume large amounts of alcohol not to exceed recommended doses of acetaminophen.

Inactive Ingredients: Cellulose, Corn Starch, Hydroxypropyl Cellulose, Hydroxypropyl Methylcellulose, Iron Oxide Black, Magnesium Stearate, Polyethylene Glycol, Sodium Citrate, Sodium Starch Glycolate, Titanium Dioxide, Yellow #6, Yellow #10.

How Supplied: Caplets: dark yellow, imprinted "TYLENOL Severe Allergy" –Blister packs of 12 and 24.
Shown in Product Identification Guide, page 513

Maximum Strength
TYLENOL® SINUS MEDICATION
Geltabs, Gelcaps, Caplets and Tablets

Description: Each Maximum Strength TYLENOL® SINUS MEDICATION Geltab, Gelcap, Caplet or Tablet contains acetaminophen 500 mg and pseudoephedrine hydrochloride 30 mg.

Actions: Maximum Strength TYLENOL SINUS MEDICATION contains a clinically proven analgesic-antipyretic and a decongestant. Maximum allowable nonprescription levels of acetaminophen and pseudoephedrine provide temporary relief of sinus headache and congestion. Acetaminophen is equal to aspirin in analgesic and antipyretic effectiveness and it is unlikely to produce many of the side effects associated with aspirin and aspirin-containing products.

Acetaminophen produces analgesia by elevation of the pain threshold and antipyresis through action on the hypothalamic heat-regulating center. Pseudoephedrine hydrochloride is a sympathomimetic amine which promotes sinus cavity drainage by reducing nasopharyngeal mucosal congestion.

Indications: Maximum Strength TYLENOL SINUS MEDICATION provides for the temporary relief of nasal and sinus congestion and sinus pain and headaches. Maximum Strength TYLENOL SINUS MEDICATION is particularly well-suited in patients with aspirin allergy, hemostatic disturbances (including anticoagulant therapy), and bleeding diatheses (e.g., hemophilia) and upper gastrointestinal disease (e.g., ulcer, gastritis, hiatus hernia).

Precautions: If a rare sensitivity occurs, the drug should be discontinued. Although pseudoephedrine is virtually without pressor effect in normotensive patients, it should be used with caution in hypertensives.

Directions: Adults and Children 12 years of Age and Older: Two Tablets, Caplets, Geltabs, or Gelcaps every 4–6 hours. Do not exceed eight Tablets, Caplets, Geltabs, or Gelcaps in any 24-hour period. Not for use in children under 12 years of age.

Warnings: Do not use if carton is opened or if blister unit is broken or if printed green neck wrap or printed foil inner seal is broken. Do not take for pain for more than 7 days or for fever for more than 3 days unless directed by a doctor if pain or fever persists. or get worse, if new symptoms occur, or if redness or swelling is present, consult a doctor because these

Continued on next page

McNeil Consumer—Cont.

could be signs of a serious condition. **Do not exceed recommended dosage.** If nervousness, dizziness or sleeplessness occur, discontinue use and consult a doctor. Do not take this product if you have heart disease, high blood pressure, thyroid disease, diabetes, or difficulty in urination due to enlargement of the prostate gland unless directed by a doctor. As with any drug, if you are pregnant or nursing a baby, seek the advice of a health professional before using this product. Keep this and all drugs out of the reach of children. In case of accidental overdose, contact a doctor or poison control center immediately. Prompt medical attention is critical for adults as well as for children even if you do not notice any signs or symptoms. Do not use with other products containing acetaminophen.

Alcohol Warning: If you generally consume 3 or more alcohol-containing drinks per day, you should consult your physician for advice on when and how you should take Maximum Strength TYLENOL® SINUS MEDICATION and other pain relievers.

Drug Interaction Precaution: Do not use this product if you are now taking a prescription monoamine oxidase inhibitor (MAOI) (certain drugs for depression, psychiatric or emotional conditions, or Parkinson's disease), or for 2 weeks after stopping the MAOI drug. If you are uncertain whether your prescription drug contains an MAOI, consult a health professional before taking this product.

PROFESSIONAL INFORMATION

Overdosage Information: Acetaminophen in massive overdosage may cause hepatic toxicity in some patients. In adults and adolescents, hepatic toxicity has rarely been reported following ingestion of acute overdoses of less than 10 grams. Fatalities are infrequent (less than 3–4% of untreated cases) and have rarely been reported with overdoses of less than 15 grams. In children, an acute overdosage of less than 150 mg/kg has not been associated with hepatic toxicity. Early symptoms following a potentially hepatotoxic overdose may include: nausea, vomiting, diaphoresis and general malaise. Clinical and laboratory evidence of hepatic toxicity may not be apparent until 48 to 72 hours postingestion. In adults and adolescents, regardless of the quantity of acetaminophen reported to have been ingested, administer acetylcysteine immediately if 24 hours or less have elapsed from the reported time of ingestion. For full prescribing information, refer to the acetylcysteine package insert. Do not await results of assays for plasma acetaminophen level before initiating treatment with acetylcysteine. The following additional procedures are recommended. The stomach should be emptied promptly by lavage or by induction of emesis with syrup of ipecac. A plasma acetaminophen assay should be obtained as early as possible, but no sooner than four hours following ingestion. If plasma level falls above the lower treatment line on the acetaminophen overdose nomogram, acetylcysteine therapy should be continued. Liver function studies should be obtained initially and repeated at 24-hour intervals.

Serious toxicity or fatalities are extremely infrequent in children, possibly due to differences in the way they metabolize acetaminophen. In children, the maximum potential amount ingested can be more easily estimated. If more than 150 mg/kg or an unknown amount was ingested, obtain a plasma acetaminophen level. The plasma acetaminophen level should be obtained as soon as possible, but no sooner than 4 hours following the ingestion. If plasma level falls above the lower treatment line on the acetaminophen overdose nomogram, the acetylcysteine therapy should be initiated and continued for a full course of therapy. If plasma acetaminophen assay capability is not available, and the estimated acetaminophen ingestion exceeds 150 mg/kg, acetylcysteine therapy should be initiated and continued for a full course of therapy.

For additional emergency information, call your regional poison center or call the Rocky Mountain Poison Center toll-free (1-800-525-6115).

Symptoms from pseodoephedrine overdose consist most often of mild anxiety, tachycardia and/or mild hypertension. Symptoms usually appear within 4 to 8 hours after ingestion and are transient, usually requiring no treatment.

Alcohol Information: Chronic heavy alcohol abusers may be at increased risk of liver toxicity from excessive acetaminophen use, although reports of this event are rare. Reports almost invariably involve cases of severe chronic alcoholics and the dosages of acetaminophen most often exceed recommended doses and often involve substantial overdose. Professionals should alert their patients who regularly consume large amounts of alcohol not to exceed recommended doses of acetaminophen.

Inactive Ingredients: Caplets—Carnuba Wax, Cellulose, Corn Starch, Hydroxypropyl Methylcellulose, Magnesium Stearate, Polyethylene Glycol, Polysorbate 80, Sodium Starch Glycolate, Titanium Dioxide, Blue #1, Red #40, Yellow #10.

Tablets—Cellulose, Corn Starch, Magnesium Stearate, Sodium Starch Glycolate, Blue #1, Yellow #6, and Yellow #10.

Gelcaps—Benzyl Alcohol, Butylparaben, Castor Oil, Cellulose, Corn Starch, Edetate Calcium Disodium, Gelatin, Hydroxypropyl Methylcellulose, Iron Oxide Black, Magnesium Stearate, Methylparaben, Propylparaben, Sodium Lauryl Sulfate, Sodium Propionate, Sodium Starch Glycolate, Titanium Dioxide, Blue #1 and Yellow #10.

Geltabs—Benzyl Alcohol, Butylparaben, Castor Oil, Cellulose, Corn Starch, Edetate Calcium Disodium, Gelatin, Hydroxypropyl Methylcellulose, Iron Oxide Black, Magnesium Stearate Methylparaben, Propylparaben, Sodium Lauryl Sulfate, Sodium Propionate, Sodium Starch Glycolate, Titanium Dioxide, D&C Yellow #10, FD&C Blue #1.

How Supplied: Tablets: (colored light green, imprinted "Maximum Strength TYLENOL SINUS")—in blister packs of 24 and tamper-resistant bottles of 50.

Caplets: (light green coating, printed "TYLENOL SINUS" in dark green) in blister packs of 24 and tamper-resistant bottles of 60.

Gelcaps: (colored green and white), printed "TYLENOL SINUS" in blister packs of 24 and tamper-resistant bottles of 60.

Geltabs: (colored green and white), printed "TYLENOL SINUS" in blister packs of 24 and tamper-resistant bottles of 60.

Shown in Product Identification Guide, page 515

Mead Johnson Nutritionals

Mead Johnson & Company
A Bristol-Myers Squibb Company
2400 W. LLOYD EXPRESSWAY
EVANSVILLE, IN 47721

Direct Inquiries to:
Product Information Section
Medical Services Department
(812) 429-5599

Enfamil® Infant Formula[1,3]
Enfamil® With Iron Infant Formula[1,3]
Enfamil® Premature Formula[3]
Enfamil® Premature Formula With Iron[3]
Enfamil® Human Milk Fortifier
Enfamil® Next Step® Toddler Formula[1]
Enfamil® Next Step® Soy Toddler Formula
Fer-In-Sol® Iron Supplement Drops, Syrup, Capsules
Lactofree® Milk-Based, Lactose-Free Formula[1,3]
Nutramigen® Hypoallergenic Protein Hydrolysate Formula[1,3]
Poly-Vi-Sol® Vitamins, Chewable Tablets and Drops (without Iron)
Poly-Vi-Sol® Vitamins, Peter Rabbit[TM2] Shaped Chewable Tablets (without Iron)
Poly-Vi-Sol® Vitamins with Iron, Peter Rabbit[TM2] Shaped Chewable Tablets
Poly-Vi-Sol® Vitamins with Iron, Drops
ProSobee® Soy Formula[1,3]

[1]Concentrated liquid, powder, and ready to use

[2]Trademark of F. Warne & Co., Inc.

Special Metabolic Diets:
Lofenalac® Iron Fortified Low Phenyl-alanine Diet Powder
Product 3200K Low Methionine Diet Powder
Product 3200AB Low PHE/TYR Diet Powder
Moducal® Dietary Carbohydrate Powder
Product 3232A Mono- and Disaccharide-Free Diet Powder
MSUD Diet Powder
Phenyl-Free® Phenylalanine-Free Diet Powder
Portagen® Iron Fortified Powder with Medium Chain Triglycerides
Pregestimil® Iron Fortified Protein Hydrolysate Formula with Medium Chain Triglycerides[3]
Infalyte® Oral Electrolyte Maintenance Solution Made With Rice Syrup Solids[3]
Kindercal™

[3] Available in Nursette® bottles

Special Metabolic Modules:
HIST 1
HIST 2
HOM 1
HOM 2
LYS 1
LYS 2
MSUD 1
MSUD 2
OS 1
OS 2
PKU 1
PKU 2
PKU 3
Product 80056 Protein-Free Diet Powder
TYR 1
TYR 2
UCD 1
UCD 2

Tri-Vi-Sol® Vitamin Drops
Tri-Vi-Sol® Vitamin Drops with Iron
Detailed information may be obtained by contacting Mead Johnson Nutritionals Medical Affairs Department at (812) 429-5599.

THERAGRAN® TABLETS
(High Potency Multivitamin Formula)
Nutrition Facts
Serving Size 1 caplet daily

Amount Per Caplet	% Daily Value
Vitamin A 5000 IU	100%
20% as Beta Carotene	
Vitamin C 90 mg	150%
Vitamin D 400 IU	100%
Vitamin E 30 IU	100%
Thiamin 3 mg	200%
Riboflavin 3.4 mg	200%
Niacin 20 mg	100%
Vitamin B₆ 3 mg	150%
Folate 400 mcg	100%
Vitamin B₁₂ 9 mcg	150%
Biotin 30 mcg	10%
Pantothenic Acid 10 mg	100%

Ingredients: Lactose, ascorbic acid, microcrystalline cellulose, dl-alpha tocopheryl acetate, niacinamide, calcium pantothenate, hydroxypropyl methylcellulose, povidone, pyridoxine hydrochloride, riboflavin, silicon dioxide, magnesium stearate, thiamin mononitrate, vitamin A acetate, polyethylene glycol, triacetin, stearic acid, titanium dioxide, annatto, beta carotene, Red 40 Lake, folic acid, biotin, vitamin D2, vitamin B12.

Warning: Close tightly and keep out of reach of children.

How Supplied: Packs of 130; and Unimatic® cartons of 100.

Storage: Store at room temperature; avoid excessive heat.

COMPLETE FORMULA THERAGRAN-M® TABLETS USP
(High Potency Multivitamin Formula with Minerals)
*USP: Theragran-M meets the USP standards of strength, quality, and purity for Oil- and Water-soluble Vitamins with Minerals Tablets.
Nutrition Facts
Serving Size 1 caplet daily

Amount Per Caplet	% Daily Value
Vitamin A 5000 IU	100%
20% as Beta Carotene	
Vitamin C 90 mg	150%
Vitamin D 400 IU	100%
Vitamin E 30 IU	100%
Vitamin K 28 mcg	*
Thiamin 3 mg	200%
Riboflavin 3.4 mg	200%
Niacin 20 mg	100%
Vitamin B₆ 3 mg	150%
Folate 400 mcg	100%
Vitamin B₁₂ 9 mcg	150%
Biotin 30 mcg	10%
Pantothenic Acid 10 mg	100%
Calcium 40 mg	4%
Iron 18 mg	100%
Phosphorus 31 mg	3%
Iodine 150 mcg	100%
Magnesium 100 mg	25%
Zinc 15 mg	100%
Selenium 21 mcg	*
Copper 2 mg	100%
Manganese 3.5 mg	*
Chromium 26 mcg	*
Molybdenum 32 mcg	*
Chloride 7.5 mg	*
Potassium 7.5 mg	Less than 1%

*Daily Value not established

Each caplet also contains 5 mcg nickel, 2 mg silicon, 150 mcg boron, 10 mcg tin, and 10 mcg vanadium.

Ingredients: Magnesium oxide, calcium phosphate, microcrystalline cellulose, ascorbic acid[1], dl-alpha tocopheryl acetate[2], ferrous fumarate, crospovidone, niacinamide[2], zinc oxide, povidone, hydroxypropyl methylcellulose, potassium chloride, calcium pantothenate[2], vitamin A acetate[2], beta carotene, manganese sulfate, vitamin D3[2], cupric sulfate, pyridoxine hydrochloride[2], silica gel, triacetin, polyethylene glycol, magnesium stearate, riboflavin[2], phytonadione, thiamin mononitrate[2], stearic acid, biotin[1], sodium borate, Red 40 Lake, Blue 2 Lake, cyanocobalamin[1], folic acid[1], potassium citrate, sodium citrate, potassium iodide, titanium dioxide, chromic chloride, sodium molybdate[1], sodium selenate[1], sodium metavandate, nickelous sulfate, stannous chloride.

[1]USP Method 2; [2]USP Method 3

Warning: Close tightly and keep out of reach of children. Contains Iron, which can be harmful or fatal to children in large doses. In case of accidental overdose, seek professional assistance or contact a poison control center immediately.

How Supplied: Packs of 90, 130, 200 and 240.

Storage: Store at room temperature; avoid excessive heat.

The Mentholatum Company, Inc
1360 NIAGARA STREET
BUFFALO, NY 14213

Direct Inquiries to:
Director of Consumer Affairs
(716) 882-7660
FAX: (716) 882-6563

For Medical Emergency Contact:
Dr. Henry Chan: (716) 882-7660
FAX: (716) 882-6563

FLETCHER'S® CASTORIA®
The Children's Laxative
Original Flavor
Alcohol Free

Natural, good-tasting Fletcher's Castoria provides gentle, effective relief from the discomfort of constipation for children of all ages. Trusted by mothers for generations.

Indications: For relief of occasional constipation. This product generally produces bowel movement in 6 to 12 hours.

Directions: SHAKE WELL BEFORE USING
Less than 2 years .... Consult a doctor
2 to 5 years .... 1 to 2 teaspoonfuls
6 to 15 years .... 2 to 3 teaspoonfuls
May be taken up to two times daily.

Warning: Do not use laxative products when abdominal pain, nausea or vomiting are present unless directed by a doctor. If you have noticed a sudden change in bowel habits that persists over a period of two weeks, consult a doctor before using a laxative. Laxative products should not be used for a period longer than 1 week unless directed by a doctor. Rectal bleeding or failure to have a bowel movement after use of a laxative may indicate a serious condition. Discontinue use and consult your doctor. **Keep this and all drugs out of the reach of children.** In case of accidental overdose seek professional assistance or

Continued on next page

Mentholatum Co.—Cont.

contact a poison control center immediately. As with any drug, if you are pregnant or nursing a baby seek the advice of a health professional before using this product.
Contains: Senna Concentrate 33.3 mg/ml.

Also contains: Citric Acid, Flavor, Glycerin, Methlyparaben, Propylparaben, Sodium Benzoate, Sucrose, Water.

How Supplied: 2½ Fl Oz (74 mL)
TAMPER RESISTANT FEATURE: USE ONLY IF NECK BAND PRINTED WITH FLETCHER'S 2½ OZ. SAFETY SEAL IS INTACT.
5 FL OZ (148 mL)
Tamper Resistant Feature: Use only if neck band printed with Fletcher's 5 oz. safety seal is intact.
The Mentholatum Co., Buffalo, NY 14213 U.S.A.

FLETCHER'S® CHERRY FLAVOR THE CHILDREN'S LAXATIVE

Good tasting Fletcher's® Cherry Flavor provides gentle effective relief from the discomforts of constipation. The convenient dosage cup lets you measure the right amount for your child's age.

Indications: For relief of occasional constipation. The product generally produces bowel movement in 6 to 12 hours.

Directions: SHAKE WELL BEFORE USING

Maximum Daily Dose

AGE	DOSAGE
6–11 Years	2–4 teaspoons
2–5 Years	1–2 teaspoons
Under 2 Years	Consult A Doctor

6-11 Years
2-5 Years

Warnings: Do not use laxative products when abdominal pain, nausea or vomiting are present unless directed by a doctor. If you have noticed a sudden change in bowel habits that persists over a period of two weeks, consult a doctor before using a laxative. Laxative products should not be used for a period longer than 1 week unless directed by a doctor. Rectal bleeding or failure to have a bowel movement after use of a laxative may indicate a serious condition. Discontinue use and consult your doctor. **Keep this and all drugs out of the reach of children. In case of accidental overdose, seek professional assistance or contact a poison control center immediately. If a skin rash appears, do not use this product or any other preparation containing phenolphthalein. As with any drug if you are pregnant or nursing a baby seek the advice of a health professional before using this**

product. Contains: Yellow Phenolphthalein 0.3%. Also contains: Citric Acid, FD&C Red No. 40, Flavor, Glycerin, Magnesium Aluminum Silicate, Methylparaben, Sodium Benzoate, Sucrose, Water, Xanthan Gum.

How Supplied: 2½ Fl Oz (74 mL)
TAMPER RESISTANT FEATURE: USE ONLY IF NECK BAND PRINTED WITH FLETCHER'S 2½ OZ. SAFETY SEAL IS INTACT.
The Mentholatum Co. Buffalo, NY 14213

MEDI-QUIK®
First Aid Antiseptic plus Pain Relief No Sting Spray

Indications: First aid to help protect against skin infection and for the temporary relief of pain and itching in minor cuts, scrapes, and burns.

Directions: Shake well. For adults and children two years of age or older: Clean the affected area. To spray hold can upright 2 to 3 inches from surface and spray a small amount of this product on the area 1 to 3 times daily. The area may be covered with a sterile bandage, however, if bandaged, let dry first.

Warnings: For external use only. Do not spray in the eyes or apply over large areas of the body, particularly over raw surfaces or blistered areas. In the case of deep or puncture wounds, animal bites, or serious burns, consult a doctor. Stop use and consult a doctor if the condition persists or gets worse, or if a rash or irritation develops. Do not use longer than 1 week unless directed by a doctor. Do not use on children under 2 years of age except under supervision of a physician. Keep this and all drugs out of reach of children. In case of accidental ingestion, seek professional assistance or contact a Poison Control Center.
Contents under pressure. Do not puncture or incinerate. Do not store at temperatures above 120°F. Use only as directed. Intentional misuse by deliberately concentrating and inhaling contents may be harmful or fatal.

Active Ingredients: Lidocaine 2% w/w, Benzalkonium Chloride 0.13% w/w of concentrate. Also contains: Benzyl Alcohol, BHA, Isobutane, Isopropyl Palmitate, Methyl Gluceth-20 Sesquistearate, Methyl Glucose Sesquistearate, Phosphoric Acid, Polyglyceryl-6 Distearate, Water.
CONTAINS NO FLUOROCARBONS

How Supplied: Net Wt. 3 oz/85g
Dist. by The Mentholatum Company, Buffalo, New York 14213 U.S.A.

MENTHOLATUM®
CHERRY CHEST RUB FOR KIDS®
Nasal Decongestant/Cough Suppressant
Aromatic Colds Medicine

Mentholatum Cherry Chest Rub for Kids is specially made for children 2 years and

older. The aromatic medicine penetrates into the nose and throat to break up congestion and ease coughs. It does not cause excitability, drowsiness or stomachache. The pleasant cherry aroma tells you it is working.

Indications: For the temporary relief of nasal congestion and coughs associated with a cold.

Directions: Children 2 years of age and older: Rub on the throat and chest as a thick layer. If desired, cover with a warm, dry cloth, but keep clothing loose to let the vapors rise to reach the nose and mouth. Repeat up to three times daily, especially at bedtime, or as directed by a doctor. Children under two years old, consult a doctor.

Warnings: For external use only. Avoid contact with the eyes. Do not take by mouth or place in nostrils. Discontinue use if irritation of the skin occurs. A persistent cough may be a sign of a serious condition. If cough persists for more than a week, tends to recur, or is accompanied by a fever, rash or persistent headache, see your doctor. Do not use this product for persistent or chronic coughs such as occurs with smoking, asthma, emphysema, or if cough is accompanied with excessive phlegm (mucus) unless directed by a doctor. Keep this and all drugs out of the reach of children. In case of accidental ingestion, seek professional assistance or contact a Poison Control Center immediately.

Contains: Camphor 4.7%, Natural Menthol 2.6%, Eucalyptus Oil 1.2% **ALSO CONTAINS:** Fragrance, Petrolatum, Steareth-2, Titanium Dioxide.

How Supplied: Net wt 1 oz (28g)
Net wt 3 oz (85g)
The Mentholatum Company, Buffalo, New York 14213

MENTHOLATUM DEEP HEATING®

Extra Strength Formula Provides Warming, Penetrating Pain Relief
- Greaseless and Stainless
- Arthritis
- Sore Muscles
- Back Pain

Directions: Apply to affected area. Repeat 3 to 4 times a day.
Massage thoroughly into affected joints to relieve arthritis pain and stiffness.

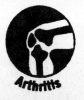

Arthritis

Rub into muscles to relieve the pain of over-exertion or for warming up before you work out.

Massage in to relieve the pain of strained back muscles and restore lost mobility.

Indications: For the temporary relief of minor aches and pains of muscles and joints associated with arthritis, simple backache, strains and sprains.

Contains: Methyl Salicylate 30%, Menthol 8%.

Also Contains: Glyceryl Stearate (and) Sodium Lauryl Sulfate, Isoceteth-20, Poloxamer 407, Quaternium-15, Sorbitan Stearate, Water.

Warning: For external use only. Do not apply to wounds or to damaged or very sensitive skin. Do not wrap, bandage or apply external heat or hot water. If you have impaired circulation or diabetes, use only upon the advice of a physician. Keep this and all drugs out of the reach of children. In case of accidental ingestion, seek professional assistance or contact a Poison Control Center immediately.

Caution: Use only as directed. If pain persists for more than 10 days, or redness is present, or in conditions affecting children under 12 years of age, consult a physician immediately. Discontinue use if excessive irritation of the skin develops. Avoid getting into the eyes or on mucous membranes.

How Supplied: Net wt 1.25 oz (35.4 g)
Net wt 3.33 oz (94.4g)
Net wt 5 oz (141 g)
Net wt 6 oz
THE MENTHOLATUM CO.
BUFFALO, NY 14213

MENTHOLATUM®
MENTHACIN™
Dual Acting Arthritis Therapy

Menthacin™ relieves the pain of arthritis in a completely new and different way than traditional creams and rubs. Its advanced, dual-acting formula provides:

● **Immediate Pain Relief**
As soon as you rub it on, Menthacin™ provides fast acting, penetrating cooling for immediate relief at the site of the pain.
[See Figure at top of next column.]

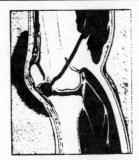

● **Long Lasting Pain Relief**
Menthacin™ contains Capsaicin, which provides long lasting warming pain relief. Over time, with repeated use, Capsaicin works to significantly reduce the sensation of pain within the affected area for long lasting relief.

Indications: For the temporary relief of minor aches and pains of muscles and joints associated with arthritis, simple backache, strains, and sprains.

Directions: Apply to affected area not more than 3 to 4 times daily. Children under 12 years of age, consult a physician. Transient irritation or burning may occur upon application, but generally disappears in several days. Wash hands with soap and water after applying.

Warnings: For external use only. Avoid contact with the eyes or mucous membranes. Do not use with a heating pad. Discontinue use if excessive irritation of the skin develops. If pain persists for 7 days or more, or clears up and occurs again within a few days, discontinue use of this product and consult a physician. Do not apply to wounds or damaged skin. Do not bandage tightly. Keep this and all drugs out of the reach of children. In case of accidental ingestion, seek professional assistance or contact a Poison Control Center immediately. Store at room temperature.

Contains: Menthol 4%, Capsaicin 0.025%.

Also Contains: Caprylic/Capric Triglyceride, Carbomer 1342, Carbomer 940, Cetyl Alcohol, Diazolidinyl Urea, Glyceryl Stearate (and) Sodium Lauryl Sulfate, Maleated Soybean Oil, Methylparaben, Polysorbate 60, Propylene Glycol, Propylparaben, Sorbitan Stearate, Trolamine, Water.

How Supplied: Net Wt 1.25 oz (35.4g)
The Mentholatum Company, Buffalo, NY 14213

MENTHOLATUM® OINTMENT
For Colds & Chapped Skin
Decongestant Analgesic
Aromotic Colds Medicine

Penetrating aromatic vapors act fast to relieve stuffy noses, chest congestion, and the distress of coughs due to colds and sinus congestion
Soothes Sore Skin and Chapped Lips
● Relieves sore skin irritated by runny noses

● Natural Moisturizer medicates and protects lips from chapping in harsh winter weather or extremely dry air
● Ideal for use with internal colds and sinus medicines
● Gentle enough for children

Indications: Colds Symptoms—Gentle aromatics help relieve stuffy noses, chest congestion, sinus congestion, head colds, chest colds and muscular aches due to coughs and colds.
Chapped Skin—Soothes chapped skin, lips, cold sores and other minor skin irritations.

Directions: For adults and children 2 years of age and older. Apply to affected area 3 to 4 times daily.
Stuffy Noses: Apply liberally below each nostril.
Chest Congestion and Muscle Aches: Rub liberally on chest, throat and back and then cover areas with warm cloth.
Chapped Skin Under Nose, Chapped Lips, Cold Sores: Liberally spread a layer over irritated areas.

Warnings: For external use only. Avoid contact with the eyes. Do not place in mouth or nostrils. For conditions that persist or are accompanied by a fever see your doctor. Keep this and all drugs out of the reach of children. In case of accidental ingestion. seek professional assistance or contact a Poison Control Center immediately.

Contains: Camphor 9%, Natural Menthol 1.3%.

Also Contains: Fragrance, Petrolatum, Titanium Dioxide.

How Supplied: Net wt 3 oz (85g)
Net wt 1 oz (28g)
The Mentholatum Company Buffalo, NY 14213

RED CROSS® TOOTHACHE
FIRST AID MEDICATION

Package includes:
● toothache medication
● cotton pellets
● metal tweezers

Indications: For the temporary relief of throbbing, persistent toothache due to a cavity until a dentist can be seen.

Directions: Rinse the tooth with water to remove any food particles from the cavity. Use tweezers to moisten pellet and place in cavity. Avoid touching tissues other than tooth cavity. Do not apply more than four times daily or as directed by a dentist.

Warnings: Do not swallow. Do not exceed recommended dosage. Not to be used for a period exceeding 7 days. Children under 2 years should not use this product. Children under 12 years should be supervised in the use of this product. If irritation persists, inflammation develops, or if fever or infection develop, discontinue use and see your dentist or physician promptly. Do not use if you are al-

Continued on next page

Mentholatum Co.—Cont.

lergic to Eugenol. Keep this and all drugs out of the reach of children. In case of accidental ingestion, seek professional assistance or contact a poison control center immediately.

Contents: Eugenol 85%. Also contains: Sesame Oil

How Supplied: Net ⅛ Fl Oz (3.7ml)
The trademarks Red Cross and the Red Cross design are registered trademarks of The Mentholatum Company. Products bearing this trademark have no connection with the American National Red Cross.
The Mentholatum Co., Buffalo, N.Y. 14213

UNGUENTINE® PLUS
First Aid Antiseptic
Pain Relieving Cream

First aid for burns, cuts, scrapes, insect bites.

Indications: First aid to help prevent infection and temporarily relieve the pain and itching associated with minor burns, sunburn, minor cuts, scrapes, insect bites, or minor skin irritations.

Directions: Adults and children 2 years of age and older: Clean the affected area. Apply a small amount of this product on the area 1 to 3 times daily. Children under 2 years of age: Consult a physician.

Contains: Lidocaine HCl 2%; Phenol 0.5%. Also Contains: Fragrance, Glyceryl Stearate, Isoceteth-20, Isopropyl Palmitate, Methylparaben, Mineral Oil, Poloxamer 407, Propylparaben, Quaternium-15, Sorbitan Stearate, Tetrasodium EDTA, Water.

Warnings: For external use only. Avoid contact with eyes. In case of deep or puncture wounds, animal bites, or serious burns, consult a doctor. If conditions worsen or if symptoms persist for more than 7 days or clear up and occur again within a few days, discontinue use of this product and consult a physician. Do not use in large quantities, particularly over raw surfaces or blistered areas. Do not apply over large areas of the body or bandage. Keep this and all medicines out of the reach of children. In case of accidental ingestion, seek professional assistance or contact a Poison Control Center immediately.

How Supplied: Net wt. 1 oz. (28.3g)
The Mentholatum Co., Buffalo, NY 14213

**IF YOU SUSPECT
AN INTERACTION...**
The 1,500-page
PDR Guide to Drug Interactions •
Side Effects • *Indications*
can help.
Use the order form
in the front of this book.

Muro Pharmaceutical, Inc.
**890 EAST STREET
TEWKSBURY, MA 01876-1496**

Direct Inquiries to:
Professional Service Department
(800) 225-0974
(508) 851-5981

BROMFED® SYRUP
**Antihistamine-Nasal Decongestant
ORANGE-LEMON FLAVOR**

Each 5 mL (1 teaspoonful) contains: 2 mg brompheniramine maleate and 30 mg pseudoephedrine hydrochloride; also contains citric acid, FD & C Yellow #6, flavor, glycerin, methylparaben, sodium benzoate, sodium citrate, sodium saccharin, sorbitol, sucrose, purified water.

Indications: For temporary relief of nasal congestion, sneezing, itching of the nose and throat, and itchy watery eyes and running nose due to common cold, hay fever or other upper respiratory allergies.

Directions: Adults and children 12 years of age and over: 2 teaspoonfuls every 4–6 hours. Children 6 to 12 years of age: 1 teaspoonful every 4–6 hours. Do not exceed 4 doses in 24 hours. Children under 6 years of age, consult a physician.

Warnings: Do not exceed recommended dosage: If nervousness, dizziness, or sleeplessness occur, discontinue use and consult a doctor. May cause excitability especially in children. A persistent cough may be a sign of a serious condition. If symptoms do not improve within 7 days or are accompanied by fever, consult a doctor. Do not take this product for persistent or chronic cough such as occurs with smoking, asthma, chronic bronchitis, emphysema, or where cough is accompanied by excessive phlegm (mucus) unless directed by a doctor. DO NOT take this product if you have heart disease, high blood pressure, thyroid disease, diabetes, or difficulty in urination due to enlargement of the prostate gland, if you have breathing problems such as emphysema or chronic bronchitis, or if you have glaucoma unless directed by a doctor. **Except under the advice and supervision of a physician:** Do not give this product to children under six years. As with any drug, if you are pregnant or nursing a baby, seek the advice of a health professional before using this product. May cause drowsiness; alcohol, sedatives, and tranquilizers may increase the drowsiness effect. Avoid alcoholic beverages while taking this product. Use caution when driving a motor vehicle or operating machinery. Keep this and all drugs out of reach of children.

Drug Interaction Precaution: Do not take this product if you are now taking a prescription monoamine oxidase inhibi-

tor (MAOI) (certain drugs for depression, psychiatric or emotional conditions, or Parkinson's disease), or for 2 weeks after stopping the MAOI drug. If you are uncertain whether your prescription drug contains an MAOI, consult a health professional before taking this product.

Overdosage: In case of accidental overdose, seek professional assistance or contact a Poison Control Center immediately.
Store at controlled room temperature between 15°C and 30°C (50°F and 86°F). Dispense in tight, light and child-resistant containers as defined in USP/NF.

How Supplied: NDC 0451-4201-16, for 16 fl. oz. (480 mL), NDC 0451-4201-04, for 4 fl. oz (120 mL).

GUAIFED® SYRUP
(Guaifenesin and Pseudoephedrine Hydrochloride)

Description:
GUAIFED® Syrup
Each 5 mL (teaspoonful) contains:
Guaifenesin, USP .... 200 mg
Pseudoephedrine
 Hydrochloride, USP .... 30 mg
This product contains ingredients of the following therapeutic classes: expectorant and nasal decongestant.

Inactive Ingredients: Benzoic Acid, Cherry Flavor, Citric Acid, Edetate Disodium, FD&C Red #40, FD&C Blue #1, Glycerin, Menthol, Polyethylene Glycol, Povidone, Propylene Glycol, Purified Water, Sodium Citrate, Sodium Saccharin, Sorbitol, Sucrose, Vanillin.

Indications: For the temporary relief of nasal congestion due to the common cold associated with sinusitis, hay fever, or other upper respiratory allergies (allergic rhinitis). Helps loosen phlegm (mucus) and thin bronchial secretions to rid the bronchial passageways of bothersome mucus, drain bronchial tubes and make coughs more productive.

Warnings: Do not exceed recommended dosage. If nervousness, dizziness or sleeplessness occur, discontinue use and consult a doctor. If symptoms do not improve within 7 days or are accompanied by fever, consult a doctor. Do not take this product if you have heart disease, high blood pressure, thyroid disease, diabetes or difficulty in urination due to enlargement of the prostate gland unless directed by a doctor. Do not take this product for persistent or chronic cough such as occurs with smoking, asthma, chronic bronchitis, or emphysema, or where cough is accompanied by excessive phlegm (mucus) unless directed by a doctor. A persistent cough may be a sign of a serious condition. If cough persists for more than one week, tends to recur, or is accompanied by a fever, rash or persistent headache, consult a doctor. As with any drug, women who are pregnant or nursing a baby should seek the advice of a health professional before using this product.

Drug Interaction Precaution: Do not use this product if you are now taking a prescription monoamine oxidase inhibitor (MAOI) (certain drugs for depression, psychiatric or emotional conditions, or Parkinson's disease) or for 2 weeks after stopping the MAOI drug. If you are uncertain whether your prescription drug contains an MAOI consult a health professional before taking this product.

Directions: Adults and Children 12 years of age and over: Two teaspoonfuls every 4–6 hours, not to exceed eight teaspoonfuls in 24 hours. Children 6 to under 12 years of age: One teaspoonful every 4–6 hours, not to exceed four teaspoonfuls in 24 hours. Children 2 to under 6 years of age: ½ teaspoonful every 4–6 hours, not to exceed two teaspoonfuls in 24 hours. Children under 2 years of age: consult a physician.

How Supplied:
GUAIFED® SYRUP is a red colored, cherry flavored syrup supplied in 473 mL (NDC# 0451-2602-16) and 118 mL (NDC# 0451-2602-04) Bottles.
Store at controlled room temperature 15°–30°C (59°–86°F).
Dispense in child resistant, tight and light resistant containers.
KEEP THIS AND ALL DRUGS OUT OF REACH OF CHILDREN, IN CASE OF ACCIDENTAL OVERDOSE, SEEK PROFESSIONAL ASSISTANCE OR CONTACT A POISON CONTROL CENTER IMMEDIATELY.

SALINEX® NASAL MIST AND DROPS
Buffered Isotonic Saline Solutions

Ingredients: Sodium Chloride 0.4%. Also contains edetate disodium, hydroxypropyl methylcellulose, sodium phosphate, polyethylene glycol, propylene glycol and purified water. Preservative used is benzalkonium chloride 0.01%.

Indications: A nasal moisturizer formulated to be physiologically compatible with nasal membranes, providing soothing relief for clogged nasal passages without stinging or burning. Salinex restores moisture to relieve dry, inflamed nasal membranes due to low humidity, colds, allergies and overuse of nasal decongestants.

Directions: Spray: Squeeze twice in each nostril as needed. Drops: Two drops in each nostril as needed or as directed by physician.

How Supplied: SPRAY: 50 ml plastic spray bottle. NDC 0451-4500-50. DROPS: 15 ml plastic dropper bottle. NDC 0451-4500-85.

Niché Pharmaceuticals, Inc.
200 N. OAK STREET
P O BOX 449
ROANOKE, TX 76262

Direct Inquiries to:
Steve F. Brandon
(817) 491-2770
FAX: (817) 491-3533

For Medical Emergencies Contact:
Gerald L. Beckloff, M.D.
(817) 491-2770
FAX: (817) 491-3533

MAGTAB® SR
[*măg-tăb*]
(Magnesium L-lactate dihydrate)
Sustained-release Magnesium Supplement

Description: MagTab® SR is a sustained release oral magnesium supplement. Each pale yellow caplet contains 7mEq (84 Mg) magnesium as magnesium L-lactate dihydrate (835 Mg in a sustained release wax matrix formulation).

Indications/Uses: As a dietary supplement, MagTab® SR is indicated for patients with, or at risk for, magnesium deficiency. Hypomagnesemia and/or magnesium deficiency can result from inadequate nutritional intake or absorption, alcoholism, or magnesium depleting drugs such as diuretics.

Warnings/Side Effects: Patients with renal disease should not take magnesium supplements without the advice and direct supervision of a physician. Excessive dosage of magnesium can cause loose stools or diarrhea.

Dosage/How Supplied: As a dietary supplement, take 1 or 2 caplets b.i.d. or as directed by a physician. MagTab® SR is available for oral administration as uncoated yellow caplets, in bottles of 60 and 100.
U.S. Patent Number: 5,002,774

UNIFIBER®
[*uni fi ' ber*]
(Powdered Cellulose)
3 grams Fiber per tablespoon

Description: Unifiber is unique in the fiber field with many patient advantages. It's an all natural bulk fiber supplement that promotes normal bowel function by adding needed bulk to the diet. Unifiber contains powdered cellulose 75%, water 5%, corn syrup 19%, and xanthan gum 1%. Unifiber mixes easily with liquids or soft foods, and is tasteless, non-gelling, and pleasant to take. One tablespoon of Unifiber provides 3 grams of concentrated dietary fiber.

Nutrition Information: Each 4 gram (1T) serving of Unifiber contains 3 grams of fiber, 4 calories, 0% fat, 0% cholesterol, 0% protein, and is free of all electrolytes or excitoxins, such as phenylalanine. Unifiber contains no other inactive ingredient and is sugar free.

Indication/Uses: As a dietary supplement, Unifiber is indicated for patients needing a concentrated source of fiber to help maintain and promote normal bowel function. Published clinical trials report that the daily use of Unifiber by institutionalized elderly patients significantly reduce the need for laxatives, suppositories, enemas, and overall nursing time. Because Unifiber is sugar free, electrolyte free and contains no phenylalanine or aspartane, it is an ideal fiber supplement for patients on a restricted diet, such as the OB patient, kidney patient on dialysis, or the diabetic patient.

Contradiction: Intestinal obstruction or fecal impaction.

Dosage: Stir one to two tablespoons once or twice daily into a glass of fruit juice, milk, coffee, or water. An advantage of Unifiber is that it can be easily mixed with soft food such as mashed potatoes, applesauce, or pudding. Best results are normally seen in 7–10 days. Liquids should be included in the daily diet.

How Supplied: Unifiber is available over the counter in powder containers of 5 oz (35 servings), 9 oz (63 servings), or 16 oz (113 servings)

Ohm Laboratories, Inc.
P.O. BOX 7397
NORTH BRUNSWICK, NJ 08902

Mailing:
P.O. Box 7397
North Brunswick, NJ 08902

Direct Inquiries to:
Allan Korn
(908) 297-3030

For Medical Emergencies Contact:
(908) 297-3030

IBUPROHM®
Ibuprofen Tablets, USP
Ibuprofen Caplets, USP

Active Ingredient: Each tablet contains Ibuprofen USP, 200 mg.

Warning: ASPIRIN SENSITIVE PATIENTS: Do not take this product if you have had a severe allergic reaction to aspirin, e.g., asthma, swelling, shock or hives, because even though this product contains no aspirin or salicylates, cross-reactions may occur in patients allergic to aspirin.

Indications: For the temporary relief of minor aches and pains associated with the common cold, headache, toothache, muscular aches, backache, for the minor pain of arthritis, for the pain of menstrual cramps, and for reduction of fever.

Continued on next page

Ohm—Cont.

Directions: *Adults:* Take 1 tablet every 4 to 6 hours while symptoms persist. If pain or fever does not respond to 1 tablet, 2 tablets may be used but do not exceed 6 tablets in 24 hours, unless directed by a doctor. The smallest effective dose should be used. Take with food or milk if occasional and mild heartburn, upset stomach, or stomach pain occurs with use. Consult a doctor if these symptoms are more than mild or if they persist. Children: Do not give this product to children under 12 except under the advice and supervision of a doctor.

Warnings: Do not take for pain for more than 10 days or for fever for more than 3 days unless directed by a doctor. If pain or fever persists or gets worse, if new symptoms occur, or if the painful area is red or swollen, consult a doctor. These could be signs of serious illness. If you are under a doctor's care for any serious condition, consult a doctor before taking this product. As with aspirin and acetaminophen, if you have any condition which requires you to take prescription drugs or if you have had any problems or serious side effects from taking any nonprescription pain reliever, do not take this product without first discussing it with your doctor. If you experience any symptoms which are unusual or seem unrelated to the condition for which you took ibuprofen, consult a doctor before taking any more of it. Although ibuprofen is indicated for the same conditions as aspirin and acetaminophen, it should not be taken with them except under a doctor's direction. Do not combine the product with any other ibuprofen-containing product. As with any drug, if you are pregnant or nursing a baby, seek the advice of a health professional before using this product. IT IS ESPECIALLY IMPORTANT NOT TO USE IBUPROFEN DURING THE LAST 3 MONTHS OF PREGNANCY UNLESS SPECIFICALLY DIRECTED TO DO SO BY A DOCTOR BECAUSE IT MAY CAUSE PROBLEMS IN THE UNBORN CHILD OR COMPLICATIONS DURING DELIVERY. Keep this and all drugs out of the reach of children. In case of accidental overdose, seek professional assistance or contact a poison control center immediately.

How Supplied: Coated tablets in bottles of 24, 50, 100, 165, 250, 500 and 1000. Coated caplets in bottles of 24, 50, 100 and 250.

Storage: Store at room temperature; avoid excessive heat 40° (104°F).

P & S Laboratories
210 WEST 131st STREET
LOS ANGELES, CA 90061

See Standard Homeopathic Company.

The Parthenon Co., Inc.
3311 W. 2400 SOUTH
SALT LAKE CITY, UTAH 84119

Direct Inquiries to:
(801) 972-5184
FAX: (801) 972-4734

For Medical Emergency Contact:
Nick G. Mihalopoulos
(801) 972-5184

DEVROM® CHEWABLE TABLETS

Description: DEVROM® is a safe and effective internal (oral) deodorant. Each tablet contains 200 mg of Bismuth Subgallate powder.

Indications: DEVROM® is indicated for the control of odors from ileostomies, colostomies and fecal incontinence.

Dosage: Take one or two tablets of DEVROM® three times a day with meals or as directed by physician. Chew or swallow whole if desired.

Note: The beneficial ingredient in DEVROM® may coat the tongue which may also darken in color. This condition is harmless and temporary. Darkening of the stool is also possible and equally harmless.

Warning: This product cannot be expected to be effective in the reduction of odor due to faulty personal hygiene. **KEEP THIS BOTTLE AND ALL MEDICATION OUT OF THE REACH OF CHILDREN.**

Inactive Ingredients: Mannitol, U.S.P., Lactose, N.F., Corn Starch, N.F., Confectioner's Sugar, N.F., Acacia Powder, N.F., Purified Water, U.S.P., Magnesium Stearate, N.F. **NO PHYSICIAN'S PRESCRIPTION IS NECESSARY**

How Supplied: DEVROM® is supplied in bottles of 100 tablets.
  DO NOT USE IF PRINTED OUTER SAFETY SEAL OR PRINTED INNER SAFETY SEAL IS BROKEN.
THE PARTHENON CO., INC./
3311 W. 2400 So./
Salt Lake City, Utah 84119

Rx DRUG INFORMATION AT THE TOUCH OF A BUTTON
Join the thousands of doctors using the handheld, electronic *Pocket PDR.®*
Use the order form in the front of this book.

Pfizer Inc.
Consumer Health Care Group
235 E. 42nd Street
NY, NY 10017-5755

Address Questions & Comments to:
Consumer Relations
(800) 723-7529
For Medical Emergencies/Information Contact:
(800) 723-7529

BENGAY® External Analgesic Products

Description: BENGAY products contain menthol in an alcohol base gel, combinations of methyl salicylate and menthol in cream and ointment bases, as well as a combination of methyl salicylate, menthol and camphor in a non-greasy cream base; all suitable for topical application.
In addition to the Original Formula Pain Relieving Ointment (methyl salicylate, 18.3%; menthol, 16%), BENGAY is offered as BENGAY Greaseless Pain Relieving Cream (methyl salicylate, 15%; menthol, 10%), an Arthritis Formula NonGreasy Pain Relieving Cream (methyl salicylate, 30%; menthol, 8%), an Ultra Strength NonGreasy Pain Relieving Cream (methyl salicylate 30%; menthol 10%; camphor 4%), and Vanishing Scent NonGreasy Pain Relieving Gel (2.5% menthol).

Action and Uses: Methyl salicylate, menthol and camphor are external analgesics which stimulate sensory receptors of warmth and/or cold. This produces a counter-irritant response which provides temporary relief of minor aches and pains of muscles and joints associated with simple backache, arthritis, strains, bruises and sprains.
Several double-blind clinical studies of BENGAY products containing menthol-methyl salicylate have shown the effectiveness of this combination in counteracting minor pain of skeletal muscle stress and arthritis.
Three studies involving a total of 102 normal subjects in which muscle soreness was experimentally induced showed statistically significant beneficial results from use of the active product vs. placebo for lowered Muscle Action Potential (spasms), greater rise in threshold of muscular pain and greater reduction in perceived muscular pain.
Six clinical studies of a total of 207 subjects suffering from minor pain due to osteoarthritis and rheumatoid arthritis showed the active product to give statistically significant beneficial results vs. placebo for greater relief of perceived pain, increased range of motion of the affected joints and increased digital dexterity. In two studies designed to measure the effect of topically applied BENGAY vs. placebo on muscular endurance, discom-

fort, onset of exercise pain and fatigue, 30 subjects performed a submaximal three-hour run and another 30 subjects performed a maximal treadmill run. BENGAY was found to significantly decrease the discomfort during the submaximal and maximal runs, and increase the time before onset of fatigue during the maximal run.

Applied before workouts, BENGAY relaxes tight muscles and increases circulation to make exercising more comfortable, longer.

To help reduce muscle ache and soreness after exercise, BENGAY can be applied and allowed to work before taking a shower.

Directions: Apply generously and gently massage into painful area until BENGAY disappears. Repeat 3 to 4 times daily.

Warnings: For external use only. Do not use with a heating pad. Keep away from children to avoid accidental poisoning. Do not bandage tightly. Do not swallow. If swallowed, induce vomiting and call a physician. Keep away from eyes, mucous membranes, broken or irritated skin. If skin redness or irritation develops, pain lasts for more than 10 days, or with arthritis—like conditions in children under 12, do not use and call a physician.
Shown in Product Identification Guide, page 515

BONINE®
(Meclizine hydrochloride)
Chewable Tablets

Action: BONINE (meclizine) is an H_1 histamine receptor blocker of the piperazine side chain group. It exhibits its action by an effect on the Central Nervous System (CNS), possibly by its ability to block muscarinic receptors in the brain.

Indications: BONINE is effective in the management of nausea, vomiting and dizziness associated with motion sickness.

Contraindications: Do not take this product, unless directed by a doctor, if you have a breathing problem such as emphysema or chronic bronchitis, or if you have glaucoma or difficulty in urination due to enlargement of the prostate gland.

Warnings: May cause drowsiness; alcohol, sedatives and tranquilizers may increase the drowsiness effect. Avoid alcoholic beverages while taking this product. Do not take this product if you are taking sedatives or tranquilizers without first consulting your doctor. Do not drive or operate dangerous machinery while taking this medication.
Usage in Children:
Clinical studies establishing safety and effectiveness in children have not been done; therefore, usage is not recommended in children under 12 years of age.

Usage in Pregnancy:
As with any drug, if you are pregnant or nursing a baby, seek advice of a health care professional before taking this product.

Adverse Reactions: Drowsiness, dry mouth, and on rare occasions, blurred vision have been reported.

Dosage and Administration: For motion sickness, take one or two tablets of Bonine once daily, one hour before travel starts, for up to 24 hours of protection against motion sickness. The tablet can be chewed with or without water or swallowed whole with water. Thereafter, the dose may be repeated every 24 hours for the duration of the travel.

How Supplied: BONINE (meclizine HCl) is available in convenient packets of 8 chewable tablets of 25 mg. meclizine HCl.

Inactive Ingredients: FD&C Red #40, Lactose, Magnesium Stearate, Purified Siliceous Earth, Raspberry Flavor, Saccharin Sodium, Starch, Talc.

DESITIN® CORNSTARCH BABY POWDER
(with Zinc Oxide)

Description: Desitin Cornstarch Baby Powder combines zinc oxide (10%) with topical starch (cornstarch) for topical application. Also contains: fragrance and tribasic calcium phosphate.

Actions and Uses: Desitin Cornstarch Baby Powder with zinc oxide and topical starch (cornstarch) is designed to protect from wetness, help prevent and treat diaper rash, and other minor skin irritations. It offers all the benefits of a talc-free, absorbent cornstarch powder, but with the addition of zinc oxide, the same protective ingredient found in Desitin Ointment. Cornstarch also prevents friction. Zinc oxide provides an additional physical barrier by forming a protective coating over the skin or mucous membranes which serves to reduce further effects of irritants on affected areas.

Directions: Prevention: Change wet and soiled diapers promptly, cleanse the diaper area, and allow to dry.
Apply powder close to the body away from child's face. Carefully shake the powder into the diaper or into the hand and apply to diaper area. Apply liberally as often as necessary with each diaper change, especially at bedtime, or anytime when exposure to wet diapers may be prolonged.

Treatment: Use liberally in all body creases, and whenever chafing, prickly heat or other minor skin irritations occur.

Warning: For external use only. Do not use on broken skin. Avoid contact with eyes. Keep powder away from child's face to avoid inhalation. If diaper rash worsens or does not improve within 7 days, consult a doctor.

How Supplied: Desitin Cornstarch Baby Powder with Zinc Oxide is available in 14 ounce (397g) containers with sifter-top caps.
Shown in Product Identification Guide, page 515

DAILY CARE® from DESITIN®
Diaper Rash Prevention Ointment
Skin Protectant (10% Zinc Oxide)

Description: Daily Care from DESITIN contains Zinc Oxide (10%) in a white petrolatum base suitable for topical application. Also contains: cyclomethicone, dimethicone, fragrance, methylparaben, mineral oil, mineral wax, propylparaben, sodium borate, sorbitan sesquioleate, white wax and purified water.

Actions and Uses: Daily Care helps treat and prevent diaper rash. It helps seal out irritating wetness that can cause diaper rash by creating a protective wetness barrier at every diaper change. Daily Care has a pleasant formula that's easy to apply, easy to clean up and has a fresh scent.

Directions: Prevention—To help prevent diaper rash, change wet and soiled diaper promptly, cleanse the diaper area and allow to dry. Apply Daily Care ointment liberally as often as necessary with each diaper change—especially at bedtime or anytime when exposure to a wet diaper may be prolonged.
Treatment—At the first sign of redness or minor skin irritation, apply Daily Care liberally over the affected area and repeat as necessary. After the rash has cleared, continue to use Daily Care at every diaper change to help protect skin from future diaper rash.

Warnings: For external use only. Avoid contact with eyes. If condition worsens or does not improve within 7 days, consult your doctor. Keep out of reach of children. In case of accidental ingestion, seek professional assistance or contact a Poison Control Center immediately. Store between 2 and 30°C (36 and 86°F).

How Supplied: Daily Care Ointment is available in 2 oz. (57g) and 4 oz. (113g) tubes.
Shown in Product Identification Guide, page 515

DESITIN® OINTMENT

Description: Desitin Ointment combines Zinc Oxide (40%) with Cod Liver Oil in a petrolatum-lanolin base suitable for topical application. Also contains: BHA, fragrances, methylparaben, talc and water.

Actions and Uses: Desitin Ointment is designed to provide relief of diaper rash, superficial wounds and burns, and other minor skin irritations. It helps pre-

Continued on next page

Pfizer Inc.—Cont.

vent incidents of diaper rash, protects against urine and other irritants, and soothes chafed skin.

Relief and protection is afforded by Zinc Oxide and Cod Liver Oil. These ingredients together with the petrolatum-lanolin base provide a physical barrier by forming a protective coating over skin or mucous membranes which serves to reduce further effects of irritants on the affected area and relieves burning, pain or itch produced by them.

Several studies have shown the effectiveness of Desitin Ointment in the relief and prevention of diaper rash.

Two clinical studies involving 90 infants demonstrated the effectiveness of Desitin Ointment in curing diaper rash. The diaper rash area was treated with Desitin Ointment at each diaper change for a period of 24 hours, while the untreated site served as controls. A significant reduction was noted in the severity and area of diaper dermatitis on the treated area.

Ninety-seven (97) babies participated in a 12-week study to show that Desitin Ointment helps prevent diaper rash. Approximately half of the infants (49) were treated with Desitin Ointment on a regular daily basis. The other half (48) received the ointment as necessary to treat any diaper rash which occurred. The incidence as well as the severity of diaper rash was significantly less among the babies using the ointment on a regular daily basis.

In a comparative study of the efficacy of Desitin Ointment vs. a baby powder, forty-five (45) babies were observed for a total of eight (8) weeks. Results support the conclusion that Desitin Ointment is a better prophylactic against diaper rash than the baby powder.

In another study, Desitin was found to be dramatically more effective in reducing the severity of medically diagnosed diaper rash than a commercially available diaper rash product in which only anhydrous lanolin and petrolatum were listed as ingredients. Fifty (50) infants participated in the study, half of whom were treated with Desitin and half with the other product. In the group (25) treated with Desitin, seventeen (17) infants showed significant improvement within 10 hours which increased to twenty-three improved infants within 24 hours. Of the group (25) treated with the other product, only three showed improvement at ten hours with a total of four improved within twenty-four hours. These results are statistically valid to conclude that Desitin Ointment reduces severity of diaper rash within ten hours.

Several other studies show that Desitin Ointment helps relieve other skin disorders, such as contact dermatitis.

Directions: Prevention: To prevent diaper rash, apply Desitin Ointment to the diaper area—especially at bedtime when exposure to wet diapers may be prolonged.

Treatment: If diaper rash is present, or at the first sign of redness, minor skin irritation or chafing, simply apply Desitin Ointment three or four times daily as needed. In superficial noninfected surface wounds and minor burns, apply a thin layer of Desitin Ointment, using a gauze dressing, if necessary. For external use only.

How Supplied: Desitin Ointment is available in 1 ounce (28g), 2 ounce (57g), and 4 ounce (114g) tubes, and 9 ounce (255g) and 1 lb. (454g) jars.

Shown in Product Identification Guide, page 515

RHEABAN® Maximum Strength FAST ACTING CAPLETS
[rē'ăban]
(attapulgite)

Description: Maximum Strength Rheaban is an anti-diarrheal medication containing activated attapulgite and is offered in caplets form.

Each white Rheaban caplets contains 750 mg. of colloidal activated attapulgite. Rheaban provides the maximum level of medication when taken as directed. Rheaban contains no narcotics, opiates or other habit-forming drugs.

Actions and Uses: Rheaban is indicated for relief of diarrhea and the cramps and pains associated with it. Attapulgite, which has been activated by thermal treatment, is a highly sorptive substance which absorbs nutrients and digestive enzymes as well as noxious gases, irritants, toxins and some bacteria and viruses that are common causes of diarrhea.

In clinical studies to show the effectiveness in relieving diarrhea and its symptoms, 100 subjects suffering from acute gastroenteritis with diarrhea participated in a double-blind comparison of Rheaban to a placebo. Patients treated with the attapulgite product showed significantly improved relief of diarrhea and its symptoms vs. the placebo.

Dosage and Administration: CAPLETS

Adults—2 caplets after initial bowel movement, 2 caplets after each subsequent bowel movement. For a maximum of 12 caplets in 24 hours.

Children 6 to 12 years—1 caplet after initial bowel movement, 1 caplet after each subsequent bowel movement. For a maximum of 6 caplets in 24 hours, or as directed by a physician.

Warnings: Do not exceed 12 caplets in 24 hours. Swallow caplets with water, do not chew. Do not use for more than two days, or in the presence of high fever. Caplets should not be used for infants or children under 6 years of age unless directed by physician. If diarrhea persists consult a physician.

How Supplied:
Caplets—Boxes of 12 caplets.

Inactive Ingredients: Carnauba Wax, Croscarmellose Sodium, D&C Yellow No. 10 Aluminum Lake, FD&C Blue No. 1 Aluminum Lake, Hydroxypropyl Cellulose, Hydroxypropyl Methylcellulose, Methylparaben, Pectin, Pharmaceutical Glaze, Propylene Glycol, Propylparaben, Sucrose, Talc Titanium Dioxide, Zinc Stearate.

RID® Spray
Lice Control Spray

PRODUCT OVERVIEW

Key Facts: Rid Lice Control Spray is a pediculicide spray for controlling lice and louse eggs on inanimate objects, to help prevent reinfestation. It contains a highly active synthetic pyrethroid that kills lice and their eggs on inanimate objects.

Major Uses: Rid Lice Control Spray effectively kills lice and louse eggs on garments, bedding, furniture and other inanimate objects that cannot be either laundered or dry cleaned.

Safety Information: Rid Lice Control Spray is intended for use on inanimate objects only; it is not for use on humans or animals. It is harmful if swallowed. It should not be sprayed in the eyes or on the skin and should not be inhaled. The product should be used only in well ventilated areas; room(s) should be vacated after treatment and ventilated before reoccupying.

PRESCRIBING INFORMATION
RID® Spray
Lice Control Spray

THIS PRODUCT IS NOT FOR USE ON HUMANS OR ANIMALS

Active Ingredient:
Permethrin* 0.5%
Inert Ingredients 99.5%
  100.00%
*(3-phenoxyphenol)methyl ± cis/trans 3-(2,2-dichloroethenyl) 2,2-dimethylcyclopropane-carboxylate, cis/trans ratio: Minimum 35% (± cis) and maximum 65% (± trans).

Actions: A highly active synthetic pyrethroid for the control of lice and louse eggs on garments, bedding, furniture and other inanimate objects.

Warnings: Avoid contamination of feed and foodstuffs. Remove pets and birds and cover fish aquaria before space spraying on surface applications. HARMFUL IF SWALLOWED. This product is not for use on humans or animals. If lice infestations should occur on humans, consult either your physician or pharmacist for a product for use on humans.

Physical And Chemical Hazards: Contents under pressure. Do not use or store near heat or open flame. Do not puncture or incinerate container. Exposure to temperatures above 130° F (54° C) may cause bursting. Store in cool, dry area. Do not store below 32° F (0° C).

CAUTION: Avoid spraying in eyes. Avoid breathing spray mist. Use only in well ventilated areas. Avoid contact with skin. In case of contact wash immediately with soap and water. Vacate room after treatment and ventilate before reoccupying.

Statement of Practical Treatment:
If inhaled: Remove affected person to fresh air. Apply artifical respiration if indicated. Get immediate medical attention.
If in eyes: Flush with plenty of water. Contact physician if irritation persists.
If on skin: Wash affected areas immediately with soap and water.

Direction For Use: It is a violation of Federal law to use this product in a manner inconsistent with its labeling.
Shake well before using.
To kill lice and louse eggs: Spray in an inconspicuous area to test for possible staining or discoloration. Inspect again after drying, then proceed to spray entire area to be treated. Hold container upright with nozzle away from you. Depress valve and spray from a distance of 8 to 10 inches.
Spray each square foot for 3 seconds. Spray only those garments, parts of bedding, including mattresses and furniture that cannot be either laundered or dry cleaned.
Allow all sprayed articles to dry thoroughly before use.
Buyer assumes all risks of use, storage or handling of this material not in strict accordance with directions given herewith.

Disposal Of Container: Wrap container in several layers of newspaper and dispose of in trash. Do not incinerate or puncture.

How Supplied: 5 ounce aerosol can. Also available in combination with RID® Lice Killing Shampoo as the RID® Lice Elimination Kit.

MAXIMUM STRENGTH RID®
Lice Killing Shampoo

PRODUCT OVERVIEW

Key Facts: Maximum Strength Rid® Lice Killing Shampoo contains a liquid pediculicide effective against head, body, and pubic (crab) lice and their eggs. The active ingredients in Rid® are pyrethrum extract and piperonyl butoxide, technical which attack the louse's nervous system. Piperonyl butoxide is a synergist. The pyrethrum extract in Rid® rinses out completely after treatment, and is poorly absorbed through the skin. Each Maximum Strength Rid® Lice Killing Shampoo package also contains a patented nit (egg) removal comb with an exclusive handle design that provides

gentle combing action to remove the nits (eggs).

Major Uses: Rid® has proved to be clinically effective in treating infestations of head lice and their eggs. It is also effective in the treatment of infestations of body lice, pubic (crab) lice and their eggs.

Safety Information: Rid® should be used with caution by ragweed sensitized persons. It is intended for external use on humans only and is harmful if swallowed. It should not be inhaled or allowed to come in contact with the eyes or mucous membranes. Contamination of feed or foodstuffs should be avoided.

PRESCRIBING INFORMATION
MAXIMUM STRENGTH RID®
Lice Killing Shampoo

Description: Rid® contains a liquid pediculicide whose active ingredients are pyrethrum extract 0.33% and piperonyl butoxide, technical 4.00%, equivalent to min. 3.2% (butylcarbityl) (6-propylpiperonyl) ether and 0.8% related compounds. Inert ingredients (95.67%) are: C13–C14 isoparaffin, fragrance, isopropyl alcohol, PEG-25 hydrogenated castor oil, water, xanthan gum.

Actions: Rid® kills head lice (Pediculus humanus capitis), body lice (Pediculus humanus humanus), and pubic (crab) lice (Phthirus pubis), and their eggs. The pyrethrum extract acts as a contact poison and affects the parasite's nervous system, resulting in paralysis and death. The efficacy of the pyrethrum extract is enhanced by a synergist, piperonyl butoxide. The pyrethrum extract rinses out completely after treatment and is not designed to leave long-acting residues. In addition, pyrethrum extract is poorly absorbed through the skin. Of the relatively minor amounts that are absorbed, they are rapidly metabolized to water-soluble compounds and eliminated from the body without ill effects.

Indications: For the treatment of head, pubic (crab), and body lice.

Warnings: Use with caution on persons allergic to ragweed. For external use only. Do not use near the eyes or permit contact with mucous membranes, such as inside the nose, mouth, or vagina, as irritation may occur. Keep out of eyes when rinsing hair. Adults and children: Close eyes tightly and do not open eyes until product is completely rinsed out. Also, protect children's eyes with washcloth, towel, or other suitable material, or by a similar method. If product gets into the eyes, immediately flush with water. If skin irritation or infection is present or develops, discontinue use and consult a doctor. Consult a doctor if infestation of eyebrows or eyelashes occurs.

Storage and Disposal: Do not store below 32°F (0°C) or above 120°F (49° C). Do not reuse empty container. Wrap in several layers of newspaper and discard in trash.

Dosage And Administration: Apply to affected area until all hair is thoroughly wet with product. Allow product to remain on area for 10 minutes but not longer. Add sufficient warm water to form a lather and shampoo as usual. Rinse thoroughly. A fine tooth comb or special lice/nit removing comb may be used to help remove dead lice or their eggs (nits) from hair. A second treatment must be done in 7 to 10 days to kill any newly hatched lice. Since there is no immunity from lice, personal cleanliness and the avoidance of infested persons and their bedding and clothes will aid in preventing infestation. These additional steps are important in order to minimize the chance of possible reinfestation.

● Inspect all family members daily for at least two weeks, and if they become infested, treat with Rid®.
● Wash all personal clothing, nightwear and bedding of any infested person in hot water, at least 130°F, or by dry cleaning.
● Soak all personal articles such as combs, brushes, etc. in Rid® solution or hot, soapy water (at least 130°F) for ten minutes. Inspect and rinse thoroughly before use.
● Tell children not to use any borrowed combs or brushes, nor to wear anyone else's clothes.

LICE WHICH INFEST HUMANS

Head Lice: Head lice live on the scalp and lay small white eggs (nits) on the hair shaft close to the scalp. The nits are most easily found on the nape of the neck or behind the ears. All personal headgear, scarfs, coats, and bed linen should be disinfected by machine washing in hot water and drying, using the hot cycle of a dryer for at least 20 minutes. Personal articles of clothing or bedding that cannot be washed may be dry-cleaned, sealed in a plastic bag for a period of about 2 weeks, or sprayed with a product specifically designed for this purpose. Personal combs and brushes may be disinfected by soaking in hot water (above 130°F) for 10 minutes. Thorough vacuuming of rooms inhabited by infected patients is recommended.

Pubic (Crab) Lice: Pubic lice may be transmitted by sexual contact; therefore, sexual partners should be treated simultaneously to avoid reinfestation. The lice are very small and look almost like brown or gray dots on the skin. Pubic lice usually cause intense itching and lay small white eggs (nits) on the hair shaft generally close to the skin surface. In hairy individuals, pubic lice may be present on the short hairs of the thighs and trunk, underarms, and occasionally on the beard and mustache. Underwear should be disinfected by machine washing in hot water, then drying, using the hot cycle for at least 20 minutes.

Body Lice: Body lice and their eggs are generally found in the seams of clothing,

Continued on next page

Pfizer Inc.—Cont.

particularly in the waistline and armpit area. They move to the skin to feed, then return to the seams of the clothing where they lay their eggs. Clothing worn and not laundered before treatment should be disinfected by the same procedure as described for head lice, except that sealing clothing in a plastic bag is not recommended because the nits (eggs) from these lice can remain dormant for a period of up to 30 days.

How Supplied: In 2, 4 and 8 fl. oz. plastic bottles. Exclusive nit (egg) removal comb that removes all nits (eggs) and patient instruction booklet (English and Spanish) are included in each package of Rid®. Also available in combination with Rid® Lice Control Spray as the Rid® Lice Elimination Kit.

MAXIMUM STRENGTH UNISOM SLEEPGELS
Nighttime Sleep Aid

Description: Maximum Strength Unisom SleepGels are liquid-filled, blue soft gelatin capsules.

Active Ingredient: Diphenhydramine Hydrochloride 50 mg.

Inactive Ingredients: FD&C Blue No. 1, Gelatin, Glycerin, Pharmaceutical Glaze, Polyethylene Glycol, Propylene Glycol, Purified Water, Sorbitol, Titanium Dioxide.

Indications: Helps to reduce difficulty falling asleep.

Action: Diphenhydramine Hydrochloride is an ethanolamine antihistamine with anticholinergic and sedative effects.

Administration and Dosage: Adults and children 12 years of age and over: Oral dosage is one softgel (50 mg.) at bedtime if needed, or as directed by a doctor.

Warnings: Do not take this product, unless directed by a doctor, if you have a breathing problem such as emphysema or chronic bronchitis, or if you have glaucoma or difficulty in urination due to enlargement of the prostate gland. Do not take this product if pregnant or nursing a baby.
- Do not give to children under 12 years of age.
- If sleeplessness persists continuously for more than two weeks, consult your doctor. Insomnia may be a symptom of serious underlying medical illness.
- Avoid alcoholic beverages while taking this product. Do not take this product if you are taking sedatives or tranquilizers, without first consulting your doctor.
- Keep this and all drugs out of the reach of children.
- In case of accidental overdose, seek professional assistance or contact a Poison Control Center immediately.

Drug Interaction: Monoamine oxidase (MAO) inhibitors prolong and intensify the anticholinergic effects of antihistamines. The CNS depressant effect is heightened by alcohol and other CNS depressant drugs.

Symptoms of Oral Overdosage: Antihistamine overdosage reactions may vary from central nervous system depression to stimulation.
Stimulation is particularly likely in children. Atropine-like signs and symptoms, such as dry mouth, fixed and dilated pupils, flushing, and gastrointestinal symptoms, may also occur.

Attention: Use only if softgel blister seals are unbroken.

How Supplied: Boxes of 16 liquid filled softgels in child resistant blisters and boxes of 8 with non-child resistant packaging. Also in a 32 count child resistant bottle.
Store between 15° and 30°C (59° and 86°F)

UNISOM®
[yu 'na-som]
Nighttime Sleep Aid
(doxylamine succinate)

PRODUCT OVERVIEW

Key Facts: Unisom is an ethanolamine antihistamine (doxylamine) which characteristically shows a high incidence of sedation. It produces a reduced latency to end of wakefulness and early onset of sleep.

Major Uses: Unisom has been shown to be clinically effective as a sleep aid when 1 tablet is given 30 minutes before retiring.

Safety Information: Unisom is contraindicated in pregnancy and nursing mothers. It is also contraindicated in patients with asthma, glaucoma, and enlargement of the prostate. Caution should be used if taken when alcohol is being consumed. Caution is also indicated when taken concurrently with other medications due to the anticholinergic properties of antihistamines.

PRESCRIBING INFORMATION
UNISOM®
[yu 'na-som]
Nighttime Sleep Aid
(doxylamine succinate)

Description: Pale blue oval scored tablets containing 25 mg. of doxylamine succinate, 2-[α-(2-dimethylaminoethoxy)α-methylbenzyl]pyridine succinate.

Action and Uses: Doxylamine succinate is an antihistamine of the ethanolamine class, which characteristically shows a high incidence of sedation. In a comparative clinical study of over 20 antihistamines on more than 3000 subjects, doxylamine succinate 25 mg. was one of the three most sedating antihistamines, producing a significantly reduced latency to end of wakefulness and comparing favorably with established hypnotic

drugs such as secobarbital and pentobarbital in sedation activity. It was chosen as the antihistamine, based on dosage, causing the earliest onset of sleep. In another clinical study, doxylamine succinate 25 mg. scored better than secobarbital 100 mg. as a nighttime hypnotic. Two additional, identical clinical studies, involving a total of 121 subjects demonstrated that doxylamine succinate 25 mg. reduced the sleep latency period by a third, compared to placebo. Duration of sleep was 26.6% longer with doxylamine succinate, and the quality of sleep was rated higher with the drug than with placebo. An EEG study on 6 subjects confirmed the results of these studies. In yet another study, no statistically significant difference was found between doxylamine succinate and flurazepam in the average time required for 200 patients with mild to moderate insomnia to fall asleep over 5 nights following a nightly dose of doxylamine succinate 25 mg. or flurazepam 30 mg., nor was any statistically significant difference found in the total time the 200 patients slept. Patients on doxylamine succinate awoke an average of 1.2 times per night while those on flurazepam awoke an average of 0.9 times per night. In either case the patients awoke rested the following morning. On a rating scale of 1 to 5, doxylamine succinate was given a 3.0, flurazepam a 3.4 by patients rating the degree of restfulness provided by their medication (5 represents "very well rested"). Although statistically significant, the difference between doxylamine succinate 25 mg. and flurazepam 30 mg. in the number of awakenings and degree of restfulness is clinically insignificant.

Administration and Dosage: One tablet 30 minutes before retiring. Not for children under 12 years of age.

Side Effects: Occasional anticholinergic effects may be seen.

Precautions: Unisom® should be taken only at bedtime.

Contraindications: Do not take this product, unless directed by a doctor, if you have a breathing problem such as emphysema or chronic bronchitis, or if you have glaucoma or difficulty in urination due to enlargement of the prostate gland. This product should not be taken by pregnant women or those who are nursing a baby.

Warnings: Should be taken with caution if alcohol is being consumed. Product should not be taken if patient is concurrently on any other drug, without prior consultation with physician. Should not be taken for longer than two weeks unless approved by physician.

How Supplied: Boxes of 8, 16, 32 or 48 tablets.

Inactive Ingredients: Dibasic Calcium Phosphate, FD&C Blue #1 Aluminum Lake, Magnesium Stearate, Microcrystalline Cellulose, Sodium Starch Glycolate.

UNISOM® WITH PAIN RELIEF®
[yu 'na-som]
Nighttime Sleep Aid and Pain Reliever

PRODUCT OVERVIEW

Key Facts: Unisom With Pain Relief (diphenhydramine sleep aid/acetaminophen pain relief formula) is a product with a dual antihistamine sleep aid/analgesic action to utilize the sedative effects of an antihistamine and relieve mild to moderate pain that may disturb normal sleep patterns. If patients have difficulty in falling asleep but are not experiencing pain at the same time, regular Unisom Sleep Aid which contains doxylamine succinate or Maximum Strength Unisom Sleepgels which contains diphenhydramine is indicated.

Major Uses: One Unisom With Pain Relief is indicated 30 minutes before retiring to help reduce difficulty in falling asleep while relieving accompanying minor aches and pains, such as headache, muscle aches or menstrual discomfort.

Safety Information: Do not take this product, unless directed by a doctor, if you have a breathing problem such as emphysema or chronic bronchitis, or if you have glaucoma or difficulty in urination due to enlargement of the prostate gland. Unisom With Pain Relief is contraindicated in pregnancy or in nursing mothers. Excessive dosing may lead to liver damage. Product is intended for patients 12 years and older. Alcoholic beverages should be avoided while taking this product. This product should not be taken without first consulting a physician if sedatives or tranquilizers are being taken.

PRESCRIBING INFORMATION
UNISOM WITH PAIN RELIEF®
[yu 'na-som]
Nighttime Sleep Aid and Pain Reliever

Description: Unisom With Pain Relief® is a pale blue, capsule-shaped, coated tablet.

Active Ingredients: 650 mg. acetaminophen and 50 mg. diphenhydramine HCl per tablet.

Indications: Unisom With Pain Relief (diphenhydramine sleep aid formula) is indicated to help reduce difficulty in falling asleep while relieving accompanying minor aches and pains such as headache, muscle ache or menstrual discomfort. If there is difficulty in falling asleep, but pain is not being experienced at the same time, regular Unisom sleep aid is indicated which contains doxylamine succinate as its active ingredient.

Administration and Dosage: One tablet at bedtime if needed, or as directed by a physician.

Contraindications: Do not take this product, unless directed by a doctor, if you have a breathing problem such as emphysema or chronic bronchitis, or if you have glaucoma or difficulty in urination due to enlargement of the prostate gland. Do not take this product if pregnant or nursing a baby.
Do not take this product for treatment of arthritis except under the advice and supervision of a physican.

Warnings: Do not exceed recommended dosage because severe liver damage may occur. If symptoms persist continuously for more than ten days, consult your physician. Insomnia may be a symptom of serious underlying medical illness. Avoid alcoholic beverages while taking this product. Do not take this product if you are taking sedatives or tranquilizers, without first consulting your doctor. For adults only. Do not give to children under 12 years of age. Keep this and all medications out of reach of children. IN CASE OF ACCIDENTAL OVERDOSE SEEK PROFESSIONAL ADVICE OR CONTACT A POISON CONTROL CENTER IMMEDIATELY.

Caution: This product contains an antihistamine and will cause drowsiness. It should be used only at bedtime.

Drug Interaction: Monoamine oxidase (MAO) inhibitors prolong and intensify the anticholinergic effects of antihistamines. The CNS depressant effect is heightened by alcohol and other CNS depressant drugs.

Attention: Use only if tablet blister seals are unbroken. Child resistant packaging.

How Supplied: Boxes of 8 and 16 tablets in child resistant blisters.

Inactive Ingredients: Crospovidone, FD&C Blue #1 Aluminum Lake, FD&C Blue #2 Aluminum Lake, Hydroxypropyl Methylcellulose, Magnesium Stearate, Polyethylene Glycol, Polysorbate 80, Povidone, Pregelatinized Starch, Stearic Acid, Titanium Dioxide.

VISINE L. R.™ EYE DROPS
(oxymetazoline hydrochloride)

Description: Visine L. R. is a sterile, isotonic, buffered ophthalmic solution containing oxymetazoline hydrochloride 0.025%, boric acid, sodium borate, sodium chloride and water. It is preserved with benzalkonium chloride 0.01% and edetate disodium 0.1%.
Visine L. R. is produced by a process that assures sterility.

Indications: Visine L. R. is a decongestant ophthalmic solution designed for the relief of redness of the eye due to minor eye irritations. Visine L. R. is specially formulated to relieve redness of the eye in minutes with effective relief that lasts up to 6 hours.

Directions: *Adults and children 6 years of age and older*—Place 1 or 2 drops in the affected eye(s). This may be repeated as needed every 6 hours or as directed by a physician.

Warning: If you experience eye pain, changes in vision, continued redness or irritation of the eye, or if the condition worsens or persists for more than 72 hours, discontinue use and consult a physician. If you have glaucoma, do not use this product except under the advice and supervision of a physician. As with any medication, if you are pregnant seek the advice of a physician before using this product. Overuse of this product may produce increased redness of the eye. If solution changes color or becomes cloudy, do not use. To avoid contamination of this product, do not touch tip of container to any surface. Replace cap after using. Remove contact lenses before using this product.

Parents: Before using with children under 6 years of age, consult your physician. Keep this and all other medications out of the reach of children. In case of accidental ingestion, seek professional assistance or contact a poison control center immediately.

Caution: Should not be used if Visine-imprinted neckband on bottle is broken or missing.

Storage: Store between 2° and 30°C (36° and 86°F).

How Supplied: In 0.5 fl. oz. and 1 fl. oz. plastic dispenser bottle.
Shown in Product Identification Guide, page 515

VISINE MAXIMUM STRENGTH ALLERGY RELIEF®
Astringent/Redness Reliever Eye Drops

Description: Visine with allergy relief is a sterile, isotonic, buffered ophthalmic solution containing tetrahydrozoline hydrochloride 0.05%, zinc sulfate 0.25%, boric acid, sodium chloride, sodium citrate and purified water. It is preserved with benzalkonium chloride 0.01% and edetate disodium 0.1%. Visine with allergy relief is an ophthalmic solution combining the effects of the vasoconstrictor tetrahydrozoline hydrochloride with the astringent effects of zinc sulfate. The vasoconstrictor provides symptomatic relief of conjunctival edema and hyperemia secondary to minor irritation due to conditions such as dust and airborne pollutants as well as so-called nonspecific or catarrhal conjunctivitis, while zinc sulfate provides relief from burning and itching, symptoms often associated with hay fever, allergies, etc. Beneficial effects include amelioration of burning, irritation, pruritis, and removal of mucus from the eye. Relief is afforded by both ingredients, tetrahydrozoline hydrochloride and zinc sulfate.
Tetrahydrozoline hydrochloride is a sympathomimetic agent, which brings about decongestion by vasoconstriction. Red-

Continued on next page

Pfizer Inc.—Cont.

dened eyes are rapidly whitened by this effective vasoconstrictor, which limits the local vascular response by constricting the small blood vessels. The onset of vasoconstriction becomes apparent within minutes. Zinc sulfate is an ocular astringent which, by precipitating protein, helps to clear mucus from the outer surface of the eye.

The effectiveness of Visine with allergy relief in relieving conjunctival hyperemia and associated symptoms induced by allergies has been clinically demonstrated. In one double-blind study allergy sufferers experienced acute episodes of minor eye irritation. Visine with allergy relief produced statistically significant beneficial results versus a placebo of normal saline solution in relieving irritation of bulbar conjunctiva, irritation of palpebral conjunctiva, and mucous build-up. Treatment with Visine with allergy relief containing zinc sulfate also significantly improved burning and itching symptoms.

Indications: For temporary relief of discomfort and redness due to minor eye irritations.

Directions: Instill 1 to 2 drops in the affected eye(s) up to 4 times daily.

Warning: To avoid contamination, do not touch tip of container to any surface. Replace cap after using. If you experience eye pain, changes in vision, continued redness or irritation of the eye, or if the condition worsens or persists for more than 72 hours, discontinue use and consult a doctor. If you have glaucoma, do not use this product except under the advice and supervision of a doctor. Overuse of this product may produce increased redness of the eye. If solution changes color or becomes cloudy, do not use. Remove contact lenses before using.

Parents: Before using with children under 6 years of age, consult your physician. Keep this and all other drugs out of the reach of children. In case of accidental ingestion, seek professional assistance or contact a poison control center immediately.

How Supplied: In 0.5 fl. oz. and 1.0 fl. oz. plastic dispenser bottle.

Shown in Product Identification Guide, page 515

VISINE MOISTURIZING
Redness Reliever/Lubricant Eye Drops

Description: Visine Moisturizing is a sterile, isotonic, buffered ophthalmic solution containing tetrahydrozoline hydrochloride 0.05%, polyethylene glycol 400 1.0%, boric acid, sodium borate, sodium chloride and water. It is preserved with benzalkonium chloride 0.013% and edetate disodium 0.1%.

Visine Moisturizing is an ophthalmic solution combining the effects of the de-

congestant tetrahydrozoline hydrochloride with the demulcent effects of polyethylene glycol. It provides symptomatic relief of conjunctival edema and hyperemia secondary to ocular allergies, minor irritations and so-called nonspecific or catarrhal conjunctivitis. Tetrahydrozoline hydrochloride is a sympathomimetic agent, which brings about decongestion by vasoconstriction. Reddened eyes are rapidly whitened by this effective vasoconstrictor, which limits the local vascular response by constricting the small blood vessels. The onset of vasoconstriction becomes apparent within minutes. Additional effects include amelioration of burning, irritation, pruritus, soreness, and excessive lacrimation. Relief is afforded by polyethylene glycol.

Polyethylene glycol is an ophthalmic demulcent which has been shown to be effective for the temporary relief of discomfort of minor irritations of the eye due to exposure to wind or sun. It is effective as a protectant and lubricant against further irritation or to relieve dryness of the eye.

The effectiveness of tetrahydrozoline hydrochloride in relieving conjunctival hyperemia and associated symptoms has been demonstrated by numerous clinicals, including several double-blind studies, involving more than 2000 subjects suffering from acute or chronic hyperemia induced by a variety of conditions. Visine Moisturizing is a product that combines the redness relieving effects of a vasoconstrictor and the soothing moisturizing and protective effects of a demulcent.

Indications: Relieves redness of the eye due to minor eye irritations. For use as a protectant against further irritation or to relieve dryness.

Directions: Instill 1 to 2 drops in the affected eye(s) up to 4 times daily.

Warning: To avoid contamination, do not touch tip of container to any surface. Replace cap after using. If you experience eye pain, changes in vision, continued redness or irritation of the eye, or if the condition worsens or persists for more than 72 hours, discontinue use and consult a doctor. If you have glaucoma, do not use this product except under the advice and supervision of a doctor. Overuse of this product may produce increased redness of the eye. If solution changes color or becomes cloudy, do not use. Remove contact lenses before using.

Parents: Before using with children under 6 years of age, consult your physician. Keep this and all other drugs out of the reach of children. In case of accidental ingestion, seek professional assistance or contact a poison control center immediately.

How Supplied: In 0.5 fl. oz. and 1.0 fl. oz. plastic dispenser bottle.

Shown in Product Identification Guide, page 515

VISINE® ORIGINAL
Tetrahydrozoline Hydrochloride
Redness Reliever Eye Drops

Description: Visine is a sterile, isotonic, buffered ophthalmic solution containing tetrahydrozoline hydrochloride 0.05%, boric acid, sodium borate, sodium chloride and water. It is preserved with benzalkonium chloride 0.01% and edetate disodium 0.1%. Visine is a decongestant ophthalmic solution designed to provide symptomatic relief of conjunctival edema and hyperemia secondary to minor irritations, due to conditions such as smoke, dust, other airborne pollutants, swimming etc. and so-called nonspecific or catarrhal conjunctivitis. Relief is afforded by tetrahydrozoline hydrochloride, a sympathomimetic agent, which brings about decongestion by vasoconstriction. Reddened eyes are rapidly whitened by this effective vasoconstrictor, which limits the local vascular response by constricting the small blood vessels. The onset of vasoconstriction becomes apparent within minutes.

The effectiveness of Visine in relieving conjunctival hyperemia has been demonstrated by numerous clinicals, including several double-blind studies, involving more than 2,000 subjects suffering from acute or chronic hyperemia induced by a variety of conditions. Visine was found to be efficacious in providing relief from conjunctival hyperemia.

Indications: Relieves redness of the eye due to minor eye irritations.

Directions: Instill 1 to 2 drops in the affected eye(s) up to four times daily.

Warning: To avoid contamination, do not touch tip of container to any surface. Replace cap after using. If you experience eye pain, changes in vision, continued redness or irritation of the eye, or if the condition worsens or persists for more than 72 hours, discontinue use and consult a doctor. If you have glaucoma, do not use this product except under the advice and supervision of a doctor. Overuse of this product may produce increased redness of the eye. If solution changes color or becomes cloudy, do not use. Remove contact lenses before using.

Parents: Before using with children under 6 years of age, consult your physician. Keep this and all other drugs out of the reach of children. In case of accidental ingestion, seek professional assistance or contact a poison control center immediately.

How Supplied: In 0.5 fl. oz., 0.75 fl. oz., and 1.0 fl. oz. plastic dispenser bottle and 0.5 fl. oz. plastic bottle with dropper.

Shown in Product Identification Guide, page 515

WART-OFF®
Liquid

Active Ingredient: Salicylic Acid 17% w/w.

Inactive Ingredients: Alcohol, 26.35% w/w, Flexible Collodion, Propylene Glycol Dipelargonate.

Indications: For the removal of common warts and plantar warts on the bottom of the foot. The common wart is easily recognized by the rough "cauliflower-like" appearance of the surface. The plantar wart is recognized by its location only on the bottom of the foot, its tenderness, and the interruption of the footprint pattern.

Warnings: For external use only. Keep this and all medications out of the reach of children to avoid accidental poisoning. In case of accidental ingestion, contact a physician or a Poison Control Center immediately. Do not use this product on irritated skin, on any area that is infected or reddened, if you are a diabetic, or if you have poor blood circulation. Do not use on moles, birthmarks, warts with hair growing from them, genital warts, or warts on the face or mucous membranes. If product gets into the eye, flush with water for 15 minutes. Avoid inhaling vapors. If discomfort persists, see your doctor.
Extremely Flammable—Keep away from fire or flame. Cap bottle tightly and store at room temperature away from heat (59°–86°F) (15°–30°C).

Instructions For Use: Read warnings and enclosed instructional brochure. Wash affected area. Dry area thoroughly. Using the special pinpoint applicator, apply one drop at a time to sufficiently cover each wart. Apply Wart-Off to warts only—not to surrounding skin. Let dry. Repeat this procedure once or twice daily as needed (until wart is removed) for up to 12 weeks. Replace cap tightly to prevent evaporation.

How Supplied: 0.45 fluid ounce (13.3mL) bottle with special pinpoint plastic applicator and instructional brochure.

Pharmaton Natural Health Products
Division of Boehringer Ingelheim Pharmaceuticals, Inc.
**900 RIDGEBURY ROAD
RIDGEFIELD, CT 06877**

Direct Inquiries to:
Customer Service: (800) 243-0127
FAX: (203) 798-5771

For Medical Emergency Contact:
Marvin Wetter, M.D.: (203) 798-4361

GINKOBA™
Ginkgo Biloba Extract
[Gĭn-kō-bă]

GINKOBA—Standardized Ginkgo Biloba Extract (50:1).
Over 30 years of extensive research results have shown that GINKOBA is a safe and natural way to supplement your diet. No other extract of the Ginkgo Biloba tree meets the standards of the one in GINKOBA.

NUTRITION FACTS:
Serving Size: 1 tablet
Each Tablet contains:
Calories: 0   Calories from Fat 0

	% Daily Value*
Total Fat 0g	0%
Cholesterol 0mg	0%
Sodium 0mg	0%
Total Carbohydrate 0g	0%
Protein 0g	0%

*Percent Daily Values are based on a 2,000 calorie diet.

Ingredients: Each GINKOBA tablet contains 40 mg of concentrated (50:1) extract from the leaves of the *Ginkgo Biloba* tree. The extract in GINKOBA is precisely standardized to 24% Ginkgo flavonoid glycosides along with other key constituents (Ginkgolides and Bilobalides) in their proven ratios.

Also Contains: Hydroxypropyl methyl cellulose, lactose, talc, polyethylene glycol, magnesium stearate, titanium dioxide, synthetic iron oxides.

Suggested Use: When taken as directed, GINKOBA is a natural way to enhance your mental focus. GINKOBA will help you maintain an overall feeling of healthy well-being, reducing normal forgetfulness and improving conentration.

Recommended Adult Intake: Adults over 12 years old should take one tablet, swallowed whole, with water three times daily at mealtimes.

Cautions: As with other supplements, please keep this product out of the reach of children. In case of accidental overdose, seek the advice of a professional immediately. If you are taking a prescription medicine, are pregnant or lactating, please contact your doctor before taking GINKOBA. No information is available on the use of ginkgo biloba extract in children under the age of 12 years old.
**The statements presented on this package have not been evaluated by the Food and Drug Administration. This product is not intended to diagnose, treat, cure or prevent any disease.
Store at room temperature and avoid excessive heat above 40°C (104°F) to maintain optimal freshness.**
Shown in Product Identification Guide, page 515

GINSANA™
G115 Ginseng Extract
[Gin-sa-na]

GINSANA—Standardized G115® Ginseng Extract (4%).
No other ginseng extract meets the quality standards of the one in GINSANA. Over 25 years of extensive research has shown that GINSANA is a safe and beneficial way to supplement your diet.

NUTRITION FACTS:
Serving Size: 1 capsule
Each Capsule contains:
Calories: 5   Calories from Fat 0

	% Daily Value*
Total Fat 0g	0%
Cholesterol 0mg	0%
Sodium 0mg	0%
Total Carbohydrate 0g	0%
Protein 0g	0%

*Percent Daily Values are based on a 2,000 calorie diet.

Ingredients: Each GINSANA capsule contains 100 mg of highly standardized, concentrated ginseng extract from the roots of the highest quality Korean Panax Ginseng, C.A. Meyer. This special standardization insures a consistent level of the eight most effective ginsenosides in their proven ratios.

Also contains: Sunflower oil, gelatin, glycerin, lecithin, beeswax, chlorophyll.

Suggested Use: When taken as directed, GINSANA is a natural way to enhance your physical endurance by improving your body's ability to utilize oxygen more efficiently. GINSANA will help you maintain your natural energy and an overall feeling of healthy well-being.

Recommended Adult Intake: Adults over 12 years old should take two soft gelatin capsules, swallowed whole, with water in the morning or one capsule in the morning and one in the afternoon. Research on doses above 200 mg per day does not substantiate any better effectiveness. Optimal effectiveness has been shown with 4 weeks of continuous use.

Precautions: As with other vitamins and supplements, please keep this product out of the reach of children. No serious or significant adverse reactions or drug interactions have been reported to date. However, as with any supplement, contact your doctor if you are taking a prescription medicine, are pregnant or lactating. There have been rare reports of mild allergic skin reactions with the use of the extract in this product. In case of accidental overdose, seek the advice of a professional immediately.
**The statements presented on this package have not been evaluated by the Food and Drug Administration. This product is not intended to diagnose, treat, cure or prevent any disease.
Store at room temperature and avoid excess heat above 40°C (104°F) to maintain optimal freshness.**
Shown in Product Identification Guide, page 515

Premier, Inc.
GREENWICH OFFICE PARK ONE
GREENWICH, CT 06831

Direct Inquiries to:
Robert Albus
(203) 622-1211
FAX: (203) 622-0773

For Medical Emergency Contact:
Sergio Nacht, Ph.D.
(415) 366-2626
FAX: (415) 368-4470
or
Subash J. Saxena, Ph.D.
(415) 366-2626
FAX: (415) 368-4470

EXACT®
[Ex-áct]
**Benzoyl Peroxide Acne Medication
Vanishing and Tinted Creams, &
Adult Acne Medication**

Vanishing Cream Active Ingredient:
Benzoyl Peroxide 5.0% in a colorless,
odorless, and greaseless cream base containing water, acrylates copolymer, glycerin, sorbitol, cetyl alcohol, glyceryl
dilaurate, stearyl alcohol, sodium lauryl
sulfate, magnesium aluminum silicate,
sodium citrate, silica, citric acid, methylparaben, xanthan gum and propylparaben.
Tinted Cream Active Ingredient:
Benzoyl Peroxide 5.0% in a flesh-toned,
odorless , and greaseless cream base containing water, acrylates copolymer, glycerin, titanium dioxide, sorbitol, cetyl alcohol, glyceryl dilaurate, stearyl alcohol,
sodium lauryl sulfate, magnesium aluminum silicate, sodium citrate, silica, iron
oxides, citric acid, methylparaben, xanthan gum and propylparaben.
**Adult Acne Medication Active
Ingredient:** Benzoyl Peroxide 2.5%
Other Ingredients: Water, Glycerin,
Acrylates Copolymer, Sorbitol, Cetyl Alcohol, Glyceryl Dilaurate, Stearyl Alcohol, Sodium Lauryl Sulfate, Magnesium
Aluminum Silicate, Sodium Citrate, Silica, Citric Acid, Methylparaben, Xanthan Gum, and Propylparaben
**Pore Treatment Gel Active Ingredi-
ent:** 2% Salicylic Acid
Other Ingredients: Water, Dimethicone, Peg-20, Polyacrylamide (and)
C13–14 Isoparaffin (and) Laureth-7,
Methyl Gluceth-20, Aloe Vera Gel, Acrylates Copolymer, Polysorbate-80, Propylene Glycol (and) Diazolindinyl Urea
(and) Methylparaben, (and) Propylparaben, Triethanolamine, Panthenol, Allantoin, Disodium Edta.

Indications: For the topical treatment
of acne vulgaris.

Actions: Exact Vanishing and Tinted
Creams contain 5% benzoyl peroxide.
ExACT Pore Gel Treatment contains 2%
Salicylic Acid. It works to absorb problem causing oil as it is released, helping
to prevent pimples and leave skin feeling
smooth. Adult Acne Medication contains
2.5% benzoyl peroxide. Each product

clears existing pimples and helps prevent new pimples from forming.
Additional Benefits: Exact utilizes a
patented Microsponge® system for super non-stop oil absorbing action. This
special Microsponge formula was designed for low irritancy and to provide
50% higher oil absorbancy than other
benzoyl peroxide medications. Exact
Tinted Cream is flesh-toned to hide acne
pimples while it treats them. Pore Gel
Treatment: Exact utilizes a patented Microsponge formula which provides super
nonstop oil absorbing action while it releases salicylic acid to unclog pores and
reduce oil buildup.

Warning: For external use only. Using
other topical acne medications at the
same time or immediately following use
of this product may increase dryness or
irritation of the skin. If this occurs, only
one medication should be used unless
directed by a doctor. Do not use this medication if you have very sensitive skin or
if you are sensitive to benzoyl peroxide.
This product may cause irritation, characterized by redness, burning, itching,
peeling, or possibly swelling. Mild irritation may be reduced by using the product
less frequently or in a lower concentration. If irritation becomes severe, discontinue use; if irritation still continues,
consult a doctor. Keep away from eyes,
lips, and mouth. This product may bleach
hair or dyed fabrics. Store at room temperature. Keep away from flame, fire
and heat.
**KEEP THIS AND ALL DRUGS OUT
OF REACH OF CHILDREN.**
In case of accidental ingestion, seek professional assistance or contact a Poison
Control Center immediately.

**Symptoms and Treatment of Inges-
tion:** These symptoms are based upon
medical judgement, not on actual experience. Theoretically, ingestion of very
large amounts may cause nausea, vomiting, abdominal discomfort and diarrhea.
Treatment is symptomatic, with bed rest
and observation.

Directions for Use: Cleanse the skin
thoroughly before applying medication.
Cover the entire affected area with a thin
layer one to three times daily. Because
excessive drying of the skin may occur,
start with one application daily, then
gradually increase to two or three times
daily if needed or as directed by a doctor.
If bothersome dryness or peeling occurs,
reduce application to once a day or every
other day.

How Supplied: 0.65 oz. (18 g) plastic
squeeze tubes. Pore Treatment Gel: 2.0
oz. (56 g) plastic squeeze tube.

Procter & Gamble
P. O. BOX 5516
CINCINNATI, OH 45201

Direct Inquiries to:
Charles Lambert
(800) 358-8707

For Medical Emergencies:
Call Collect: (513) 558-4422

ALEVE®
[ə lēv ']
**Naproxen Sodium Tablets, USP
Pain Reliever/Fever Reducer**

Allergy Warning: Do not take this
product if you have had either hives or a
severe allergic reaction after taking any
pain reliever. Even though this product
may not contain the same ingredient,
ALEVE could cause similar reactions in
patients allergic to other pain relieving
drugs.

Alcohol Warning: If you generally
consume 3 or more alcohol-containing
drinks per day, you should consult your
doctor for advice on when and how you
should take ALEVE and other pain relievers.

Active Ingredient: Each [tablet] [cap-
let] contains naproxen sodium 220 mg
(naproxen 200 mg and sodium 20 mg).

Inactive Ingredients: Magnesium Stearate, Microcrystalline Cellulose, Povidone, Talc, Opadry YS-1-4215.

Indications: For the temporary relief
of minor aches and pains associated with
the common cold, headache, toothache,
muscular aches, backache, for the minor
pain of arthritis, for the pain of menstrual cramps and for the reduction of
fever.

Dosage and Administration:
Adults: Take 1 [tablet] [caplet] every 8
to 12 hours while symptoms persist. With
experience, some people may find that an
initial dose of 2 [tablets] [caplets] followed by 1 [tablet] [caplet] 12 hours later,
if necessary, will give better relief. *Do not
exceed 3 [tablets] [caplets] in 24 hours unless directed to do so by a doctor.* The
smallest effective dose should be used. A
full glass of water or other liquid is
recommended with each dose.
Adults over age 65: Do not take more
than 1 [tablet] [caplet] every 12 hours,
unless directed to do so by a doctor.
Children under age 12: Do not give this
product to children under 12, except under the advice and supervision of a
doctor.

General Warnings: Do not take
ALEVE for more than 10 days for pain,
or for more than 3 days for fever, unless
directed by a doctor.
Consult a doctor if:
*your pain or fever persists or gets worse
*the painful area is red or swollen
*you take any other drugs on a regular
basis

*you have had serious side effects from any pain reliever

*you have any new or unusual symptoms

*more than mild heartburn, upset stomach, or stomach pain occurs with use of this product or if even mild symptoms persist

Although naproxen sodium is indicated for the same conditions as aspirin, ibuprofen and acetaminophen, it should not be taken with them or other naproxen-containing products except under a doctor's direction. As with any drug, if you are pregnant or nursing a baby, seek the advice of a health professional before using this product. IT IS ESPECIALLY IMPORTANT NOT TO USE NAPROXEN SODIUM DURING THE LAST 3 MONTHS OF PREGNANCY UNLESS SPECIFICALLY DIRECTED TO DO SO BY A DOCTOR BECAUSE IT MAY CAUSE PROBLEMS IN THE UNBORN CHILD OR COMPLICATIONS DURING DELIVERY.

Keep this and all drugs out of the reach of children. In case of accidental overdose, seek professional assistance or contact a poison control center immediately. If you have questions, comments or problems, call 1-800-395-0689 to report them.

How Supplied: Light blue round tablets or oval-shaped caplets debossed with "ALEVE". Child-resistant "Safety SquEASE" bottles of 24, 50, 100, and 150 (200 available in caplets) tablets or caplets, with fold-out back label containing important information on the 24 and 50 count bottles.

Storage: Store at room temperature. Avoid excessive heat (104°F or 40°C).
Shown in Product Identification Guide, page 515

CREST® Sensitivity Protection Toothpaste for sensitive teeth and cavity prevention

Active Ingredients: Potassium Nitrate (5%), Sodium Fluoride (0.15% w/v fluoride ion).

Actions: Builds protection against sensitive tooth pain. Contains **Fluoride** for cavity prevention. Gentle on tooth enamel, leaves teeth feeling clean.
WHAT ARE SENSITIVE TEETH?
If you experience flashes of tooth pain or discomfort from cold or hot foods and drinks, or even when you touch your teeth with your toothbrush, you may suffer from **Dentinal Hypersensitivity** (or "sensitive teeth.") **Hypersensitivity** can occur when dentin, which surrounds the pulp cavity and tooth nerve, is not protected. Dentin can become exposed when gums recede and the protective layer covering the root surface is worn away, leaving dentin exposed. Crest Sensitivity Protection helps relieve the pain of sensitive teeth by soothing the nerves in your teeth when the dentin is exposed.
This product has been given the Seal of Acceptance from the Council on Scientific Affairs–ADA.

Uses: When used regularly, builds increasing protection against painful sensitivity of the teeth to cold, heat, acids, sweets, or contact, and aids in the prevention of cavities.

Directions: Adults and children 12 years of age and older: Apply at least a 1-inch strip of the product onto a soft bristle toothbrush. Brush teeth thoroughly for at least 1 minute twice a day (morning and evening) or as recommended by a dentist or physician. Make sure to brush all sensitive areas of the teeth. Do not swallow. Children under 12 years of age: ask a dentist or physician.

Warnings: Sensitive teeth may indicate a serious problem that may need prompt care by a dentist. See your dentist if the problem persists or worsens. Do not use this product longer than four weeks unless recommended by a dentist or physician. **Keep this and all drugs out of the reach of children.**

Inactive Ingredients: Water, Hydrated Silica, Glycerin, Sorbitol, Trisodium Phosphate, Sodium Lauryl Sulfate, Cellulose Gum, Flavor, Xanthan Gum, Sodium Saccharin, Titanium Dioxide.

How Supplied: 6.2 OZ (175g), 2.5 OZ (70g) and 1.0 OZ (28g) tubes in cartons.

HEAD & SHOULDERS® INTENSIVE TREATMENT DANDRUFF AND SEBORRHEIC DERMATITIS SHAMPOO

Head & Shoulders Intensive Treatment Dandruff and Seborrheic Dermatitis Shampoo offers effective control of persistent dandruff, and beautiful hair from a pleasant-to-use formula. Double-blind and expert-graded testing have proven that Intensive Treatment Dandruff and Seborrheic Dermatitis Shampoo reduces persistent dandruff. It is also gentle enough to use every day for clean, manageable hair.

Active Ingredient: 1% selenium sulfide suspended in a mild surfactant base. Shampoo also includes mild conditioning agents.

Indications: For effective control of seborrheic dermatitis and dandruff of the scalp.

Actions: Selenium sulfide is substantive to the scalp and remains after rinsing. Its mechanism is believed to be antiproliferative, and to also control the microorganisms associated with persistent dandruff flaking and itching.

WARNINGS: For external use only. Avoid contact with eyes—if this happens, rinse thoroughly with water. If scalp condition worsens, or does not improve, consult a doctor. Keep out of reach of children.

Caution: If used on light, gray, or chemically treated hair, rinse **VIGOROUSLY** for 5 minutes.

Dosage and Administration: For best results in controlling persistent dandruff, Head & Shoulders Intensive Treatment Dandruff and Seborrheic Dermatitis Shampoo should be used regularly. It is gentle enough to use for every shampoo.

Ingredients: Selenium sulfide in a shampoo base of water, ammonium laureth sulfate, ammonium lauryl sulfate, cocamide MEA, glycol distearate, ammonium xylenesulfonate, dimethicone, fragrance, tricetylmonium chloride, cetyl alcohol, DMDM hydantoin, sodium chloride, stearyl alcohol, hydroxypropyl methylcellulose, FD&C Red No. 4.

How Supplied: Intensive Treatment Dandruff and Seborrheic Dermatitis Shampoo is available in 15 FL OZ unbreakable plastic bottles.

METAMUCIL®
[met uh-mū sil]
(psyllium husk fiber)

Description: Metamucil contains a bulk forming natural therapeutic fiber for restoring and maintaining regularity as recommended by a physician. It contains psyllium husk, a highly efficient fiber from the plant Plantago ovata. Metamucil contains no chemical stimulants and does not disrupt normal bowel function. Each dose contains approximately 3.4 grams of psyllium. Inactive ingredients, sodium, potassium, calories, carbohydrate, fat and phenylalanine content are shown in Table 1 for all forms and flavors. Phenylketonurics should be aware that phenylalanine is present in Metamucil products that contain aspartame. Metamucil Sugar-Free Regular Flavor contains no sugar and no artificial sweetners.
Metamucil in powdered forms is gluten-free. Wafers contain gluten: Apple Crisp contains 0.7g/dose, Cinnamon Spice contains 0.5g/dose.

Actions: The active ingredient in Metamucil is psyllium, a natural fiber which promotes elimination due to its bulking effect in the colon. This bulking effect is due to both the water-holding capacity of undigested fiber and the increased bacterial mass following partial fiber digestion. These actions result in enlargement of the lumen of the colon, and softer stool, thereby decreasing intraluminal pressure and straining, and speeding colonic transit in constipated patients.

Indications: Metamucil is indicated in the management of chronic constipation, irritable bowel syndrome, as adjunctive therapy in the constipation of diverticular disease, the bowel management of patients with hemorrhoids, for constipation associated with convalescence and senility and for occasional constipation during pregnancy when under the care of a physician. Pregnancy: Category B.

Continued on next page

Procter & Gamble—Cont.

TABLE 1

Forms/ Flavors	Inactive Ingredients	Sodium mg/ Dose	Potassium mg/ Dose	Calories per Dose	Carbohydrate g/ Dose	Fat g/ Dose	Phenylalanine mg/Dose	Dosage 1–3 Times Daily. Each Dose Contains 3.4 g Psyllium Husk Fiber	How Supplied
Smooth Texture Orange Flavor **METAMUCIL** Powder	Citric acid, D&C Yellow No. 10, FD&C Yellow No. 6, Flavoring, Sucrose	<5	30	35	12	—	—	1 rounded tablespoonful 12 g	Canisters: 13, 20.3, 30.4 and 48 ozs. (Doses: 30, 48, 72 and 114); Cartons: 30 single-dose packets (OTC)
Smooth Texture Sugar-Free Orange Flavor **METAMUCIL** Powder	Aspartame, Citric acid, D&C Yellow No. 10, FD&C Yellow No. 6, Flavoring, Maltodextrin	<5	30	10	5	—	25	1 rounded teaspoonful 5.8 g	Canisters: 10, 15, 23.3 ozs. and 36.8 ozs. (Doses: 48, 72, 114 and 180); Cartons: 30 single-dose packets (OTC) 100 single-dose packets (Institutional)
Smooth Texture Citrus Flavor **METAMUCIL** Powder	Citric acid, D&C Yellow No. 10, FD&C Yellow No. 6, Flavoring, Sucrose	<5	40	35	12	—	—	1 rounded tablespoonful 12 g	Canisters: 13, 20.3, 30.4 and 48 ozs. (Doses: 30, 48, 72 and 114); Cartons: 30 single-dose packets (OTC) 100 single-dose packets (Institutional)
Smooth Texture Sugar-Free Citrus Flavor **METAMUCIL** Powder	Aspartame, Citric acid, D&C Yellow No. 10, FD&C Yellow No. 6, Flavoring, Maltodextrin	<5	30	10	5	—	25	1 rounded teaspoonful 5.8 g	Canisters: 10, 15 and 23.3 ozs. (Doses: 48, 72 and 114); Cartons: 30 single-dose packets (OTC)
Smooth Texture Sugar-Free Regular Flavor **METAMUCIL** Powder	Citric Acid (less than 1%), Magnesium sulfate*, Maltodextrin	<5	30	10	5	—	—	1 rounded teaspoonful 5.8 g	Canisters: 10, 15 and 23.3 ozs. (Doses: 48, 72 and 114)
Original Texture Regular Flavor **METAMUCIL** Powder	Dextrose	<5	30	14	6	—	—	1 rounded teaspoonful 7 g	Canisters: 13, 19 and 29 ozs. (Doses: 48, 72 and 114)

Contraindications: Intestinal obstruction, fecal impaction. Known allergy to any component.

Warnings: Patients are advised they should not use the product without consulting a doctor when abdominal pain, nausea, or vomiting are present or if they have noticed a sudden change in bowel habits that persists over a period of two weeks, or rectal bleeding. Patients are advised to consult a physician if constipation persists for longer than one week, as this may be a sign of a serious medical condition. **PATIENTS ARE CAUTIONED THAT TAKING THIS PRODUCT WITHOUT ADEQUATE FLUID MAY CAUSE IT TO SWELL AND BLOCK THE THROAT OR ESOPHAGUS AND MAY CAUSE CHOKING. THEY SHOULD NOT TAKE THE PRODUCT IF THEY HAVE DIFFICULTY IN SWALLOWING. IF THEY EXPERIENCE CHEST PAIN, VOMITING, OR DIFFICULTY IN SWALLOWING OR BREATHING AFTER TAKING THIS PRODUCT, THEY ARE ADVISED TO SEEK IMMEDIATE MEDICAL ATTENTION.** Psyllium products may cause allergic reaction in people sensitive to inhaled or ingested psyllium. Keep this and all medications out of the reach of children.

Precaution: Notice to Health Care Professionals: To minimize the potential for allergic reaction, health care professionals who frequently dispense powdered psyllium products should avoid inhaling airborne dust while dispensing these products. Handling and Dispensing: To minimize generating airborne dust, spoon product from the canister into a glass according to label directions.

Dosage and Administration: The usual adult dosage is 1 rounded teaspoonful or 1 rounded tablespoonful depending on product form. Generally the sugar-free products are dosed by the teaspoonful, sucrose-containing products by the tablespoonful. Some forms are available in packets. The appropriate dose should be mixed with 8 oz. of liquid (e.g., cool water, fruit juice, milk) following the labeled instructions. Metamucil wafers should be consumed with 8 oz. of liquid. **THE PRODUCT (CHILD OR ADULT DOSE) SHOULD BE TAKEN WITH AT LEAST 8 OZ (A FULL GLASS) OF WATER OR OTHER FLUID. TAKING THIS PRODUCT WITHOUT ENOUGH LIQUID MAY CAUSE CHOKING (SEE WARNINGS).** Metamucil can be taken orally one to three times a day, depend-

TABLE 1 (continued)

Forms/ Flavors	Inactive Ingredients	Sodium mg/ Dose	Potas- sium mg/ Dose	Calo- ries per Dose	Carbo- hy- drate g/ Dose	Fat g/ Dose	Phenyl- alanine mg/Dose	Dosage 1–3 Times Daily. Each Dose Contains 3.4 g Psyllium Hydrophilic Mucilloid	How Supplied
Original Texture Orange Flavor **METAMUCIL** Powder	Citric acid, FD&C Yellow No. 6, Flavoring, Sucrose	<5	35	30	10	—	—	1 rounded tablespoonful 11 g	Canisters: 13, 19, 29 and 44.2 ozs. (Doses: 30, 48, 72 and 114)
Sugar-Free Lemon-Lime Flavor **METAMUCIL** Effervescent Powder	Aspartame, Calcium carbonate, Citric acid, Flavoring, Potassium bicarbonate, Silicon dioxide, Sodium bicarbonate	10	280	6	4	—	30	1 packet 5.4 g	Cartons: 30 single-dose packets (OTC), 100 single-dose packets (Institutional)
Sugar-Free Orange-Flavor **METAMUCIL** Effervescent Powder	Aspartame, Citric acid, FD&C Yellow No. 6, Flavoring, Potassium bicarbonate, Silicon dioxide, Sodium bicarbonate	5	280	6	4	—	28	1 packet 5.2 g	Cartons: 30 single-dose packets (OTC)
Apple Crisp **METAMUCIL** Wafers	Ascorbic acid, Brown sugar, Cinnamon, Corn oil, Flavors, Fructose, Lecithin, Modified food starch, Molasses, Oat hull fiber, Sodium bicarbonate, Sucrose, Water, Wheat flour	20	50	100	19	5	—	2 wafers 25 g	Cartons: 12 doses; 24 doses
Cinnamon Spice **METAMUCIL** Wafers	Ascorbic acid, Cinnamon, Corn oil, Flavors, Fructose, Lecithin, Modified food starch, Molasses, Nutmeg, Oat hull fiber, Oats, Sodium bicarbonate, Sucrose, Water, Wheat flour	15	45	100	18	5	—	2 wafers 25 g	Cartons: 12 doses; 24 doses

*Metamucil Sugar-Free Regular Flavor contains 26 mg of magnesium per dose.

ing on the need and response. It may require continued use for 2 to 3 days to provide optimal benefit. Generally produces effect in 12–72 hours. For children (6 to 12 years old), use ½ the adult dose in/ with 8 oz. of liquid, 1 to 3 times daily. Children under 6 consult a doctor.

New Users: (Label statement)
Your doctor can recommend the right dosage of Metamucil to best meet your needs. In general, start by taking one dose each day. Gradually increase to three doses per day, if needed or recommended by your doctor. If minor gas or bloating occurs when you increase doses, try slightly reducing the amount you are taking.

How Supplied: Powder: canisters (OTC) and cartons of single-dose packets (OTC and Institutional). Wafers: cartons of single-dose packets (OTC). (See Table 1).
[See table at top of preceding page.]
[See table above.]

Shown in Product Identification Guide, page 515

OIL OF OLAY®—Daily UV Protectant SPF 15 Beauty Fluid—Original & Fragrance Free Versions (Olay Co., Inc.)

Oil of Olay Daily UV Protectant Beauty Fluid is a light, greaseless lotion that is specially formulated to provide effective moisturization and SPF 15 protection with minimal migration to reduce the likelihood of eye sting. Oil of Olay Daily UV Protectant is PABA free. It is non-comedogenic and is suitable for daily use under facial make-up.

Active Ingredients: Octyl Methoxy-cinnamate, Phenylbenzimidazole Sulfonic Acid

Inactive Ingredients: Water, Isohexadecane, Butylene Glycol, Triethanolamine, Glycerin, Stearic Acid, Cetyl Alcohol, Cetyl Palmitate, DEA-Cetyl Phosphate, Aluminum Starch Octenyl-succinate, Titanium Dioxide, Imidazolidinyl Urea, Methylparaben,

Propylparaben, Carbomer, Acrylates/ C10–30 Alkyl Acrylate Crosspolymer, PEG-10 Soya Sterol, Disodium EDTA, Castor Oil, Fragrance, FD&C Red No. 4, FD&C Yellow No. 5.
Available in both lightly scented original version and a 100% color free and fragrance free version.

Indications: Filters out the sun's harmful rays to help prevent skin damage. Provides SPF 15 protection in a light, greaseless moisturizer. Regular use over the years may reduce the chance of skin damage, some types of skin cancer, and other harmful effects due to the sun.

Directions: Adults and children 6 months of age and over: Apply liberally as often as necessary. Children under 6 months of age: Consult a doctor.

WARNINGS: For external use only, not to be swallowed. Avoid contact with the eyes. If contact occurs, rinse eyes

Continued on next page

Procter & Gamble—Cont.

thoroughly with water. Discontinue use if signs of irritation or rash appear. If irritation or rash persists, consult a doctor. **KEEP OUT OF REACH OF CHILDREN.**

How Supplied: Available in 3.5 fl. oz. and 5.25 fl. oz. plastic bottles.

PEPTO-BISMOL®
ORIGINAL LIQUID,
ORIGINAL AND CHERRY TABLETS
AND EASY-TO-SWALLOW
CAPLETS
For upset stomach, indigestion, diarrhea, heartburn and nausea.

Multi-symptom Pepto-Bismol contains bismuth subsalicylate and is the only leading OTC stomach remedy clinically proven effective for both upper and lower GI symptoms. Pepto-Bismol is in more households than any other stomach remedy, making it a convenient recommendation with a name your patients will know. It has been clinically proven in double-blind placebo-controlled trials for relief of upset stomach symptoms and diarrhea.

Description: Each tablespoon (15 ml) of Pepto-Bismol Liquid contains 262 mg bismuth subsalicylate. Each tablespoonful of liquid contains a total of 130 mg non-aspirin salicylate. Pepto-Bismol liquid contains no sugar and is very low in sodium (less than 3 mg/tablespoonful). Inactive ingredients: benzoic acid, D&C Red No. 22, D&C Red No. 28, flavor, magnesium aluminum silicate, methylcellulose, saccharin sodium, salicylic acid, sodium salicylate, sorbic acid and water. Each Pepto-Bismol Tablet contains 262 mg bismuth subsalicylate. Each tablet contains a total of 102 mg non-aspirin salicylate (99 mg non-aspirin salicylate for Cherry). Pepto-Bismol tablets contain no sugar and are very low in sodium (less than 2 mg/tablet). Inactive ingredients include: adipic acid (in Cherry only), calcium carbonate, D&C Red No. 27, FD&C Red No. 40 (in Cherry only), flavors, magnesium stearate, mannitol, povidone, saccharin sodium and talc. Each Pepto-Bismol Caplet contains 262 mg bismuth subsalicylate. Each caplet contains a total of 99 mg non-aspirin salicylate. Caplets contain no sugar and are low in sodium (less than 2 mg/caplet). Inactive ingredients include: calcium carbonate, D&C Red No. 27, magnesium stearate, mannitol, microcrystalline cellulose, polysorbate 80, povidone, silicon dioxide, and sodium starch glycolate.

Indications: Pepto-Bismol controls diarrhea within 24 hours, relieving associated abdominal cramps; soothes heartburn and indigestion without constipating; and relieves nausea and upset stomach.

Actions: For upset stomach symptoms (i.e., indigestion, heartburn, nausea and fullness caused by over-indulgence), the active ingredient is believed to work via a topical effect on the stomach mucosa. For diarrhea, it is believed to work by several mechanisms in the gastrointestinal tract, including: 1) normalizing fluid movement via an antisecretory mechanism, 2) binding bacterial toxins and 3) antimicrobial activity.

Warnings: Children and teenagers who have or are recovering from chicken pox or flu should not use this medicine to treat nausea or vomiting. If nausea or vomiting is present, patients are advised to consult a doctor because this could be an early sign of Reye syndrome, a rare but serious illness.
This product contains non-aspirin salicylates. If taken with aspirin and ringing in the ears occurs, discontinue use. This product does not contain aspirin, but should not be administered to those patients who have a known allergy to aspirin or non-aspirin salicylates as an adverse reaction may occur. Caution is advised in the administration to patients taking medication for anticoagulation, diabetes and gout.
If diarrhea is accompanied by a high fever or continues more than 2 days, patients are advised to consult a physician. As with any drug, caution is advised in the administration to pregnant or nursing women.
Keep all medicine out of the reach of children.

Note: This medication may cause a temporary and harmless darkening of the tongue and/or stool. Stool darkening should not be confused with melena.

Overdosage: In case of overdose, patients are advised to contact a physician or Poison Control Center. Emesis induced by ipecac syrup is indicated in large ingestions provided ipecac can be administered within one hour of ingestion. Activated charcoal should be administered after gastric emptying. Patients should be evaluated for signs and symptoms of salicylate toxicity.

Dosage and Administration:
Liquid: Shake well before using.
Adults—2 tablespoonsful
(1 dose cup, 30 ml)
Children (according to age)—
9–12 yrs. 1 tablespoonful
(½ dose cup, 15 ml)
6–9 yrs. 2 teaspoonsful
(⅓ dose cup, 10 ml)
3–6 yrs. 1 teaspoonful
(⅙ dose cup, 5 ml)

Repeat dosage every ½ to 1 hour, if needed, to a maximum of 8 doses in a 24-hour period. Drink plenty of clear fluids to help prevent dehydration which may accompany diarrhea.

For children under 3 years of age, consult a physician.
Tablets:
Adults—Two tablets
Children (according to age)—
9–12 yrs. 1 tablet
6–9 yrs. ⅔ tablet
3–6 yrs. ⅓ tablet

Chew or dissolve in mouth. Repeat every ½ to 1 hour as needed, to a maximum of 8 doses in a 24-hour period. Drink plenty of clear fluids to help prevent dehydration, which may accompany diarrhea. For children under 3 years of age, consult a physician.

Caplets:
Adults—Two caplets
Children (according to age)—
9–12 yrs. 1 caplet
6–9 yrs. ⅔ caplet
3–6 yrs. ⅓ caplet

Swallow caplet(s) with water, do not chew. Repeat every ½ to 1 hour as needed, to a maximum of 8 doses in a 24-hour period. Drink plenty of clear fluids to help prevent dehydration, which may accompany diarrhea. For children under 3 years of age, consult a physician.

How Supplied: Pepto-Bismol Liquid is available in: 4, 8, 12, 16 and 20 FL OZ bottles. Pepto-Bismol Tablets are pink, round, chewable tablets imprinted with a debossed triangle and "Pepto-Bismol" on one side. Tablets are available in: boxes of 30 and 48 (Original only). Tablets are available in bottles of 24 and 40. Caplets are imprinted with "Pepto-Bismol" on one side.

PEPTO-BISMOL®
MAXIMUM STRENGTH LIQUID
For upset stomach, indigestion, diarrhea, heartburn and nausea.

Multi-symptom Pepto-Bismol contains bismuth subsalicylate and is the only leading OTC stomach remedy clinically proven effective for both upper and lower GI symptoms. Pepto-Bismol is in more households than any other stomach remedy, making it a convenient recommendation with a name your patients will know. It has been clinically-proven in double-blind placebo-controlled trials for relief of upset stomach symptoms and diarrhea.

Description: Each tablespoonful (15 ml) of Maximum Strength Pepto-Bismol Liquid contains 525 mg bismuth subsalicylate (236 mg non-aspirin salicylate). Maximum Strength Pepto-Bismol Liquid contains no sugar and is low in sodium (less than 3 mg/tablespoonful). Inactive ingredients include: benzoic acid, D&C

Red No. 22, D&C Red No. 28, flavor, magnesium aluminum silicate, methylcellulose, saccharin sodium, salicylic acid, sodium salicylate, sorbic acid and water.

Indications: Maximum Strength Pepto-Bismol soothes upset stomach and indigestion without constipating; controls diarrhea within 24 hours, relieving associated abdominal cramps; and relieves heartburn and nausea.

Actions: For upset stomach symptoms (i.e. indigestion, heartburn, nausea and fullness caused by over-indulgence), the active ingredient is believed to work via a topical effect on the stomach mucosa. For diarrhea, it is believed to work by several mechanisms in the gastrointestinal tract, including: 1) normalizing fluid movement via an antisecretory mechanism, 2) binding bacterial toxins, and 3) antimicrobial activity.

Warnings: Children and teenagers who have or are recovering from chicken pox or flu should not use this medicine to treat nausea or vomiting. If nausea or vomiting is present, patients are advised to consult a doctor because this could be an early sign of Reye syndrome, a rare but serious illness.
This product contains non-aspirin salicylates. If taken with aspirin and ringing in the ears occurs, discontinue use. This product does not contain aspirin, but should not be administered to those patients who have a known allergy to aspirin or other non-aspirin salicylates as an adverse reaction may occur. Caution is advised in the administration to patients taking medication for anticoagulation, diabetes and gout.
If diarrhea is accompanied by a high fever or continues more than 2 days, patients are advised to consult a physician. As with any drug, caution is advised in the administration to pregnant or nursing women.
Keep all medicine out of the reach of children.
Note: This medication may cause a temporary and harmless darkening of the tongue and/or stool. Stool darkening should not be confused with melena.

Overdosage: In case of overdose, patients are advised to contact a physician or Poison Control Center. Emesis induced by ipecac syrup is indicated in large ingestions provided ipecac can be administered within one hour of ingestion. Activated charcoal should be administered after gastric emptying. Patients should be evaluated for signs and symptoms of salicylate toxicity.

Dosage and Administration: Shake well before using.
Adults—2 tablespoonful
    (1 dose cup, 30 ml)
Children (according to age)—
9–12 yrs.   1 tablespoonful
             (½ dose cup, 15 ml)
6–9 yrs.   2 teaspoonsful
             (⅓ dose cup, 10 ml)
3–6 yrs.   1 teaspoonful
             (⅙ dose cup, 5 ml)

Repeat dosage every hour, if needed, to a maximum of 4 doses in a 24-hour period. Drink plenty of clear fluids to help prevent dehydration, which may accompany diarrhea.

How Supplied: Maximum Strength Pepto-Bismol is available in: 4, 8, and 12 FL OZ bottles.

PEPTO DIARRHEA CONTROL®
Loperamide Hydrochloride
Caplets

Description: Each caplet of Pepto Diarrhea Control contains 2 mg of Loperamide Hydrochloride and is scored and colored white.

Actions: Pepto Diarrhea Control contains a clinically proven antidiarrheal medication, Loperamide Hydrochloride, that works in many cases with just one dose. Loperamide Hydrochloride acts by slowing intestinal motility and by affecting water and electrolyte movement through the bowel.

Indication: Pepto Diarrhea Control controls the symptoms of diarrhea.

Directions: Drink plenty of clear fluids to help prevent dehydration, which may accompany diarrhea.

Usual Dosage: Adults and children 12 years of age and older: Two caplets after first loose bowel movement followed by one caplet after each subsequent loose bowel movement but no more than four caplets a day for no more than two days. Children 9–11 years old (60–95 lbs.): One caplet after first loose bowel movement, followed by one-half caplet after each subsequent loose bowel movement, but no more than three caplets a day for no more than two days.
Children 6–8 years old (48–59 lbs.): One caplet after first loose bowel movement, followed by one-half caplet after each subsequent loose bowel movement, but no more than two caplets a day for no more than two days.
Under 6 years old (up to 47 lbs.): Consult a physician. Not intended for children under 6 years old.

Warnings: DO NOT USE FOR MORE THAN TWO DAYS UNLESS DIRECTED BY A PHYSICIAN. Do not use if diarrhea is accompanied by high fever (greater than 101°F), or if blood is present in the stool, or if you have had a rash or other allergic reaction to Loperamide Hydrochloride. If you are taking antibiotics or have a history of liver disease, consult a physician before using this product. As with any drug, caution is advised in the administration to pregnant and nursing women. Keep this and all drugs out of the reach of children. In case of accidental overdose, seek professional assistance or contact a poison control center immediately.

Overdosage: Overdosage of Loperamide Hydrochloride in humans may result in constipation, CNS depression and nausea. A slurry of activated charcoal

administered promptly after ingestion of Loperamide Hydrochloride can reduce the amount of drug which is absorbed. If vomiting occurs spontaneously upon ingestion, a slurry of 100 grams of activated charcoal may be administered orally as soon as fluids can be retained. If vomiting has not occurred, and CNS depression is evident, gastric lavage should be performed followed by administration of 100 grams of the activated charcoal slurry through the gastric tube. In the event of overdosage, patients should be monitored for signs of CNS depression for at least 24 hours. Children may be more sensitive to central nervous system effects than adults. If CNS depression is observed, naloxone may be administered. If responsive to naloxone, vital signs must be monitored carefully for recurrence of symptoms of drug overdose for at least 24 hours after the last dose of naloxone.

Inactive Ingredients: Corn starch, lactose, magnesium stearate, microcrystalline cellulose.

How Supplied: White scored caplets in 6's and 12's blister packaging which is tamper-evident and child-resistant. Caplets are imprinted with "Pepto DC" on one side, "2" and "MG" separated by score mark on other side.

PERCOGESIC®
[pĕrkō-jē'zĭk]
Analgesic Tablets
Pain Reliever/Fever Reducer

Active Ingredients: Each tablet contains:
Acetaminophen, 325 mg; Phenyltoloxamine citrate, 30 mg.

Inactive Ingredients: Cellulose, FD&C Yellow No. 6, Flavor, Hydroxypropyl Methylcellulose, Magnesium stearate, Polyethylene, glycol, Povidone, Silica gel, Starch, Stearic acid, Sucrose.

Indications: For temporary relief of minor aches and pains associated with headaches, muscular aches, backaches, premenstrual and menstrual periods, colds, the flu, toothaches, as well as for minor pain from arthritis, and to reduce fever.

Dosage and Administration: Adults (12 years and over)—1 or 2 tablets every four hours. Maximum daily dose—8 tablets.
Children (6 to under 12 years)—1 tablet every 4 hours. Maximum daily dose—4 tablets.
Children under 6 years of age: consult a doctor.

Warnings: Do not take this product for pain for more than 10 days (adults) or 5 days (children), and do not take for fever for more than 3 days unless directed by a doctor. If pain or fever persists or worsens, new symptoms occur or redness or swelling is present, consult a doctor as

Continued on next page

Procter & Gamble—Cont.

these could be signs of a serious condition. Do not give to children for arthritis pain unless directed by a doctor. May cause excitability especially in children. Do not take this product unless directed by a doctor, if you have a breathing problem such as emphysema or chronic bronchitis, or if you have glaucoma or difficulty in urination due to enlargement of the prostate gland. May cause marked drowsiness; alcohol, sedatives, and tranquilizers may increase the drowsiness effect. Avoid alcoholic beverages while taking this product. Do not take this product if you are taking sedatives or tranquilizers without first consulting your doctor. Use caution when driving a motor vehicle or operating machinery. **KEEP THIS AND ALL DRUGS OUT OF THE REACH OF CHILDREN.** In case of accidental overdose, seek professional assistance or contact a poison control center immediately. Prompt medical attention is critical for adults as well as for children even if you do not notice any signs or symptoms. As with any drug, if you are pregnant or nursing a baby, seek the advice of a health professional before using this product.

How Supplied: Light orange tablets engraved with "Percogesic". Child-resistant bottles of 24 and 90 tablets, and non-child-resistant bottles of 50 tablets.

VICKS® 44 COUGH RELIEF
Dextromethorphan HBr/
Cough Suppressant

Active Ingredient per 3 tsp. (15 ml): Dextromethorphan Hydrobromide 30 mg

Inactive Ingredients: Alcohol 5%, Carboxymethylcellulose Sodium, Citric Acid, FD&C Blue No. 1, FD&C Red No. 40, Flavor, High Fructose Corn Syrup, Polyethylene Oxide, Polyoxyl 40 Stearate, Propylene Glycol, Purified Water, Saccharin Sodium, Sodium Benzoate, Sodium Citrate.

Use: Temporary relieves coughs due to minor throat and bronchial irritation associated with a cold.

Directions: Use teaspoon (tsp) or dose cup.

Ask a doctor before using in children under 6 yrs. of age.

6–11 yrs.	(48–95 lbs.)	1½ tsp or 7½ ml
12 yrs. & older	(Over 95 lbs.)	3 tsp or 15 ml

A total of 4 doses may be given per day, each 6 hours apart, or use as directed by a doctor.

Warnings: A persistent cough may be a sign of a serious condition. If cough persists for more than 1 week, tends to recur, or is accompanied by fever, rash, or persistent headache, ask a doctor. Do not take this product for persistent or chronic cough such as occurs with smoking, asthma, emphysema, or if cough is accompanied by excessive phlegm (mucus) unless directed by a doctor. **Keep this and all drugs out of the reach of children.**
In case if accidental overdose, seek professional advice or contact a poison control center immediately. As with any drug, if you are pregnant or nursing a baby, seek the advice of a health professional before using this product.
Drug Interaction Precaution: Do not use this product without first asking a doctor if you take a prescription monoamine oxidase inhibitor (MAOI) (certain drugs for depression, psychiatric or emotional conditions, or Parkinson's disease), or for 2 weeks after stopping the MAOI drug or if you are uncertain whether your prescription drug contains an MAOI.

How Supplied: Available in 4 FL OZ (115 ml) plastic bottle. A calibrated dose cup accompanies each bottle.

**VICKS® 44D
COUGH & HEAD CONGESTION RELIEF**
Cough Suppressant/
Nasal Decongestant

Active Ingredients per 3 tsp. (15 ml): Dextromethorphan Hydrobromide 30 mg, Pseudoephedrine Hydrochloride 60 mg.

Inactive Ingredients: Alcohol 5%, Carboxymethylcellulose Sodium, Citric Acid, FD&C Blue No. 1, FD&C Red No.40, Flavor, High Fructose Corn Syrup, Polyethylene Oxide, Polyoxyl 40 Stearate, Propylene Glycol, Purified Water, Saaccharin Sodium, Sodium Benzoate, Sodium Citrate.

Uses: Temporary relieves coughs and nasal congestion due to a common cold.

Directions: Use teaspoon (tsp) or dose cup.

Ask a doctor before using in children under 6 yrs. of age.

6–11 yrs.	(48–95 lbs.)	1½ tsp or 7½ ml
12 yrs. & older	(Over 95 lbs.)	3 tsp or 15 ml

A total of 4 doses may be given per day, each 6 hours apart, or use as directed by a doctor.

Warnings: Do not exceed recommended dosage.
If nervousness, dizziness, or sleeplessness occur, discontinue use and ask a doctor. *Do not take unless directed by a doctor if you have:*

- heart disease
- asthma
- emphysema
- thyroid disease
- diabetes
- high blood pressure
- excessive phlegm (mucus)
- persistent or chronic cough
- cough associated with smoking
- difficulty in urination due to enlarged prostate gland

Keep this and all drugs out of the reach of children. In the case of accidental overdose, seek professional advice or contact a poison control center immediately. As with any drug, if you are pregnant or nursing a baby, seek the advice of a health professional before using this product.
Drug Interaction Precaution: Do not use this product without first asking a doctor if you take a prescription monoamine oxidase inhibitor (MAOI) (certain drugs for depression, psychiatric or emotional conditions, or Parkinson's disease), or for 2 weeks after stopping the MAOI drug or if you are uncertain whether your prescription drug contains an MAOI.
Dosing Duration: Do not use over 7 days. *Ask a Doctor:*
- If symptoms do not improve or are accompanied by fever.
- If a cough persists for more than 7 days, recurs, or is accompanied by fever, rash or persistent headache. A persistent cough may be the sign of a serious condition.

How Supplied: Available in 4 FL OZ (115 ml) and 8 FL OZ (235 ml) plastic bottles. A calibrated dose cup accompanies each bottle.

VICKS® 44 LIQUICAPS® COUGH, COLD & FLU RELIEF
Cough Suppressant • Nasal Decongestant • Antihistamine • Pain Reliever/Fever Reducer

Active Ingredient (per softgel): Dextromethorphan Hydrobromide 10 mg, Pseudoephedrine Hydrochloride 30 mg, Chlorpheniramine Maleate 2 mg, Acetaminophen 250 mg.

Inactive Ingredients: D&C Red No. 33 Lake, FD&C Blue No. 1 Lake, Gelatin, Glycerin, Polyethylene Glycol, Povidone, Propylene Glycol, Purified Water, Edible Ink.

Indications: Vicks® 44 LiquiCaps® Cough, Cold & Flu Relief provides temporary relief of coughing, nasal congestion, runny nose and sneezing due to a cold. Also for temporary relief of headache, fever, muscular aches and sore throat pain due to a cold or flu.

Directions: Adults and Children 12 years and older: Swallow 2 softgels with water.
Children (6 to under 12 years): Swallow 1 softgel with water. Do not chew. Repeat every 4 hours not to exceed 4 doses per day. Not recommended for children under 6 years.

WARNINGS: Do not take this product for persistent or chronic cough such as occurs with smoking, asthma, emphysema, or if cough is accompanied by excessive phlegm (mucus) unless directed by a doctor. **Do not exceed recommended dosage.** If nervousness, dizziness, or sleeplessness occurs, discontinue use and consult a doctor. Do not take this product if you have heart disease, high blood pressure, thyroid disorder, diabetes, glaucoma, or difficulty in urination due to enlargement of the prostate gland unless directed by a doctor. *Drug Interaction Precaution:* Do not use this product if you are now taking a prescription monoamine oxidase inhibitor (MAOI) (certin drugs for depression, psychiatric or emotional conditions, or Parkinson's disease), or for take two weeks after stopping the MAOI drug. If you are uncertain whether your prescription drug contains an MAOI, consult a health professional before taking this product. May cause excitability especially in children. Do not take this product, unless directed by a doctor, if you have a breathing problem such as emphysema or chronic bronchitis. May cause marked drowsiness; alcohol, sedatives and tranquilizers may increase the drowsiness effect. Avoid alcoholic beverages while taking this product. Do not take this product if you are taking sedatives or tranquilizers, without first consulting your doctor. Use caution when driving a motor vehicle or operating machinery. Do not take this product for more than 7 days (for adults) or 5 days (for children). A persistent cough may be a sign of a serious condition. If cough persists for more than 7 days, tends to recur, or is accompanied by rash, or persistent headache, fever that lasts for more than three days or if new symptoms occur, consult a doctor. If sore throat is severe, persists for more than 2 days, is accompanied or followed by fever, headache, rash, nausea, or vomiting, consult a doctor promptly. **Keep this and all drugs out of the reach of children.** In case of accidental overdose, seek professional assistance or contact a poison control center immediately. Prompt medical attention is critical for adults as well as for children even if you do not notice any signs or symptoms. As with any drug, if you are pregnant or nursing a baby, seek the advice of a health professional before using this product.

How Supplied: Available in 12-count child-resistant blister packages. Each blue softgel is imprinted: "44".

**VICKS® 44
LIQUICAPS®NON-DROWSY
COUGH & COLD RELIEF
Cough Suppressant/
Nasal Decongestant**

Active Ingredient (per softgel): Dextromethorphan Hydrobromide 30 mg, Pseudoephedrine Hydrochloride 60 mg.

Inactive Ingredients: D&C Red No. 33, FD&C Blue No. 1, FD&C Red No. 40, Gelatin, Glycerin, Polyethylene Glycol, Povidone, Purified Water, Sorbitol, Edible Ink.

Indications: VICKS® 44 LiquiCaps® Non-Drowsy Cough & Cold Relief provides temporary relief of coughs and nasal congestion due to the common cold.

Directions: Adults and children 12 years of age and over: Swallow 1 softgel with water. Do not chew. Repeat every 6 hours, not to exceed 4 softgels per day. Not recommended for children under 12.

WARNINGS: A persistent cough may be a sign of a serious condition. If cough persists for more than 1 week, tends to recur, or is accompanied by fever, rash, or persistent or chronic headache, consult a doctor. Do not take this product for persistent or chronic cough such as occurs with smoking, asthma, emphysema, or if cough is accompanied by excessive phlegm (mucus) unless directed by a doctor. **Do not exceed recommended dosage.** If nervousness, dizziness, or sleeplessness occurs, discontinue use and consult a doctor. Do not take this product for more than 7 days. If symptoms do not improve or are accompanied by fever, consult a doctor. Do not take this product if you have heart disease, high blood pressures, thyroid disease, diabetes, or difficulty; in urination due to enlargement of the prostate gland. *Drug Interaction Precaution:* Do not use this product if you are now taking a prescription monoamine oxidase inhibitor (MAOI) (certain drugs for depression, psychiatric or emotional conditions, or Parkinson's disease), or for 2 weeks after stopping the MAOI drug. If you are uncertain whether your prescription drug contains an MAOI, consult a health professional before taking this product. **Keep this and all drugs out of the reach of children.** In case of accidental overdose, seek professional assistance or contact a poison control center immediately. As with any drug, if you are pregnant or nursing a baby, seek the advice of a health professional before using this product.

How Supplied: Available in 10 count blister packages. Each red softgel is imprinted "44".

**VICKS® 44E
Cough & Chest Congestion Relief
Cough Suppressant/Expectorant**

Active Ingredients: per 3 teaspoons (15 ml): Dextromethorphan Hydrobromide 20 mg, Guaifenesin 200 mg

Inactive Ingredients: Alcohol 5%, Carboxymethylcellulose Sodium, Citric Acid, FD&C Blue No. 1, FD&C Red No. 40, Flavor, High Frutose Corn Syrup, Polyethylene Oxide, Polyoxyl 40 Stearate, Propylene Glycol, Purified Water, Saaccharin Sodium, Sodium Benzoate, Sodium Citrate.

Uses: Temporarily relieves coughs due to a common cold. Helps loosen phlegm to rid the bronchial passageways of bothersome mucus.

Directions: Use teaspoon (tsp) or dose cup.

Ask a doctor before using in children under 6 yrs. of age.

6–11 yrs.	(48–95 lbs.)	1½ tsp or 7½ ml
12 yrs. & older	(Over 95 lbs.)	3 tsp or 15 ml

A total of 6 doses may be given per day, each 4 hours apart, or use as directed by a doctor.

Warnings: *Do not take unless directed by a doctor if you have:*
● asthma
● emphysema
● excessive phlegm (mucus)
● persistent or chronic cough
● chronic bronchitis
● cough associated with smoking
Keep this and all drugs out of the reach of children.
In the case of accidental overdose, seek professional advice or contact a poison control center immediately. As with any drug, if you are pregnant or nursing a baby, seek the advice of a health professional before using this product.
Drug Interaction Precaution: Do not use this product without first asking a doctor if you take a prescription monoamine oxidase inhibitor (MAOI) (certain drugs for depression, psychiatric or emotional conditions, or Parkinson's disease), or for 2 weeks after stopping the MAOI drug or if you are uncertain whether your prescription drug contains an MAOI.
Dosing Duration & When to Ask a Doctor:
● If a cough persists for more than 7 days, recurs, or is accompanied by fever, rash or persistent headache. A persistent cough may be the sign of a serious condition.

How Supplied: Available in 4 FL OZ (115 ml) and 8 FL OZ (235 ml) plastic bottles. A calibrated dose cup accompanies each bottle.

**VICKS® 44M
COUGH, COLD & FLU RELIEF
Cough Suppressant/Nasal
Decongestant/Antihistamine/
Pain Reliever–Fever Reducer**

Active Ingredients: per 4 tsp. (20 ml): Dextromethorphan Hydrobromide 30 mg, Pseudoephedrine Hydrochloride 60 mg, Chlorpheniramine Maleate 4 mg, Acetaminophen 650 mg

Inactive Ingredients: Alcohol 10%, Carboxymethylcellulose Sodium, Citric Acid, FD&C Blue No. 1, FD&C Red No. 40, Flavor, High Fructose Corn Syrup,

Continued on next page

Procter & Gamble—Cont.

Polyethylene Glycol, Polyethylene Oxide, Propylene Glycol, Purified Water, Saccharin Sodium, Sodium Citrate.

Uses: Temporarily relieves cough/cold/flu symptoms:
- cough
- nasal congestion
- runny nose
- sneezing
- headache
- fever
- muscular aches
- sore throat pain

Directions: Use teaspoon (tsp) or dose cup.

Ask a doctor before using in children under 12 yrs. of age.

12 yrs. & older	4 tsp or 20 ml

Repeat every 6 hours, not to exceed 4 doses per day, or use as directed by a doctor.

Warnings: Do not exceed recommended dosage.
If nervousness, dizziness, or sleeplessness occur, discontinue use and ask a doctor. May cause marked drowsiness. May cause excitability in children.
Do not take unless directed by a doctor if you have:
- heart disease
- asthma
- emphysema
- thyroid disease
- diabetes
- glaucoma
- high blood pressure
- excessive phlegm (mucus)
- breathing problems
- chronic bronchitis
- difficulty in breathing
- persistent or chronic cough
- cough associated with smoking
- difficulty in urination due to enlarged prostate gland

Keep this and all drugs out of the reach of children. In the case of accidental overdose, seek professional advice or contact a poison control center immediately. Prompt medical attention is critical for adults as well as for children even if you do not notice any signs or symptoms. As with any drug, if you are pregnant or nursing a baby, seek the advice of a health professional before using this product.
Alcohol, sedatives, and tranquilizers may increase the drowsiness effect. Avoid alcoholic beverages while taking this product. Use caution when driving a motor vehicle or operating machinery.
Drug Interaction Precaution: Do not use this product without first asking a doctor if you take:
- sedatives
- tranquilizers
- a prescription monoamine oxidase inhibitor (MAOI) (certain drugs for depression, psychiatric or emotional conditions, or Parkinson's disease), or for 2 weeks after stopping the MAOI drug or if you are uncertain whether your prescription drug contains an MAOI.

Dosing Duration: Do not use over 7 days. *Ask a Doctor:*
- If sore throat is severe, persists for more than 2 days, is accompanied or followed by fever, headache, rash, nausea, or vomiting.
- If symptoms do not improve or are accompanied by a fever that lasts more than 3 days, or if new symptoms occur.
- If a cough presists for more than 7 days, recurs, or is accompanied by a rash or persistent headache. A persistent cough may be the sign of a serious condition.

How Supplied: Available in 4 FL OZ (115 ml) and 8 FL OZ (235 ml) plastic bottles. A calibrated dose cup accompanies each bottle.

CHILDREN'S VICKS® CHLORASEPTIC® SORE THROAT LOZENGES
Benzocaine/Oral Anesthetic
(Grape Flavor)

Active Ingredient: Benzocaine 5 mg per lozenge.

Inactive Ingredients: Corn syrup, FD&C Blue No. 1, FD&C Red No. 40, flavor, and sucrose.

Uses: Temporarily relieves:
- sore mouth
- sore throat
- occasional minor mouth irritation and pain
- pain associated with canker sores

Directions: Adults and Children 5 years and older: Allow 1 lozenge to dissolve slowly in mouth. May be repeated every 2 hours as needed or as directed by a physician or dentist.
Children under 5 years: ask a physician or dentist.

Warnings: *Do not use this product if you have a history of allergy to local anesthetics like:*
- procaine
- butacaine
- benzocaine
- other 'caine' anesthetics
Keep this and all drugs out of the reach of children.
In the case of accidental overdose, seek professional advice or contact a poison control center immediately. As with any drug, if you are pregnant or nursing a baby, seek the advice of a health professional before using this product.
Dosing Duration and When to Ask a Doctor:
- If sore throat is severe, persists for more than 2 days, or is accompanied by difficulty in breathing.
- If sore throat is accompanied or followed by fever, headache, rash, swelling, nausea, or vomiting.
- If sore mouth symptoms do not improve in 7 days, or if irritation, pain, or redness persists or worsens.

How Supplied: Cartons of 18. Each purple lozenge is debosed with "CC".

CHILDREN'S VICKS® CHLORASEPTIC® SORE THROAT SPRAY
Phenol/Oral
Anesthetic/Antiseptic

Children's Chloraseptic® is specially formulated with a reduced concentration of phenol, the active ingredient in Chloraseptic®, to provide fast, effective relief in a great-tasting grape flavor your child will like.

Active Ingredient: Phenol 0.5%

Inactive Ingredients: FD&C Blue No. 1, FD&C Red No. 40, flavor, glycerin, purified water, saccharin sodium, and sorbitol.

Indications: For temporary relief of occasional minor sore throat pain and sore mouth. Also, for temporary relief of pain due to canker sores, minor irritation or injury of the mouth and gums, minor dental procedures, or orthodontic appliances.

Directions—Children 2 Years of Age and Older: Spray 5 times directly into throat or affected area and swallow. Repeat every two hours or as directed by a physician or dentist. Children under 12 years of age should be supervised in product use.
Children Under 2 Years of Age: Consult a physician or dentist.

WARNINGS: If sore throat is severe, or is accompanied by difficulty in breathing, or persists for more than 2 days, do not use, and consult a doctor promptly. If sore throat is accompanied or followed by fever, headache, rash, swelling, nausea or vomiting, consult a doctor promptly. If sore mouth symptoms do not improve in 7 days, or if irritation, pain, or redness persists or worsens, see your doctor promptly. **Keep this and all drugs out of the reach of children.** In case of accidental overdose, seek professional assistance or contact a poison control center immediately. As with any drug, if you are pregnant or nursing a baby, seek the advice of a health professional before using this product.

How Supplied: Available in 6 FL. OZ. (177 mL) plastic bottles with sprayer.

CHILDREN'S VICKS® DAYQUIL® ALLERGY RELIEF
Antihistamine/Nasal Decongestant

Children's Vicks DayQuil Allergy Relief was specially formulated with two effective ingredients to relieve allergy symptoms and head colds without coughs.

Active Ingredients per 1 TBSP: Chlorpheniramine Maleate 2 mg, Pseudoephedrine HCl 30 mg.

Inactive Ingredients: Citric Acid, FD&C Blue No. 1, FD&C Red No. 40, Flavor, Methylparaben, Potassium Sorbate, Propylene Glycol, Purified Water, Sodium Citrate, Sorbitol and Sucrose.

Uses: Temporarily relieves:
- nasal and sinus congestion
- runny nose
- sneezing
- itchy, watery eyes due to hay fever or other upper respiratory allergies

Directions: Use Tablespoon (TBSP) or dose cup.

Under 6 yrs.	(Under 48 lbs.)	Ask a doctor.
6–11 yrs.	(48–95 lbs.)	1 TBSP or 15 ml
12 yrs. & older	(Over 95 lbs.)	2 TBSP or 30 ml

*Professional Labeling: Children under 6 years of age: Use only as directed by a physician. Suggested doses for children under 6 years of age:

Age	Weight	Dose
6–11 mo.	17–21 lbs.	1 teaspoon (tsp.) (5 ml)
12–23 mo.	22–27 lbs.	1¼ teaspoon (tsp.) (6.25 ml)
2–5 yrs.	28–47 lbs.	½ TABLESPOON (TBSP.) (7.5 ml)

Repeat every 6 hours, not to exceed 4 doses in 24 hours, or use as directed by doctor.
*Based on extrapolation from studies on the safety and efficacy of active ingredients conducted among older children and adults. Use caution in treating children under 2 years of age who were born prematurely.

Warnings: Do not exceed recommended dosage.
If nervousness, dizziness or sleeplessness occur, discontinue use and ask a doctor. May cause drowsiness. May cause excitability in children.
Do not take unless directed by a doctor if you have:
- heart disease
- emphysema
- glaucoma
- thyroid disease
- diabetes
- high blood pressure
- breathing problems
- chronic bronchitis
- difficulty in urination due to enlarged prostate gland

Keep this and all drugs out of the reach of children. In the case of accidental overdose, seek professional advice or contact a poison control center immediately. As with any drug, if you are pregnant or nursing a baby, seek the advice of a health professional before using this product.
Alcohol, sedatives, and tranquilizers may increase the drowsiness effect. Avoid alcoholic beverages while taking this product. Use caution when driving a motor vehicle or operating machinery.
Drug Interaction Precaution: Do not take this product without first asking a doctor if you take:
- sedatives
- tranquilizers
- a prescription monoamine oxidase inhibitor (MAOI) (certain drugs for depression, psychiatric or emotional conditions, or Parkinson's disease), or for weeks after stopping the MAOI drug or if you are uncertain whether your prescription drug contains an MAOI.

Dosing Duration: Do not use over 7 days.
Ask a Doctor: If symptoms do not improve within 7 days or are accompanied by a fever.

How Supplied: Available in 4 FL OZ (115 ml) plastic bottles with child-resistant, tamper-evident cap and a calibrated medicine cup.

CHILDREN'S VICKS® NYQUIL® COLD/COUGH RELIEF
Antihistamine/Nasal Decongestant/ Cough Suppressant

Children's NyQuil was specially formulated with three effective ingredients to relieve nighttime cough, nasal congestion, and runny nose so children can rest. Children's NyQuil® is alcohol free and analgesic free and has a pleasant cherry flavor.

Active Ingredients: Per 1 TBSP.: Chlorpheniramine Maleate 2 mg, Pseudoephedrine HCl 30 mg, Dextromethorphan Hydrobromide 15 mg.

Inactive Ingredients: Citric Acid, FD&C Red No. 40, Flavor, Potassium Sorbate, Propylene Glycol, Purified Water, Sodium Citrate, Sucrose.

Uses: Temporarily relieves cold symptoms:
- nasal congestion
- runny nose
- sneezing
- cough

Directions: Use Tablespoon (TBSP) or dose cup.

Under 6 yrs.	(Under 48 lbs.)	Ask a doctor
6–11 yrs.	(48–95 lbs.)	1 TBSP or 15 ml
12 yrs. & older	(Over 95 lbs.)	2 TBSP or 30 ml

*Professional Labeling: Children under 6 years of age: Use only as directed by a physician. Suggested doses for children under 6 years of age:

Age	Weight	Dose
6–11 mo.	17–21 lbs.	1 teaspoon (tsp.) (5 ml)
12–23 mo.	22–27 lbs.	1¼ teaspoon (tsp.) (6.25 ml)
2–5 yrs.	28–47 lbs.	½ TABLESPOON (TBSP.) (7.5 ml)

Repeat every 6 hours, not to exceed 4 doses in 24 hours, or use as directed by doctor.
*Based on extrapolation from studies on the safety and efficacy of active ingredients conducted among older children and adults. Use caution in treating children under 2 years of age who were born prematurely.

Warnings: Do not exceed recommended dosage.
If nervousness, dizziness, or sleeplessness occur, discontinue use and ask a doctor. May cause marked drowsiness. May cause excitability in children.
Do not take unless directed by a doctor if you have:
- heart disease
- asthma
- emphysema
- thyroid disease
- diabetes
- glaucoma
- high blood pressure
- excessive phelgm (mucus)
- breathing problems
- chronic bronchitis
- difficulty in breathing
- persistent or chronic cough
- cough associated with smoking
- difficulty in urination due to enlarged prostate gland

Keep this and all drugs out of the reach of children. In the case of accidental overdose, seek professional advice or contact a poison control center immediately. As with any drug, if you are pregnant or nursing a baby, seek the advice of a health professional before using this product.
Alcohol, sedatives, and tranquilizers may increase the drowsiness effect. Avoid alcoholic beverages while taking this product. Use caution when driving a motor vehicle or operating machinery.
Drug Interaction Precaution: Do not take this product without first asking a doctor if you take:
- sedatives
- tranquilizers
- a prescription monoamine oxidase inhibitor (MAOI) (certain drugs for depression, psychiatric or emotional conditions, or Parkinson's disease), or for 2 weeks after stopping the MAOI drug or if you are uncertain whether your prescription drug contains an MAOI.

Dosing Duration: Do not use over 7 days.
Ask a Doctor:
- If symptoms do not improve within 7 days or are accompanied by a fever.

Continued on next page

Procter & Gamble—Cont.

- If a cough persists for more than 7 days, recurs, or is accompanied by a fever, rash or persistent headache. A persistent cough may be the sign of a serious condition.

How Supplied: Available in 4 FL OZ (115 ml) plastic bottles with child-resistant, tamper-evident cap and a calibrated medicine cup.

VICKS® CHLORASEPTIC® COUGH & THROAT DROPS
Menthol Cough Suppressant/Oral Anesthetic

Active Ingredients: Menthol Flavor: Menthol 8.4 mg, Cherry and Honey Lemon: Menthol 10 mg.

Inactive Ingredients: Menthol Flavor: Corn Syrup, FD&C Blue No. 1, Flavor, Sucrose. Cherry Flavor: Corn Syrup, FD&C Blue No. 2, FD&C Red No. 40, Flavor, Sucrose. Honey Lemon: Citric Acid, Corn Syrup, D&C Yellow No. 10, FD&C Yellow No. 6, Flavor, Sucrose.

Indications: Temporarily relieves sore throat and coughs due to colds or inhaled irritants.

Directions: Adults and children 5 to 12 years: Allow drop to dissolve slowly in mouth. **Cough:** may be repeated every hour as needed or as directed by a doctor. **Sore Throat:** may be repeated every 2 hours as needed or as directed by a doctor. **Children under 5 years of age:** consult a doctor.

WARNINGS: A persistent cough may be a sign of a serious condition. If cough persists for more than 1 week, tends to recur, or is accompanied by fever, rash, or persistent headache, consult a doctor. Do not take this product for persistent or chronic cough such as occurs with smoking, asthma, emphysema, or if cough is accompanied by excessive phlegm (mucus), unless directed by a doctor. If sore throat is severe, or is accompanied by difficulty in breathing, or persists for more than 2 days, do not use, and consult a doctor promptly. If sore throat is accompanied or followed by fever, headache, rash, swelling, nausea, or vomiting, consult a doctor promptly. **Keep this and all drugs out of the reach of children.** As with any drug, if you are pregnant or nursing a baby, seek the advice of a health professional before using this product.

How Supplied: Vicks® Chloraseptic® Cough & Throat Drops are available in single sticks of 9 drops each and bags of 25 drops. Each drop is debossed with "V".

VICKS® CHLORASEPTIC® SORE THROAT LOZENGES
Menthol/Benzocaine
Oral Anesthetic
Menthol and Cherry Flavors

Active Ingredients: Benzocaine 6 mg, Menthol 10 mg (per lozenge).

Inactive Ingredients: Menthol Lozenges: Corn syrup, D&C Yellow No. 10, FD&C Blue No. 1, FD&C Yellow No. 6, flavor and sucrose. Cherry Lozenges: Corn syrup, FD&C Blue No. 1, FD&C Red No. 40, flavor and sucrose.

Uses: Temporary relieves:
- sore mouth
- sore throat
- occasional minor mouth irritation and pain
- pain associated with canker sores

Directions: Adults and Children 5 years & older: Allow 1 lozenge to dissolve slowly in mouth. May be repeated every 2 hours as needed or as directed by a physician or dentist. **Children under 5 years:** ask a physician or dentist.

Warnings: *Do not use this product if you have a history of allergy to local anesthetics like:*
- procaine
- butacaine
- benzocaine
- other 'caine' anesthetics

Keep this and all drugs out of the reach of children. In case of accidental overdose, seek professional advice or contact a poison control center immediately. As with any drug if you are pregnant or nursing a baby, seek the advice of a health professional before using this product. *Dosing Duration and When to Ask a Doctor:*
- If sore throat is severe, persists for more than 2 days, or is accompanied by difficulty in breathing.
- If sore throat is accompanied or followed by fever, headache, rash, swelling, nausea, or vomiting.
- If sore mouth symptoms do not improve in 7 days, or if irritation, pain, or redness persists or worsens.

How Supplied: Available in Menthol and Cherry, lozenges in packages of 18. Each green or red lozenge is debossed with "VC".

VICKS® CHLORASEPTIC®
SORE THROAT SPRAY
GARGLE & MOUTH RINSE
Phenol/oral anesthetic/antiseptic
Menthol and Cherry Flavors

Active Ingredient: Gargle and Spray—Phenol 1.4%.

Inactive Ingredients: Menthol Liquid: D&C Green No. 5, D&C Yellow No. 10, FD&C Green No. 3, flavor, glycerin, purified water, saccharin sodium. Cherry

Liquid: FD&C Red No. 40, flavor, glycerin, purified water, saccharin sodium.

Uses: Temporarily relieves:
- sore mouth
- sore throat pain
- minor irritation or injury of the mouth and gums
- pain due to minor dental procedures, dentures or orthodontic appliances
- pain associated with canker sores

Directions: Adults and Children 12 years & older: Spray 5 times directly into throat or affected area. **Children 2–12 years:** Spray 3 times and swallow. Children under 12 years should be supervised in product use. Repeat every 2 hours or as directed by a physician or dentist. **Children under 2 years:** ask a physician or dentist.

Warnings: Keep this and all drugs out of the reach of children. In case of accidental overdose, seek professional advice or contact a poison control center immediately. As with any drug, if you are pregnant or nursing a baby, seek the advice of a health professional before using this product. *Dosing Duration and When to Ask a Doctor:*
- If sore throat is severe, persists for more than 2 days, or is accompanied by difficulty in breathing.
- If sore throat is accompanied or followed by fever, headache, rash, swelling, nausea, or vomiting.
- If sore mouth symptoms do not improve in 7 days, or if irritation, pain, or redness persists or worsens.

How Supplied: Available in Menthol and Cherry flavors in 6 FL OZ (175 mL) plastic bottles with sprayer. Menthol Flavor is also available in 12 FL OZ (355 mL) gargle.

VICKS® Cough Drops
Menthol Cough Suppressant/
Oral Anesthetic
Menthol and Cherry Flavors

Active Ingredient: Menthol 3.3mg (Menthol), 1.7mg (Cherry)

Inactive Ingredients: [Menthol] Ascorbic Acid, Caramel, Corn Syrup, Eucalyptus Oil, Sucrose. [Cherry] Ascorbic Acid, Citric Acid, Corn Syrup, Ecualyptus Oil, FD&C Blue No. 1, FD&C Red No. 40, Flavor, Sucrose.

Directions: Adults and children 5 to 12 years of age:
Menthol: Allow 2 drops to dissolve slowly in mouth.
Cherry: Allow 3 drops to dissolve slowly in mouth.
COUGH: May be repeated every hour as needed or as directed by a doctor.
SORE THROAT: May be repeated every 2 hours as needed or as directed by a doctor.
Children under 5 years of age: Ask a doctor.

Warnings: A persistent cough may be a sign of a serious condition. If cough persists for more than 1 week, tends to recur, or is accompanied by fever, rash, or persistent headache, ask a doctor. Do not take this product for persistent or chronic cough such as occurs with smoking, asthma, emphysema, or if cough is accompanied by excessive phlegm (mucus) unless directed by a doctor. If sore throat is severe, or is accompanied by difficulty in breathing, or persists for more than 2 days, do not use, and ask a doctor promptly. If sore throat is accompanied or followed by fever, headache, rash, swelling, nausea, or vomiting, ask a doctor promptly. **Keep this and all drugs out of the reach of children.** As with any drug, if you are pregnant or nursing a baby, seek the advice of a health professional before using this product.

How Supplied: Vicks® Cough Drops are available in cartons of 20 triangular drops. Each red or green drop is debossed with "V."

ORIGINAL VICKS® COUGH DROPS
Menthol Cough Suppressant/ Oral Anesthetic

Active Ingredient: Menthol 6.6 mg (menthol), 3.1 mg (cherry) Menthol and Cherry Flavors.

Inactive Ingredients: Menthol Flavor: Benzyl Alcohol, Camphor, Caramel, Corn Syrup, Eucalyptus Oil, Flavor, Sucrose, Tolu Balsam, Thymol. Cherry Flavor: Citric Acid, Corn Syrup, FD&C Blue No. 1, FD&C Red No. 40, Flavor, Sucrose.

Uses: Temporarily relieves sore throat and coughs due to colds or inhaled irritants.

Directions: **Adults and children 5 to 12 years:** [Menthol] Allow drop to dissolve slowly in mouth. [Cherry] Allow 2 drops to dissolve slowly in mouth. **Cough:** may be repeated every hour as needed or as directed by a doctor. **Sore Throat:** may be repeated every 2 hours —as needed or as directed by a doctor. **Children under 5 years of age:** ask a doctor.

Warnings: A persistent cough may be a sign of a serious condition. If cough persists for more than 1 week, tends to recur, or is accompanied by fever, rash, or persistent headache, ask a doctor. Do not take this product for persistent or chronic cough such as occurs with smoking, asthma, emphysema, or if cough is accompanied by excessive phlegm (mucus), unless directed by a doctor. If sore throat is severe, or is accompanied by difficulty in breathing, or persists for more than 2 days, do not use, and ask a doctor promptly. If sore throat is accompanied or followed by fever, headache, rash, swelling, nausea, or vomiting, ask a doctor promptly. **Keep this and all**

drugs out of the reach of children. As with any drug, if you are pregnant or nursing a baby, seek the advice of a health professional before using this product.

How Supplied: Original Vicks® Cough Drops are available in bags of 30 oval drops. Each red or green drop is debossed with "V".

VICKS® DAYQUIL® ALLERGY RELIEF 4 HOUR TABLETS
Nasal Decongestant/Antihistamine

Active Ingredients: Each tablet contains: 25 mg Phenylpropanolamine Hydrochloride, 4 mg Brompheniramine Maleate.

Inactive Ingredients: FD&C Blue No. 1 Aluminum Lake, Magnesium Stearate, Microcrystalline Cellulose, Starch.

Uses: Temporarily relieves nasal congestion due to:
- a cold
- hay fever
- upper respiratory allergies
- or associated with sinusitis
Temporarily relieves:
- runny nose
- sneezing
- itchy, watery eyes as may occur in allergic rhinitis
Temporarily restores freer breathing through the nose.

Directions: **Adults and Children 12 yrs. and older:** 1 tablet every 4 hours. Maximum: 6 tablets per day. Children under 12 yrs: Ask a doctor.

Warnings: Do not exceed recommended dosage. If nervousness, dizziness, or sleeplessness occur, discontinue use and ask a doctor. May cause drowsiness. May cause excitability in children. *Do not take unless directed by a doctor if you have:*
- thyroid disease
- emphysema
- diabetes
- heart disease
- glaucoma
- chronic bronchitis
- high blood pressure
- breathing problems
- difficulty in urination due to enlarged prostate gland
Keep this and all drugs out of the reach of children. In the case of accidental overdose, seek professional advice or contact a poison control center immediately. As with any drug, if you are pregnant or nursing a baby, seek the advice of a health professional before using this product. *Dosing Duration:* Do not use over 7 days. *Ask a Doctor:*
- If symptoms do not improve within 7 days or are accompanied by a fever. Alcohol, sedatives, and tranquilizers may increase the drowsiness effect. Avoid alcoholic beverages while taking

this product. Use caution when driving a motor vehicle or operating machinery. *Drug Interaction Precaution:* Do not take this product without first asking a doctor if you take:
- sedatives
- tranquilizers
- a prescription monoamine oxidase inhibitor (MAOI) (certain drugs for depression, psychiatric or emotional conditions, or Parkinson's disease), or for 2 weeks after stopping the MAOI drug or if you are uncertain whether your prescription drug contains an MAOI.

How Supplied: Available in 24 count blister packages. Each blue tablet is imprinted with "D4".

VICKS® DAYQUIL® ALLERGY RELIEF 12 HOUR EXTENDED RELEASE TABLETS
Nasal Decongestant/Antihistamine

Active Ingredients: Each Extended Release Tablet Contains: 75 mg Phenylpropanolamine Hydrochloride, 12 mg Brompheniramine Maleate

Inactive Ingredients: Dimethyl Polysiloxane Oil, FD&C Blue No. 1 Aluminum Lake, Hydroxypropyl Methylcellulose, Lactose, Magnesium Stearate, Polyethylene Glycol, Talc, Titanium Dioxide.

Uses: For the temporary relief of nasal congestion due to the common cold, hay fever or other upper respiratory allergies, or associated with sinusitis; temporarily relieves runny nose, sneezing, and itchy and watery eyes as may occur in allergic rhinitis (such as hay fever). Temporarily restores freer breathing through the nose.

Directions: Adults and children 12 years of age and older: One tablet every 12 hours. DO NOT EXCEED 1 TABLET EVERY 12 HOURS, OR 2 TABLETS IN A 24-HOUR PERIOD. Children under 12 years of age: ask a doctor.

Warnings: This product may cause excitability, especially in children. Do not take this product if you have heart disease, high blood pressure, thyroid disease, diabetes, glaucoma, or difficulty in urination due to enlargement of the prostate gland, except under the advice and supervision of a doctor. Do not take this product, unless directed by a doctor, if you have a breathing problem such as emphysema or chronic bronchitis. Do not give this product to children under 12 years, except under the advice and supervision of a doctor. May cause drowsiness. Do not exceed recommended dosage because at higher doses nervousness, dizziness, or sleeplessness may occur. If symptoms do not improve within 7 days or are accompanied by fever, ask a doctor before continuing use. Do not take if hypersensitive to any of the ingredients. As with any drug, if you are pregnant or nursing a baby, seek the advice of a

Continued on next page

Procter & Gamble—Cont.

health professional before using this product. **CAUTION:** Avoid driving a motor vehicle or operating machinery and avoid alcoholic beverages while taking this product. **DRUG INTERACTION PRECAUTION:** Do not take this product if you are presently taking a prescription antihypertensive or antidepressant drug containing a monoamine oxidase inhibitor, except under the advice and supervision of a doctor. KEEP THIS AND ALL DRUGS OUT OF THE REACH OF CHILDREN. IN CASE OF ACCIDENTAL OVERDOSE, SEEK PROFESSIONAL ASSISTANCE OR CONTACT A POISON CONTROL CENTER IMMEDIATELY.

How Supplied: Available in 24 count blister packages. Each blue tablet is imprinted with the letter "A" inside the Vicks shield.

VICKS® DAYQUIL® LIQUID
VICKS® DAYQUIL® LIQUICAPS®
**Multi-Symptom Cold/Flu Relief
Nasal Decongestant/Expectorant/
Pain Reliever/Cough
Suppressant/Fever Reducer**

Active Ingredients: LIQUID—per 2 TBSP or LIQUICAPS—per two softgels, contains: Pseudoephedrine Hydrochloride 60 mg, Guaifenesin 200 mg, Acetaminophen 650 mg (Liquid) or 500 mg (softgels), Dextromethorphan Hydrobromide 20 mg.

Inactive Ingredients: Liquid: Citric Acid, FD&C Yellow No. 6, Flavor, Glycerin, Polyethylene Glycol, Propylene Glycol, Purified Water, Saccharin Sodium, Sodium Citrate, Sucrose. Softgels: FD&C Red No. 40, FD&C Yellow No. 6, Gelatin, Glycerin, Polyethylene Glycol, Povidone, Propylene Glycol, Purified Water and Sorbitol Special.

Uses: Temporarily relieves common cold/flu symptoms:
• minor aches
• pains
• headache
• muscular aches
• sore throat pain
• fever
• nasal congestion
• cough
Helps loosen phlegm (muscus and thin secretions to drain bronchial tubes and make coughs more productive.

Liquid

Directions: Use measuring spoon or dose cup.

Under 6 years	Ask a doctor.
6–11 years	1 Tablespoon (TBSP) or 15 ml
12 yrs. and older	2 Tablespoons (TBSP) or 30 ml

A total of 4 doses may be given per day, each 4 hours apart, or use as directed by a doctor.

LiquiCaps

Directions: Under 6 years—Ask a doctor.

6–11 years	Swallow 1 softgel with water.
12 yrs. and older	Swallow 2 softgels with water.

Repeat every 4 hours, not to exceed 4 doses per day, or use as directed by a doctor.

Warnings: Do not exceed recommended dosage.
If nervousness, dizziness, or sleeplessness occur, discontinue use and ask a doctor.
Do not take unless directed by a doctor if you have:
• heart disease
• asthma
• emphysema
• thyroid disease
• diabetes
• high blood pressure
• chronic bronchitis
• persistent or chronic cough
• cough associated with smoking
• excessive phlegm (mucus)
• breathing problems
• difficulty in urination due to enlarged prostate gland
DRUG INTERACTION PRECAUTION:
Do not take this product without first asking a doctor if you take:
• a prescription monoamine oxidase inhibitor (MAOI) (certain drugs for depression, psychiatric or emotional conditions, or Parkinson's disease), or for 2 weeks after stopping the MAOI drug or if you are uncertain whether your prescription drug contains an MAOI.
Keep this and all drugs out of the reach of children. In the case of accidental overdose, seek professional advice or contact a poison control center immediately. Prompt medical attention is critical for adults as well as for children even if you do not notice any signs or symptoms. As with any drug, if you are pregnant or nursing a baby, seek the advice of a health professional before using this product.
DOSING DURATION: Do not use over 7 days (for adults) or 5 days (for children).
ASK A DOCTOR:
• If sore throat is severe, persists for more than 2 days, is accompanied or followed by fever, headache, rash, nausea, or vomiting.
• If symptoms do not improve or are accompanied by a fever that lasts more than 3 days, or if new symptoms occur.
• If a cough persists for more than 7 days (adults) or 5 days (children), recurs, or is accompanied by a rash or persistent headache. A persistent cough may be the sign of a serious condition.

How Supplied: Available in: **LIQUID** 6 FL OZ (175 ml) plastic bottles with child-resistant, tamper-evident cap and a calibrated medicine cup.
LIQUICAP: in 12-count child-resistant packages and 20-count nonchild-resistant packages. Each softgel is imprinted: "DayQuil."

VICKS® DAYQUIL® SINUS PRESSURE & CONGESTION RELIEF
Nasal Decongestant/Expectorant

Active Ingredients (per caplet): Guaifenesin 200 mg, Phenylpropanolamine Hydrochloride 25 mg.

Inactive Ingredients: Colloidal Silicone Dioxide, Crospovidone, FD&C Yellow No. 6 Aluminum Lake, Hydroxypropyl Methylcellulose, Microcrystalline Cellulose, Polyethylene Glycol, Polysorbate 80, Povidone, Stearic Acid, Titanium Dioxide.

Uses: For the temporary relief of nasal/sinus congestion and pressure associated with sinusitis, hay fever, upper respiratory allergies or the common cold. Also helps to loosen phlegm and thin bronchial secretions to relieve chest congestion.

Directions: Adult and Children (12 yrs. and older): 1 caplet every 4 hours. Maximum: 6 caplets per day.
Not recommended for children under 12 years of age.

Warnings: Do not exceed recommended dosage.
If nervousness, dizziness, or sleeplessness occur, discontinue use and ask a doctor.
Do not take unless directed by a doctor if you have:
• heart disease
• asthma
• emphysema
• thyroid disease
• diabetes
• high blood pressure
• excessive phlegm (mucus)
• persistent or chronic cough
• cough associated with smoking
• chronic bronchitis
• difficulty in urination due to enlarged prostate gland
Keep this and all drugs out of the reach of children. In the case of accidental overdose, seek professional advice or contact a poison control center immediately. As with any drug, if you are pregnant or nursing a baby, seek the advice of a health professional before using this product.
Drug Interaction Precaution: Do not use this product without first asking a doctor if you take a prescription monoamine oxidase inhibitor (MAOI) (certain drugs for depression, psychiatric or emotional conditions, or Parkinson's disease), or for 2 weeks after stopping the MAOI drug or if you are uncertain whether your prescription drug contains an MAOI.
Dosing Duration: Do not use over 7 days. *Ask a Doctor:*

- If symptoms do not improve or are accompanied by fever.
- If a cough persists for more than 7 days, recur, or is accompanied by fever, rash or persistent headache. A persistent cough may be the sign of a serious condition.

How Supplied: Available in 12 and 24 count blister packages.
Each caplet is imprinted with "DQ SC"

VICKS® DAYQUIL® SINUS Pressure & PAIN Relief WITH IBUPROFEN*
IBUPROFEN/PSEUDOEPHEDRINE HCL
Pain Reliever/Fever Reducer/ Nasal Decongestant
*NEW FORMULA—SEE NEW WARNINGS

Warning: ASPIRIN SENSITIVE PATIENTS. Do not take this product if you have had a severe reaction to aspirin (e.g., asthma, swelling, shock or hives) because even though this product contains no aspirin or salicylates, cross-reactions may occur in patients allergic to aspirin.

Uses: For temporary relief of symptoms associated with the common cold, sinusitis or flu including nasal congestion, headache, fever, body aches, and pains.

Directions: Adults: Take 1 caplet every 4 to 6 hours while symptoms persist. If symptoms do not respond to 1 caplet, 2 caplets may be used but do not exceed 6 caplets in 24 hours, unless directed by a doctor. The smallest effective dose should be used. Take with food or milk if occasional and mild heartburn, upset stomach, or stomach pain occurs with use. Ask a doctor if these symptoms are more than mild or they persist.
Children: Do not give this product to children under 12 years of age except under the advice and supervision of a doctor.

Warnings: Do not take for colds for more than 7 days or for fever for more than 3 days unless directed by a doctor. If the cold or fever persists or gets worse or if new symptoms occur, ask a doctor. These could be signs of serious illness. As with aspirin and actaminophen, if you have any condition which requires you to take prescription drugs or if you have had problems or serious side effects from taking any non-prescription pain reliever, do not take this product without first discussing it with your doctor. IF YOU EXPERIENCE ANY SYMPTOMS WHICH ARE UNUSUAL OR SEEM UNRELATED TO THE CONDITION FOR WHICH YOU TOOK THIS PRODUCT, CONSULT A DOCTOR BEFORE TAKING ANY MORE OF IT. If you are under a doctor's care for any serious condition, ask a doctor before taking this product. **Do not exceed recommended dosage.** If nervousness, dizziness or sleeplessness occur, discontinue use and ask a doctor. Do not take this product if

you have high blood pressure, heart disease, diabetes, thyroid disease or difficulty in urination due to enlargement of the prostate gland, unless directed by of a doctor. Do not combine this product with other non-prescription pain relievers. Do not combine this product with any other ibuprofen-containing product. As with any drug, if you are pregnant or nursing a baby, seek the advice of a health professional before using this product. IT IS ESPECIALLY IMPORTANT NOT TO USE THIS PRODUCT DURING THE LAST 3 MONTHS OF PREGNANCY UNLESS SPECIFICALLY DIRECTED TO DO SO BY A DOCTOR BECAUSE IT MAY CAUSE PROBLEMS IN THE UNBORN CHILD OR COMPLICATIONS DURING DELIVERY. Keep this and all drugs out of reach of children. In case of accidental overdose, seek professional assistance or contact a poison control center immediately. DRUG INTERACTION PRECAUTION: Do not take this product if you are taking a prescription monoamine oxidase inhibitor (MAOI) (certain drugs for depression, psychiatric or emotional conditions, or Parkinson's disease), or for 2 weeks after stopping the MAOI drug. If you are uncertain whether your prescription drug contains an MAOI, ask a health professional before taking this product.

Active Ingredients: each caplet contains Ibuprofen 200 mg, Pseudoephedrine Hydrochloride 30 mg.

Inactive Ingredients: Carnuba or Equivalent Wax, Croscarmellose Sodium, Iron Oxide, Methylparaben, Microcrystalline Cellulose, Propylparaben, Silicon Dioxide, Sodium Benzoate, Sodium Lauryl Sulfate, Starch, Stearic Acid, Sucrose, Titanium Dioxide.

How Supplied: Available in 20 count blister package and 40 count bottle. Each white caplet is imprinted: "DAYQUIL Sinus Pain".

VICKS® NYQUIL®
HOT THERAPY®
ADULT NIGHTTIME COLD/FLU HOT LIQUID MEDICINE
Honey Lemon Hot Liquid Drink
Antihistamine/Cough Suppressant/ Pain Reliever/Nasal Decongestant/ Fever Reducer

Active Ingredients: (per packet) Doxylamine Succinate 12.5 mg, Dextromethorphan Hydrobromide 30 mg, Acetaminophen 1000 mg, Pseudoephedrine Hydrochloride 60 mg.

Inactive Ingredients: Citric Acid, Flavor, and Sucrose.

Uses: For temporary relief of minor aches, pains, headache, muscular aches, sore throat pain, and fever associated with a cold or flu. Temporarily relieves nasal congestion, cough due to minor throat and bronchial irritations, runny nose and sneezing associated with the common cold.

Directions: Adults and Children 12 years and over: Take one dose at bedtime. DISSOLVE ONE PACKET IN 6 OZ. CUP OF HOT WATER. SIP PROMPTLY WHILE HOT. If your cold or flu symptoms keep you confined to bed or at home, a total of 4 doses may be taken per day, each 6 hours apart, or as directed by a doctor. **MICROWAVE HEATING INSTRUCTIONS:** Add contents of packet and 6 ounces of cool water to a microwave-safe cup and stir briskly. Microwave on high 1½ minutes or until hot. Drink promptly. **DO NOT BOIL.** Sweeten to taste if desired.

Warnings: Do not exceed recommended dosage. If nervousness, dizziness, or sleeplessness occurs, discontinue use and ask a doctor. Do not take this product if you have heart disease, high blood pressure, thyroid disease, diabetes, glaucoma, or difficulty in urination due to enlargement of the prostate gland unless directed by a doctor. *Drug Interaction Precaution:* Do not use this product if you are now taking a prescription monoamine oxidase inhibitor (MAOI) (certain drugs for depression, psychiatric or emotional conditions, or Parkinson's disease), or for two weeks after stopping the MAOI drug. If you are uncertain whether your prescription drug contains an MAOI, ask a health professional before taking this product. Do not take this product for persistent or chronic cough such as occurs with smoking, asthma, emphysema, or if cough is accompanied by excessive phlegm (mucus) unless directed by a doctor. May cause excitability especially in children. Do not take this product, unless directed by a doctor, if you have a breathing problem such as emphysema or chronic bronchitis. May cause marked drowsiness; alcohol, sedatives and tranquilizers may increase the drowsiness effect. Avoid alcoholic beverages while taking this product. Do not take this product if you are taking sedatives or tranquilizers without first asking your doctor. Use caution when driving a motor vehicle or operating machinery. Do not take this product for more than 7 days. A persistent cough may be a sign of a serious condition. If cough persists for more than 7 days, tends to recur, or is accompanied by rash, or persistent headache, ask a doctor. If symptoms do not improve or are accompanied by fever that lasts for more than 3 days, or if new symptoms occur, ask a doctor. If sore throat is severe, persists for more than 2 days, is accompanied or followed by fever, headache, rash, nausea or vomiting, ask a doctor promptly. **Keep this and all drugs out of the reach of children.** In case of accidental overdose, seek professional assistance or contact a poison control center immediately. Prompt medical attention is critical for adults as well as for children even if you do not notice any signs or symptoms. As with any drug, if you are pregnant or nursing a baby, seek the advice of

Continued on next page

Procter & Gamble—Cont.

a health professional before using this product.

How Supplied: Available in child-resistant packages of 6 single-dose packets.

VICKS® NYQUIL® LIQUICAPS®
VICKS® NYQUIL® LIQUID
(Original and Cherry)
Multi-Symptom Cold/Flu Relief
Antihistamine/Cough
Suppressant/Pain Reliever/
Nasal Decongestant/
Fever Reducer

Active Ingredients (per softgel): Doxylamine Succinate 6.25 mg, Dextromethorphan HBr 10 mg, Acetaminophen 250 mg, Pseudoephedrine HCl 30 mg. **(per 2 TBSP):** Doxylamine succinate 12.5 mg, Dextromethorphan HBr 30 mg, Acetaminophen 1000 mg, Pseudoephedrine HCl 60 mg.

Inactive Ingredients: (per softgel): D&C Yellow No. 10, FD&C Blue No. 1, Gelatin, Glycerin, Polyethylene Glycol, Povidone, Propylene Glycol and Purified Water. May contain Sorbitol Special. **(Liquid):** Alcohol 10%, Citric Acid, Flavor, High Fructase Corn Syrup, Polyethylene Glycol, Propylene Glycol, Purified Water, Saccharin Sodium, Sodium Citrate.
Original flavor also has D&C Yellow No. 10, FD&C Green No. 3, FD&C Yellow No. 6.
Cherry flavor also has FD&C Blue No. 1, FD&C Red No. 40.

Uses: Temporary relieves common cold/flu symptoms:
● minor aches
● pains
● headache
● muscular aches
● sore throat pain
● fever
● runny nose and sneezing
● nasal congestion
● cough due to minor throat and bronchial irritation

Liquid

Directions: **Adults Dose (12 yrs. and older):**
Take 2 Tablespoons (TBSP) or 30 ml in dose cup provided. A total of 4 doses may be taken per day, each 6 hours apart, or as directed by a doctor.
Ask a doctor for use in children under 12 yrs. of age.

LiquiCaps

Directions: **Adults 12 yrs. and older:** Swallow two softgels with water. A total of 4 doses may be taken per day, each 4 hours apart or as directed by a doctor. **NOT RECOMMENDED FOR CHILDREN.**

Warnings: Do not exceed recommended dosage.
If nervousness, dizziness, or sleeplessness occur, discontinue use and ask a doctor.

May caused marked drowsiness. May cause excitability in children. *Do not take unless directed by a doctor if you have:*
● heart disease
● asthma
● emphysema
● thyroid disease
● diabetes
● glaucoma
● high blood pressure
● excessive phlegm (muscus)
● breathing problems
● chronic bronchitis
● difficulty in breathing
● persistent or chronic cough
● cough associated with smoking
● difficulty in urination due to enlarged prostate gland
Keep this and all drugs out of the reach of children. In the case of accidental overdose, seek professional advice or contact a poison control center immediately. Prompt medical attention is critical for adults as well as for children even if you do not notice any signs or symptoms. As with any drug, if you are pregnant or nursing a baby, seek the advice of a health professional before using this product.
Drug Interaction Precaution: Do not take this product without first asking a doctor if you take:
● sedatives
● tranquilizers
● a prescription monoamine oxidase inhibitor (MAOI) (certain drugs for depression, psychiatric or emotional conditions, or Parkinson's disease), or for 2 weeks after stopping the MAOI drug or if you are uncertain whether your prescription drug contains an MAOI.
DOSING DURATION: Do not use over 7 days. *ASK A DOCTOR:*
● If sore throat is severe, persists for more than 2 days, is accompanied or followed by fever, headache, rash, nausea, or vomiting.
● If symptoms do not improve or are accompanied by a fever that lasts more than 3 days, or if new symptoms occur.
● If a cough persists for more than 7 days, recur, or is accompanied by a rash or persistent headache. A persistent cough may be the sign of a serious condition.
Alcohol, sedatives, and tranquilizers may increase the drowsiness effect. Avoid alcoholic beverages while taking this product. Use caution when driving a motor vehicle or operating machinery.

How Supplied: (LiquiCaps®) Available in 12-count child-resistant blister packages and 20-count non-child resistant blister packages. Each softgel is imprinted: "NyQuil".
(Liquid) Available in 6 and 10 FL OZ (175 and 295 ml, respectively) plastic bottles with child-resistant, tamper-evident cap and calibrated medicine cup.

PEDIATRIC VICKS® 44d
Cough & Head Congestion Relief

Active Ingredients: Per 1 tablespoon (TBSP.) (15 ml): Dextromethorphan Hydrobromide 15 mg, Pseudoephedrine Hydrochloride 30 mg.

CONTAINS NO ALCOHOL

Inactive Ingredients: Carboxymethylcellulose Sodium, Cellulose, Citric Acid, FD&C Red No. 40, Flavor, Glycerin, Polysorbate 80, Potassium Sorbate, Propylene Glycol, Purified Water, Sodium Citrate, Sorbitol, Sucrose.

Uses: Temporarily relieves:
● coughs
● nasal congestion due to the common cold.

Directions: **Use Tablespoon (TBSP) or dose cup.**

Under 2 yrs.	(Under 28 lbs.)	Ask a doctor
2–5 yrs.	(28–47 lbs.)	½ TBSP or 7½ ml
6–11 yrs.	(48–95 lbs.)	1 TBSP or 15 ml
12 yrs. & older	(Over 95 lbs.)	2 TBSP or 30 ml

Repeat every 6 hours, no more than 4 doses in 24 hours, or as directed by a doctor.

***Professional Dosage:**
Physicians: Suggested doses for children under 2 years of age.

Age	Weight	Dose
* 6–11 mo.	17–21 lbs.	1 teaspoon (tsp.) (5 ml)
*12–23 mo.	22–27 lbs.	1¼ teaspoon (tsp.) (6.25 ml)

Repeat every 6 hours. No more than 4 doses in 24 hours, or as directed by doctor.

*Based on extrapolation from studies on the safety and efficacy of active ingredients conducted among older children and adults. Use caution in treating children under 2 years who were born prematurely.

Warnings: Do not exceed recommended dosage.
If nervousness, dizziness, or sleeplessness occur, discontinue use and ask a doctor.
Do not take unless directed by a doctor if you have:
● heart disease
● asthma
● emphysema
● thyroid disease
● diabetes
● high blood pressure
● excessive phlegm (muscus)
● persistent or chronic cough
● cough associated with smoking

• difficulty in urination due to enlarged prostate gland

Keep this and all drugs out of the reach of children. In the case of accidental overdose, seek professional advice or contact a poison control center immediately. As with any drug, if you are pregnant or nursing a baby, seek the advice of a health professional before using this product.

Drug Interaction Precaution: Do not use this product without first asking a doctor if you take a prescription monoamine oxidase inhibitor (MAOI) (certain drugs for depression, psychiatric or emotional conditions, or Parkinson's disease), or for 2 weeks after stopping the MAOI drug or if you are uncertain whether your prescription drug contains an MAOI

Dosing Duration: Do not use over 7 days. *Ask a Doctor:*

• If symptoms do not improve or are accompanied by fever.

• If cough persists for more than 7 days, recurs, or is accompanied by fever, rash, or persistent headache. A persistent cough may be a sign of a serious condition.

How Supplied: 4 FL OZ (115 ml) plastic bottle. A calibrated dose cup accompanies each bottle.

PEDIATRIC VICKS® 44e
Cough & Chest Congestion Relief

Active Ingredients per 1 tablespoon (TBSP.) (15 ml):
Dextromethorphan Hydrobromide 10 mg, Guaifenesin 100 mg.

CONTAINS NO ALCOHOL

Inactive Ingredients: Carboxymethylcellulose Sodium, Cellulose, Citric Acid, FD&C Red No. 40, Flavor, Glycerin, Polysorbate 80, Potassium Sorbate, Propylene Glycol, Purified Water, Sodium Citrate, Sorbitol, Sucrose.

Uses: Temporary relief of coughs due to a common cold and helps loosen phlegm to rid the bronchial passageways of bothersome mucus.

Directions: Use Tablespoon (TBSP) or dose cup.

Under 2 yrs.	(Under 28 lbs.)	Ask a doctor.
2–5 yrs.	(28–47 lbs.)	½ TBSP or 7½ ml
6–11 yrs.	(48–95 lbs.)	1 TBSP or 15 ml
12 yrs. & older	(Over 95 lbs.)	2 TBSP or 30 ml

Repeat every 4 hours. No more than 6 doses in 24 hours, or as directed by a doctor.

***Professional Dosage:**

Physicians: Suggested doses for children under 2 years of age.

Age	Weight	Dose
* 6–11 mo.	17–21 lbs.	1 teaspoon (tsp.) (5 ml)
*12–23 mo.	22–27 lbs.	1¼ teaspoon (tsp.) (6.25 ml)

Repeat every 4 hours. No more than 6 doses in 24 hours, or as directed by doctor.

* Based on extrapolation from studies on the safety and efficacy of active ingredients conducted among older children and adults. Use caution in treating children under 2 years who were born prematurely.

Warnings:
Do not take unless directed by a doctor if you have:
• asthma
• emphysema
• excessive phlegm (mucus)
• persistent or chronic cough
• chronic bronchitis
• cough associated with smoking
Keep this and all drugs out of the reach of children.
In the case of accidental overdose, seek professional advice or contact a poison control center immediately. As with any drug, if you are pregnant or nursing a baby, seek the advice of a health professional before using this product.
Drug Interaction Precaution: Do not use this product without first asking a doctor if you are take a prescription monoamine oxidase inhibitor (MAOI) (certain drugs for depression, psychiatric or emotional conditions, or Parkinson's disease), or for 2 weeks after stopping the MAOI drug. If you are uncertain whether your prescription drug contains an MAOI.
Dosing Duration & When to Ask a Doctor:
• If a cough persists for more than 7 days, recurs, or is accompanied by fever, rash or persistent headache. A persistent cough may be the sign of a serious condition.

How Supplied: 4 FL OZ (115 ml) plastic bottles. A calibrated dose cup accompanies each bottle.

PEDIATRIC VICKS® 44m
Cough & Cold Relief
Cough Suppressant/Nasal Decongestant/Antihistamine

Active Ingredients Per 1 tablespoon (TBSP) (15 ml): Dextromethorphan Hydrobromide 15 mg, Pseudoephedrine Hydrochloride 30 mg, Chlorpheniramine Maleate 2 mg

CONTAINS NO ALCOHOL

Inactive Ingredients: Carboxymethylcellulose Sodium, Cellulose, Citric Acid, FD&C Red No. 40, Flavor, Glycerin, Polysorbate 80, Potassium Sorbate, Propylene Glycol, Purified Water, Sodium Citrate, Sorbitol, Sucrose.

Uses: Temporary relieves cough/cold symptoms:
• cough
• nasal congestion
• runny nose
• sneezing

Directions: Use Tablespoon (TBSP) or dose cup.

Under 6 yrs.	(Under 48 lbs.)	Ask a doctor.
6–11 yrs.	(48–95 lbs.)	1 TBSP or 15 ml
12 yrs. & older	(Over 95 lbs.)	2 TBSP or 30 ml

Repeat every 6 hours. No more than 4 doses in 24 hours, or as directed by a doctor.

Professional Dosage:

*Physicians: Suggested doses for children under 6 years of age.

Age	Weight	Dose
* 6–11 mo.	17–21 lbs.	1 teaspoon (tsp.) (5 ml)
*12–23 mo.	22–27 lbs.	1¼ teaspoon (tsp.) (6.25 ml)
2–5 yrs.	28–47 lbs.	½ TABLE-SPOON (TBSP.) (7.5 ml)

Repeat every 6 hours, no more than 4 doses in 24 hours, or as directed by doctor.

*Based on extrapolation from studies on the safety and efficacy of active ingredients conducted among older children and adults. Use caution in treating children under 2 years of age who were born prematurely.

Warnings: Do not exceed recommended dosage.
If nervousness, dizziness, or sleeplessness occur, discontinue use and ask a doctor. May cause marked drowsiness. May cause excitability in children.
Do not take unless directed by a doctor if you have:
• heart disease
• asthma
• emphysema
• thyroid disease
• diabetes
• glaucoma
• high blood pressure
• excessive phlegm (mucus)
• breathing problems
• chronic bronchitis
• difficulty in breathing
• persistent or chronic cough
• cough associated with smoking
• difficulty in urination due to enlarged prostate gland
Keep this and all drugs out of the reach of children. In case of accidental overdose, seek professional advice or contact a poison control center immediately. As with any drug, if you are pregnant or nursing a baby, seek the advice of a

Continued on next page

Procter & Gamble—Cont.

health professional before using this product.

Alcohol, sedatives, and tranquilizers may increase the drowsiness effect. Avoid alcoholic beverages while taking this product. Use caution when driving a motor vehicle or operating machinery. *Drug Interaction Precaution:* Do not take this product without first asking a doctor if you take:

• sedatives
• tranquilizers
• a prescription monoamine oxidase inhibitor (MAOI) (certain drugs for depression, psychiatric or emotional conditions, or Parkinson's disease), or for 2 weeks after stopping the MAOI drug or if you are uncertain whether your prescription drug contains an MAOI.

Dosing Duration: Do not use over 7 days. *Ask a Doctor:*

• If symptoms do not improve within 7 days or are accompanied by a fever.
• If a cough persists for more than 7 days, recurs, or is accompanied by fever, rash or persistent headache. A persistent cough may be a sign of a serious condition.

How Supplied: 4 FL OZ (115 ml) plastic bottles. A calibrated dose cup accompanies each bottle.

VICKS® SINEX® NASAL SPRAY
[sī′něx]
Nasal Decongestant Spray and Ultra Fine Mist

Active Ingredient: Phenylephrine Hydrochloride 0.5%.

Inactive Ingredients: Aromatic Vapors (Camphor, Eucalyptol, Menthol), Citric Acid, Disodium EDTA, Purified Water, Tyloxapol. Preservatives: Benzalkonium Chloride, Chlorhexidine Gluconate.

Use: For temporary relief of sinus/nasal congestion due to colds, hay fever, upper respiratory allergies or sinusitis.

Dosage: Ultra Fine Mist: Remove protective cap. Before using for the first time, prime the pump by firmly depressing its rim several times. Hold container with thumb at base and nozzle between first and second fingers. Without tilting your head, insert nozzle into nostril. Fully depress rim with a firm even stroke and inhale deeply. Adults and Children—age 12 and over: 2 or 3 sprays in each nostril not more often than every 4 hours. Do not give to children under 12 years of age unless directed by a doctor. Squeeze Bottle: Adults and Children—age 12 and over: 2 or 3 sprays in each nostril without tilting your head, not more often than every 4 hours. Do not give to children under 12 years of age unless directed by a doctor.

Warnings: Do not exceed recommended dosage. This product may cause temporary discomfort such as

burning, stinging, sneezing, or an increase of nasal discharge. The use of this container by more than one person may spread infection. Do not use this product for more than 3 days. Use only as directed. Frequent or prolonged use may cause nasal congestion to recur or worsen. If symptoms persist, ask a doctor. Do not use this product if you have heart disease, high blood pressure, thyroid disease, diabetes, or difficulty in urination due to enlargement of the prostate gland unless directed by a doctor. **Keep this and all drugs out of the reach of children.** In case of accidental ingestion, seek professional assistance or contact a poison control center immediately.

How Supplied: Available in ½ FL OZ (15 ml) plastic squeeze bottle and ½ FL OZ (15 ml) measured dose Ultra Fine mist pump.

VICKS® SINEX®
[sī′něx]
12-HOUR Nasal Decongestant Spray and Ultra Fine Mist

Active Ingredient: Oxymetazoline Hydrochloride 0.05%.

Inactive Ingredients: Aromatic Vapors (Camphor, Eucalyptol, Menthol), Disodium EDTA, Potassium Phosphate, Purified Water, Sodium Chloride, Sodium Phosphate, Tyloxapol. Preservatives: Benzalkonium Chloride, Chlorhexidine Gluconate.

Use: For temporary relief of nasal congestion due to colds, hay fever, upper respiratory allergies or sinusitis.

Dosage and Administration: Keep head and dispenser upright. May be used twice daily (morning and evening) or as directed by a physician.
Ultra Fine Mist: Remove protective cap. Before using for the first time, prime the pump by firmly depressing its rim several times. Hold container with thumb at base and nozzle between first and second fingers. Without tilting head, insert nozzle into nostril. Fully depress rim with a firm even stroke and inhale deeply. Adults and children 6 years of age and over (with adult supervision): 2 or 3 sprays in each nostril not more often than every 10 to 12 hours. Do not exceed 2 applications in any 24-hour period. Children under 6 years of age: ask a doctor. Squeeze Bottle: Adults and children 6 years of age and over (with adult supervision): 2 or 3 sprays in each nostril without tilting your head, not more often than every 10 to 12 hours. Do not exceed 2 applications in any 24-hour period. Children under 6 years of age: ask a doctor.

Warnings: Do not exceed recommended dosage. This product may cause temporary discomfort such as burning, stinging, sneezing or an increase of nasal discharge. The use of this

container by more than one person may spread infection. Do not use this product for more than 3 days. Use only as directed. Frequent or prolonged use may cause nasal congestion to recur or worsen. If symptoms persist, ask a doctor. Do not use this product if you have heart disease, high blood pressure, thyroid disease, diabetes, or difficulty in urination due to enlargement of the prostate gland unless directed by a doctor. **Keep this and all drugs out of the reach of children.** In case of accidental ingestion, seek professional assistance or contact a poison control center immediately.

How Supplied: Available in ½ FL OZ (15 ml) plastic squeeze bottle and ½ FL OZ (15 ml) measured-dose Ultra Fine mist pump.

VICKS® VAPOR INHALER
l-Desoxyephedrine/Nasal Decongestant

Active Ingredient per inhaler: *l*-Desoxyephedrine 50 mg.

Inactive Ingredients: Special Vicks Vapors (bornyl acetate, camphor, lavender oil, menthol).

Indications: For the temporary relief of nasal congestion due to the common cold, hay fever, upper respiratory allergies or sinusitis.

Directions: Adults: 2 inhalations in each nostril not more often than every 2 hours. **Children 6 to under 12 years of age** (with adult supervision): 1 inhalation in each nostril not more often than every 2 hours. Children under 6 years of age: ask a doctor.

Warnings: Do not exceed recommended dosage. This product may cause temporary discofort such as burning, stinging, sneezing, or an increase of nasal discharge. The use of this container by more than one person may spread infection. Do not use this product for more than 3 days. Frequent or prolonged use may cause nasal congestion to recur or worsen. If symptoms persist, ask a doctor. **Keep this and all drugs out of the reach of children.** In case of accidental ingestion, seek professional assistance or contact a poison control center immediately.

VICKS® VAPOR INHALER is effective for a minimum of 3 months after first use. Keep tightly closed.

How Supplied: Available as a cylindrical plastic nasal inhaler. Net weight: 0.007 OZ (200 mg).

VICKS® VAPORUB®
VICKS® VAPORUB® CREAM
[vā'pō-rub]
**Nasal Decongestant/Cough
Suppressant/Topical Analgesic**

Active Ingredients: Camphor (5.2% cream) 4.8% oint.), Menthol (2.8% cream) 2.6% oint.), Eucalyptus Oil 1.2%.
USE on Chest & Throat: For temporary relief of nasal congestion and coughs associated with a cold.

Active Ingredients: Camphor (5.2% cream) 4.8% oint.), Menthol (2.8% cream) 2.6% oint.).
USE: For temporary relief of minor aches and pains of muscles.

Inactive Ingredients: (ointment) Cedarleaf Oil, Nutmeg Oil, Special Petrolatum, Spirits of Turpentine, Thymol. **(cream)** Carbomer, Cedarleaf Oil, Cetyl Alcohol, Cetyl Palmitate, Cyclomethicone and Dimethicone Copolyol, Dimethicone, EDTA, Glycerin, Imidazolidinyl Urea, Isopropyl Palmitate, Methylparaben, Nutmeg Oil, PEG-100, Stearate, Propylparaben, Purified Water, Sodium Hydroxide, Spirits of Turpentine, Stearic Acid, Stearyl Alcohol, Thymol, Titanium Dioxide.

Directions: Adults and children 2 years of age and over:
Chest & Throat: rub on a thick layer. [If desired, cover with a dry, soft cloth, but keep clothing loose to let vapors rise to the nose and mouth. (oint.)]
Rub on sore area.
Repeat up to three times daily or as directed by a doctor.
Children under 2 years of age: consult a doctor.
Do not heat. Never expose VapoRub to flame, microwave, or place in any container in which you are heating water. [Such improper use may cause the mixture to splatter. (oint.)]

Warnings: For external use only. Do not take by mouth or place in nostrils. A persistent cough may be a sign of a serious condition. If cough persists for more than 1 week, recur, or are accompanied by fever, rash, or persistent headache, discontinue using this product and consult a doctor. Do not apply to wounds or damaged skin. **Keep this and all drugs out of the reach of children.** In case of accidental ingestion, seek professional assistance or contact a poison control center immediately.

How Supplied: (ointment) Available in 1.5 OZ (40 g), 3.0 OZ (90 g) and 6.0 OZ (170 g) plastic jars. **(cream)** 2.0 OZ (60 g) tube.

VICKS® VAPOSTEAM®
[vā'pō"stēm]
**Liquid Medication for
Hot Steam Vaporizers.
Nasal Decongestant/Cough
Suppressant**

Active Ingredients: Camphor 6.2%, Menthol 3.2%, Eucalyptus Oil 1.5%.

Inactive Ingredients: Alcohol 74%, Cedarleaf Oil, Nutmeg Oil, Poloxamer 124, Polyoxyethylene Dodecanol, Silicone.

Indications: For temporary relief of nasal congestion due to colds, hay fever, or other upper respiratory allergies. Temporarily relieves cough occurring with a cold.

Directions:
Adults and children 2 years of age and older: Use VAPOSTEAM only in hot/warm steam vaporizers, as described below. Follow directions for use carefully. Breathe in medicated vapors. May be repeated up to 3 times daily or as directed by a doctor.
Children under 2 years of age: consult a doctor.
In Hot/Warm Steam Vaporizers: VAPOSTEAM is formulated to be added directly to the water in your hot/warm steam vaporizer. Add one tablespoon of VAPOSTEAM with each quart of water added to the vaporizer. Do not direct steam from vaporizer close to face. For best performance, vaporizer should be thoroughly cleaned after each use according to manufacturer's instructions. To promote steaming, follow directions of vaporizer manufacturer.
Never expose VAPOSTEAM to flame, microwave, or place in any container in which you are heating water except for a hot-warm steam vaporizer. Never use VAPOSTEAM in any bowl or washbasin with hot water. Improper use may cause the mixture to splatter and cause burns.

Warnings: For hot/warm steam vaporizers only. Do not use in cold steam vaporizers or humidifiers. **Not to be taken by mouth.** A persistent cough may be a sign of a serious condition. If cough persists for more than one week, tends to recur or is accompanied by fever, rash, or persistent headache, consult a doctor. Do not use this product for persistent or chronic cough such as occurs with smoking, asthma, emphysema, or if cough is accompanied by excessive phlegm (mucus) unless directed by a doctor. **Keep this and all drugs out of the reach of children.**

Accidental Ingestion: In case of accidental ingestion, seek professional assistance or contact a poison control center immediately.

How Supplied: Available in 4 FL OZ (118 mL) and 8 FL OZ (236 mL) bottles.

EDUCATIONAL MATERIAL

Procter & Gamble offers to health care professionals a variety of journal reprints and patient education materials on:
• pain management (Aleve),
• fiber therapy and related bowel disorders (Metamucil),
• H. pylori research and healthy traveling advice (Pepto-Bismol),
• caffeine reduction (Folgers), and
• pharmacy practice issues (Pharmacy Digest newsletter).

Additionally, selected professional samples of Procter & Gamble Health Care and Skin Care products are available to targeted health care specialists.
For these materials, please call 1-800/358-8707, or write:
Charles Lambert
Manager, Scientific Communications
The Procter & Gamble Company
Two Procter & Gamble Plaza
Cincinnati, OH 45201

Quintex Pharmaceuticals, Ltd.
ONE EXECUTIVE DRIVE
FORT LEE, NJ 07024

Direct Inquiries to:
Customer Service
(201) 947-8700
FAX: (201) 947-8779

For Medical Emergencies Contact:
Professional Services
(201) 947-8700
FAX: (201) 947-8779

ALCOMED® 2-60 TABLETS
Allergy & Cold Medication

Dexbrompheniramine Maleate 2 mg. and Pseudoephedrine HCl 60 mg.

How Supplied: Blister Packs of 24

CAP-Z® ROLL-ON
Arthritis Pain Formula

Purified Capsaicin 0.03% (0.09% HP) with Aloe & Vitamin E

How Supplied: 2 Fl. Oz. Roll-On

EXPRESSIN® 400 CAPLETS
Breathe Easier Formula

Guaifenesin 400 mg. and Pseudoephedrine HCl 60 mg.

How Supplied: Blister Packs of 20

INSPIRE® L.A. NASAL SPRAY
Extra Soothing Formula

Xylometazoline HCl .01%, with Aloe & Vitamin E

How Supplied: 0.5 Fl. Oz. & 1 Fl. Oz.

ISOHIST® 2.0 TABLETS
Antihistamine–Allergy & Hay Fever

Dexbrompheniramine Maleate 2 mg.

How Supplied: Blister Packs of 24

Continued on next page

Quintex Pharmaceutical—Cont.

IVY SOOTHE™ DERMA SPRAY
ITCH & PAIN RELIEF

Zinc Acetate 1.6%, Pramoxine HCl 1% with Hydrolyzed Oatmeal, Aloe Vera, Vit. A,D,E & Benzylkonium Chloride

How Supplied: 2 Fl. Oz. Pump Spray

PEDIA-PRESSIN® DM DROPS
Pediatric Cough and Cold Drops

Pseudoephedrine HCl 15 mg.
Dextromethorphan HBr 5 mg.
Guaifenesin 50 mg (per 1 mL.)

How Supplied: 1 Fl. Oz. with Dropper

RESTYN® 76 CAPLETS
Sleep Aid

Diphenhydramine Citrate 76 mg.

How Supplied: Blister Packs of 21

SUPRESSIN® DM CAPLETS
Cough Suppressant—Expectorant

Dextromethorphan HBr 15 mg. and Guaifenesin 200 mg.

How Supplied: Blister Packs of 20

Requa, Inc.
BOX 4008
1 SENECA PLACE
GREENWICH, CT 06830

Direct Inquiries to:
J. Geils
(203) 869-2445
(800) 321-1085
FAX: (203) 661-5630

CharcoAid 2000
Emergency Poison Adsorbent with super activated charcoal.

Active Ingredient: Super Activated Charcoal U.S.P., 50g

Indication: For the emergency treatment of acute ingested poison.

Action: Adsorbent

Dosage and Administration: Shake bottle vigorously for at least 15 seconds. Drink entire contents, or for children use as directed by a health professional.

How Supplied: 240 ml bottle contains 50g charcoal in water suspension
For information concerning the use of this product please call 1-800-321-1085. Dist. by Regua, Inc. Greenwich, CT.

CHARCOCAPS®
HOMEOPATHIC FORMULA
Relieves Gas Pain Bloat, Flatus
Symptoms of Intestinal Gas

Indications: For symptomatic relief of intestinal gas.

Dosage: 2 caplets after eating or at first sign of discomfort. Hold caplets in mouth 15–30 seconds to dissolve outer coating before swallowing. Repeat in ½ to 1 hour as needed but do not exceed 8 doses per day.

Active Ingredients: CARBO VEGETABILIS 5C (VEGETABLE CHARCOAL), LYCOPODIUM CLAVATUM 5C (CLUBMOSS), CINCHONA OFFICINALIS 5C (CINCHONA BARK), SULPHUR 5C (SUBLIMED SULPHUR). For information concerning the use of this product please call 1-800-321-1085. Dist. by Requa, Inc., Greenwich, CT

Warning: May adsorb other medication, space at least one hour apart.

Richardson-Vicks Inc.
(See Procter & Gamble.)

Roberts Pharmaceutical Corporation
4 INDUSTRIAL WAY WEST
EATONTOWN, NJ 07724

Direct Inquiries to:
Customer Service Department:
(908) 389-1182
(800) 828-2088
FAX: (908) 389-1014

For Medical Emergencies Contact:
Medical Services Department
(800) 992-9306

CHERACOL® Nasal Spray Pump
Cherry Scented

Description: CHERACOL® NASAL SPRAY PUMP is a cherry scented long acting topical nasal decongestant. One application lasts up to 12 hours.

How Supplied: Available in 1 fluid ounce bottles fitted with a metered pump (NDC 54092-880-30).
Manufactured for
Roberts Laboratories Inc.,
a subsidiary of
ROBERTS PHARMACEUTICAL CORPORATION
Eatontown, NJ 07724 USA

CHERACOL® SINUS
12 Hour Formula

Description: Cheracol® SINUS sustained-action tablets combine a nasal decongestant with an antihistamine in a special continuous-acting timed-release tablet to provide temporary relief of nasal congestion due to the common cold, and associated with sinusitis. Also alleviates running nose and sneezing due to hay fever.

How Supplied: 10 sustained-action release tablets. NDC 54092-045-10
Manufactured for
Roberts Laboratories Inc., a subsidiary of
ROBERTS PHARMACEUTICAL CORPORATION
Eatontown, NJ 07724, USA

CHERACOL® Sore Throat Spray
Anesthetic/Antiseptic Liquid

Description: A pleasant tasting cherry flavored liquid spray with anesthetic and antiseptic properties.

How Supplied: Available in 6 fluid ounce spray pump bottle (NDC 54092-340-06).
Manufactured for
Roberts Laboratories Inc.,
a subsidiary of
ROBERTS PHARMACEUTICAL CORPORATION
Eatontown, NJ 07724 USA

CHERACOL D® Cough Formula
Maximum Strength Cough Relief

Description: CHERACOL D® is a non-narcotic cough formula which combines two important medicines in one safe, fast-acting pleasant tasting liquid:
- The highest level of cough suppressant available without prescription.
- A clinically proven expectorant to help loosen phlegm and drain bronchial tubes.

Indications: CHERACOL D® cough formula helps quiet dry, hacking coughs, and helps loosen phlegm and mucus. Recommended for adults and children 6 years of age and older.

Active Ingredients: Each teaspoonful (5 ml) contains dextromethorphan hydrobromide, 10 mg; guaifenesin, 100 mg; **Inactive Ingredients:** alcohol, 4.75%, benzoic acid, FD&C Red #40, flavors, fragrances, fructose, glycerin, propylene glycol, sodium chloride, sucrose, and purified water.

Dosage—Adults and children 12 years of age and over: Oral dosage is 2 teaspoonfuls every 4 hours, not to exceed 12 teaspoonfuls in 24 hours, or as directed by a doctor. **Children 6 to under 12 years of age:** Oral dosage is 1 teaspoonful every 4 hours, not to exceed 6 teaspoonfuls in 24 hours, or as directed by a doctor. **Children under 6 years of age:** Consult a doctor.

Warnings: Keep this and all medication out of the reach of children. Do not give this product to children under 6 years of age except under the advice and supervision of a physician. Do not use this product for persistent or chronic cough such as occurs with smoking, asthma, or emphysema or where cough is accompanied by excessive secretions except under the advice and supervision of a physician. As with any drug, pregnant or nursing women should seek the advice of a health professional before using this product.

Caution: A persistent cough may be a sign of a serious condition. If cough persists for more than 1 week, tends to recur or is accompanied by high fever, rash or persistent headache, consult a physician.

Overdose: In case of accidental overdose contact a physician or a poison control center immediately.

Drug Interaction Precaution: Do not use this product if you are now taking a prescription monoamine inhibitor (maoi) (certain drugs for depression, psychiatric or emotional conditions, or Parkinson's Disease), or for two weeks after stopping the maoi drug. If you are uncertain whether your prescription drug contains an maoi, consult a health professional before taking this product.

How Supplied: Available 4 oz bottle (NDC 54092-400-04), and 6 oz bottle (NDC 54092-400-06).
Manufactured for
Roberts Laboratories Inc.,
a subsidiary of
ROBERTS PHARMACEUTICAL CORPORATION
Eatontown, NJ 07724 USA
Shown in Product Identification Guide, page 515

CHERACOL PLUS® Cough Syrup
Multisymptom cough/cold formula

Description: CHERACOL PLUS® Cough Syrup is a pleasant tasting 3-ingredient non-narcotic liquid formulation.

Indications: Cheracol Plus® syrup is an effective 3-ingredient, maximum strength formula for the temporary relief of head cold symptoms and cough (without narcotic side effects).

Active Ingredients: Each tablespoonful (15ml) contains phenylpropanolamine HCl, 25 mg; dextromethorphan hydrobromide, 20 mg; chlorpheniramine maleate, 4 mg; and alcohol, 8%.

Inactive Ingredients: Flavors, glycerin, methylparaben, propylene glycol, propylparaben, FD&C Red No. 40, sodium chloride, sorbitol solution, and purified water.

Dosage and Administration: Adults and children over 12 years of age: 1 tablespoonful (15ml) every 4 hours or as directed by a physician. Do not take more than 6 tablespoonfuls in a 24 hour period. Do not administer to children under 12 years of age.

Uses: Cheracol Plus® multisymptom head cold/cough formula provides cough suppressant and decongestant activity and controls runny nose associated with the common cold ("flu").

Warnings: Do not take this product for persistent or chronic cough such as occurs with smoking, asthma, or emphysema or where cough is accompanied by excessive secretions or if you have high blood pressure, heart or thyroid disease, diabetes, asthma, glaucoma, or difficulty in urination due to enlargement of the prostate gland except under the advice and supervision of a physician. If symptoms do not improve within 7 days or are accompanied by high fever, consult a physician before continuing use. May cause excitability, especially in children. Do not give this product to children under 12 years except under the advice and supervision of a physician. May cause marked drowsiness. Avoid alcoholic beverages, driving a motor vehicle or operating heavy machinery while taking this product. As with any drug, if you are pregnant or nursing a baby consult a health professional before using this product. Keep this and all medication out of the reach of children.

Drug Interaction Precaution: Do not use this product if you are now taking a prescription monoamine oxidase inhibitor (MAOI) (certain drugs for depression, psychiatric or emotional conditions, or Parkinson's disease), or for 2 weeks after stopping the MAOI drug. If you are uncertain whether your prescription drug contains an MAOI, consult a health professional before taking this product.

Overdose: In case of accidental overdose contact a physician or a poison control center immediately.

How Supplied: Available in 4 oz bottle (NDC 54092-401-04), 6 oz bottle (54092-401-06).
Manufactured for
Roberts Laboratories Inc.,
a subsidiary of
ROBERTS PHARMACEUTICAL CORPORATION
Eatontown, NJ 07724 USA

COLACE®
[kōlās]
docusate sodium,
capsules • syrup • liquid (drops)

Description: Colace® (docusate sodium) is a stool softener.
Colace® Capsules, 50 mg, contain the following inactive ingredients: citric acid, D&C Red No. 33, FD&C Red No. 40, nonporcine gelatin, edible ink, polyethylene glycol, propylene glycol, and purified water.
Colace® Capsules, 100 mg, contain the following inactive ingredients: citric acid, D&C Red No. 33, FD&C Red No. 40, FD&C Yellow No. 6, nonporcine gelatin, edible ink, polyethylene glycol, propylene glycol, titanium dioxide, and purified water.
Colace® Liquid, 1%, contains the following inactive ingredients: citric acid, D&C Red No. 33, methylparaben, poloxamer, polyethylene glycol, propylene glycol, propylparaben, sodium citrate, vanillin, and purified water.
Colace® Syrup, 20 mg/5 mL, contains the following inactive ingredients: alcohol (not more than 1%), citric acid, D&C Red No. 33, FD&C Red No. 40, flavor (natural), menthol, methylparaben, peppermint oil, poloxamer, polyethylene glycol, propylparaben, sodium citrate, sucrose, and purified water.

Actions and Uses: Colace®, a surface-active agent, helps to keep stools soft for easy, natural passage and is not a laxative, thus, not habit forming. Useful in constipation due to hard stools, in painful anorectal conditions, in cardiac and other conditions in which maximum ease of passage is desirable to avoid difficult or painful defecation, and when peristaltic stimulants are contraindicated.
Note: When peristaltic stimulation is needed due to inadequate bowel motility, see Peri-Colace® (laxative and stool softener).

Contraindications: There are no known contraindications to Colace®.

Warning: As with any drug, pregnant or nursing women should seek the advice of a health professional before using this product. Keep this and all medication out of the reach of children.

Side Effects: The incidence of side effects—none of a serious nature—is exceedingly small. Bitter taste, throat irritation, and nausea (primarily associated with the use of the syrup and liquid) are the main side effects reported. Rash has occurred.

Administration and Dosage: *Orally*—Suggested daily Dosage: *Adults and older children:* 50 to 200 mg *Children 6 to 12:* 40 to 120 mg *Children 3 to 6:* 20 to 60 mg. *Infants and children under 3:* 10 to 40 mg. The higher doses are recommended for initial therapy. Dosage should be adjusted to individual response. The effect on stools is usually apparent 1 to 3 days after the first dose. Colace® liquid or syrup must be given in a 6 oz. to 8 oz. glass of milk or fruit juice or in infant's formula to prevent throat irritation. In *enemas*—Add 50 to 100 mg Colace® (5 to 10 mL Colace® liquid) to a retention or flushing enema.

How Supplied: Colace® capsules, 50 mg
   NDC 54092-052-30 Bottles of 30
   NDC 54092-052-60 Bottles of 60
   NDC 54092-052-52 Cartons of 100 single unit packs
Colace® capsules, 100 mg
   NDC 54092-053-30 Bottles of 30
   NDC 54092-053-60 Bottle of 60
   NDC 54092-053-02 Bottles of 250
   NDC 54092-053-10 Bottles of 1000
   NDC 54092-053-52 Cartons of 100 single unit packs
Note: Colace® capsules should be stored at controlled room temperature (59°–86°F or 15°–30°C)

Continued on next page

Roberts—Cont.

Colace® liquid, 1% solution; 10 mg/mL (with calibrated dropper)
NDC 54092-414-16 Bottles of 16 fl oz
NDC 54092-414-30 Bottles of 30 mL
Colace® syrup, 20 mg/5 mL teaspoon; contains not more than 1% alcohol
NDC 54092-415-08 Bottles of 8 fl oz
NDC 54092-415-16 Bottles of 16 fl oz
Manufactured for
Roberts Laboratories Inc.,
a subsidiary of
ROBERTS PHARMACEUTICAL CORPORATION
Eatontown, NJ 07724 USA
Shown in Product Identification Guide, page 515

**PERI-COLACE® capsules • syrup
(casanthranol and docusate sodium)**

Description: Peri-Colace® is a combination of the mild stimulant laxative casanthranol, and the stool-softener Colace® (docusate sodium). Each capsule contains 30 mg of casanthranol and 100 mg of Colace®; the syrup contains 30 mg of casanthranol and 60 mg of Colace® per 15-mL tablespoon (10 mg of casanthranol and 20 mg of Colace® per 5-mL teaspoon) and 10% alcohol.
Peri-Colace® Capsules contain the following inactive ingredients: D&C Red No. 33, FD&C Red No. 40, non-porcine gelatin, edible ink, polyethylene glycol, propylene glycol, titanium dioxide, and purified water.
Peri-Colace® Syrup contains the following inactive ingredients: alcohol (10% v/v), citric acid, flavors, methyl salicylate, methylparaben, poloxamer, polyethylene glycol, propylparaben, sodium citrate, sorbitol solution, sucrose, and purified water.

Action and Uses: Peri-Colace® provides gentle peristaltic stimulation and helps to keep stools soft for easier passage. Bowel movement is induced gently—usually overnight or in 8 to 12 hours. Nausea, griping, abnormally loose stools, and constipation rebound are minimized. Useful in management of chronic or temporary constipation.
Note: To prevent hard stools when laxative stimulation is not needed or undesirable, see Colace® (stool softener).

Warnings: Do not use when abdominal pain, nausea, or vomiting is present. Frequent or prolonged use of this preparation may result in dependence on laxatives.
As with any drug, pregnant or nursing women should seek the advice of a health professional before using this product. Keep this and all medication out of the reach of children.

Side Effects: The incidence of side effects—none of a serious nature—is exceedingly small. Nausea, abdominal cramping or discomfort, diarrhea, and rash are the main side effects reported.

Administration and Dosage:
Adults—1 or 2 capsules, or 1 or 2 tablespoons syrup at bedtime, or as indicated. In severe cases, dosage may be increased to 2 capsules or 2 tablespoons twice daily, or 3 capsules at bedtime. *Children*—1 to 3 teaspoons of syrup at bedtime, or as indicated. Peri-Colace® syrup must be given in a 6 oz. to 8 oz. glass of milk or fruit juice or in infant's formula to prevent throat irritation.

Overdosage: In addition to symptomatic treatment, gastric lavage, if timely, is recommended in cases of large overdosage.

How Supplied: Peri-Colace® Capsules
NDC 54092-054-30 Bottles of 30
NDC 54092-054-60 Bottles of 60
NDC 54092-054-02 Bottles of 250
NDC 54092-054-10 Bottles of 1000
NDC 54092-054-52 Cartons of 100 single unit packs
Note: Peri-Colace® capsules should be stored at controlled room temperatures (59°–86°F or 15°–30°C).
Peri-Colace® Syrup
NDC 54092-418-08 Bottles of 8 fl oz
NDC 54092-418-16 Bottles of 16 fl oz
Manufactured for
Roberts Laboratories Inc.,
a subsidiary of
ROBERTS PHARMACEUTICAL CORPORATION
Eatontown, NJ 07724 USA
Shown in Product Identification Guide, page 515

**PYRROXATE® Caplets
Extra Strength Decongestant/
Antihistamine/
Analgesic Caplets**

Description: *Pyrroxate®* provides single-caplet, multisymptom relief for colds, allergies, nasal/sinus congestion, runny nose, sneezing, and watery eyes. Because it contains the non-aspirin analgesic **acetaminophen**, *Pyrroxate®* gives temporary relief of occasional minor aches, pains, headache, and helps in the reduction of fever. *Pyrroxate®* is caffeine and aspirin-free.

Active Ingredients: Each *Pyrroxate®* Caplet contains: chlorpheniramine maleate, 4 mg; phenylpropanolamine HCl, 25 mg; acetaminophen, 650 mg.

Inactive Ingredients: Croscarmellose Sodium NF; Powdered Cellulose, Stearic Acid, Hydroxypropyl Methyl Cellulose, Titanium Dioxide, D&C Yellow #10 Lake, Polyethylene Glycol, Polysorbate 80, FD&C Yellow #6 Lake, Synthetic Black Iron Oxide, Lecithin. Also may contain other ingredients.

Indications: *Pyrroxate®* Caplets are for the temporary relief of runny nose, sneezing, itching of the nose or throat; for the temporary relief of nasal congestion due to the common cold, allergies (hay fever), sinus congestion and for the temporary relief of occasional minor aches, pains, headache, and for the reduction of fever.

Actions: Chlorpheniramine maleate is an antihistamine effective in controlling runny nose, sneezing, watery eyes, and itching of the nose and throat. Phenylpropanolamine HCl is an oral nasal decongestant effective in relieving nasal/sinus congestion due to the common cold or allergies (hay fever). Acetaminophen is a clinically effective analgesic and antipyretic without aspirin side effects.

Warnings: Do not take this product for more than 7 days. If symptoms persist, do not improve, or new ones occur, or if fever persists for more than 3 days, discontinue use and consult your physician. Do not take this product if you have asthma, glaucoma, difficulty in urination due to the enlargement of the prostate gland, high blood pressure, diabetes, thyroid disease, or if you are presently taking a prescription antihypertensive or antidepressant drug containing a monoamine oxidase inhibitor, except under the advice and supervision of a physician. As with any drug, if you are pregnant or nursing a baby, seek the advice of a health professional before using this product. Do not exceed recommended dosage because severe liver damage may occur and at higher doses, nervousness, dizziness or sleeplessness may occur. Do not take other medications containing acetaminophen simultaneously, to avoid the risk of overdosage. Do not take this product for the treatment of arthritis except under the advice and supervision of a physician.

Cautions: Avoid alcoholic beverages, driving a motor vehicle, or operating heavy machinery while taking this product. This product may cause drowsiness or excitability, especially in children. Keep this and all medication out of the reach of children. In case of accidental overdose, seek professional assistance or contact a poison control center immediately.

Dosage and Administration: Take 1 caplet every 4 hours or as directed by a physician. Do not take more than 6 caplets in a 24-hour period. Do not administer to children under 12 years of age.

How Supplied: Yellow caplets available in bottles of 24 (NDC 54092-041-24) and 500 (NDC 54092-041-05).
Manufactured for
Roberts Laboratories Inc.,
a subsidiary of
ROBERTS PHARMACEUTICAL CORPORATION
Eatontown, NJ 07724 USA
Shown in Product Identification Guide, page 516

A. H. Robins Consumer Products

American Home Products Corporation
FIVE GIRALDA FARMS
MADISON, NJ 07940-0871

For information on A.H. Robins Consumer Products see product listings under Whitehall-Robins Healthcare.

Ross Products Division Abbott Laboratories

COLUMBUS, OHIO 43215-1724

Direct Inquiries to:
1-800-227-5767

PEDIATRIC NUTRITIONAL PRODUCTS

Alimentum® Protein Hydrolysate Formula With Iron

Isomil® Soy Formula With Iron

Isomil® DF Soy Formula For Diarrhea

Isomil® SF Sucrose-Free Soy Formula With Iron

PediaSure® Complete Liquid Nutrition

PediaSure® With Fiber Complete Liquid Nutrition

RCF® Ross Carbohydrate Free Soy Formula Base With Iron

Similac® Low-Iron Infant Formula

Similac® NeoCare™ Infant Formula With Iron

Similac® PM 60/40 Low-Iron Infant Formula

Similac® Special Care® With Iron 24 Premature Infant Formula

Similac® Toddler's Best™ Nutritional Beverage With Iron

Similac® With Iron Infant Formula

For most current information, refer to product labels.

CLEAR EYES®
[klēr īz]
Lubricant Eye Redness Reliever Eye Drops

Description: Clear Eyes is a sterile, isotonic buffered solution containing the active ingredients naphazoline hydrochloride (0.012%) and glycerin (0.2%). It also contains boric acid, purified water and sodium borate. Edetate disodium and benzalkonium chloride are added as preservatives. Clear Eyes is a lubricating, decongestant ophthalmic solution specially designed for temporary relief of redness and drying due to minor eye irritation caused by dust, smoke, smog, sun glare, wearing contact lenses or swimming. Clear Eyes contains laboratory-tested and scientifically blended ingredients, including an effective vasoconstrictor which narrows swollen blood vessels and rapidly whitens reddened eyes in a formulation which also contains a lubricant and produces a refreshing, soothing effect. Clear Eyes is a sterile, isotonic solution compatible with the natural fluids of the eye.

Indications: For the temporary relief of redness due to minor eye irritation AND for protection against further irritation or dryness of the eye.

Warnings: To avoid contamination, do not touch tip of container to any surface. Replace cap after using. If you experience eye pain, changes in vision, continued redness or irritation of the eye, or if the condition worsens or persists for more than 72 hours, discontinue use and consult a doctor. If you have glaucoma, do not use this product except under the advice and supervision of a doctor. Overuse of this product may produce increased redness of the eye. If solution changes color or becomes cloudy, do not use. Keep this and all drugs out of the reach of children. In case of accidental ingestion, seek professional assistance or contact a Poison Control Center immediately.

Directions: Instill 1 or 2 drops in the affected eye(s), up to four times daily.

How Supplied: In 0.5-fl-oz (15 mL) and 1.0-fl-oz (30 mL) plastic dropper bottles. (FAN 3178)

CLEAR EYES® ACR
[klēr īz]
Astringent/Lubricant Redness Reliever Eye Drops

Description: Clear Eyes ACR is a sterile, isotonic buffered solution containing the active ingredients naphazoline hydrochloride (0.012%), zinc sulfate (0.25%) and glycerin (0.2%). It also contains boric acid, purified water, sodium chloride and sodium citrate. Edetate disodium and benzalkonium chloride are added as preservatives. Clear Eyes ACR is a triple-action formula that: (1) has an extra ingredient to clear away mucus buildup and relieve itching associated with exposure to airborne allergens, (2) immediately removes redness and (3) moisturizes irritated eyes. Clear Eyes ACR contains laboratory-tested and scientifically blended ingredients, including an effective vasoconstrictor which narrows swollen blood vessels and rapidly whitens reddened eyes in a formulation which also contains a lubricant and produces a refreshing, soothing effect. Clear Eyes ACR also contains an ocular astringent (zinc sulfate) that precipitates the sticky mucus buildup on the eye often associated with exposure to airborne allergens, and this helps clear the mucus from the outer surface of the eye. Clear Eyes ACR is a sterile, isotonic solution compatible with the natural fluids of the eye.

Indications: For the temporary relief of redness due to minor eye irritation AND for protection against further irritation or dryness of the eye.

Warnings: To avoid contamination, do not touch tip of container to any surface. Replace cap after using. If you experience eye pain, changes in vision, continued redness or irritation of the eye, or if the condition worsens or persists for more than 72 hours, discontinue use and consult a doctor. If you have glaucoma, do not use this product except under the advice and supervision of a doctor. Overuse of this product may produce increased redness of the eye. If solution changes color or becomes cloudy, do not use. Keep this and all drugs out of the reach of children. In case of accidental ingestion, seek professional assistance or contact a Poison Control Center immediately.

Directions: Instill 1 or 2 drops in the affected eye(s), up to four times daily.

How Supplied: In 0.5-fl-oz (15 mL) and 1.0-fl-oz (30 mL) plastic dropper bottles. (FAN 3178)

EAR DROPS BY MURINE®
[myūr'ēn]
See Murine Ear Wax Removal System/Murine Ear Drops.

MURINE® EAR WAX REMOVAL SYSTEM/MURINE® EAR DROPS
[myūr'ēn]
Carbamide Peroxide
Ear Wax Removal Aid

Description: MURINE EAR DROPS contains the active ingredient carbamide peroxide, 6.5%. It also contains alcohol (6.3%), anhydrous glycerin, polysorbate 20 and other ingredients in a buffered vehicle. The MURINE EAR WAX REMOVAL SYSTEM includes a 1.0-fl-oz soft bulb ear syringe. This system is a complete, medically approved system to safely remove ear wax. Application of carbamide peroxide drops followed by warm-water irrigation is an effective, medically recommended way to help loosen excessive and/or hardened ear wax.

Actions: The carbamide peroxide formula in MURINE EAR DROPS is an aid in the removal of wax from the ear canal. Anhydrous glycerin penetrates and softens wax while the release of oxygen from carbamide peroxide provides a mechanical action resulting in the loosening of

Continued on next page

Ross—Cont.

the softened wax accumulation. It is usually necessary to remove the loosened wax by gently flushing the ear with warm water, using the soft bulb ear syringe provided.

Indications: The MURINE EAR WAX REMOVAL SYSTEM is indicated for occasional use as an aid to soften, loosen and remove excessive ear wax.

Warnings: DO NOT USE if you have ear drainage or discharge, ear pain, irritation or rash in the ear or are dizzy: Consult a doctor. DO NOT USE if you have an injury or perforation (hole) of the eardrum or after ear surgery, unless directed by a doctor.
DO NOT USE for more than 4 days; if excessive ear wax remains after use of this product, consult a doctor. Avoid contact with the eyes. If accidental contact with eyes occurs, flush eyes with water and consult a doctor. KEEP THIS AND ALL MEDICINES OUT OF THE REACH OF CHILDREN. In case of accidental ingestion, seek professional assistance or contact a Poison Control Center immediately.

Directions: FOR USE IN THE EAR ONLY. Adults and children over 12 years of age: Tilt head sideways and place 5 to 10 drops in ear. Tip of applicator should not enter ear canal. Keep drops in ear for several minutes by keeping head tilted or placing cotton in the ear. Use twice daily for up to 4 days if needed, or as directed by a doctor. Any wax remaining after treatment may be removed by gently flushing the ear with warm water, using a soft bulb ear syringe. Children under 12 years: Consult a doctor.
Note: When the ear canal is irrigated, the tip of the ear syringe should not obstruct the flow of water leaving the ear canal.

How Supplied: The MURINE EAR WAX REMOVAL SYSTEM contains 0.5-fl-oz (15 mL) drops and a 1.0-fl-oz (30 mL) soft bulb ear syringe.
Also available in 0.5-fl-oz (15 mL) drops only, MURINE EAR DROPS.
(FAN 3178)

MURINE TEARS™
[myūr´ēn ´ti(ə)rs]
Lubricant Eye Drops

Description: Murine Tears eye lubricant is a sterile, buffered solution containing the active ingredients 0.5% polyvinyl alcohol and 0.6% povidone. Also contains benzalkonium chloride, dextrose, disodium edetate, potassium chloride, purified water, sodium bicarbonate, sodium chloride, sodium citrate and sodium phosphate (mono- and dibasic). Murine Tears is a sterile, hypotonic solution formulated to more closely match the natural tear fluid of the eye for gentle, soothing relief from minor eye irritation while moisturizing and relieving dryness. Use as desired to temporarily relieve minor eye irritation, dryness and burning.

Indications: For the temporary relief or prevention of further discomfort due to minor eye irritations and symptoms related to dry eyes.

Warnings: To avoid contamination, do not touch tip of container to any surface. Replace cap after using. If you experience eye pain, changes in vision, continued redness or irritation of the eye, or if the condition worsens or persists for more than 72 hours, discontinue use and consult a doctor. If solution changes color or becomes cloudy, do not use. Keep this and all drugs out of the reach of children. In case of accidental ingestion, seek professional assistance or contact a Poison Control Center immediately.

Directions: Instill 1 or 2 drops in the affected eye(s) as needed.

How Supplied: In 0.5-fl-oz (15 mL) and 1.0-fl-oz (30 mL) plastic dropper bottles. (FAN 3249)

MURINE TEARS™ PLUS
[myūr´ēn ´ti(ə)rs]
Lubricant Redness Reliever Eye Drops

Description: Murine Tears Plus is a sterile, non-staining, buffered solution containing the active ingredients 0.5% polyvinyl alcohol, 0.6% povidone and 0.05% tetrahydrozoline hydrochloride. Also contains benzalkonium chloride, dextrose, disodium edetate, potassium chloride, purified water, sodium bicarbonate, sodium chloride, sodium citrate and sodium phosphate (mono- and dibasic). Murine Tears Plus is a sterile, hypotonic, ophthalmic solution formulated to more closely match the natural fluid of the eye. It contains demulcents for gentle, soothing relief from minor eye irritation as well as the sympathomimetic agent, tetrahydrozoline hydrochloride, which produces local vasoconstriction in the eye. Thus, the drug effectively narrows swollen blood vessels locally and provides symptomatic relief of edema and hyperemia of conjunctival tissues due to eye allergies, minor local irritations and conjunctivitis. Use up to four times daily, to remove redness due to minor eye irritation. The effect of Murine Tears Plus is prompt (apparent within minutes).

Indications: For the temporary relief or prevention of further discomfort due to minor eye irritations and symptoms related to dry eyes PLUS removal of redness.

Warnings: To avoid contamination, do not touch tip of container to any surface. Replace cap after using. If you experience eye pain, changes in vision, continued redness or irritation of the eye, or if the condition worsens or persists for more than 72 hours, discontinue use and consult a doctor. If you have glaucoma, do not use this product except under the advice and supervision of a doctor. Overuse of this product may produce increased redness of the eye. If solution changes color or becomes cloudy, do not use. Keep this and all drugs out of the reach of children. In case of accidental ingestion, seek professional assistance or contact a Poison Control Center immediately.

Directions: Instill 1 or 2 drops in the affected eye(s), **up to four times daily.**

How Supplied: In 0.5-fl-oz (15 mL) and 1.0-fl-oz (30 mL) plastic dropper bottles. (FAN 3249)

PEDIALYTE®
[pē´dē-ah-līt″]
Oral Electrolyte Maintenance Solution

Usage: To quickly restore fluid and minerals lost in diarrhea and vomiting; for maintenance of water and electrolytes following corrective parenteral therapy for severe diarrhea.
Features:
● Ready To Use—no mixing or dilution necessary.
● Balanced electrolytes to replace stool losses and provide maintenance requirements.
● Provides glucose to promote sodium and water absorption.
● Unflavored form available for younger infants; Bubble Gum, Fruit and Grape-flavored forms available to enhance compliance in older infants and children.
● Plastic liter bottles are resealable and easy to pour.
● Widely available in grocery, drug and convenience stores.

Availability:
1 quart 1.8 fl oz (1 liter) plastic bottles; 8 per case; Unflavored, No. 336; Fruit-flavored, No. 365; Bubble Gum-flavored, No. 51752; Grape-flavored, No. 240.
8-fl-oz (237 mL) bottles; 4 six-packs per case; Unflavored, No. 160. For hospital use, Pedialyte is available in the Ross Hospital Formula System.

Dosage: See Administration Guide to restore fluids and minerals lost in diarrhea and vomiting (Pedialyte Unflavored, Bubble Gum-flavored, Fruit-flavored or Grape-flavored) and management of mild to moderate dehydration secondary to moderate to severe diarrhea (Rehydralyte® Oral Electrolyte Rehydration Solution).
Pedialyte (Unflavored, Bubble Gum-flavored, Fruit-flavored or Grape-flavored) or Rehydralyte should be offered frequently in amounts tolerated. Total daily intake should be adjusted to meet individual needs, based on thirst and response to therapy. The following suggested intakes for maintenance are based on water requirements for ordinary energy expenditure.[1] For dehydrated children, the suggested intakes

Pedialyte, Rehydralyte Administration Guide*

For Infants and Young Children

Age	2 Weeks	3	6 Months	9	1	1½	2	2½ Years	3	3½	4	5	6
Approximate Weight†													
(lb)	7	13	17	20	23	25	28	30	32	35	38	41	46
(kg)	3.2	6.0	7.8	9.2	10.2	11.4	12.6	13.6	14.6	16.0	17.0	18.7	20.7
PEDIALYTE UNFLAVORED, BUBBLE GUM-FLAVORED, FRUIT OR GRAPE-FLAVORED fl oz/day for maintenance**	13 to 16	28 to 32	34 to 40	38 to 44	41 to 46	45 to 50	48 to 53	51 to 56	54 to 58	56 to 60	57 to 62	59 to 66	62 to 69
REHYDRALYTE fl oz/day for Replacement for 5% Dehydration (including maintenance)**	18 to 21	38 to 42	47 to 53	53 to 59	58 to 63	64 to 69	69 to 74	74 to 79	78 to 82	83 to 87	85 to 90	90 to 97	96 to 104
REHYDRALYTE fl oz/day for Replacement for 10% Dehydration (including maintenance)**	23 to 26	48 to 52	60 to 66	68 to 74	75 to 80	83 to 88	90 to 95	97 to 102	102 to 106	110 to 114	113 to 118	121 to 128	131 to 138

* Administration Guide does not apply to infants less than 1 week of age.

**Fluid intakes do not take into account ongoing stool losses. Fluid loss in the stool should be replaced by consumption of an extra amount of Pedialyte or Rehydralyte equal to stool losses, in addition to the amounts indicated in this Administration Guide.

† Weight based on the 50th percentile of weight for age of the National Center for Health Statistics (NCHS) reference growth data. Hamill PVV, Drizd TA, Johnson CL, et al: Physical growth: National Center for Health Statistics percentiles. *Am J Clin Nutr* 1979; 32:607-629.

---

are for replacement and for maintenance, based on a fluid deficit of 5% or 10% of body weight (including maintenance requirement). The fluid deficit should be replaced as quickly as possible, usually in the first 4 to 6 hours. [See table above.]

Reference:
1. Extrapolated from Barness L: Nutrition and nutritional disorders, in Behrman RE, Kliegman RM, Nelson WE, Vaughan VC III: *Nelson Textbook of Pediatrics*, ed 14. Philadelphia: WB Saunders Co, 1992, pp 105-107.

Composition: Unflavored Pedialyte (Bubble Gum-flavored, Fruit-flavored, and Grape-flavored Pedialyte have similar composition and nutrient values. Fruit-Flavored and Grape-Flavored Pedialyte contain fructose. For specific information, including artificial colors in flavored products, see product labels.)

Ingredients: (Pareve, Ⓤ) Water, dextrose, potassium citrate, sodium chloride and sodium citrate.

Provides:	Per 8 Fl Oz	Per Liter	Per 32 Fl Oz
Sodium (mEq)	10.6	45	42.4
Potassium (mEq)	4.7	20	18.8
Chloride (mEq)	8.3	35	33.2
Citrate (mEq)	7.1	30	28.4
Dextrose (g)	5.9	25	23.6
Calories	24	100	96

(FAN 3250-01)
Shown in Product Identification Guide, page 516

PEDIASURE® And PEDIASURE® WITH FIBER

[pē 'dē -ah-shur "]

Complete Liquid Nutrition For Children 1 to 10 years old.

Usage: As a liquid food providing complete, balanced nutrition for children 1 to 10 years of age. May be used for total nutritional support or as a nutritional supplement with and between meals.

Features: PediaSure and PediaSure With Fiber
- Doctor recommended and hospital used
- Nutrition to help recover from illness
- For unpredictable/"picky" eaters
- Ideal for busy, active lifestyles
- A dietary source of fiber (PediaSure With Fiber only)
- Lactose free, * easily digested
- Convenient, ready to drink, great tasting

---

*Not for patients with galactosemia.

PediaSure and PediaSure With Fiber contain 100% or more of the NAS-NRC Recommended Dietary Allowances (RDA) for protein, vitamins and minerals in 1000 mL (approx. 34 fl oz) for children 1 to 6 years of age and in 1300 mL (approx. 44 fl oz) for children 7 to 10 years of age.

Availability: Ready To Use 8-fl-oz (237 mL) cans in 6-packs; 24 cans per case. PediaSure: Vanilla, No. 373; Chocolate, No. 51812; Strawberry, No. 51810; Banana Cream, No. 51808. PediaSure With Fiber: Vanilla, No. 50652.

Directions for Use: Shake very well. Delicious chilled. Do not add water. Suggest 1 to 3 cans per day for supplemental use. Once opened, cover, refrigerate and use within 48 hours. Consult your health care professional regarding your child's specific needs. Not intended for infants under 1 year of age unless specified by a physician.

Continued on next page

If desired, additional information on any Ross product will be provided upon request to Ross Products Division, Abbott Laboratories, Columbus, Ohio 43215-1724.

Ross—Cont.

Ingredients[†] PediaSure and PediaSure With Fiber (Vanilla flavor): Ⓤ-D Water, hydrolyzed cornstarch, sugar (sucrose), sodium caseinate, high-oleic safflower oil, soy oil, fractionated coconut oil (medium-chain triglycerides), whey protein concentrate, soy fiber (PediaSure With Fiber only), calcium phosphate tribasic, natural and artificial flavor, potassium citrate, magnesium chloride, potassium phosphate dibasic, potassium chloride, soy lecithin, mono- and diglycerides, choline chloride, carrageenan, ascorbic acid, m-inositol, taurine, ferrous sulfate, zinc sulfate, niacinamide, alpha-tocopheryl acetate, L-carnitine, calcium pantothenate, manganese sulfate, thiamine chloride hydrochloride, pyridoxine hydrochloride, riboflavin, cupric sulfate, vitamin A palmitate, folic acid, biotin, potassium iodide, sodium selenite, sodium molybdate, phylloquinone, vitamin D₃ and cyanocobalamin.

Nutrients (grams/8 fl oz): Protein, 7.1; Fat, 11.8; Carbohydrate, 26 (26.9[‡], PediaSure With Fiber); L-Carnitine, 0.004; Taurine, 0.017; Water, 200. Calories per mL, 1.0; Calories per fl oz, 29.6.

[†] For Vanilla product; minor differences exist in other PediaSure flavors. For specific information, see product labels.

[‡] Includes soy fiber (a source of dietary fiber that provides 3.4 Calories and 1.2 g of total dietary fiber).

(FAN 3139-02) (PediaSure)
(FAN 3139-01) (PediaSure With Fiber)

Shown in Product Identification Guide, page 516

REHYDRALYTE®
[rē-hī'drǝ-līt″]
Oral Electrolyte Rehydration Solution

Usage: To restore fluid and minerals lost during moderate to severe diarrhea.

Features:
- Ready To Use—no mixing or dilution necessary.
- Safe, economical alternative to IV therapy.
- 75 mEq of sodium per liter for effective replacement of fluid deficits.
- 2½% glucose solution to promote sodium and water absorption and provide energy.
- Available in pharmacies.

Availability: 8-fl-oz (237 mL) bottles; 4 six-packs per case; No. 162.

Dosage: (See Administration Guide under Pedialyte®.)

Ingredients: (Pareve, Ⓤ) Water, dextrose, sodium chloride, potassium citrate and sodium citrate.

Provides:	Per 8 Fl Oz	Per Liter
Sodium (mEq)	17.7	75
Potassium (mEq)	4.7	20
Chloride (mEq)	15.4	65
Citrate (mEq)	7.1	30
Dextrose (g)	5.9	25
Calories	24	100

(FAN 3106-01)

SELSUN BLUE®
[sel'sun blü]
**Dandruff Shampoo
(selenium sulfide lotion, 1%)**

Description: Selsun Blue is a non-prescription anti-dandruff shampoo containing the active ingredient selenium sulfide, 1%, in a freshly scented, pH-balanced formula to leave hair clean and manageable. Available in Balanced Treatment, Moisturizing Treatment, Medicated Treatment and 2-in-1 Treatment formulas.

Inactive Ingredients:

Balanced Treatment formula —Ammonium laureth sulfate, ammonium lauryl sulfate, citric acid, cocamide DEA, cocamidopropyl betaine, DMDM hydantoin, FD&C blue No. 1, fragrance, hydroxypropyl methylcellulose, magnesium aluminum silicate, purified water, sodium chloride and titanium dioxide.

Moisturizing Treatment formula — Aloe, ammonium laureth sulfate, ammonium lauryl sulfate, citric acid, cocamide DEA, di (hydrogenated) tallow phthalic acid amide, dimethicone, DMDM hydantoin, FD&C blue No. 1, fragrance, hydroxypropyl methylcellulose, purified water, sodium citrate, sodium isostearoyl lactylate and titanium dioxide.

Medicated Treatment formula — Ammonium laureth sulfate, ammonium lauryl sulfate, citric acid, cocamide DEA, cocamidopropyl betaine, DMDM hydantoin, D&C red No. 33, FD&C blue No. 1, fragrance, hydroxypropyl methylcellulose, magnesium aluminum silicate, menthol, purified water, sodium chloride and TEA-lauryl sulfate.

2-in-1 Treatment formula — Ammonium lauryl sulfate, ammonium laureth sulfate, citric acid, cocamide DEA, di (hydrogenated) tallow phthalic acid amide, dimethicone, DMDM hydantoin, hydroxypropyl methylcellulose, purified water, sodium citrate and fragrance.

Clinical testing has shown Selsun Blue to be as safe and effective as other leading shampoos in helping control dandruff symptoms with regular use. May be used on color-treated or permed hair, if used as directed.

Directions: Shake well. Shampoo and rinse thoroughly. For best results, use regularly, at least twice a week or as directed by a doctor.

Warnings: For external use only. Avoid contact with the eyes. If contact occurs, rinse eyes thoroughly with water. If condition worsens or does not improve after regular use of this product as directed, consult a doctor. Keep this and all drugs out of the reach of children. In case of accidental ingestion, seek professional assistance or contact a Poison Control Center immediately.

How Supplied: 4 (118 mL), 7 (207 mL) and 11 (325 mL) fl oz plastic bottles. (FAN 3225)

SIMILAC® Toddler's Best™
[sim'e-lak täd'lǝrs best]
Nutritional Beverage With Iron

Usage: As an iron-fortified, milk-based alternative to cow's milk or juice for children over 12 months of age.

Features:
- Caloric density: 20 Cal/fl oz
- 2.9 mg of iron per 8 fl oz to help avoid iron deficiency
- Iron content per 8 fl oz is 30% of the Daily Value (DV)
- Contains 40% of the DV for vitamin C per 8 fl oz (6 times the amount in whole cow's milk)
- Contains 50% of the DV for vitamin E per 8 fl oz (17 times the amount in whole cow's milk)
- Higher in many essential nutrients than whole cow's milk

Availability: Ready To Use 8-fl-oz (237 mL) drink box; 27 8-fl-oz drink boxes per case (9 units of 3 drink boxes); Vanilla, No. 52154; Chocolate, No. 52152; Berry, No. 52156.

Directions for Use: Shake well before using. Serve one 8-fl-oz drink box as an alternative to cow's milk or fruit juice with or between regular meals. Delicious at room temperature or chilled. Once opened, refrigerate unused portion and use within 24 hours.

Composition: Ready To Use Vanilla (Chocolate and Berry flavors have similar composition and nutrient values. For specific information, see product labels.)

Ingredients: Ⓤ-D Water, nonfat milk, sugar (sucrose), high-oleic safflower oil, coconut oil, soy oil, natural and artificial flavor, calcium carbonate, ascorbic acid, lactose, soy lecithin, choline chloride, ferrous sulfate, taurine, m-inositol, alpha-tocopheryl acetate, zinc sulfate, niacinamide, calcium pantothenate, vitamin A palmitate, cupric sulfate, thiamine chloride hydrochloride, riboflavin, pyridoxine hydrochloride, folic acid, manganese sulfate, phylloquinone, biotin, sodium selenite, vitamin D₃ and cyanocobalamin.

[See table at top of next page.]
(FAN 3293-02)

Shown in Product Identification Guide, page 516

TRONOLANE®
[tron'ǝ-lān]
Anesthetic Cream for Hemorrhoids

Description: The active ingredient in Tronolane cream is the topical anesthetic agent, pramoxine hydrochloride, 1% (chemically unrelated to the benzoate esters of the "caine" type), which is

Similac® Toddler's Best™ Compared With Whole Cow's Milk: Selected Nutrients

Nutrient	NLEA* Labeling Daily Values (DV)	Similac Toddler's Best		Whole Cow's Milk	
	Children <4 years of age	8 fl oz	% DV	8 fl oz	% DV
Protein, g	16	5.6	35	8.0	50
Fat, g	NA	7.5	NA	8.2	NA
Carbohydrate, g	NA	17.6	NA	11.5	NA
Iron, mg	10	2.9	30	0.12	2
Vitamin E, IU	10	4.8	50	0.28	2
Vitamin C, mg	40	15.2	40	2.24	6

*Nutrition Labeling and Education Act, 1990
NA Not applicable

chemically designated as a 4-n-butoxy-phenyl gammamor-pholinopropyl-ether hydrochloride. Also contains the following inactive ingredients: A nongreasy cream base containing beeswax, cetyl alcohol, cetyl esters wax, glycerin, methylparaben, propylparaben, sodium lauryl sulfate and zinc oxide.

Tronolane cream contains a rapidly acting topical anesthetic producing analgesia that lasts up to 5 hours. Because the drug is chemically unrelated to other anesthetics, cross-sensitization is unlikely. Patients who are already sensitized to the "caine" anesthetics can generally use Tronolane cream.

The emollient/emulsion base of Tronolane cream provides soothing lubrication. Tronolane cream is in a nondrying base that is nongreasy and nonstaining to undergarments.

Indications: Tronolane cream is indicated for the temporary relief of pain, itching, burning and soreness associated with hemorrhoids.

Warnings: If condition worsens or does not improve within 7 days, consult a doctor. Do not exceed the recommended daily dosage, unless directed by a doctor. In case of bleeding, consult a doctor promptly. Do not put this product into the rectum by using fingers or any mechanical device or applicator. Certain persons can develop allergic reactions to ingredients in this product. If the symptom being treated does not subside, or if redness, irritation, swelling, pain or other symptoms develop or increase, discontinue use and consult a doctor. As with any drug, if you are pregnant or nursing a baby, seek the advice of a health care professional before using this product. Keep this and all drugs out of the reach of children. In case of accidental ingestion, seek professional assistance or contact a Poison Control Center.

Dosage and Administration (Directions): Adults—When practical, cleanse the affected area with mild soap and warm water and rinse thoroughly or cleanse by patting or blotting with an appropriate cleansing pad. Gently dry by patting or blotting with toilet tissue or a soft cloth before application of this product. Apply externally to the affected area up to five times daily. Children under 12 years of age—Consult a doctor.

How Supplied: Tronolane cream is available in 1-oz (28g) and 2-oz (57g) tubes.
(FAN 2393)

TRONOLANE®
[tron 'ə-lān]
Hemorrhoidal Suppositories

Description: The active ingredients in Tronolane suppositories are zinc oxide, 5%, and hard fat, 95%. Zinc oxide (an astringent) and hard fat (a skin protectant) afford temporary relief of hemorrhoidal itching and burning and protect irritated hemorrhoidal areas.

Indications: Tronolane suppositories are indicated for the temporary relief of the itching, burning and irritation associated with hemorrhoids.

Warnings: If condition worsens or does not improve within 7 days, consult a doctor. Do not exceed the recommended daily dosage, unless directed by a doctor. In case of bleeding, consult a doctor promptly. As with any drug, if you are pregnant or nursing a baby, seek the advice of a health care professional before using this product. **Do not store above 86°F.** Keep this and all drugs out of the reach of children. In case of accidental ingestion, seek professional assistance or contact a Poison Control Center immediately.

Dosage and Administration (Directions): Adults—When practical, cleanse the affected area with mild soap and warm water and rinse thoroughly or cleanse by patting or blotting with an appropriate cleansing pad. Gently dry by patting or blotting with toilet tissue or a soft cloth before application of this product. Remove foil wrapper before inserting into the rectum. Use up to six times daily or after each bowel movement. Children under 12 years of age—Consult a doctor.

How Supplied: Tronolane suppositories are available in 10- and 20-count boxes.
(FAN 2393)

Sandoz Pharmaceuticals Corporation/ Consumer Division
59 ROUTE 10
EAST HANOVER, NJ 07936

Direct Inquiries to:
(201) 503-7500
FAX: (201) 503-8265

For Medical Information Contact:
Medical Department
Sandoz Pharmaceuticals Corporation
East Hanover, NJ 07936
(201) 503-7500

ACID MANTLE® CREME
[ă 'sĭd-mănt 'l]
Acid pH

Description: Restores and maintains protective acidity of the skin. Provides relief of mildly irritated skin due to exposure to soaps, detergents, chemicals and alkalis. Aids in the treatment of diaper rash; bath dermatitis; winter eczema and dry, rough, scaly skin of varied causes.

Ingredients: Water, cetostearyl alcohol, white petrolatum, glycerin, synthetic beeswax, light mineral oil, sodium lauryl sulfate, aluminum sulfate, calcium acetate, methylparaben, white potato dextrin.

Caution: For external use only. Avoid contact with the eyes.

Directions: Apply several times daily, especially after wet work.

How Supplied: 1 oz. tubes; 4 oz. and 1 lb. jars.

BiCOZENE® Creme External Analgesic
[bī-cō-zēn]

Active Ingredients: Benzocaine 6%, resorcinol 1.67% in a specially prepared cream base.

Inactive Ingredients: Castor Oil, Chlorothymol, Glycerin, Glyceryl Monostearate, Parachlorometaxylenol, Perfume, Polysorbate 80, Sodium Borate,

Continued on next page

Sandoz—Cont.

Stearic Acid, Triglycerol Diisostearate, Trolamine, Water.

Indications: For the temporary relief of pain and itching associated with minor burns, sunburn, minor cuts, scrapes, insect bites or minor skin irritations.

Actions: Benzocaine is a topical anesthetic and resorcinol is a topical antipruritic, at the concentrations used in BiCozene Creme. Both exert their actions by depressing cutaneous sensory receptors.

Warnings: Do not apply this product to large areas of the body. Caution: Use only as directed. Keep away from the eyes. Not for prolonged use. If the symptoms persist for more than seven days or clear up and reoccur within a few days, or if a rash or irritation develops, discontinue use and consult a physician. For external use only. **KEEP THIS AND ALL DRUGS OUT OF THE REACH OF CHILDREN.** In case of accidental ingestion, seek professional assistance or contact a poison control center immediately.

Drug Interaction Precautions: No known drug interaction.
Resorcinol is an antipruritic in solutions of 0.5 to 3.0 percent.

Dosage: For adults and children 2 years of age and older: Apply a 0.5 to 3.0 percent concentration of resorcinol to affected area not more than 3 to 4 times daily. For children under 2 years of age, there is no recommended dosage except under the advice and supervision of a physician.
Do not apply this product to extensive areas of the body or under compresses or bandages.
Do not apply this product to large areas of the body.

How Supplied: BiCozene Creme is available in 1-ounce tubes.
Shown in Product Identification Guide, page 516

CAMA® ARTHRITIS PAIN RELIEVER
[kă'măh]

Description: Each CAMA Inlay-Tab contains: aspirin USP 500 mg; magnesium oxide USP 150 mg; dried aluminum hydroxide gel USP, equivalent to 125 mg aluminum hydroxide. **Other ingredients:** colloidal silicon dioxide, croscarmellose sodium, hydrogenated vegetable oil, methylcellulose, methylparaben, microcrystalline cellulose, polyethylene glycol, povidone, pregelatinized starch, starch, Yellow 6, Yellow 10.

Indications: For the temporary relief of minor arthritic pain.

Warnings: Children and teenagers should not use this medicine for chicken pox or flu symptoms before a doctor is consulted about Reye syndrome, a rare but serious illness reported to be associ-

ated with aspirin. If pain persists for more than 10 days consult a physician immediately. If redness or swelling is present, consult a doctor because these could be signs of a serious condition. As with any drug, if you are pregnant or nursing a baby, seek the advice of a health professional before using this product. **IMPORTANT: IT IS ESPECIALLY IMPORTANT NOT TO USE ASPIRIN DURING THE LAST 3 MONTHS OF PREGNANCY UNLESS SPECIFICALLY DIRECTED TO DO SO BY A DOCTOR BECAUSE IT MAY CAUSE PROBLEMS IN THE UNBORN CHILD OR COMPLICATIONS DURING DELIVERY.** Stop taking this product if ringing in the ears, loss of hearing, or dizziness occur. Do not take this product if you are presently taking a prescription drug for diabetes, anticoagulation (thinning the blood), or gout, or if you have an aspirin allergy. Do not take this product if you have asthma or stomach problems (such as heartburn, upset stomach, or stomach pain) that persist or recur, or if you have ulcers or bleeding problems, unless directed by a doctor. Keep this and all medicines out of the reach of children. In case of accidental overdose, contact a physician immediately.

Directions For Use: Adults: 2 tablets with a full glass of water every 6 hours. Not to exceed 8 tablets in 24 hours unless directed by a physician. Do not use in children under 12 years of age except under the advice and supervision of a physician.

How Supplied: CAMA Arthritis Pain Reliever Tablets (white with salmon inlay), imprinted "Cama 500" on one side, "Dorsey" on the other, in bottles of 100.

DORCOL® CHILDREN'S COUGH SYRUP
[door'call]

Description: Each teaspoonful (5 ml) of DORCOL Children's Cough Syrup contains guaifenesin 50 mg, pseudoephedrine hydrochloride 15 mg, dextromethorphan hydrobromide 5 mg. Other ingredients: benzoic acid, Blue 1, edetate disodium, flavors, glycerin, propylene glycol, purified water, Red 40, sodium hydroxide, sucrose, tartaric acid.

Indications: Temporarily relieves your child's cough due to minor throat and bronchial irritation as may occur with the common cold. Helps loosen phlegm (mucus) and thin bronchial secretions to rid the bronchial passageways of bothersome mucus. Helps drain bronchial tubes and makes coughs more productive. Temporarily relieves nasal stuffiness due to the common cold, hay fever or other upper respiratory allergies. Promotes nasal and/or sinus drainage.

Warnings: Keep this and all drugs out of the reach of children. In case of accidental overdose, seek professional assis-

tance or contact a Poison Control Center immediately.
Do not exceed recommended dosage. If nervousness, dizziness, or sleeplessness occur, discontinue use and consult a doctor. If symptoms do not improve within 7 days or are accompanied by fever, consult a doctor. Do not give this product to a child who has heart disease, high blood pressure, thyroid disease, or diabetes unless directed by a doctor. A persistent cough may be a sign of a serious condition. If cough persists for more than 1 week, tends to recur, or is accompanied by fever, rash, or persistent headache, consult a doctor. Do not give this product for persistent or chronic cough, such as occurs with asthma or if cough is accompanied by excessive phlegm (mucus), unless directed by a doctor.

Drug Interactions Precaution: Do not give this product to a child who is taking a prescription monoamine oxidase inhibitor (MAOI) (certain drugs for depression, psychiatric or emotional conditions) or for 2 weeks after stopping the MAOI drug. If you are uncertain whether your child's prescription drug contains a MAOI, consult a health professional before giving this product.

Directions For Use: Dosing to children under 2 yrs. of age is to be under the direction of a physician.
By age:
Children 2 to under 6 years: 1 teaspoonful every 4 hours.
Children 6 to under 12 years: 2 teaspoonfuls every 4 hours.
By weight:
Children 24 to 47 pounds: 1 teaspoonful every 4 hours.
Children 48 to 95 pounds: 2 teaspoonfuls every 4 hours.
Do not exceed 4 doses in 24 hours, or as directed by a doctor.

Professional Labeling: The suggested dosage for pediatric patients is:

4–12 months	3 drops/Kg of body weight every 4 hours
12–24 months	7 drops (0.2 ml)/Kg of body weight every 4 hours

Maximum 4 doses in 24 hours.

How Supplied: DORCOL Children's Cough Syrup (grape colored), in 4 fl oz plastic bottles with tamper-evident band around child-resistant cap.
Shown in Product Identification Guide, page 516

EX–LAX® Chocolated Laxative Tablets

Active Ingredient: Yellow phenolphthalein, 90 mg. phenolphthalein per tablet.

Inactive Ingredients: Cocoa, Confectioner's Sugar, Hydrogenated Palm Kernel Oil, Lecithin, Nonfat Dry Milk, Vanillin.

Indication: For relief of occasional constipation (irregularity).

Caution: Do not take any laxative when abdominal pain, nausea, or vomiting are present. Frequent or prolonged use of this or any other laxative may result in dependence on laxatives. If skin rash appears, do not use this or any other preparation containing phenolphthalein.

Warnings: Keep this and all drugs out of the reach of children. In case of accidental overdose, seek professional assistance or contact a poison control center immediately. As with any drug, if you are pregnant or nursing a baby, seek the advice of a health care professional before using this product.

Dosage and Administration: Adults and children 12 years old and over: Chew 1 or 2 tablets, preferably at bedtime. Children over 6 years: Chew ½ tablet.

How Supplied: Available in boxes of 6, 18, 48, and 72 chewable chocolated tablets.
Shown in Product Identification Guide, page 516

EX–LAX® Laxative Pills

Regular Strength Ex-Lax®
Laxative Pills
Extra Gentle Ex-Lax® Laxative Pills
Maximum Relief Formula Ex-Lax®
Laxative Pills
Ex-Lax® Gentle Nature® Laxative Pills

Active Ingredients: Regular Strength Ex-Lax Laxative Pills—Yellow phenolphthalein USP, 90 mg. phenolphthalein per pill. **Extra Gentle Ex-Lax Laxative Pills**—Docusate sodium USP, 75 mg. and yellow phenolphthalein USP, 65 mg. per pill. **Maximum Relief Formula Ex-Lax Laxative Pills**—Yellow phenolphthalein USP, 135 mg. per pill. **Ex-Lax Gentle Nature Laxative Pills**—Sennosides, 20 mg. per pill.

Inactive Ingredients: Regular Strength Ex-Lax Laxative Pills—Acacia, Alginic Acid, Carnauba Wax, Colloidal Silicon Dioxide, Dibasic Calcium Phosphate, Iron Oxides, Magnesium Stearate, Microcrystalline Cellulose, Sodium Benzoate, Sodium Lauryl Sulfate, Starch, Stearic Acid, Sucrose, Talc, Titanium Dioxide. **Extra Gentle Ex-Lax Laxative Pills**—Acacia, Croscarmellose Sodium, Dibasic Calcium Phosphate, Colloidal Silicon Dioxide, Magnesium Stearate, Microcrystalline Cellulose, Red 7, Stearic Acid, Sucrose, Talc, Titanium Dioxide. **Maximum Relief Formula Ex-Lax Laxative Pills**—Acacia, Alginic Acid, Blue No. 1, Carnauba Wax, Colloidal Silicon Dioxide, Dibasic Calcium Phosphate, Magnesium Stearate, Microcrystalline Cellulose, Povidone, Sodium Benzoate, Sodium Lauryl Sulfate, Starch, Stearic Acid, Sucrose, Talc, Titanium Dioxide. **Ex-Lax Gentle Nature Laxative Pills**—Alginic Acid, Colloidal Silicon Dioxide, Dibasic Calcium Phosphate, Magnesium Stearate, Microcrystalline Cellulose, Pregelati-

nized Starch, Sodium Lauryl Sulfate, Stearic Acid.

Indication: For relief of occasional constipation (irregularity).

Caution: Do not take any laxative when abdominal pain, nausea, or vomiting are present. Frequent or prolonged use of this or any other laxative may result in dependence on laxatives. If skin rash appears, do not use this or any other preparation containing phenolphthalein.

Warnings: Keep this and all drugs out of the reach of children. In case of accidental overdose, seek professional assistance or contact a Poison Control Center immediately. As with any drug, if you are pregnant or nursing a baby, seek the advice of a health care professional before using this product.

Dosage and Administration: Regular Strength Ex-Lax Laxative Pills, Extra Gentle Ex-Lax Laxative Pills, and Maximum Relief Formula Ex-Lax Laxative Pills—Adults and children 12 years of age and over: Take 1 to 2 pills with a glass of water, preferably at bedtime. Consult with a physician for children under 12 years of age. **Ex-Lax Gentle Nature Laxative Pills**—Adults and children 12 years of age and over: Take 1 or 2 pills with a glass of water, preferably at bedtime.
Children 6 to under 12 years of age: Take 1 pill with a glass of water, preferably at bedtime.

How Supplied: Regular Strength Ex-Lax Laxative Pills—Available in boxes of 8, 30, and 60 pills. **Extra Gentle Ex-Lax Laxative Pills and Maximum Relief Formula Ex-Lax Laxative Pills**—Available in boxes of 24 pills. **Ex-Lax Gentle Nature Laxative Pills**—Available in boxes of 16 pills.
Shown in Product Identification Guide, page 516

GAS–X®
EXTRA STRENGTH GAS-X®
Antiflatulent, Anti-Gas Chewable Tablets
Extra Strength Softgels

Active Ingredients: GAS-X®—Each chewable tablet contains 80 mg. simethicone.
EXTRA STRENGTH GAS-X®—Each chewable tablets and Softgels contain 125 mg. simethicone.

Inactive Ingredients: Chewables: calcium phosphates tribasic, calcium carbonate, colloidal silicon dioxide, microcrystalline cellulose, maltodextrin dextrose, flavors. GAS-X cherry creme flavored tablets also contain Red 30. Extra Strength GAS-X peppermint creme and Extra Strength GAS-X cherry creme flavored tablets also contain Red 30 and Yellow 10.
Softgels: Blue #1, gelatin, glycerin, peppermint oil, Red #40, sorbitol, titanium dioxide, water, Yellow #10.

Indications: For relief of the pain and pressure symptoms of excess gas in the digestive tract, which is often accompanied by complaints of bloating, distention, fullness, pressure, pain, cramps or excess anal flatus.

Actions: GAS-X acts in the stomach and intestines to disperse and reduce the formation of mucus-trapped gas bubbles. The GAS-X defoaming action reduces the surface tension of gas bubbles so that they are more easily eliminated.

Warning: Keep this and all drugs out of the reach of children.

Drug Interaction Precautions: No known drug interaction.

Dosage and Administration: Adults: Chew thoroughly and swallow one or two tablets as needed after meals and at bedtime. Do not exceed six GAS-X tablets or four EXTRA STRENGTH GAS-X tablets in 24 hours. Do not increase dosage unless recommended by your physician.
For Extra Strength GAS-X Softgels: swallow whole with water, follow dosing instructions for Extra Strength Gas-X Chewables.

Professional Labeling: GAS-X may be used in the alleviation of postoperative gas pain, and for use in endoscopic examination.

How Supplied: GAS-X Chewable tablets are available in peppermint creme and cherry creme flavored, chewable, scored tablets in boxes of 36 tablets and 12 tablets.
EXTRA STRENGTH GAS-X Chewable tablets are available in peppermint creme and cherry creme flavored, chewable, scored tablets in boxes of 18 tablets and 48 tablets.
Extra Strength Gas-X Softgels are available in easy-to-swallow softgels in boxes of 10 pills and 30 pills.
Shown in Product Identification Guide, page 516

TAVIST-1® TABLETS

Description: Active Ingredients: clemastine fumarate, USP 1.34 mg (equivalent to 1 mg clemastine). **Inactive Ingredients:** lactose, povidone, starch, stearic acid, and talc.

Indications: Temporarily reduces runny nose and relieves sneezing, itching of the nose or throat, and itchy, watery eyes due to hay fever or other upper respiratory allergies.

Warnings: May cause drowsiness; alcohol, sedatives, and tranquilizers may increase the drowsiness effect. Avoid alcoholic beverages while taking this product. Do not take this product if you are taking sedatives or tranquilizers without first consulting your doctor. Use caution when driving a motor vehicle or operating machinery. May cause excitability especially in children. Do not take this

Continued on next page

Sandoz—Cont.

product if you have glaucoma, a breathing problem such as emphysema or chronic bronchitis, or difficulty in urination due to enlargement of the prostate gland unless directed by a doctor. As with any drug, if you are pregnant or nursing a baby, seek the advice of a health professional before using this product. Keep this and all drugs out of reach of children. In case of accidental overdose, seek professional assistance or contact a Poison Control Center immediately.

Directions: Adults and children 12 years of age and over: Take one tablet every 12 hours, not to exceed 2 tablets in 24 hours, or as directed by a doctor. Children under 12 years of age: Consult a doctor.

How Supplied: Tavist-1 tablets (white) imprinted "Tavist-1" on both sides in blister packs of 8, 16, and 32.

Shown in Product Identification Guide, page 516

TAVIST-D® TABLETS

Description: Active Ingredients: clemastine fumarate, USP 1.34 mg (equivalent to 1 mg clemastine) immediate release and 75 mg phenylpropanolamine hydrochloride, USP extended release. **Inactive Ingredients:** Colloidal silicon dioxide, dibasic calcium phosphate, lactose, magnesium stearate, methylcellulose, polyethylene glycol, povidone, starch, synthetic polymers, titanium dioxide and Yellow 10.

Indications: For the temporary relief of nasal congestion associated with upper respiratory allergies or sinusitis when accompanied by other symptoms of hay fever or allergies, including runny nose, sneezing, itchy nose or throat or itchy, watery eyes.

Warnings: May cause drowsiness; alcohol, sedatives, and tranquilizers may increase the drowsiness effect. Avoid alcoholic beverages while taking this product. Do not take this product if you are taking sedatives or tranquilizers without first consulting your doctor. Use caution when driving a motor vehicle or operating machinery. May cause excitability especially in children. **Do not exceed recommended dosage because at higher doses nervousness, dizziness, or sleepiness may occur.** Do not take this product for more than 7 days. If symptoms do not improve or are accompanied by fever, consult a doctor. Do not take this product if you have heart disease, high blood pressure, thyroid disease, diabetes, glaucoma, a breathing problem such as emphysema or chronic bronchitis, or difficulty in urination due to enlargement of the prostate gland unless directed by a doctor. As with any drug, if you are pregnant or nursing a baby, seek the advice of a health profes-

sional before using this product. Keep this and all drugs out of reach of children. In case of accidental overdose, seek professional assistance or contact a Poison Control Center immediately.

Drug Interaction Precaution: Do not take this product if you are presently taking a decongestant or prescription drug for high blood pressure or depression, without first consulting your doctor.

Directions: Adults and children 12 years of age and over: Take one tablet swallowed whole every 12 hours, not to exceed 2 tablets in 24 hours, or as directed by a doctor. Children under 12 years of age: Consult a doctor.

How Supplied: Tavist-D tablets (white) imprinted "Tavist-D" on both sides, in blister packs of 8, 16, and 32; and Bottles of 50

Shown in Product Identification Guide, page 517

THERAFLU®
Flu and Cold Medicine
Flu, Cold & Cough Medicine

Description: Each packet of TheraFlu Flu and Cold Medicine contains: acetaminophen 650 mg, pseudoephedrine hydrochloride 60 mg, and chlorpheniramine maleate 4 mg. Each packet of TheraFlu Flu, Cold & Cough Medicine also contains dextromethorphan hydrobromide 20 mg. Other ingredients: ascorbic acid (vitamin C), citric acid, natural lemon flavors, pregelatinized starch, silicon dioxide, sodium citrate, sucrose, titanium dioxide, tribasic calcium phosphate, Yellow 6, and Yellow 10.

Indications: Provides temporary relief of the symptoms associated with flu, common cold and other upper respiratory infections including: headache, body aches, fever, minor sore throat pain, nasal and sinus congestion, runny nose and sneezing. TheraFlu Flu, Cold & Cough Medicine also suppresses coughs due to minor throat and bronchial irritation.

Warnings: Keep this and all drugs out of the reach of children. In case of accidental overdose, seek professional assistance or contact a poison control center immediately. Prompt medical attention is critical for adults as well as children even if you do not notice any signs or symptoms.
Do not exceed recommended dosage. If nervousness, dizziness, or sleeplessness occur, discontinue use and consult a doctor. If symptoms do not improve within 7 days or are accompanied by fever, consult a doctor. May cause excitability especially in children. Do not take this product if you have heart disease, high blood pressure, thyroid disease, diabetes, glaucoma, a breathing problem such as emphysema or chronic bronchitis, or difficulty in urination due to enlargement of the prostate gland, unless directed by a doctor.

Do not take this product for pain for more than 10 days or for fever for more than 3 days unless directed by a doctor. If pain or fever persists or gets worse, if new symptoms occur, or if redness or swelling is present, consult a doctor because these could be signs of a serious condition. If sore throat is severe, persists for more than 2 days, is accompanied or followed by fever, headache, rash, nausea, or vomiting, consult a doctor promptly.

May cause marked drowsiness; alcohol, sedatives, and tranquilizers may increase the drowsiness effect. Avoid alcoholic beverages while taking this product. Do not take this product if you are taking sedatives or tranquilizers, without first consulting your doctor. Use caution when driving a motor vehicle or operating machinery.

A persistent cough may be a sign of a serious condition. If cough persists for more than 1 week, tends to recur, or is accompanied by a fever, rash, or persistent headache, consult a doctor. Do not take the Flu, Cold & Cough formula for persistent or chronic cough such as occurs with smoking, asthma, or emphysema, or if cough is accompanied by excessive phlegm (mucus) unless directed by a doctor.

As with any drug, if you are pregnant or nursing a baby, seek the advice of a health professional before using this product.

Drug Interaction Precaution: Do not take this product if you are now taking a prescription monoamine oxidase inhibitor (MAOI) (certain drugs for depression, psychiatric or emotional conditions, or Parkinson's disease), or for 2 weeks after stopping the MAOI drug. If you are uncertain whether your prescription drug contains an MAOI, consult a health professional before taking this product.

Directions: Adults and children 12 years of age and over—dissolve one packet in 6 oz. hot water; sip while hot. One packet every 4 to 6 hours, not to exceed 4 packets in 24 hours, or as directed by a doctor. Children under 12 years of age: consult a doctor. **Microwave heating instructions:** Add contents of packet and 6 oz. of cool water to a microwave-safe cup and stir briskly. Microwave on high 1½ minutes or until hot. Do not boil water or overheat, and remember to stir liquid between reheatings. Sweeten to taste if desired.

How Supplied: TheraFlu Flu and Cold Medicine powder in foil packets, 6 or 12 packets per carton. TheraFlu Flu, Cold & Cough Medicine powder in foil packets, 6 or 12 packets per carton.
Shown in Product Identification Guide, page 517

THERAFLU® MAXIMUM STRENGTH
Flu and Cold Medicine
For Sore Throat

Each packet of Therflu Maximum Strength Sore Throat formula contains: acetaminophen 1000 mg, pseudophedrine HCl 60 mg, chlorphenramine maleate 4 mg. **Other Ingredients:** Acesulfame K, natural apple and cinnamon flavors, ascorbic acid, aspartame, Blue 1, citric acid, maltodextrin, Red 40, silicon dioxide, sodium citrate, sucrose, tribasic calcium phosphate, and Yellow 10.

Indications: Provides temporary relief of minor sore throat pain, body aches, pains, and headaches and reduces fever. Temporarily relieves runny nose, sneezing and nasal congestion due to flu, the common cold, hay fever or other upper respiratory allergies.

Warnings: Keep this and all drugs out of the reach of children. In case of accidental overdose, contact a doctor or a poison control center immediately. Prompt medical attention is critical for adults as well as children even if you do not notice any signs or symptoms. **DO NOT EXCEED RECOMMENDED DOSAGE.** If nervousness, dizziness, or sleeplessness occur, discontinue use and consult a doctor. If symptoms do not improve within 7 days or are accompanied by fever, consult a doctor. May cause excitability, especially in children. Do not take this product if you have heart disease, high blood pressure, thyroid disease, diabetes, glaucoma, a breathing problem such as emphysema or chronic bronchitis, or difficulty in urination due to enlargement of the prostate gland, unless directed by a doctor. Unless directed by a doctor, do not take this product for fever for more than 3 days. If pain or fever persists or gets worse, if new symptoms occur, or if redness or swelling is present, consult a doctor because these could be signs of a serious condition. If sore throat is severe, persists for more than 2 days, is accompanied or followed by fever, headache, rash, nausea, or vomiting, consult a doctor promptly. May cause drowsiness. Alcohol, sedatives and tranquilizers may increase the drowsiness effect. Avoid alcoholic beverages while taking this product. Do not take this product if you are taking sedatives or tranquilizers without first consulting your doctor. Use caution when driving a motor vehicle or operating machinery. As with any drug, if you are pregnant or nursing a baby, seek the advice of a health professional before using this product.

Drug Interaction Precaution: Do not use this product if you are now taking a prescription monoamine oxidase inhibitor [MAOI] (certain drugs for depression, psychiatric or emotional conditions, or Parkinson's Disease), or for 2 weeks after stopping the MAOI drug. If you are uncertain whether your prescription drug contains an MAOI, consult a health professional before taking this product. Phenylketonurics: Contains Phenylalanine 25 mg per adult dose.

Directions: Adults and children 12 years of age and over: Dissolve one packet in 6 oz. of hot water; sip while hot. **Microwave Heating Instructions:** Add contents of packet and 6 oz. of cool water to a microwave-safe cup and stir briskly. Microwave on high 1 ½ minutes or until hot. Do not boil water or overheat, and remember to stir liquid between reheatings.
Sweeten to taste if desired. May repeat every 6 hours, but not to exceed 4 doses in 24 hours.

How Supplied: Theraflu Maximum Strength flu and Cold Medicine for Sore Throat powder in foil packets, 6 packets per carton.

Shown in Product Identification Guide, page 517

THERAFLU®
MAXIMUM STRENGTH NIGHTTIME
Flu, Cold & Cough Medicine

Description: Each packet of TheraFlu Maximum Strength Nighttime Flu, Cold & Cough Medicine contains: acetaminophen 1000 mg, dextromethorphan HBr 30 mg, pseudoephedrine HCl 60 mg, and chlorpheniramine maleate 4 mg. Other ingredients: ascorbic acid (Vitamin C), citric acid, natural lemon flavors, maltol, pregelatinized starch, silicon dioxide, sodium citrate, sucrose, titanium dioxide, tribasic calcium phosphate, Yellow 6 and Yellow 10.

Indications: Provides temporary relief of the symptoms associated with flu, common cold and other upper respiratory infections including: headache, body aches, fever, minor sore throat pain, nasal and sinus congestion, runny nose and sneezing. TheraFlu Maximum Strength Flu, Cold, & Cough Medicine also suppresses coughs due to minor throat and bronchial irritation.

Warnings: Keep this and all drugs out of the reach of children. In case of accidental overdose, seek professional assistance or contact a poison control center immediately. Prompt medical attention is critical for adults as well as children even if you do not notice any signs or symptoms. **Do not exceed recommended dosage.** If nervousness, dizziness, or sleeplessness occur, discontinue use and consult a doctor. If symptoms do not improve within 7 days or are accompanied by fever, consult a doctor. May cause excitability, especially in children. Do not take this product if you have heart disease, high blood pressure, thyroid disease, diabetes, glaucoma, a breathing problem such as emphysema or chronic bronchitis, or difficulty in urination due to enlargement of the prostate gland, unless directed by a doctor. A persistent cough may be a sign of a serious condition. If cough persists for more than 1 week, tends to recur, or is accompanied by a fever, rash, or persistent headache, consult a doctor. Do not take this product for persistent or chronic cough such as occurs with smoking, asthma, or emphysema, or if cough is accompanied by excessive phlegm (mucus) unless directed by a doctor.
Do not take this product for pain for more than 10 days or for fever for more than 3 days unless directed by a doctor. If pain or fever persists or gets worse, if new symptoms occur, or if redness or swelling is present, consult a doctor because these could be signs of a serious condition. If sore throat is severe, persists for more than 2 days, is accompanied or followed by fever, headache, rash, nausea, or vomiting, consult a doctor promptly.
May cause marked drowsiness; alcohol, sedatives, and tranquilizers may increase the drowsiness effect. Avoid alcoholic beverages while taking this product. Do not take this product if you are taking sedatives or tranquilizers, without first consulting your doctor. Use caution when driving a motor vehicle or operating machinery.
As with any drug, if you are pregnant or nursing a baby, seek the advice of a health professional before using this product.

Drug Interaction Precaution: Do not use this product if you are now taking a prescription monoamine oxidase inhibitor [MAOI] (certain drugs for depression, psychiatric or emotional conditions, or Parkinson's disease), or for 2 weeks after stopping the MAOI drug. If you are uncertain whether your prescription drug contains an MAOI, consult a health professional before taking this product.

Directions: Adults and children 12 years of age and over: Dissolve contents of one packet in 6 oz. cup of hot water. Sip while hot. One packet every 6 hours, not to exceed 4 packets in 24 hours, or as directed by a doctor. Children under 12 years of age: consult a doctor. Microwave heating instructions: Add contents of packet and 6 oz. of cool water to a microwave-safe cup and stir briskly. Microwave on high 1½ minutes or until water is hot. Do not boil water or overheat, and remember to stir liquid between reheatings. Sweeten to taste if desired.

How Supplied: TheraFlu Maximum Strength Nighttime Flu, Cold, & Cough Medicine powder in foil packets, 6, or 12, or 18 packets per carton.

Shown in Product Identification Guide, page 517

THERAFLU®
MAXIMUM STRENGTH
NON-DROWSY FORMULA
Flu, Cold & Cough Medicine

Description: Each packet of TheraFlu Maximum Strength Non-Drowsy Formula contains: acetaminophen 1000 mg,

Continued on next page

Sandoz—Cont.

dextromethorphan 30 mg, pseudoephedrine HCl 60 mg. Other Ingredients: ascorbic acid (Vitamin C), citric acid, natural lemon flavors, maltol, pregelatinized starch, silicon dioxide, sodium citrate, sucrose, titanium dioxide, tribasic calcium phosphate, Yellow 6 and Yellow 10.

Indications: Provides temporary relief of the symptoms associated with flu, common cold, and other upper respiratory infections including: headache, body aches, fever, minor sore throat pain, nasal and sinus congestion. TheraFlu Maximum Strength Non-Drowsy Formula also suppresses coughs due to minor throat and bronchial irritation.

Warnings: Keep this and all drugs out of the reach of children. In case of accidental overdose, seek professional assistance or contact a poison control center immediately. Prompt medical attention is critical for adults as well as children even if you do not notice any signs or symptoms. **Do not exceed recommended dosage.** If nervousness, dizziness, or sleeplessness occur, discontinue use and consult a doctor. If symptoms do not improve within 7 days or are accompanied by fever, consult a doctor. Do not take this product if you have heart disease, high blood pressure, thyroid disease, diabetes, or difficulty in urination due to enlargement of the prostate gland unless directed by a physician.
A persistent cough may be a sign of a serious condition. If cough persists for more than 1 week, tends to recur, or is accompanied by a fever, rash, or persistent headache, consult a doctor. Do not take this product for persistent or chronic cough such as occurs with smoking, asthma, or emphysema, or if cough is accompanied by excessive phlegm (mucus) unless directed by a doctor.
Do not take this product for pain for more than 10 days or for fever for more than 3 days unless directed by a doctor. If pain or fever persists or gets worse, if new symptoms occur, or if redness or swelling is present, consult a doctor, because these could be signs of a serious condition. If sore throat is severe, persists for more than 2 days, is accompanied or followed by fever, headache, rash, nausea, or vomiting, consult a doctor promptly.
As with any drug, if you are pregnant or nursing a baby, seek the advice of a health professional before using this product.

Drug Interaction Precaution: Do not take this product if you are now taking a prescription monoamine oxidase inhibitor (MAOI) (certain drugs for depression, psychiatric or emotional conditions, or Parkinson's disease), or for 2 weeks after stopping the MAOI drug. If you are uncertain whether your prescription drug contains an MAOI, consult a health professional before taking this product.

Directions: Adults and children 12 years of age and over: Dissolve one packet in 6 oz. cup of hot water; sip while hot. One packet every 6 hours, not to exceed 4 packets in 24 hours, or as directed by a doctor. Children under 12 years of age: consult a doctor. Microwave Heating Instructions: Add contents of packet and 6 oz. of cool water to a microwave-safe cup and stir briskly. Microwave on high 1 1/2 minutes or until hot. Do not boil or overheat, and remember to stir liquid between reheatings. Sweeten to taste if desired.

Shown in Product Identification Guide, page 517

THERAFLU® MAXIMUM STRENGTH NON-DROWSY FORMULA CAPLETS

Description: Each TheraFlu Maximum Strength Non-Drowsy caplet contains: Acetaminophen 500 mg, dextromethorphan HBr 15 mg, and pseudoephedrine HCl 30 mg. Other ingredients: colloidal silicon dioxide, croscarmellose sodium, gelatin, hydroxypropyl cellulose, hydroxpropyl methylcellulose, lactose, magnesium stearate, methylparaben, polydextrose, polyethylene glycol, pregelatinized starch, Red 40, titanium dioxide, triacetin, Yellow 6, Yellow 10.

Indications: Provides temporary relief of the symptoms associated with flu, common cold, and other upper respiratory allergies including: headache, body aches, fever, minor sore throat pain, nasal and sinus congestion. TheraFlu Maximum Strength Non-Drowsy Formula Caplets also suppress coughs due to minor throat and bronchial irritation.

Warnings: Keep this and all drugs out of the reach of children. In case of accidental overdose, seek professional assistance or contact a poison control center immediately. Prompt medical attention is critical for adults as well as children even if you do not notice any signs or symptoms. **Do not exceed recommended dosage.** If nervousness, dizziness or sleeplessness occur, discontinue use and consult a doctor. If symptoms do not improve within 7 days or are accompanied by fever, consult a doctor. Do not take this product if you have heart disease, high blood pressure, thyroid disease, diabetes, or difficulty in urination due to enlargement of the prostate gland, unless directed by a doctor.
A persistent cough may be a sign of a serious condition. If cough persists for more than 1 week, tends to recur, or is accompanied by fever, rash, or persistent headache, consult a doctor. Do not take this product for persistent or chronic cough such as occurs with smoking, asthma, emphysema, or if cough is accompanied by excessive phlegm (mucus) unless directed by a doctor.
Do not take this product for pain for more than 10 days or for fever for more than 3 days unless directed by a doctor. If pain or fever persists or gets worse, if new symptoms occur, or if redness or swelling is present, consult a doctor because these could be signs of a serious condition. If sore throat is severe, persists for more than 2 days, is accompanied or followed by fever, headache, rash, nausea, or vomiting, consult a doctor promptly.
As with any drug, if you are pregnant or nursing a baby, seek the advice of a health professional before using this product.

Drug Interaction Precaution: Do not use this product if you are now taking a prescription monoamine oxidase inhibitor [MAOI] (certain drugs for depression, psychiatric or emotional conditions, or Parkinson's disease), or for 2 weeks after stopping the MAOI drug. If you are uncertain whether your prescription drug contains an MAOI, consult a health professional before taking this product.

Directions: Adults and children 12 years of age and over: Two caplets every 6 hours, not to exceed eight caplets in 24 hours. Children under 12 years of age—Consult a doctor.

How Supplied: TheraFlu Maximum Strength Non-Drowsy Formula gelatin film coated caplets (yellow) in blister packs of 12 and 24.

Shown in Product Identification Guide, page 517

THERAFLU® MAXIMUM STRENGTH SINUS NON-DROWSY FORMULA

Description: Each Theraflu Maximum Strength Sinus Non-Drowsy formula caplet contains: 500 mg acetaminophen and 30 mg pseudoephedrine HCl.
Other Ingredients: Colloidal silicon dioxide, croscarmellose sodium, hydroxypropyl cellulose, lactose, magnesium stearate, methylcellulose, methylparaben, polyethylene glycol, povidone, pregelatinized starch, titanium dioxide.

Indications: Each dose provides the maximum allowable levels of these active ingredients in easy-to-swallow coated caplets for temporary relief of these symptoms without drowsiness: Sinus Pain & Headache (Analgesic—acetaminophen 500 mg per caplets). Nasal and Sinus Congestion Pressure (Nasal Decongestant—pseudoephedrin HCl, 30 mg per caplet).

Warnings: Keep this and all drugs out of the reach of children. In case of accidental overdose, contact a doctor or poison control center immediately. Prompt medical attention is critical for adults as well as children even if you do not notice any signs or symptoms.
Do not exceed recommended dosage. If nervousness, dizziness or sleeplessness occur, discontinue use and consult a doctor. If symptoms do not improve within 7 days or are accompanied by fever, consult a doctor. Do not take this product if you have heart disease, high blood pressure, thyroid disease, diabetes or diffi-

culty in urination due to enlargement of the prostate gland, unless directed by a doctor. Do not take this product for pain for more than 10 days or for fever for more than 3 days unless directed by a doctor. If pain or fever persists or gets worse, if new symptoms occur, or if redness or swelling is present, consult a doctor because these could be signs of a serious condition. As with any drug, if you are pregnant or nursing a baby, seek the advice of a health professional before using this product.

Drug Interaction Precaution: Do not use this product if you are now taking a prescription monoamine oxidase inhibitor [MAOI] (certain drugs for depression, psychiatric or emotional conditions or Parkinson's Disease), or for 2 weeks after stopping the MAOI drug. If you are uncertain whether your prescription drug contain an MAOI, consult a health professional before taking this product. Store in a dry place at controlled room temperature 15°–30°C (59°–86°F).

Directions: Adults and children 12 years of age and over: Two caplets every six hours, not to exceed eight caplets in 24 hours. Children under 12 years of age: Consult a doctor.

How Supplied: Theraflu Maximum Strength Sinus gelatin coated caplets (white) in blister packs of 24.
Shown in Product Identification Guide, page 517

TRIAMINIC® AM COUGH AND DECONGESTANT FORMULA

Description: Each teaspoonful (5 ml) of TRIAMINIC AM COUGH AND DECONGESTANT FORMULA contains: pseudoephedrine hydrochloride, USP 15 mg and dextromethorphan hydrobromide, USP 7.5 mg in a palatable, orange flavored, dye-free, non-drowsy, alcohol-free liquid. Other ingredients: Benzoic acid, citric acid, dibasic sodium phosphate, edetate disodium, flavors, propylene glycol, purified water, sorbitol, sucrose.

Indications: Temporarily quiets coughs due to minor throat and bronchial irritations and relieves stuffy noses.

Warnings: Keep this and all drugs out of the reach of children. In case of accidental overdose, seek professional assistance or contact a Poison Control Center immediately.
Do not exceed recommended dosage. If nervousness, dizziness, or sleeplessness occur, discontinue use and consult a doctor. If symptoms do not improve within 7 days or are accompanied by fever, consult a doctor. Do not take this product if you have heart disease, high blood pressure, thyroid disease, diabetes, or difficulty in urination due to enlargement of the prostate gland, unless directed by a doctor.
A persistent cough may be a sign of a serious condition. If cough persists for

more than 1 week, tends to recur, or is accompanied by fever, rash or persistent headache, consult a doctor. Do not take this product for persistent or chronic cough such as occurs with smoking, asthma, or emphysema or if cough is accompanied by excessive phlegm (mucus) unless directed by doctor.
As with any drug, if you are pregnant or nursing a baby, seek the advice of a health professional before using this product.

Drug Interaction Precaution: Do not use this product if you are now taking a prescription monoamine oxidase inhibitor (MAOI) (certain drugs for depression, psychiatric or emotional conditions, or Parkinson's disease) or for 2 weeks after stopping the MAOI drug. If you are uncertain whether your prescription drug contains an MAOI, consult a health professional before taking this product.

Dosage and Administration: Adults and children 12 and over (96+ lbs)—4 teaspoons every 6 hours. Children 6 to under 12 years (48–95 lbs)—2 teaspoons every 6 hours. Children 2 to under 6 years (24–47 lbs)—1 teaspoon every 6 hours. Do not exceed 4 doses in 24 hours, or as directed by a doctor. Dosing to children under 2 years of age is to be under the direction of a physician. For convenience, a True-Dose® dosage cup is provided with each 4 fl. oz. and 8 fl. oz. bottle.
Professional Labeling: The suggested dosage for pediatric patients is:

4–12 months	1.25 ml (1/4 tsp)	
(12–17 lbs)	every 6 hours	
12–24 months	2.5 ml (1/2 tsp)	
(18–23 lbs)	every 6 hours	

Do not exceed 4 doses in 24 hours.

How Supplied: TRIAMINIC AM COUGH AND DECONGESTANT FORMULA (clear liquid) in 4 fl. oz. and 8 fl. oz. plastic bottles with tamper-evident band around child-resistant cap. Orange flavored. Alcohol-free. Dye-free. Non-drowsy.
Shown in Product Identification Guide, page 517

TRIAMINIC® AM DECONGESTANT FORMULA

Description: Each teaspoonful (5 ml) of TRIAMINIC AM DECONGESTANT FORMULA contains: Pseudoephedrine hydrochloride, USP 15 mg. in a palatable, orange flavored, dye-free, non-drowsy, alcohol-free liquid. Other ingredients: Benzoic acid, edetate disodium, flavors, purified water, sodium hydroxide, sorbitol, sucrose

Indications: For temporary relief of nasal congestion due to the common cold, hay fever or upper respiratory allergies, or associated with sinusitis. Reduces swelling of nasal passages; shrinks swollen membranes.

Warnings: Keep this and all drugs out of the reach of children. In case of accidental overdose, seek professional assis-

tance or contact a Poison Control Center immediately.
Do not exceed recommended dosage. If nervousness, dizziness, or sleeplessness occur, discontinue use and consult a doctor. If symptoms do not improve within 7 days or are accompanied by fever, consult a doctor. Do not take this product if you have heart disease, high blood pressure, thyroid disease, diabetes, or difficulty in urination due to enlargement of the prostate gland, unless directed by a doctor.
As with any drug, if you are pregnant or nursing a baby, seek the advice of a health professional before using this product.

Drug Interaction Precaution: Do not use this product if you are now taking a prescription monoamine oxidase inhibitor (MAOI) (certain drugs for depression, psychiatric or emotional conditions, or Parkinson's disease) or for 2 weeks after stopping the MAOI drug. If you are uncertain whether your prescription drug contains an MAOI, consult a health professional before taking this product.

Dosage and Administration: Adults and children 12 and over (96+ lbs)—4 teaspoons every 4–6 hours. Children 6 to under 12 years (48–95 lbs)—2 teaspoons every 4–6 hours. Children 2 to under 6 years (24–47 lbs)—1 teaspoon every 4–6 hours. Do not exceed 4 doses in 24 hours, or as directed by a doctor. Dosing to children under 2 years of age is to be under the direction of a physician. For convenience, a True-Dose® dosage cup is provided with each 4 fl. oz. and 8 fl. oz. bottle.
Professional Labeling: The suggested dosage for pediatric patients is:

4–12 months	1.25 ml (1/4 tsp)	
(12–17 lbs)	every 4 to 6 hours	
12–24 months	2.5 ml (1/2 tsp)	
(18–23 lbs)	every 4 to 6 hours	

Do not exceed 4 doses in 24 hours.

How Supplied: TRIAMINIC AM DECONGESTANT FORMULA (clear liquid) in 4 fl oz and 8 fl oz plastic bottles with tamper-evident band around child-resistant cap. Orange flavored. Alcohol-free. Dye-free. Non-drowsy.
Shown in Product Identification Guide, page 517

TRIAMINIC® EXPECTORANT
[trī"ah-mĭn'ĭc]

Description: Each teaspoonful (5 ml) of TRIAMINIC Expectorant contains: guaifenesin, USP 50 mg, and phenylpropanolamine hydrochloride, USP 6.25 mg in a palatable, citrus-flavored alcohol-free liquid. Other ingredients: benzoic acid, edetate disodium, flavors, glycerin, polyethylene glycol, propylene glycol, purified water, sorbitol, sucrose, Yellow 6, Yellow 10.

Indications: Relieves chest congestion by loosening phlegm to help clear bron-

Continued on next page

Sandoz—Cont.

chial passageways. Temporarily relieves stuffy nose.

Warnings: Keep this and all drugs out of the reach of children. In case of accidental overdose, seek professional assistance or contact a Poison Control Center immediately.

Do not exceed recommended dosage. If nervousness, dizziness, or sleeplessness occur, discontinue use and consult a doctor. If symptoms do not improve within 7 days or are accompanied by fever, consult a doctor. A persistent cough may be a sign of a serious condition. If cough persists for more than 1 week, tends to recur, or is accompanied by fever, rash, or persistent headache, consult a doctor. Do not take this product: 1) if cough is accompanied by excessive phlegm (mucus), 2) for persistent or chronic cough such as occurs with smoking, asthma, chronic bronchitis or emphysema. 3) if you have heart disease, high blood pressure, thyroid disease, diabetes, difficulty in urination due to enlargement of the prostate gland, or 4) if you are presently taking another product containing phenylpropanolamine, unless directed by a doctor. As with any drug, if you are pregnant or nursing a baby, seek the advice of a health professional before using this product.

Drug Interaction Precaution: Do not use this product if you are now taking a prescription monoamine oxidase inhibitor (MAOI) (certain drugs for depression, psychiatric or emotional conditions, or Parkinson's disease) or for 2 weeks after stopping the MAOI drug. If you are uncertain whether your prescription drug contains an MAOI, consult a health professional before taking this product.

Dosage and Administration: Adults and children 12 and over (96+ lbs)— 4 teaspoons every 4 hours. Children 6 to under 12 years (48–95 lbs)—2 teaspoons every 4 hours. Children 2 to under 6 years (24–47 lbs)—1 teaspoon every 4 hours. Do not exceed 6 doses in 24 hours, or as directed by a doctor. Dosing to children under 2 years of age is to be under the direction of a physician. For convenience, a True-Dose® dosage cup is provided with each 4 fl. oz. and 8 fl. oz. bottle.

Professional Labeling: The suggested dosage for pediatric patients is:
4–12 months   1.25 ml (¼ tsp)
(12–17 lbs)   every 4 hours
12–24 months   2.5 ml (½ tsp)
(18–23 lbs)   every 4 hours
Do not exceed 6 doses in 24 hours.

How Supplied: TRIAMINIC Expectorant (yellow), in 4 fl oz and 8 fl oz plastic bottles with tamper-evident band around child-resistant cap. Citrus flavored, Alcohol free.

Shown in Product Identification Guide, page 517

TRIAMINIC® INFANT
Oral Decongestant Drops

Description: Each dropperful (0.8mL) of Triaminic Infant Oral Decongestant Drops contains: pseudoephedrine hydrochloride, USP 7.5 mg in a palatable, grape-flavored alcohol-free, dye-free liquid. **Other ingredients:** benzoic acid, edetate disodium, flavors, purified water, sodium chloride, sorbitol solution, sucrose.

Indications: For temporary relief of nasal congestion due to the common cold, hay fever, other upper respiratory allergies, or nasal congestion associated with sinusitis. The decongestant is provided in an alcohol-free and antihistamine-free formula.

Warnings: Keep this and all drugs out of the reach of children. In case of accidental overdose, seek professional assistance or contact a poison control center immediately.
Do not exceed recommended dosage. If nervousness, dizziness, or sleeplessness occur, discontinue use and consult a doctor. If symptoms do not improve within 7 days or are accompanied by fever, consult a doctor. Do not give this product to a child who has heart disease, high blood pressure, thyroid disease, or diabetes unless directed by a doctor.

Drug Interaction Precaution: Do not give this product to a child who is taking a prescription monoamine oxidase inhibitor [MAOI] (certain drugs for depression, psychiatric or emotional conditions) or for 2 weeks after stopping the MAOI drug. If you are uncertain whether your child's prescription drug contains an MAOI, consult a health professional before giving this product.

Dosage and Administration: Children 2 to 3 years of age (24–35 lbs.): Two dropperfuls (1.6mL) every 4–6 hours (or as directed by a doctor). Children under 2 years of age: consult a doctor. Do not exceed 4 doses in a 24-hour period. **Give by mouth only.** Not for use in the nose. For convenience, a True-Dose® dosing child-resistant dropper is provided.
Professional Labeling: The suggested dosage for pediatric patients is:

Age	Weight	Amount
4–11 months	12–17 lbs.	1 dropperful (0.8mL)
12–23 months	18–23 lbs.	1½ dropperfuls (1.2mL)
2–3 years	24–35 lbs.	2 dropperfuls (1.6mL)

The dose may be repeated every 4 to 6 hours, not to exceed 4 doses in 24 hours or as directed by a doctor.

How Supplied: Triaminic Infant Oral Decongestant Drops (clear), in a ½ fl. oz. (15mL) glass bottle with tamper evident band around cap. True-Dose® dosing child-resistant dropper is also provided. Grape flavored, alcohol-free, antihista-mine-free, crystal clear, non-staining formula.

TRIAMINIC® Night Time
Maximum Strength
Nighttime Cough and Cold Medicine for Children
[tri "ah-min 'ic]

Description: Each teaspoonful (5 ml) of Triaminic® Night Time contains: Pseudoephedrine hydrochloride USP 15 mg, dextromethorphan hydrobromide, USP 7.5 mg, chlorpheniramine maleate, USP 1 mg, in a palatable, grape-flavored, alcohol-free liquid.
Other ingredients: Benzoic acid, Blue 1, citric acid, dibasic sodium phosphate, flavors, propylene glycol, purified water, Red 33, sorbitol, sucrose.

Indications: Temporarily relieves cold and allergy symptoms, including coughs due to minor throat and bronchial irritation, runny nose, stuffy nose, sneezing, itching nose or throat, and itchy, watery eyes.

Warnings: Keep this and all drugs out of the reach of children. In case of accidental overdose, seek professional assistance or contact a poison control center immediately.
Do not exceed recommended dosage. If nervousness, dizziness, or sleeplessness occur, discontinue use and consult a doctor. If symptoms do not improve within 7 days or are accompanied by fever, consult a doctor. A persistent cough may be a sign of a serious condition. If cough persists for more than 1 week, tends to recur, or is accompanied by fever, rash, or persistent headache, consult a doctor. Do not take this product: 1) if cough is accompanied by excessive phlegm (mucus), 2) for persistent or chronic cough such as occurs with smoking, asthma or emphysema, 3) if you have heart disease, high blood pressure, thyroid disease, diabetes, glaucoma, a breathing problem such as emphysema or chronic bronchitis, or difficulty in urination due to enlargement of the prostate gland, or 4) if you are taking sedatives or tranquilizers, unless directed by a doctor. May cause excitability especially in children. May cause drowsiness; alcohol, sedatives or tranquilizers may increase the drowsiness effect. Avoid alcoholic beverages while taking this product. Use caution when driving a motor vehicle or operating machinery. As with any drug, if you are pregnant or nursing a baby, seek the advice of a health professional before using this product.

Drug Interaction Precaution: Do not use this product if you are now taking a prescription monoamine oxidase inhibitor (MAOI) (certain drugs for depression, psychiatric or emotional conditions, or Parkinson's disease) or for 2 weeks after stopping the MAOI drug. If you are uncertain whether your prescription drug contains an MAOI, consult a health professional before taking this product.

Dosage and Administration: Adults and children 12 and over (96+ lbs.)—4 teaspoons every 6 hours. Children 6 to under 12 years (48–95 lbs.)—2 teaspoons every 6 hours. Do not exceed 4 doses in 24 hours, or as directed by a doctor. Dosing to children under 6 years of age is to be under the direction of a physician. For convenience, a True-Dose® dosage cup is provided with each 4 fl. oz. and 8 fl. oz. bottle.

Professional Labeling: The suggested dosage for pediatric patients is:

4 to under 12 months (12–17 lbs.)	¼ teaspoon or 1.25 ml	every 6 hours
12 months to under 2 years (18–23 lbs.)	½ teaspoon or 2.5 ml	every 6 hours
2 to under 6 years	1 teaspoon or 5 ml	every 6 hours

Not to exceed 4 doses in 24 hours

How Supplied: Triaminic® Night Time Cough and Cold Medicine for Children (purple), in 4 fl. oz. and 8 fl. oz. plastic bottles packaged in cartons with tamper-evident band around child-resistant cap. Grape flavored. Alcohol free.
Shown in Product Identification Guide, page 517

TRIAMINIC®
Sore Throat Formula
[trī "ah-mĭn 'ĭc]

Description: Each teaspoonful (5 ml) of Triaminic Sore Throat Formula contains: acetaminophen, USP 160 mg, dextromethorphan hydrobromide, USP 7.5 mg, and pseudoephedrine hydrochloride, USP 15 mg. in a palatable, grape-flavored, alcohol-free liquid. Other ingredients: benzoic acid, Blue 1, dibasic sodium phosphate, edetate disodium, flavors, glycerin, polyethylene glycol, propylene glycol, purified water, Red 33, Red 40, sucrose, tartaric acid.

Indications: Temporarily relieves sore throat pain and other minor aches and pains, quiets coughs due to minor throat and bronchial irritations, relieves stuffy nose, and reduces fever.

Warnings: Keep this and all drugs out of the reach of children. In case of accidental overdose, seek professional assistance or contact a Poison Control Center immediately. Prompt medical attention is critical for adults as well as for children even if you do not notice any signs or symptoms.
Do not exceed recommended dosage. If nervousness, dizziness, or sleeplessness occur, discontinue use and consult a doctor. Do not take this product for more than 7 days (for adults) or 5 days (for children). Do not take for sore throat pain for more than 2 days, and for fever for more than 3 days. If pain or fever persists or gets worse, if new symptoms occur, or if redness or swelling is present, consult a doctor because these could be signs of a serious condition. If sore throat is severe,

persists for more than 2 days, is accompanied or followed by fever, headache, rash, nausea, or vomiting, consult a doctor promptly. If symptoms do not improve within 7 days or are accompanied by fever, consult a doctor. A persistent cough may be a sign of a serious condition. If cough persists for more than 1 week, tends to recur, or is accompanied by rash, persistent headache, fever that lasts for more than 3 days, or if new symptoms occur, consult a doctor. Do not take this product: 1) if cough is accompanied by excessive phlegm (mucus), 2) for persistent or chronic cough such as occurs with smoking, asthma or emphysema, or 3) if you have heart disease, high blood pressure, thyroid disease, diabetes, difficulty in urination due to enlargement of the prostate gland, unless directed by a doctor. As with any drug, if you are pregnant or nursing a baby, seek advice from a health professional before using this product.

Drug Interaction Precaution: Do not use this product if you are now taking a prescription monoamine oxidase inhibitor (MAOI) (certain drugs for depression, psychiatric or emotional conditions, or Parkinson's disease) or for 2 weeks after stopping the MAOI drug. If you are uncertain whether your prescription drug contains an MAOI, consult a health professional before taking this product.

Dosage and Administration: Adults and children 12 and over (96+lbs)—4 teaspoons every 6 hours. Children 6 to under 12 years (48–95 lbs)—2 teaspoons every 6 hours. Children 2 to under 6 years (24–47 lbs)—1 teaspoon every 6 hours. Do not exceed 4 doses in 24 hours, or as directed by a doctor. Dosing to children under 2 years of age is to be under the direction of a physician. For convenience, a True-Dose® dosage cup is provided with each 4 fl. oz and 8 fl. oz. bottle.

Professional Labeling: The suggested dosage for pediatric patients is:

4–12 months (12–17 lbs)	1.25 ml (¼ tsp)	every 6 hours
12–24 months (18–23 lbs)	2.5 ml (½ tsp)	every 6 hours
2–6 years (24–47 lbs)	5 ml (1 tsp)	every 6 hours

Do not exceed 4 doses in 24 hours.

How Supplied: Triaminic Sore Throat Formula (purple), in 4 fl. oz. and 8 fl. oz. plastic bottles with tamper-evident band around child resistant cap. Grape flavored, alcohol-free.
Shown in Product Identification Guide, page 517

TRIAMINIC® SYRUP
[trī "ah-mĭn 'ĭc]

Description: Each teaspoonful (5 ml) of TRIAMINIC Syrup contains: phenylpropanolamine hydrochloride USP 6.25 mg and chlorpheniramine maleate USP 1 mg in a palatable, orange-flavored, alcohol-free liquid. Other ingredients: benzoic acid, edetate disodium, flavors,

purified water, sodium hydroxide, sorbitol, sucrose, and Yellow No. 6.

Indications: Temporarily relieves cold and allergy symptoms, including runny nose, stuffy nose, sneezing, itching of the nose or throat, and itchy, watery eyes.

Warnings: Keep this and all drugs out of the reach of children. In case of accidental overdose, seek professional assistance or contact a Poison Control Center immediately.
Do not exceed recommended dosage. If nervousness, dizziness or sleeplessness occur, discontinue use and consult a doctor. If symptoms do not improve within 7 days or are accompanied by fever, consult a doctor. Do not take this product: 1) if you have heart disease, high blood pressure, thyroid disease, diabetes, glaucoma, a breathing problem such as emphysema or chronic bronchitis, or difficulty in urination due to enlargement of the prostate gland, 2) if you are taking sedatives or tranquilizers, or 3) if you are presently taking another product containing phenylpropanolamine, unless directed by a doctor. May cause excitability, especially in children. May cause drowsiness; alcohol, sedatives or tranquilizers may increase the drowsiness effect. Avoid alcoholic beverages while taking this product. Use caution when driving a motor vehicle or operating machinery.
As with any drug, if you are pregnant or nursing a baby, seek the advice of a health professional before using this product.

Drug Interaction Precaution: Do not use this product if you are now taking a prescription monoamine oxidase inhibitor (MAOI) (certain drugs for depression, psychiatric or emotional conditions, or Parkinson's disease) or for 2 weeks after stopping the MAOI drug. If you are uncertain whether your prescription drug contains an MAOI, consult a health professional before taking this product.

Dosage and Administration: Adults and children 12 and over (96+ lbs)— 4 teaspoons every 4 to 6 hours. Children 6 to under 12 years (48–95 lbs)—2 teaspoons every 4 to 6 hours. Do not exceed 6 doses in 24 hours, or as directed by a doctor. Dosing to children under 6 years of age is to be under the direction of a physician. For convenience, a True-Dose® dosage cup is provided with each 4 fl. oz. and 8 fl. oz. bottle.

Professional Labeling: The suggested dosage for pediatric patients is:

4–12 months (12–17 lbs)	1.25 ml (¼ tsp)	every 4 to 6 hours
12–24 months (18–23 lbs)	2.5 ml (½ tsp)	every 4 to 6 hours
2–6 years (24–47 lbs)	5 ml (1 tsp)	every 4 to 6 hours

Do not exceed 6 doses in 24 hours.

How Supplied: TRIAMINIC Syrup (orange), in 4 fl oz and 8 fl oz plastic bottles with tamper-evident band around

Continued on next page

Sandoz—Cont.

child-resistant cap. Orange flavored. Alcohol-free.

Shown in Product Identification Guide, page 517

TRIAMINIC DM® SYRUP
[trī"ah-mĭn'ĭc]

Description: Each teaspoonful (5 ml) of TRIAMINIC DM Syrup contains: phenylpropanolamine hydrochloride, USP 6.25 mg and dextromethorphan hydrobromide USP 5 mg in a palatable, berry-flavored alcohol-free liquid. Other ingredients: benzoic acid, Blue 1, flavors, propylene glycol, purified water, Red 40, sodium chloride, sorbitol, sucrose.

Indications: Temporarily quiets coughs due to minor throat and bronchial irritation, and relieves stuffy nose.

Warnings: Keep this and all drugs out of the reach of children. In case of accidental overdose, seek professional assistance or contact a Poison Control Center immediately. **Do not exceed recommended dosage.** If nervousness, dizziness, or sleeplessness occur, discontinue use and consult a doctor. If symptoms do not improve within 7 days or are accompanied by fever, consult a doctor. A persistent cough may be a sign of a serious condition. If cough persists for more than 1 week, tends to recur, or is accompanied by fever, rash, or persistent headache, consult a doctor. Do not take this product: 1) if cough is accompanied by excessive phlegm (mucus), 2) for persistent or chronic cough such as occurs with smoking, asthma or emphysema, 3) if you have heart disease, high blood pressure, thyroid disease, diabetes, difficulty in urination due to enlargement of the prostate gland, or 4) if you are presently taking another product containing phenylpropanolamine, unless directed by a doctor.
As with any drug, if you are pregnant or nursing a baby, seek the advice of a health professional before using this product.

Drug Interaction Precaution: Do not use this product if you are now taking a prescription monoamine oxidase inhibitor (MAOI) (certain drugs for depression, psychiatric or emotional conditions, or Parkinson's disease) or for 2 weeks after stopping the MAOI drug. If you are uncertain whether your prescription drug contains an MAOI, consult a health professional before taking this product.

Dosage and Administration: Adults and children 12 and over (96+ lbs)—4 teaspoons every 4 hours. Children 6 to under 12 years (48–95 lbs)—2 teaspoons every 4 hours. Children 2 to under 6 years (24–47 lbs) 1 teaspoon every 4 hours. Do not exceed 6 doses in 24 hours, or as directed by a doctor. Dosing to children under 2 years of age is to be under the direction of a physician. For conve-

nience, a True-Dose® dosage cup is provided with each 4 fl. oz. and 8 fl. oz. bottle.

Professional Labeling: The suggested dosage for pediatric patients is:
4–12 months   1.25 ml (¼ tsp)
(12–17 lbs)   every 4 hours
12–24 months   2.5 ml (½ tsp)
(18–23 lbs)   every 4 hours
Do not exceed 6 doses in 24 hours.

How Supplied: TRIAMINIC DM Syrup (dark red), in 4 fl oz and 8 fl oz plastic bottles with tamper-evident band around child-resistant cap. Berry flavored. Alcohol-free.

Shown in Product Identification Guide, page 517

TRIAMINICIN® TABLETS
[trī"ah-mĭn'ĭ-sĭn]

Description: Each tablet contains: acetaminophen 650 mg., phenylpropanolamine hydrochloride 25 mg, and chlorpheniramine maleate 4 mg. Other ingredients: colloidal silicon dioxide, croscarmellose sodium, hydroxypropyl cellulose, lactose, magnesium stearate, methylcellulose, methylparaben, polyethylene glycol, povidone, pregelatinized starch, Red 40, titanium dioxide, Yellow 10.

Indications: Temporarily relieves minor aches, pains, headache, muscular aches, and fever associated with the common cold, nasal congestion associated with sinusitis, or nasal congestion, runny nose, sneezing, itching of the nose or throat and itchy, watery eyes due to hay fever (allergic rhinitis) or other upper respiratory allergies.

Warnings: Keep this and all drugs out of the reach of children. In case of accidental overdose, seek professional assistance or contact a poison control center immediately. Prompt medical attention is critical for adults as well as children even if you do not notice any signs or symptoms. **Do not exceed recommended dosage.** If nervousness, dizziness or sleeplessness occur, discontinue use and consult a doctor. Do not take this product for pain for more than 10 days or for fever for more than 3 days unless directed by a doctor. If pain or fever persists or gets worse, if new symptoms occur, or if redness or swelling is present, consult a doctor because these could be signs of a serious condition. May cause excitability especially in children. Do not take this product if you have heart disease, high blood pressure, thyroid disease, diabetes, glaucoma, a breathing problem such as emphysema or chronic bronchitis, difficulty in urination due to enlargement of the prostate gland, or you are now taking another product containing phenylpropanolamine, unless directed by a doctor. May cause drowsiness; alcohol, sedatives and tranquilizers may increase the drowsiness effect. Avoid alcoholic beverages while taking this product. Do not take this product if you are taking sedatives or tranquilizers, without first consulting

your doctor. Use caution when driving a motor vehicle or operating machinery. As with any drug, if you are pregnant or nursing a baby, seek the advice of a health professional before using this product.

Drug interaction precaution: Do not use this product if you are now taking a prescription monoamine oxidase inhibitor (MAOI) (certain drugs for depression, psychiatric or emotional conditions, or Parkinson's disease), or for 2 weeks after stopping the MAOI drug. If you are uncertain whether your prescription drug contains an MAOI, consult a health professional before taking this product.

Directions: Adults and children 12 years of age and over: 1 tablet every 4 to 6 hours, not to exceed 6 tablets in 24 hours, or as directed by a doctor. Children under 12 years of age: consult a doctor.

How Supplied: TRIAMINICIN Tablets (yellow) imprinted "DORSEY" on one side, "TRIAMINICIN" on the other, in blister packs of 12, 24 and 48, and bottles of 100 tablets.

Shown in Product Identification Guide, page 518

TRIAMINICOL® Cold & Cough
[trī"ah-mĭn'ĭ-call]

Description: Each teaspoonful (5 ml) of TRIAMINICOL Cold & Cough contains: phenylpropanolamine hydrochloride, USP 6.25 mg, dextromethorphan hydrobromide, USP 5 mg, chlorpheniramine maleate, USP 1 mg in a palatable, cherry flavored alcohol-free liquid. Other ingredients: benzoic acid, flavor, propylene glycol, purified water, Red 40, sodium chloride, sorbitol, sucrose.

Indications: Temporarily relieves cold and allergy symptoms, including coughs due to minor throat and bronchial irritation, runny nose, stuffy nose, sneezing, itching of the nose or throat and itchy, watery eyes.

Warnings: Keep this and all drugs out of the reach of children. In case of accidental overdose, seek professional assistance or contact a Poison Control Center immediately. **Do not exceed recommended dosage.** If nervousness, dizziness, or sleeplessness occur, discontinue use and consult a doctor. If symptoms do not improve within 7 days or are accompanied by fever, consult a doctor. A persistent cough may be a sign of a serious condition. If cough persists for more than 1 week, tends to recur, or is accompanied by fever, rash, or persistent headache, consult a doctor. Do not take this product: 1) if cough is accompanied by excessive phlegm (mucus), 2) for persistent or chronic cough such as occurs with smoking, asthma or emphysema, 3) if you have heart disease, high blood pressure, thyroid disease, diabetes, glaucoma, a breathing problem such as emphysema or chronic bronchitis, or difficulty in urination due to enlargement of the prostate gland, 4) if you are presently taking another product containing, phenylpropanolamine, or 5) if you are taking sedatives or tranquilizers, unless directed by a doctor. May cause excitability, especially in children. May cause drowsiness; alcohol, sedatives and tranquilizers may increase the drowsiness effect. Avoid alcoholic beverages while taking this product. Use caution when driving a motor vehicle or operating machinery.

As with any drug, if you are pregnant or nursing a baby, seek the advice of a health professional before using this product.

Drug Interaction Precaution: Do not use this product if you are now taking a prescription monoamine oxidase inhibitor (MAOI) (certain drugs for depression, psychiatric or emotional conditions, or Parkinson's disease) or for 2 weeks after stopping the MAOI drug. If you are uncertain whether your prescription drug contains an MAOI, consult a health professional before taking this product.

Dosage and Administration: Adults and children 12 and over (96+ lbs)— 4 teaspoons every 4 to 6 hours. Children 6 to under 12 years (48–95 lbs)—2 teaspoons every 4 to 6 hours. Unless directed by physician, do not exceed 6 doses in 24 hours or give to children under 6 years of age. For convenience, a True-Dose® Dosage cup is provided with each 4 fl. oz. and 8 fl. oz. bottle.

Professional Labeling: The suggested dosage for pediatric patients is:

4–12 months	1.25 ml (¼ tsp)
(12–17 lbs)	every 4 to 6 hours
12–24 months	2.5 ml (½ tsp)
(18–23 lbs)	every 4 to 6 hours
2–6 years	5 ml (1 tsp)
(24–47 lbs)	every 4 to 6 hours

Do not exceed 4 doses in 24 hours

How Supplied: TRIAMINICOL (red), in 4 fl oz and 8 fl oz plastic bottles with tamper-evident band around child-resistant cap. Cherry flavored. Alcohol-free.
Shown in Product Identification Guide, page 517

Scandinavian Natural Health & Beauty Products, Inc.
Scandinavian Pharmaceuticals, Inc.
**13 NORTH SEVENTH STREET
PERKASIE, PA 18944**

Direct Inquiries to:
Catherine Peklak
(215) 453-2505

**SALIX SST Lozenges
Saliva Stimulant**

Active Ingredients: Sorbitol, malic acid, sodium citrate, dicalcium phosphate, citric acid.

Indications and Usage: SALIX is an aid for mild oral dryness or severe xerostomia conditions such as in autoimmune conditions/Sjogren's, post-irradiation or side effect from dozens of medications. Also helpful in oral candidiasis. Helps defend against dental and denture wear, caries, gum disease, halitosis, swallowing difficulties, reduced oral defense.... SALIX helps provide a regulated stimulation to salivary glands with buffering action to protect the teeth and balance the oral ph.
Note: Primary or secondary saliva cells must be functioning to some degree. The acidic content, although quickly buffered, may irritate conditions of active localized oral tissue inflammation.

Dosage: As needed or up to 1 per hour in severe xerostomia conditions.

**Schering-Plough HealthCare Products
LIBERTY CORNER, NJ 07938**

Direct Product Requests to:
Public Relations
(908) 604-1836

For Medical Emergencies Contact:
Clinical Department
(901) 320-2998

A AND D® MEDICATED DIAPER RASH OINTMENT

Description: An ointment containing White Petrolatum and Zinc Oxide. Also contains: Benzoic Acid, Benzyl Alcohol, Cholecalciferol, Cod Liver Oil, Cyclomethicone, Glyceryl Monostearate, Light Mineral Oil, Magnesium Aluminum Silicate, Ozokerite, Propylparaben.

Indications: Helps treat and prevent diaper rash. Protects chafed skin due to diaper rash and helps seal out wetness. Also for the temporary protection of minor burns, chafed skin, and abrasions.

Directions: Change wet and soiled diapers promptly, cleanse the diaper area and allow to dry. Apply ointment liberally as often as necessary, with each diaper change, especially at bedtime or anytime when exposure to wet diapers may be prolonged.
Warning: For external use only. Avoid contact with eyes. If condition worsens or does not improve within 7 days, consult a doctor. Keep this and all drugs out of the reach of children. In case of accidental ingestion, seek professional assistance or contact a Poison Control Center immediately.

How Supplied: A and D® Medicated Ointment is available in 1 ½-ounce (42.5g) and 4-ounce (113g) tubes.
Store between 15° and 25°C (59° and 77°F).
Shown in Product Identification Guide, page 518

A and D® Ointment

Description: An ointment containing the emollients, lanolin and petrolatum. Also contains: Cholecalciferol, Fish Liver Oil, Fragrance, Mineral Oil, Paraffin.

Indications: *Diaper rash—***A and D Ointment** provides prompt, soothing relief for diaper rash and helps heal baby's tender skin; forms a moisture-proof shield that helps protect against urine and detergent irritants; comforts baby's skin and helps prevent chafing. *Chafed Skin—***A and D Ointment** helps skin retain its vital natural moisture; quickly soothes chafed skin in adults and children and helps prevent abnormal dryness. *Abrasions and Minor Burns—***A and D Ointment** soothes and helps relieve the smarting and pain of abrasions and minor burns, encourages healing and prevents dressings from sticking to the injured area.

Warning: Keep this and all drugs out of the reach of children. In case of accidental ingestion, seek professional assistance or contact a poison control center immediately.

Dosage and Administration: Apply as needed or consult your physician.

How Supplied: A and D Ointment is available in 1½-ounce (42.5 g) and 4-ounce (113 g) tubes and 1-pound (454 g) jars and 2.5 oz. pumps.
Shown in Product Identification Guide, page 518

AFRIN®
[a 'frin]
**Nasal Spray 0.05%
Nasal Spray Pump 0.05%
Sinus Nasal Spray 0.05%
Cherry Scented Nasal Spray 0.05%
Menthol Nasal Spray 0.05%
Extra Moisturizing Nasal Spray 0.05%
Nose Drops 0.05%**

Description: AFRIN products contain oxymetazoline hydrochloride, the longest acting topical nasal decongestant available.
Each mL of **AFRIN Nasal Spray, Nasal Spray Pump, and Nose Drops** contains Oxymetazoline Hydrochloride, 0.05%.
Also contains: Benzalkonium Chloride,

Continued on next page

Information on Schering-Plough HealthCare Products appearing on these pages is effective as of November 1995.

Schering-Plough—Cont.

Edetate Disodium, Polyethlene Glycol 1450, Povidone, Propylene Glycol, Sodium Phosphate Dibasic, Sodium Phosphate Monobasic, Water.

Each mL of **AFRIN Sinus** contains Oxymetazoline Hydrochloride 0.05%. **Also contains:** Benzalkonium Chloride, Benzyl Alcohol, Edetate Disodium, Mentanase-12™ (Camphor, Eucalyptol, Menthol), Polysorbate 80, Propylene Glycol, Sodium Phosphate Dibasic, Sodium Phosphate Monobasic, Water.

AFRIN Extra Moisturizing Nasal Spray is specially formulated to sooth dry, irritated nasal passages.

AFRIN Menthol Nasal Spray contains cooling aromatic vapors of menthol, eucalyptol, camphor and polysorbate in addition to the ingredients of AFRIN Nasal Spray.

AFRIN Cherry Scented Nasal Spray contains artificial cherry flavor in addition to the ingredients in regular AFRIN.

Indications: For the temporary relief of nasal congestion due to a cold, hay fever or other upper respiratory allergies, or associated with sinusitis. Reduces swelling of nasal passages; shrinks swollen membranes. Temporarily restores freer breathing through the nose.

Actions: The sympathomimetic action of AFRIN products constricts the smaller arterioles of the nasal passages, producing a prolonged, gentle and predictable decongesting effect. In just a few minutes a single dose, as directed, provides prompt, temporary relief of nasal congestion that lasts up to 12 hours. AFRIN products last up to 3 or 4 times longer than most ordinary nasal sprays.

Warnings: Do not exceed recommended dosage. This product may cause temporary discomfort such as burning, stinging, sneezing, or an increase in nasal discharge. Do not use this product for more than 3 days. Use only as directed. Frequent or prolonged use may cause nasal congestion to recur or worsen. If symptoms persist, consult a doctor. The use of this container by more than one person may spread infection. Do not use this product if you have heart disease, high blood pressure, thyroid disease, diabetes, or difficulty in urination due to enlargement of the prostate gland unless directed by a doctor. As with any drug, if you are pregnant or nursing a baby, seek the advice of a health professional before using this product. Keep this and all medicines out of the reach of children. In case of accidental ingestion, seek professional assistance or contact a Poison Control Center immediately.

Directions: Adults and children 6 to under 12 years of age (with adult supervision): 2 or 3 sprays in each nostril not more often than every 10 to 12 hours. Do not exceed 2 doses in any 24-hour period. **Children under 6 years of age:** consult a doctor. To spray, squeeze bottle quickly and firmly. Do not tilt head backward while spraying. Wipe nozzle clean after use.

How Supplied: AFRIN Nasal Spray 0.05%, 15 ml and 30 ml plastic squeeze bottles.
AFRIN Nasal Spray Pump 0.05% (1:2000), 15 ml spray pump bottles.
AFRIN Sinus Nasal Spray 0.05%, 15 ml plastic squeeze bottles.
AFRIN Extra Moisturizing Nasal Spray 0.05%, 15 ml and 30 ml plastic squeeze bottles.
AFRIN Cherry Scented Nasal Spray 0.05% (1:2000), 15 ml plastic squeeze bottle.
AFRIN Menthol Nasal Spray 0.05% (1:2000), 15 ml plastic squeeze bottle.
AFRIN Nose Drops 0.05% (1:2000), 20 ml dropper bottle.
Store all nasal sprays and nose drops between 2° and 30°C (36° and 86°F)

Shown in Product Identification Guide, page 518

AFRIN®
[a΄frin]
Saline Mist

Ingredients: Water, PEG-32, Sodium Chloride, PVP, Disodium Phosphate, Sodium Phosphate, Benzalkonium Chloride, Disodium EDTA.

Indications: Provides soothing moisture to dry, inflamed nasal membranes due to colds, allergies, low humidity, and other minor nasal irritations. Afrin Saline Mist loosens and thins mucus secretions to aid removal of mucus from nose and sinuses. Afrin Saline Mist can be used as often as needed, and is safe to use with cold, allergy, and sinus medications. It is also safe for infants.

Directions: For infants, children, and adults, 2 to 6 sprays/drops in each nostril as often as needed or as directed by a physician. For a fine mist, keep bottle upright; for nose drops, keep bottle upside down; for a stream, keep bottle horizontal. Wipe nozzle clean after use.

Keep out of the reach of children.
The use of this dispenser by more than one person may spread infection.

CONTAINS NO ALCOHOL

CHLOR-TRIMETON®
[klor-tri΄mĕ-ton]
4 Hour Allergy Tablets
8 Hour Allergy Tablets
12 Hour Allergy Tablets

Active Ingredients: Each 4 Hour Allergy Tablet contains: 4 mg chlorpheniramine maleate, USP; also contains: Corn Starch, D&C Yellow No. 10 Aluminum Lake, Lactose, Magnesium Stearate. **Each 8 Hour Allergy Tablet contains:** 8 mg chlorpheniramine maleate; also contains: Acacia, Butylparaben, Calcium Phosphate, Calcium Sulfate, Carnauba Wax, Corn Starch, D&C Yellow No. 10 Aluminum Lake, FD&C Yellow No. 6 Aluminum Lake, FD&C Yellow No. 6, Lactose, Magnesium Stearate, Neutral Soap, Oleic Acid, Potato Starch, Rosin, Sugar, Talc, White Wax, Zein.
Each 12 Hour Allergy Tablet contains: 12 mg chlorpheniramine maleate; also contains: Acacia, Butylparaben, Calcium Phosphate, Calcium Sulfate, Carnauba Wax, Corn Starch, D&C Yellow No. 10 Aluminum Lake, FD&C Blue No. 2 Aluminum Lake, FD&C Yellow No. 6, FD&C Yellow No. 6 Aluminum Lake, Lactose, Magnesium Stearate, Neutral Soap, Oleic Acid, Potato Starch, Rosin, Sugar, Talc, White Wax, Zein.

Indications: For effective relief of sneezing, itchy, watery eyes, itchy throat, and runny nose due to hay fever and other upper respiratory allergies.

Warnings: May cause excitability especially in children. Do not give the 8 Hour or 12 Hour Allergy Tablets to children under 12 years, or 4 Hour Allergy Tablets to children under 6 years except under the advice and supervision of a doctor. Do not take this product, unless directed by a doctor, if you have a breathing problem such as emphysema or chronic bronchitis, or if you have glaucoma, difficulty in urination due to enlargement of the prostate gland. May cause drowsiness; alcohol may increase the drowsiness effect. Avoid alcoholic beverages while taking this product. Do not take this product if you are taking sedatives or tranquilizers, without first consulting your doctor. Use caution when driving a motor vehicle or operating machinery. As with any drug, if you are pregnant or nursing a baby, seek the advice of a health professional before using this product. Keep this and all drugs out of the reach of children. In case of accidental overdose, seek professional assistance or contact a Poison Control Center immediately.

Dosage and Administration: 4 Hour Allergy Tablets—Adults and Children 12 years of age and over: Oral dosage is one tablet (4 mg) every 4 to 6 hours, not to exceed 6 tablets in 24 hours. Children 6 to under 12 years of age: Oral dosage is one half the adult dose (2 mg) (break tablet in half) every 4 to 6 hours, not to exceed 3 whole tablets (12 mg) in 24 hours, or as directed by a doctor. Children under 6 years of age: consult a doctor.

8 Hour Allergy Tablets—Adults and Children 12 years and over—One tablet every 8 to 12 hours. Do not take more than one tablet every 8 hours or 3 tablets in 24 hours.

12 Hour Allergy Tablets—Adults and children 12 years and over—One tablet every 12 hours. Do not exceed 2 tablets in 24 hours.

How Supplied: CHLOR-TRIMETON 4 Hour Allergy Tablets, box of 24, bottles of 100.
CHLOR-TRIMETON 8 Hour Allergy Tablets, boxes of 15, bottles of 100.
CHLOR-TRIMETON 12 Hour Allergy Tablets, boxes of 10 and 24, bottles of 100.

Store between 2° and 30°C (36° and 86°F). Protect from excessive moisture.
Shown in Product Identification Guide, page 518

CHLOR–TRIMETON®
[klortri 'mĕ-ton]
4 Hour Allergy/Decongestant Tablets
12 Hour Allergy/Decongestant Tablets

Active Ingredients: Each 4 Hour Allergy/Decongestant Tablet contains: 4 mg chlorpheniramine maleate, USP and 60 mg pseudoephedrine sulfate; also contains: Corn Starch, FD&C Blue No. 1, Lactose, Magnesium Stearate, Povidone. **Each 12 Hour Allergy/Decongestant Tablet contains:** 8 mg chlorpheniramine maleate and 120 mg pseudoephedrine sulfate; also contains: Acacia, Butylparaben, Calcium Sulfate, Carnauba Wax, Corn Starch, D&C Yellow No. 10 Aluminum Lake, FD&C Blue No. 1 Aluminum Lake, FD&C Yellow No. 6 Aluminum Lake, Gelatin, Lactose, Magnesium Stearate, Neutral Soap, Oleic Acid, Povidone, Rosin, Sugar, Talc, White Wax, Zein.

Indications: For effective temporary relief of sneezing, itchy, watery eyes, itchy throat, and runny nose due to hay fever and other upper respiratory allergies. Helps decongest sinus openings and sinus passages; relieves sinus pressure. Temporarily restores freer breathing through the nose.

Warnings: CHLOR-TRIMETON 4 HOUR ALLERGY/DECONGESTANT: Do not exceed recommended dosage. If nervousness, dizziness, or sleeplessness occur, discontinue use and consult a doctor. If symptoms do not improve within 7 days or are accompanied by fever, consult a doctor. Do not take this product if you have a breathing problem such as emphysema, chronic bronchitis, or if you have glaucoma, heart disease, high blood pressure, thyroid disease, diabetes, or difficulty in urination due to enlargement of the prostate gland unless directed by a doctor. May cause excitability, especially in children. May cause drowsiness; alcohol, sedatives, and tranquilizers may increase the drowsiness effect. Avoid alcoholic beverages while taking this product. Do not take this product if you are taking sedatives or tranquilizers, without first consulting your doctor. Use caution when driving a motor vehicle or operating machinery. As with any drug, if you are pregnant or nursing a baby, seek the advice of a health professional before using this product. Keep this and all drugs out of the reach of children. In case of accidental overdose, seek professional assistance or contact a Poison Control Center immediately.

Drug Interaction Precaution: Do not use this product if you are taking a prescription monoamine oxidase inhibitor (MAOI) (certain drugs for depression, psychiatric or emotional conditions, or Parkinson's disease), or for 2 weeks after stopping the MAOI drug. If you are uncertain whether your prescription drug contains an MAOI, consult a health professional before taking this product.

CHLOR-TRIMETON 12 HOUR ALLERGY/DECONGESTANT: Do not exceed recommended dosage. If nervousness, dizziness, or sleeplessness occur, discontinue use and consult a doctor. If symptoms do not improve within 7 days or are accompanied by fever, consult a doctor. Do not take this product if you have a breathing problem such as emphysema, chronic bronchitis, or if you have glaucoma, heart disease, high blood pressure, thyroid disease, diabetes, or difficulty in urination due to enlargement of the prostate gland, or give this product children under 12 years of age, unless directed by a doctor. May cause excitability especially in children. May cause drowsiness; alcohol, sedatives, and tranquilizers may increase the drowsiness effect. Avoid alcoholic beverages while taking this product. Do not take this product if you are taking sedatives or tranquilizers without first consulting a doctor. Use caution when driving a motor vehicle or operating machinery. As with any drug, if you are pregnant or nursing a baby, seek the advice of a health professional before using this product. Keep this and all drugs out of the reach of children. In case of accidental overdose, seek professional assistance or contact a Poison Control Center immediately.

Drug Interaction Precaution: Do not use this product if you are taking a prescription monoamine oxidase inhibitor (MAOI) (certain drugs for depression, psychiatric or emotional conditions, or Parkinson's disease), or for 2 weeks after stopping the MAOI drug. If you are uncertain whether your prescription drug contains an MAOI, consult a health professional before taking this product.

Dosage and Administration: 4 Hour Allergy/Decongestant Tablets — ADULTS AND CHILDREN 12 YEARS OF AGE AND OVER: Oral dosage is one tablet every 4 to 6 hours, not to exceed 4 tablets in 24 hours, or as directed by a doctor. CHILDREN 6 TO UNDER 12 YEARS OF AGE: Oral dosage is one half the adult dose (break tablet in half) every 4 to 6 hours, not to exceed 2 whole tablets in 24 hours, or as directed by a doctor. CHILDREN UNDER 6 YEARS OF AGE: Consult a doctor. **12 Hour Allergy/Decongestant Tablets—**ADULTS AND CHILDREN 12 YEARS AND OVER: one tablet every 12 hours. Do not exceed 2 tablets in 24 hours.

How Supplied: CHLOR-TRIMETON 4 Hour Allergy/Decongestant Tablets—boxes of 24. CHLOR-TRIMETON 12 Hour Allergy/Decongestant Tablets boxes of 10. Store these CHLOR-TRIMETON Products between 2° and 30°C (36°and 86°F); and protect from excessive moisture.
Shown in Product Identification Guide, page 518

COPPERTONE® SKIN SELECTS™ SUNSCREEN LOTION SPF 15 For Dry Skin

Active Ingredients: Ethylhexyl p-Methoxycinnamate, Oxybenzone.

Other Ingredients: Water, Caprylic/Capric Trigylceride, Propylene Glycol, Squalane, PVP/Eicosene Copolymer, Glyceryl Stearate, PEG-50 Stearate, Cetyl Alcohol, Dimethicone, Glycol Stearate, Myristyl Myristate, DEA-Cetyl Phosphate, Acrylates/C10–30 Alkyl Acrylate Cross-polymer, Diazolidinyl Urea. Methylparaben, Disodium EDTA, Sodium Hydroxide. BHT

Indications: Coppertone® Skin Selects™ Sun Protecting Lotion for Dry Skin SPF 15 contains deeply hydrating emollients to counter the effects of the sun on dry skin. Its extra rich moisturizers replenish moisture lost during sun exposure. Coppertone Skin Selects Lotion also provides 15 times a patient's natural protection against sunburn. It blocks UVB rays that are primarily responsible for sunburn. It also protects a patient's skin against the deeper penetrating UVA rays that have been associated with skin damage resulting in premature aging and wrinkling.
Coppertone Skin Selects Lotion has been clinically tested by Dermatologists to be HYPOALLERGENIC and NON-COMEDOGENIC (will not clog pores) and it is FRAGRANCE-FREE and PABA-FREE making it appropriate for daily facial use. It is also WATER-RESISTANT so it will maintain its degree of protection for 40 minutes or more in water making it appropriate for full body use.

Directions for Use: Apply liberally to all exposed areas. For best results, let dry at least 15 minutes before exposure to the sun and reapply often, especially after toweling. Avoid contact with eyes. If skin irritation or rash develops, discontinue use. Keep this and all drugs out of the reach of children. In case of accidental ingestion, seek professional assistance or contact a Poison Control Center immediately.

How Supplied: 4 oz plastic bottle packaged in box
Shown in Product Identifcation Guide page 518

Continued on next page

Information on Schering-Plough HealthCare Products appearing on these pages is effective as of November 1995.

Schering-Plough—Cont.

COPPERTONE® SKIN SELECTS™ SUNSCREEN LOTION SPF 15 for Oily Skin

Active Ingredients: Ethylhexyl p-Methoxycinnamate, Oxybenzone.

Other Ingredients: Water, Aluminum Starch Octenylsuccinate, PEG-8, PVP/Eicosene Copolymer, Tocopheryl Acetate (Vitamin E Acetate), Aloe Extract, Triethanolamine, Propylene Glycol, Acrylates/C$_{10-30}$ Alkyl Acrylate Crosspolymer, Diazolidinyl Urea, Methylparaben, Propylparaben, Disodium EDTA.

Indications: Coppertone® Skin Selects™ Sun Protecting Lotion for Oily Skin SPF 15 is 100% oil free so it won't clog pores or cause greasy build-up like some sunscreens. This light, non-greasy formula absorbs quickly and feels clean and dry. Coppertone Skin Selects Lotion also provides 15 times a patient's natural protection against sunburn. It blocks UVB rays that are primarily responsible for sunburn. It also protects a patient's skin against the deeper penetrating UVA rays that have been associated with skin damage resulting in premature aging and wrinkling. Coppertone Skin Selects Lotion has been clinically tested by Dermatologists to be HYPOALLERGENIC and NON-COMEDOGENIC (will not clog pores) and it is FRAGRANCE-FREE and PABA-FREE making it appropriate for daily facial use. It is also WATER-RESISTANT so it will maintain its degree of protection for 40 minutes or more in water making it appropriate for full body use.

Directions for Use: Apply liberally to all exposed areas. For best results, let dry at least 15 minutes before exposure to the sun and reapply often, especially after toweling. Avoid contact with eyes. If skin irritation or rash develops, discontinue use. Keep this and all drugs out of the reach of children. In case of accidental ingestion, seek professional assistance or contact a Poison Control Center immediately.

How Supplied: 4 oz. plastic bottle packaged in box
Shown in Product Identification Guide, page 518

COPPERTONE® SKIN SELECTS™ SUNSCREEN LOTION SPF 15 for Sensitive Skin

Active Ingredients: Titanium Dioxide, Ethylhexyl p-Methoxycinnamate.

Other Ingredients: Water, Cyclomethicone, Propylene Glycol, C$_{12-15}$ Alkyl Benzoate, PVP/Eicosene Copolymer, Glyceryl Stearate, PEG-$_{50}$ Stearate, Cetyl Alcohol, Dimethicone, Glycol Stearate, Myristyl Myristate, DEA-Cetyl Phosphate, Acrylates/C$_{10-30}$ Alkyl Acrylate Crosspolymer, Diazolidinyl Urea, Methylparaben, Disodium EDTA. Sodium Hydroxide, BHT, Iron Oxides.

Indications: Coppertone® Skin Selects™ Sun Protecting Lotion for Sensitive Skin SPF 15 contains titanium dioxide, a gentle, natural sunscreen that won't irritate sensitive skin. This extra gentle formula is proven to be non-stinging and irritant-free. Coppertone Skin Selects Lotion also provides 15 times a patient's natural protection against sunburn. It blocks UVB rays that are primarily responsible for sunburn. It also protects a patient's skin against the deeper penetrating UVA rays that have been associated with skin damage resulting in premature aging and wrinkling. Coppertone Skin Selects Lotion has been clinically tested by Dermatologists to be HYPOALLERGENIC and NON-COMEDOGENIC (will not clog pores) and it is FRAGRANCE-FREE and PABA-FREE making it appropriate for daily facial use. It is also WATER-RESISTANT so it will maintain its degree of protection for 40 minutes or more in water making it appropriate for full body use.

Directions for Use: Shake well before using. Apply liberally to all exposed areas. For best results, let dry at least 15 minutes before exposure to the sun and reapply often, especially after toweling. Avoid contact with eyes. If skin irritation or rash develops, discontinue use. Keep this and all drugs out of the reach of children. In case of accidental ingestion, seek professional assistance or contact a Poison Control Center immediately.

How Supplied: 4 oz. plastic bottle packaged in box
Shown in Product Identification Guide, page 518

CORICIDIN® Cold & Flu Tablets
[*kor-a-see 'din*]
CORICIDIN® Cough & Cold Tablets
CORICIDIN 'D'® Decongestant Tablets

Active Ingredients: CORICIDIN Cold & Flu Tablets—2 mg chlorpheniramine maleate, 325 mg (5 gr) acetaminophen. CORICIDIN® Cough & Cold Tablets—4 mg chlorpheniramine maleate, 30 mg dextromethorphan hydrobromide. CORICIDIN 'D' Decongestant Tablets—2 mg chlorpheniramine maleate, 12.5 mg phenylpropanolamine hydrochloride, 325 mg (5 gr) acetaminophen.

Inactive Ingredients: CORICIDIN Cold & Flu Tablets—Acacia, Butylparaben, Calcium Sulfate, Carnauba Wax, Cellulose, Corn Starch, FD&C Red No. 40 Aluminum Lake, FD&C Yellow No. 6 Aluminum Lake, Lactose, Magnesium Stearate, Povidone, Sugar, Talc, Titanium Dioxide, White Wax. CORICIDIN® Cough & Cold Tablets—Acacia, Calcium Sulfate, Carnauba Wax, Croscarmellose Sodium, D&C Red No. 27 Aluminum Lake, FD&C Yellow No. 6 Aluminum Lake, Lactose, Magnesium Stearate, Microcrystalline Cellulose, Povidone, Sodium Benzoate, Sugar, Talc, Titanium Dioxide, White Wax. CORICIDIN 'D' Decongestant Tablets—Acacia, Butylparaben, Calcium Sulfate, Carnauba Wax, Cellulose, Corn Starch, Magnesium Stearate, Povidone, Sugar, Talc, Titanium Dioxide, White Wax.

Indications: CORICIDIN Cold & Flu Tablets temporarily relieve minor aches, pains and headache, and reduce the fever associated with colds or flu; temporarily relieve sneezing, runny nose and itchy watery eyes due to hay fever, other upper respiratory allergies or the common cold. **Unlike other cold remedies, CORICIDIN Cold & Flu Tablets do not contain a decongestant and therefore are suitable for hypertensive patients.** CORICIDIN Cough & Cold Tablets temporarily relieve coughs due to minor throat irritations as may occur with a cold; temporarily relieve sneezing, runny nose and itchy, watery eyes due to the common cold, hayfever or other respiratory allergies. **Unlike other cold remedies, CORICIDIN Cough & Cold Tablets do not contain a decongestant and therefore are suitable for hypertensive patients.** CORICIDIN 'D' Tablets temporarily relieve minor aches and pains, and reduces the fever associated with a cold or flu. Provides temporary relief of: sneezing and runny nose; nasal congestion due to the common cold and associated with sinusitis; stuffy nose; sinus congestion and pressure. Helps decongest sinus openings and passages. **CORICIDIN 'D' Tablets do contain a decongestant.**

Warnings: CORICIDIN Cold & Flu Tablets—Do not take this product for pain for more than 10 days (adults) or 5 days (children 6 to under 12 years of age) and do not take for fever for more than 3 days unless directed by a doctor. If pain or fever persists or gets worse, if new symptoms occur, or if redness or swelling is present, consult a doctor because these could be signs of a serious condition. May cause excitability especially in children. Do not take this product, unless directed by a doctor, if you have a breathing problem such as emphysema or chronic bronchitis, or if you have glaucoma or difficulty in urination due to enlargement of the prostate gland. May cause drowsiness; alcohol, sedatives, and tranquilizers may increase the drowsiness effect. Avoid alcoholic beverages while taking this product. Do not take this product if you are taking sedatives or tranquilizers without first consulting your doctor. Use caution when driving a motor vehicle or operating machinery. As with any drug if you are pregnant or nursing a baby, seek the advice of a health professional before using this product. Keep this and all drugs out of the reach of children. In case of accidental overdose, seek professional assistance or contact a Poison Control Center immediately. Prompt medical attention is critical for adults as well as for children even if you do not notice any signs or symptoms.

CORICIDIN Cough & Cold Tablets—A persistent cough may be a sign of a serious condition. If cough persists for more than 1 week, tends to recur, or is accompanied by fever, rash or persistent headache, consult a doctor. Do not take this product for persistent or chronic cough such as occurs with smoking, asthma, emphysema, or if cough is accompanied by excessive phlegm (mucus) unless directed by a doctor. May cause excitability, especially in children. Do not take this product, unless directed by a doctor, if you have a breathing problem such as emphysema or chronic bronchitis, or if you have glaucoma or difficulty in urination due to enlargement of the prostate gland. May cause marked drowsiness; alcohol, sedatives, and tranquilizers may increase the drowsiness effect. Avoid alcoholic beverages while taking this product. Do not take this product if you are taking sedatives or tranquilizers, without first consulting your doctor. Use caution when driving a motor vehicle or operating machinery. As with any drug, if you are pregnant or nursing a baby, seek the advice of a health professional before using this product. Keep this and all drugs out of the reach of children. In case of accidental overdose, seek professional assistance or contact a Poison Control Center immediately.

DRUG INTERACTION PRECAUTION: Do not use this product if you are now taking a prescription monoamine oxidase inhibitor (MAOI) (certain drugs for depression, psychiatric or emotional conditions, or Parkinson's disease), or for 2 weeks after stopping the MAOI drug. If you are uncertain whether your prescription drug contains an MAOI, consult a health professional before taking this product.

CORICIDIN 'D' Decongestant Tablets— Do not exceed recommended dosage. If nervousness, dizziness, or sleeplessness occur, discontinue use and consult a doctor. If congestion does not improve within 7 days, consult a doctor. Do not take this product for pain for more than 10 days (adults) or 5 days (children 6 to under 12 years) or for fever for more than 3 days unless directed by a doctor. If pain or fever persists or gets worse, if new symptoms occur, or if redness or swelling is present, consult a doctor because these could be signs of a serious condition. May cause excitability, especially in children. Do not take this product, unless directed by a doctor if you have a breathing problem such as emphysema or chronic bronchitis, or if you have glaucoma, heart disease, high blood pressure, thyroid disease, diabetes, or difficulty in urination due to enlargement of the prostate gland. May cause drowsiness; alcohol, sedatives, and tranquilizers may increase the drowsiness effect. Avoid alcoholic beverages while taking this product. Do not take this product if you are taking sedatives or tranquilizers without first consulting your doctor. Use caution when driving a motor vehicle or operating machinery.

As with any drug, if you are pregnant or nursing a baby, seek the advice of a health professional before using this product. Keep this and all drugs out of the reach of children. In case of accidental overdose, seek professional assistance or contact a Poison Control Center immediately. Prompt medical attention is critical for adults as well as for children even if you do not notice any signs or symptoms.

Drug Interaction Precaution: Do not use this product if you are now taking a prescription monoamine oxidase inhibitor (MAOI) (certain drugs for depression, psychiatric or emotional conditions, or Parkinson's disease), or for 2 weeks after stopping the MAOI drug. If you are uncertain whether your prescription drug contains an MAOI, consult a health professional before taking this product. Do not use this product if you are now taking an appetite-controlling medication containing phenylpropanolamine.

Dosage and Administration: CORICIDIN Cold & Flu Tablets—**Adults and children 12 years of age and over:** oral dosage is 2 tablets every 4 to 6 hours, not to exceed 12 tablets in 24 hours, or as directed by a doctor. **Children 6 to under 12 years of age:** oral dosage is 1 tablet every 4 to 6 hours, not to exceed 5 tablets in 24 hours, or as directed by a doctor. **Children under 6 years of age:** consult a doctor.

CORICIDIN Cough & Cold Tablets **—Adults and Children 12 years of age and over:** one tablet every 6 hours, not to exceed 4 tablets in 24 hours. This product is not for children under 12 years of age.

CORICIDIN 'D' Decongestant Tablets **—Adults and children 12 years of age and over:** oral dosage is 2 tablets every 4 hours not to exceed 12 tablets in 24 hours, or as directed by a doctor. **Children 6 to under 12 years of age:** oral dosage is 1 tablet every 4 hours not to exceed 5 tablets in 24 hours, or as directed by a doctor. **Children under 6 years of age:** consult a doctor.

How Supplied: CORICIDIN Cold & Flu Tablets— Bottles of 48, and 100 tablets, blisters of 12 and 24.
CORICIDIN Cough & Cold Tablets— blisters of 16.
CORICIDIN 'D' Decongestant Tablets— Bottles of 48, and 100 tablets, blisters of 12 and 24.
Store between 2° and 30°C (36° and 86°F).

Shown in Product Identification Guide, page 518

CORRECTOL®
Herbal Tea
Laxative
Honey Lemon Flavor
Cinnamon Spice Flavor

Active Ingredient: Senna (30 mg Total Sennosides per tea bag)

Inactive Ingredients: Natural Flavors

Indications: For gentle, overnight relief of occasional constipation. **Correctol Herbal Tea Laxative** generally produces a bowel movement in 6–12 hours.

Warnings: Do not reuse individual tea bags. Do not use concurrently with other laxative products or when abdominal pain, nausea, or vomiting are present unless directed by a doctor. Keep this and all drugs out of the reach of children. In case of accidental overdose, seek professional assistance, or contact a Poison Control Center immediately.

General Warnings about Laxatives: If you have noticed a sudden change in bowel habits that persist over two weeks, consult a doctor before using a laxative. Laxative products should not be used for longer than 1 week unless directed by a doctor. Rectal bleeding or failure to have a bowel movement after use of a laxative may indicate a serious condition. Discontinue use and consult a doctor.

Recommended Dosage: Adults and children 12 years of age and over: 1 cup of tea once a day (maximum: 3 cups of tea per day). In most cases, one 6 oz. cup should be just right. However, you can easily adjust the laxative effect by varying the amount of tea you drink, as long as you don't exceed the recommended dosage. For example, to lessen the laxative effect, brew as directed above but only drink ⅔ of a full 6 oz. cup (4 oz.). To increase the laxative effect, prepare a second 6 oz. cup and drink as much as you feel necessary. For children under 12 years of age, consult your doctor.

Directions: Place one tea bag into a cup and add 6 oz. of boiling water. Let steep for 5 minutes and remove the bag. For iced tea, use 3 oz. of boiling water and add ice cubes after steeping. Sweeten to taste. Take at bedtime for morning results.

How Supplied: 15 individual tea bags per box.

Shown in Product Identification Guide, page 519

CORRECTOL®
Laxative Tablets and Caplets

Active Ingredient: Bisacodyl, 5 mg.

Inactive Ingredients: Acetylated monoglycerides, calcium sulfate, carnauba wax, corn starch, D&C Red #7 calcium lake, gelatin, hydroxypropyl-menthylcellulose phthalate, lactose, magnesium stearate, povidone, sugar, talc, titanium dioxide, white wax.

Indications: For gentle, overnight relief of occasional constipation and irregu-

Continued on next page

Information on Schering-Plough HealthCare Products appearing on these pages is effective as of November 1995.

Schering-Plough—Cont.

larity. Correctol Laxative generally produces a bowel movement in 6 to 12 hours.

Warnings: Do not chew tablets or caplets. Do not give to children under 6 years of age, or to persons who cannot swallow without chewing, unless directed by a doctor. Do not take this product within 1 hour after taking an antacid or milk. Do not use laxative products when abdominal pain, nausea, or vomiting are present unless directed by a doctor. If you have noticed a sudden change in bowel habits that persists over a period of 2 weeks, consult a doctor before using a laxative. Laxative products should not be used for a period longer than 1 week unless directed by a doctor. Rectal bleeding or failure to have a bowel movement after use of a laxative may indicate a serious condition. Discontinue use and consult a doctor. This product may cause abdominal discomfort, faintness, and cramps. As with any drug, if you are pregnant or nursing a baby, seek the advice of a health professional before using this product. Keep this and all drugs out of the reach of children. In case of accidental overdose, seek professional assistance or contact a Poison Control Center immediately. Store at temperatures not above 86°F (30°C).

Directions: Adults and children 12 years of age and older: Take 1 to 3 tablets or caplets in a single dose once daily. **Children 6 to under 12 years of age:** Take 1 tablet or caplet once daily. **Children under 6 years of age:** consult a doctor. **Do not chew or crush tablets or caplets.**

How Supplied: Tablets: Individual foil-backed safety sealed blister packaging in boxes of 5, 10, 30, 60, & 90 tablets. Caplets: Individual foil-backed safety sealed blister packaging in boxes of 30 caplets.

Shown in Product Identification Guide, page 518

CORRECTOL® STOOL SOFTENER
Laxative

Active Ingredient: Docusate sodium 100 mg. per soft gel.
Also Contains—D&C Red No. 33, FD&C Red No. 40, FD&C Yellow No. 6, gelatin, glycerin, polyethylene glycol 400, propylene glycol, sorbitol.

Indications: For relief of constipation without cramps for sensitive systems. Correctol Stool Softener will work gradually to return you to regularity in 12 to 72 hours.

Warning: Do not use laxative products when abdominal pain, nausea, or vomiting are present unless directed by a doctor. If you have noticed a sudden change in bowel habits that persists over two weeks, consult a doctor before using a laxative. Laxative products should not be used for longer than 1 week unless di-

rected by a doctor. Rectal bleeding or failure to have a bowel movement after use of a laxative may indicated a serious condition. Discontinue use and consult your doctor. Keep this and all drugs out of the reach of children. In case of accidental overdose, seek professional assistance or contact a Poison Control Center immediately.

Drug Interaction Precaution: Do not take this product if you are presently taking mineral oil, unless directed by a doctor.

Directions: Adults: For gradual relief of constipation, take 2 soft gels daily, as needed. Children 6–12: Take 1 daily, as needed.

How Supplied: Tablets—individual foil-backed safety sealed blister packaging in boxes of 30 tablets.
Store below 86°F. Protect from freezing.

Shown in Product Identification Guide, page 518

DI-GEL®
Antacid · Anti-Gas
Tablets/Liquid

DI-GEL Tablets: Active Ingredients: (Per Tablet)—Simethicone 20 mg., Calcium Carbonate 280 mg., Magnesium Hydroxide 128 mg. **Inactive Ingredients:** D & C yellow No. 10 aluminum lake, dextrin, FD&C yellow No. 6 aluminum lake, flavor, magnesium stearate, mannitol, povidone, stearic acid, sucrose, talc.
Dietetically sodium free, calcium rich.

DI-GEL Liquid: Active Ingredients—per teaspoonful (5 ml): Simethicone 20 mg., aluminum hydroxide (equivalent to aluminum hydroxide dried gel USP 200 mg.), magnesium hydroxide 200 mg. **Also contains:** Flavor, hydroxypropyl methylcellulose, methylcellulose, methylparaben, propylparaben, sodium saccharin, sorbitol, water.
Dietetically sodium free.

Indications: For fast, temporary relief of acid indigestion, heartburn, sour stomach and accompanying symptoms of gas.

Actions: When excess acid and bubbles of gas are trapped in the stomach, they can cause heartburn and acid indigestion.
The white layer of Di-Gel goes to work fast to neutralize excess acid. And unlike plain antacids, the Simethicone in the yellow layer breaks up gas bubbles rapidly.

Warnings: Do not take more than 20 teaspoonfuls or 24 tablets in a 24 hour period, or use the maximum dosage of this product for more than 2 weeks, except under the advice and supervision of a physician. In case of kidney disease do not use this product except under the advice and supervision of a physician. Tablets may cause constipation or have a

laxative effect. Keep this and all drugs out of the reach of children.

Drug Interaction: (Liquid Only) This product should not be taken if patient is presently taking a prescription antibiotic drug containing any form of tetracycline.

Dosage and Administration: Two teaspoonfuls or tablets every 2 hours, or after or between meals and at bedtime, not to exceed 20 teaspoonfuls or 24 tablets per day, or as directed by a physician.

How Supplied:
DI-GEL Liquid in Mint Flavor - 6 and 12 fl. oz. bottles, safety sealed and Lemon/Orange Flavor - 12 fl. oz. bottles, safety sealed.
DI-GEL Tablets in Mint and Lemon/Orange Flavor - In boxes of 30 and 90 in handy portable safety sealed blister packaging. Also available in Mint 60-tablet bottles.

DRIXORAL® COUGH Liquid Caps
Cough Suppressant
Liquid Caps

Description: Each DRIXORAL® COUGH Liquid Cap contains 30 mg Dextromethorphan Hydrobromide. **Also contains:** FD&C Blue No. 1, FD&C Red No. 40, Gelatin, Glycerin, Polyethylene Glycol 400, Povidone, Propylene Glycol, Sorbitol, Water.

Indications: Temporarily relieves coughs due to minor throat and bronchial irritations as may occur with a cold. Each DRIXORAL® COUGH Liquid Cap contains a maximum strength dose of cough suppressant to control daytime and nighttime coughs without narcotic side effects. Safe for individuals with diabetes.

Warnings: A persistent cough may be a sign of a serious condition. If cough persists for more than 1 week, tends to recur, or is accompanied by fever, rash or persistent headache, consult a doctor. Do not take this product for persistent or chronic cough such as occurs with smoking, asthma, emphysema, or if cough is accompanied by excessive phlegm (mucus) unless directed by a doctor. As with any drug, if you are pregnant or nursing a baby, seek the advice of a health professional before using this product. Keep this and all drugs out of the reach of children. In case of accidental overdose, seek professional assistance or contact a Poison Control Center immediately.

Drug Interaction Precaution: Do not use this product if you are now taking a prescription monoamine oxidase inhibitor (MAOI) (certain drugs for depression, psychiatric or emotional conditions, or Parkinson's disease), or for 2 weeks after stopping the MAOI drug. If you are uncertain whether your prescription drug contains an MAOI, consult a health professional before taking this product.

Dosage and Administration: Adults: Swallow one liquid cap (30 mg.) with water every 6 to 8 hours, not to exceed 4 liq-

uid caps (120 mg.) in 24 hours, or as directed by a doctor. This product is not for children under 12 years of age.
Store below 86°. Protect from freezing. Protect from excessive moisture.

How Supplied: DRIXORAL® COUGH Caps are available in boxes of 10's and 20's.

Shown in Product Identification Guide, page 519

DRIXORAL® COLD & ALLERGY
[*dricks-or 'al*]
Sustained-Action Tablets

Description: EACH DRIXORAL® COLD & ALLERGY SUSTAINED-ACTION TABLET CONTAINS: 120 mg of pseudoephedrine sulfate and 6 mg of dexbrompheniramine maleate. Half of the medication is released after the tablet is swallowed and the remaining amount of medication is released hours later providing continuous long-lasting relief for 12 hours. Also contains: Acacia, Butylparaben, Calcium Sulfate, Carnauba Wax, Corn Starch, D&C Yellow No. 10 Aluminum Lake, FD&C Blue No. 1 Aluminum Lake, FD&C Yellow No. 6 Aluminum Lake, Gelatin, Lactose, Magnesium Stearate, Neutral Soap, Oleic Acid, Povidone, Rosin, Sugar, Talc, White Wax, Zein.

Indications: The decongestant (pseudoephedrine sulfate) temporarily relieves nasal congestion due to the common cold, hay fever or other upper respiratory allergies, and associated with sinusitis. Helps decongest sinus openings and sinus passages. Reduces swelling of nasal passages; shrinks swollen membranes; and temporarily restores freer breathing through the nose. The antihistamine (dexbrompheniramine maleate) alleviates runny nose, sneezing, itching of the nose or throat and itchy and watery eyes as may occur in allergic rhinitis (such as hay fever).

Warnings: Do not exceed recommended dosage. If nervousness, dizziness, or sleeplessness occur, discontinue use and consult a doctor. If symptoms do not improve within 7 days, or are accompanied by fever, consult a doctor. May cause excitability especially in children. Do not take this product if you have a breathing problem such as emphysema or chronic bronchitis, or if you have glaucoma, heart disease, high blood pressure, thyroid disease, diabetes, or difficulty in urination due to enlargement of the prostate gland or give this product to children under 12 years of age, unless directed by a doctor. May cause drowsiness; alcohol, sedatives, and tranquilizers may increase the drowsiness effect. Avoid alcoholic beverages while taking this product. Do not take this product if you are taking sedatives or tranquilizers without first consulting your doctor. Use caution when driving a motor vehicle or operating machinery. As with any drug, if you are pregnant or nursing a baby,

seek the advice of a health professional before using this product. Keep this and all drugs out of the reach of children. In case of accidental overdose, seek professional assistance or contact a Poison Control Center immediately.

Drug Interaction Precaution: Do not use this product if you are now taking a prescription monoamine oxidase inhibitor (MAOI) (certain drugs for depression, psychiatric or emotional conditions, or Parkinson's disease),or for 2 weeks after stopping the MAOI drug. If you are uncertain whether your prescription drug contains an MAOI, consult a health professional before taking this product.

Dosage and Administration: ADULTS AND CHILDREN 12 YEARS AND OVER—one tablet every 12 hours. Do not exceed two tablets in 24 hours.

How Supplied: DRIXORAL® Cold & Allergy Sustained-Action Tablets, green, sugar-coated tablets branded in black with the product name, boxes of 10, 20, and 40, bottle of 100.
Store between 2° and 25°C (36° and 77°F).
Protect from excessive moisture.
Shown in Product Identification Guide, page 519

DRIXORAL® COUGH & CONGESTION Liquid Caps
Cough Suppressant/Nasal Decongestant
Liquid Caps

Description: Each DRIXORAL® COUGH & CONGESTION Liquid Cap contains 30 mg Dextromethorphan Hydrobromide, and 60 mg Pseudoephedrine Hydrochloride. **Also contains:** D&C Red No. 33 Aluminum Lake, FD&C Blue No. 1 Aluminum Lake, Gelatin, Glycerin, Polyethylene Glycol 400, Povidone, Propylene Glycol, Sorbitol, Water.

Indications: The **cough suppressant** temporarily relieves coughs due to minor throat and bronchial irritations as may occur with a cold. The **decongestant** temporarily relieves nasal congestion due to the common cold.

Warnings: A persistent cough may be a sign of a serious condition. If cough persists for more than 1 week, tends to recur, or is accompanied by fever, rash, or persistent headache, consult a doctor. Do not take this product for persistent or chronic cough such as occurs with smoking, asthma, emphysema, or if cough is accompanied by excessive phlegm (mucus), unless directed by a doctor. Do not exceed recommended dosage because at higher doses nervousness, dizziness, or sleeplessness may occur. Do not take this product for more than 7 days. If symptoms do not improve, or are accompanied by a fever, consult a doctor. Do not take this product if you have heart disease, high blood pressure, thyroid disease, diabetes, or difficulty in urination due to the enlargement of the prostate gland unless

directed by a doctor. As with any drug, if you are pregnant or nursing a baby, seek the advice of a health professional before using this product. Keep this and all drugs out of reach of children. In case of accidental overdose, seek professional assistance or contact a Poison Control Center immediately.

Drug Interaction Precaution: Do not use this product if you are now taking a prescription drug containing a monoamine oxidase inhibitor (MAOI) (certain drugs for depression, psychiatric or emotional conditions or Parkinson's disease), or for 2 weeks after stopping the MAOI drug. If you are uncertain whether your prescription contains an MAOI consult a health professional before taking this product.

Dosage and Administration: Adults (12 yrs and older): Swallow one liquid cap with water every 6 hours, not to exceed 4 liquid caps in 24 hours, or as directed by a doctor. This product is not for children under 12 years of age.
Store below 86°F. Protect from freezing. Protect from excessive moisture.

How Supplied: DRIXORAL® COUGH & CONGESTION Liquid Caps are available in boxes of 10's.
Shown in Product Identification Guide, page 519

DRIXORAL® COUGH & SORE THROAT Liquid Caps
Cough Suppressant/Pain Reliever-Fever Reducer
Liquid Caps

Description: Each DRIXORAL® COUGH & SORE THROAT Liquid Cap contains 15 mg. Dextromethorphan Hydrobromide, and 325 mg Acetaminophen. **Also contains:** Colloidal Silicon Dioxide, D&C Red No. 33, FD&C Blue No. 1, Gelatin, Glycerin, Polyethylene Glycol 400, Providone, Propylene Glycol, Sorbitol, Titanium Dioxide.

Indications: The **cough suppressant** temporarily relieves coughs due to minor throat and bronchial irritations as may occur with a cold. The **pain reliever-fever reducer** temporarily relieves minor aches, pains, fever and sore throat. **Safe for individuals with diabetes.**

Warnings: A persistent cough may be a sign of a serious condition. If cough persists for more than 1 week, tends to recur, or is accompanied by fever, rash, or persistent headache, consult a doctor. Do not take this product for persistent or chronic cough such as occurs with smoking, asthma, emphysema, or if cough is accompanied by excessive phlegm (mucus), unless directed by a doctor. Do not

Continued on next page

Information on Schering-Plough HealthCare Products appearing on these pages is effective as of November 1995.

Schering-Plough—Cont.

take this product for pain for more than 10 days (adults) or 5 days (children 6 to under 12 years of age) or for fever for more than 3 days unless directed by a doctor. If pain or fever persists or gets worse, if new symptoms occur, or if redness or swelling is present, consult a doctor because these could be signs of a serious condition. If sore throat is severe, persists for more than 2 days, is accompanied or followed by fever, headache, rash, nausea, or vomiting, consult a doctor promptly. As with any drug, if you are pregnant or nursing a baby, seek the advice of a health professional before using this product. Keep this and all drugs out of reach of children. In case of accidental overdose, seek professional assistance or contact a Poison Control Center immediately. Prompt medical attention is critical for adults as well as children, even if you do not notice any signs or symptoms.

Drug Interaction Precaution: Do not use this product if you are now taking a prescription drug containing a monoamine oxidase inhibitor (MAOI) (certain drugs for depression, psychiatric or emotional conditions or Parkinson's disease), or for 2 weeks after stopping the MAOI drug. If you are uncertain whether your prescription contains an MAOI consult a health professional before taking this product.

Dosage and Administration: Adults (12 yrs and older): Swallow two liquid caps with water every 6 to 8 hours, not to exceed 8 liquid caps in 24 hours, or as directed by a doctor. **Children (6 to under 12 yrs old):** Swallow one liquid cap with water every 6 to 8 hours, not to exceed 4 liquid caps in 24 hours or as directed by a doctor.
Store below 86°F. Protect from freezing. Protect from excessive moisture.

How Supplied: DRIXORAL® COUGH & SORE THROAT Liquid Caps are available in boxes of 10's.
Shown in Product Identification Guide, page 519

DRIXORAL® NON-DROWSY FORMULA
[*dricks-or 'al*]
Long-Acting Nasal Decongestant

DRIXORAL® NON-DROWSY FORMULA Long-Acting Nasal Decongestant Tablets contain 120 mg pseudoephedrine sulfate, a nasal decongestant, in an extended-release tablet providing up to 12 hours of continuous relief ... without drowsiness. Also contains: Acacia, Butylparaben, Calcium Sulfate, Carnauba Wax, Corn Starch, FD&C Blue No. 1 Aluminum Lake, Gelatin, Lactose, Magnesium Stearate, Neutral Soap, Oleic Acid, Povidone, Rosin, Sugar, Talc, White Wax, Zein.

Indications: For temporary relief of nasal congestion due to the common cold, hay fever or other upper respiratory al-

lergies, and nasal congestion associated with sinusitis. Helps decongest sinus openings and sinus passages.

Directions: Adults and Children 12 Years and Over—One tablet every 12 hours. Do not exceed two tablets in 24 hours. DRIXORAL® NON-DROWSY FORMULA is not recommended for children under 12 years of age.

Warnings: Do not exceed recommended dosage. If nervousness, dizziness, or sleeplessness occur, discontinue use and consult a doctor. If symptoms do not improve within 7 days or are accompanied by fever, consult a doctor. Do not take this product if you have heart disease, high blood pressure, thyroid disease, diabetes, or difficulty in urination due to enlargement of the prostate gland, or give this product to children under 12 years of age, unless directed by a doctor. As with any drug, if you are pregnant or nursing a baby, seek the advice of a health professional before using this product. Keep this and all drugs out of the reach of children. In case of accidental overdose, seek professional assistance or contact a Poison Control Center immediately.

Drug Interaction Precaution: Do not use this product if you are now taking a prescription monoamine oxidase inhibitor (MAOI) (certain drugs for depression, psychiatric or emotional conditions, or Parkinson's disease), or for 2 weeks after stopping the MAOI drug. If you are uncertain whether your prescription drug contains an MAOI, consult a health professional before taking this product.

How Supplied: DRIXORAL® NON-DROWSY FORMULA Long-Acting Nasal Decongestant Tablets are available in boxes of 10's and 20's.
Store between 2° and 25°C (36° and 77°F).
Protect from excessive moisture.
Shown in Product Identification Guide, page 519

DRIXORAL® COLD & FLU
[*dricks-or 'al*]
Extended-Release Tablets

Active Ingredients: 500 mg Acetaminophen, 3 mg Dexbrompheniramine Maleate, 60 mg Pseudoephedrine Sulfate.

Also Contains: Calcium Phosphate, Carnauba Wax, D&C Yellow No. 10 Aluminum Lake, FD&C Blue No. 1 Aluminum Lake, FD&C Yellow No. 6 Aluminum Lake, Hydroxypropyl Methylcellulose, Magnesium Stearate, Methylparaben, PEG, Propylparaben, Stearic Acid. DRIXORAL® COLD & FLU Extended-Release Tablets combine a nasal decongestant and an antihistamine with a nonaspirin analgesic in a special 12-hour continuous-acting timed-release tablet.

Indications: The *decongestant* temporarily relieves nasal congestion due to the common cold, hay fever or other up-

per respiratory allergies, and associated with sinusitis. Reduces swelling of nasal passages; shrinks swollen membranes; and temporarily restores freer breathing through the nose. Also helps decongest sinus openings, sinus passages. The *non-aspirin analgesic* temporarily relieves minor aches, pains, and headache and reduces fever due to the common cold. The *antihistamine* alleviates running nose, sneezing, itching of the nose or throat, and itchy and watery eyes as may occur in allergic rhinitis (such as hay fever).

Directions: ADULTS AND CHILDREN 12 YEARS AND OVER—two tablets every 12 hours. Do not exceed four tablets in 24 hours. **CHILDREN UNDER 12 YEARS OF AGE:** consult a doctor.

Warnings: Do not exceed recommended dosage. If nervousness, dizziness, or sleeplessness occur, discontinue use and consult a doctor. If symptoms do not improve within 7 days , or are accompanied by fever that lasts for more than 3 days or recurs, consult a doctor before continuing use. If pain or fever persists or gets worse, if new symptoms occur, or if redness or swelling is present, consult a doctor because these could be signs of a serious condition. May cause excitability especially in children. Do not take this product if you have a breathing problem such as emphysema or chronic bronchitis, or if you have glaucoma, heart disease, high blood pressure, thyroid disease, diabetes, or difficulty in urination due to enlargement of the prostate gland, or give this product to children under 12 years of age, unless directed by a doctor. May cause drowsiness; alcohol, sedatives, and tranquilizers may increase the drowsiness effect. Avoid alcoholic beverages while taking this product. Do not take this product if you are taking sedatives or tranquilizers without first consulting your doctor. Use caution when driving a motor vehicle or operating machinery. As with any drug, if you are pregnant or nursing a baby, seek the advice of a health professional before using this product. Keep this and all drugs out of the reach of children. In case of accidental overdose, seek professional assistance or contact a Poison Control Center immediately. Prompt medical attention is critical for adults as well as for children even if you do not notice any signs or symptoms.

Drug Interaction Precaution: Do not use this product if you are now taking a prescription monoamine oxidase inhibitor (MAOI) (certain drugs for depression, psychiatric or emotional conditions, or Parkinson's disease), or for 2 weeks after stopping the MAOI drug. If you are uncertain whether your prescription drug contains an MAOI, consult a health professional before taking this product.

How Supplied: DRIXORAL® COLD & FLU Extended-Release Tablets are available in boxes of 12's and 24's.

Store between 2° and 25°C (36° and 77°F).
Protect from excessive moisture.
Shown in Product Identification Guide, page 519

DRIXORAL® ALLERGY/SINUS

[*dricks-or'al*]
Nasal decongestant/Pain reliever/ Antihistamine

DRIXORAL® ALLERGY/SINUS Extended-Release Tablets combine a nasal decongestant, a non-aspirin analgesic, and an antihistamine in a 12-hour timed-release tablet.

Indications: The *decongestant* temporarily relieves nasal congestion due to sinusitis, the common cold, and hay fever or other upper respiratory allergies. Helps decongest sinus openings, sinus passages; relieves sinus pressure. Reduces swelling of nasal passages; shrinks swollen membranes; and temporarily restores freer breathing through the nose. The *non-aspirin analgesic* temporarily relieves headaches, and minor aches and pains. The *antihistamine* alleviates runny nose, sneezing, itching of the nose or throat, and itchy and watery eyes as may occur in allergic rhinitis (such as hay fever).

Each DRIXORAL® ALLERGY/SINUS Extended-Release Tablet Contains: 60 mg of pseudoephedrine sulfate, 3 mg of dexbrompheniramine maleate, and 500 mg of acetaminophen. These ingredients are released continuously, providing long-lasting relief for 12 hours. Also contains: Calcium Phosphate, Carnauba Wax, D&C Yellow No. 10 Aluminum Lake, FD&C Yellow No. 6 Aluminum Lake, Hydroxypropyl Methylcellulose, Magnesium Stearate, Methylparaben, PEG, Propylparaben, Stearic Acid.

Directions: ADULTS AND CHILDREN 12 YEARS AND OVER—two tablets every 12 hours. Do not exceed four tablets in 24 hours. **CHILDREN UNDER 12 YEARS OF AGE:** consult a physician.
Store between 2° and 25°C (36° and 77°F).

Warnings: Do not exceed recommended dosage. If nervousness, dizziness, or sleeplessness occur, discontinue use and consult a doctor. If symptoms do not improve within 7 days, or are accompanied by fever that lasts for more than 3 days or recurs, consult a doctor before continuing use. If pain or fever persists or gets worse, if new symptoms occur, or if redness or swelling is present, consult a doctor because these could be signs of a serious condition. May cause excitability especially in children. Do not take this product if you have a breathing problem such as emphysema or chronic bronchitis, or if you have glaucoma, heart disease, high blood pressure, thryoid disease, diabetes, or difficulty in urination due to enlargement of the prostate gland, or give this product to children under 12 years of age, unless directed by a doctor. May cause drowsiness; alcohol, sedatives, and tranquilizers may increase the drowsiness effect. Avoid alcoholic beverages while taking this product. Do not take this product if you are taking sedatives or tranquilizers without first consulting your doctor. Use caution when driving a motor vehicle or operating machinery. As with any drug, if you are pregnant or nursing a baby, seek the advice of a health professional before using this product. Keep this and all drugs out of the reach of children. In case of accidental overdose, seek professional assistance or contact a Poison Control Center immediately. Prompt medical attention is critical for adults as well as for children even if you do not notice any signs or symptoms.

Drug Interaction Precaution: Do not use this product if you are now taking a prescription monoamine oxidase inhibitor (MAOI) (certain drugs for depression, psychiatric or emotional conditions, or Parkinson's disease), or for 2 weeks after stopping the MAOI drug. If you are uncertain whether your prescription drug contains an MAOI, consult a health professional before taking this product.

How Supplied: DRIXORAL® ALLERGY/SINUS Extended-Release Tablets are available in boxes of 12's and 24's.
Shown in Product Identification Guide, page 519

DUOFILM® LIQUID
Wart Remover

Active Ingredient: Salicylic Acid 17% (w/w).

Inactive Ingredients: Alcohol 15.8% w/w, castor oil, ether 42.6% w/w, ethyl lactate, and polybutene in flexible collodion.

Indications: For the removal of common and plantar warts. Common warts can be easily recognized by the rough, cauliflower-like appearance of the surface. Plantar warts are found on the bottom of the foot.

Warnings: For external use only. Do not use this product on irritated skin, on any area that is infected or reddened, if you are a diabetic, or if you have poor blood circulation. If discomfort persists, see your doctor. Do not use on moles, birthmarks, warts with hair growing from them, genital warts, or warts on the face or mucous membranes. Keep this and all drugs out of the reach of children. If product gets in eyes, flush with water for 15 minutes. Avoid inhaling vapors. HIGHLY FLAMMABLE. Keep away from fire or flame. Cap bottle tightly when not in use. Store at room temperature away from heat. In case of accidental ingestion, seek professional assistance or contact a Poison Control Center immediately.

Directions: Wash affected area. May soak wart in warm water for 5 minutes. Dry area thoroughly. Apply one thin layer (with brush applicator) at a time to sufficiently cover each wart. Let dry. Repeat this procedure once or twice daily as needed (until wart is removed) for up to 12 weeks.
Note: Adhesive bandage may be used to cover treated area.

How Supplied: DuoFilm Liquid is available in ½ fluid oz. spill-resistant bottles with brush applicator for pinpoint application.
Shown in Product Identification Guide, page 519

DUOFILM®PATCH FOR CHILDREN
Wart Remover

Active Ingredient: Salicylic Acid 40% in a rubber-based vehicle.

Indications: For the concealment and removal of common warts. Common warts can be easily recognized by the rough, cauliflower-like appearance of the surface.

Warnings: For external use only. Do not use this product on irritated skin, on any area that is infected or reddened, if you are a diabetic, or if you have poor blood circulation. If discomfort persists, see your doctor. Do not use on moles, birthmarks, warts with hair growing from them, genital warts, or warts on the face or mucous membranes. Keep this and all drugs out of the reach of children. In case of accidental ingestion, seek professional assistance or contact a Poison Control Center immediately.

Directions: Wash affected area. May soak wart in warm water for five minutes. Dry area thoroughly. Apply Medicated Patch (packet A). If necessary, cut patch to fit wart. Repeat procedure every 48 hours as needed (until wart is removed) for up to 12 weeks.
Note: Self-adhesive cover-up patches (packet B) may be used to conceal Medicated Patch and wart.

How Supplied: DuoFilm Patch includes 54 Medicated Patches of varying sizes, with 20 self-adhesive Cover-Up patches for concealment while treatment is ongoing.
Shown in Product Identification Guide, page 519

DUOPLANT® GEL
Plantar Wart Remover

Active Ingredient: Salicylic Acid 17% (w/w).

Continued on next page

Information on Schering-Plough HealthCare Products appearing on these pages is effective as of November 1995.

Schering-Plough—Cont.

Inactive Ingredients: Alcohol 57.6% w/w, ether 16.42% w/w, ethyl lactate, hydroxypropyl cellulose, and polybutene in flexible collodion, USP.

Indications: For the removal of plantar and common warts. Plantar warts are found on the bottom of the foot. Common warts can be easily recognized by the rough, cauliflower-like appearance of the surface.

Warnings: For external use only. Do not use this product on irritated skin, on any area that is infected or reddened, if you are a diabetic, or if you have poor blood circulation. If discomfort persists, see your doctor. Do not use on moles, birthmarks, warts with hair growing from them, genital warts, or warts on the face or mucous membranes. Keep this and all drugs out of the reach of children. If product gets in eyes, flush with water for 15 minutes. Avoid inhaling vapors. DuoPlant Gel is extremely flammable. Keep away from fire or flame. Cap tube tightly and store at room temperature away from heat. In case of accidental ingestion, seek professional assistance or contact a Poison Control Center immediately.

Directions: Wash affected area. May soak wart in warm water for five minutes. Dry area thoroughly. Apply a thin layer to sufficiently cover each wart. Let dry. Repeat this procedure once or twice daily as needed (until wart is removed) for up to 12 weeks.
Note: Adhesive bandage may be used to cover treated area.

How Supplied: DuoPlant Gel is available in ½ oz. tubes with applicator tip for pinpoint application.
Shown in Product Identification Guide, page 519

DURATION
12 Hour Nasal Spray 0.05%

Description: DURATION products contain oxymetazoline hydrochloride, the longest acting topical nasal decongestant available. Each ml of DURATION Nasal Spray contains Oxymetazoline Hydrochloride, USP 0.5 mg (0.05%). **Also Contains:** Benzalkonium Chloride, Edetate Disodium, Polyethylene Glycol 1450, Povidone, Propylene Glycol, Sodium Phosphate Dibasic, Sodium Phosphate Monobasic, Water.

Indications: For prompt, temporary relief for up to 12 hours of nasal congestion due to colds, hay fever and sinusitis, and other upper respiratory allergies.

Actions: The sympathomimetic action of DURATION products constricts the smaller arterioles of the nasal passages, producing a prolonged, gentle and predictable decongesting effect. In just a few minutes a single dose, as directed, provides prompt, temporary relief of nasal congestion that lasts up to 12 hours.

Warnings: Do not exceed recommended dosage. This product may cause temporary discomfort such as burning, stinging, sneezing, or an increase in nasal discharge. Do not use this product for more than 3 days. Use only as directed. Frequent or prolonged use may cause nasal congestion to recur or worsen. If symptoms persist, consult a doctor. The use of this container by more than one person may spread infection. Do not use this product if you have heart disease, high blood pressure, thyroid disease, diabetes, or difficulty in urination due to enlargement of the prostate gland unless directed by a doctor. As with any drug, if you are pregnant or nursing a baby, seek the advice of a health professional before using this product. Keep this and all medicines out of the reach of children. In case of accidental ingestion, seek professional assistance or contact a Poison Control Center immediately.

Directions: Adults and children 6 to under 12 years of age (with adult supervision): 2 or 3 sprays in each nostril not more often than every 10 to 12 hours. Do not exceed 2 doses in any 24-hour period. **Children under 6 years of age:** consult a doctor. To spray squeeze bottle quickly and firmly. Do not tilt head backward while spraying. Wipe nozzle clean after use.

How Supplied: DURATION 12 Hour Nasal Spray 0.05%—½ oz and 1 oz plastic squeeze bottles

---

LOTRIMIN® AF ANTIFUNGAL
[lo-tre-min]
Clotrimazole
Cream 1%
Solution 1%
Lotion 1%

Description: Lotrimin® AF Cream 1% is a white fully vanishing homogeneous cream containing 1% clotrimazole. The cream contains no sensitizing parabens and is totally grease free and nonstaining.
Lotrimin® AF Solution 1% is a nonaqueous liquid, containing polyethylene glycol.
Lotrimin® AF Lotion 1% is a light penetrating buffered emulsion also containing no common sensitizing agents and is greaseless and nonstaining.

Indications: Lotrimin® AF Cream, Solution and Lotion contain 1% clotrimazole, a synthetic broad-spectrum antifungal agent. Clotrimazole is used for the treatment of dermal infections caused by a variety of pathogenic dermatophytes, yeasts and *Malassezia furfur*. The primary action of clotrimazole is against dividing and growing organisms. Lotrimin® AF was first made available as an over-the-counter drug in 1990 and is indicated for superficial dermatophyte infections: athlete's foot (tinea pedis), jock itch (tinea cruris) and ringworm (tinea corporis). Lotrimin® remains on prescription for topical candidiasis due to *Candida albicans* and tinea versicolor due to *Malassezia furfur*.

Directions: Cleanse skin with soap and water and dry thoroughly. Apply a thin layer over affected area morning and evening or as directed by a physician. For athlete's foot, pay special attention to the spaces between the toes. It is also helpful to wear well-fitting, ventilated shoes and to change shoes and socks at least once daily. Best results in athlete's foot and ringworm are usually obtained with 4 weeks use of this product, and in jock itch, with 2 weeks use. If satisfactory results have not occurred within these times, consult a physician or pharmacist. Children under 12 years of age should be supervised in the use of this product. This product is not effective on the scalp or nails.

How Supplied: Lotrimin® AF Antifungal Cream is available in a 0.42 oz. tube (12 grams) and a 0.84 oz. tube (24 grams).
Inactive ingredients include: benzyl alcohol, cetearyl alcohol, cetyl esters wax, octyldodecanol, polysorbate, sorbitan monostearate and water.
Lotrimin® AF Antifungal Solution is available in a 0.33 fl. oz. (10 milliliters) bottle. Inactive ingredients include PEG.
Lotrimin® AF Antifungal Lotion is available in a 0.66 fl. oz. (20 milliliters) bottle. Inactive ingredients include benzyl alcohol, cetearyl alcohol, cetyl esters wax, octyldodecanol, polysorbate, sodium biphosphate, sodium phosphate dibasic, sorbitan monostearate and water.

Storage: Keep Lotrimin® AF products between 2° and 30°C (36° and 86°F).
Shown in Product Identification Guide, page 519

LOTRIMIN® AF ANTIFUNGAL
Miconazole Nitrate 2%
Athlete's Foot Spray Liquid
Athlete's Foot Spray Powder
Athlete's Foot Spray Deodorant Powder
Athlete's Foot Powder
Jock Itch Spray Powder

Active Ingredients:
SPRAY LIQUID contains Miconazole Nitrate 2%. Also contains: Alcohol SD-40 (17% w/w), Cocamide DEA, Isobutane, Propylene Glycol, Tocopherol (vitamin E).
SPRAY POWDER (Athlete's Foot/Jock Itch) contains Miconazole Nitrate 2%. Also contains: Alcohol SD-40 (10% w/w), Isobutane, Stearalkonium Hectorite, Talc.
SPRAY DEODORANT POWDER contains Miconazole Nitrate 2%. Also contains: Isobutane, Alcohol SD-40 (10% w/w), Talc, Stearalkonium Hectorite, Fragrance.
POWDER contains Miconazole Nitrate 2%. Also contains: Talc.

Indications: LOTRIMIN AF Athlete's Foot Spray Liquid, Spray Powder, Spray Deodorant Powder and Powder are proven clinically effective in the treatment of athlete's foot (tinea pedis), jock itch (tinea cruris) and ringworm (tinea corporis). For effective relief of the itching, cracking, burning, scaling and discomfort that can accompany these conditions.

LOTRIMIN AF Powder also aids in the drying of naturally moist areas.

LOTRIMIN AF Jock Itch Spray Powder cures jock itch (tinea cruris). For effective relief of the itching, burning, scaling and discomfort associated with jock itch.

Warnings: For Athlete's Foot Spray Powder, Spray Liquid, Spray Deodorant Powder and Jock Itch Spray Powder: Do not use on children under 2 years of age unless directed by a doctor. For external use only. If irritation occurs or if there is no improvement within 4 weeks (for athlete's foot and ringworm) or 2 weeks (for jock itch), discontinue use and consult a doctor. Flammable. Do not use while smoking or near heat or flame. Avoid spraying in eyes. Contents under pressure. Do not puncture or incinerate. Do not store at temperature above 120°F. Use only as directed. Intentional misuse by deliberately concentrating and inhaling contents can be harmful or fatal. Keep this and all drugs out of the reach of children. In case of accidental ingestion, seek professional assisatnce or contact a Poison Control Center immediately.

Lotrimin AF Powder: Do not use on children under 2 years of age unless directed by a doctor. For external use only. If irritation occurs, or if there is no improvement within 4 weeks (for athlete's foot or ringworm) or within 2 weeks (for jock itch) discontinue use and consult a doctor. Keep this and all drugs out of reach of children. In case of accidental ingestion, seek professional assistance or contact a Poison Control Center immediately.

Directions: For Athlete's Foot Spray Liquid, Spray Powder, Spray Deodorant Powder and Jock Itch Spray Powder: Wash affected area and dry thoroughly. Shake can well. Spray a thin layer of product over affected area twice daily (morning and night) or as directed by a doctor. Supervise children in the use of this product. For athlete's foot, pay special attention to the spaces between the toes; wear well-fitting, ventilated shoes and change shoes and socks at least once daily. For athlete's foot and ringworm use daily for 4 weeks; for jock itch use daily for 2 weeks. If condition persists longer, consult a doctor. This product is not effective on the scalp or nails.

Powder: Wash affected area and dry throughly. Sprinkle a thin layer of product over affected area twice daily (morning and night) or as directed by a doctor. Supervise children in the use of this product. For athlete's foot, pay special attention to the spaces between the toes; wear well-fitting, ventilated shoes and change shoes and socks at least once daily. For athlete's foot and ringworm use daily for 4 weeks; for jock itch use daily for 2 weeks. If condition persists longer, consult a doctor. This product is not effective on the scalp or nails.
Store between 2° and 30° C (36° and 86°F).

How Supplied: LOTRIMIN AF Athlete's Foot Spray Powder and Jock Itch Spray Powder—3.5 oz. cans. LOTRIMIN AF Spray Liquid—4 oz. can. LOTRIMIN AF POWDER—3 oz. plastic bottle. LOTRIMIN AF Spray Deodorant Powder—3.5 oz. cans.
Shown in Product Identification Guide, page 519

SHADE® SUNBLOCK GEL SPF 30

Active Ingredients: Ethylhexyl p-methoxycinnamate, homosalate, oxybenzone.

Other Ingredients: SD alcohol 40 (73% V/V), water, PVP/VA copolymer, tetrahydroxypropyl ethylenediamine, acrylates/C10-30 alkyl acrylate crosspolymer, acrylates/octylacrylamide copolymer.

Indications: PABA-FREE Shade SPF 30 Oil-Free Clear Gel is clinically tested to protect your skin from the sun's burning UVA and UVB rays. This clean, clear gel vanishes quickly without any greasy residue. It leaves your skin feeling fresh and clean while providing 30 times your natural protection against sunburn. This unique formula blocks UVB rays that are primarily responsible for sunburn and long-term skin damage caused by overexposure to the sun. It also protects your skin against the deeper penetrating UVA rays that have been associated with skin damage resulting in premature aging and wrinkling. Regular use of Shade 30 Oil-Free Clear Gel may help prevent skin cancer caused by long-term overexposure to the sun.

Non-greasy/Non-oily: Fresh, clear, lightweight greaseless formula that absorbs quickly—feels cool. Specially formulated for people with normal to oily skin.

Waterproof: Maintains its degree of protection (SPF 30) for 80 minutes or more in the water.

Non-acnegenic/Non-comedogenic: Won't clog pores or cause blemishes.

Fragrance-free: Free of fragrances that may irritate those with sensitive skin.

Hypoallergenic: Won't irritate or sting sensitive skin like some protective sunscreens. Gentle enough for children's delicate skin.

Warnings: Flammable, do not use near heat or flame.

Directions for Use: Apply liberally to all exposed areas. For best results, let dry 15 minutes before exposure to sun and reapply after prolonged swimming, excessive perspiration and toweling. Avoid contact with eyes. If skin irritation or rash develops, discontinue use. For children under 6 months consult your doctor. Keep this and all drugs out of the reach of children. In case of accidental ingestion, seek professional assistance or contact a Poison Control Center immediately.

How Supplied: 4 oz. plastic bottles.
Shown in Product Identification Guide, page 519

SHADE® SUNBLOCK LOTION SPF 45

Active Ingredients: Ethylhexyl p-Methoxycinnamate, 2-Ethylhexyl Salicylate, Oxybenzone, Homosalate.

Other Ingredients: Water, Sorbitan Isostearate, Sorbitol, Polyglyceryl-3 Distearate, Octadecene/MA Copolymer, Triethanolamine, Stearic Acid, Barium Sulfate, Benzyl Alcohol, Dimethicone, Aloe Extract, Jojoba Oil, Methylparaben, Tocopherol (Vitamin E), Propylparaben, Carbomer, Disodium EDTA, Imidazolidinyl Urea, Phenethyl Alcohol.

Indications: PABA-FREE Shade SPF 45 is clinically tested to protect your skin from the sun's burning UVA and UVB rays. This ultra moisturizing formula keeps your skin feeling soft yet provides 45 times your natural protection against sunburn. It blocks UVB rays that are primarily responsible for sunburn and long-term skin damage caused by overexposure to the sun. It also protects your skin against the deeper penetrating UVA rays that have been associated with skin damage resulting in premature aging and wrinkling. Regular use of Shade 45 may help prevent skin cancer caused by long-term overexposure to the sun.

Moisturizing: Rich moisturizing formula helps keep your skin feeling smooth, soft and supple.

Waterproof: Maintains its degree of protection (SPF 45) for 80 minutes or more in the water.

Non-comedogenic: Won't clog pores.

Non-Irritating: Won't irritate sensitive skin like some protective sunscreens.

Fragrance Free: Free of fragrances that may irritate those with sensitive skin.

Directions: Apply liberally to all exposed areas. For best results, let dry at least 15 minutes before exposure to the sun and reapply often, especially after

Continued on next page

Information on Schering-Plough HealthCare Products appearing on these pages is effective as of November 1995.

Schering-Plough—Cont.

toweling. Avoid contact with eyes. If skin irritation or rash develops, discontinue use. For children under 6 months, consult your doctor. In case of accidental ingestion, seek professional assistance or contact a Poison Control Center immediately. Keep this and all drugs out of the reach of children.

How Supplied: 4 oz. plastic bottles
Shown in Product Identification Guide, page 519

SHADE® UVAGUARD™
SPF 15 Sunscreen Lotion

Active Ingredients: Octyl methoxycinnamate, 7.5%; avobenzone (Parsol® 1789), 3%; oxybenzone, USP, 3%.

Other Ingredients: Benzyl alcohol, carbomer-941, dimethicone, edetate disodium, glyceryl stearate SE, isopropyl myristate, methylparaben, octadecene/MA copolymer, propylparaben, purified water, sorbitan monooleate, sorbitol, stearic acid and trolamine.

Indications: While all sunscreens protect your skin from the sun's burning rays, Shade® UVAGUARD™ sunscreen, with the patented ingredient Parsol®1789, offers extra protection from the UVA rays that may contribute to skin damage and premature aging of the skin. Shade UVAGUARD is clinically tested to provide 15 times your natural sunburn protection (UVB). And the moisturizing formula of Shade UVAGUARD keeps your skin feeling soft and is PABA-free. Regular use of Shade UVAGUARD may help reduce the chance of acute and long-term skin damage associated with exposure to UVA and UVB rays. Overexposure to the sun may lead to premature aging of the skin and skin cancer.

Water-resistant: Maintains its degree of protection (SPF 15) for 40 minutes or more in water.

Fragrance-free: Free of fragrance that may irritate those with sensitive skin.

Moisturizing: Moisturizing formula helps keep your skin feeling smooth and soft.

Non-comedogenic: Won't clog pores.

Warnings: Do not use if sensitive to cinnamates, benzophenones or any other ingredient in this product. Avoid contact with the eyes, if contact occurs, rinse eyes thoroughly with water. For external use only, not to be swallowed. Discontinue use if signs of irritation or rash appear. Keep this and all drugs out of the reach of children. In case of accidental ingestion, seek professional assistance or contact a Poison Control Center immediately.

Directions for Use: Shake well before using. Before sun exposure, apply evenly and liberally on all exposed areas and

reapply after 40 minutes in the water or after excessive sweating. There is no recommended dosage for children under six (6) months of age except under the advice and supervision of a physician.

How Supplied: 4 oz. plastic bottles.
Shown in Product Identification Guide, page 519

ST. JOSEPH®
ADULT CHEWABLE ASPIRIN
Low Strength Tablets (81 mg. each)

Active Ingredient: Each St. Joseph Adult Chewable Aspirin Tablet contains 81 mg. aspirin in a chewable, orange flavored form.

Inactive Ingredients: Corn Starch, D&C Yellow No. 10 Aluminum Lake, FD&C Yellow No. 6 Aluminum Lake, Flavor, Hydrogenated Vegetable Oil, Maltodextrin, Mannitol, Saccharin.

Indications: St. Joseph® Adult Chewable Aspirin Tablets provide safe, effective, temporary relief from: headaches, muscular aches and pains; and pain associated with a cold, menstrual cramps, backaches and for reducing fever due to colds.

Warnings: Children and teenagers should not use this medicine for chicken pox or flu symptoms before a doctor is consulted about Reye Syndrome, a rare but serious illness reported to be associated with aspirin. Do not take this product for pain for more than 10 days or for fever for more than 3 days unless directed by a doctor. If pain or fever persists or gets worse, if new symptoms occur, or if redness or swelling is present, consult a doctor because these could be signs of serious conditions. Do not take this product for at least 7 days after tonsillectomy or oral surgery unless directed by a doctor. Do not take this product if you are allergic to aspirin, have asthma, have stomach problems (such as heartburn, upset stomach or stomach pain) that persist or recur, or have ulcers or bleeding problems, unless directed by a doctor. If ringing in the ears or loss of hearing occurs, consult a doctor before taking any more of this prodcut. As with any drug, if you are pregnant or nursing a baby, seek the advice of a health professional before using this product. **IT IS ESPECIALLY IMPORTANT NOT TO USE ASPIRIN DURING THE LAST 3 MONTHS OF PREGNANCY UNLESS SPECIFICALLY DIRECTED TO DO SO BY A DOCTOR BECAUSE IT MAY CAUSE PROBLEMS IN THE UNBORN CHILD OR COMPLICATIONS DURING DELIVERY.** Keep this and all drugs out of the reach of children. In case of accidental overdose, seek professional assistance or contact a Poison Control Center immediately.

Drug Interaction Precaution: Do not take this product if you are taking a prescription drug for anticoagulation (thin-

ning the blood), diabetes, gout, or arthritis unless directed by a doctor.

Directions: Adults chew from 4 to 8 tablets (325 to 650 mg) every 4 hours as needed. Do not exceed 48 tablets in 24 hours or as directed by a doctor. Drink a full glass of water with each dose. Do not give to children under 12 years of age unless directed by a doctor.

Professional Labeling: Aspirin for Myocardial Infarction.

Indication: Aspirin is indicated to reduce the risk of death and/or nonfatal myocardial infarction in patients with a previous infarction or unstable angina pectoris.

Clinical Trials: The indication is supported by the results of six large randomized, multicenter, placebo-controlled studies[1–7] involving 10,816 predominantly male post–myocardial infarction (MI) patients and one randomized placebo-controlled study of 1,266 men with unstable angina. Therapy with aspirin was begun at intervals after the onset of acute MI varying from less than three days to more than five years and continued for periods of from less than one year to four years. In the unstable angina study, treatment was started within one month after the onset of unstable angina and continued for 12 weeks, and complicating conditions, such as congestive heart failure, were not included in the study. Aspirin therapy in MI patients was associated with about a 20% reduction in the risk of subsequent death and/or nonfatal reinfarction, a median absolute decrease of 3% from the 12% to 22% event rates in the placebo groups. In the aspirin-treated unstable angina patients, the reduction in risk was about 50%, a reduction in the event rate of 5% from the 10% rate in the placebo group over the 12 weeks of study.

Daily dosage of aspirin in the post–myocardial infarction studies was 300 mg in one study and 900–1,500 mg in five studies. A dose of 325 mg was used in the study of unstable angina.

Adverse Reactions: Gastrointestinal Reactions: Doses of 1,000 mg per day of aspirin caused gastrointestinal symptoms and bleeding that, in some cases, were clinically significant. In the largest postinfarction study (the Aspirin Myocardial Infarction Study [AMIS] with 4,500 people), the percentage of incidences of gastrointestinal symptoms for the aspirin (1,000 mg of a standard, solid-tablet formulation) and placebo-treated subjects, respectively, were stomach pain (14.5%, 4.4%), heartburn, (11.9%, 4.8%), nausea and/or vomiting (7.6%, 2.1%), hospitalization for GI disorder (4.9%, 3.5%). In the AMIS and other trials, aspirin-treated patients had increased rates of gross gastrointestinal bleeding. Symptoms and signs of gastrointestinal irritation were not significantly increased in subjects treated for unstable angina with buffered aspirin in solution.

Cardiovascular and Biochemical: In the AMIS trial, the dosage of 1,000 mg per day of aspirin was associated with small increases in systolic blood pressure (BP) (average 1.5 to 2.1 mm) and diastolic BP (0.5 to 0.6 mm), depending upon whether maximal or last available readings were used. Blood urea nitrogen and uric acid levels were also increased, but by less than 1.0 mg percent. Subjects with marked hypertension or renal insufficiency had been excluded from the trial so that the clinical importance of these observations for such subjects or for any subjects treated over more prolonged periods is not known. It is recommended that patients placed on long-term aspirin treatment, even at doses of 300 mg per day, be seen at regular intervals to assess changes in these measurements.

Dosage and Administration: Although most of the studies used dosage exceeding 300 mg, two trials used only 300 mg daily and pharmacologic data indicate that this dose inhibits platelet function fully. Therefore, 300 mg or 325 mg (4 tablets) aspirin dose daily is a reasonable routine dose that would minimize gastrointestinal adverse reactions.

References:

1. Elwood PC, et al: A randomized controlled trial of acetylsalicylic acid in the secondary prevention of mortality from myocardial infarction, *BR Med J.* 1974;1;436–440.
2. The Coronary Drug Project Research Group: Aspirin in coronary heart disease. *J Chronic Dis.* 1976;29:625–642.
3. Breddin K, et al: Secondary prevention of myocardial infarction: a comparison of acetylsalicylic acid, phenprocoumon or placebo. *Homeostasis.* 1979;470:263–268.
4. Aspirin Myocardial Infarction Study Research Group: A randomized, controlled trial of aspirin in persons recovered from myocardial infarction, *JAMA.* 1980;245:661–669.
5. Elwood PC, and Sweetnam, PM: Aspirin and secondary mortality after myocardial infarction. *Lancet.* December 22–29, 1979, pp 1313–1315.
6. The Persantine-Aspirin Reinfarction Study Research Group: Persantine and aspirin in coronary heart disease. *Circulation.* 1980;62:449–460.
7. Lewis HD. et al: Protective effects of aspirin against acute myocardial infarction and death in men with unstable angina: Results of a Veterans Administration Cooperative Study, *N Engl J Med* 1983;309:396–403.

How Supplied: Chewable, orange flavored tablets in plastic bottles of 36 tablets each.

Shown in Product Identification Guide, page 519

Similasan Corporation Homeopathic OTC Medications
1321 S. CENTRAL AVENUE SUITE D KENT, WA 98032

Direct Inquiries to:
Brian S. Banks
1-800-426-1644
FAX: 206-859-9102

For Medical Emergency Contact:
Alfred Knaus
(206) 859-9072
FAX: (206) 859-9102

SIMILASAN®
Eye Drops #1

Similasan® natural eye drops #1, provide fast relief for dryness and redness due to smog, overwork, contact lens wear etc. The solution is immediately soothing and does not sting upon application. Packaged in a quality glass bottle with a unique dropper.
Suitable for adults and children.

Indications: According to homeopathic principles the ingredients of this medication give you temporary relief from symptoms of:
● Dry, red, irritated eyes
● Inflammation of eyelids
● Sensation of grittiness, hypersensitivity to light, watery eyes
● Tired, strained eyes
Directions for use:
● One to several times daily, place 1–2 drops in each eye.
● Squeeze plastic outlet of bottle with two fingers and allow preparation to drip into the eye.
● Replace cap immediately after using.
● Use before expiration date.

Contraindications: None

Adverse Reactions: None

Drug Interactions: None
Safety packaging:
Use only if bottle seal is intact.

Warning: To avoid contamination of this product, do not touch tip of container to any surface. Replace cap after using. If solution changes color or becomes cloudy, do not use. If you experience eye pain, changes in vision, continued redness or irritation of the eye, or if the condition worsens or persists, consult a physician. Keep this and all medicines out of the reach of children.
Active Ingredients (in homeopathic microdilutions—call for details): 1-800-426-1644. Belladonna HPUS 6X, Euphrasia HPUS 6X, Mercurius sublimatus HPUS 6X
Inactive ingredients: SoluSept® 0.001%, Natrium chloratum 0.9%, Purified water
Similasan® and **SoluSept®** are registered Trademarks of Similasan AG, Switzerland

Manufactured by:
Similasan AG, Switzerland
Imported and Distributed by:
Similasan Corp., Kent, WA 98032
1-800-426-1644
Made in Switzerland
NDC 59262-345-11
10 ml/0.33 fl oz

SIMILASAN®
Eye Drops #2

Similasan® natural allergy eye drops provide fast, soothing relief for itching and burning due to allergic reactions caused by pollen, animal hair, dust etc. The solution is immediately soothing and does not sting upon application. Packaged in a quality glass bottle with a unique dropper.
Suitable for adults and children.

Indications: According to homeopathic principles the ingredients of this medication give you temporary relief from symptoms of:
● Hayfever
● Allergic reactions of the eyes and eyelids, such as:
— Redness
— Itching and burning sensations
— Excessive tearing
Directions for use:
● One to several times daily, place 1–2 drops in each eye.
● Squeeze plastic outlet of bottle with two fingers and allow preparation to drip into the eye.
● Replace cap immediately after using.
● Use before expiration date.

Contraindications: None

Adverse Reactions: None

Drug Interactions: None
Safety packaging:
Use only if bottle seal is intact.

Warning: To avoid contamination of this product, do not touch tip of container to any surface. Replace cap after using. If solution changes color or becomes cloudy, do not use. If you experience eye pain, changes in vision, continued redness or irritation of the eye, or if the condition worsens or persists, consult a physician. Keep this and all medicines out of the reach of children.
Active Ingredients (in homeopathic microdilutions—call for details): 1-800-426-1644. Apis HPUS 6X, Euphrasia HPUS 6X, Sabadilla HPUS 6X
Inactive ingredients: SoluSept® 0.001%, Natrium chloratum 0.9%, Purified water
Similasan® and **SoluSept®** are registered Trademarks of Similasan AG, Switzerland
Manufactured by:
Similasan AG, Switzerland
Imported and Distributed by:
Similasan Corp., Kent, WA 98032
1-800-426-1644
Made in Switzerland
NDC 59262-346-11
10 ml/0.33 fl oz

SmithKline Beecham Consumer Healthcare, L.P.

POST OFFICE BOX 1467
PITTSBURGH, PA 15230

For Medical Information Contact:
(800) 245-1040 (Consumer Inquiries)
(800) 378-4055 (Healthcare Professional Inquiries)

Direct Healthcare Professional Sample Requests to:
(800) BEECHAM

CĒPASTAT®
[sē 'pə-stăt]
Sore Throat Lozenges
Cherry Flavor and Extra Strength

Description: Cherry Flavor lozenge:
Active Ingredient: Each lozenge contains Phenol 14.5mg.
Inactive Ingredients: Antifoam Emulsion, D&C Red #33, FD&C Yellow #6, Flavor, Gum Crystal, Menthol, Saccharin Sodium, and Sorbitol.
Extra Strength lozenge:
Active Ingredient: Each lozenge contains Phenol 29mg.
Inactive Ingredients: Antifoam Emulsion, Caramel, Eucalyptus Oil, Gum Crystal, Menthol, Saccharin Sodium, and Sorbitol.

Actions: Phenol is a recognized topical anesthetic. The sugar-free formula should not promote tooth decay as sugar-based lozenges can.

Indications: For fast, temporary relief of minor sore throat pain.

Warnings: If sore throat is severe, persists for more than 2 days, is accompanied or followed by fever, headache, rash, swelling, nausea, or vomiting, consult a doctor promptly. If sore mouth symptoms do not improve in 7 days or if irritation, pain, or redness persists or worsens, see your dentist or doctor promptly. Do not exceed recommended dosage. KEEP THIS AND ALL MEDICINES OUT OF THE REACH OF CHILDREN. In case of accidental overdose, seek professional assistance or contact a poison control center immediately. As with any drug, if you are pregnant or nursing a baby seek the advice of a health professional before using this product.
Note to Diabetics: Each lozenge contributes approximately 8 calories from 2 grams of sorbitol.

Dosage and Administration:
Lozenges–Cherry Flavor
Adults and children 12 years of age and older: Allow the lozenge to dissolve slowly in the mouth. May be repeated every 2 hours, not to exceed 18 lozenges per day, or as directed by a dentist or physician. Children 6 to under 12 years of age: Allow lozenge to dissolve slowly in

the mouth. May be repeated every 2 hours, not to exceed 10 lozenges per day, or as directed by a dentist or physician. Children under 6 years of age: Consult a dentist or physician.
Lozenges–Extra Strength
Adults and children 12 years of age and older: Allow the lozenge to dissolve slowly in the mouth. May be repeated every 2 hours, or as directed by a dentist or physician. Children 6 to under 12 years of age: Allow lozenge to dissolve slowly in the mouth. May be repeated every 2 hours, not to exceed 10 lozenges per day, or as directed by a dentist or physician. Children under 6 years of age: Consult a dentist or physician.

How Supplied:
Lozenges–Cherry Flavor
Trade package: Boxes of 18 lozenges as 2 pocket packs of 9 lozenges each.
Lozenges–Extra Strength
Trade package: Boxes of 18 lozenges as 2 pocket packs of 9 lozenges each.
Store at room temperature, below 86°F (30°C). Protect contents from humidity.
Shown in Product Identification Guide, page 519

Orange Flavor
CITRUCEL®
[sĭt 'rə-sĕl]
(Methylcellulose)
Bulk-forming Fiber Laxative

Description: Each 19 g adult dose (approximately one heaping measuring tablespoonful) contains Methylcellulose 2 g. Each 9.5 g child's dose (one-half the adult dose) contains Methylcellulose 1 g. Methylcellulose is a nonallergenic fiber. Also contains: Citric Acid, FD&C Yellow No. 6, Orange Flavors (natural and artificial), Potassium Citrate, Riboflavin, Sucrose, and other ingredients. Each adult dose contains approximately 3 mg of sodium, 105 mg of potassium, and contributes 60 calories from Sucrose.

Actions: Promotes elimination by providing additional fiber (bulk) to the diet. This product generally produces bowel movement in 12 to 72 hours.

Indications: For relief of constipation (irregularity). May also be used for relief of constipation associated with other bowel disorders such as irritable bowel syndrome, diverticular disease, and hemorrhoids as well as for bowel management during postpartum, postsurgical, and convalescent periods when recommended by a physician.

Contraindications: Intestinal obstruction, fecal impaction, known hypersensitivity to formula ingredients.

Warnings: Patients should be instructed to consult their physician before using any laxative if they have noticed a sudden change in bowel habits which persists for two weeks. Unless directed by a physician, patients should be ad-

vised not to use laxative products when abdominal pain, nausea, or vomiting is present. Patients should also be advised to discontinue use and consult a physician if rectal bleeding or failure to have a bowel movement occurs after use of any laxative product. Unless recommended by a physician, patients should not exceed the recommended maximum daily dose. Patients should not use laxative products for a period longer than one week unless directed by a physician. **TAKING THIS PRODUCT WITHOUT ADEQUATE FLUID MAY CAUSE IT TO SWELL AND BLOCK YOUR THROAT OR ESOPHAGUS AND MAY CAUSE CHOKING. DO NOT TAKE THIS PRODUCT IF YOU HAVE DIFFICULTY IN SWALLOWING. IF YOU EXPERIENCE CHEST PAIN, VOMITING, OR DIFFICULTY IN SWALLOWING OR BREATHING AFTER TAKING THIS PRODUCT, SEEK IMMEDIATE MEDICAL ATTENTION. KEEP THIS AND ALL DRUGS OUT OF THE REACH OF CHILDREN.**

Dosage and Administration: Adult Dose: *one rounded tablespoonful* (19 g) stirred briskly into at least 8 ounces of cold water up to three times daily at the first sign of constipation. Children age 6 to 12 years of age: *one-half the adult dose* stirred briskly into at least 8 ounces of cold water, once daily at the first sign of constipation. The mixture should be administered promptly and drinking another glass of water is highly recommended (see warnings). Children under 6 years of age: *Use only as directed by a physician.* Continued use for 12 to 72 hours may be necessary for full benefit. **TAKE THIS PRODUCT (CHILD OR ADULT DOSE) WITH AT LEAST 8 OZ. (A FULL GLASS) OF WATER OR OTHER FLUID. TAKING THIS PRODUCT WITHOUT ENOUGH LIQUID MAY CAUSE CHOKING. SEE WARNINGS.**

How Supplied: 16 oz. and 30 oz. containers.
Boxes of 20-single-dose packets.
Store below 86°F (30°C). Protect contents from humidity; keep tightly closed.
Shown in Product Identification Guide, page 519

Sugar Free Orange Flavor
CITRUCEL®
[sĭt 'rə-sĕl]
(Methylcellulose)
Bulk-forming Fiber Laxative

Description: Each 10.2 g adult dose (approximately one rounded measuring tablespoonful) contains Methylcellulose 2 g. Each 5.1 g child's dose (one-half the adult dose) contains Methylcellulose 1 g. Methylcellulose is a nonallergenic fiber. Also contains: Aspartame*, Dibasic Calcium Phosphate, FD&C Yellow No. 6, Malic Acid, Maltodextrin, Orange Flavors (natural and artificial), Potassium

Citrate and Riboflavin. Each 10.2 g dose contributes 24 calories from Maltodextrin.

Actions: Promotes elimination by providing additional fiber (bulk) to the diet. This product generally produces bowel movement in 12 to 72 hours.

Indications: For relief of constipation (irregularity). May also be used for relief of constipation associated with other bowel disorders such as irritable bowel syndrome, diverticular disease, and hemorrhoids as well as for bowel management during postpartum, postsurgical, and convalescent periods when recommended by a physician.

Contraindications: Intestinal obstruction, fecal impaction, known hypersensitivity to formula ingredients.

Warnings: Patients should be instructed to consult their physician before using any laxative if they have noticed a sudden change in bowel habits which persists for two weeks. Unless directed by a physician, patients should be advised not to use laxative products when abdominal pain, nausea, or vomiting is present. Patients should also be advised to discontinue use and consult a physician if rectal bleeding or failure to have a bowel movement occurs after use of any laxative product. Unless recommended by a physician, patients should not exceed the recommended maximum daily dose. Patients should not use laxative products for a period longer than one week unless directed by a physician. **TAKING THIS PRODUCT WITHOUT ADEQUATE FLUID MAY CAUSE IT TO SWELL AND BLOCK YOUR THROAT OR ESOPHAGUS AND MAY CAUSE CHOKING. DO NOT TAKE THIS PRODUCT IF YOU HAVE DIFFICULTY IN SWALLOWING. IF YOU EXPERIENCE CHEST PAIN, VOMITING, OR DIFFICULTY IN SWALLOWING OR BREATHING AFTER TAKING THIS PRODUCT, SEEK IMMEDIATE MEDICAL ATTENTION. KEEP THIS AND ALL DRUGS OUT OF THE REACH OF CHILDREN. Phenylketonurics:** CONTAINS PHENYLALANINE 52 mg per adult dose. Individuals with phenylketonuria and other individuals who must restrict their intake of phenylalanine should be warned that each 10.2 g adult dose contains aspartame which provides 52 mg of phenylalanine.

Dosage and Administration: Adult Dose: *one rounded tablespoonful* (10.2 g) stirred briskly into at least 8 ounces of cold water up to three times daily at the first sign of constipation. Children age 6 to 12 years of age: *one-half the adult dose* stirred briskly into at least 8 ounces of cold water, once daily at the first sign of constipation. The mixture should be administered promptly and drinking another glass of water is highly recommended (see warnings). Children under 6 years of age: *Use only as directed by a*

physician. Continued use for 12 to 72 hours may be necessary for full benefit. **TAKE THIS PRODUCT (CHILD OR ADULT DOSE) WITH AT LEAST 8 OZ. (A FULL GLASS) OF WATER OR OTHER FLUID. TAKING THIS PRODUCT WITHOUT ENOUGH LIQUID MAY CAUSE CHOKING. SEE WARNINGS.**

How Supplied:
8.6 oz and 16.9 oz containers.
Boxes of 20 single-dose packets.
Store below 86°F (30°C). Protect contents from humidity; keep tightly closed.

---

*NutraSweet and the NutraSweet symbol are trademarks of the NutraSweet Company.

Shown in Product Identification Guide, page 519

CONTAC
Day & Night Allergy/Sinus

Product Information: Contac Day & Night Allergy/Sinus includes 15 day caplets and 5 night caplets in each package to provide:
- 5 days of relief from stuffy nose, sinus pressure and headache pain without drowsiness.
- 5 nights of relief from stuffy, runny nose, sinus pressure, sneezing and headache pain to let your rest.

Day Caplets
Product Benefits: Contac Day Caplets provide an ANALGESIC and a DECONGESTANT.

Indications: Temporarily relieves headache pain and nasal congestion due to hay fever or other upper respiratory allergies or associated with sinusitis. Promotes nasal and/or sinus drainage; temporarily relieves sinus congestion and pressure.

Directions: Adults (12 years and older): Take one White Day Caplet every 6 hours, or as directed by a doctor. DO NOT EXCEED A TOTAL OF 4 CAPLETS (whether all Day or all Night or combination of each) IN 24 HOURS. ALL CAPLETS SHOULD BE TAKEN AT LEAST 6 HOURS APART. Children under 12 years of age: Consult a doctor.

Night Caplets
Product Benefits: Contac Night Caplets provide an ANALGESIC, an ANTIHISTAMINE, and a DECONGESTANT

Indication: Temporarily relieves headache pain and nasal congestion, runny nose, sneezing and itchy, watery eyes due to hay fever or other upper respiratory allergies or associated with sinusitis. Promotes nasal and/or sinus drainage; temporarily relieves sinus congestion and pressure.

Directions: Adults (12 years and older): Take one Green Night Caplet every 6 hours, or as directed by a doctor. DO NOT EXCEED A TOTAL OF 4 CAPLETS (whether all Day or all Night or combination of each) IN 24 HOURS. ALL

CAPLETS SHOULD BE TAKEN AT LEAST 6 HOURS APART. Children under 12 years of age: Consult a doctor.

Warnings for Day and Night Caplets: Do not take this product for more than 10 days. If symptoms do not improve or are accompanied by fever that lasts for more than 3 days, or if new symptoms occur, consult a doctor. Do not take this product, unless directed by a doctor, if you have a breathing problem such as emphysema or chronic bronchitis, or if you have heart disease, high blood pressure, thyroid disease, diabetes, glaucoma or difficulty in urination due to enlargement of the prostate gland. **Do not exceed recommended dosage.** If nervousness, dizziness, or sleeplessness occur, discontinue use and consult a doctor. **KEEP THIS AND ALL DRUGS OUT OF THE REACH OF CHILDREN.** Prompt medical attention is critical for adults as well as for children even if you do not notice any signs or symptoms. In case of accidental overdose, seek professional assistance or contact a Poison Control Center immediately. As with any drug, if you are pregnant or nursing a baby, seek the advice of a health professional before using this product.

Additional Warnings for Night Caplets: May cause excitability especially in children. May cause marked drowsiness; alcohol, sedatives, and tranquilizers may increase the drowsiness effect. Avoid alcoholic beverages while taking this product. Do not take this product if you are taking sedatives or tranquilizers, without first consulting your doctor. Use caution when driving a motor vehicle or operating machinery.

Drug Interaction Precaution: Do not use this product if you are now taking a prescription monoamine oxidase inhibitor (MAOI) (certain drugs for depression, psychiatric or emotional conditions, or Parkinson's disease), or for 2 weeks after stopping the MAOI drug. If you are uncertain whether your prescription drug contains an MAOI, consult a health professional before taking this product.

Active Ingredients: EACH DAY AND NIGHT CAPLET CONTAINS: Acetaminophen 650 mg, Pseudoephedrine Hydrochloride 60 mg. NIGHT CAPLETS ALSO CONTAIN: Diphenhydramine Hydrochloride 50 mg.

Inactive Ingredients: EACH DAY AND NIGHT CAPLET CONTAINS: Hydroxpropyl Methylcellulose, Magnesium Stearate, Microcrystalline Cellulose, Polyethylene Glycol, Polysorbate 80, Silicon Dioxide, Starch, Stearic Acid, Titanium Dioxide. NIGHT CAPLETS ALSO CONTAIN: D&C Yellow 10, FD&C Blue 1, FD&C Yellow 6.

How Supplied: Consumer package of 5 Night Caplets and 15 Day Caplets (see previous Day Caplet listing).

Continued on next page

SmithKline Beecham—Cont.

Note: There are other CONTAC products. Make sure this is the one you are interested in.

Shown in Product Identification Guide, page 520

CONTAC
Day & Night Cold/Flu

Composition: [See table on page 774.]

Product Information: Contac Day & Night Cold/Flu includes 15 day caplets and 5 night caplets in each package to provide:

- 5 days of relief from stuffy nose, coughing and aches and pains without drowsiness
- 5 nights of relief from stuffy runny, nose, sneezing and aches and pains to let you rest.

Day Caplets

Product Benefits: Contac Day Caplets provide an ANALGESIC, a DECONGESTANT, and a COUGH SUPPRESSANT.

Indications: For the temporary relief of headache, minor aches and pains, fever, nasal congestion and coughs due to the common cold or flu.

Directions: Adults (12 years and older): Take one Yellow Day Caplet every 6 hours, or as directed by a doctor. DO NOT EXCEED A TOTAL OF 4 CAPLETS (whether all Day or all Night or combination of each) IN 24 HOURS. ALL CAPLETS SHOULD BE TAKEN AT LEAST 6 HOURS APART. Children under 12 years of age: Consult a doctor.

Night Caplets

Product Benefits: Contac Night Caplets provide an ANALGESIC, an ANTIHISTAMINE, and a DECONGESTANT.

Indications: For the temporary relief of headache minor aches and pains, fever, nasal congestion, runny nose, and sneezing due to the common cold and flu.

Directions: Adults (12 years and older): Take one Blue Night Caplet every 6 hours, or as directed by a doctor. DO NOT EXCEED A TOTAL OF 4 CAPLETS (whether all Day or all Night or combination of each) IN 24 HOURS. ALL CAPLETS SHOULD BE TAKEN AT LEAST 6 HOURS APART. Children under 12 years of age: Consult a doctor.

Warnings for Day and Night Caplets: Do not take this product for more than 10 days. If symptoms do not improve or are accompanied by fever that lasts for more than 3 days, or if new symptoms occur, consult a doctor. Do not take this product, unless directed by a doctor, if you have a breathing problem such as emphysema or chronic bronchitis, or if you have heart disease, high blood pressure, thyroid disease, diabetes, glaucoma or difficulty in urination due to enlargement of the prostate gland. **Do not exceed recommended dosage.** If ner-vousness, dizziness, or sleeplessness occur, discontinue use and consult a doctor. **KEEP THIS AND ALL DRUGS OUT OF THE REACH OF CHILDREN.** Prompt medical attention is critical for adults as well as for children even if you do not notice any signs or symptoms. In case of accidental overdose, seek professional assistance or contact a Poison Control Center immediately. As with any drug, if you are pregnant or nursing a baby, seek the advice of a health professional before using this product.

Additional Warnings for Day Caplets: A persistent cough may be a sign of a serious condition. If cough persists for more than 7 days, tends to recur, or is accompanied by rash, persistent headache, fever that lasts for more than 3 days, or if new symptoms occur, consult a doctor. Do not take this product for persistent or chronic cough such as occurs with smoking, asthma, emphysema, or if cough is accompanied by excessive phlegm (mucus) unless directed by a doctor.

Additional Warnings for Night Caplets: May cause excitability especially in children. May cause marked drowsiness; alcohol, sedatives, and tranquilizers may increase the drowsiness effect. Avoid alcoholic beverages while taking this product. Do not take this product if you are taking sedatives or tranquilizers, without first consulting your doctor. Use caution when driving a motor vehicle or operating machinery.

Drug Interaction Precaution: Do not use this product if you are now taking a prescription monoamine oxidase inhibitor (MAOI) (certain drugs for depression, psychiatric or emotional conditions, or Parkinson's disease), or for 2 weeks after stopping the MAOI drug. If you are uncertain whether your prescription drug contains an MAOI, consult a health professional before taking this product.

Active Ingredients: EACH DAY CAPLET CONTAINS: Acetaminophen 650 mg, Pseudoephedrine Hydrochloride 60 mg. Dextromethorphan Hydrobromide 30 mg. EACH NIGHT CAPLET CONTAINS: Acetaminophen 650 mg, Pseudoephedrine Hydrochloride 60 mg, Diphenhydramine Hydrochloride 50 mg.

Inactive Ingredients: EACH DAY AND NIGHT CAPLET CONTAINS: Hydroxypropyl Methylcellulose, Magnesium Stearate, Microcrystalline Cellulose, Polyethylene Glycol, Polysorbate 80, Silicon Dioxide, Starch, Stearic Acid, Titanium Dioxide. DAY CAPLETS ALSO CONTAIN: D&C Yellow 10, FD&C Yellow 6. NIGHT CAPLETS ALSO CONTAIN: FD&C Blue 1.

How Supplied: Consumer package of 5 Night Caplets and 15 Day Caplets (see previous Day Caplet listing).

Note: There are other CONTAC products. Make sure this is the one you are interested in.

Shown in Product Identification Guide, page 520

CONTAC®
MAXIMUM STRENGTH
Continuous Action Nasal
Decongestant/Antihistamine
12 Hour Caplets

Composition: [See table on page 774.]

Product Information: Each CONTAC Maximum Strength timed release caplet provides up to 12 hours of relief. Part of the caplet goes to work right away for fast relief; the rest is released gradually to provide up to 12 hours of prolonged relief. With just *one* caplet in the morning and *one* at bedtime, you feel better all day, sleep better at night, breathing freely without congestion. CONTAC Maximum Strength provides:

- A NASAL DECONGESTANT which helps clear nasal passages, shrinks swollen membranes and helps decongest sinus openings.
- AN ANTIHISTAMINE at the maximum level to help relieve itchy, watery eyes, sneezing, and runny nose.

Indications: For temporary relief of nasal congestion due to the common cold, hay fever or other upper respiratory allergies, and nasal congestion associated with sinusitis.

Directions: Adults and children 12 years of age and older: One caplet every 12 hours, not to exceed 2 caplets in 24 hours, or as directed by a doctor. Children under 12 years of age: consult a doctor.

NOTE: The nonactive portion of the caplet that supplies the active ingredients may occasionally appear in your stool as a soft mass.

TAMPER-RESISTANT PACKAGING FEATURES FOR YOUR PROTECTION:
Each caplet is encased in a plastic cell with a foil back; do not use if cell or foil is broken. The name CONTAC appears on each caplet; do not use this product if the CONTAC name is missing.
This carton is protected by a clear overwrap printed with "safety-sealed"; do not use if overwrap is missing or broken.

Warnings: Do not exceed recommended dosage. If nervousness, dizziness or sleeplessness occur, discontinue use and consult a doctor. If symptoms do not improve within 7 days or are accompanied by fever, consult a physician before continuing use. Do not take this product unless directed by a doctor, if you have a breathing problem such as emphysema, heart disease, high blood pressure, thyroid disease, diabetes, or chronic bronchitis, or if you have glaucoma or difficulty in urination due to enlargement of the prostate gland. Do not take this product if you are taking another medication containing phenylpropanolamine. May cause drowsiness; alcohol, sedatives and tranquilizers may increase the drowsiness effect. Avoid alcoholic beverages while taking this product. Do not take this product if you are taking sedatives or tranquilizers, without first consulting your doctor. Do not drive or operate heavy machinery. May cause excitability, especially in children. Keep this and all drugs out of reach of children. In case of accidental overdose, seek professional assistance or contact a poison control center immediately. As with any drug, if you are pregnant or nursing a baby, seek the advice of a health professional before using this product. Store at controlled room temperature (59°–86°F).

Drug Interaction Precaution: Do not use this product if you are now taking a prescription monoamine oxidase inhibitor (MAOI) (certain drugs for depression, psychiatric or emotional conditions or Parkinson's disease), or for 2 weeks after stopping the MAOI drug. If you are uncertain whether your prescription drug contains an MAOI, consult a health professional before taking this product.

Formula: Active Ingredients: Each Maximum Strength caplet contains Phenylpropanolamine Hydrochloride 75 mg.; Chlorpheniramine Maleate 12 mg. (which is a higher dose of antihistamine than CONTAC capsules). **Inactive Ingredients (listed for individuals with specific allergies):** Acetylated Monoglycerides, Carnauba Wax, Colloidal Silicon Dioxide, Ethylcellulose, Hydroxypropyl Methylcellulose, Lactose, Stearic Acid, Titanium Dioxide.

How Supplied: Consumer packages of 10, 20 and 40 caplets.
Note: There are other CONTAC products. Make sure this is the one you are interested in.
Shown in Product Identification Guide, page 519

CONTAC®
Continuous Action Nasal Decongestant/Antihistamine
12 Hour Capsules

Composition: [See table on next page.]

Product Information: Each CONTAC time release capsule contains over 600 "tiny time pills." Some go to work right away. The rest are scientifically timed to dissolve slowly to give up to 12 hours of relief.

Indications: Temporarily relieves nasal congestion due to the common cold, hay fever or other upper respiratory allergies and associated with sinusitis. Temporarily relieves runny nose and reduces sneezing, itching of the nose or throat and itchy, watery eyes due to hay fever or other upper respiratory allergies. Helps clear nasal passages; shrinks swollen membranes. Helps decongest sinus openings and passages; temporarily relieves sinus congestion and pressure.

Directions: Adults and children over 12 years of age: One capsule every 12 hours, not to exceed 2 capsules in 24 hours, or as directed by a doctor. Children under 12 years of age: consult a doctor.

TAMPER-RESISTANT PACKAGING FEATURES FOR YOUR PROTECTION:
Each capsule is encased in a plastic cell with a foil back; do not use if cell or foil is broken. Each CONTAC capsule is protected by a red Perma-Seal™ band which bonds the two capsule halves together; do not use if capsule or band is broken.
This carton is protected by a clear overwrap printed with "safety-sealed"; do not use if overwrap is missing or broken.

Warnings: Do not exceed the recommended dosage. If nervousness, dizziness, or sleeplessness occur, discontinue use and consult a doctor. If symptoms do not improve within 7 days or are accompanied by high fever, consult a doctor. Do not take this product, unless directed by a doctor, if you have a breathing problem such as emphysema or chronic bronchitis, or if you have heart disease, high blood pressure, thyroid disease, diabetes, glaucoma or difficulty in urination due to enlargement of the prostate gland. Do not take this product if you are taking another medication containing phenylpropanolamine. Use caution when driving a motor vehicle or operating machinery. May cause drowsiness; alcohol, sedatives and tranquilizers may increase the drowsiness effect. Avoid alcoholic beverages while taking this product. Do not take this product if you are taking sedatives or tranquilizers, without first consulting your doctor. May cause excitability especially in children. KEEP THIS AND ALL DRUGS OUT OF REACH OF CHILDREN. IN CASE OF ACCIDENTAL OVERDOSE, SEEK PROFESSIONAL ASSISTANCE OR CONTACT A POISON CONTROL CENTER IMMEDIATELY. As with any drug, if you are pregnant or nursing a baby, seek the advice of a health professional before using this product. Store in a dry place at controlled room temperature 15°–30°C (59°–86°F).

Drug Interaction Precaution: Do not use this product if you are now taking a prescription monoamine oxidase inhibitor (MAOI) (certain drugs for depression, psychiatric or emotional conditions, or Parkinson's disease), or for 2 weeks after stopping the MAOI drug. If you are uncertain whether your prescription drug contains an MAOI, consult a health professional before taking this product.

Each Capsule Contains: Phenylpropanolamine Hydrochloride 75 mg. and Chlorpheniramine Maleate 8 mg. Also Contains: Benzyl Alcohol, Butylparaben, D&C Red No. 33, D&C Yellow No. 10, Edetate Calcium Disodium, FD&C Red No. 3, FD&C Yellow No. 6, Gelatin, Methylparaben, Pharmaceutical Glaze, Propylparaben, Sodium Lauryl Sulfate, Sodium Propionate, Starch, Sucrose and other ingredients, may also contain: Polysorbate 80.

How Supplied: Consumer packages of 10, 20 and 40 capsules.

Note: There are other CONTAC products. Make sure this is the one you are interested in.
Shown in Product Identification Guide, page 519

CONTAC®
Severe Cold and Flu
Caplets
Analgesic ● Decongestant
Antihistamine ● Cough Suppressant

Composition:
[See table at bottom of next page.]

Product Information: Two caplets every 6 hours to help relieve the discomforts of severe colds with flu-like symptoms.

Product Benefits: CONTAC Severe Cold and Flu contains a Non-Aspirin Analgesic, a Decongestant, an Antihistamine and a Cough Suppressant.

Indications: Provides temporary relief from nasal and sinus congestion, runny nose, sneezing, coughing, fever, headache and minor aches assoicated with the common cold, sore throat and the flu.

Directions: Adults (12 years and over): Two caplets every 6 hours, not to exceed 8 caplets in any 24-hour period, or as directed by a doctor.

TAMPER-RESISTANT PACKAGING FEATURES FOR YOUR PROTECTION:
Caplets are encased in a plastic cell with a foil back; do not use if cell or foil is broken. The letters SCF appear on each caplet; do not use this product if these letters are missing.
This carton is protected by a clean overwrap printed with "safety-sealed"; do not use if overwrap is missing or broken.

Warnings: Do not take this product for more than 10 days. If symptoms do not improve or are accompanied by fever that lasts for more than 3 days, or if new symptoms occur, consult a doctor. If sore throat is severe, persists for more than 2 days, is accompanied or followed by fever, headache, rash, nausea, or vomiting, consult a doctor promptly. A persistent cough may be a sign of a serious condition. If cough persists for more than 7 days, tends to recur, or is accompanied by rash, persistent headache, fever that lasts for more than 3 days, or if new symptoms occur, consult a doctor. Do not take this product for persistent or chronic cough such as occurs with smoking, asthma, emphysema, or if cough is accompanied by excessive phlegm (mucus) unless directed by a doctor. May cause excitability especially in children. Do not take this product, unless directed by a doctor, if you have a breathing problem such as emphysema or chronic bronchitis, or if you have heart disease, high blood pressure, thyroid disease, diabetes, glaucoma or difficulty in urination due to enlargement of the prostate gland. May cause marked drowsiness: alcohol,

Continued on next page

SmithKline Beecham—Cont.

sedatives, and tranquilizers may increase the drowsiness effect. Avoid taking alcoholic beverages while taking this product. Do not take this product if you are taking sedatives or tranquilizers, without first consulting your doctor. Use caution when driving a motor vehicle or operating machinery. **Do not exceed recommended dosage.** If nervousness, dizziness, or sleeplessness occur, discontinue use and consult a doctor. **KEEP THIS AND ALL DRUGS OUT OF THE REACH OF CHILDREN.** Prompt medical attention is critical for adults as well as for children even if you do not notice any signs or symptoms. In case of accidental overdose, seek professional assistance or contact a Poison Control Center immediately. As with any drug, if you are pregnant or nursing a baby, seek the advice of a health professional before using this product.

Drug Interaction Precaution: Do not use this product if you are now taking a prescription monoamine oxidase inhibitor (MAOI) (certain drugs for depression, psychiatric or emotional conditions, or Parkinson's disease), or for 2 weeks after stopping the MAOI drug. If you are uncertain whether your prescription drug contains an MAOI, consult a health professional before taking this product.

Formula: Active Ingredients: Each caplet contains Acetaminophen, 500 mg., Dextromethorphan Hydrobromide, 15 mg.; Phenylpropanolamine Hydrochloride, 12.5 mg.; Chlorpheniramine Maleate, 2 mg. **Inactive Ingredients (listed for individuals with specific allergies):** Cellulose, FD&C Blue 1, Hydroxypropyl Methylcellulose, Polyethylene Glycol, Polysorbate 80, Povidone, Sodium Starch Glycolate, Starch, Stearic Acid, Titanium Dioxide.
Avoid storing at high temperature (greater than 100°F).

How Supplied: Consumer packages of 16 and 30 caplets.

Note: There are other CONTAC products. Make sure this is the one you are interested in.
Shown in Product Identification Guide, page 520

CONTAC
Severe Cold and Flu
Non-Drowsy
Caplets
Decongestant * Analgesic
Cough Suppressant

Product Information: Two caplets every 6 hours to help relieve, without drowsiness, the discomfort of severe colds with flu-like symptoms.
Product Benefits: Contac Severe Cold and Flu Non-Drowsy contains a NON-ASPIRIN ANALGESIC, a DECONGESTANT, and a COUGH SUPPRESSANT.

Indications: Temporarily relieves nasal congestion and coughing due to the common cold. Provides temporary relief of fever, sore throat, headache and minor aches associated with the common cold or the flu.

Directions: Adults (12 years and older): Two caplets every 6 hours, not to exceed 8 caplets in any 24-hour period, or as directed by a doctor. Children under 12 years of age: consult a doctor.

Warnings: Do not take this product for more than 10 days. If symptoms do not improve or are accompanied by fever that lasts for more than 3 days, or if new symptoms occur, consult a doctor. If sore throat is severe, persists for more than 2 days, is accompanied or followed by fever, headache, rash, nausea, or vomiting, consult a doctor promptly. A persistent cough may be a sign of a serious condition. If cough persists for more than 7 days, tends to recur, or is accompanied by rash, persistent headache, fever that lasts for more than 3 days, or if new symptoms occur, consult a doctor. Do not take this product for persistent or chronic cough such as occurs with smoking, asthma, emphysema, or if cough is accompanied by excessive phlegm (mucus) unless directed by a doctor. Do not take this product if you have heart disease, high blood pressure, thyroid disease, diabetes, or difficulty in urination due to enlargement of the prostate gland unless directed by a doctor. **Do not exceed recommended dosage.** If nervousness, dizziness, or sleeplessness occur, discontinue use and consult a doctor. **KEEP THIS AND ALL DRUGS OUT OF THE REACH OF CHILDREN.** In case of accidental overdose, seek professional assistance or contact a Poison Control Center immediately. Prompt medical attention is critical for adults as well as for children even if you do not notice any signs or symptoms. As with any drug, if you are pregnant or nursing a baby, seek the advice of a health professional before using this product.

Drug Interaction Precaution: Do not use this product if you are now taking a prescription monoamine oxidase inhibitor (MAOI) (certain drugs for depression, psychiatric or emotional conditions, or Parkinson's disease), or for 2 weeks after stopping the MAOI drug. If you are uncertain whether your prescription drug contains an MAOI, consult a health professional before taking this product.

Active Ingredients: Acetaminophen 325 mg, Pseudoephedrine Hydrochloride 30 mg and Dextromethorphan Hydrobromide 15 mg.

Inactive Ingredients: Carnuba Wax, Colloidal Silicon Dioxide, Hydroxypropyl Methylcellulose, Magnesium Stearate, Microcrystalline Cellulose, Polyethylene Glycol, Polysorbate 80, Starch, Stearic Acid and Titanium Dioxide.
Store at controlled room temperature (59° to 86°F).
Retain outer carton for complete directions and warnings.

How Supplied: Consumer package of 16 and 30 caplets.
Note: There are other Contact products. Make sure this is the one you are interested in.
Shown in Product Identification Guide, page 520

PDR For Nonprescription Drugs

	CONTACT 12 Hour Cold Caplets	CONTACT 12 Hour Cold Capsules	CONTAC Severe Cold and Flu Caplets (each 2 caplet dose)	CONTAC Severe Cold and Flu Non-Drowsy Caplet (each 2 caplet dose)	CONTAC Day & Night Cold & Flu Day Caplets	CONTAC Day & Night Cold & Flu Night Caplets
Phenylpropanolamine HCl	75.0 mg	75.0 mg	25.0 mg	—	—	—
Chlorpheniramine Maleate	12.0 mg	8.0 mg	4.0 mg	—	—	—
Pseudoephedrine HCl	—	—	—	60.0 mg	60.0 mg	60.0 mg
Acetaminophen	—	—	1000.0 mg	650.0 mg	650.0 mg	650.0 mg
Dextromethorphan Hydrobromide	—	—	30.0 mg	30.0 mg	30.0 mg	—
Diphenhydramine HCl	—	—	—	—	—	50.0 mg

DEBROX® Drops
Ear Wax Removal Aid

Description: Carbamide peroxide 6.5%. Also contains citric acid, glycerin, propylene glycol, sodium stannate, water, and other ingredients.

Actions: DEBROX®, used as directed, cleanses the ear with sustained microfoam. DEBROX Drops foam on contact with earwax due to the release of oxygen (there may be an associated crackling sound). DEBROX Drops provide a safe, nonirritating method of softening and removing ear wax.

Indications: For occasional use as an aid to soften, loosen, and remove excessive earwax.

Directions: FOR USE IN THE EAR ONLY. Adults and children over 12 years of age: tilt head sideways and place 5 to 10 drops into ear. Tip of applicator should not enter ear canal. Keep drops in ear for several minutes by keeping head tilted or placing cotton in the ear. Use twice daily for up to four days if needed, or as directed by a doctor. Any wax remaining after treatment may be removed by gently flushing the ear with warm water, using a soft rubber bulb ear syringe. Children under 12 years of age: consult a doctor.

Warnings: Do not use if you have ear drainage or discharge, ear pain, irritation or rash in the ear, or are dizzy; consult a doctor. Do not use if you have an injury or perforation (hole) of the eardrum or after ear surgery unless directed by a doctor. Do not use for more than four days. If excessive earwax remains after use of this product, consult a doctor. Avoid contact with the eyes.

Cautions: Avoid exposing bottle to excessive heat and direct sunlight. Keep tip on bottle when not in use. Keep this and all drugs out of the reach of children. In case of accidental ingestion, seek professional assistance or contact a poison control center immediately.

How Supplied: DEBROX Drops are available in ½- or 1-fl-oz (15 or 30 ml) plastic squeeze bottles with applicator spouts.

Shown in Product Identification Guide, page 520

ECOTRIN®
Enteric-Coated Aspirin
Antiarthritic, Antiplatelet

Description: 'Ecotrin' is enteric-coated aspirin (acetylsalicylic acid, ASA) available in tablet and caplet forms in 81 mg, 325 mg and 500 mg dosage units. The enteric coating covers a core of aspirin and is designed to resist disintegration in the stomach, dissolving in the more neutral-to-alkaline environment of the duodenum. Such action helps to protect the stomach from injury that may result from ingestion of plain, buffered or highly buffered aspirin (see SAFETY).

Indications: 'Ecotrin' is indicated for:
- conditions requiring chronic or long-term aspirin therapy for pain and/or inflammation, e.g., rheumatoid arthritis, juvenile rheumatoid arthritis, systemic lupus erythematosus, osteoarthritis (degenerative joint disease), ankylosing spondylitis, psoriatic arthritis, Reiter's syndrome and fibrositis,
- antiplatelet indications of aspirin (see the ANTIPLATELET-EFFECT section) and
- situations in which compliance with aspirin therapy may be affected because of the gastrointestinal side effects of plain, i.e., non-enteric-coated, or buffered aspirin.

Dosage: For analgesic indications, the OTC maximum dosage for aspirin is 4000 mg per day in divided doses, i.e., up to 650 mg every 4 hours or 1000 mg every 6 hours.
For antiplatelet effect dosage: see the ANTIPLATELET EFFECT section.
Under a physician's direction, the dosage can be increased or otherwise modified as appropriate to the clinical situation. When 'Ecotrin' is used for anti-inflammatory effect, the physician should be attentive to plasma salicylate levels, and may also caution the patient to be alert to the development of tinnitus as an indicator of elevated salicylate levels. It should be noted that patients with a high frequency hearing loss (such as may occur in older individuals) may have difficulty perceiving the tinnitus. Tinnitus would then not be a reliable indicator in such individuals.

Inactive Ingredients:
ECOTRIN 81 mg—Carnauba Wax, D&C Yellow #10, FD&C Blue #2, FD&C Red #40, FD&C Yellow #6, Hydroxypropyl Methylcellulose, Iron Oxide, Methacrylic Acid Copolymer, Microcrystalline Cellulose, Polyethylene Glycol, Polysorbate 80, Propylene Glycol, Silicon Dioxide, Starch, Stearic Acid, Talc, Titanium Dioxide, Triethyl Citrate.
ECOTRIN 325 mg and 500 mg—Carnauba Wax, Cellulose Acetate Phthalate, Diethyl Phthalate, D&C Yellow #10, FD&C Blue #2, FD&C Red #40, FD&C Yellow #6, Iron Oxide, Microcrystalline Cellulose, Silicon Dioxide, Sodium Starch Glycolate, Starch, Stearic Acid, Titanium Dioxide.

Bioavailability: The bioavailability of aspirin from 'Ecotrin' has been demonstrated in a number of salicylate excretion studies. The studies show levels of salicylate (and metabolites) in urine excreted over 48 hours for 'Ecotrin' do not differ statistically from plain, i.e., non-enteric-coated, aspirin.
Plasma studies, in which 'Ecotrin' has been compared with plain aspirin in steady-state studies over eight days, also demonstrate that 'Ecotrin' provides plasma salicylate levels not statistically different from plain aspirin.
Information regarding salicylate levels over a range of doses was generated in a study in which 24 healthy volunteers (12

male and 12 female) took daily (divided) doses of either 2600 mg, 3900 mg, or 5200 mg of 'Ecotrin'. Plasma salicylate levels generally acknowledged to be anti-inflammatory (15 mg/dL.) were attained at daily doses of 5200 mg, on Day 2 by females and Day 3 by males. At 3900 mg, anti-inflammatory levels were attained at Day 3 by females and Day 4 by males. Dissolution of the enteric coating occurs at a neutral-to-basic pH and is therefore dependent on gastric emptying into the duodenum. With continued dosing, appropriate plasma levels are maintained.

Safety: The safety of 'Ecotrin' has been demonstrated in a number of endoscopic studies comparing 'Ecotrin', plain aspirin, buffered aspirin and highly buffered aspirin preparations. In these studies, all forms of aspirin were dosed to the OTC maximum (3900–4000 mg per day) for up to 14 days. The normal healthy volunteers participating in these studies were gastroscoped before and after the courses of treatment and 14-day drug-free periods followed active drug. Compared to all the other preparations, there was less gastric damage at a statistically significant level during the 'Ecotrin' courses. There was also statistically less duodenal damage when compared with the plain, i.e., non-enteric-coated, aspirin.
Details of studies demonstrating the safety and bioavailability of 'Ecotrin' are available to health care professionals. Write: Professional Services Department, SmithKline Beecham Consumer Healthcare, L.P., P.O. Box 1467, Pittsburgh, Pa. 15230.

WARNINGS: Children and teenagers should not use this product for chicken pox or flu symptoms before a doctor is consulted about Reye Syndrome, a rare but serious illness reported to be associated with aspirin. Do not take this product for pain for more than 10 days or for fever for more than 3 days unless directed by a doctor. If pain or fever persists or gets worse, if new symptoms occur, or if redness or swelling is present, consult a doctor because these could be signs of a serious condition. Do not take this product if you are allergic to aspirin, have asthma, or if you have stomach problems that persist or recur, or if you have ulcers or bleeding problems unless directed by a doctor. If ringing in the ears or a loss of hearing occurs, consult a doctor before taking any more of this product. **Keep this and all drugs out of the reach of children.** In case of accidental overdose, seek professional assistance or contact a poison control center immediately. As with any medicine, if you are pregnant or nursing a baby, seek the advice of a health professional before using this product. **IT IS ESPECIALLY IMPORTANT NOT TO USE ASPIRIN DURING THE LAST 3 MONTHS OF PREGNANCY UNLESS SPECIFICALLY DIRECTED TO DO SO BY A DOCTOR BECAUSE IT MAY CAUSE PROBLEMS IN THE UNBORN CHILD**

Continued on next page

SmithKline Beecham—Cont.

OR COMPLICATIONS DURING DELIVERY.

Drug Interaction Precaution: Do not take this product if you are taking a prescription drug for anticoagulation (thinning of the blood), diabetes, gout, or arthritis unless directed by a doctor.

Professional Warning: There have been occasional reports in the literature concerning individuals with impaired gastric emptying in whom there may be retention of one or more enteric coated aspirin tablets over time. This unusual phenomenon may occur as a result of outlet obstruction from ulcer disease alone or combined with hypotonic gastric peristalsis. Because of the integrity of the enteric coating in an acidic environment, these tablets may accumulate and form a bezoar in the stomach. Individuals with this condition may present with complaints of early satiety or of vague upper abdominal distress. Diagnosis may be made by endoscopy or by abdominal films which show opacities suggestive of a mass of small tablets *(Ref.: Bogacz, K. and Caldron, P.: Enteric-coated Aspirin Bezoar: Elevation of Serum Salicylate Level by Barium Study. Amer. J. Med. 1987:83, 783–6.).* Management may vary according to the condition of the patient. Options include: gastrotomy and alternating slightly basic and neutral lavage *(Ref.: Baum, J.: Enteric-Coated Aspirin and the Problem of Gastric Retention. J. Rheum., 1984:11, 250–1.).* While there have been no clinical reports, it has been suggested that such individuals may also be treated with parenteral cimetidine (to reduce acid secretion) and then given sips of slightly basic liquids to effect gradual dissolution of the enteric coating. Progress may be followed with plasma salicylate levels or via recognition of tinnitus by the patient. It should be kept in mind that individuals with a history of partial or complete gastrectomy may produce reduced amounts of acid and therefore have less acidic gastric pH. Under these circumstances, the benefits offered by the acid-resistant enteric coating may not exist.

Antiplatelet Effect Aspirin may be recommended to reduce the risk of death and/or nonfatal myocardial infarction (MI) in patients with a previous infarction or unstable angina pectoris and its use in reducing the risk of transient ischemic attacks in men.
Labeling for both indications follows:

ASPIRIN FOR MYOCARDIAL INFARCTION

Indication: Aspirin is indicated to reduce the risk of death and/or nonfatal myocardial infarction in patients with a previous infarction or unstable angina pectoris.

Clinical Trials: The indication is supported by the results of six, large, randomized multicenter, placebo-controlled studies involving 10,816 predominantly male, post-myocardial infarction (MI) patients and one randomized placebo-controlled study of 1,266 men with unstable angina.[1–7] Therapy with aspirin was begun at intervals after the onset of acute MI varying from less than three days to more than five years and continued for periods of from less than one year to four years. In the unstable angina study, treatment was started within one month after the onset of unstable angina and continued for 12 weeks, and patients with complicating conditions such as congestive heart failure were not included in the study.

Aspirin therapy in MI patients was associated with about a 20 percent reduction in the risk of subsequent death and/or nonfatal reinfarction, a median absolute decrease of 3 percent from the 12 to 22 percent event rates in the placebo groups. In aspirin-treated unstable angina patients, the reduction in risk was about 50 percent, a reduction in event rate to 5% from the 10% in the placebo group over the 12 weeks of the study. Daily dosage of aspirin in the post-myocardial infarction studies was 300 mg in one study and 900 to 1500 mg in five studies. A dose of 325 mg was used in the study of unstable angina.

Adverse Reactions

Gastrointestinal Reactions: Doses of 1000 mg per day of plain aspirin caused gastrointestinal symptoms and bleeding that in some cases were clinically significant. In the largest postinfarction study (the Aspirin Myocardial Infarction Study [AMIS] with 4,500 people), the percentage incidences of gastrointestinal symptoms of a standard, solid-tablet formulation and placebo-treated subjects, respectively, were: stomach pain (14.5%; 4.4%); heartburn (11.9%; 4.8%); nausea and/or vomiting (7.6%; 2.1%); hospitalization for gastrointestinal disorder (4.9%; 3.5%). In the AMIS and other trials, plain aspirin-treated patients had increased rates of gross gastrointestinal bleeding. Symptoms and signs of gastrointestinal irritation were not significantly increased in subjects treated for unstable angina with buffered aspirin in solution.

Cardiovascular and Biochemical: In the AMIS trial, the dosage of 1000 mg per day of plain aspirin was associated with small increases in systolic blood pressure (BP) (average 1.5 to 2.1 mmHg) and diastolic BP (0.5 to 0.6 mmHg), depending upon whether maximal or last available readings were used. Blood urea nitrogen and uric acid levels were also increased, but by less than 1.0 mg%. Subjects with marked hypertension or renal insufficiency had been excluded from the trial so that the clinical importance of these observations for such subjects or for any subjects treated over more prolonged periods is not known. It is recommended that patients placed on long-term aspirin treatment, even at doses of 300 mg per day, be seen at regular intervals to assess changes in these measurements.

Sodium in Buffered Aspirin for Solution Formulations: One tablet daily of buffered aspirin in solution adds 553 mg of sodium to that in the diet and may not be tolerated by patients with active sodium-retaining states such as congestive heart or renal failure. This amount of sodium adds about 30 percent to the 70 to 90 meq intake suggested as appropriate for dietary hypertension in the 1984 Report of the Joint National Committee on Detection, Evaluation, and Treatment of High Blood Pressure.[8]

Dosage and Administration: Although most of the studies used dosages exceeding 300 mg daily, two trials used only 300 mg and pharmacologic data indicate that this dose inhibits platelet function fully. Therefore, 300 mg or a conventional 325 mg aspirin dose daily is a reasonable, routine dose that would minimize gastrointestinal adverse reactions for both solid oral dosage forms (buffered and plain aspirin) and buffered aspirin in solution.

References:
1. Elwood, P.C., et al.: A Randomized Controlled Trial of Acetylsalicylic Acid in the Secondary Prevention of Mortality from Myocardial Infarction, *Br. Med. J.* 1:436–440, 1974.
2. The Coronary Drug Project Research Group: Aspirin in Coronary Heart Disease, *J. Chronic Dis.* 29:625–642, 1976.
3. Breddin, K., et al.: Secondary Prevention of Myocardial Infarction: A Comparison of Acetylsalicylic Acid, Phenprocoumon or Placebo, *Homeostasis* 470:263–268, 1979.
4. Aspirin Myocardial Infarction Study Research Group: A Randomized Controlled Trial of Aspirin in Persons Recovered from Myocardial Infarction, *J.A.M.A.* 243:661–669, 1980.
5. Elwood, P.C., and Sweetnam, P.M.: Aspirin and Secondary Mortality After Myocardial Infarction, *Lancet* pp. 1313–1315, Dec. 22–29, 1979.
6. The Persantine-Aspirin Reinfarction Study Research Group, Persantine and Aspirin in Coronary Heart Disease, *Circulation* 62: 449–469, 1980.
7. Lewis, H.D., et al.: Protective Effects of Aspirin Against Acute Myocardial Infarction and Death in Men with Unstable Angina, Results of a Veterans Administration Cooperative Study, *N. Engl. J. Med.* 309:396–403, 1983.
8. 1984 Report of the Joint National Committee on Detection, Evaluation, and Treatment of High Blood Pressure, U.S. Department of Health and Human Services and U.S. Public Health Service, National Institutes of Health. NIH Pub. No. 84–1088.

Aspirin for Transient Ischemic Attacks

Indication For reducing the risk of recurrent transient ischemic attacks (TIAs) or stroke in men who have had transient ischemia of the brain due to fibrin platelet emboli. There is inadequate evidence that aspirin or buffered aspirin is effective in reducing TIAs in women at the recommended dosage. There is no evidence that aspirin or buffered aspirin is of benefit in the treatment of completed strokes in men or women.

Clinical Trials The indication is supported by the results of a Canadian study[1] in which 585 patients with threatened stroke were followed in a randomized clinical trial for an average of 26 months to determine whether aspirin or sulfinpyrazone, singly or in combination, was superior to placebo in preventing transient ischemic attacks, stroke or death. The study showed that, although sulfinpyrazone had no statistically significant effect, aspirin reduced the risk of continuing transient ischemic attacks, stroke or death by 19 percent and reduced the risk of stroke or death by 31 percent. Another aspirin study carried out in the United States with 178 patients showed a statistically significant number of "favorable outcomes," including reduced transient ischemic attacks, stroke and death.[2]

Precautions Patients presenting with signs and/or symptoms of TIAs should have a complete medical and neurologic evaluation. Consideration should be given to other disorders that resemble TIAs. Attention should be given to risk factors: it is important to evaluate and treat, if appropriate, other diseases associated with TIAs and stroke, such as hypertension and diabetes.

Concurrent administration of absorbable antacids at therapeutic doses may increase the clearance of salicylates in some individuals. The concurrent administration of nonabsorbable antacids may alter the rate of absorption of aspirin, thereby resulting in a decreased acetylsalicylic acid/salicylate ratio in plasma. The clinical significance of these decreases in available aspirin is unknown. Aspirin at dosages of 1,000 mg per day has been associated with small increases in blood pressure, blood urea nitrogen, and serum uric acid levels. It is recommended that patients placed on long-term aspirin treatment be seen at regular intervals to assess changes in these measurements.

Adverse Reactions: At dosages of 1,000 mg or higher of aspirin per day, gastrointestinal side effects include stomach pain, heartburn, nausea and/or vomiting, as well as increased rates of gross gastrointestinal bleeding.

Dosage and Administration Adult dosage for men is 1,300 mg a day, in divided doses of 650 mg twice a day or 325 mg four times a day.

References:
1. The Canadian Cooperative Study Group: Randomized Trial of Aspirin and Sulfinpyrazone in Threatened Stroke, *N. Engl. J. Med.* 299:53, 1978.
2. Fields, W. S., et al.: Controlled Trial of Aspirin in Cerebral Ischemia, *Stroke* 8:301–316, 1980.

How Supplied:
'Ecotrin' Tablets
  81 mg in bottle of 36
  325 mg in bottles of 100*, 250
  500 mg in bottles of 60*, 150

'Ecotrin' Caplets
  500 mg in bottles of 60.
* Without child-resistant caps.

TAMPER-RESISTANT PACKAGE FEATURES FOR YOUR PROTECTION:
- Bottle has imprinted seal under cap.
- The words ECOTRIN LOW or ECOTRIN REG or ECOTRIN MAX appear on each tablet or caplet (see product illustration printed on carton).
- **DO NOT USE THIS PRODUCT IF ANY OF THESE TAMPER-RESISTANT FEATURES ARE MISSING OR BROKEN.**

Comments or Questions? Call Toll-Free 800-245-1040 weekdays.
Shown in Product Identification Guide, page 520

FEOSOL® CAPSULES
Hemantinic
Iron Supplement

Description: 'Feosol' Capsules provide the body with ferrous sulfate—iron in its most efficient form—for simple iron deficiency and iron-deficiency anemia when the need for such therapy has been determined by a physician. The special targeted-release capsule formulation—ferrous sulfate in pellets—reduces stomach upset, a common problem with iron.

Formula:
INGREDIENTS
Dried ferrous sulfate 159 mg (50 mg iron) per capsule. Sugar Spheres, Glycerin, Confectioner's Sugar, Starch, Povidone, White Wax, Gelatin, D&C Red 7, Polyethylene Glycol, Glyceryl Distearate, Ferric Oxide, FD&C Red 40, FD&C Blue 1, D&C Red 33, D&C Yellow 10, and trace amounts of other ingredients.

NUTRITION FACTS
Serving Size: 1 Capsule

Amount Per Capsule	% Daily Value
Iron 50 mg	278%

Directions: Adults and children 12 years and over—One capsule daily or as directed by a physician. Children under 12 years—consult a physician.

TAMPER-RESISTANT PACKAGING FEATURES:
- The carton is protected by a clear overwrap printed with "safety sealed", do not use if overwrap is missing or broken.
- Each capsule is encased in a plastic cell with a foil back; do not use if cell or foil is broken.
- Each FEOSOL capsule is protected by a red Perma-Seal™ band which bonds the two capsule halves together; do not use if capsule is broken or band is missing or broken.

Warnings: Do not exceed recommended dosage. The treatment of any anemic condition should be under the advice and supervision of a physician. Since oral iron products interfere with absorption of oral tectrac cline antibiotics, these products should not be taken

within two hours of each other. Iron-containing medication may occasionally cause constipation or diarrhea. **Keep away from children. Close tightly. Contains iron, which can be harmful or fatal to children in large doses. In case of accidental overdose, seek professional assistance or contact a Poison Control Center immediately.** If you are pregnant or nursing a baby, seek the advice of a health professional before using this product.

Warning: Manufactured with methylchloroform, a substance which harms public health and environment by destroying ozone in the upper atmosphere.

Store at room temperature (59°–86°F.). Avoid excessive heat or humidity.

How Supplied: Packages of 30 and 60 capsules; in Single Unit Packages of 100 capsules (intended for institutional use only).

Also available in Tablets and Elixir.
Shown in Product Identification Guide, page 520

FEOSOL® ELIXIR
Iron Supplement

Description: 'Feosol' Elixir, an unusually palatable iron elixir, provides the body with ferrous sulfate—iron in its most efficient form. The standard elixir for simple iron deficiency and iron-deficiency anemia when the need for such therapy has been determined by a physician.

NUTRITION FACTS
Serving Size: 1 teaspoonful
Servings per Container: 94

Amount per teaspoonful	% Daily Value
Iron 44 mg	244%

Formula:
INGREDIENTS
Purified Water, Sucrose, Glucose, Alcohol 5%, Ferrous Sulfate, Citric Acid, Saccharin Sodium, FD&C Yellow #6, Flavors.

Directions: Adults—1 teaspoonful daily or as directed by a doctor. Children under 12 years—Consult a physician. Mix with water or fruit juice to avoid temporary staining of teeth; do not mix with milk or wine-based vehicles.

TAMPER-RESISTANT PACKAGE FEATURE:
IMPRINTED SEAL AROUND BOTTLE CAP: DO NOT USE IF BROKEN.

Warnings: Do not exceed recommended dosage. The treatment of any anemic condition should be under the advice and supervision of a physician. Since oral iron products interfere with absorption of oral tetracycline antibiotics, these products should not be taken within two hours of each other. Occasional gastrointestinal discomfort (such

Continued on next page

SmithKline Beecham—Cont.

as nausea) may be minimized by taking with meals and by beginning with one teaspoonful the first day, two the second, etc., until the recommended dosage is reached. Iron-containing medication may occasionally cause constipation or diarrhea and liquids may cause temporary staining of the teeth (this is less likely when diluted). **Keep away from children. Close tightly. Contains iron, which can be harmful or fatal to children in large doses. In case of accidental overdose, seek professional assistance or contact a Poison Control Center immediately.** If you are pregnant or nursing a baby, seek the advice of a health professional before using this product.
Store at room temperature (59°–86°F). Protect from freezing.

How Supplied: A clear orange liquid in 16 fl. oz. bottle.

Also available: 'Feosol' Tablets, 'Feosol' Capsules
NOTE: There are other Feosol products. Make sure this is the one you are interested in.
Shown in Product Identification Guide, page 520

FEOSOL® TABLETS
Iron Supplement

Description: 'Feosol' Tablets provide the body with ferrous sulfate, iron in its most efficient form, for iron deficiency and iron-deficiency anemia when the need for such therapy has been determined by a physician. The distinctive triangular-shaped tablet has a coating to prevent oxidation and improve palatability.

NUTRITION FACTS
Serving Size: 1 Tablet
Amount per Tablet   **% Daily Value**
Iron 65 mg   361%

Formula: Each tablet contains 200 mg. of dried ferrous sulfate USP (65 mg. of elemental iron), equivalent to 325 mg. (5 grains) of ferrous sulfate USP: calcium sulfate, starch, glucose, hydroxypropyl methylcellulose, talc, stearic acid, polyethylene glycol, sodium lauryl sulfate, mineral oil, titanium dioxide, D&C Yellow 10, FD&C Blue 2.

Directions: Adults and children 12 years and over—One tablet daily or as directed by a physician. Children under 12 years—Consult a physician.
TAMPER-RESISTANT PACKAGE FEATURES:
• Bottle has imprinted seal under cap. Do not use if missing or broken.
• FEOSOL Tablets are triangular shaped (see product illustration printed on carton).
CAUTION: DO NOT USE THIS PRODUCT IF ANY OF THESE TAMPER-RE-

**SISTANT FEATURES ARE MISSING OR BROKEN.
Comments or Questions?
Call toll-free 800-245-1040 weekdays.**

Warnings: Do not exceed recommended dosage. The treatment of any anemic condition should be under the advice and supervision of a physician. Since oral iron products interfere with absorption of oral tetracycline antibiotics, these products should not be taken within two hours of each other. Occasional gastrointestinal discomfort (such as nausea) may be minimized by taking with meals and by beginning with one tablet the first day, two the second, etc., until the recommended dosage is reached. Iron-containing medication may occasionally cause constipation or diarrhea. **Keep away from children. Close tightly. Contains iron, which can be harmful or fatal to children in large doses. In case of accidental overdose, seek professional assistance or contact a Poison Control Center immediately.** If you are pregnant or nursing a baby, seek the advice of a health professional before using this product.
Store at room temperature (59°–86°F). Not USP for dissolution.

How Supplied: Bottles of 100 tablets. Also available in Capsules and Elixir.
Shown in Product Identification Guide, page 520

GAVISCON® Antacid Tablets
[găv 'ĭs-kŏn]

Composition: Each chewable tablet contains the following active ingredients:
Aluminum hydroxide dried gel... 80 mg
Magnesium trisilicate .... 20 mg
and the following inactive ingredients: alginic acid, calcium stearate, flavor, sodium bicarbonate, starch (may contain cornstarch), and sucrose.

Actions: Unique formulation produces soothing foam which floats on stomach contents. Foam containing antacid precedes stomach contents into the esophagus when reflux occurs to help protect the sensitive mucosa from further irritation. GAVISCON® acts locally without neutralizing entire stomach contents to help maintain integrity of the digestive process. Endoscopic studies indicate that GAVISCON Antacid Tablets are equally as effective in the erect or supine patient.

Indications: GAVISCON is specifically formulated for the temporary relief of heartburn (acid indigestion) due to acid reflux. GAVISCON is not indicated for the treatment of peptic ulcers.

Directions: Chew two to four tablets four times a day or as directed by a physician. Tablets should be taken after meals and at bedtime or as needed. For best results follow by a half glass of water or other liquid. DO NOT SWALLOW WHOLE.

Warnings: Do not take more than 16 tablets in a 24-hour period or 16 tablets daily for more than 2 weeks, except under the advice and supervision of a physician. Do not use this product except under the advice and supervision of a physician if you are on a sodium-restricted diet. Each GAVISCON Tablet contains approximately 0.8 mEq sodium.

Drug Interaction Precaution: Antacids may interact with certain prescription drugs. If you are presently taking a prescription drug, do not take this product without checking with your physician or other health professional.
Store at a controlled room temperature in a dry place.
Keep this and all drugs out of the reach of children. In case of accidental overdose, seek professional assistance or contact a poison control center immediately.

How Supplied: Available in bottles of 100 tablets and in foil-wrapped 2s in boxes of 30 tablets.
Issued 2/87
Shown in Product Identification Guide, page 520

GAVISCON® EXTRA STRENGTH RELIEF FORMULA Antacid Tablets
[găv 'ĭs-kŏn]

Composition: Each chewable tablet contains the following active ingredients:
Aluminum hydroxide .... 160 mg
Magnesium carbonate .... 105 mg
and the following inactive ingredients: alginic acid, calcium stearate, flavor, sodium bicarbonate, and sucrose. May contain stearic acid. Contains sorbitol or mannitol. May contain starch.

Directions: Chew 2 to 4 tablets four times a day or as directed by a physician. Tablets should be taken after meals and at bedtime or as needed. For best results follow by a half glass of water or other liquid. DO NOT SWALLOW WHOLE.

Indications: For the relief of heartburn, sour stomach, acid indigestion and upset stomach associated with these conditions.

Warnings: Do not take more than 16 tablets in a 24-hour period or 16 tablets daily for more than 2 weeks, except under the advice and supervision of a physician. Do not use this product except under the advice and supervision of a physician if you are on a sodium-restricted diet. Each tablet contains approximately 1.3 mEq sodium.

Drug Interaction Precaution: Antacids may interact with certain prescription drugs. If you are presently taking a prescription drug, do not take this product without checking with you physician or other health professional.
Store at a controlled room temperature in a dry place.
Keep this and all drugs out of the reach of children.

In case of accidental overdose, seek professional assistance or contact a poison control center immediately.

How Supplied: Available in bottles of 100 tablets and in foil-wrapped 2s in boxes of 30.

Shown in Product Identification Guide, page 520

GAVISCON® EXTRA STRENGTH RELIEF FORMULA
Liquid Antacid
[găv 'ĭs-kŏn]

Composition: Each 2 teaspoonfuls (10 mL) contains the following active ingredients:
Aluminum hydroxide.................. 508 mg
Magnesium carbonate................. 475 mg
And the following inactive ingredients: benzyl alcohol, edetate disodium, flavor, glycerin, saccharin sodium, simethicone emulsion, sodium alginate, sorbitol solution, water, and xanthan gum.

Indications: For the relief of heartburn, sour stomach, acid indigestion & upset stomach associated with these conditions.

Directions: SHAKE WELL BEFORE USING. Take 2 to 4 teaspoonfuls four times a day or as directed by a physician. GAVISCON Extra Strength Relief Formula Liquid should be taken after meals and at bedtime, followed by half a glass of water. Dispense product only by spoon or other measuring device.

Warnings: Except under the advice and supervision of a physician, do not take more than 16 teaspoonfuls in a 24-hour period or 16 teaspoonfuls daily for more than 2 weeks. May have laxative effect. Do not use this product if you have a kidney disease; do not use this product if you are on a sodium-restricted diet. Each teaspoonful contains approximately 0.9 mEq sodium.

Drug Interaction Precaution: Antacids may interact with certain prescription drugs. If you are presently taking a prescription drug, do not take this product without checking with your physician or other health professional.
Keep tightly closed. Avoid freezing. Store at a controlled room temperature.
Keep this and all drugs out of the reach of children.
In case of accidental overdose, seek professional assistance or contact a poison control center immediately.

How Supplied: Available in 12 fl oz (355 mL) bottles.

Shown in Product Identification Guide, page 520

GAVISCON® Liquid Antacid
[găv 'ĭs-kŏn]

Composition: Each tablespoonful (15 ml) contains the following active ingredients:

Aluminum hydroxide .... 95 mg
Magnesium carbonate .... 358 mg
And the following inactive ingredients: benzyl alcohol, D&C Yellow #10, edetate disodium, FD&C Blue #1, flavor, glycerin, saccharin sodium, sodium alginate, sorbitol solution, water, and xanthan gum.

Indications: For the relief of heartburn, sour stomach, acid indigestion & upset stomach associated with these conditions.

Directions: SHAKE WELL BEFORE USING. Take 1 or 2 tablespoonfuls four times a day or as directed by a physician. GAVISCON Liquid should be taken after meals and at bedtime, followed by half a glass of water. Dispense product only by spoon or other measuring device.

Warnings: Except under the advice and supervision of a physician, do not take more than 8 tablespoonfuls in a 24-hour period or 8 tablespoonfuls daily for more than 2 weeks. May have laxative effect. Do not use this product if you have a kidney disease; do not use this product if you are on a sodium-restricted diet. Each tablespoonful of GAVISCON Liquid contains approximately 1.7 mEq sodium.

Drug Interaction Precaution: Antacids may interact with certain prescription drugs. If you are presently taking a prescription drug, do not take this product without checking with your physician or other health professional.
Keep tightly closed. Avoid freezing. Store at a controlled room temperature.
Keep this and all drugs out of the reach of children.
In case of accidental overdose, seek professional assistance or contact a poison control center immediately.

How Supplied: Bottles of 12 fluid ounce (355 ml) and 6 fluid ounce (177 ml).

Shown in Product Identification Guide, page 520

GAVISCON®-2 Antacid Tablets
[găv 'ĭs-kŏn]

Composition: Each chewable tablet contains the following active ingredients:
Aluminum hydroxide dried gel...160 mg
Magnesium trisilicate .... 40 mg
and the following inactive ingredients: alginic acid, calcium stearate, flavor, sodium bicarbonate, starch (may contain cornstarch), and sucrose.

Indications: GAVISCON® is specifically formulated for the temporary relief of heartburn (acid indigestion) due to acid reflux. GAVISCON is not indicated for the treatment of peptic ulcers.

Directions: Chew one to two tablets four times a day or as directed by a physician. Tablets should be taken after meals and at bedtime or as needed. For best results follow by a half glass of water or other liquid. DO NOT SWALLOW WHOLE.

Warnings: Do not take more than eight tablets in a 24-hour period or eight

tablets daily for more than 2 weeks, except under the advice and supervision of a physician. Do not use this product except under the advice and supervision of a physician if you are on a sodium-restricted diet. Each GAVISCON-2 Tablet contains approximately 1.6 mEq sodium.

Drug Interaction Precaution: Antacids may interact with certain prescription drugs. If you are presently taking a prescription drug, do not take this product without checking with your physician or other health professional.
Store at a controlled room temperature in a dry place.
Keep this and all drugs out of the reach of children. In case of accidental overdose, seek professional assistance or contact a poison control center immediately.

How Supplied: Boxes of 48 foil-wrapped tablets.

Issued 2/87
Shown in Product Identification Guide, page 520

GLY-OXIDE® Liquid

Description: GLY-OXIDE® Liquid contains carbamide peroxide 10%.

Actions: GLY-OXIDE® Liquid has an oxygen-rich formula that works to relieve the pain of canker sores by cleaning and debriding damaged tissue so natural healing can occur. GLY-OXIDE Liquid's dense oxygenating microfoam helps destroy odor-forming germs and flushes out food particles that ordinary brushing can miss.

Administration: Do not dilute. Apply directly from bottle. Replace tip on bottle when not in use.

Indications and Usage: For local treatment and hygienic prevention of minor oral inflammation such as canker sores, denture irritation, and postdental procedure irritation. Place several drops on affected area four times daily, after meals and at bedtime, or as directed by a dentist or physician; expectorate after two or three minutes. Or place 10 drops onto tongue, mix with saliva, swish for several minutes, and expectorate.
As an adjunct to oral hygiene (orthodontics, dental appliances) after regular brushing, swish 10 or more drops vigorously. Continue for two to three minutes; expectorate.
When normal oral hygiene is inadequate or impossible (total care geriatrics, etc), swish 10 or more drops vigorously after meals and expectorate.

Precautions: Severe or persistent oral inflammation, denture irritation, or gingivitis may be serious. If these conditions or unexpected side effects occur, consult a dentist or physician immediately. Avoid contact with eyes. Protect from heat and direct light. Keep this and all drugs out of the reach of children. In case of accidental overdose, seek professional

Continued on next page

SmithKline Beecham—Cont.

assistance or contact a poison control center immediately.

How Supplied: GLY-OXIDE® Liquid is available in ½-fl-oz and 2-fl-oz non-spill, plastic squeeze bottles with applicator spouts.

Shown in Product Identification Guide, page 520

MASSENGILL® Douches,
Towelettes and Cleansing Wash
[mas'sen-gil]

PRODUCT OVERVIEW

Key Facts: Massengill is the brand name for a line of douches which are recommended for routine cleansing and for temporary relief of vaginal itching and irritation. Massengill disposable douches are available in two Vinegar & Water formulas (Extra Mild and Extra Cleansing), a Baking Soda formula, four Cosmetic solutions (Country Flowers, Fresh Baby Powder Scent, Mountain Breeze, and Spring Rain Freshness), and a Medicated formula (with povidone-iodine). Massengill also is available in a Non-Medicated liquid concentrate and powder form. Massengill also has products specially designed to safely and gently cleanse the external vaginal area: Massengill Soft Cloth Towelettes (Unscented and Baby Powder), Massengill Medicated Soft Cloth Towelettes and Massingill Feminine Cleansing Wash.

Major Uses: Massengill's Vinegar & Water, Baking Soda & Water, and Cosmetic douches are recommended for routine douching, or for cleansing following menstruation, prescribed use of vaginal medication or use of contraceptives. Massengill Medicated is recommended in a seven day regimen for the symptomatic relief of minor itching and irritation associated with vaginitis due to Candida albicans, Trichomonas vaginalis, and Gardnerella vaginalis. Massengill Feminine Cleansing Wash is a gentle soapfree way to clean the external vaginal area. Massengill Non-medicated Soft Cloth Towelettes are a convenient and portable way to cleanse the external vaginal area and wash odor away. Massengill Medicated Soft Cloth Towelettes provide temporary relief of minor external itching associated with irritation or skin rashes.

Safety Information: Do not douche during pregnancy unless directed by a physician. Douching does not prevent pregnancy. Do not use this product and consult your physician if you are experiencing any of the following symptoms: unusual vaginal discharge, vaginal bleeding, painful and/or frequent urination, lower abdominal/pelvis pain, or you or your sex partner has genital sores or ulcers.
Massengill Vinegar & Water, Baking Soda & Water, and Cosmetic Douches—If

vaginal dryness or irritation occurs, discontinue use.
Massengill Medicated — Women with iodine-sensitivity should not use this product. If symptoms persist after seven days, or if redness, swelling or pain develop, consult a physician. Do not use while nursing unless directed by a physician.

PRODUCT INFORMATION

MASSENGILL®
[mas'sen-gil]
Disposable Douches
MASSENGILL®
Liquid Concentrate
MASSENGILL® Powder

Ingredients: DISPOSABLES: Extra Mild Vinegar and Water—Purified Water and Vinegar.
Extra Cleansing Vinegar and Water—Purified Water, Vinegar, Puraclean™ (Cetylpyridinium Chloride), Diazolidinyl Urea, Disodium EDTA.
*Puraclean is a trademark for cetylpyridinium chloride, a safe, special cleansing ingredient not found in any other vinegar & water douche.
Baking Soda and Water—Sanitized Water, Sodium Bicarbonate (Baking Soda).
Fresh Baby Powder Scent—Water, SD Alcohol 40, Lactic Acid, Sodium Lactate, Octoxynol-9, Cetylpyridinium Chloride, Propylene Glycol (and) Diazolidinyl Urea (and) Methylparaben (and) Propylparaben, Disodium EDTA, Fragrance, FD&C Blue #1.
Country Flowers—Water, SD Alcohol 40, Lactic Acid, Sodium Lactate, Octoxynol-9, Cetylpyridinium Chloride, Propylene Glycol (and) Diazolidinyl Urea (and), Methylparaben (and) Propylparaben, Disodium EDTA, Fragrance, D&C Red #28, FD&C Blue #1.
Mountain Breeze—Water, SD Alcohol 40, Lactic Acid, Sodium Lactate, Octoxynol-9, Cetylpyridinium Chloride, Propylene Glycol (and) Diazolidinyl Urea (and) Methylparaben (and) Propylparaben, Disodium EDTA, Fragrance, D&C Yellow #10, FD&C Blue #1.
Spring Rain Freshness—Water, SD Alcohol 40, Lactic Acid, Sodium Lactate, Octoxynol-9, Cetylpyridinium Chloride, Propylene Glycol (and) Diazolidinyl Urea (and) Methylparaben (and) Propylparaben, Disodium EDTA, Fragrance.
LIQUID CONCENTRATE: Water, SD Alcohol 40, Lactic Acid, Sodium Bicarbonate, Octoxynol-9, Methyl Salicylate, Eucalyptol, Menthol, Thymol, D&C Yellow #10, FD&C Yellow #6 (Sunset Yellow).
POWDER: Sodium Chloride, Ammonium alum, PEG-8, Phenol, Methyl Salicylate, Eucalyptus Oil, Menthol, Thymol, D&C Yellow #10, FD&C Yellow #6 (Sunset Yellow).

Indications: Recommended for routine cleansing at the end of menstruation, after use of contraceptive creams or jellies (check the contraceptive package instructions first) or to rinse out the residue of prescribed vaginal medication (as directed by physician).

Actions: The buffered acid solutions of Massengill Douches are valuable adjuncts to specific vaginal therapy following the prescribed use of vaginal medication or contraceptives and in feminine hygiene.

Directions: DISPOSABLES: Twist off flat, wing-shaped tab from bottle containing premixed solution, attach nozzle supplied and use. The unit is completely disposable.
LIQUID CONCENTRATE: Fill cap ¾ full, to measuring line, and pour contents into douche bag containing 1 quart of warm water. Mix thoroughly.
POWDER Packettes: Dissolve the contents of 1 packet in a quart of warm water. Mix thoroughly in a separate container or douche bag.
Container: Dissolve two rounded teaspoonfuls in a douche bag containing 1 quart of warm water. Mix thoroughly.

Warning: Douching does not prevent pregnancy. Do not use during pregnancy except under the advice and supervision of your physician. If vaginal dryness or irritation occurs, discontinue use. Use this product only as directed for routine cleansing. You should douche no more than twice a week except on the advice of your doctor.
An association has been reported between douching and pelvic inflammatory disease (PID), a serious infection of your reproductive system which can lead to sterility and/or ectopic (tubal) pregnancy. PID requires immediate medical attention.
PID's most common symptoms are pain and/or tenderness in the lower part of the abdomen and pelvis. You may also experience a vaginal discharge, vaginal bleeding, nausea or fever. Other sexually transmitted diseases (STDs) have similar symptoms and/or frequent urination, genital sores, or ulcers. Douches should not be used for the self treatment of any STDs or PID. If you suspect you have one of these infections or PID, stop using this product and see your doctor immediately.
See the enclosed insert for important health information concerning sexually transmitted diseases and PID.

How Supplied: Disposable—6 oz. disposable plastic bottle.
Liquid Concentrate—4 oz. plastic bottles.
Powder—4 oz., Packettes—12's.
Shown in Product Identification Guide, page 520

MASSENGILL Feminine Cleansing Wash
[mas'sen-gil]

Ingredients: Water, sodium laureth sulfate, magnesium laureth sulfate, sodium laureth-8 sulfate, magnesium laureth-8 sulfate, sodium oleth sulfate, magnesium oleth sulfate, lauramidopropyl betaine, myristamine oxide, lactic acid, PEG-120 methyl glucose dioleate, fragrance, sodium methylparaben, sodium ethylparaben, sodium propylparaben, methylchloroisothiazolinone, methylisothiazolinone, D&C Red #33.

Indications: For cleansing and refreshing of external vaginal area.

Actions: Massengill feminine cleansing wash safely and gently cleanses the external vaginal area.

Directions: Pour small amount into palm of hand or wash cloth and lather into wet skin. Rinse clean. Safe to use daily. For external use only.

How Supplied: 8 fl. oz plastic flip-top bottle.

MASSENGILL®
[mas 'sen-gil]
Fragrance-Free Soft Cloth Towelette and Baby Powder Scent

Ingredients: <u>Unscented</u>
Water, Octoxynol-9, Lactic Acid, Sodium Lactate, Potassium Sorbate, Disodium EDTA, and Cetylpyridinium Chloride.
<u>Baby Powder Scent</u>
Water, Lactic Acid, Sodium Lactate, Potassium Sorbate, Octoxynol-9, Disodium EDTA, Cetylpyridinium Chloride, and Fragrance.

Indications: For cleansing and refreshing the external vaginal area.

Actions: Massengill Baby Powder Scent and Fragrance-Free Soft Cloth Towelettes safely cleanse the external vaginal area. The towelette delivery system makes the application soft and gentle.

Directions: Remove towelette from foil packet, unfold, and gently wipe. Throw away towelette after it has been used once.

How Supplied: Sixteen individually wrapped, disposable towelettes per carton.

MASSENGILL® Medicated
[mas 'sen-gil]
Disposable Douche

Active Ingredient: Cepticin™ (povidone-iodine)

Indications: For symptomatic relief of minor vaginal irritation or itching associated with vaginitis due to Candida albicans, Trichomonas vaginalis, and Gardnerella vaginalis.

Action: Povidone-iodine is widely recognized as an effective broad spectrum microbicide against both gram negative and gram positive bacteria, fungi, yeasts and protozoa. While remaining active in the presence of blood, serum or bodily secretions, it possesses virtually none of the irritating properties of iodine.

Warning: Douching does not prevent pregnancy. Do not use during pregnancy or while nursing except under the advice and supervision of your physician. If vaginal dryness or irritation occurs discontinue use. Use this product only as directed. Do not use this product for routine cleansing.

An association has been reported between douching and pelvic inflammatory disease (PID), a serious infection of your reproductive system, which can lead to sterility and/or ectopic (tubal) pregnancy. PID requires immediate medical attention.
PID's most common symptoms are pain and/or tenderness in the lower part of the abdomen and pelvis. You may also experience a vaginal discharge, vaginal bleeding, nausea or fever. Other sexually transmitted diseases (STDs) have similar symptoms and/or frequent urination, genital sores, or ulcers. Douches should not be used for self-treatment of any STDs or PID. If you suspect you have one of these infections or PID, stop using this product and see your doctor immediately.
See the enclosed insert for important health information concerning sexually transmitted diseases and PID. Women with iodine sensitivity should not use this product.
Keep out of the reach of children.
Avoid storing at high temperature (greater than 100°F).
Protect from freezing.

Dosage and Administration: Dosage is provided as a single unit concentrate to be added to 6 oz. of sanitized water supplied in a disposable bottle. A specially designed nozzle is provided. After use, the unit is discarded. Use one bottle a day for seven days. Although symptoms may be relieved earlier, for maximum relief, treatment should be continued for the full seven days.

How Supplied: 6 oz. bottle of sanitized water with 0.17 oz. vial of povidone-iodine and nozzle.
Shown in Product Identification Guide, page 520

MASSENGILL® Medicated
[mas 'sen-gil]
Soft Cloth Towelette

Active Ingredient: Hydrocortisone (0.5%).

Inactive Ingredients: Diazolidinyl Urea, DMDM Hydantoin, Isopropyl Myristate, Methylparaben, Polysorbate 60, Propylene Glycol, Propylparaben, Sorbitan Stearate, Steareth-2, Steareth-21, Water.
Also available in non-medicated Baby Powder Scent and Unscented formulas to freshen and cleanse the external vaginal area.

Indications: For soothing relief of minor external feminine itching or other itching associated with minor skin irritations, and rashes. Other uses of this product should be only under the advice and supervision of a physician.

Action: Massengill Medicated Soft Cloth Towelettes contain hydrocortisone, a proven anti-inflammatory, anti-pruritic ingredient. The towelette delivery system makes the application soothing, soft, and gentle.

Warnings: For external use only. Avoid contact with eyes. If condition worsens, symptoms persist for more than seven days, or symptoms recur within a few days, do not use this or any other hydrocortisone product unless you have consulted a physician. If experiencing a vaginal discharge, see a physician. Do not use this product for the treatment of diaper rash.
Keep this and all drugs out of the reach of children. As with any drug, if pregnant or nursing a baby, seek the advice of a health professional before using this product. In case of accidental ingestion, seek professional assistance or contact a Poison Control Center immediately.

Directions: Adults and Children two years of age and older—apply to the affected area not more than three to four times daily. Remove towelette from foil packet, gently wipe, and discard. Throw away towelette after it has been used once. Children under 2 years of age: DO NOT USE.

How Supplied: Ten individually wrapped, disposable towelettes per carton.

EDUCATIONAL MATERIAL

"The facts about Vaginal Infections and STDs"
A guide for women on vaginal infections and sexually transmitted diseases (STDs).
Free to physicians, pharmacists and patients in Limited quantities by writing SmithKline Beecham Consumer Healthcare, L.P. or calling 1-800-233-2426.
"A Personal Guide to Feminine Freshness"
A pamphlet on vaginal infections, feminine hygiene and douching. (BiLingual) free to physicians, pharmacists and patients in limited quantities by writing SmithKline Beecham Consumer Healthcare, L.P. or calling 1-800-233-2426

N'ICE® Medicated Sugarless Sore Throat and Cough Lozenges
[nis]

Active Ingredient: <u>Cherry</u>—Each lozenge contains 5.0 mg. menthol in a sorbitol base. <u>Citrus</u>—Each lozenge contains 5.0 mg. menthol in a sorbitol base. <u>Menthol Eucalyptus</u>—Each lozenge contains 5.0 mg. menthol in a sorbitol base. <u>Cool Peppermint</u>—Each lozenge contains 5.0 mg. menthol in a sorbitol base. N'ICE 'N CLEAR <u>Cherry Eucalyptus</u>—Each loz-

Continued on next page

SmithKline Beecham—Cont.

enge contains 7.0 mg. menthol in a sorbitol base. N'ICE 'N CLEAR. Menthol Eucalyptus—Each lozenge contains 5.0 mg. menthol in a sorbitol base.

Inactive Ingredients: Cherry—Flavors, D&C Red 33, Sorbitol, Tartaric Acid, FD&C Yellow 6. Citrus—Citric Acid, Flavors, Saccharin Sodium, Sodium Citrate, Sorbitol, Yellow 10. Menthol Eucalyptus—Citric Acid, Flavors, Sorbitol. Cool Peppermint—Blue 1, Flavor, Maltitol Solution, Sorbitol, Yellow 10. N'ICE 'N CLEAR Cherry Eucalyptus —Flavors, D&C Red 33, Sorbitol, Tartaric Acid, FD&C Yellow 6. N'ICE 'N CLEAR Menthol Eucalyptus—Citric Acid, Flavors, Sorbitol.

Indications: Temporarily suppresses cough due to minor throat and bronchial irritation associated with a cold or inhaled irritants. Temporarily relieves minor sore throat pain.

Warnings: Do not exceed recommended dosage. Excess consumption may have a laxative effect. A persistent cough may be a sign of a serious condition. If cough persists for more than 1 week, tends to recur, or is accompanied by fever, rash, or persistent headache, consult a doctor. Do not take this product for persistent or chronic cough such as occurs with smoking, asthma, emphysema, or if cough is accompanied by excessive phlegm (mucus) unless directed by a doctor. If sore throat is severe, persists for more than 2 days, is accompanied or followed by fever, headache, rash, nausea, or vomiting, consult a doctor promptly. If sore mouth symptoms do not improve in 7 days or if irritation, pain, or redness persists or worsens, see your dentist or doctor promptly. Do not exceed recommended dosage. KEEP THIS AND ALL DRUGS OUT OF THE REACH OF CHILDREN.

Drug Interaction: No known drug interaction.

Dosage and Administration: Cherry, Citrus, Menthol Eucalyptus, Cool Peppermint, N'ICE 'N CLEAR Cherry Eucalyptus, N'ICE 'N CLEAR Menthol Eucalyptus—Adults and children six and older: Let lozenge dissolve slowly in the mouth. Repeat every hour as needed, or as directed by a doctor, up to 10 lozenges per day.

Professional Labeling: For the temporary relief of pain associated with tonsillitis, pharyngitis, throat infections or stomatitis.

How Supplied: Available in packages of 16 lozenges. N'ICE Cherry available in packages of 8 and 16 lozenges.

NOVAHISTINE® DMX
[nō"vă-hĭs'tēn]
Cough/Cold Formula & Decongestant

Active Ingredients: Each 5 ml teaspoonful contains Dextromethorphan Hydrobromide 10 mg., Guaifenesin 100 mg., Pseudoephedrine Hydrochloride 30 mg.

Inactive Ingredients: Alcohol 10%, FD & C Red No. 40, FD & C Yellow No. 6, Flavors, Glycerin, Hydrochloric Acid, Invert Sugar, Saccharin Sodium, Sodium Chloride, Sorbitol and Water.

Indications: For temporary relief from cough and nasal congestion due to the common cold. Helps loosen phlegm (sputum) and thin bronchial secretions to rid the bronchial passageways of bothersome mucus. Helps decongest sinus openings and passages; temporarily relieves sinus congestion and pressure.

Warnings: If symptoms do not improve within 7 days or are accompanied by fever, consult a doctor. A persistent cough may be a sign of a serious condition. If cough persists for more than 7 days, tends to recur, or is accompanied by fever, rash, or persistent headache, consult a doctor. Do not take this product for persistent or chronic cough such as occurs with smoking, asthma, chronic bronchitis or emphysema, or where cough is accompanied by excessive phlegm (mucus) unless directed by a doctor. Do not take this product if you have heart disease, high blood pressure, thyroid disease, diabetes, or difficulty in urination due to enlargement of the prostate gland, unless directed by a doctor. **Do not exceed recommended dosage.** If nervousness, dizziness, or sleeplessness occur, discontinue use and consult a doctor. **KEEP THIS AND ALL DRUGS OUT OF THE REACH OF CHILDREN.** In case of accidental overdose, seek professional assistance or contact a Poison Control Center immediately. As with any drug, if you are pregnant or nursing a baby, seek the advice of a health professional before using this product.

Drug Interaction Precaution: Do not use this product if you are now taking a prescription monoamine oxidase inhibitor (MAOI) (certain drugs for depression, psychiatric or emotional conditions, or Parkinson's Disease), or for 2 weeks after stopping the MAOI drug. If you are uncertain whether your prescription drug contains an MAOI, consult a health professional before taking this product.

Contraindications: NOVAHISTINE DMX is contraindicated in patients with severe hypertension, severe coronary artery disease, and in patients on MAOI therapy. Patient idiosyncrasy to adrenergic agents may be manifested by insomnia, dizziness, weakness, tremor, or arrhythmias.
Nursing mothers: Pseudoephedrine is contraindicated in nursing mothers because of the higher than usual risk for infants from sympathomimetic amines.

Hypersensitivity: NOVAHISTINE DMX is contraindicated in patients with hypersensitivity or idiosyncrasy to sympathomimetic amines, dextromethorphan, or to other formula ingredients.

Adverse Reactions: Adverse reactions occur infrequently with usual oral doses of NOVAHISTINE DMX. When they occur, adverse reactions may include gastrointestinal upset and nausea. Because of the pseudoephedrine in NOVAHISTINE DMX, hyperreactive individuals may display ephedrine-like reactions such as tachycardia, palpitations, headache, dizziness or nausea. Sympathomimetic drugs have been associated with certain untoward reactions including fear, anxiety, tenseness, restlessness, tremor, weakness, pallor, respiratory difficulty, dysuria, insomnia, hallucinations, convulsions, CNS depression, arrhythmias, and cardiovascular collapse with hypotension.
Note: Guaifenesin interferes with the colorimetric determination of 5-hydroxyindoleacetic acid (5-HIAA) and vanillylmandelic acid (VMA).

Directions For Use: Adults and children 12 years and older: 2 teaspoonfuls every 4 hours, not to exceed 8 teaspoonfuls in 24 hours, or as directed by a doctor. Children 6 to under 12 years: 1 teaspoonful every 4 hours, not to exceed 4 teaspoonfuls in 24 hours, or as directed by a doctor. Consult a doctor for the use in children under 6 years of age.

How Supplied: NOVAHISTINE DMX, in 4 fluid ounce bottles. Keep tightly closed. Protect from excessive heat and light. Avoid freezing.
Shown in Product Identification Guide, page 521

NOVAHISTINE® Elixir
[nō"vă-hĭs'tēn]
Cold & Hay Fever Formula

Active Ingredients: Each 5 ml teaspoonful of NOVAHISTINE Elixir contains: Chlorpheniramine Maleate 2 mg. and Phenylephrine Hydrochloride 5 mg.

Inactive Ingredients: Alcohol 5%, D & C Yellow No. 10, FD & C Blue No. 1, Flavors, Glycerin, Sodium Chloride, Sorbitol and Water. Although considered sugar-free, each 5 ml contributes approximately 7 calories from sorbitol.

Indications: For the temporary relief of nasal congestion, runny nose, sneezing, itching of the nose or throat, and itchy watery eyes due to the common cold, hay fever, or other upper respiratory allergies.

Warnings: If symptoms do not improve within 7 days or are accompanied by a fever, consult a doctor. May cause excitability especially in children. Do not take this product, unless directed by a doctor, if you have a breathing problem such as emphysema or chronic bronchitis, or if you have heart disease, high blood pressure, thyroid disease, diabetes, glaucoma, or difficulty in urination due to enlargement of the prostate gland. May cause drowsiness; alcohol, sedatives, and tranquilizers may increase the drowsiness effect. Avoid alcoholic beverages while taking this product. Do not take this product if you are taking sedatives or tranquilizers, without first consulting your doctor. Use caution when driving a motor vehicle or operating machinery. **Do not exceed recommended dosage.** If nervousness, dizziness, or sleeplessness occur, discontinue use and consult a doctor. **KEEP THIS AND ALL DRUGS OUT OF THE REACH OF CHILDREN.** In case of accidental overdose, seek professional assistance or contact a Poison Control Center immediately. As with any drug, if you are pregnant or nursing a baby, seek the advice of a health professional before using this product.

Drug Interaction Precaution: Do not use this product if you are now taking a prescription monoamine oxidase inhibitor (MAOI) (certain drugs for depression, psychiatric or emotional conditions, or Parkinson's Disease), or for 2 weeks after stopping the MAOI drug. If you are uncertain whether your prescription drug contains an MAOI, consult a health professional before taking this product.

Contraindications: NOVAHISTINE Elixir is contraindicated in patients with severe hypertension, severe coronary artery disease, and in patients on MAOI therapy. Patient idiosyncrasy to adrenergic agents may be manifested by insomnia, dizziness, weakness, tremor, or arrhythmias.
NOVAHISTINE Elixir is also contraindicated in patients with narrow-angle glaucoma, urinary retention, peptic ulcer, asthma, emphysema, chronic pulmonary disease, shortness of breath, or difficulty in breathing.
Nursing Mothers: Phenylephrine is contraindicated in nursing mothers.
Hypersensitivity: NOVAHISTINE Elixir is also contraindicated in patients with hypersensitivity or idiosyncrasy to sympathomimetic amines, antihistamines, or to other formula ingredients.

Adverse Reactions: Drugs containing sympathomimetic amines have been associated with certain untoward reactions, including fear, anxiety, tenseness, restlessness, tremor, weakness, pallor, respiratory difficulty, dysuria, insomnia, hallucinations, convulsions, CNS depression, arrhythmias, and cardiovascular collapse with hypotension. Individuals hyperreactive to phenylephrine may display ephedrine-like reactions such as tachycardia, palpitations, headache, dizziness, or nausea.
Phenylephrine is considered safe and relatively free of unpleasant side effects when taken at recommended dosage. Patients sensitive to antihistamine drugs may experience mild sedation. Other side effects from antihistamines may include dry mouth, dizziness, weakness, anorexia, nausea, vomiting, headache,

nervousness, polyuria, heartburn, diplopia, dysuria, and very rarely dermatitis.

Directions For Use: Adults (12 years and older): 2 teaspoonfuls every 4 hours, not to exceed 12 teaspoonfuls in 24 hours, or as directed by a doctor. Children 6 to under 12 years: 1 teaspoonful ever 4 hours, not to exceed 6 teaspoonfuls in 24 hours, or as directed by a doctor. Consult a doctor for use in chldren under 6 years of age.

How Supplied: NOVAHISTINE Elixir, in 4 fluid ounce bottles. Keep tightly closed. Protect from excessive heat and light. Avoid freezing.
Shown in Product Identification Guide, page 521

PANADOL®
Acetaminophen
Tablets and Caplets

Description: Each Maximum Strength PANADOL Caplet or Tablet contains acetaminophen 500 mg.

Indications: For the fast, temporary relief of minor aches, and pains associated with headaches, backaches, muscle aches, toothache, menstrual pain and colds and flu. Also to reduce fever and for temporary relief of minor arthritis pain.

Directions: Adults and children 12 years and over: 2 tablets or caplets every 4 hours as needed, not to exceed 8 tablets or caplets in 24 hours or as directed by a doctor.
Children under 12 years: Consult a doctor.

Warnings: Do not take this product for pain for more than 10 days or for fever for more than 3 days unless directed by a doctor. If pain or fever persists or gets worse, if new symptoms occur, or if redness or swelling is present, consult a doctor because these could be signs of a serious condition. Keep this and all drugs out of the reach of children. In case of accidental overdose, seek professional assistance or contact a poison control center immediately. Prompt medical attention is critical for adults as well as for children even if you do not notice any signs or symptoms. As with any drug, if you are pregnant or nursing a baby, seek the advice of a health professional before using this product.

Active Ingredient: Acetaminophen 500 mg per tablet or caplet.

Inactive Ingredients: Hydroxypropyl Methylcellulose, Potassium Sorbate, Povidone, Pregelatinized Starch, Starch, Stearic Acid, Talc, and Triacetin.

How Supplied: Tablets (white with "P" and "500" imprint) in bottles of 30 and 60. Caplets (white with "P" and "500" imprint) in bottle of 24.
Shown in Product Identification Guide, page 521

Children's PANADOL®
Acetaminophen Chewable Tablets, Liquid, Drops

Description: Each Children's PANADOL Chewable Tablet contains 80 mg acetaminophen in a fruit-flavored sugar-free tablet. Children's PANADOL Acetaminophen Liquid is fruit-flavored, red in color, and is alcohol-free, sugar-free and aspirin-free. Each ½ teaspoonful contains 80 mg of acetaminophen. Infant's PANADOL Drops are fruit-flavored, red in color, and are alcohol-free, sugar-free and aspirin-free. Each 0.8 mL (one calibrated dropperful) contains 80 mg acetaminophen.

Indications: Acetaminophen, the active ingredient in Children's PANADOL, is the analgesic/antipyretic most widely recommended by pediatricians for fast, effective relief of children's fevers. It also relieves the aches and pains of colds and flu, earaches, headaches, teething, immunizations, tonsillectomy, and childhood illnesses.
Children's PANADOL Tablets, Liquid, and Drops are aspirin-free and contain no alcohol or sugar. The pleasant-tasting formulations are not likely to upset or irritate children's stomachs.

Usual Dosage: Dosing is based on single doses in the range of 10–15 mg/kg body weight. Doses may be repeated every four hours up to 4 or 5 times daily, but not to exceed 5 doses in 24 hours. To be administered to children under 2 years only on advice of a physician.
Children's PANADOL Chewable Tablets: 2–3 yr, 24–35 lb, 2 tablets; 4–5 yr, 36–47 lb, 3 tablets; 6–8 yr, 48–59 lb, 4 tablets; 9–10 yr, 60–71 lb, 5 tablets; 11 yr, 72–95 lb, 6 tablets. May be repeated every 4 hours, up to 5 times in a 24-hour period.
Children's PANADOL Liquid: 4–11 mo, 12–17 lb, ½ teaspoonful; 12–23 mo, 18–23 lb, ¾ teaspoonful; 2–3 yr, 24–35 lb, 1 teaspoonful; 4–5 yr, 36–47 lb, 1½ teaspoonfuls; 6–8 yr, 48–59 lb, 2 teaspoonfuls; 9–10 yr, 60–71 lb, 2½ teaspoonfuls; 11 yr, 72–95 lb, 3 teaspoonfuls. May be repeated every 4 hours up to 5 times in a 24-hour period. May be administered alone or mixed with formula, milk, juice, cereal, etc.
Infant's PANADOL Drops: 0–3 mo, 6–11 lb, ½ dropperful (0.4 mL); 4–11 mo, 12–17 lb, 1 dropperful (0.8 mL); 12–23 mo, 18–23 lb, 1½ dropperfuls (1.2 mL); 2–3 yr, 24–35 lb, 2 dropperfuls (1.6 mL); 4–5 yr, 36–47 lb, 3 dropperfuls (2.4 mL); 6–8 yr, 48–59 lb, 4 dropperfuls (3.2 mL). May be repeated every 4 hours, up to 5 times in a 24-hour period. May be administered alone or mixed with formula, milk, juice, cereal, etc.

Warnings: Do not give this product for pain for more than 5 days or for fever for more than 3 days unless directed by a doctor. If pain or fever persists or gets worse, if new symptoms occur, or if redness or swelling is present, consult a doc-

Continued on next page

SmithKline Beecham—Cont.

tor because these could be signs of a serious condition. Keep this and all drugs out of the reach of children. In case of accidental overdose, seek professional assistance or contact a poison control center immediately. Prompt medical attention is critical for adults as well as for children even if you do not notice any signs or symptoms. As with any drug, if you are pregnant or nursing a baby, seek the advice of a health professional before using this product.

Composition:
Chewable Tablets: Active Ingredient: Acetaminophen, 80 mg per tablet. Inactive Ingredients: FD&C Red No. 28, FD&C Red No. 40, flavor, Mannitol, Saccharin Sodium, Starch, Stearic Acid and other ingredients.
Liquid: Active Ingredient: Acetaminophen, 80 mg per ½ teaspoon. Inactive Ingredients: Benzoic acid, FD&C Red No. 40, Flavor, Glycerin, Polyethylene Glycol, Potassium Sorbate, Propylene Glycol, Purified Water, Saccharin Sodium, Sorbitol solution. May also contain Sodium Chloride or Sodium Hydroxide.
Drops: Active Ingredient: Acetaminophen, 80 mg per 0.8mL dropper. Inactive Ingredients: Citric Acid, FD&C Red No. 40, Flavors, Glycerin, Parabens, Polyethylene Glycol, Propylene Glycol, Purified Water, Saccharin Sodium, Sodium Chloride, Sodium Citrate.

How Supplied: Chewable Tablets (colored pink and scored)—bottles of 30. Liquid (colored red)—bottles of 2 fl. oz. and 4 fl. oz. Drops (colored red)—bottles of ½ oz. (15 mL).
All packages listed above have child-resistant safety caps and tamper-resistant features.

Shown in Product Identification Guide, page 521

SINE–OFF®
No Drowsiness Formula
Caplets

Active Ingredients: Each caplet contains: Pseudoephedrine Hydrochloride 30 mg., Acetaminophen 500 mg.

Inactive Ingredients: Crospovidone, FD & C Red 40, Hydroxypropyl Methylcellulose, Magnesium Stearate, Microcrystalline Cellulose, Polyethylene Glycol, Polysorbate 80, Povidone, Starch, and Titanium Dioxide.

Indications: For temporary relief of sinus and headache pain and nasal congestion associated with sinusitis or due to a cold, hay fever or other upper respiratory allergies (allergic rhinitis). Temporarily restores freer breathing through the nose. Helps decongest sinus openings and passages; temporarily relieves sinus congestion and pressure.

Directions For Use: Adults (12 years and older): 2 caplets every 6 hours, not to exceed 8 caplets in any 24-hour period, or

as directed by a doctor. Children under 12 years of age: Consult a doctor.

Warnings: Do not take this product for more than 10 days. If symptoms do not improve or are accompanied by fever that lasts for more than 3 days, or if new symptoms occur, consult a doctor. Do not take this product if you have heart disease, high blood pressure, thyroid disease, diabetes, or difficulty in urination due to enlargement of the prostate gland unless directed by a doctor. **Do not exceed recommended dosage.** If nervousness, dizziness, or sleeplessness occur, discontinue use and consult a doctor. **KEEP THIS AND ALL DRUGS OUT OF THE REACH OF CHILDREN.** In case of accidental overdose, seek professional assistance or contact a Poison Control Center immediately. Prompt medical attention is critical for adults as well as for children even if you do not notice any signs or symptoms. As with any drug, if you are pregnant or nursing a baby, seek the advice of a health professional before using this product.

Drug Interaction Precaution: Do not use this product if you are now taking a prescription monoamine oxidase inhibitor (MAOI) (certain drugs for depression, psychiatric or emotional conditions, or Parkinson's disease), or for 2 weeks after stopping the MAOI drug. If you are uncertain whether your prescription drug contains an MAOI, consult a health profesional before taking this product.
Note: There are other SINE-OFF products. Make sure this is the one you are interested in.
Also Available: SINE-OFF Sinus Medicine Caplets, 24 and 100 count.

Tamper-Evident Package Features
● Each caplet is encased in a clear plastic cell with a foil back.
● The name SINE-OFF appears on each caplet.
● DO NOT USE THIS PRODUCT IF ANY OF THESE TAMPER-EVIDENT FEATURES ARE MISSING OR BROKEN.
Comments or Questions? Call Toll-Free 1-800-245-1040 Weekdays.
Avoid storing at high temperature (greater than 100°F).

Shown in Product Identification Guide, page 521

SINE–OFF® Sinus Medicine
Caplets
Relieves sinus headache, pain, pressure, congestion, runny nose, sneezing & itchy, watery eyes.

Active Ingredients: Each caplet contains: Chlorpheniramine 2 mg, Pseudoephedrine Hydrochloride 30 mg., Acetaminophen 500 mg.

Inactive Ingredients: Carnauba Wax, Hydroxypropyl Methylcellulose, Magnesium Stearate, Microcrystalline Cellulose, Polydextrose, Polyethylene Glycol, Povidone, Sodium Starch Glycolate, Starch, Stearic Acid, Titanium Dioxide,

Triacetin, FD & C Yellow #6, D & C Yellow 10.

Indications: For temporary relief of sinus and headache pain and nasal congestion associated with sinusitis or due to a cold, hay fever or other upper respiratory allergies. Promotes nasal and/or sinus drainage; temporarily relieves sinus congestion and pressure. Also temporarily relieves runny nose, sneezing, itching of the nose or throat, and itchy, watery eyes due to hay fever or other upper respiratory allergies.

Directions: Adults (12 years and older): 2 caplets every 6 hours, not to exceed 8 caplets in any 24-hour period, or as directed by a doctor. Children under 12 of age: Consult a doctor.

Warnings: Do not take this product for more than 10 days. If symptoms do not improve or are accompanied by fever that lasts for more than 3 days, or if new symptoms occur, consult a doctor. Do not take this product, unless directed by a doctor, if you have a breathing problem such as emphysema or chronic bronchitis, or if you have heart disease, high blood pressure, thyroid disease, diabetes, glaucoma or difficulty in urination due to enlargement of the prostate gland. May cause excitability, especially in children. May cause drowsiness; alcohol, sedatives, and tranquilizers may increase the drowsiness effect. Avoid alcoholic beverages while taking this product. Do not take this product if you are taking sedatives or tranquilizers, without first consulting your doctor. Use caution when driving a motor vehicle or operating machinery. **Do not exceed recommended dosage.** If nervousness, dizziness, or sleeplessness occur, discontinue use and consult a doctor. **KEEP THIS AND ALL DRUGS OUT OF THE REACH OF CHILDREN.** Prompt medical attention is critical for adults as well as for children even if you do not notice any signs or symptoms. In case of accidental overdose, seek professional assistance or contact a Poison Control Center immediately. As with any drug, if you are pregnant or nursing a baby, seek the advice of a health professional before using this product.

Drug Interaction Precaution: Do not use this product if you are now taking a prescription monoamine oxidase inhibitor (MAOI) (certain drugs for depression, psychiatric or emotional conditions, or Parkinson's disease), or for 2 weeks after stopping the MAOI drug. If you are uncertain whether your prescription drug contains an MAOI, consult a health professional before taking this product.

How Supplied: Consumer packages of 24 and 100 caplets.
Note: There are other SINE-OFF products. Make sure this is the one you are interested in.
Also Available: SINE-OFF® Maximum Strength No Drowsiness Formula Caplets 24's .

Tamper-Resistant Package Features For Your Protection:

- Outer carton is sealed.
- Each blister unit is sealed in printed foil.
- DO NOT USE THIS PRODUCT IF ANY OF THESE TAMPER-EVIDENT FEATURES ARE MISSING OR BROKEN.

Comments or Questions? Call Toll-Free 1-800-245-1040 Weekdays.
Store at controlled room temperature (59–86°F).

Shown in Product Identification Guide, page 521

SINGLET® For Adults
Nasal Decongestant/Antihistamine/ Analgesic (pain reliever)/Antipyretic (fever reducer)

Indications: For temporary relief of nasal congestion and sinus and headache pain associated with sinusitis or due to a cold, hay fever or other upper respiratory allergies. Also temporarily relieves nasal congestion, sinus headache, runny nose, sneezing, itching of the nose or throat, and itchy, watery eyes due to hay fever or other upper respiratory allergies. Also temporarily relieves fever due to the common cold.

Directions: Adults (12 years and older): 1 caplet every 4 to 6 hours, **not to exceed 4 caplets in any 24-hour period,** or as directed by a doctor. Children under 12 years of age: Consult a doctor.

Warnings: Do not take this product for more than 10 days. If symptoms do not improve or are accompanied by fever that lasts for more than 3 days, or if new symptoms occur, consult a doctor. Do not take this product, unless directed by a doctor, if you have a breathing problem such as emphysema or chronic bronchitis, or if you have heart disease, high blood pressure, thyroid disease, diabetes, glaucoma or difficulty in urination due to enlargement of the prostate gland. May cause excitability especially in children. May cause drowsiness; alcohol, sedatives, and tranquilizers may increase the drowsiness effect. Avoid alcoholic beverages while taking this product. Do not take this product if you are taking sedatives or tranquilizers, without first consulting your doctor. Use caution when driving a motor vehicle or operating machinery. **Do not exceed recommended dosage.** If nervousness, dizziness, or sleeplessness occur, discontinue use and consult a doctor. **KEEP THIS AND ALL DRUGS OUT OF THE REACH OF CHILDREN.** Prompt medical attention is critical for adults as well as for children even if you do not notice any signs or symptoms. In case of accidental overdose, seek professional assistance or contact a Poison Control Center immediately. As with any drug, if you are pregnant or nursing a baby, seek the advice of a health professional before using this product.

Drug Interaction Precaution: Do not use this product if you are now taking a prescription monoamine oxidase inhibitor (MAOI) (certain drugs for depression, psychiatric or emotional conditions, or Parkinson's disease), or for 2 weeks after stopping the MAOI drug. If you are uncertain whether your prescription drug contains an MAOI, consult a health professional before taking this product.

Active Ingredients: Each caplet contains: Pseudoephedrine Hydrochloride 60 mg, Chlorpheniramine Maleate 4 mg, Acetaminophen 650 mg.

Inactive Ingredients: D&C Red 27, D&C Yellow 10, FD&C Blue 1, Hydroxypropyl Cellulose, Hydroxypropyl Methylcellulose, Magnesium Stearate, Microcrystalline Cellulose, Polyethylene Glycol, Pregelatinized Corn Starch, Sodium Starch Glycolate, Sucrose and Titanium Dioxide.
Protect from excessive heat and moisture.
Comments or Questions? Call toll-free 1-800-245-1040 weekdays
Distributed by: SmithKline Beecham Consumer Healthcare, L.P.
Pittsburgh, PA 15230. Made in U.S.A.
Lot No. 00/00 Exp. 00/00
New NDC# 0135-0107-26

SUCRETS® Maximum Strength Wintergreen
SUCRETS® Wild Cherry Regular Strength
SUCRETS® Children's Cherry Flavored
Sore Throat Lozenges
[su 'krets]
SUCRETS® Regular Strength Original Mint
SUCRETS® Regular Strength Vapor Lemon
SUCRETS® Maximum Strength Vapor Black Cherry

Active Ingredient: Maximum Strength Wintergreen: Dyclonine Hydrochloride 3.0 mg. per lozenge. Wild Cherry, Regular Strength: Dyclonine Hydrochloride 2.0 mg. per lozenge. Children's Cherry: Dyclonine Hydrochloride 1.2 mg. per lozenge. Regular Strength–Original Mint: Hexylresorcinol 2.4 mg. per lozenge. Regular Strength–Vapor Lemon: Dyclonine Hydrochloride 2.0 mg. per lozenge. Maximum Strength–Vapor Black Cherry: Dyclonine Hydrochloride 3.0 mg. per lozenge.

Inactive Ingredients: Maximum Strength Wintergreen: Citric Acid, Corn Syrup, Silicon Dioxide, Sucrose, Mineral Oil, Yellow 10. Wild Cherry Regular Strength: Blue 1, Corn Syrup, Flavor, Red 40, Silicon Dioxide, Sucrose, Tartaric Acid. Children's Cherry: Blue 1, Citric Acid, Corn Syrup, Red 40, Silicon Dioxide, Sucrose. Regular Strength–Original Mint: Blue 1, Corn Syrup, Flavors, Silicon Dioxide, Sucrose, Mineral Oil, Yellow 10. Regular Strength–Vapor Lemon: Citric Acid, Corn Syrup, Flavors,

Silicon Dioxide, Sucrose, Mineral Oil, Yellow 10. Maximum Strength–Vapor Black Cherry: Blue 1, Corn Syrup, Flavor, Menthol, Red 40, Silicon Dioxide, Sucrose, Tartaric Acid.

Indications: For temporary relief of occasional minor sore throat pain and mouth irritations.

Actions: Dyclonine Hydrochloride's soothing anesthetic action relieves minor throat irritations.

Warnings: If sore throat is severe, persists for more than 2 days, is accompanied or followed by fever, headache, rash, swelling, nausea, or vomiting, do not use and consult a doctor promptly. If sore mouth symptoms do not improve in 7 days or if irritation, pain, or redness persists or worsens, see your dentist or doctor promptly. Do not exceed recommended dosage. KEEP THIS AND ALL MEDICINES OUT OF THE REACH OF CHILDREN. In case of accidental overdose, seek professional assistance or contact a poison control center immediately.

Drug Interaction: No known drug interaction.

Symptoms and Treatment of Oral Overdosage: Reactions due to large overdosage are systemic and involve the central nervous system and cardiovascular system. Central nervous system reactions are characterized by excitation and/or depression. Nervousness, dizziness, blurred vision or tremors may occur. Reactions involving the cardiovascular system include depression of the myocardium, hypotension or bradycardia. Should a large overdose be suspected seek professional assistance. Call your physician, local poison control center or the Rocky Mountain Poison Control Center at 303-592-1710 (Collect), 24 hours a day.

Dosage and Administration: Adults and children 2 years of age or older: Allow one lozenge to dissolve slowly in the mouth. May be repeated every two hours as needed. Children under 2 years of age: Consult a dentist or doctor.

Professional Labeling: For the temporary relief of pain associated with tonsillitis, pharyngitis, throat infections or stomatitis.

How Supplied: Available in plastic packages of 18 lozenges.
Shown in Product Identification Guide, page 521

SUCRETS® 4 HOUR COUGH SUPPRESSANT
[su 'krets]
dextromethorphan hydrobromide

Active Ingredient:
Each cough lozenge contains Dextromethorphan Hydrobromide 15 mg.
Inactive Ingredients:
Menthol Eucalyptus—Corn Syrup, D&C Yellow #10, FD&C Blue #1 Flavor,

Continued on next page

SmithKline Beecham—Cont.

Magnesium Trisilicate, Menthol, Mineral Oil, Sucrose.

Wild Cherry—Corn Syrup, FD&C Blue #1, FD&C Red #40, Flavor, Magnesium Trisilicate, Menthol, Mineral Oil, Sucrose.

Indications For Use: For effective temporary relief of coughs due to minor sore throat and bronchial irritation associated with colds or inhaled irritants.

Directions: Adults and children twelve years of age and over: Take one (1) cough lozenge every 4 hours as needed. Do not exceed maximum dosage of 6 lozenges in any 24-hour period unless directed by a physician.
Children over six years of age: Take one (1) cough lozenge every 6 hours as needed. Do not exceed maximum dosage of 4 lozenges in any 24-hour period unless directed by a physician.
This product not intended for children under 6 years of age.
Avoid storing at high temperature (greater than 100°F).

Drug Interaction Precaution: Do not use this product (or give this product to your child) if you (or your child) are now taking a prescription monoamine oxidase inhibitor (MAOI) (certain drugs for depression, psychiatric or emotional conditions, or Parkinson's disease), or for 2 weeks after stopping MAOI drug. If you are uncertain whether you or your child's prescription drug contains a MAOI, consult a health professional before taking this product.

Warnings: A persistent cough may be a sign of a serious condition. If cough persists for more than 1 week, tends to recur, or is accompanied by fever, rash or persistent headache, consult a physician. Do not take this product for persistent or chronic cough such as occurs with smoking, asthma, emphysema, or if cough is accompanied by excessive phlegm (mucus) unless directed by a physician. Do not administer to children under 6 years of age unless directed by a physician. As with any drug, if you are pregnant or nursing a baby, seek the advice of a health professional before using this product.
In case of accidental overdose, seek professional assistance or contact a poison control center immediately.
Keep this and all medication out of the reach of children.
Shown in Product Identification Guide, page 521

TAGAMET® HB™   OTC
Acid Reducer/Cimetidine Tablets 100 mg

Tagamet® HB™ provides relief from heartburn, acid indigestion and sour stomach when used as directed. It contains the same ingredient found in prescription strength Tagamet.

Tagamet HB reduces the production of stomach acid.
ACTIVE INGREDIENT Cimetidine Tablets, 100 mg. Acid Reducer.
INACTIVE INGREDIENTS Cellulose, hydroxypropyl methylcellulose, magnesium stearate, polyethylene glycol, polysorbate 80, povidone, sodium lauryl sulfate, sodium starch glycolate, starch titanium dioxide.
USES Relieves heartburn acid indigestion, and sour stomach.

Directions: Take 2 tablets with water as symptoms occur or as directed by a doctor. Tagamet HB can be used up to twice daily (up to 4 tablets in 24 hours). This product should not be given to children under 12 years old unless directed by a doctor.

Warnings:
● Consult your doctor if you are taking theophylline (oral asthma medicine), warfarin (blood thinning medicine), or phenytoin (seizure medicine) before taking Tagamet HB. If you are not sure whether your medication contains one of these drugs or have any other questions about medicines you are taking, call our consumer affairs specialist at 1-800-482-4394.
● Do not take the maximum daily dosage for more than 2 weeks continuously except under the advice and supervision of a doctor.
● As with any drug, if you are pregnant or nursing a baby, seek the advice of a health professional before using this product.
● If you have trouble swallowing, or persistent abdominal pain, see your doctor promptly. You may have a serious condition that may need a different treatment.
● Keep this and all drugs out of the reach of children.
● In case of accidental overdose, seek professional assistance or contact a poison control center immediately.
READ THE LABEL
Read the directions and warnings before taking this medication.
Store at room temperature (59–86°F).
Comments or questions? Call Toll-Free 1-800-482-4394 Weekdays
PHARMACOKINETIC INTERACTIONS
Cimetidine at prescription doses is known to inhibit various P450 metabolizing isoenzymes, which could affect metabolism of other drugs and increase their blood concentration. Investigation of pharmacokinetic interactions at the recommended OTC doses of cimetidine have thus far shown only small effects. A pharmacokinetic study conducted in 26 normal male subjects (mean age, 38 years) at steady state using the maximum recommended OTC dose level (200 mg twice a day), showed that Tagamet HB, on average, increased the 24 hour AUC of theophylline by 14% and increased peak theophylline levels by 15%. This interaction should be borne in mind in advising patients on the use of Tagamet HB. At the prescription doses

of cimetidine, clinically significant pharmacokinetic interactions between cimetidine and warfarin, phenytoin, and theophylline have been reported. At prescription doses, pharmacokinetic interactions have been reported for a number of other drugs as well, such as with dihydropyridine calcium channel blockers or short acting benzodiazepines. At the maximum recommended OTC dose level (200 mg twice a day), a pharmacokinetic study conducted in 21 normal male subjects (mean age, 38 years) showed that Tagamet HB, on average, increased the total AUC of triazolam by 26–28% and increased peak triazolam levels by 11–23%. Tagamet HB did not alter the apparent terminal elimination half-life of triazolam.
This labeling information is current as of Nov. 1, 1995.

How Supplied: Tagamet HB (cimetidine Tablets 100 mg) is available in boxes of blister strips in 16, 32 & 64 tablet sizes.
Shown in Product Identification Guide, page 521

TELDRIN®
Chlorpheniramine Maleate/ Phenylpropanolamine Hydrochloride Timed-Release 12 hour Allergy Relief Capsules

IMPROVED!
Now relieves congestion too!
PLEASE NOTE: This description replaces the previous formulation of TELDRIN—Timed Release Allergy Capsules which contained Chlorpheniramine 12 mg. per capsule.

Active Ingredients: Each capsule contains Chlorpheniramine Maleate 8 mg. and Phenylpropanolamine Hydrochloride 75 mg.

Inactive Ingredients: Benzyl Alcohol, Butylparaben, D & C Red No. 33, Edetate Calcium Disodium, FD & C Red No. 3, FD & C Yellow No. 6, Gelatin, Methylparaben, Pharmaceutical Glaze, Propylparaben, Sodium Lauryl Sulfate, Sodium Propionate, Starch, Sucrose, and other ingredients. May also contain Polysorbate 80.

Indications: Temporarily relieves runny nose and reduces sneezing, itching of the nose or throat, and itchy, watery eyes due to hay fever or other upper respiratory allergies. Temporarily relieves nasal congestion due to the common cold, hay fever, or associated with sinusitis.

Direction For Use: Adults and children over 12 years of age: One capsule every 12 hours, not to exceed 2 capsules in 24 hours, or as directed by a doctor. Children under 12 years of age, consult a doctor.

Warnings: Do not exceed recommended dosage. If nervousness, dizziness, or sleeplessness occur, discontinue use and consult a doctor. If symptoms do not improve within 7 days or are accompanied by fever, consult a doctor. Do not take this product unless directed by a doctor, if you have a breathing problem such as emphysema or chronic bronchitis, or if you have heart disease, high blood pressure, thyroid disease, diabetes, glaucoma, or difficulty in urination due to enlargement of the prostate gland. Do not take this product if you are taking another medication containing phenylpropanolamine. May cause excitability, especially in children. May cause drowsiness; alcohol, sedatives, and tranquilizers may increase the drowsiness effect. Avoid alcoholic beverages while taking this product. Do not take this product if you are taking sedatives or tranquilizers without first consulting your doctor. Use caution when driving a motor vehicle or operating machinery. **KEEP THIS AND ALL DRUGS OUT OF THE REACH OF CHILDREN.** In case of accidental overdose, seek professional assistance or contact a Poison Control Center immediately. As with any drug, if you are pregnant or nursing a baby, seek the advice of a health professional before using this product.

Drug Interaction Precaution: Do not use this product if you are now taking a prescription monoamine oxidase inhibitor (MAOI) (certain drugs for depression, psychiatric or emotional conditions, or Parkinson's Disease), or for 2 weeks after stopping the MAOI drug. If you are uncertain whether your prescription drug contains an MAOI, consult a health professional before taking this product.

Tamper-Evident Package Features
- Each capsule is encased in a plastic cell with a foil back.
- Each capsule is protected by a red Perma Seal™ band which bonds the two capsule halves together.
- DO NOT USE THIS PRODUCT IF ANY OF THESE TAMPER-EVIDENT FEATURES ARE MISSING OR BROKEN.

Comments or Questions? Call Toll-Free 1-800-245-1040 Weekdays.
Store in a dry place, at controlled room temperature 15°–30°C (59–86°F).
Shown in Product Identification Guide, page 521

TUMS® Antacid/Calcium Supplement Tablets
TUMS E–X® Antacid/Calcium Supplement Tablets
TUMS ULTRA® Antacid/Calcium Supplement Tablets

Indications: For fast relief of acid indigestion, heartburn, sour stomach, and upset stomach associated with these symptoms.

Professional Labeling: Indicated for the symptomatic relief of hyperacidity associated with the diagnosis of peptic ulcer, gastritis, peptic esophagitis, gastric hyperacidity, and hiatal hernia.

Active Ingredient:
Tums, Calcium Carbonate 500 mg
Tums E-X, Calcium Carbonate 750 mg
Tums ULTRA, Calcium Carbonate 1000 mg

Actions: Tums provides rapid neutralization of stomach acid. Each Tums tablet has an acid-neutralizing capacity (ANC) of 10 mEq. Each Tums E-X tablet has an ANC of 15 mEq and each Tums ULTRA tablet, an ANC of 20 mEq. This high neutralization capacity makes Tums tablets an ideal antacid for management of conditions associated with hyperacidity. It effectively neutralizes free acid yet does not cause systemic alkalosis in the presence of normal renal function. A double-blind placebo-controlled clinical study demonstrated that calcium carbonate taken at a dosage of 16 Tums tablets daily for a two-week period was non-constipating/non-laxative.

Warnings: Tums: Do not take more than 16 tablets in a 24-hour period or use the maximum dosage of this product for more than 2 weeks, except under the advice and supervision of a physician. If symptoms persist for 2 weeks, stop using this product and see a physician. Keep this and all drugs out of the reach of children.

Tums E-X: Do not take more than 10 tablets in a 24-hour period or use the maximum dosage of this product for more than two weeks, except under the advice and supervision of a physician. If symptoms persist for two weeks, stop using this product and see a physician. Keep this and all drugs out of the reach of children.

Tums ULTRA: Do not take more than 8 tablets in 24-hour period or use the maximum dosage of this product for more than two weeks, except under the advice and supervision of a physician. If symptoms persist for two weeks, stop using and see a physician. Keep this and all drugs out of the reach of children.

Drug Interaction Precaution: Antacids may interact with certain prescription drugs. If you are presently taking a prescription drug, do not take this product without checking with your physician or other health professional.

Dosage and Administration:
Tums: Chew 2-4 tablets as symptoms occur. Repeat hourly if symptoms return, or as directed by physician.
Tums E-X: Chew 2-4 tablets as symptoms occur. Repeat hourly if symptoms return, or as directed by a physician.
Tums ULTRA: Chew 2-3 tablets as symptoms occur. Repeat hourly if symptoms return, or as directed by a physician.

As a Dietary Supplement
Calcium Supplement Directions
Tums, Tums E-X & Tums ULTRA: Chew 2 tablets after meals or as directed by a physician.

Nutritional Information:
Tums

Nutrition Facts
Serving Size: 2 Tablets

Amount Per Serving

Calories 5

	% Daily Value
Sugars 1g	
Calcium 400 mg	40%

Tums tablets are sodium free (the ingredient sodium polyphosphate adds a dietary insignificant amount of sodium).

Tum E-X

Nutrition Facts
Serving Size: 2 Tablets

Amount Per Serving

Calories 10

	% Daily Value
Sugars 2 g	
Calcium 600 mg	60%
Sodium 5 mg	less than 1%

Tums E-X tablets are very low sodium

Tums ULTRA

Nutrition Facts
Serving Size: 2 Tablets

Amount Per Serving

Calories 10

	% Daily Value
Sugars 3g	
Calcium 800 mg	80%
Sodium 10mg	less than 1%

Tums ULTRA tablets are very low sodium.

Ingredients: Sucrose, Starch, Talc, Mineral Oil, Flavors, Sodium Polyphosphate. May also contain 1% or less of Adipic Acid, FD&C Blue 1, FD&C Yellow 6, D&C Yellow 10, D&C Red 27, D&C Red 30.

How Supplied:
Tums: Peppermint flavor is available in 12-tablet rolls, 3-roll wraps, and bottles of 75 and 150. **Assorted Flavors** (Cherry, Lemon, Orange, and Lime), are available in 12-tablet rolls, 3-roll wraps, and bottles of 75, 150, and 400.
Tums E-X: Wintergreen, Cherry, Assorted Fruit and **Assorted Tropical Fruit Flavors;** 8-tablet rolls, 3-roll wraps and bottles of 48 and 96 tablets. Tropical fruit is also available in bottles of 250 tablets.
Tums ULTRA: Assorted Fruit and **Assorted Mint Flavors;** bottles of 36 and 72 tablets.

Continued on next page

SmithKline Beecham—Cont.

This labeling information is current as of November 1, 1995.

Shown in Product Identification Guide, page 521

TUMS® Anti-gas /Antacid Formula

Active Ingredients: 500 mg of calcium carbonate and 20 mg of simethicone per tablet.
Tums Anti-gas/Antacid formula Assorted Fruit Flavor Inactive Ingredients: Adipic Acid, Corn Syrup, D&C Red 27, D&C Red 30, D&C Yellow 10, FD&C Blue 1, FD&C Yellow 6, Flavors, Microcrystalline Cellulose, Mineral Oil, Sodium Polyphosphate, Starch, Sucrose, Talc, Triglycerol Monooleate.
Each tablet contains not more than 2 mg of sodium and is considered dietetically sodium free.
Non-laxative/non-constipating.

Indications: For fast relief of acid indigestion, heartburn, and sour stomach accompanied by gas and upset stomach associated with these symptoms.

Professional Labeling: Indicated for the symptomatic relief of hyperacidity associated with the diagnosis of peptic ulcer, gastritis, peptic esophagitis, gastric hyperacidity, and hiatal hernia.

Actions: Calcium carbonate, when tested in vitro neutralizes 10 mEq of 0.1N HCl. This neutralization capacity combined with a rapid rate of reaction makes calcium carbonate an ideal antacid for management of conditions associated with hyperacidity. It effectively neutralizes free acid yet does not cause systemic alkalosis in the presence of normal renal function.

Warnings: Do not take more than 16 tablets in a 24-hour period or use the maximum dosage of this product for more than 2 weeks, except under the advice and supervision of a doctor. Keep this and all drugs out of the reach of children.

Drug Interaction Precaution: Antacids may interact with certain prescription drugs. If you are presently taking a prescription drug, do not take this product without checking with your physician or other health professional.

Dosage and Administration: Chew 1 or 2 tablets as symptoms occur. Repeat hourly if symptoms return, or as directed by a doctor. No water is required.

How Supplied: 60 tablet bottles 4770D

TUMS 500™
Calcium Supplement

Each Tablet Contains: 1,250 mg calcium carbonate, which provides 500 mg elemental calcium (50% of the U.S. RDA, or Daily Value). Each tablet contains less than 4 mg sodium.

Ingredients: Sucrose, Calcium Carbonate, Starch, Talc, Mineral Oil and Sodium Polyphosphate. May also contain Adipic Acid, FD&C Blue 1, FD&C Yellow 6, D&C Yellow 10, D&C Red 27, D&C Red 30.

Directions: Chew one tablet with meals, two to three times a day or as recommended by a physician.
IMPORTANT INFORMATION ON OSTEOPOROSIS
Osteoporosis affects older persons, especially middle-aged, white and Asian women and those whose families tend to have fragile bones in later years. A lifetime of regular exercise and eating a healthful diet that includes enough calcium, especially during teen and early adult years, builds and maintains good bone health and may reduce the risk of osteoporosis later in life. Adequate calcium intake is important, but intakes above 2,000 mg elemental calcium are not likely to provide any additional benefit.
This labeling information is current as of Nov. 1, 1995.

How Supplied: Tums 500™ is available in **Assorted Fruit and Peppermint,** Flavors, in bottles of 60 tablets.

Standard Homeopathic Company
**210 WEST 131st STREET
BOX 61067
LOS ANGELES, CA 90061**

Direct Inquiries to:
Jay Borneman
(800) 624-9659

HYLAND'S ARNICAID™ TABLETS
100% natural temporary relief of symptoms of pain and soreness from muscle overexertion or injury.

Indications: Hyland's Arnicaid Tablets are a homeopathic product indicated for the control and symptomatic relief of acute bruising and soreness due to falls, blows, and muscle strain. Arnicaid provides a 100% natural relief for children and adults. Use after minor accidents or after sports workouts. Arnicaid contains no sucrose, dextrose or fillers. Like all homeopathic products, Arnicaid has no known contraindications or side effects.

Directions: Adults—1–2 tablets every 4 hours, or as needed.
Children over 3 years of age—½ adult dose.

Active Ingredients: Arnica Montana 30X HPUS in a base of lactose USP.

Warnings: Do not use if cap band is broken or missing. If symptoms persist for more than seven days or worsen, contact a licensed health care professional. Do not use in children under three years of age without consulting a licensed health care professional. As with any drug, if you are pregnant or nursing a baby, seek the advice of a licensed health care professional before using this product. Keep this and all medications out of reach of children. In case of accidental overdose, contact a poison control center or the manufacturer at the number provided below.
P&S Laboratories
Los Angeles, CA 90061
Questions? Call us: 800/624-9659
MADE IN USA
Arnicaid and Hyland's are trademarks of Standard Homeopathic Co.

HYLAND'S BEDWETTING TABLETS

Active Ingredients: *Equisetum hyemale* (Scouring Rush) 2X HPUS, *Rhus aromatica* (Fragrant Sumac) 3X HPUS, *Belladonna* 3X HPUS (0.0003% Alkaloids).

Inactive Ingredients: Lactose USP.

Indications: A homeopathic combination for the temporary relief of involuntary urination (common bedwetting) in children.

Directions: Children 3 to 12 years: 2 to 3 tablets before meals and at bedtime, or as directed by a licensed health care practitioner. Children over 12 years: double the above recommended dose.

Warnings: If symptoms persist for more than seven days or worsen, consult a Health Care Professional. As with any drug, if you are pregnant or nursing a baby, seek the advice of a health professional before using this product. Keep this and all medication out of the reach of children.

How Supplied: Bottles of 125—one grain sublingual tablets (NDC 54973-7501-01). Store at room temperature.

HYLAND'S CALMS FORTÉ TABLETS

Active Ingredients: *Passiflora* (Passion Flower) 1X triple strength HPUS, *Avena sativa* (Oat) 1X triple strength HPUS, *Humulus lupulus* (Hops) 1X double strength HPUS, *Chamomilla* (Chamomile) 2X HPUS, *Calcarea Phosphorica* (Calcium Phosphate) 3X HPUS, *Ferrum Phosphorica* (Iron Phosphate) 3X HPUS, *Kali Phosphoricum* (Potassium Phosphate) 3X HPUS, *Natrum Phosphoricum* (Sodium Phosphate) 3X HPUS, *Magnesia Phosphoricum* (Magnesium Phosphate) 3X HPUS.

Inactive Ingredients: Lactose USP.

Indications: Temporary symptomatic relief of simple nervous tension and insomnia.

Directions: Adults, As a relaxant: 1 to 2 tablets as needed or 3 times daily between meals. In insomnia: 1 to 3 tablets ½ to 1 hour before retiring. Repeat as needed without danger of side effects. Children, As a relaxant: 1 tablet as needed or 3 times daily before meals. In insomnia: 1 to 2 tablets 1 hour before retiring. Non-habit-forming.

Warnings: If symptoms persist for more than seven days or worsen, consult a Health Care Professional. As with any drug, if you are pregnant or nursing a baby, seek the advice of a health professional before using this product. Keep this and all medication out of the reach of children.

How Supplied: Bottles of 100 four grain tablets (NDC 54973-1121-02). Store at room temperature. Bottles of 50 four grain tablets (NDC 54973-1121-01). Store at room temperature.

HYLAND'S CLEARAC™ TABLETS
All natural ClearAc helps clear up acne, pimples, and acne blemishes.

Indications: Hyland's ClearAc Tablets are a homeopathic combination indicated for the management and symptomatic relief of symptoms of pimples, blackheads, and blemishes associated with common acne (acne vulgaris). ClearAc Tablets provide a 100% natural approach. Like all homeopathic products, ClearAc Tablets have no known contraindications or side effects. Use in conjunction with a high-quality skin cleanser, such as 100% Natural Hyland's ClearAc Cleanser with Calendula.

Directions: Adults—2-3 tablets every 4 hours, or as needed.

Active Ingredients: Echinacea Ang. 6X HPUS, Berberis Vulg. 6X HPUS, Sulphur Iod. 6X HPUS, Hepar Sulph. 6X HPUS in a base of lactose USP.

Warnings: Do not use if cap band is broken or missing. If symptoms persist or worsen, contact a licensed health care professional. As with any drug, if you are pregnant or nursing a baby, seek the advice of a licensed health care professional before using this product. Keep this and all medications out of reach of children. In case of accidental overdose, contact a poison control center or the manufacturer at the number provided below. P&S Laboratories Los Angeles, CA 90061 Questions? Call us: 800/624-9659 MADE IN USA ClearAc and Hyland's are trademarks of Standard Homeopathic Co.

HYLAND'S COLIC TABLETS

Active Ingredients: *Disocorea* (Wild Yam) 2X HPUS, *Chamomilla* (Chamomile) 3X HPUS, *Colocynth* (Bitter Apple) 3X HPUS.

Inactive Ingredients: Lactose USP.

Indications: A homeopathic combination for the temporary relief of colic and gas pains caused by irritating food, feeding too quickly, swallowing air and similar conditions during teething, colds and other minor upset periods in children.

Directions: For children to 2 years of age: administer 2 tablets dissolved in a teaspoon of water on the tongue every 15 minutes until relieved; then every 2 hours as required. Children over 2 years: 3 tablets dissolved on the tongue as above; or as recommended by a licensed health care practitioner.

Warnings: If symptoms persist for more than seven days or worsen, consult a Health Care Professional. Keep this and all medication out of the reach of children.

How Supplied: Bottles of 125—one grain sublingual tablets (NDC 54973-7502-01). Store at room temperature.

HYLAND'S COUGH SYRUP WITH HONEY™

Active Ingredients: Each fluid ounce contains: *Ipecacuanha* (Ipecac) 3X HPUS, *Aconitum napellus* (Aconite) 3X HPUS, *Spongia Tosta* (Sponge) 3X HPUS, *Antimonium Tartaricum* (Potassium Antimony Tartrate) 6X HPUS.

Inactive Ingredients: Simple syrup and honey.

Indications: A homeopathic combination for the temporary relief of symptoms of simple, dry, tight or tickling coughs due to colds in children.

Directions: Children 1 to 12 years: 1 to 3 teaspoonfuls as required. Children over 12 years and adults: 3 to 4 teaspoonfuls as required. May be taken with or without water. Repeat as often as necessary to relieve symptoms. For children under 1 year of age, consult a licensed health care practitioner.

Warnings: Do not use this product for persistent or chronic cough such as occurs with asthma, smoking or emphysema; or if cough is accompanied with excessive mucus, unless directed by a licensed health care practitioner. If symptoms persist for more than seven days, tend to recur, or are accompanied by a high fever, rash, or persistent headache, consult a Health Care Professional. As with any drug, if you are pregnant or nursing a baby, seek the advice of a health professional before using this product. Keep this and all medication out of the reach of children.

How Supplied: Bottles of 4 fluid ounces (120 ml) (NDC 54973-7503-02). Store at room temperature.

HYLAND'S C-PLUS™ COLD TABLETS

Active Ingredients: *Eupatorium perfoliatum* (Boneset) 2X HPUS, *Euphrasia officinalis* (Eyebright) 2X HPUS, *Gelsemium sempervirens* (Yellow Jasmine) 3X HPUS, *Kali Iodatum* (Potassium Iodide) 3X HPUS.

Inactive Ingredients: Lactose USP, Natural Raspberry Flavor.

Indications: A homeopathic combination for the temporary relief of symptoms of runny nose and sneezing due to common head colds in children.

Directions: Children 1 to 3 years: 2 tablets every 15 minutes for 4 doses, then hourly until relieved. For children 3 to 6 years: 3 tablets as above; for children 6 and older: 6 tablets as above or as directed by a licensed health care practitioner.

Warnings: If symptoms persist for more than seven days or worsen, consult a Health Care Professional. As with any drug, if you are pregnant or nursing a baby, seek the advice of a health professional before using this product. Keep this and all medication out of the reach of children.

How Supplied: Bottles of 125—one grain sublingual tablets (NDC 54973-7505-01). Store at room temperature.

HYLAND'S ENURAID™ TABLETS
100% natural temporary relief of symptoms of common incontinence in adults.

Indications: Hyland's EnurAid Tablets are a homeopathic combination indicated for the control and symptomatic relief of involuntary urination (common incontinence) in adults. EnurAid provides a 100% natural approach which aids in relief of symptoms of bladder control and related symptoms. Like all homeopathic products, EnurAid has no known contraindications or side effects.

Directions: Adults—2-3 tablets every 4 hours, or as needed.

Active Ingredients: Belladonna 6X HPUS, Cantharis 6X HPUS, Apis Mell. 6X HPUS, Arnica Mont. 6X HPUS, Allium Cepa 6X HPUS, Rhus Arom. 6X HPUS, Equisetum Hyem. 6X HPUS in a base of lactose USP.

Warnings: Do not use if cap band is broken or missing. If symptoms persist for more than seven days or worsen, contact a licensed health care professional. Discontinue use if symptoms are accompanied by a high fever (greater than 101°F), or if blood is present in urine and contact a licensed health care professional. As with any drug, if you are pregnant or nursing a baby, seek the advice of a licensed health care professional before using this product. Keep this and all medications out of reach of children. In case of accidental overdose, contact a poison control center or the manufacturer at the number provided below.

Continued on next page

Standard Homeopathic—Cont.

P&S Laboratories
Los Angeles, CA 90061
Questions? Call us: 800/624-9659
MADE IN USA
EnurAid and Hyland's are trademarks of
Standard Homeopathic Co.

HYLAND'S HEADACHE TABLETS

Active Ingredients: Iris Versicolor
3X, HPUS; Gelsemium Sempervirens
3X, HPUS; Ipecac 3X, HPUS; Belladonna 6X, HPUS.

Inactive Ingredients: Lactose USP.

Indications: Relief of symptoms of
headache due to stress and "nervous or
sick" headache. Headache may be either
right or left sided and may extend to the
base of the neck.

Directions: Adults: Dissolve 2–3 tablets under tongue every 4 hours as
needed. Children 6 to 12 years old: ½
adult dose.

Warnings: Do not use if imprinted cap
band is missing or broken. If symptoms
persist for more than seven days or
worsen, contact a licensed health care
professional. As with any drug, if you are
pregnant or nursing a baby, seek the advice of a licensed health care professional
before using this product. Keep this and
all medications out of the reach of children. In case of accidental overdose, contact a poison control center immediately.

How Supplied: Bottles of 100 three-
grain sublingual tablets (NDC 54973-
2950-02). Store at room temperature.

HYLAND'S LEG CRAMPS TABLETS

Active Ingredients: Viscum Album
3X, HPUS; Gnaphalium Polycephalum
3X, HPUS; Rhus Toxicodendron 6X,
HPUS; Aconitum Napellus 6X, HPUS;
Ledum Palustre 6X, HPUS; Magnesia
Phosphorica 6X, HPUS.

Inactive Ingredients: Lactose USP.

Indications: Formerly Hyland's #22,
Hyland's Leg Cramps is a traditional homeopathic formula for the relief of symptoms of cramps and pains in lower back
and legs often made worse by damp
weather. Working without contraindications or side effects, Hyland's Leg
Cramps stimulates your body's natural
healing response to relieve symptoms.
Hyland's Leg Cramps is safe for adults
and children and can be used in conjuc-
tion with other medications.

Directions: Adults: Dissolve 2–3 tablets under tongue every 4 hours as
needed. Children 6 to 12 years old: ½
adult dose.

Warnings: Do not use if imprinted cap
band is missing or broken. If symptoms
persist for more than seven days or
worsen, contact a licensed health care

professional. As with any drug, if you are
pregnant or nursing a baby, seek the advice of a licensed health care professional
before taking this product. Keep this and
all medications out of the reach of children. In case of accidental overdose, contact a poison control center immediately.

How Supplied: Bottles of 100 three-
grain sublingual tablets (NDC 54973-
2956-02), Bottles of 50 three-grain sublingual tablets (NDC 54973-2956-01). Store
at room temperature.

HYLAND'S TEETHING TABLETS

Active Ingredients: *Calcarea Phosphorica* (Calcium Phosphate) 3X HPUS,
Chamomilla (Chamomile) 3X HPUS, *Cof-
fea Cruda* (Coffee) 3X HPUS, *Belladonna*
3X HPUS (Alkaloids 0.0003%).

Inactive Ingredients: Lactose USP.

Indications: A homeopathic combination for the temporary relief of symptoms of simple restlessness and wakeful
irritability due to cutting of teeth.

Directions: 2 to 3 tablets in a teaspoon
of water or on the tongue, 4 times per
day. If the child is restless or wakeful,
2 tablets every hour for 6 doses or
as directed by a licensed health care
practitioner.

Warnings: If symptoms persist for
more than seven days or worsen, consult
a Health Care Professional. As with any
drug, if you are pregnant or nursing a
baby, seek the advice of a health professional before using this product. Keep
this and all medication out of the reach
of children.

How Supplied: Bottles of 125—one
grain sublingual tablets (NDC 54973-
7504-01). Store at room temperature.

EDUCATIONAL MATERIAL

Booklets—Brochures
"Homeopathy—What it is, How it
Works," A Consumer's Guide to Homeopathic Medicine, Free
"Homeopathy—A Guide for Pharmacists," An ACPE (0.2 CEU) program on
the basic principles of homeopathy.

UNKNOWN DRUG?
Consult the
Product Identification Guide
(Gray Pages)
for full-color photos of
leading over-the-counter
medications

Stellar Pharmacal Corp.
Div./Star Pharmaceuticals, Inc.
1990 N.W. 44TH STREET
POMPANO BEACH, FL
33064-8712

Direct Inquiries to:
Scott Davidson
1-800-845-7827

For Medical Emergencies:
Scott Davidson
1-800-845-7827

STAR–OTIC® EAR SOLUTION
**Antibacterial, Antifungal,
Nonaqueous Ear Solution**

Active Ingredients: Acetic acid nonaqueous, Burow's solution, Boric acid, in
a propylene glycol vehicle, with an acid
pH and a low surface tension.

Indications: For the prevention of oti-
tis externa, commonly called "Swim-
mer's Ear". To inhibit bacterial and fun-
gal growth and maintain the external
ear canal's normal acid mantle following
swimming or showering.

Actions: Star-Otic Ear Solution is antibacterial, antifungal, hydrophilic, has an
acid pH and a low surface tension. Acetic
acid and boric acid inhibit the rapid mul-
tiplication of microorganisms and help
maintain the lining mantle of the ear
canal in its normal acid state. Burow's
solution (aluminum acetate) is a mild
astringent. Propylene glycol reduces
moisture in the ear canal.

Warning: Do not use in ear if tympanic
membrane (ear drum) is perforated or
punctured.

**Symptoms and Treatment of Over-
dosage:** Discontinue use if undue irritation or sensitivity occurs.

Dosage and Administration: Adults
and Children: To help restore normal pH
to the outer ear canal. In susceptible persons, instill 3–5 drops of Star-Otic Ear
Solution in each ear before and after
swimming or bathing, or as directed by
physician.

Professional Labeling: Same as those
outlined under Indications.

How Supplied: Available in ½ oz
measured drop, safety tip, plastic bottle.

**Rx DRUG INFORMATION
AT THE TOUCH OF A BUTTON**
Join the thousands of doctors
using the handheld, electronic
Pocket PDR.
Use the order form
in the front of this book.

Sterling Health
See Bayer Corporation
Consumer Care Division

Sunsource International, Inc.
535 LIPOA PARKWAY
SUITE #110
KIHEI, MAUI HI 96753

Direct Inquiries to:
Preston Zoller
Director of Marketing
Sunsource International, Inc.
535 Lipoa Parkway, Suite 110
Kihei, HI 96753
(808) 874-6733, ext. 277

GARLIQUE™
"One Per Day" Garlic Formula
30 Odor-Free Tablets

Each 400 mg tablet of *Garlique* contains the equivalent of 1200 mg of fresh garlic (approx. 1 clove).
Garlique tablets are enteric coated (absorbed in the small intestine not in the stomach)—odor-free, tasteless, easy to swallow, and easy to digest. *Garlique* has none of the 'unsocial' qualities associated with fresh garlic cloves.

"One Per Day" Garlic Formula
Each 400 mg tablet of Garlique contains the equivalent of 1200mg of fresh garlic (approximately 1 clove). One tablet per day will bring you all the healthful benefits of garlic.

Enteric Coated—For Your Comfort
Garlique is odor-free, easy to swallow and easy to digest. Each tablet is enteric and film coated. These safe and effective coatings assure maximum potency and freshness. Enteric coating allows absorption to occur in the small intestine rather than the stomach where powerful digestive juices would destroy the allicin.

Directions: As a dietary supplement, take one Garlique™ tablet daily with a meal. Store in a dry place at a controlled room temperature (59°–86°F). Keep out of reach of children.

Each tablet contains: 400 mg of high allicin potential garlic. Additional (inactive) ingredients: cellulose (binder and disintegrant), stearic acid and magnesium stearate (lubricant), silica (drying agent) and aqueous enteric coating.

Guaranteed: No sugar, starch, yeast, sodium, preservatives, artificial colors, dyes or flavors. Garlique is blister packed for your convenience and tamper resistant for your protection.
If you have any questions or comments about Garlique™ or any of our other fine Sunsource® products, please contact our **Customer Service Department,** toll free, at **800-666-6505, ext. 203.**

Shown in Product Identification Guide, page 521

MELATONEX™
melatonin with vitamin B6
Dietary supplement for a natural sleep cycle

- time-release formula
- antioxidant action
- finest pure melatonin

melatonex™ is a dietary supplement containing melatonin, a substance produced by our own bodies that regulates the body's natural sleep/wake cycle. After we reach maturity, melatonin production declines with age, which can make restful sleep more difficult to achieve. Melatonin production can also diminish through our use of substances like alcohol, tobacco, caffeine, aspirin and many common medications. Dietary supplementation can help to restore the melatonin we need for restful natural sleep.
melatonex™ uses a unique time-release delivery system that releases melatonin the way the body does, gradually while we sleep.
RESEARCH has also shown melatonin to be a highly effective antioxidant against hydroxyl free radicals, toxic by-products of normal metabolism that can cause cell damage.*
melatonex™ contains the finest pure melatonin (not of animal origin).

*This statement has not been evaluated by the Food and Drug Administration. This product is not intended to diagnose, treat, cure or prevent any disease.

Tamper Evident: Double safety-sealed: outer tamper tape and inner bubble seal. Do not use if either seal or foil backing is missing or broken.

Each tablet supplies: % Daily Value
Vitamin B6
(Pyridoxine HCL) 10 mg 500%
Melatonin 3 mg *
*Daily Value not established

Additional (inactive) ingredients: Dicalcium phosphate (binder and hardening agent), microcrystalline cellulose (binder and disintegrant), glyceryl monostearate (binder and distintegration retardant), magnesium stearate (lubricant).
Contains: NO sugar, starch, yeast, sodium, dairy, artifical colors or preservatives.
Satisfaction Guaranteed: See insert for details.
Suggested use: Adults: As a dietary supplement, take one (1) tablet, swallowed whole with water, one-half (½) hour before bedtime. Fractional portions of a tablet may be taken if desired.
Cautions: If you are taking prescription medicine, are pregnant or lactating, or have an autoimmune, seizure or endocrine disorder, please consult your doctor before taking **melatonex™**. Do not take **melatonex™** when operating a motor vehicle or machinery. As with any adult supplement, keep this product out of the reach of children. **Store in a dry place**

at room temperature, avoiding excessive heat over 86°F (30°C).

How Supplied: 30 tablets; 60 tablets. Tamper-evident blister packs.
Shown in Product Identification Guide, page 521

For Women—During and After Menopause
REJUVEX
Dietary supplement for the mature woman
30 or 50 ONE PER DAY CAPLETS
Net. Wt. 1.45 oz. (41.2g)

Directions:
Serving Size 1 tablet
Servings Per Container 30

Amount Per Tablet	% Daily Value
Vitamin E (as d l-Alpha Tocopherol Acetate) 30 iu	100%
Thiamin HCL (Vitamin B₁) 2 mg	133%
Riboflavin (Vitamin B₂) 2 mg	117%
Niacin (Vitamin B₃) 10 mg	50%
Vitamin B₆ (Pyridoxine HCL) 10 mg	500%
Pantothenic Acid (d-Calcium Pantothenate) 10 mg	100%
Magnesium (as Oxide) 500 mg	125%
Selenium (as Sodium Selenate) 25 mcg	*
Manganese (as Sulfate) 2 mg	*

*Daily Value not established

Additional Ingredients: 200 mg Dong Quai; raw glandular powders from bovine source: 25 mg mammary, 19 mg ovary, 10 mg uterus, 10 mg adrenal, 5 mg pituitary; 3 mg Boron (as chelate, citrate, and aspartate); microcrystalline cellulose (binder and disintegrant); croscarmellose sodium (disintegrant); colloidal silica (drying agent); stearic acid and magnesium stearate (lubricants).

Guaranteed: NO sugar, starch, yeast, dairy, caffeine, preservatives, artificial colors, dyes or flavors.

Directions: As a dietary supplement, take one **REJUVEX** caplet daily, with a meal. For best results, do not take **REJUVEX** at the same time as a calcium supplement. Take **REJUVEX** in the morning and the calcium supplement at night. Keep out of reach of children. Store in a dry place at controlled room temperature (59°–86°F).
Double safety sealed: tamper tape and inner bubble seal. Do not use if either seal or foil backing is missing or broken.

REJUVEX is not a replacement for any medically prescribed treatment. Do not discontinue the use of any medications, or alter the time at which you normally take them, when you add REJUVEX to your daily regimen. If you have any questions related to REJUVEX and any medications, consult

Continued on next page

Sunsource Int'l—Cont.

with your health care professional.

Shown in Product Identification Guide, page 521

SUNSOURCE® ALLERGY RELIEF
All Natural Homeopathic Medicine

Homeopathy is a highly effective, natural system of healing whose origins date back more than 200 years. Its present worldwide rise in popularity parallels consumer preference for all natural, effective health care alternatives. SUNSOURCE Traditional Homeopathic Medicines are formulated to stimulate the body's own innate healing powers to temporarily relieve symptoms without side effects.

Indications: For the temporary relief of sneezing, runny nose, watery eyes, sinus pressure and headache, cough and congestion due to hayfever and seasonal allergies.

Directions/Dosage: Adults: Chew one tablet slightly and allow to dissolve in the mouth every ½ hour for the first 2 hours; then decrease to 1 tablet every four hours, or as needed. For continued relief, take 3–4 tablets daily. Children 4–12 years: Use ½ the adult dosage.

Each Tablet Contains: Active: Chamomilla (Chamomile) 1X, Echinacea angustifolia (Purple Cone Flower) 1X, Alliumcepa (Red Onion) 6X, Sabadilla (Cevadilla Seed) 6X, Sanguinaria canadensis (Blood Root) 6X, Ambrosia artemisiaefolia (Rag Weed) 12X, Arsenicum iodatum (Arsenic Iodide Salt) 12X, Histaminum (Histamine) 12X, Kali iodatum (Potassium Iodide Salt) 12X, Solidago vigaurea (Golden Rod) 12X. Inactive: Lactose Magnesium Stearate.

Warnings: If symptoms persist for more than 7 days, worsen or are accompanied by a fever, consult your physician. As with any drug, if you are pregnant or nursing a baby, seek the advice of a health professional before using this product. Keep this and all medication out of the reach of children.

Sunsource homeopathic tablets are individually blister sealed. Do not use if paper backing is punctured. Paper backing is printed with the product name, lot number and expiration date. Boxes are safety sealed with tamper tape at both ends for your protection. Do not purchase if either seal is missing or broken.

Guaranteed: No starch, yeast, sodium, preservatives, artificial colors or flavors. Store in a cool, dry place.

Shown in Product Identification Guide, page 522

SUNSOURCE® ARTHRITIS RELIEF
All Natural Homeopathic Medicine

Indications: For the temporary relief of minor pain, inflammation, stiffness, swelling, redness and joint pain from arthritis.

Directions/Dosage: Adults: Chew one tablet slightly and allow to dissolve in the mouth every ½ hour for the first 2 hours; then decrease to 1 tablet every four hours, or as needed. For continued relief, take 4 tablets daily. Children 4–12 years: Use ½ the adult dosage.

Each Tablet Contains: Active: Lappa major (Burdock) 3X, Sarsaparilla (Sarsaparilla) 3X, Cimicifuga racemosa (Black Snakeroot) 4X, Pulsatilla vulgaris (Wind Flower) 4X, Berberis vulgaris (Barberry) 6X, Rhus toxicodendron (Poison Ivy) 6X, Calcarea carbonica (Calcium Carbonate) 12X, Causticum (Hahnemann's Causticum) 12X, Lycopodium clavatum (Club Moss) 12X. Inactive: Lactose, Magnesium Stearate.

Warnings: Adults: If pain persists for more than 10 days or worsens, consult your physician. Children: Do not give this product for more than five days unless directed by a physician. If pain persists, worsens or new symptoms appear, consult a physician. As with any drug, if you are pregnant or nursing a baby, seek the advice of a health professional before using this product. Keep this and all medication out of the reach of children.

Sunsource homeopathic tablets are individually blister sealed. Do not use if paper backing is punctured. Paper backing is printed with the product name, lot number and expiration date. Boxes are safety sealed with tamper tape at both ends for your protection. Do not purchase if either seal is missing or broken.

Guaranteed: No starch, yeast, sodium, preservatives, artificial colors or flavors. Store in a cool, dry place.

Shown in Product Identification Guide, page 522

SUNSOURCE® COLD RELIEF
All Natural Homeopathic Medicine

Indications: For the temporary relief of runny nose, sneezing, congestion, headache, sore scratchy throat, cough, stuffiness, minor fever and chills.

Directions/Dosage: Adults: Chew one tablet slightly and allow to dissolve in the mouth every ½ hour for the first 2 hours; then decrease to 1 tablet every four hours, or as needed. Children 4–12 years: Use ½ adult dosage.

Each Tablet Contains: Active: Zingiber officinalis (Ginger) 1X, Echinacea angustifolia (Purple Cone Flower) 3X, Allium cepa (Red Onion) 6X, Gelsemium sempervirens (Yellow Jasmine) 6X, Nux vomica (Poison Nut) 6X, Sanguinaria canadensis (Blood Root) 6X, Kali bichromicum (Potassium Bromide Salt) 9X, Mercurius solubilis (Hahnemann's Soluble Mercury) 12X, Hepar sulphuris calcareum (Calcium Sulfide) 12X. Inactive: Lactose, Magnesium Stearate.

Warnings: A persistent cough or high fever may be a sign of a serious condition. If fever persists for more than 3 days, consult a physician. If cough persists for more than one week, tends to recur, or is accompanied by a fever, rash, or persistent headache, consult a physician. Do not take this product for consistent or chronic cough such as occurs with smoking, asthma, or emphysema, or if cough is accompanied by excessive phlegm (mucus) unless directed by a physican. As with any drug, if you are pregnant or nursing a baby, seek the advice of a health professional before using this product. Keep this and all medication out of the reach of children.

Sunsource homeopathic tablets are individually blister sealed. Do not use if paper backing is punctured. Paper backing is printed with the product name, lot number and expiration date. Boxes are safety sealed with tamper tape at both ends for your protection. Do not purchase if either seal is missing or broken.

Guaranteed: No starch, yeast, sodium, preservatives, artificial colors or flavors. Store in a cool, dry place.

Shown in Product Identification Guide, page 522

SUNSOURCE® FLU RELIEF
All Natural Homeopathic Medicine

Indications: For the temporary relief of body aches, minor fever, chills, sore throat, headache, cough, congestion, nausea and vomiting.

Directions/Dosage: Adults: Chew one tablet slightly and allow to dissolve in the mouth every ½ hour for the first 2 hours: then decrease to 1 tablet every four hours, or as needed. For continued relief, take 4 tablets daily for 7 days. Children 4–12 years: Use ½ the adult dosage.

Each Tablet Contains: Active: Echinacea angustifolia (Purple Cone Flower) 3X, Aconitum napellus, (Aconite) 4X, Baptisia tinctoria (Wild Indigo) 4X, Bryonia alba (Wild Hops) 4X. Pulsatilla vulgaris (Wind Flower) 4X, Gelsemium sempervirens (Yellow Jessamine) 6X, Ipecacuanha (Ipecac) 6X, Influenzium (Influenza Nosode) 12X. Inactive: Lactose, Magnesium Stearate.

Warnings: A persistent cough or high fever may be a sign of a serious condition. If fever persists for more than 3 days, consult a physician. If cough persists for more than one week, tends to recur, or is accompanied by a fever, rash, or persistent headache, consult a physician. Do not take this product for consistent or chronic cough such as occurs with smoking, asthma, or emphysema, or if cough is accompanied by excessive phlegm (mucus) unless directed by a physician. As with any drug, if you are pregnant or nursing a baby, seek the advice of a health professional before using this product. Keep this and all medication out of the reach of children.

Sunsource homeopathic tablets are individually blister sealed. Do not use if paper backing is punctured. Paper backing is printed with the product name, lot number and expiration date. Boxes are safety sealed with tamper tape at both ends for your protection. Do not purchase if either seal is missing or broken.

Guaranteed: No starch, yeast, sodium, preservatives, artifical colors or flavors. Store in a cool, dry place.

Shown in Product Identification Guide, page 522

SUNSOURCE® INSOMNIA RELIEF
All Natural Homeopathic Medicine

Indications: For the temporary relief of occasional sleeplessness. Helps to reduce difficulty falling asleep.

Directions/Dosage: Adults: Chew two tablets and allow to dissolve in the mouth ½ hour before bedtime, and two tablets at bedtime as needed. Children under 12 years: Use ½ the adult dosage.

Each Tablet Contains: Active: Humulus lupulus (Hops) 1X, Passiflora incarnata (Passion Flower) 3X, Valeriana officinalis (Valeriana) 3X, Aconitum napellus (Aconite) 4X, Avena sativa (Oat) 4X, Absinthinum (Common Wormwood) 6X, Kali bromatum (Potassium Bromide Salt) 6X, Ambra grisea (Ambergris) 12X. Inactive: Lactose, Magnesium Stearate.

Warnings: If sleeplessness persists continuously for more than 2 weeks, consult your physician. Insomnia may be a symptom of serious underlying medical illness. As with any drug, if you are pregnant or nursing a baby, seek the advice of a health professional before using this product. Keep this and all medication out of the reach of children. Avoid alcoholic beverages while taking this product. Do not take this product if you are taking sedatives or tranquilizers, without first consulting your physician.

Sunsource homeopathic tablets are individually blister sealed. Do not use if paper backing is punctured. Paper backing is printed with the product name, lot number and expiration date. Boxes are safety sealed with tamper tape at both ends for your protection. Do not purchase if either seal is missing or broken.

Guaranteed: No starch, yeast, sodium, preservatives, artifical colors or flavors. Store in a cool, dry place.

Shown in Product Identification Guide, page 522

SUNSOURCE® SINUS RELIEF
All Natural Homeopathic Medicine

Indications: For the temporary relief of sinus pain; sinus pressure; sinus headache; nasal congestion; sneezing; burning; watery eyes and runny nose.

Directions/Dosage: Adults: Chew one tablet slightly and allow to dissolve in the mouth every ½ hour for the first 2 hours, then decrease to 1 tablet every four hours, or as needed. For continued relief, take 4 tablets daily for 7 days. Children 4–12 years: Use ½ the adult dosage.

Each Tablet Contains: Active: Pulsatilla vulgaris (Wind Flower) 4X, Teucrium marum (Cat Thyme) 4X, Euphorbium officinarum (Euphorbium) 6X, Hydrastis canadensis (Golden Seal) 6X, Kali iodatum (Potassium Iodide) 6X, Sanguinaria canadensis (Blood Root) 6X, Phosphorus (Phosphorus) 9X, Sabadilla (Cevadilla Seed) 9X, Ambrosia artemisiafolia (Rag Weed) 12X, Calcarea carbonica (Calcium Carbonate) 12X, Mercurius solubilis (Mercuric Oxide) 12X.
Inactive: Lactose, Magnesium Stearate.

Warnings: If symptoms persist for more than 7 days, worsen or are accompanied by a fever, consult your physician. As with any drug, if you are pregnant or nursing a baby, seek the advice of a health professional before using this product. Keep this and all medication out of the reach of children.

Sunsource homeopathic tablets are individually blister sealed. Do not use if paper backing is punctured. Paper backing is printed with the product name, lot number and expiration date. Boxes are safety sealed with tamper tape at both ends for your protection. Do not purchase if either seal is missing or broken.

Guaranteed: No starch, yeast, sodium, preservatives, artificial colors or flavors. Store in a cool, dry place.

Shown in Product Identification Guide, page 522

ARTHRITIS RELIEF CREAM
Homeopathic Arthritis Relief/Topical Analgesic Cream
Fast, Effective Relief of Pain and Stiffness due to Arthritis
Odor-Free! Non-Greasy, Non-Staining Formula

Indications: For the temporary relief of minor aches, pains and stiffness of muscles and joints due to arthritis.

Directions for use: For adults & children over 2 years of age: Rubbing gently, apply generously to the affected area 2–3 times daily or as needed. Children under 2 years of age: Consult a physician.

Warnings: For external use only. If symptoms persist for more than 5 days, worsen, or if a rash develops, discontinue use and consult a physician. Keep this and all medicines out of the reach of children.

Active Ingredients: Arnica montana (Leopard's Bane) 1X, Berberis vulgaris (Barberry) 1X, Cimicifuga racemosa (Black Snakeroot) 1X, Kalmia latifolia (Mountain Laurel) 1X, Pilsatilla nigricans (Wind Flower) 1X, Rhus toxicodendron (Poison Ivy) 1X, Ruta graveolens (Rue) 1X, Causticum (Hahnemann's Causticum) 2X.

Inactive Ingredients: Acrylates, BHT (Butylated Hydroxy Toluene), Cetyl-Alcohol, Cholesterol, Dimethicone Copolyol, Glycerin, Glycol Stearate, Imidazolidinyl Urea, Isopropyl Myristate, Lecithin, Methyl Gluceth-20, Methyl & Propyl Parabens, PEG 100 Stearate, Panthenol, Propylene Glycol, Stearic Acid, Sodium Hydroxide, Tetra Sodium EDTA, Tocopheryl Acetate, Water.

Tamper Evident: Sunsource Arthritis Relief Cream has a tube mouth seal. Do not use if seal is punctured. Boxes are safety sealed with tamper tape at both ends for your protection. Do not purchase if either seal is missing or broken.
Lot number and expiration date are stamped at end of tube. Store at controlled room temperature (59°–86°F).

How Supplied: Net Contents: 2.0 OUNCES
NDC 60348-107-02
Shown in Product Identification Guide, page 522

PSORIASIS/ECZEMA RELIEF CREAM
Homeopathic Psoriasis/Eczema Topical Anti-Itch Cream
Fast, Effective Relief of Itching, Pain and Inflammation due to Psoriasis and Eczema
Odor-Free! Non-Greasy, Non-Staining Formula

Indications: For the temporary relief of itching, pain and inflammation due to psoriasis or eczema.

Directions for use: For adults & children over 2 years of age: Rubbing gently, apply generously to the affected area 2–3 times daily or as needed. Children under 2 years of age: Consult a physician.

Warnings: For external use only. If symptoms persist for more than 5 days, worsen, or if a rash develops, discontinue use and consult a physician. Keep this and all medicines out of the reach of children.

Active Ingredients: Cicuta virosa (Water Hemlock) 1X, Pix Liquida (Pine tar) 1X, Stillingia sylvatica (Queen's Delight) 1X, Thuja Occidentalis (White Cedar) 1X, Graphites (Graphite) 4X, Sepia (Sepia) 4X, Arsenicum Album (Arsenous Oxide) 6X, Cuprum Metallicum (Copper) 6X.

Inactive Ingredients: Acrylates, BHT (Butylated Hydroxy Toluene), Cetyl-Alcohol, Cholesterol, Dimethicone Copolyol, Glycerin, Glycol Stearate, Imidazolidinyl Urea, Isopropyl Myristate, Lecithin, Methyl Gluceth-20,

Continued on next page

Sunsource Int'l—Cont.

Methyl & Propyl Parabens, PEG 100 Stearate, Panthenol, Propylene Glycol, Stearic Acid, Sodium Hydroxide, Tetra Sodium EDTA, Tocopheryl Acetate, Water.

Tamper Evident: Sunsource Psoriasis/Eczema Relief Cream has a tube mouth seal. Do not use if seal is punctured. Boxes are safety sealed with tamper tape at both ends for your protection. Do not purchase if either seal is missing or broken.

Lot number and expiration date are stamped at end of tube. Store at controlled room temperature (59°–86°F).

How Supplied: Net Contents: 2.0 ounces
NDC 60348-109-02
Shown in Product Identification Guide, page 522

SPORTS INJURY RELIEF CREAM
Homeopathic Sports Injury/Topical Analgesic Cream Fast, Effective Relief of Pain due to Sprains, Bruises, Muscle Pulls and Other Minor Muscle Injuries
Odor-Free! Non-Greasy, Non-Staining Formula

Indications: For the temporary relief of minor aches and pains of muscles and joints due to sprains, bruises, pulled muscles and other minor muscle injuries.

Directions for use: For adults & children over 2 years of age: Rubbing gently, apply generously to the affected area 2–3 times daily or as needed. Children under 2 years of age: Consult a physician.

Warnings: For external use only. If symptoms persist for more than 5 days, worsen, or if a rash develops, discontinue use and consult a physician. Keep this and all medicines out of the reach of children.

Active Ingredients: Aconitum napellus (Aconite) 1X, Arnica montana (Leopard's Bane) 1X, Bellis perennis (Daisy) 1X, Calendula officinalis (Garden Marigold) 1X, Echinacea angustifolia (Cone Flower) 1X, Hypericum perforatum (St. John's-Wort) 1X, Rhus toxicodendron (Poison Ivy) 1X.

Inactive Ingredients: Acrylates, BHT (Butylated Hydroxy Toluene), Cetyl-Alcohol, Cholesterol, Dimethicone Copolyol, Glycerin, Glycol Stearate, Imidazolidinyl Urea, Isopropyl Myristate, Lecithin, Methyl Gluceth-20, Methyl & Propyl Parabens, PEG 100 Stearate, Panthenol, Propylene Glycol, Stearic Acid, Sodium Hydroxide, Tetra Sodium EDTA, Tocopheryl Acetate, Water.

Tamper Evident: Sunsource Sports Injury Relief Cream has a tube mouth seal. Do not use if seal is punctured. Boxes are safety sealed with tamper tape at both ends for your protection. Do not purchase if either seal is missing or broken.

Lot number and expiration date are stamped at end of tube. Store at controlled room temperature (59°–86°F).

How Supplied: Net Contents: 2.0 OUNCES
NDC 60348-108-02
Shown in Product Identification Guide, page 522

Thompson Medical Company, Inc.
222 LAKEVIEW AVENUE
WEST PALM BEACH
FLORIDA 33401

Direct Inquiries to:
Consumer Services: (407) 820-9900
Fax: (407) 832-2297

ASPERCREME®
[ăs-per-crēme]
External Analgesic Rub With Aloe

Description: ASPERCREME® is available as an odor-free creme and lotion for use as a topical massage rub that temporarily relieves minor muscle aches and pains.
Aspercreme does not contain aspirin.

Active Ingredient: Salycin® 10% (Thompson Medical's brand of Trolamine Salicylate).

Other Ingredients: Creme: Aloe Vera Gel, Cetyl Alcohol, Glycerin, Methylparaben, Mineral Oil, Potassium Phosphate, Propylparaben, Stearic Acid, Triethanolamine, Water. Lotion: Aloe Vera Gel, Cetyl Alcohol, Glyceryl Stearate, Isopropyl Palmitate, Lanolin, Methylparaben, Potassium Phosphate, Propylene Glycol, Propylparaben, Sodium Lauryl Sulfate, Stearic Acid, Water.

Actions: External analgesic rub.

Indications: Analgesic rub for temporary relief of minor aches and pains of muscles associated with simple strains and sprains.

Warnings: Use only as directed. If prone to allergic reaction from aspirin or salicylate, consult a physician before using. If redness is present or condition worsens, or if pain persists for more than 7 days or clears up and occurs again within a few days, discontinue use and consult a physician. For external use only. Avoid contact with eyes. As with any drug, if you are pregnant or nursing a baby, seek the advice of a health professional before using this product. **Do not use:** On children under 10 years of age. If skin is irritated or if irritation develops. **KEEP THIS AND ALL MEDICINES OUT OF THE REACH OF CHILDREN.** In case of accidental ingestion seek professional assistance or contact a poison control center immediately.

Dosage and Administration: Apply generously to affected area. Massage into painful area until thoroughly absorbed into skin. Repeat as necessary, but not more than 4 times daily.

How to Store: Store at controlled room temperature 59°–86°F (15°–30°C).

How Supplied: Creme: 1¼ oz., 3 oz. and 5 oz. tubes. Lotion: 6 oz. bottle.
Shown in Product Identification Guide, page 522

CAPZASIN-P
[Căp-zā-sĭn-P]
Topical Analgesic Creme

Description: Capzasin-P contains purified capsaicin, a natural ingredient that penetrates deep to temporarily relieve minor aches and pains of muscles and joints associated with arthritis, simple backache, strains and sprains. Capsaicin is so effective that doctors recommend it more than all other topical analgesic ingredients combined.

Active Ingredient: Capsaicin 0.025% w/w.

Other Ingredients: Benzyl Alcohol, Cetyl Alcohol, Glyceryl Monostearate, Isopropyl Myristate, Polyoxyl 40 Stearate, Purified Water, Sorbitol Solution, White Petrolatum.

Actions: External analgesic rub.

Indications: For the temporary relief of minor aches and pains of muscles and joints associated with arthritis, simple backache, strains and sprains.

Warnings: For external use only. Transient burning may occur upon application, but generally disappears in several days. Avoid contact with the eyes and mucous membranes. If condition worsens, or if symptoms persist for more than 7 days or clear up and occur again within a few days, discontinue use of this product and consult a physician. Do not apply to wounds, damaged or broken (open), irritated skin or if excessive irritation develops. Do not bandage tightly. Do not use with a heating pad. As with any drug, if you are pregnant or nursing a baby, seek the advice of a health professional before using this product. **KEEP THIS AND ALL MEDICINES OUT OF THE REACH OF CHILDREN.** In case of accidental ingestion, seek professional assistance or contact a poison control center immediately.

Dosage and Administration: Adults: Apply to affected area not more than 3 to 4 times daily. **WASH HANDS WITH SOAP AND WATER AFTER APPYLING. Children under 12 years of age:** Consult a physician. Read package insert before using.
How to Store: Store at controlled room temperature 15°–30°C (59°–86°F)
How Supplied: 1.5 oz. creme tube.
Shown in Product Identification Guide, page 522

CORTIZONE-5®
Creme and Ointment

CORTIZONE FOR KIDS™ Creme
Anti-itch
(0.5% hydrocortisone)

Description: CORTIZONE-5® creme and ointment are topical anti-itch preparations containing aloe.

Active Ingredient: Hydrocortisone 0.5%.

Other Ingredients: Creme: Aloe Vera Gel, Aluminum Sulfate, Calcium Acetate, Cetearyl Alcohol, Glycerin, Light Mineral Oil, Methylparaben, Potato Dextrin, Propylparaben, Sodium C12–15 Alcohols Sulfate, Sodium Lauryl Sulfate, Water, White Petrolatum, White Wax. Ointment: Aloe Extract, White Petrolatum.

Indications: CORTIZONE-5® is recommended for the temporary relief of itching associated with minor skin irritations, inflammation and rashes due to: eczema, insect bites, poison ivy, oak, sumac, soaps, detergents, cosmetics, jewelry, seborrheic dermatitis, psoriasis, external anal and genital itching. Other uses of this product should be only under the advice and supervision of a physician.

Warnings: For external use only. Avoid contact with the eyes. If condition worsens, or if symptoms persist for more than 7 days or clear up and occur again within a few days, stop use of this product and do not begin use of any other hydrocortisone product unless you have consulted a physician. Do not use in genital area if you have a vaginal discharge, consult a physician. Do not use for the treatment of diaper rash, or for the treatment of chicken pox, consult a physician.
Warnings For External Anal Itching Users: Do not exceed the recommended daily dosage unless directed by a physician. In case of bleeding, consult a physician promptly. Do not put this product into the rectum by using fingers or any mechanical device or applicator.
KEEP THIS AND ALL MEDICINES OUT OF THE REACH OF CHILDREN. In case of accidental ingestion, seek professional assistance or contact a poison control center immediately.

Dosage and Administration: Adults and children 2 years of age and older: Apply to affected area not more than 3 to 4 times daily. Children under 2 years of age: Do not use, consult a physician.
Directions For External Anal Itching Users: Adults: When practical, cleanse the affected area with mild soap and warm water and rinse thoroughly. Gently dry by patting or blotting with toilet tissue or a soft cloth before application of this product. Children under 12 years of age: Consult a physician.

How to Store: Store at controlled room temperature 15°–30°C (59°–86°F).

How Supplied: CORTIZONE-5® creme: 1 oz. and 2 oz. tubes. CORTIZONE for KIDS™ creme: ½ oz. and 1 oz. tubes. CORTIZONE-5® ointment: 1 oz. tube.
Shown in Product Identification Guide, page 522

CORTIZONE-10®
Creme and Ointment

CORTIZONE-10® EXTERNAL ANAL ITCH RELIEF Creme

CORTIZONE-10® SCALP ITCH FORMULA™ Liquid
Anti-itch
(1.0% hydrocortisone)

Description: CORTIZONE-10® creme with aloe, ointment and liquid are topical anti-itch preparations. Maximum Strength available without a prescription.

Active Ingredient: Hydrocortisone 1.0%.

Other Ingredients: Creme: Aloe Vera Gel, Aluminum Sulfate, Calcium Acetate, Cetearyl Alcohol, Glycerin, Light Mineral Oil, Methylparaben, Potato Dextrin, Propylparaben, Sodium C12-15 Alcohols Sulfate, Sodium Lauryl Sulfate, Water, White Petrolatum, White Wax. Ointment: White Petrolatum. Liquid: Benzyl Alcohol, Propylene Glycol, Purified Water, SD Alcohol 40-2 (60% v/v)

Indications: Cortizone-10® is recommended for the temporary relief of itching associated with minor skin irritations, inflammation and rashes due to: eczema, insect bites, poison ivy, oak, sumac, soaps, detergents, cosmetics, jewelry, seborrheic dermatitis, psoriasis, external anal and genital itching. Other uses of this product should be only under the advice and supervision of a physician.

Warnings: For external use only. Avoid contact with the eyes. If condition worsens, or if symptoms persist for more than 7 days or clear up and occur again within a few days, stop use of this product and do not begin use of any other hydrocortisone product unless you have consulted a physician. Do not use in genital area if you have a vaginal discharge, consult a physician. Do not use for the treatment of diaper rash, consult a physician. **Warnings For External Anal Itching Users:** Do not exceed the recommended daily dosage unless directed by a physician. In case of bleeding, consult a physician promptly. Do not put this product into the rectum by using fingers or any mechanical device or applicator.
KEEP THIS AND ALL MEDICINES OUT OF THE REACH OF CHILDREN. In case of accidental ingestion, seek professional assistance or contact a poison control center immediately.

Dosage and Administration: Adults and children 2 years of age and older: Apply to affected area not more than 3 to 4 times daily. Children under 2 years of age: Do not use, consult a physician.

Directions For External Anal Itching Users: Adults: When practical, cleanse the affected area with mild soap and warm water. Rinse thoroughly. Gently dry by patting or blotting with tissue or a soft cloth before application of this product. Children under 12 years of age: Consult a physician.

How to Store: Store at controlled room temperature 15°–30°C (59°–86°F).

How Supplied: CORTIZONE-10® creme: 1 oz. and 2 oz. tubes. CORTIZONE-10® ointment: 1 oz. and 2 oz. tubes. CORTIZONE-10® External Anal Itch Relief creme: 1 oz. tube. CORTIZONE-10® Scalp Itch Formula™ liquid: 1.5 fl. oz.
Shown in Product Identification Guide, page 522

DEXATRIM® Caplets and Tablets
[dĕx-a-trĭm]
Prolonged action anorectic for weight control

DEXATRIM® Maximum Strength Plus Vitamin C/Caffeine Free Caplets

Active Ingredient: Phenylpropanolamine HCl 75 mg. (appetite suppressant time release)

Inactive Ingredients: Vitamin C (Ascorbic Acid) 180 mg., Carnauba Wax, Croscarmellose Sodium, Ethylcellulose, FD & C Red No. 40 Aluminum Lake, FD & C Yellow No. 6 Aluminum Lake, Hydroxypropyl Methylcellulose, Magnesium Stearate, Microcrystalline Cellulose, Polyethylene Glycol, Polysorbate 80, Povidone, Silicon Dioxide, Stearic Acid, Titanium Dioxide.

DEXATRIM® Maximum Strength Caffeine Free Caplets

Active Ingredient: Phenylpropanolamine HCl 75 mg. (appetite suppressant time release)

Inactive Ingredients: Carnauba Wax, D&C Yellow No. 10 Aluminum Lake, FD&C Yellow No. 6 Aluminum Lake, Hydroxypropyl Methylcellulose, Iron Oxide, Magnesium Stearate, Microcrystalline Cellulose, Polyethylene Glycol, Polysorbate 80, Povidone, Silicon Dioxide, Stearic Acid, Titanium Dioxide.

Extended Duration DEXATRIM® Maximum Strength Caffeine Free Tablets

Active Ingredient: Phenylpropanolamine HCl 75 mg. (appetite suppressant time release)

Inactive Ingredients: Calcium Sulfate, Carnauba Wax, D&C Yellow No. 10 Aluminum Lake, Ethylcellulose, FD&C Yellow No. 6 Aluminum Lake, Hydroxypropyl Methylcellulose, Iron Oxide, Magnesium Stearate, Propylene Glycol, Povidone, Stearic Acid, Titanium Dioxide, Triacetin.

Continued on next page

Thompson Medical—Cont.

Indication: DEXATRIM® is an aid for effective appetite control to assist weight reduction. It is available in a time release dosage form.

Directions: Adult oral dosage is **one caplet** at mid-morning with a full glass of water. **Exceeding the recommended dose has not been shown to result in greater weight loss.** (This product's effectiveness is directly related to the degree to which you reduce your usual daily food intake.) The use of this product should be limited to periods not exceeding 3 months, because this should be enough time to establish new eating habits. Read and follow the important Diet Plan enclosed.

Warnings: DO NOT TAKE MORE THAN 1 DEXATRIM CAPLET PER DAY (24 HOURS). Exceeding the recommended dose may cause serious health problems. FOR ADULT USE ONLY. Do not give this product to children under 12 years of age. Persons between 12 and 18 or over 60 are advised to consult their physician before using this product.

There have been reports that stroke, seizure, heart attack, arrhythmia, psychosis, and death might be associated with the ingestion of phenylpropanolamine. If you are being treated for depression, an eating disorder or have heart disease, diabetes, thyroid or any other disease, do not take this product except under the supervision of a physician. If nervousness, dizziness, sleeplessness, palpitations or headache occurs, stop taking this medication and consult your physician. Check your blood pressure regularly. If you have high blood pressure, do not use this product and consult your physician. As with any drug, if you are pregnant or nursing a baby, seek the advice of a health professional before using this product. Do not take this product if you are hypersensitive to any of its ingredients.

Drug Interaction Precaution: If you are taking a cough/cold or allergy medication containing any form of phenylpropanolamine, or any oral nasal decongestant, do not take this product. Do not use this product if you are taking any prescription drug, except under the advice and supervision of a physician. Do not use this product if you are presently taking a prescription monoamine oxidase inhibitor (MAOI) for depression or for two weeks after stopping use of an MAOI without first consulting a physician. KEEP THIS AND ALL MEDICATIONS OUT OF THE REACH OF CHILDREN. In case of accidental overdose, seek professional assistance or contact a poison control center immediately.

Dosage and Administration:
Caplet Dosage Forms: DEXATRIM® Maximum Strength Plus Vitamin C/Caffeine Free, DEXATRIM® Maximum Strength/Caffeine Free.

Tablet Dosage Form: DEXATRIM® Maximum Strength Extended Duration Time Tablets.
Administration: One caplet or tablet at midmorning with a full glass of water.

How Supplied: All Dexatrim products are supplied in tamper-evident blister packages. Do not use if individual seals are broken.
DEXATRIM® Maximum Strength Plus Vitamin C/Caffeine Free Caplets: Packages of 20 and 40 with 1250 calorie DEXATRIM Diet Plan.
DEXATRIM® Maximum Strength Extended Duration Time Tablets: Packages of 20 and 40 with 1250 calorie DEXATRIM Diet Plan.

References: Schteingerrt, DE et. al., *Int J Obesity,* 1992;16, 487-493.
Atkinson, RL, Dannels SA, Marlin RL; *Am J Clin Nutr,* 56 (4); 755; Oct. 1992.
Blackburn, G.L., et. al., *JAMA,* 1989; 261:3267-3272.
Morgan, J.P., et. al., *J Clin Psychopharm,* 1989;9(1):33-38.
All referenced materials available on request.

Shown in Product Identification Guide, page 522

DEXATRIM® PLUS VITAMINS
[*Dĕx-ă-trĭm Plus Vitamins*]
Prolonged action anorectic for weight control plus a multi-vitamin.

Indication: DEXATRIM® is an aid for effective appetite control to assist weight reduction. It is available in a time release dosage form. The multi-vitamin, in caplet form, is for dietary supplementation.

Active Ingredient: Each Dexatrim Caplet Contains: Phenylpropanolamine HCl 75 mg. (appetite suppressant time release)

Each Vitamin/Mineral Caplet Contains:	%U.S.RDA[1]
Vitamin A (as Acetate & Beta Carotene)	5,000 IU 100%
Vitamin E (di-Alpha Tocopheryl Acetate)	30 IU 100%
Vitamin C (as Ascorbic Acid)	60 mg. 100%
Folic Acid	0.4 mg. 100%
Vitamin B1 (as Thiamine Mononitrate)	1.5 mg. 100%
Vitamin B2 (as Riboflavin)	1.7 mg. 100%
Niacinamide	20 mg. 100%
Vitamin B6 (as Pyridoxine Hydrochloride)	2 mg. 100%
Vitamin B12 (as Cyanocobalamin)	6 mcg. 100%
Vitamin D	400 IU 100%
Biotin	30 mcg. 10%
Pantothenic Acid (as Calcium Pantothenate)	10 mg. 100%
Calcium (as Dibasic Calcium Phosphate)	162 mg. 16%
Phosphorus (as Dibasic Calcium Phosphate)	125 mg. 13%
Iodine (as Potassium Iodide)	150 mcg. 100%
Iron (as Ferrous Fumarate)	18 mg. 100%
Magnesium (as Magnesium Oxide)	100 mg. 25%
Copper (as Cupric Oxide)	2 mg. 100%
Zinc (as Zinc Oxide)	15 mg. 100%
Manganese (as Manganese Sulfate)	2.5 mg. *
Potassium (as Potassium Chloride)	40 mg. *
Chloride (as Potassium Chloride)	36.3 mg. *
Chromium (as Chromium Chloride)	25 mcg. *
Molybdenum (as Sodium Molybdate)	25 mcg. *
Selenium (as Sodium Selenate)	25 mcg. *
Vitamin K1 (as Phytonadione)	25 mcg. *
Nickel (as Nickel Sulfate)	5 mcg. *
Tin (as Stannous Chloride)	10 mcg. *
Silicon (as Sodium Metasilicate & Oxides)	2 mg. *
Vanadium (as Sodium Metavanadate)	10 mcg. *
Boron (as Borates)	150 mcg. *

[1] U.S. RECOMMENDED DAILY ALLOWANCE (U.S. RDA) FOR ADULTS AND CHILDREN 4 OR MORE YEARS OF AGE.
*NO U.S. RDA HAS BEEN ESTABLISHED.

Inactive Ingredients: Vitamin C (Ascorbic Acid) 180 mg., Carnauba Wax, Cellulose, Croscarmellose Sodium Ethylcellulose, FD & C Blue No. 1, FD & C Red No. 40 Aluminum Lake, FD & C Yellow No. 6, FD & C Yellow No. 6 Aluminum Lake, Hydroxypropyl Methylcellulose, Magnesium Stearate, Methylcellulose, Microcrystalline Cellulose, Polyethylene Glycol, Polysorbate 80, Povidone, Propylene Glycol, Silica, Silicon Dioxide, Starch, Stearic Acid, Titanium Dioxide.

Directions: Adult oral dosage is **one red caplet marked "dexatrim" and one vitamin/mineral caplet marked "Complete Vitamin"** at mid-morning with a full glass of water. Exceeding the recommended dose has not been shown to result in greater weight loss. (This product's effectiveness is directly related to the degree to which you reduce your usual daily food intake.) The use of this product should be limited to periods not exceeding 3 months, because this should be enough time to establish new eating habits. Read and follow important Diet Plan enclosed.

WARNINGS: FOR ADULT USE ONLY. DO NOT TAKE MORE THAN 1 DEXATRIM CAPLET PER DAY (24 HOURS). Exceeding the recommended dose may cause serious health problems. FOR ADULT USE ONLY. Do not give this product to children under 12 years of age. Persons between 12 and 18 or over 60 are advised to consult their physician before using this product.
There have been reports that stroke, seizure, heart attack, arrhythmia, psychosis, and death might be associated with the ingestion of phenylpropanolamine. If

you are being treated for depression, an eating disorder or have heart disease, diabetes, thyroid or any other disease, do not take this product except under the supervision of a physician. If nervousness, dizziness, sleeplessness, palpitations or headache occurs, stop taking this medication and consult your physician. Check your blood pressure regularly. If you have high blood pressure, do not use this product and consult your physician. As with any drug, if you are pregnant or nursing a baby, seek the advice of a health professional before using this product. Do not take this product if you are hypersensitive to any of its ingredients.

Drug Interaction Precaution: If you are taking a cough/cold or allergy medication containing any form of phenylpropanolamine, or any oral nasal decongestant, do not take this product. Do not use this product if you are taking any prescription drug, except under the advice and supervision of a physician. Do not use this product if you are presently taking a prescription monoamine oxidase inhibitor (MAOI) for depression or for two weeks after stopping use of an MAOI without first consulting a physician.
KEEP THIS AND ALL MEDICATIONS OUT OF THE REACH OF CHILDREN. In case of accidental overdose, seek professional assistance or contact a poison control center immediately.

How Supplied: Dexatrim Plus Vitamins is supplied in tamper-evident blister packaging containing 14 Dexatrim caplets and 14 multi-vitamin/mineral caplets or containing 28 Dexatrim caplets and 28 multi-vitamin/mineral caplets.
Shown in Product Identification Guide, page 522

ENCARE®
[en'kar]
Vaginal Contraceptive Suppositories

Description: Encare is a safe and effective contraceptive in a convenient vaginal suppository form available without a prescription. Encare is reliable because it offers two-way protection: (1) Encare kills sperm on contact by releasing a precise dose of nonoxynol 9, the spermicide most recommended by doctors. (2) Encare gently disperses a physical barrier of protection against the cervix to help prevent pregnancy.
Encare is colorless and odorless; it is as pleasant to use as it is effective.
Encare is an effective contraceptive in vaginal suppository form.

Active Ingredient: Each Suppository contains 100 mg Nonoxynol 9.

Other Ingredients: Polyethylene Glycols, Sodium Bicarbonate, Sodium Citrate, Tartaric Acid.

Indications: Encare is effective in the prevention of pregnancy.

Action: Encare is 100% free of hormones and free of the serious side effects associated with oral contraceptives.
Encare is convenient and easy to use. Women like Encare because each insert is individually wrapped and can be easily carried in a pocket or purse. Encare is approximately as effective as vaginal foam contraceptives in actual use, yet there is no applicator, so there is nothing to fill, remove, or clean. For added protection, Encare may be used in conjunction with other contraceptive methods, such as a condom or as a second application with a diaphragm.
Because Encare can be inserted as much as an hour before intercourse, it does not interfere with spontaneity. Encare has been used successfully by millions of women throughout Europe and America.

Special Warning: Spermicidal contraceptives should not be used during pregnancy. Some experts believe that there may be an increased risk of birth defects occurring in children whose mothers used a spermicidal contraceptive at the time of conception or during pregnancy. If you believe you may be pregnant, have a pregnancy test before using a spermicidal contraceptive. If you have used a spermicidal contraceptive after becoming pregnant, or used a spermicidal contraceptive when you became pregnant, discuss this issue with your doctor.

Cautions: If your doctor has told you that you should not become pregnant, consult your doctor as to which method, (including Encare), is best for you.
If you or your partner experience irritation, discontinue use. If irritation persists, consult your doctor. This product has not been shown to protect against HIV (AIDS) and other sexually transmitted diseases.
Do not take orally. **KEEP THIS AND ALL DRUGS OUT OF THE REACH OF CHILDREN.** In case of accidental ingestion, call a poison control center, emergency medical facility or a doctor immediately.
Keep away from excessive heat and moisture. Store at controlled room temperature: 15°C–30°C (59°–86°F).

Dosage and Administration: For best protection against pregnancy, it is essential to follow package instructions. At least 10 minutes before intercourse, place one Encare insert with your fingertip as far as possible into the vagina, towards the small of your back. Best protection will occur when Encare is placed deep into the vagina. You may feel a pleasant sensation of warmth as Encare effervesces and distributes the spermicide, nonoxynol 9, within the vagina. This is a natural attribute of the active ingredient.

IMPORTANT: It is essential to insert Encare at least 10 minutes before intercourse. If one chooses, Encare can be inserted up to one hour before intercourse. If intercourse has not taken place within one hour after insertion, use a new En-

care insert. Use a new Encare insert each time intercourse is repeated. Encare can be used safely and as frequently as needed.
Douching after use of Encare is not required; however, should you desire to do so, wait at least six hours after intercourse.
Instructions enclosed in package are in both English and Spanish.

How Supplied: Boxes of 12 and 18.

References: Barwin, B., *Contraceptive Delivery System,* 4, 331–334, 1983. Masters, W., et. al. *Fertility and Sterility,* 32, 161–165, 1979.
Dimpfl J., et. al. *Sexualmedizin* 1984; 2: 95-8. Schill WB, Wolff HH. *Andrologia* 1981; 13(1): 42-9. Stone SC, Cardinale F. Am J Obstet Gynecol 1979; 133: 635-8.

HEMORID®
Hemorrhoidal Creme, Ointment, Suppositories, and Personal Cleansing Lotion

Description: HEMORID® is available in Creme, Ointment, Suppositories and Cleanser.

Ingredients:
Creme: Active Ingredients: White Petrolatum 30.0%, Mineral Oil 20.0%, Pramoxine Hydrochloride 1.0%, Phenylephrine Hydrochloride 0.25%. Other Ingredients: Aloe Vera Gel, Cetyl Alcohol, Methylparaben, Polysorbate 80, PPG-15 Stearyl Ether, Propylparaben, Purified Water, Sorbitan Monooleate, Stearyl Alcohol.
Ointment: Active Ingredients: White Petrolatum 82.15%, Light Mineral Oil 12.5%, Pramoxine Hydrochloride 1.0%, Phenylephrine Hydrochloride .25%. Other Ingredients: Aloe Extract, White Wax.
Suppositories: Active Ingredients: Zinc Oxide USP 11.0%, Phenylephrine Hydrochloride USP 0.25%, Hard Fat 88.25%.
Other Ingredients: Aloe Vera
Cleanser: Contains: Water, Mineral Oil, Petrolatum, Glyceryl Stearate, PEG-100 Stearate, Glycerin, Stearic Acid, Triethanolamine, Squalane, Methylparaben, Cetyl Alcohol, Diazolidinyl Urea, Propylparaben, Orange Blossom Extract.

Indications:
Creme/Ointment: Temporarily shrinks swollen hemorrhoidal tissue and helps relieve the local pain, burning, itching and discomfort associated with hemorrhoids or anorectal inflammation.
Suppositories: Temporarily shrinks swollen hemorrhoidal tissue and helps relieve the local itching, discomfort, and burning associated with hemorrhoids or anorectal inflammation.
Cleanser: Specifically formulated to cleanse, refresh, and soothe the perianal area. Also may be used for the external vaginal area.

Continued on next page

Thompson Medical—Cont.

Warnings:
Creme/Ointment: Do not use in the eyes or nose. If condition worsens or does not improve within 7 days, consult a physician. Do not exceed the recommended daily dosage, unless directed by a physician. Do not apply to large areas of the body. In case of bleeding, consult a physician promptly. Do not put this product into the rectum by using fingers or any mechanical device or applicator. Certain persons can develop allergic reactions to ingredients in this product. If the symptom being treated does not subside or if redness, irritation, swelling, pain or other symptoms develop or increase, discontinue use and consult a physician. Do not use this product if you have heart disease, high blood pressure, thyroid disease, diabetes or difficulty in urination due to enlargement of the prostate gland, unless directed by a physician. As with any drug, if you are pregnant or nursing a baby, seek the advice of a health professional before using this product. Do not use this product if you are presently taking a prescription drug for high blood pressure or depression, without first consulting your physician.
Suppositories: If condition worsens or does not improve within 7 days, consult a physician. Do not exceed the recommended daily dosage, unless directed by a physician. In case of bleeding, consult a physician promptly. Do not use this product if you have heart disease, high blood pressure, thyroid disease, diabetes or difficulty in urination due to enlargement of the prostate gland, unless directed by a physician. As with any drug, if you are pregnant or nursing a baby, seek the advice of a health professional before using this product. Do not use this product if you are presently taking a prescription drug for high blood pressure or depression, without first consulting your physician.
Cleanser: If irritation persists or worsens, discontinue use and consult a physician. In case of bleeding, consult a physician promptly.

Dosage and Administration:
Creme/Ointment: **Adults:** When practical, cleanse the affected area with mild soap and warm water and rinse thoroughly. Gently dry by patting or blotting with toilet tissue or a soft cloth before application of this product. Apply externally to the affected area up to 4 times daily. **Children under 12 years of age:** Consult a physician.
Suppositories: Adults: When practical, cleanse the affected area with mild soap and warm water and rinse thoroughly. Gently dry by patting or blotting with toilet tissue or a soft cloth before application of this product. Detach one suppository from strip of suppositories. Holding one suppository upright, carefully remove the wrapper by peeling down both sides starting from the pointed end. Insert into the rectum pointed end first. Avoid excessive han-

dling of the suppository. May be used up to 4 times daily. **Children under 12 years of age:** Consult a physician.
Cleanser: Apply a small amount of the cleanser onto bathroom tissue and wipe skin around the perianal area after bowel movements or when discomfort occurs. To soothe and refresh the external vaginal area, apply a small amount of cleanser onto bathroom tissue and cleanse as needed.
How to Store: Store at controlled room temperature 15°-30°C (59°–86°F).

How Supplied: HEMORID® Creme: 1 oz. tube. HEMORID® Ointment: 1 oz. tube. HEMORID® Suppositories: 12's. HEMORID® For Women Cleanser: 4 oz. bottle.
Shown in Product Identification Guide, page 522

SLEEPINAL®
Night-time Sleep Aid Capsules and Softgels
(Diphenhydramine HCl)

Description: SLEEPINAL is a night-time sleep aid. When taken prior to bedtime, it helps to relieve sleeplessness and aids in falling asleep.

Active Ingredient: Diphenhydramine HCl 50 mg.

Other Ingredients: Capsules: FD&C Blue No. 1, Gelatin, Lactose, Magnesium Stearate, Povidone, Talc.
Softgels: D&C Yellow No. 10, Gelatin, Glycerin, Polyethylene Glycol 400, Povidone, Propylene Glycol, Purified Water, Sorbitol. May also contain: FD&C Blue No. 1, FD&C Green No. 3.

Indications: For relief of occasional sleeplessness.

Action: SLEEPINAL is an antihistamine with anticholinergic and sedative action.

Warnings: Read before using. Do not exceed recommended dosage. Do not give to children under 12 years of age. If sleeplessness persists continuously for more than 2 weeks, consult your physician. Insomnia may be a symptom of serious underlying medical illness. Do not take this product, unless directed by a physician, if you have a breathing problem such as emphysema or chronic bronchitis, or if you have glaucoma or difficulty in urination due to the enlargement of the prostate gland. Avoid alcoholic beverages while taking this product. Do not take this product if you are taking sedatives or tranquilizers, without first consulting your physician. As with any drug, if you are pregnant or nursing a baby, seek the advice of a health professional before using this product.
KEEP THIS AND ALL MEDICATIONS OUT OF THE REACH OF CHILDREN. In case of accidental overdose, seek professional assistance or contact a poison control center immediately.

Dosage and Administration: Capsules and Softgels: Adults and children 12

years of age and over: Oral dosage, one at bedtime if needed, or as directed by a physician.

How to Store: Store in a dry place at controlled room temperature 15° C–30° C (59° F–86° F). Protect softgels from light, retain product in box until administered.

How Supplied: Capsules and Softgels: Sleepinal is supplied in tamper-evident blister packages. Do not use if individual seals are broken. Packages of 16 and 32 capsules and 8 and 16 softgels.
Shown in Product Identification Guide, page 522

SPORTSCREME®
[*sports-crēme*]
External Analgesic Rub

Description: SPORTSCREME® is available as a creme and lotion for use as a topical massage rub that temporarily relieves minor muscle aches and pains. Sportscreme has a clean, fresh scent.

Active Ingredient: Salycin® 10% (Thompson Medical's brand of Trolamine Salicylate).

Other Ingredients: Cetyl Alcohol, FD&C Blue No. 1, FD&C Yellow No. 5, Fragrance, Glycerin, Methylparaben, Mineral Oil, Potassium Phosphate Monobasic, Propylparaben, Stearic Acid, Triethanolamine, Water.

Actions: External analgesic rub.

Indications: Analgesic rub for temporary relief of minor aches and pains of muscles associated with simple strains and sprains.

Warnings: Use only as directed. If prone to allergic reaction from aspirin or salicylates, consult a physician before using. If redness is present or if condition worsens, or if pain persists for more than 7 days, discontinue use and consult a physician. Do not use on children under ten years of age. Do not apply if skin is irritated or if irritation develops. As with any drug, if you are pregnant or nursing a baby, seek the advice of a health professional before using this product. For external use only. Avoid contact with eyes. **KEEP THIS AND ALL MEDICINES OUT OF THE REACH OF CHILDREN.** In case of accidental ingestion, seek professional assistance or contact a poison control center immediately.

Dosage and Administration: Apply generously to affected area. Massage into painful area until thoroughly absorbed into skin. Repeat as needed, especially before retiring and in the morning, but not more than 4 times daily.

How to Store: Store at controlled room temperature 15°–30°C (59°–86°F).

How Supplied: Cream: 1.25 oz. and 3 oz. tubes: Lotion: 6 oz. bottle.

TEMPO®
[tem-pō]
Soft Antacid

Description: Tempo is a unique, chewable soft antacid that provides fast, effective relief from acid indigestion, heartburn, and gas. Tempo is pleasant tasting, not chalky or gritty.

Active Ingredients: Each drop contains Calcium Carbonate 414 mg., Aluminum Hydroxide 133 mg., Magnesium Hydroxide 81 mg., Simethicone 20 mg.

Other Ingredients: Corn Syrup, Deionized Water, FD&C Blue No. 1, Flavor, Sorbitol, Soy Protein, Starch, Titanium Dioxide, [3.0 mg. Sodium per drop (dietetically sodium free)].

Indication: For the relief of heartburn, sour stomach, acid indigestion, gas, and upset stomach associated with these symptoms.

Warnings: Do not take more than 12 drops in a 24-hour period or use the maximum dosage for more than two weeks except under the advice and supervision of a doctor. **KEEP THIS AND ALL MEDICATIONS OUT OF THE REACH OF CHILDREN.**

Drug Interaction Precaution: Antacids may interact with certain prescription drugs. If you are presently taking a prescription drug, do not take this product without checking with your physician or other health professional.

Dosage and Administration: One tablet dosage. Not to exceed more than 12 tablets in a 24-hour period.

How to Store: Store at controlled room temperature 15°–30°C (59°–86°F).

How Supplied: 10, 30, and 60 Pieces
Shown in Product Identification Guide, page 522

Tishcon Corp.
**30 NEW YORK AVENUE
WESTBURY, NY 11590**

Direct Inquiries to:
Product Information Director 516-333-3050
FAX 516-997-1052

LUMITENE™ BETA CAROTENE
**30 mg beadlets
(Pharmaceutical grade Dry Beta Carotene beadlets, 10%)**

Description: Lumitene™ (beta-carotene) is available in capsules for oral administration. Each capsule is composed of beadlets containing 30 mg beta-carotene, ascorbyl palmitate, corn starch, dl-alpha-tocopherol, gelatin, peanut oil and sucrose. Gelatin capsule shells may contain parabens (methyl and propyl), potassium sorbate, FD&C Blue No. 1, D&C Yellow No. 10, FD&C Red No. 3, FD&C Green No. 3 and titanium dioxide.

Beta-carotene, precursor of vitamin A, is a carotenoid pigment occurring naturally in green and yellow vegetables. Chemically, beta-carotene has the empirical formula $C_{40}H_{56}$ and a calculated molecular weight of 536.85. Trans-beta-carotene is a red, crystalline compound which is insoluble in water. Its structural formula is as follows:

Clinical Pharmacology: Beta-carotene, a pro-vitamin A, belongs to the class of carotenoid pigments. In terms of its vitamin activity, 6 μg of dietary beta-carotene is considered equivalent to 1 μ9 of vitamin A (retinol). Bio-availability of beta-carotene depends on the presence of fat in the diet to act as a carrier, and bile in the intestinal tract for its absorption. Beta-carotene is metabolized, primarily in the intestine, to vitamin A at a rate of approximately 50% to 60% of normal dietary intake and falls off rapidly as intake goes up. In humans, an appreciable amount of unchanged beta-carotene is absorbed and stored in various tissues, especially the depot fat. Small amounts may be converted to vitamin A in the liver. The vitamin A derived from beta-carotene follows the same metabolic pathway as that from dietary sources. The major route of elimination is fecal excretion. Excessive ingestion of carotenes is not harmful, but it may cause yellow coloration of the skin, which disappears upon reduction or cessation of intake.

Contraindications: Lumitene™ is contraindicated in patients with known hypersensitivity to beta-carotene.

Warnings: Lumitene™ has not been shown to be effective as a sunscreen.

Precautions: General: Lumitene™ should be used with caution in patients with impaired renal or hepatic function because safe use in the presence of these conditions has not been established.
Information for Patients: Patients receiving Lumitene™ should be advised against taking supplementary vitamin A since Lumitene™ administration will fulfill normal vitamin A requirements. They should be cautioned to continue sun protection, and forewarned that their skin may appear slightly yellow while receiving Lumitene™.
Carcinogenesis, Mutagenesis, Impairment of Fertility: Long-term studies in animals to determine carcinogenesis have not been completed. *In vitro* and *in vivo* studies to evaluate mutagenic potential were negative. No effects on fertility in male rats were observed at doses as high as 500 mg/kg/day (100 times the recommended human dose).
Pregnancy: Teratogenic Effects: Pregnancy Category C. Beta-carotene has been shown to be fetotoxic (i.e., cause an increase in resorption rate), but not tera-togenic when given to rats at doses 300 to 400 times the maximum recommended human dose. No such fetotoxicity was observed at 75 times the maximum recommended human dose or less. A generation reproduction study in rats receiving beta-carotene at a dietary concentration of 0.1% (1000 ppm) has revealed no evidence of impaired fertility or effect on the fetus. There are no adequate and well-controlled studies in pregnant women. Lumitene™ should be used during pregnancy only if the potential benefit justifies the potential risk to the fetus.
Nursing Mothers: It is not known whether this drug is excreted in human milk. Because many drugs are excreted in human milk, caution should be exercised when Lumitene™ is administered to a nursing mother.

Adverse Reactions: Some patients may have occasional loose stools while taking Lumitene™. This reaction is sporadic and may not require discontinuance of medication. Other reactions which have been reported rarely are ecchymoses and arthralgia.

Overdosage: There are no reported cases of overdosage. The oral LD_{50} of beta-carotene (suspended in 5% gum acacia solution) in mice and rats is greater than 20,000 mg/kg. No lethality was observed in mice following administration of 30-mg beadlet capsules (ground and suspended in 5% gum acacia) at a dose of 1200 mg/kg beta-carotene.

Dosage and Administration: Lumitene™ may be administered either as a single daily dose or in divided doses, preferably with meals.
Usage in Children: The usual dosage for children under 14 is 30 to 150 mg (1 to 5 capsules) per day. Capsules may be opened and the contents mixed in orange or tomato juice to aid administration.
Usage in Adults: The usual adult dosage is 30 to 300 mg (1 to 10 capsules) per day.
Dosage should be adjusted depending on the severity of the symptoms and the response of the patient. Several weeks of therapy are necessary to accumulate enough Lumitene™ in the skin to exert its effect. Patients should be instructed not to increase exposure to sunlight until they appear carotenemic (first seen as yellowness of palms and soles). This usually occurs after two to six weeks of therapy. Exposure to the sun may then be increased gradually. The protective effect is not total and each patient should establish his or her own limits of exposure.

How Supplied: Lumitene™ is available in blue and green capsules, each containing 30 mg of beta-carotene—bottles of 100 (NDC 1465-4658-08).

Triton Consumer Products, Inc.
561 W. GOLF ROAD
ARLINGTON HEIGHTS, IL 60005

Direct Inquiries to:
Karen Shrader
(800) 942-2009

For Medical Emergencies Contact:
(800) 942-2009

MG 217® PSORIASIS/DANDRUFF MEDICATION
Skin Care: Ointment and Lotion
Scalp: Shampoo

Active Ingredients: Ointment—Coal Tar Solution USP 10%. **Lotion**—Coal Tar Solution USP 5%. **Sal-Acid Ointment**—Salicylic acid 3%. **Tar Shampoo**—Coal Tar Solution USP 15%. **Tar-Free Shampoo**—Sulfur 5% and salicylic acid 3%.

Action/Uses: Relief for itching, scaling and flaking of psoriasis, seborrheic dermatitis and/or dandruff.

Warnings: For external use only. Keep out of the reach of children. Avoid contact with eyes. If undue skin irritation occurs, discontinue use.

Administration: **Ointment or Lotion** —Apply to affected area one to four times daily. **Shampoo**—Wet hair, then massage shampoo into scalp and leave on for several minutes. Rinse thoroughly. Use at least twice a week or as directed by a physician.

How Supplied: Ointment—3.8 oz. jars. **Lotion**—4 oz. bottles. **Sal-Acid Ointment**—2 oz. jars. **Shampoo**—4 oz. and 8 oz. bottles.

UAS Laboratories
5610 ROWLAND RD #110
MINNETONKA, MN 55343

Direct Inquiries To:
Dr. S.K. Dash: (612) 935-1707
Fax: (612) 935-1650

Medical Emergency Contact:
Dr. S.K. Dash: (612) 935-1707
Fax: (612) 935-1650

DDS-ACIDOPHILUS
Capsule, Tablet & Powder free of dairy products, corn, soy, and preservatives

Description: DDS-Acidophilus is the source of a special strain of Lactobacillus acidophilus free of dairy products, corn, soy and preservatives. Each capsule or tablet contains one billion viable DDS-1 L.acidophilus at the time of manufacturing. One gram of powder contains two billion viable DDS-1 L.acidophilus.

Indications and Usages: An aid in implanting the gut with beneficial Lacto-bacillus acidophilus under conditions of digestive disorders, acne, yeast infections, and following antibiotic therapy.

Administration: One to two capsules or tablets twice daily before meals. One-fourth teaspoon powder can be substituted for two capsules or tablets.

How Supplied: Bottles of 100 capsules or tablets. 12 bottles per case. Powder is available in 2 oz. bottle; 12 bottles per case.

Storage: Keep refrigerated under 40°F.

EDUCATIONAL MATERIAL

DDS-Acidophilus
Booklet describing superior-strain Acidophilus without dairy products, corn, soy, or preservatives. Two billion viable DDS-L. acidopohilus per gram.

The Upjohn Company
KALAMAZOO, MI 49001

For Medical and Pharmaceutical Information, Including Emergencies:
(616) 329-8244
(616) 323-6615

CORTAID®
Maximum Strength, Sensitive Skin Formula, and FastStick.
Cream, Ointment, Spray and Roll-on Stick
(hydrocortisone 1% and ½%)
Anti-itch products

Indications: Use CORTAID for the temporary relief of itching associated with minor skin irritations, inflammation, and rashes due to eczema, psoriasis, seborrheic dermatitis, poison ivy, poison oak, or poison sumac, insect bites, soaps, detergents, cosmetics, jewelry, and for external feminine and anal itching. Other uses of this product should be only under the advice and supervision of a physician.

Description: CORTAID provides safe, effective relief of many different types of itches and rashes and is the brand recommended most by physicians and pharmacists. Maximum Strength CORTAID is the same strength and form of hydrocortisone relief formerly available only with a prescription. CORTAID Sensitive Skin Formula has been specially formulated with aloe and ½% hydrocortisone. CORTAID FastStick provides the relief of Maximum Strength CORTAID in a convenient roll-on-stick—Great for insect bites. CORTAID is available in 1) a greaseless, odorless vanishing cream that leaves no residue; 2) a soothing, lubricating ointment; 3) a quick-drying non-staining, non-aerosol spray and roll-on stick (Maximum Strength only).

Active Ingredients: CORTAID Cream and CORTAID Ointment: 1% or ½% hydrocortisone.
CORTAID Spray and FastStick: hydrocortisone 1%.

Other Ingredients:
Maximum Strength Products:
Maximum Strength Cream: Aloe vera gel, ceteareth-20, ceteareth alcohol, cetyl palmitate, glycerin, isopropyl myristate, isostearyl neopentanoate, methylparaben, and purified water.
Maximum Strength Ointment: butylparaben, cholesterol, methylparaben, microcrystalline wax, mineral oil, and white petrolatum.
Maximum Strength Spray and Fast-Stick: alcohol, glycerin, methylparaben, and purified water.
Sensitive Skin Products:
Sensitive Skin Formula Cream: aloe vera, butylparaben, cetyl palmitate, glyceryl stearate, methylparaben, polyethylene glycol, stearamidoethyl diethylamine, and purified water.
Sensitive Skin Formula Ointment: aloe vera, butylparaben, cholesterol, methylparaben, mineral oil, white petrolatum, and microcrystalline wax.

Uses: The vanishing action of CORTAID Cream makes it cosmetically acceptable when the skin itch or rash treated is on exposed parts of the body such as the hands or arms. CORTAID Ointment is best used where protection lubrication and soothing of dry and scaly lesions is required. The ointment is also recommended for treating itchy genital and anal areas. CORTAID Spray is a quick-drying, non-staining formulation suitable for covering large areas of the skin. CORTAID FastStick delivers quick-drying, non-staining medicine via a convenient and highly portable roll-on stick.

Warnings: For external use only. Avoid contact with the eyes. If condition worsens, or if symptoms persist for more than 7 days or clear up and occur again within a few days, stop use of this product and do not begin use of any other hydrocortisone product unless you have consulted a physician. Do not use for the treatment of diaper rash. Consult a physician. For external feminine itching, do not use if you have a vaginal discharge. Consult a physician. For external anal itching, do not exceed the recommended daily dosage unless directed by a physician. In case of bleeding, consult a physician promptly. Do not put this product into the rectum by using fingers or any mechanical device or applicator.
Keep this and all drugs out of the reach of children. In case of accidental ingestion, seek professional assistance or contact a poison control center immediately.

Dosage and Administration: *Adults and children 2 years of age and older:* Apply to affected area not more than 3 to 4 times daily. *Children under 2 years of age:* Do not use, consult a physician. *Adults:* For external anal itching, when practical, cleanse the affected area with mild soap and warm water and rinse thoroughly by patting or blotting with an appropriate cleansing pad. Gently dry by patting or blotting with toilet tissue or a soft cloth before application of this product. *Children under 12 years of age:* For external anal itching, consult a physician.

How Supplied:
Cream: ½ oz. and 1 oz. tubes
Ointment: ½ oz. and 1 oz. tubes
Non-Aerosol Spray: 1.5 fluid oz.
FastStick: ½ oz.
Shown in Product Identification Guide, page 522

DOXIDAN® LIQUI-GELS®
Stimulant/Stool Softener Laxative

Indications: DOXIDAN is a safe reliable laxative for the relief of occasional constipation. The combination of a stimulant/stool softener laxative allows positive laxative action on a softened stool for gentle evacuation without straining. DOXIDAN generally produces a bowel movement in 6 to 12 hours.

Active Ingredients: Each soft gelatin Liqui-gel contains 65 mg yellow phenolphthalein and 60 mg docusate calcium.

Inactive Ingredients: Also contains corn oil, FD&C Blue #1 and Red #40, gelatin, glycerin, hydrogenated vegetable oil, lecithin, parabens, sorbitol, titanium dioxide, vegetable shortening, yellow wax, and other ingredients.

Dosage and Administration: Adults and children 12 years of age and over: one or two Liqui-gels by mouth daily. For children over 6, one Liqui-gel daily. For use in children 6 and under, consult a physician.

Warnings: Do not use laxative products when abdominal pain, nausea, or vomiting are present unless directed by a doctor. If you have noticed a sudden change in bowel habits that persists over a period of 2 weeks, consult a doctor before using a laxative. Laxative products should not be used for a period longer than 1 week unless directed by a doctor. Rectal bleeding or failure to have a bowel movement after use of a laxative may indicate a serious condition. Discontinue use and consult your doctor. If skin rash appears, do not use this product or any other preparation containing phenolphthalein. Keep this and all drugs out of the reach of children. In case of accidental overdose, seek professional assistance or contact a poison control center immediately. As with any drug, if you are pregnant or nursing a baby, seek the advice of a health professional before using this product.

Drug Interaction Precaution: Do not take this product if you are presently taking mineral oil, unless directed by a doctor.

How Supplied: Packages of 10, 30, 100 and 1,000 maroon soft gelatin capsules, and Unit Dose 100s (10 × 10 strips). LIQUI-GELS® Reg TM R P Scherer Corp
Shown in Product Identification Guide, page 522

DRAMAMINE® Tablets
(dimenhydrinate USP)
DRAMAMINE® Chewable Tablets
(dimenhydrinate USP)
DRAMAMINE® Children's Liquid
(dimenhydrinate syrup USP)

Indications: For the prevention and treatment of the nausea, vomiting, or dizziness associated with motion sickness.

Description: Dimenhydrinate is the chlorotheophylline salt of the antihistaminic agent diphenhydramine. Dimenhydrinate contains not less than 53% and not more than 56% of diphenhydramine, and not less than 44% and not more than 47% of 8-chlorotheophylline, calculated on the dried basis.

Active Ingredients:
DRAMAMINE Tablets and Chewable Tablets: Dimenhydrinate 50 mg.
DRAMAMINE Children's: Dimenhydrinate 12.5 mg. per 5 ml.

Inactive Ingredients:
DRAMAMINE Tablets: Acacia, Carboxymethylcellulose Sodium, Corn Starch, Magnesium Stearate, and Sodium Sulfate.
DRAMAMINE Children's: FD&C Red No. 40, Flavor, Glycerin, Methylparaben, Sucrose, and Water.
DRAMAMINE Chewable Tablets: Aspartame, Citric Acid, FD&C Yellow No. 6, Flavor, Magnesium Stearate, Methacrylic Acid Copolymer, Sorbitol.
Phenylketonurics: Contains Phenylalanine 1.5 mg per tablet.
Contains FD&C Yellow No. 5 (tartrazine) as a color additive.

Actions: While the precise mode of action of dimenhydrinate is not known, it is thought to have a depressant action on hyperstimulated labyrinthine function.

Directions:
DRAMAMINE Tablets and Chewable Tablets: To prevent motion sickness, the first dose should be taken one half to one hour before starting activity.
ADULTS: 1 to 2 tablets every 4 to 6 hours, not to exceed 8 tablets in 24 hours or as directed by a doctor.
CHILDREN 6 TO UNDER 12: ½ to 1 tablet every 6 to 8 hours, not to exceed 3 tablets in 24 hours or as directed by a doctor.
CHILDREN 2 to UNDER 6: ¼ to ½ tablet every 6 to 8 hours not to exceed 1½ tablets in 24 hours or as directed by a doctor.
Children may also be given DRAMAMINE Cherry Flavored Liquid in accordance with directions for use.

DRAMAMINE Children's: To prevent motion sickness, the first dose should be taken one half to one hour before starting activity. CHILDREN 2 TO UNDER 6: 1 to 2 teaspoonfuls every 6 to 8 hours not to exceed 6 teaspoonfuls in 24 hours or as directed by a doctor. Use of a measuring device is recommended for all liquid medication. CHILDREN 6 TO UNDER 12: 2 to 4 teaspoonfuls every 6 to 8 hours, not to exceed 12 teaspoonfuls in 24 hours or as directed by a doctor. CHILDREN 12 YEARS OR OLDER: 4 to 8 teaspoons (5 ml per teaspoonful) every 4 to 6 hours, not to exceed 32 teaspoonfuls in 24 hours or as directed by a doctor.

Warnings: Do not take this product, unless directed by a doctor, if you have a breathing problem such as emphysema or chronic bronchitis, or if you have glaucoma or difficulty in urination due to enlargement of the prostate gland. Do not give to children under 2 years of age unless directed by a doctor. May cause marked drowsiness; alcohol, sedatives, and tranquilizers may increase the drowsiness effect. Avoid alcoholic beverages while taking this product. Do not take this product if you are taking sedatives or tranquilizers, without first consulting your doctor. Use caution when driving a motor vehicle or operating machinery. Not for frequent or prolonged use except on advice of a doctor. Do not exceed recommended dosage. Keep this and all drugs out of the reach of children. In case of accidental overdose, seek professional assistance or contact a poison control center immediately. As with any drug, if you are pregnant or nursing a baby, seek the advice of a health professional before using this product.

How Supplied: *Tablets* —scored, white tablets available in packets of 12 and 36 and bottles of 100; *Chewables* —scored, orange tablets available in packets of 8 and 24; *Liquid* —Available in bottles of 4 fl oz).
Shown in Product Identification Guide, page 522

DRAMAMINE II™
(Meclizine hydrochloride)

Indications: For the prevention and treatment of the nausea, vomiting, or dizziness associated with motion sickness.

Description: Meclizine hydrochloride is an antihistamine of the piperazine class with antiemetic action.

Actions: While the precise mode of action of meclizine hydrochloride is not known, it is thought to have a depressant action on hyperstimulated labyrinthine function.

Active Ingredients: Each tablet contains 25 mg. meclizine hydrochloride.

Inactive Ingredients: Colloidal silicon dioxide, croscarmellose sodium, di-

Continued on next page

Upjohn—Cont.

basic calcium phosphate, D&C yellow no. 10 aluminum lake, microcrystalline cellulose, magnesium stearate.

Directions: To prevent motion sickness, the first dose should be taken one hour before starting your activity. **Adults:** Take 1 to 2 tablets daily or as directed by a doctor. Do not exceed 2 tablets in 24 hours.

Warnings: Do not take this product, unless directed by a doctor, if you have a breathing problem such as emphysema or chronic bronchitis, or if you have glaucoma or difficulty in urination due to enlargement of the prostate gland. Do not give to children under 12 years of age unless directed by a doctor. May cause drowsiness; alcohol, sedatives, and tranquilizers may increase the drowsiness effect. Avoid alcoholic beverages while taking this product. Do not take this product if you are taking sedatives or tranquilizers without first consulting your doctor. Use caution when driving a motor vehicle or operating machinery. Not for frequent or prolonged use except on the advice of a doctor. Do not exceed recommended dosage. Keep this and all drugs out of reach of children. In case of accidental overdose, seek professional assistance or contact a poison control center immediately. As with any drug, if you are pregnant or nursing a baby, seek the advice of a health professional before using this product.

How Supplied: Dramamine II is supplied as a yellow tablet in packages of 8.
Shown in Product Identification Guide, page 523

KAOPECTATE®
Anti-Diarrheal,
Regular Flavor, Peppermint Flavor and Children's Cherry Flavored Liquids. Maximum Strength Caplets.

Indications: For the fast relief of diarrhea and cramping.

Active Ingredients: Each tablespoon or caplet contains 750 mg attapulgite.

Inactive Ingredients: Liquids: flavors, gluconodelta-lactone, magnesium, aluminum silicate, methylparaben, sorbic acid, sucrose, titanium dioxide, xanthan gum and purified water; Peppermint flavor and Children's Cherry flavor contain FD&C Red #40. Maximum Strength Caplets: Carnauba Wax, Croscarmellose Sodium, Hydroxypropyl Cellulose, Hydroxypropyl Methylcellulose, Methylparaben, Pectin, Propylene Glycol, Propylparaben, Sucrose, Titanium Dioxide, Zinc Stearate. May also contain Talc.

Dosage and Administration: Liquids: For best results, take full recommended dose at first sign of diarrhea and after each subsequent bowel movement. (Maximum 6 times in 24 hours.) Adults and

children 12 years of age and over: 2 tablespoons. Children 6 to under 12 years of age: 1 tablespoon. Children 3 to 6 years of age: ½ tablespoon. Maximum Strength Tablets: Swallow whole caplets with water; do not chew. For best results, take full recommended dose. Adults: Take 2 caplets after the initial bowel movement and 2 caplets after each subsequent bowel movement, not to exceed 12 caplets in 24 hours. Children 6 to 12 years of age: Take 1 caplet after the initial bowel movement and 1 caplet after each subsequent movement, not to exceed 6 caplets in 24 hours. Children 3 to under 6 years of age: Use Children's Cherry Flavored Liquid or Advanced Formula KAOPECTATE Liquid.

Warnings: Unless directed by a physician, do not use Kaopectate Liquids in infants and children under 3 years of age or Kaopectate Caplets in infants or children under 6 years of age or for more than two days in the presence of high fever. Keep this and all drugs out of the reach of children. In case of accidental overdose, seek professional assistance or contact a poison control center immediately.

How Supplied: Regular flavor available in 8 oz., 12 oz. and 16 oz. bottles. Peppermint flavor available in 8 oz. and 12 oz. bottles. Children's Cherry flavor available in 6 oz. bottle. Maximum Strength Caplets available in blister packs of 12 and 20 caplets.
Shown in Product Identification Guide, page 523

MOTRIN® IB
Caplets, Tablets and Gelcaps
(ibuprofen, USP)
Pain Reliever/Fever Reducer

WARNING: ASPIRIN-SENSITIVE PATIENTS. Do not take this product if you have had a severe allergic reaction to aspirin, eg—asthma, swelling, shock or hives because even though this product contains no aspirin or salicylates, cross-reactions may occur in patients allergic to aspirin.

Indications: For the temporary relief of headache, muscular aches, minor pain of arthritis, toothache, backache, minor aches and pains associated with the common cold, pain of menstrual cramps, and for reduction of fever.

Directions: Adults: Take 1 caplet, tablet or gelcap every 4 to 6 hours while symptoms persist. If pain or fever does not respond to 1 caplet, tablet or gelcap, 2 caplets, tablets or gelcaps may be used, but do not exceed 6 caplets, tablets or gelcaps in 24 hours, unless directed by a doctor. The smallest effective dose should be used. Take with food or milk, if stomach or stomach pain occurs with use. Consult a doctor if these symptoms are more than mild or if they persist. Children: Do not give this product to children under 12 except under the advice and supervision of a doctor.

Warnings: Do not take for pain for more than 10 days or for fever for more than 3 days unless directed by a doctor. If pain or fever persists or gets worse, if new symptoms occur, or if the painful area is red or swollen, consult a doctor. These could be signs of serious illness. If you are under a doctor's care for any serious condition, consult a doctor before taking this product. As with aspirin and acetaminophen, if you have any condition which requires you to take prescription drugs or if you have had any problems or serious side effects from taking any nonprescription pain reliever, do not take MOTRIN® IB without first discussing it with your doctor. If you experience any symptoms which are unusual or seem unrelated to the condition for which you took ibuprofen, consult a doctor before taking any more of it.

Although ibuprofen is indicated for the same conditions as aspirin and acetaminophen, it should not be taken with them except under a doctor's direction. Do not combine this product with any other ibuprofen-containing product.

As with any drug, if you are pregnant or nursing a baby, seek the advice of a health professional before using this product. IT IS ESPECIALLY IMPORTANT NOT TO USE IBUPROFEN DURING THE LAST 3 MONTHS OF PREGNANCY UNLESS SPECIFICALLY DIRECTED TO DO SO BY A DOCTOR BECAUSE IT MAY CAUSE PROBLEMS IN THE UNBORN CHILD OR COMPLICATIONS DURING DELIVERY.

Keep this and all drugs out of the reach of children. In case of accidental overdose, seek professional assistance or contact a poison control center immediately. **Store at room temperature. Avoid excessive heat 40°C (104°F).**

Active Ingredient: Each caplet, tablet or gelcap contains ibuprofen 200 mg.

Other Ingredients: Carnauba wax, cornstarch, hydroxypropyl methylcellulose, propylene glycol, silicon dioxide, pregelatinized starch, stearic acid, titanium dioxide. Gelcaps also contain benzyl alcohol, butylparaben, butyl alcohol, castor oil, colloidal silicon dioxide, edetate calcium disodium, FDC Yellow No. 6, gelatin, iron oxide black, magnesium stearate, methylparaben, microcrystalline cellulose, povidone, propylparaben, SDA 3A starch, propylparaben, SDA 3A alcohol, sodium lauryl sulfate, sodium propionate, and sodium starch glycolate.

How Supplied: Bottles of 24, 50, 100, 130 and 165 Caplets or Tablets. Bottles of 24 and 50 Gelcaps. Vial of 8 caplets.
Shown in Product Identification Guide, page 523

Maximum Strength
MYCITRACIN®
Triple Antibiotic First Aid Ointment
MYCITRACIN® Plus Pain Reliever

Indications: Maximum Strength MYCI-TRACIN and MYCITRACIN Plus Pain Reliever are first aid ointments to help prevent infection in minor burns, cuts, nicks, scrapes, scratches and abrasions.

Description: MYCITRACIN combines three topical antibiotics in a soothing, non-irritating petrolatum base that does not sting, aids healing, and helps prevent infection. MYCITRACIN Plus Pain Reliever also temporarily relieves pain.

Directions: *For adults and children (all ages):* Clean the affected area. Apply a small amount of MYCITRACIN (an amount equal to the surface area of the tip of a finger) on the affected area 1 to 3 times daily. If desired, cover the affected area with a sterile bandage.

Warnings: For external use only. Do not use in the eyes or apply over large areas of the body. In case of deep or puncture wounds, animal bites, or serious burns, consult a physician. Stop use and consult a physician if the condition persists or gets worse. Do not use longer than 1 week unless directed by a physician. Keep this and all medications out of the reach of children. In case of accidental ingestion, seek professional assistance or contact a poison control center immediately.

Active Ingredients:
Maximum Strength MYCITRACIN:
Each Gram Contains: Bacitracin Zinc 500 units; Neomycin Sulfate equiv. to 3.5 mg neomycin; Polymyxin B Sulfate, 10,000 units;
MYCITRACIN Plus Pain Reliever: *Each Gram Contains: Bacitracin Zinc, 500 units; Neomycin Sulfate equiv. to 3.5 mg neomycin; Polymyxin B Sulfate, 10,000 units; Lidocaine, 40 mg.*

Other Ingredients:
Maximum Strength MYCITRACIN: *Also contains butylparaben, cholesterol, methylparaben, microcrystalline wax, mineral oil, and white petrolatum.*
MYCITRACIN Plus Pain Reliever: *Also contains butylparaben, cholesterol, methylparaben, microcrystalline wax, mineral oil, and white petrolatum.*

How Supplied:
½ oz. tubes, 1 oz. tubes and ¹⁄₃₂ oz. foil packets (144 per carton)
Shown in Product Identification Guide, page 523

SURFAK® LIQUI-GELS®
Stool Softener Laxative

Indications: Surfak®, a stool softener, is indicated for the relief of occasional constipation. Unlike some other types of laxatives, Surfak contains no harsh stimulants that can upset your stomach or cause cramps. Instead, Surfak works gently by drawing water into the stool, making it softer and easier to pass. With Surfak you can expect to return to regularity in 12 to 72 hours.

Active Ingredients: Each soft gelatin Liqui-gel contains 240 mg docusate calcium.

Inactive Ingredients: Also contains corn oil, FD&C Blue #1 and Red #40, gelatin, glycerin, parabens, sorbitol, and other ingredients.

Dosage and Administration: Adults and children 12 years of age and over: one capsule by mouth daily for several days or until bowel movements are normal. For use in children under 12, consult a physician.

Warnings: Do not use laxative products when abdominal pain, nausea, or vomiting are present unless directed by a doctor. If you have noticed a sudden change in bowel habits that persists over a period of 2 weeks, consult a doctor before using a laxative. Laxative products should not be used for a period longer than 1 week unless directed by a doctor. Rectal bleeding or failure to have a bowel movement after use of a laxative may indicate a serious condition. Discontinue use and consult your doctor. Keep this and all drugs out of the reach of children. In case of accidental overdose, seek professional assistance or contact a poison control center immediately. As with any drug, if you are pregnant or nursing a baby, seek the advice of a health professional before using this product.

Drug Interaction Precaution: Do not take this product if you are presently taking mineral oil, unless directed by a doctor.

How Supplied: Packages of 10, 30, 100 and 500 red soft gelatin capsules and Unit Dose 100s (10 × 10 strips).
LIQUI-GELS® Reg TM R P Scherer Corp
Shown in Product Identification Guide, page 523

Wallace Laboratories
P.O. BOX 1001
HALF ACRE ROAD
CRANBURY, NJ 08512

Direct Inquiries to:
Wallace Laboratories
Div. of Carter-Wallace, Inc.
P.O. Box 1001
Cranbury, NJ 08512
(609) 655-6000

For Medical Emergencies Contact:
(800) 526-3840

MALTSUPEX®
(malt soup extract)
Powder, Liquid, Tablets

Composition: MALTSUPEX is a non-diastatic extract from barley malt, which is available in powder, liquid, and tablet form. Each MALTSUPEX product has a gentle laxative action and promotes soft, easily passed stools. Each **Tablet** contains 750 mg of Malt Soup Extract. Other Ingredients: D&C Yellow No. 10, FD&C Red No. 40, flavor (artificial), hydroxypropyl methylcellulose, methylparaben, polyethylene glycol, propylparaben, povidone, simethicone emulsion, stearic acid, talc, titanium dioxide.
Powder: Each level scoop provides approximately 8 g of Malt Soup Extract.
Liquid: Each tablespoonful (½ fl. oz.) contains approximately the equivalent of 16 g Malt Soup Extract Powder. Other ingredients: Sodium propionate and potassium sorbate.

EFFECTIVE, NON-HABIT-FORMING

Indications: For relief of occasional constipation. This product generally produces a bowel movement in 12 to 72 hours.

Warnings: Do not use laxative products when abdominal pain, nausea or vomiting are present unless directed by a physician. If constipation persists, consult a physician.
If you have noticed a sudden change in bowel habits that persists over a period of 2 weeks, consult a physician before using a laxative.
Keep this and all medications out of the reach of children.
Laxative products should not be used for a period longer than one week unless directed by a physician. Rectal bleeding or failure to have a bowel movement after use of a laxative may indicate a serious condition. Discontinue use and consult a physician.
MALTSUPEX Liquid and Tablet only —Do not use this product if you are on a low salt diet unless directed by a physician. Maltsupex Liquid contains approximately 36 mg of sodium per tablespoon. Maltsupex Tablets contain approximately 7 mg of sodium per tablet. Maltsupex Powder contains approximately 5 mg of sodium per scoop.
As with any drug, if you are pregnant or nursing a baby, seek the advice of a health professional before using this product.
Note: Allow for carbohydrate content in diabetic diets and infant formulas.
Liquid: (67%, 14 g/tablespoon, or 56 calories/tablespoon)
Powder: (83%, 6 g or 24 calories per scoop)
Tablets: (Approximately 83%, 0.6 g or 2.5 calories per tablet).

Directions: General—Drink a full glass (8 ounces) of liquid with each dose. The recommended daily dosage of MALTSUPEX may vary. Use the smallest dose that is effective and lower dosage as improvement occurs.
MALTSUPEX **Powder**—Each bottle contains a scoop. Each scoopful (which is the equivalent of a standard measuring tablespoon) should be levelled with a knife.

Continued on next page

Wallace—Cont.

AGE	CORRECTIVE*		MAINTENANCE
12 years to ADULTS	Up to 4 scoops twice a day (Take a full glass [8 oz.] of liquid with each dose.)		2 to 4 scoops at bedtime
CHILDREN 6–12 years of age	Up to 2 scoops twice a day (Take a full glass [8 oz.] of liquid with each dose.)		
CHILDREN 2–6 years of age	1 scoop twice a day (Take a full glass [8 oz.] of liquid with each dose.)		
BOTTLE FED INFANTS (Over 1 month)	1 to 2 scoops per day in formula		½ to 1 scoop per day in formula
BREAST FED INFANTS (Over 1 month)	½ scoop in 2–4 oz. of water or fruit juice twice a day		

* Full corrective dosage should be used for 3 or 4 days or until relief is noted. Then continue on maintenance dosage as needed. Use a clean, dry scoop to remove powder. Replace cover tightly to keep out moisture.

AGE	CORRECTIVE*	MAINTENANCE
12 years to ADULTS	2 tablespoonfuls twice a day (Take a full glass [8 oz.] of liquid with each dose.)	1 to 2 tablespoonfuls at bedtime
CHILDREN 6–12 years of age	1 to 2 tablespoonfuls once or twice a day (Take a full glass [8 oz.] of liquid with each dose.)	
CHILDREN 2–6 years of age	½ tablespoonful twice a day (Take a full glass [8 oz.] of liquid with each dose.)	
BOTTLE FED INFANTS (Over 1 month)	½ to 2 tablespoonfuls per day in formula	1 to 2 teaspoonfuls per day in formula
BREAST FED INFANTS (Over 1 month)	1 to 2 teaspoonfuls in 2 to 4 oz. water or fruit juice once or twice a day	

* Full corrective dosage should be used for 3 or 4 days or until relief is noted. Then continue on maintenance dosage as needed. Use a clean, dry scoop to remove the liquid. Replace cover tightly after use.

Usual Dosage—Powder:
[See first table above.]
Usual Dosage—Liquid:
[See second table above.]
MALTSUPEX **Tablets:** Adult Dosage: Start with four tablets (3 g) four times daily (with meals and at bedtime) and adjust dosage according to response up to 12 tablets (36 g) four times daily, not to exceed 48 tablets daily. Drink a full glass (8 oz.) of liquid with each dose.
Preparation Tips: Powder—Add dosage to milk, water, or fruit juice and stir until dissolved. Mixing is easier if added to warm milk or warm water. May be flavored with vanilla or cocoa to make "malteds." Excellent with warm milk at bedtime. Also available in tablet and liquid forms.
Note: Although shade, texture, taste, and height of contents may vary between bottles, action remains the same.
Liquid: Mixing is easier if MALTSUPEX Liquid is added to an ounce or two of warm water and stirred. Then add milk, water, or fruit juice and stir until dissolved. May be flavored with vanilla or cocoa to make "malteds." Excellent with warm milk at bedtime. Also available in tablet and powder forms.

How Supplied: MALTSUPEX is supplied in 8 ounce (NDC 0037-9101-12) and 16 ounce (NDC 0037-9101-08) jars of MALTSUPEX Powder; 8 fluid ounce (NDC 0037-9051-12) and 1 pint (NDC 0037-9051-08) bottles of MALTSUPEX Liquid; and in bottles of 100 MALTSUPEX Tablets (NDC 0037-9201-01).
Storage: Store at controlled room temperature 15°–30°C (59°–86°F). Protect MALTSUPEX powder and tablets from moisture.
MALTSUPEX **Powder** and **Liquid** are Distributed by

WALLACE LABORATORIES
Division of
CARTER-WALLACE, INC.
Cranbury, New Jersey 08512

MALTSUPEX **Tablets** are Manufactured by

WALLACE LABORATORIES
Division of
CARTER-WALLACE, INC.
Cranbury, New Jersey 08512
Rev. 10/95
Shown in Product Identification Guide, page 523

RYNA®
(Liquid)
RYNA–C® ℂ
(Liquid)
RYNA–CX® ℂ
(Liquid)

Description:
RYNA Liquid—Each 5 mL (one teaspoonful) contains:
Chlorpheniramine maleate .... 2 mg
Pseudoephedrine hydrochloride....30 mg
Other ingredients: flavor (artificial), glycerin, malic acid, purified water, sodium benzoate, sorbitol in a clear, colorless to slightly yellow-colored, lemon-vanilla flavored demulcent base containing no sugar, dyes, or alcohol.
RYNA-C Liquid—Each 5 mL (one teaspoonful) contains, in addition:
Codeine phosphate ....10 mg
(WARNING: May be habit-forming)
Other ingredients: flavor (artificial), glycerin, malic acid, purified water, saccharin sodium, sodium benzoate, sorbitol in a clear, colorless to slightly yellow, cinnamon flavored demulcent base containing no sugar, dyes, or alcohol.
RYNA-CX Liquid—Each 5 mL (one teaspoonful) contains:
Codeine phosphate ....10 mg
(WARNING: May be habit-forming)
Pseudoephedrine hydrochloride....30 mg
Guaifenesin ....100 mg
Other ingredients: flavors (artificial), glycerin, glycine, malic acid, povidone, propylene glycol, purified water, saccharin sodium, sorbitol in a clear, colorless to slightly yellow or straw-colored, cherry-vanilla-menthol flavored demulcent base containing no sugar, dyes, or alcohol.

Actions:
Chlorpheniramine maleate in RYNA and RYNA-C is an antihistamine that antagonizes the effects of histamine.
Codeine phosphate in RYNA-C and RYNA-CX is a centrally-acting antitussive that relieves cough.
Pseudoephedrine hydrochloride in RYNA, RYNA-C and RYNA-CX is a sympathomimetic nasal decongestant that acts to shrink swollen mucosa of the respiratory tract.
Guaifenesin in RYNA-CX is an expectorant, the action of which promotes or

facilitates the removal of secretions from the respiratory tract. By increasing sputum volume and making sputum less viscous, guaifenesin facilitates expectoration of retained secretions.

Indications:
RYNA: For the temporary relief of nasal congestion due to the common cold, hay fever or other upper respiratory allergies. Temporarily relieves runny nose, sneezing, itching of the nose or throat, and itchy, watery eyes due to hay fever or other respiratory allergies such as allergic rhinitis.

RYNA-C: Temporarily relieves cough, nasal congestion, runny nose and sneezing as may occur with the common cold.

RYNA-CX: Temporarily relieves cough due to minor throat and bronchial irritation and nasal congestion as may occur with the common cold or inhaled irritants. Calms the cough control center and relieves coughing. Helps loosen phlegm (mucus) and thin bronchial secretions to rid the bronchial passageways of bothersome mucus, drain bronchial tubes, and make coughs more productive.

Warnings:
For RYNA:
Do not give this product to children taking other medication or to children under 6 years except under the advice and supervision of a doctor. Do not exceed recommended dosage because nervousness, dizziness or sleeplessness may occur. Do not take this product for more than 7 days. If symptoms do not improve or are accompanied by fever, consult a doctor. Do not take this product except under the advice and supervision of a doctor if you have any of the following symptoms or conditions: high blood pressure; heart disease; thyroid disease; diabetes; asthma; glaucoma; emphysema; chronic pulmonary disease; shortness of breath; difficulty in breathing; or difficulty in urination due to enlargement of the prostate.

For RYNA-C and RYNA-CX:
Adults and children who have a chronic pulmonary disease or shortness of breath, or children who are taking other drugs, should not take these products unless directed by a doctor. Do not give these products to children under 6 years of age except under the advice and supervision of a doctor. A persistent cough may be a sign of a serious condition. If cough persists for more than one week, tends to recur, or is accompanied by fever, rash or persistent headache, consult a doctor. Do not take these products for persistent or chronic cough such as occurs with smoking, asthma, emphysema, or if cough is accompanied by excessive phlegm (mucus) unless directed by a doctor. Do not take these products if you have glaucoma, asthma, emphysema, difficulty in breathing, difficulty in urination due to enlargement of the prostate gland, heart disease, high blood pressure, thyroid disease, or diabetes unless directed by a doctor. May cause or aggravate constipation.

Do not take these products or give to children for more than 7 days. If symptoms do not improve or are accompanied by fever, consult a doctor. Unless directed by a doctor, do not exceed recommended dosage because nervousness, dizziness or sleeplessness may occur at higher doses.

For RYNA and RYNA-C:
These products contain an antihistamine which may cause excitability, especially in children, or may cause drowsiness. Alcohol may increase the drowsiness effect. Do not drive motor vehicles, operate machinery, or drink alcoholic beverages while taking these products.

As with any drug, if you are pregnant or nursing a baby, seek the advice of a health professional before using these products.

Drug Interaction Precaution: Do not use these products without first consulting your doctor if you are presently taking a prescription drug for high blood pressure or depression. [Do not use this product if you are now taking a prescription monoamine oxidase inhibitor (MAOI) (certain drugs for depression, psychiatric or emotional conditions, or Parkinson's disease), or for 2 weeks after stopping the MAOI drug. If you are uncertain whether your prescription drug contains an MAOI, consult a health professional before taking this product.]

Dosage and Administration:
Adults: 2 teaspoonfuls every 6 hours
Children 6 to under 12 years: 1 teaspoonful every 6 hours.
Children under 6 years: Do not take except under the advice and supervision of a doctor.
DO NOT EXCEED 4 DOSES IN 24 HOURS.
Ryna-C and Ryna-CX:
A special measuring device should be used to give an accurate dose of these products to children under 6 years of age. Giving a higher dose than recommended by a doctor could result in serious side effects for the child.

How Supplied:
RYNA: bottles of 4 fl oz (NDC 0037-0638-66) and one pint (NDC 0037-0638-68).
RYNA-C: bottles of 4 fl oz (NDC 0037-0522-66) and one pint (NDC 0037-0522-68).
RYNA-CX: bottles of 4 fl oz (NDC 0037-0801-66) and one pint (NDC 0037-0801-68).
TAMPER-RESISTANT BAND ON CAP PRINTED "WALLACE LABORATORIES." DO NOT USE IF BAND IS MISSING OR BROKEN.

Storage:
RYNA: Store at controlled room temperature 15°–30°C (59°–86°F).
RYNA-C and RYNA-CX: Store at controlled room temperature 15°–30°C (59°–86°F). Dispense in a tight, light-resistant container.
KEEP THESE AND ALL DRUGS OUT OF THE REACH OF CHILDREN. IN CASE OF ACCIDENTAL OVERDOSE, SEEK PROFESSIONAL ASSISTANCE

OR CONTACT A POISON CONTROL CENTER IMMEDIATELY.

WALLACE LABORATORIES
Division of
CARTER-WALLACE, Inc.
Cranbury, New Jersey 08512
Rev. 11/94
Shown in Product Identification Guide, page 523

Warner-Lambert Company
Consumer Health Products Group
201 TABOR ROAD
MORRIS PLAINS, NJ 07950

Direct Inquiries to:
1-(800) 223-0182

For Medical Emergencies Contact:
1-(800) 524-2854
1-(800) 223-0182

CELESTIAL SEASONINGS® SOOTHERS™ Herbal Throat Drops

Active Ingredients: Menthol and pectin.

Inactive Ingredients: HONEY-LEMON CHAMOMILE–Chamomile Flower Extract; Citric Acid; Corn Syrup; Honey; Lemon Juice; Natural Flavoring; Oils of Angelica Root, Anise Star, Ginger, Lemon grass, Sage and White Thyme; Sucrose; Tea Extract. HARVEST CHERRY–Cherry, Elderberry and Pineapple Juices; Citric Acid; Corn Syrup; Natural Flavoring; Oils of Angelica Root, Anise Star, Ginger, Lemon Grass, Sage and White Thyme; Sucrose. HERBAL ORANGE SPICE–Beta Carotene; Citric Acid; Corn Syrup; Natural Flavoring; Oils of Angelica Root, Anise Star, Cassia Bark, Ginger, Lemon Grass, Sage and White Thyme; Orange Juice; Sucrose.

Indications: For temporary relief of occasional minor irritation, pain, sore mouth and sore throat. Provides temporary protection of irritated areas in sore mouth and sore throat.

Warnings: If sore throat is severe, persists for more than 2 days, is accompanied or followed by fever, headache, rash, nausea, or vomiting, consult a doctor promptly. If sore mouth symptoms do not improve in 7 days, see your dentist or doctor promptly. Keep this and all drugs out of the reach of children.

Dosage and Administration: Adults and children 5 years and over: Dissolve 2 drops (one at a time) slowly in the mouth. May be repeated every 2 hours as needed or as directed by a dentist or doctor. Children under 5 years: Consult a dentist or doctor.

How Supplied: Celestial Seasonings Soothers Throat Drops are available in bags of 24 drops. They are available in three flavors: Honey-Lemon Chamomile, Harvest Cherry and Herbal Orange Spice. Boxes of 8 drops are also available

Continued on next page

Warner-Lambert—Cont.

in Honey-Lemon Chamomile & Harvest Cherry.

Shown in Product Identification Guide, page 523

HALLS® JUNIORS SUGAR FREE
Cough Suppressant Drops
[Hols]

Active Ingredient: Menthol 2.5 mg per drop.

Inactive Ingredients: ORANGE: Acesulfame Potassium, Eucalyptus Oil, Isomalt, Natural Flavoring and Yellow 6. GRAPE: Acesulfame Potassium, Blue 1, Eucalyptus Oil, Isomalt, Natural Flavoring and Red 40.

Indications: For temporary relief of minor throat irritation and coughs due to colds or inhaled irritants.

Warnings: A persistent cough may be a sign of a serious condition. If cough persists for more than 1 week, tends to recur, or is accompanied by fever, rash, or persistent headache, consult a doctor. Do not take this product for persistent or chronic cough such as occurs with smoking, asthma, or emphysema, or if cough is accompanied by excessive phlegm (mucus) unless directed by a doctor. If sore throat is severe, persists for more than 2 days, is accompanied or followed by fever, headache, rash, swelling, nausea, or vomiting, consult a doctor promptly. KEEP THIS AND ALL DRUGS OUT OF THE REACH OF CHILDREN.

Dosage and Administration: Adults and children 5 years and over: dissolve 2 drops (one at a time) slowly in mouth. Repeat every hour as needed or as directed by a doctor. Children under 5 years: consult a doctor.

Additional Information: Diabetics: This product may be useful in your diet on the advice of a physician.

Exchange Information*:
2 Drops = Free Exchange
22 Drops = 2 Fruits

*The dietary exchanges are based on the *Exchange Lists for Meal Planning*, Copyright © 1989 by the American Diabetes Association, Inc. and the American Dietetic Association.

How Supplied: Halls Juniors Sugar Free Cough Suppressant Drops are available in Grape and Orange flavors in bags of 22 drops each.

Shown in Product Identification Guide, page 523

HALLS® MENTHO–LYPTUS®
Cough Suppressant Drops
[Hols]

Active Ingredient: MENTHO-LYPTUS and CHERRY: Menthol 6.1 mg per drop. HONEY LEMON: Menthol 8.4 mg per drop. ICE BLUE PEPPERMINT: Menthol 12 mg per drop. SPEARMINT: Menthol 5 mg per drop.

Inactive Ingredients: MENTHOLYPTUS: Citric Acid, Corn Syrup, Eucalyptus Oil and Sucrose. CHERRY: Carmine Color, Corn Syrup, Eucalyptus Oil, Flavoring and Sucrose. HONEY-LEMON: Corn Syrup, Eucalyptus Oil, Flavoring, Sucrose, Yellow 6 and Yellow 10. ICE BLUE PEPPERMINT: Blue 1, Corn Syrup, Eucalyptus Oil, Flavoring and Sucrose. SPEARMINT: Blue 1, Corn Syrup, Eucalyptus Oil, Flavoring, Sucrose and Yellow 10.

Indications: For temporary relief of minor throat irritation and coughs due to colds or inhaled irritants.

Warnings: A persistent cough may be a sign of a serious condition. If cough persists for more than 1 week, tends to recur, or is accompanied by fever, rash or persistent headache, consult a doctor. Do not take this product for persistent or chronic cough such as occurs with smoking, asthma, or emphysema, or if cough is accompanied by excessive phlegm (mucus) unless directed by a doctor. If sore throat is severe, persists for more than 2 days, is accompanied or followed by fever, headache, rash, swelling, nausea, or vomiting, consult a doctor promptly. KEEP THIS AND ALL DRUGS OUT OF THE REACH OF CHILDREN.

Dosage and Administration: Adults and children 5 years and over: dissolve 1 drop slowly in mouth. Repeat every hour as needed or as directed by a doctor. Children under 5 years: consult a doctor.

How Supplied: Halls Mentho-Lyptus Cough Suppressant Drops are available in single sticks of 9 drops each and in bags of 30 and 60 drops. They are available in five flavors: Regular Mentho-Lyptus, Cherry, Honey-Lemon, Ice Blue Peppermint and Spearmint. Mentho-Lyptus & Cherry flavors are also available in bags of 230 drops.

Shown in Product Identification Guide, page 523

HALLS® SUGAR FREE MENTHO-LYPTUS®
Cough Suppressant Drops
[Hols]

Active Ingredients: BLACK CHERRY and CITRUS BLEND: Menthol 5 mg per drop. MOUNTAIN MENTHOL: Menthol 6 mg per drop.

Inactive Ingredients: BLACK CHERRY: Acesulfame Potassium, Blue 1, Citric Acid, Eucalyptus Oil, Flavoring, Isomalt and Red 40. CITRUS BLEND: Acesulfame Potassium, Citric Acid, Eucalyptus Oil, Flavoring, Isomalt and Yellow 5 (Tartrazine). MOUNTAIN MENTHOL: Acesulfame Potassium, Eucalyptus Oil, Flavoring and Isomalt.

Indications: For temporary relief of minor throat irritation and coughs due to colds or inhaled irritants.

Warnings: A persistent cough may be a sign of a serious condition. If cough persists for more than 1 week, tends to recur, or is accompanied by fever, rash, or persistent headache, consult a doctor. Do not take this product for persistent or chronic cough such as occurs with smoking, asthma, or emphysema, or if cough is accompanied by excessive phlegm (mucus) unless directed by a doctor. If sore throat is severe, persists for more than 2 days, is accompanied or followed by fever, headache, rash, swelling, nausea, or vomiting, consult a doctor promptly. KEEP THIS AND ALL DRUGS OUT OF THE REACH OF CHILDREN.

Dosage and Administration: Adults and children 5 years and over: dissolve 1 drop slowly in mouth. Repeat every hour as needed or as directed by a doctor. Children under 5 years: consult a doctor.

Additional Information: Diabetics: This product may be useful in your diet on the advice of a physician.

Exchange Information*:
1 Drop = Free Exchange
10 Drops = 1 Fruit

*The dietary exchanges are based on the *Exchange Lists for Meal Planning*, Copyright © 1989 by the American Diabetes Association, Inc. and the American Dietetic Association.

How Supplied: Halls Sugar Free Mentho-Lyptus Cough Suppressant Drops are available in bags of 25 drops. They are available in three flavors: Black Cherry, Citrus Blend and Mountain Menthol.

Shown in Product Identification Guide, page 523

MAXIMUM STRENGTH HALLS® PLUS
Cough Suppressant Drops
[Hols]

Active Ingredient: Menthol 10 mg per centerfilled drop.

Inactive Ingredients: MENTHO-LYPTUS: Citric Acid, Corn Syrup, Eucalyptus Oil, Glycerin, High Fructose Corn Syrup and Sucrose. CHERRY: Blue 2, Corn Syrup, Eucalyptus Oil, Flavoring, Glycerin, High Fructose Corn Syrup, Red 40 and Sucrose. HONEY-LEMON: Acesulfame Potassium, Corn Syrup, Eucalyptus Oil, Flavoring, Glycerin, High Fructose Corn Syrup, Honey, Sucrose, Yellow 6 and Yellow 10.

Indications: For temporary relief of minor throat irritation and coughs due to colds or inhaled irritants.

Warnings: A persistent cough may be a sign of a serious condition. If cough persists for more than 1 week, tends to recur, or is accompanied by fever, rash or persistent headache, consult a doctor. Do not take this product for persistent or chronic cough such as occurs with smoking, asthma, or emphysema, or if cough is accompanied by excessive phlegm (mucus) unless directed by a doctor. If sore throat is severe, persists for more than 2 days, is accompanied or followed by fever, headache, rash, swelling, nausea, or vomiting, consult a doctor promptly. KEEP THIS AND ALL DRUGS OUT OF THE REACH OF CHLDREN.

Dosage and Administration: Adults and children 5 years and over: for cough dissolve 1 drop slowly in mouth—repeat every hour as needed or as directed by a doctor; for sore throat dissolve either 1 drop or 2 drops (one at a time) slowly in mouth—repeat every 2 hours as needed or as directed by a doctor. Children under 5 years; consult a doctor.

How Supplied: Maximum Strength Halls Plus Cough Suppressant Drops are available in single sticks of 10 drops each and in bags of 25 drops. They are available in three flavors: Regular Mentho-Lyptus, Cherry and Honey-Lemon.
Shown in Product Identification Guide, page 524

HALLS® Vitamin C Drops
[Hols]

Ingredients: ASSORTED CITRUS FLAVORS: Sugar, Corn Syrup, Citric Acid, Sodium Ascorbate, Natural Flavoring, Ascorbic Acid, Color Added and Red 40.

Description: Halls® Vitamin C Drops are a delicious way to get 100% of the Daily Value of Vitamin C. Each drop provides 60 mg. of Vitamin C (100% of the Daily Value).

Indication: Dietary Supplementation.

How Supplied: Halls® Vitamin C Drops are available in single sticks of 9 drops each and in bags of 30 drops. They are available in an all-natural citrus flavor assortment (lemon, sweet grapefruit and orange).
Shown in Product Identification Guide, page 524

ROLAIDS® Antacid Tablets
Original Flavor and Spearmint

Active Ingredient: Calcium Carbonate 412 mg. and Magnesium Hydroxide 80 mg.

Inactive Ingredients: Flavoring, Light Mineral Oil, Magnesium Stearate, Mannitol, Microcrystalline Cellulose, Polyethylene Glycol, Pregelatinized Starch, Silicon Dioxide and Sucrose.

Indications: For the relief of heartburn, sour stomach or acid indigestion and upset stomach associated with these symptoms.

Actions: Rolaids® provides rapid neutralization of stomach acid. Each tablet has acid-neutralizing capacity of 11 mEq and the ability to maintain the pH of stomach contents to 3.5 or greater for a significant period of time. Each tablet provides 16% of the nutritional Daily Value for calcium and 8% of the nutri-

tional Daily Value for magnesium and contains less than 0.4 mg. of sodium.

Warnings: Do not take more than 14 tablets in a 24-hour period or use the maximum dosage of this product for more than 2 weeks except under the advice and supervision of a physician. Keep this and all drugs out of the reach of children.

Drug Interaction Precaution: Antacids may interact with certain prescription drugs. If you are presently taking a prescription drug, do not take this product without checking with your physician or other health professional.

Dosage and Administration: Chew 1 or 2 tablets as symptoms occur. Repeat hourly if symptoms return or as directed by a physician.

How Supplied: One roll contains 12 tablets; 3-pack contains three 12-tablet rolls; one bottle contains 75 tablets; one bottle contains 150 tablets.
Shown in Product Identification Guide, page 524

CALCIUM RICH/SODIUM FREE
ROLAIDS® Antacid Tablets
Cherry and Assorted Fruit Flavors

Active Ingredient: Calcium Carbonate 550 mg. per tablet.

Inactive Ingredients:
Cherry Flavor: Colors (Red 27 and Titanium Dioxide), Corn Starch, Flavoring, Light Mineral Oil, Magnesium Stearate, Mannitol, Pregelatinized Starch, Silicon Dioxide and Sucrose.
Assorted Fruit Flavors: Colors (Blue 1, Red 27, Red 40, Titanium Dioxide, Yellow 5 [Tartrazine] and Yellow 6), Corn Starch, Flavoring, Light Mineral Oil, Magnesium Stearate, Mannitol, Pregelatinized Starch, Silicon Dioxide and Sucrose.

Indications: For the relief of heartburn, sour stomach or acid indigestion and upset stomach associated with these symptoms.

Actions: Calcium Rich/Sodium Free Rolaids provides rapid neutralization of stomach acid. Each tablet has an acid-neutralizing capacity of 11 mEq and the ability to maintain the pH of stomach contents at 3.5 or greater for a significant period of time. Each tablet provides 22% of the nutritional Daily Value for calcium and contains less than 0.4 mg. of sodium.

Warnings: Do not take more than 14 tablets in a 24-hour period or use the maximum dosage of this product for more than 2 weeks except under the advice and supervision of a physician. Keep this and all drugs out of the reach of children.

Drug Interaction Precaution: Antacids may interact with certain prescription drugs. If you are presently taking a prescription drug, do not take this prod-

uct without checking with your physician or other health professional.

Dosage and Administration: Chew 1 or 2 tablets as symptoms occur. Repeat hourly if symptoms return or as directed by a physician.

How Supplied: One roll contains 12 tablets; 3-pack contains three 12-tablet rolls; one bottle contains 75 tablets; one bottle contains 150 tablets.
Shown in Product Identification Guide, page 524

Warner Wellcome
Consumer HealthCare Products
Warner-Lambert Company
201 TABOR ROAD
MORRIS PLAINS, NJ 07950
(See also Warner-Lambert)

Direct Inquiries to:
1-(800) 223-0182
For Medical Information Contact:
1-(800) 524-2624
1-(800) 562-0266
1-(800) 773-1554
1-(800) 547-8374
1-(800) 378-1783
1-(800) 337-7266

ACTIFED® Cold & Allergy Tablets
[ăk 'tuh-fěd]

Active Ingredients: Pseudoephedrine Hydrochloride 60 mg and Triprolidine Hydrochloride 2.5 mg.

Inactive Ingredients: Flavor, Hydroxypropyl Methylcellulose, Lactose, Magnesium Stearate, Polyethylene Glycol, Potato Starch, Povidone, Sucrose, and Titanium Dioxide.

Product Benefits: Each ACTIFED® Cold & Allergy Tablet contains two maximum strength ingredients for temporary relief from symptoms of the common cold, seasonal allergies (hay fever) and sinus congestion.
The **ANTIHISTAMINE** (triprolidine) temporarily dries runny nose and relieves sneezing associated with the common cold, hay fever or other upper respiratory allergies. Also relieves itching of the nose or throat, and itchy, watery eyes due to hay fever.
The **DECONGESTANT** (pseudoephedrine) temporarily relieves nasal congestion due to the common cold, hay fever or other upper respiratory allergies, or as-

Continued on next page

This product information was prepared in November 1995. On these and other Warner Wellcome Consumer HealthCare Products, detailed information may be obtained by addressing Warner Wellcome Consumer HealthCare Products, Warner-Lambert, Morris Plains, NJ 07950

Warner Wellcome—Cont.

sociated with sinusitis. Temporarily relieves nasal stuffiness. Reduces the swelling of nasal passages; shrinks swollen membranes; and temporarily restores freer breathing through the nose. Also, helps to decongest sinus openings and passages; relieves sinus pressure.

Directions: Adults and children 12 years of age and over, 1 tablet every 4 to 6 hours. Children 6 to under 12 years of age, ½ tablet every 4 to 6 hours. Do not exceed 4 doses in 24 hours. Children under 6 years of age, consult a doctor.

Warnings: Do not exceed recommended dosage. If nervousness, dizziness, or sleeplessness occur, discontinue use and consult a doctor. If symptoms do not improve within 7 days or are accompanied by fever, consult a doctor. Do not take this product, unless directed by a doctor, if you have heart disease, high blood pressure, thyroid disease, diabetes, a breathing problem such as emphysema or chronic bronchitis, or if you have glaucoma or difficulty in urination due to enlargement of the prostate gland. May cause excitability especially in children. May cause drowsiness; alcohol, sedatives, and tranquilizers may increase the drowsiness effect. Avoid alcoholic beverages while taking this product. Do not take this product if you are taking sedatives or tranquilizers, without first consulting your doctor. Use caution when driving a motor vehicle or operating machinery. As with any drug, if you are pregnant or nursing a baby, seek the advice of a health professional before using this product. **KEEP THIS AND ALL DRUGS OUT OF THE REACH OF CHILDREN.** In case of accidental overdose, seek professional assistance or contact a Poison Control Center immediately.

Drug Interaction Precaution: Do not take this product if you are now taking a prescription monoamine oxidase inhibitor (MAOI) (certain drugs for depression, psychiatric or emotional conditions, or Parkinson's disease), or for 2 weeks after stopping the MAOI drug. If you are uncertain whether your prescription drug contains an MAOI, consult a health professional before taking this product.

How Supplied: Boxes of 12, 24, 48, and bottles of 100.
Store at 15° to 25°C (59° to 77°F) in a dry place and protect from light.
Shown in Product Identification Guide, page 524

ACTIFED® ALLERGY DAYTIME/ NIGHTTIME CAPLETS
[ăk 'tuh-fěd]

This package contains 2 separate products: Actifed® Allergy DAYTIME (white caplets) is a no-drowsiness product. Actifed® Allergy NIGHTTIME (blue caplets) may cause marked drowsiness. Read directions carefully for both products.

ACTIFED® ALLERGY DAYTIME
(white caplets)
ANTIHISTAMINE-FREE. NON-DROWSY

Active Ingredients for Actifed Allergy Daytime Caplet: Pseudoephedrine Hydrochloride 30 mg.

Inactive Ingredients: Carnauba Wax, Crospovidone, Hydroxypropyl Methylcellulose, Lactose, Magnesium Stearate, Microcrystalline cellulose, Polyethylene Glycol, and Titanium Dioxide.

Product Benefits: The **DAYTIME** no-drowsiness product (white caplets) contains a nasal decongestant (pseudoephedrine) that provides temporary relief of nasal congestion due to hay fever or other upper respiratory allergies. Helps decongest sinus openings and passages; relieves sinus pressure; reduces swollen nasal passages.

Directions: Adults and children 12 years and over, 2 caplets every 4 to 6 hours during waking hours. **Do not exceed a total of 8 caplets (Daytime or Nighttime) in 24 hours. Do not take Actifed Allergy Daytime within 4 hours of Actifed Allergy Nighttime.** Children under 12 years of age: consult a doctor.

ACTIFED® ALLERGY NIGHTTIME
(blue caplets) **MAY CAUSE MARKED DROWSINESS.**

Active Ingredients for Actifed Allergy Nighttime Caplet: Diphenhydramine Hydrochloride 25 mg and Pseudoephedrine Hydrochloride 30 mg.

Inactive Ingredients: Carnauba Wax, Crospovidone, FD&C Blue No. 1 Lake, Hydroxypropyl Methylcellulose, Lactose, Magnesium Stearate, Microcrystalline Cellulose, Polyethylene Glycol, Polysorbate 80, and Titanium Dioxide.

ACTIFED DAYTIME/NIGHTTIME products do not contain triprolidine hydrochloride, the antihistamine found in other ACTIFED products.

Product Benefits: The **NIGHTTIME** product (blue caplets) contains a nasal decongestant (pseudoephedrine) and an antihistamine (diphenhydramine) that provide temporary relief of nasal congestion, sinus pressure, swollen nasal passages, runny nose, and sneezing due to hay fever or other upper respiratory allergies. Also relieves itching of the nose or throat and itchy, watery eyes due to hay fever.

Directions: Adults and children 12 years and over, 2 caplets at bedtime or as directed by a doctor. Due to potential marked drowsiness, do not take during waking hours unless confined to bed or resting at home; 2 caplets then may be taken every 4 to 6 hours. **Do not exceed a total of 8 caplets (Daytime and/or Nighttime) in 24 hours. Do not take Actifed Allergy Nighttime within 4** hours of Actifed Daytime. Not recommended for children under 12.

Warnings for both the daytime and nighttime caplets: Do not exceed recommended dosage. If nervousness, dizziness, or sleeplessness occur, discontinue use and consult a doctor. If symptoms do not improve within 7 days or are accompanied by fever, consult a doctor. Do not take this product, unless directed by a doctor, if you have heart disease, high blood pressure, thyroid disease, diabetes, a breathing problem such as emphysema or chronic bronchitis, or if you have glaucoma or difficulty in urination due to enlargement of the prostate gland. As with any drug, if you are pregnant or nursing a baby, seek the advice of a health professional before using this product. **KEEP THIS AND ALL DRUGS OUT OF THE REACH OF CHILDREN.** In case of accidental overdose, seek professional assistance or contact a Poison Control Center immediately.

Additional warnings for the nighttime caplet: May cause excitability especially in children. May cause drowsiness; alcohol, sedatives, and tranquilizers may increase the drowsiness effect. Avoid alcoholic beverages while taking this product. Do not take this product if you are taking sedatives or tranquilizers, without first consulting your doctor. Use caution when driving a motor vehicle or operating machinery.

Drug Interaction Precaution: Do not use this product if you are now taking a prescription monoamine oxidase inhibitor (MAOI) (certain drugs for depression, psychiatric or emotional conditions, or Parkinson's disease), or for 2 weeks after stopping the MAOI drug. If you are uncertain whether your prescription drug contains an MAOI, consult a health professional before taking this product.

How Supplied: Package contains 24 Daytime Caplets and 8 Nighttime Caplets.
Store at 15° to 25°C (59° to 77°F) in a dry place and protect from light.
Shown in Product Identification Guide, page 524

ACTIFED® Cold & Sinus Caplets and Tablets
[ăk 'tuh-fěd]

Active Ingredients: Acetaminophen 500 mg, Pseudoephedrine Hydrochloride 30 mg and Triprolidine Hydrochloride 1.25 mg.

Inactive Ingredients: Carnauba Wax, Crospovidone, FD&C Blue No. 1 Aluminum Lake, D&C Yellow No. 10 Aluminum Lake, Hydroxypropyl Methylcellulose, Magnesium Stearate, Microcrystalline Cellulose, Polyethylene Glycol, Polysorbate 80, Povidone, Pregelatinized Starch, Stearic Acid, and Titanium Dioxide.

Product Benefits: Each dose of ACTIFED® Cold & Sinus contains three maximum strength ingredients for temporary relief from symptoms of the common cold, seasonal allergies (hay fever) and sinus congestion.

The **ANTIHISTAMINE** (triprolidine) temporarily dries runny nose and relieves sneezing associated with the common cold, hay fever or other upper respiratory allergies. Also relieves itching of the nose or throat, and itchy, watery eyes due to hay fever.

The **DECONGESTANT** (pseudoephedrine) temporarily relieves nasal congestion due to the common cold, hay fever or other upper respiratory allergies, or associated with sinusitis. Temporarily relieves nasal stuffiness. Reduces the swelling of nasal passages; shrinks swollen membranes; and temporarily restores freer breathing through the nose. Also, helps to decongest sinus openings and passages; relieves sinus pressure.

The non-aspirin **ANALGESIC** (acetaminophen) temporarily relieves occasional minor aches, pains and headache, and reduces fever due to the common cold.

Directions: Adults and children 12 years of age and over, 2 caplets or tablets every 6 hours. While symptoms persist, not to exceed 8 caplets or tablets in 24 hours, or as directed by a doctor. Children under 12 years of age: consult a doctor.

Warnings: Do not exceed recommended dosage. If nervousness, dizziness, or sleeplessness occur, discontinue use and consult a doctor. Do not take this product for more than 10 days. If symptoms do not improve or are accompanied by fever that lasts for more than 3 days, or if new symptoms occur, consult a doctor. Do not take this product, unless directed by a doctor, if you have heart disease, high blood pressure, thyroid disease, diabetes, a breathing problem such as emphysema or chronic bronchitis, or if you have glaucoma or difficulty in urination due to enlargement of the prostate gland. May cause excitability especially in children. May cause drowsiness; alcohol, sedatives, and tranquilizers may increase the drowsiness effect. Avoid alcoholic beverages while taking this product. Do not take this product if you are taking sedatives or tranquilizers, without first consulting your doctor. Use caution when driving a motor vehicle or operating machinery. As with any drug, if you are pregnant or nursing a baby, seek the advice of a health professional before using this product. **KEEP THIS AND ALL DRUGS OUT OF THE REACH OF CHILDREN.** In case of accidental overdose, seek professional assistance or contact a Poison Control Center immediately. Prompt medical attention is critical for adults as well as for children even if you do not notice any signs or symptoms.

Drug Interaction Precaution: Do not use this product if you are now taking a prescription monoamine oxidase inhibitor (MAOI) (certain drugs for depression, psychiatric or emotional conditions, or Parkinson's disease), or for 2 weeks after stopping the MAIO drug. If you are uncertain whether your prescription drug contains an MAIO, consult a health professional before taking this product.

How Supplied: Boxes of 20.
Store at 15° to 25°C (59° to 77°F) in a dry place and protect from light.
Shown in Product Identification Guide, page 524

ACTIFED® SINUS DAYTIME/NIGHTTIME Tablets and Caplets
[ak'tuh-fĕd]

This package contains 2 separate products: Actifed® Sinus DAYTIME (white tablets or caplets) is a no-drowsiness product; Actifed® Sinus NIGHTTIME (blue tablets or caplets) may cause marked drowsiness. Read directions carefully for both products.

ACTIFED® SINUS DAYTIME (white tablets and caplets)
NON-DROWSY.

Active Ingredients for Actifed Sinus Daytime Tablets or Caplets: Acetaminophen 500 mg and Pseudoephedrine Hydrochloride 30 mg.

Inactive Ingredients: Carnauba Wax, Crospovidone, Hydroxypropyl Methylcellulose, Magnesium Stearate, Microcrystalline Cellulose, Polyethylene Glycol, Povidone, Pregelatinized Starch, Stearic Acid, and Titanium Dioxide.

Product Benefits: The **DAYTIME** no-drowsiness product (white tablets or caplets) contains a non-aspirin pain reliever (acetaminophen) and nasal decongestant (pseudoephedrine) that provide temporary relief of sinus headache pain, sinus pressure and nasal congestion due to the common cold, hay fever, or other allergies.

Directions: Adults and children 12 years and over, 2 caplets or tablets every 6 hours during waking hours while symptoms persist, or as directed by a doctor. **Do not exceed a total of 8 caplets or tablets (Daytime and/or Nighttime) in 24 hours. Do not take Actifed Sinus Daytime within 6 hours of Actifed Sinus Nighttime.** Children under 12 years of age: consult a doctor.

ACTIFED® SINUS NIGHTTIME (blue tablets and caplets)
MAY CAUSE MARKED DROWSINESS.

Active Ingredients for Actifed Sinus Nighttime Tablet or Caplet: Acetaminophen 500 mg, Diphenhydramine Hydrochloride 25 mg and Pseudoephedrine Hydrochloride 30 mg.

Inactive Ingredients: Carnauba Wax, Crospovidone, FD&C Blue No. 1 Lake, Hydroxypropyl Methylcellulose, Magnesium Stearate, Microcrystalline Cellulose, Polyethylene Glycol, Polysorbate 80, Povidone, Pregelatinized Starch, Sodium Starch Glycolate, Stearic Acid, and Titanium Dioxide.

Product Benefits: The **NIGHTTIME** product (blue tablets or caplets) contains a non-aspirin pain reliever (acetaminophen), a nasal decongestant (pseudoephedrine), and an antihistamine (diphenhydramine) that provide temporary relief of sinus headache pain, sinus pressure, nasal congestion, runny nose, and sneezing due to the common cold, hay fever, or other allergies. Also relieves itching of the nose or throat and itchy, watery eyes due to hay fever.

Directions: Adults and children 12 years and over, 2 tablets or caplets at bedtime while symptoms persist, or as directed by a doctor. Due to potential marked drowsiness, do not take during waking hours unless confined to bed or resting at home; 2 tablets or caplets then may be taken every 6 hours. **Do not exceed a total of 8 tablets or caplets (Daytime and/or Nighttime) in 24 hours. Do not take Actifed Sinus Nighttime within 6 hours of Actifed Sinus Daytime.** Children under 12 years of age: consult a doctor.
ACTIFED DAYTIME/NIGHTTIME products do not contain triprolidine hydrochloride, the antihistamine found in other ACTIFED products.

Warnings for both the daytime and nighttime caplets/tablets: Do not exceed recommended dosage. If nervousness, dizziness, or sleeplessness occur, discontinue use and consult a doctor. Do not take this product for more than 10 days. If symptoms do not improve or are accompanied by fever that lasts for more than 3 days, or if new symptoms occur, consult a doctor. Do not take this product, unless directed by a doctor, if you have heart disease, high blood pressure, thyroid disease, diabetes, a breathing problem such as emphysema or chronic bronchitis, or if you have glaucoma or difficulty in urination due to enlargement of the prostate gland. As with any drug, if you are pregnant or nursing a baby, seek the advice of a health professional before using this products. **KEEP THIS AND ALL DRUGS OUT OF THE REACH OF CHILDREN.** In case of accidental overdose, seek professional assistance or contact a Poison Control Center immediately. Prompt medical attention is critical for adults as well as children even if you do not notice any signs or symptoms.

Continued on next page

This product information was prepared in November 1995. On these and other Warner Wellcome Consumer HealthCare Products, detailed information may be obtained by addressing Warner Wellcome Consumer HealthCare Products, Warner-Lambert, Morris Plains, NJ 07950

Warner Wellcome—Cont.

Additional warnings for the nighttime caplets/tablets: May cause excitability especially in children. May cause drowsiness; alcohol, sedatives, and tranquilizers may increase the drowsiness effect. Avoid alcoholic beverages while taking this product. Do not take this product if you are taking sedatives or tranquilizers, without first consulting your doctor. Use caution when driving a motor vehicle or operating machinery.

Drug Interaction Precaution: Do not use this product if you are now taking a prescription monoamine oxidase inhibitor (MAOI) (certain drugs for depression, psychiatric or emotional conditions, or Parkinson's disease), or for 2 weeks after stopping the MAOI drug. If you are uncertain whether your prescription drug contains an MAOI, consult a health professional before taking this product.

How Supplied: Package contains 18 Daytime Tablets or Caplets and 6 Nighttime Tablets or Caplets.
Store at 15° to 25°C (59° to 77°F) in a dry place and protect from light.
Shown in Product Identification Guide, page 524

ANUSOL®
Hemorrhoidal Suppositories/ Ointment
[ă'nū-sōl"]

Description:
Anusol Suppositories: **Active Ingredient:** Topical Starch 51%. Also contains: Benzyl Alcohol, Partially Hydrogenated Soy Bean Oil with Sorbitan Tristearate, Tocopheryl Acetate.
Anusol Ointment: **Active ingredients:** Pramoxine HCl 1%, Mineral Oil and Zinc Oxide 12.5%. Also contains: Benzyl Benzoate, Calcium Phosphate Dibasic, Cocoa Butter, Glyceryl Monooleate, Glyceryl Monostearate, Kaolin, Peruvian Balsam and Polyethylene Wax.

Actions: Anusol Suppositories and Anusol Ointment help to relieve burning, itching and discomfort arising from irritated anorectal tissues. They have a soothing, lubricant action on mucous membranes. Pramoxine Hydrochloride in Anusol Ointment is a rapidly acting local anesthetic for the skin and mucous membranes of the anus and rectum. Pramoxine HCl is also chemically distinct from procaine, cocaine, and dibucaine and can often be used in the patient previously sensitized to other surface anesthetics. Surface analgesia lasts for several hours.

Indications: Anusol Ointment: Temporarily relieves the pain, soreness, and burning of hemorrhoids and other anorectal disorders while it forms a temporary protective coating over inflamed tissues to help prevent the drying of tissues. Anusol Ointment is to be applied externally or in the lower portion of the anal canal (The enclosed dispensing cap is designed to control dispersion of the ointment to the affected area in the lower portion of the anal canal only.)
Anusol Suppositories: Gives temporary relief from the itching, burning and discomfort of hemorrhoids and other anorectal disorders, and temporarily provides a coating for relief of anorectal discomforts and protects the irritated areas.

Contraindications: Anusol Suppositories and Anusol Ointment are contraindicated in those patients with a history of hypersensitivity to any of the components of the preparations. Upon application of Anusol Ointment, which contains Pramoxine HCl, a patient may occasionally experience burning, especially if the anoderm is not intact. Sensitivity reactions have been rare; discontinue medication if suspected. Certain persons can develop allergic reactions to ingredients in this product.

Warnings: Anusol Ointment: If condition worsens or does not improve within 7 days, consult a physician. Certain persons can develop allergic reactions to ingredients in this product. If the symptom being treated does not subside or if redness, irritation, swelling, pain or other symptoms develop or increase, discontinue use and consult a phsyician. In case of bleeding, consult a physician promptly. Do not exceed the recommended daily dosage unless directed by a physician. Do not put this product into the rectum by using fingers or any mechanical device or applicator. Keep this and all drugs out of the reach of children. In case of accidental ingestion seek professional assistance or contact a Poison Control Center immediately. Anusol Suppositories: Do not exceed recommended daily dosage unless directed by a physician. If condition worsens or does not improve within 7 days, consult a physician. In case of bleeding, consult a physician promptly. Keep this and all drugs out of the reach of children. In case of accidental ingestion seek professional assistance or contact a Poison Control Center immediately. As with any drug, if you are pregnant or nursing a baby, seek the advice of a health professional before using this product.

Directions: Anusol Suppositories: Adults: When practical, cleanse the affected area with Tucks® Hemorrhoidal Pads or mild soap and warm water. Rinse thoroughly. Gently dry by patting or blotting with toilet tissue or soft cloth before application of this product.
1. Detach one suppository from the strip of suppositories.
2. Remove wrapper before inserting into the rectum as follows: Hold suppository upright (with words "pull apart" at top) and carefully separate foil by inserting tip of fingernail at foil split.
3. Peel foil slowly and evenly down both sides, exposing suppository.
4. Avoid excessive handling of suppository which is designed to melt at body temperature. If suppository seems soft, hold in foil wrapper under cold water for 2 or 3 minutes.
5. Insert one (1) suppository rectally up to six (6) times daily or after each bowel movement.
Children under 12 years of age: consult a physician.
Anusol Ointment: Adults: When practical, cleanse the affected area with mild soap and warm water and rinse thoroughly. Gently dry by patting or blotting with toilet tissue or a soft cloth before application of this product. Apply externally to the affected area up to five (5) times daily. To use dispensing cap, attach it to tube, lubricate well, then gently insert part way into the anus. Squeeze tube to deliver medication. Thoroughly cleanse dispensing cap after use. Children under 12 years of age: Consult a physician.

How Supplied: Anusol Suppositories— boxes of 12 or 24 in silver foil strips.
Anusol Ointment—1-oz tubes and 2-oz tubes with plastic applicator.
Ointment: Store between 15° and 30°C (59° and 86°F).
Suppositories: Do not store above 86°F or suppositories may melt.
Shown in Product Identification Guide, page 524

ANUSOL HC-1
Hydrocortisone Anti-Itch Ointment
[ă'nū-sōl"]

Active Ingredient: Hydrocortisone Acetate (equivalent to 1% Hydrocortisone).

Inactive Ingredients: Diazolidinyl Urea, Methylparaben, Microcrystalline Wax, Mineral Oil, Propylene Glycol, Propylparaben, Sorbitan Sesquioleate and White Petrolatum.

Indications: For temporary relief of minor skin irritations and for external itching. Other uses of this product should be only under the advice and supervision of a physician.

Warnings: For external use only. Avoid contact with the eyes. If condition worsens, or if symptoms persist for more than 7 days or clear up and occur again within a few days, stop use of this product and do not begin use of any other hydrocortisone product unless you have consulted a physician. Do not exceed the recommended daily dosage unless directed by a physician. In case of bleeding, consult a physician promptly. Do not put this product into the rectum by using fingers or any mechanical device or applicator. Do not use for treatment of diaper rash. Consult a physician. KEEP THIS AND ALL DRUGS OUT OF THE REACH OF CHILDREN. In case of accidental ingestion seek professional assistance or contact a Poison Control Center immediately.

Directions: Adults: when practical cleanse affected area with mild soap and warm water and rinse thoroughly.

Gently dry by patting or blotting with tissue or soft cloth before application of this product. Apply to affected area not more than 3 to 4 times daily. Children under 12 years of age: consult a physician.

How Supplied: Anusol HC-1 Ointment in 0.7 oz tube. Store at Room Temperature 59°–86°F.

Shown in Product Identification Guide, page 524

BENADRYL® Allergy Tablets and Kapseals®
[bĕ'nă-drĭl]

Active Ingredients: Each Tablet/Kapseal contains: Diphenhydramine Hydrochloride 25 mg.

Inactive Ingredients: Each Tablet contains: Candelilla Wax, Croscarmellose Sodium, Dibasic Calcium Phosphate Dihydrate, D&C Red No. 27 Aluminum Lake, Hydroxypropyl Methylcellulose, Microcrystalline Cellulose, Polyethylene Glycol, Polysorbate 80, Corn Starch, Stearic Acid, Titanium Dioxide, and Zinc Stearate.
Each Kapseal contains: Lactose and Magnesium Stearate. The Kapseals capsule shell contains: FD&C Red No. 3, FD&C Red No. 40, FD&C Blue No. 1, Gelatin, Glyceryl Monooleate, and Titanium Dioxide.

Indications: Temporarily relieves runny nose and sneezing, itching of the nose or throat, and itchy, watery eyes due to hay fever or other upper respiratory allergies, and runny nose and sneezing associated with the common cold.

Warnings: May cause excitability especially in children. Do not take this product, unless directed by a doctor, if you have a breathing problem such as emphysema or chronic bronchitis, or if you have glaucoma or difficulty in urination due to enlargement of the prostate gland. May cause marked drowsiness; alcohol, sedatives, and tranquilizers may increase the drowsiness effect. Avoid alcoholic beverages while taking this product. Do not take this product if you are taking sedatives or tranquilizers, without first consulting your doctor. Use caution when driving a motor vehicle or operating machinery. Do not use any other products containing diphenhydramine while using this product. As with any drug, if you are pregnant or nursing a baby, seek the advice of a health professional before using this product. KEEP THIS AND ALL DRUGS OUT OF THE REACH OF CHILDREN. In case of accidental overdose, seek professional assistance or contact a Poison Control Center immediately.

Directions: Adult and children 12 years of age and over: 25 to 50 mg (1 to 2 tablets/kapseals) every 4 to 6 hours. Not to exceed 12 tablets/kapseals in 24 hours. Children 6 to under 12 years of age: oral dosage is 12.5 mg* to 25 mg (1 tablet/kapseal) every 4 to 6 hours, not to exceed 6 tablets/kapseals in 24 hours. For children under 6 years of age consult your doctor.

How Supplied: Benadryl tablets are supplied in boxes of 24 and 100, kapseals are supplied in boxes of 24 and 48. Store at room temperature 15°–30° C (59°–86° F). Protect from moisture.

---

* This dosage is not available in this package. Do not attempt to break tablet/kapseal. This dosage is available in a pleasant tasting Benadryl Allergy Liquid Medication.

Shown in Product Identification Guide, page 524

BENADRYL® ALLERGY/COLD TABLETS
[bĕ'nă-drĭl]

Active Ingredients: Each tablet contains: Diphenhydramine Hydrochloride 12.5 mg, Pseudoephedrine Hydrochloride 30 mg and Acetaminophen 500 mg.

Inactive Ingredients: Candelilla Wax, Croscarmellose Sodium, Hydroxypropyl Cellulose, Hydroxypropyl Methylcellulose, Magnesium Stearate, Microcrystalline Cellulose, Polyethylene Glycol, Pregelatinized Starch, Propylene Glycol, Sodium Starch, Glycolate, Starch, Stearic Acid, Titanium Dioxide, and Zinc Stearate.

Indications: For the temporary relief of minor aches, pains, headache, muscular aches, sore throat, fever, runny nose and sneezing, itching of the nose or throat, and itchy, watery eyes due to hay fever, and nasal congestion due to the common cold.

Warnings: **Do not exceed recommended dosage.** If nervousness, dizziness, or sleeplessness occur, discontinue use and consult a doctor. Do not take this product for more than 10 days. If symptoms do not improve or are accompanied by fever that lasts more than 3 days, or if new symptoms occur, consult a doctor. If sore throat is severe, persists for more than 2 days, is accompanied or followed by fever, headache, rash, nausea, or vomiting, consult a doctor promptly. Do not take this product, unless directed by a doctor, if you have a breathing problem such as emphysema or chronic bronchitis, heart disease, high blood pressure, thyroid disease, diabetes, or if you have glaucoma or difficulty in urination due to enlargement of the prostate gland. May cause excitability especially in children. May cause marked drowsiness; alcohol, sedatives, and tranquilizers may increase the drowsiness effect. Avoid alcoholic beverages while taking this product. Do not take this product if you are taking sedatives or tranquilizers, without first consulting your doctor. Use caution when driving a motor vehicle or operating machinery. Do not use any other products containing diphenhydramine

while using this product. As with any drug, if you are pregnant or nursing a baby, seek the advice of a health professional before using this product. KEEP THIS AND ALL DRUGS OUT OF THE REACH OF CHILDREN. In case of accidental overdose, seek professional assistance or contact a Poison Control Center immediately. Prompt medical attention is critical for adults as well as for children even if you do not notice any signs or symptoms.

Directions: Adults and children 12 years of age and over: two (2) tablets every 6 hours while symptoms persist. Not to exceed 8 tablets in 24 hours. Children under 12 years of age: consult a doctor.

How Supplied: Benadryl® Allergy/Cold tablets are supplied in boxes of 24 tablets. Store at room temperature 59°–86°F. Protect from moisture.

Shown in Product Identification Guide, page 524

BENADRYL® ALLERGY CHEWABLES
[bĕ'nă-drĭl]

Active Ingredients: Each chewable tablet contains: Diphenhydramine Hydrochloride 12.5 mg.

Inactive Ingredients: Aspartame, Dextrates, D&C Red No. 27 Aluminum Lake, FD&C Blue No. 1 Aluminum Lake, Flavors, Magnesium Stearate, Magnesium Trisilicate, and Tartaric Acid.

Indications: Temporarily relieves runny nose and sneezing, itching of the nose or throat, and itchy, water eyes due to hay fever or other upper respiratory allergies, and runny nose and sneezing associated with the common cold.

Warnings: May cause excitability especially in children. Do not take this product, unless directed by a doctor, if you have a breathing problem such as emphysema or chronic bronchitits, or if you have glaucoma or difficulty in urination due to enlargement of the prostate gland. May cause marked drowsiness; alcohol, sedatives, and tranquilizers may increase the drowsiness effect. Avoid alcoholic beverages while taking this product. Do not take this product if you are taking sedatives or tranquilizers, without first consulting your doctor. Use caution when driving a motor vehicle or operating machinery. Do not use any other products containing diphenhydramine

Continued on next page

This product information was prepared in November 1995. On these and other Warner Wellcome Consumer HealthCare Products, detailed information may be obtained by addressing Warner Wellcome Consumer HealthCare Products, Warner-Lambert, Morris Plains, NJ 07950

Warner Wellcome—Cont.

while using this product. As with any drug, if you are pregnant or nursing a baby, seek the advice of a health professional before using this product. KEEP THIS AND ALL DRUGS OUT OF THE REACH OF CHILDREN. In case of accidental overdose, seek professional assistance or contact a Poison Control Center immediately. **Phenylketonurics: Contains Phenylalanine 4.2 mg. Per Tablet.**

Directions: Chew tablets thoroughly before swallowing. Adult and children 12 years of age and over: 2 to 4 tablets (25 to 50 mg.) every 4 to 6 hours. Not to exceed 24 tablets in 24 hours. Children 6 to under 12 years of age: 1 to 2 tablets (12.5 to 25 mg.) every 4 to 6 hours. Not to exceed 12 tablets in 24 hours. For children under 6 years of age: consult a doctor.

How Supplied: Benadryl® Allergy Chewables are supplied in boxes of 24 tablets. Store at room temperature 59°–77°F. Protect from heat and humidity.

Shown in Product Identification Guide, page 524

BENADRYL®
Allergy Decongestant Tablets
[bĕ'nă-drĭl]

Active Ingredients: Each tablet contains: Diphenhydramine Hydrochloride 25 mg and Pseudoephedrine Hydrochloride 60 mg.

Inactive Ingredients: Each tablet contains: Croscarmellose Sodium, Dibasic Calcium Phosphate Dihydrate, FD&C Blue No. 1 Aluminum Lake, Hydroxypropyl Methylcellulose, Microcrystalline Cellulose, Polyethylene Glycol, Polysorbate 80, Pregelatinized Starch, Stearic Acid, Titanium Dioxide and Zinc Stearate.

Indications: Temporarily relieves nasal congestion; runny nose and sneezing, itching of the nose or throat, and itchy, watery eyes due to hay fever or other upper respiratory allergies, and runny nose, sneezing, and nasal congestion associated with the common cold.

Warning: Do not exceed recommended dosage. If nervousness, dizziness, or sleeplessness occur, discontinue use and consult a doctor. If symptoms do not improve within 7 days or are accompanied by fever, consult a doctor. Do not take this product, unless directed by a doctor, if you have a breathing problem such as emphysema or chronic bronchitis, heart disease, high blood pressure, thyroid disease, diabetes, or if you have glaucoma or difficulty in urination due to enlargement of the prostate gland. May cause excitability especially in children. May cause marked drowsiness; alcohol, sedatives, and tranquilizers may increase the drowsiness effect. Avoid alcoholic beverages while taking this product. Do not take this product if you are taking sedatives or tranquilizers, without first consulting your doctor. Use caution when driving a motor vehicle or operating machinery. Do not use any other products containing diphenhydramine while using this product. As with any drug, if you are pregnant or nursing a baby, seek the advice of a health professional before using this product. KEEP THIS AND ALL DRUGS OUT OF THE REACH OF CHILDREN. In case of accidental overdose, seek professional assistance or contact a Poison Control Center immediately.

Drug Interaction Precaution: Do not use this product if you are now taking a prescription monoamine oxidase inhibitor (MAOI) (certain drugs for depression, psychiatric or emotional conditions, or Parkinson's disease), or for 2 weeks after stopping the MAOI drug. If you are uncertain whether your prescription drug contains an MAOI, consult a health professional before taking this product.

Directions: Follow dosage recommendations below, or use as directed by your doctor. Adults and children 12 years of age and over: one (1) tablet every 4 to 6 hours, not to exceed 4 tablets in 24 hours. Children under 12 years of age: consult a doctor.

How Supplied: Benadryl Allergy Decongestant Tablets are supplied in boxes of 24.
Store at room temperature 59°–86° F. Protect from moisture.

Shown in Product Identification Guide, page 524

BENADRYL®
Allergy Decongestant Liquid Medication
[bĕ'nă-drĭl]

Active Ingredients: Each teaspoonful (5 mL) contains: Diphenhydramine Hydrochloride) 12.5 mg and Pseudoephedrine Hydrochloride 30 mg.

Inactive Ingredients: Citric Acid, FD&C Blue No. 1, FD&C Red No. 40, Flavors, Glycerin, Poloxamer 407, Polysorbate 20, Purified Water, Saccharin Sodium, Sodium Benzoate, Sodium Chloride, Sodium Citrate and Sorbitol Solution.

Indications: Temporarily relieves nasal congestion, runny nose, and sneezing, itching of the nose or throat, and itchy, watery eyes due to hay fever or other upper respiratory allergies, and runny nose, sneezing and nasal congestion associated with the common cold.

Directions: Follow dosage recommendations below, or use as directed by your doctor.

Benadryl® Allergy Decongestant Liquid Medication

AGE	DOSAGE
Children Under 6 years of age	Consult a Doctor
Children 6 to under 12 years of age	One (1) teaspoonful every 4 to 6 hours. Not to exceed 4 teaspoonfuls in 24 hours.
Adults and Children 12 years of age and over	Two (2) teaspoonfuls every 4 to 6 hours. Not to exceed 8 teaspoonfuls in 24 hours.

Warnings: Do not exceed recommended dosage. If nervousness, dizziness, or sleeplessness occur, discontinue use and consult a doctor. If symptoms do not improve within 7 days or are accompanied by fever, consult a doctor. Do not take this product, unless directed by a doctor, if you have a breathing problem such as emphysema or chronic bronchitis, heart disease, high blood pressure, thyroid disease, diabetes, or if you have glaucoma or difficulty in urination due to enlargement of the prostate gland. May cause excitability, especially in children. May cause marked drowsiness; alcohol, sedatives, and tranquilizers may increase the drowsiness effect. Avoid alcoholic beverages while taking this product. Do not take this product if you are taking sedatives or tranquilizers, without first consulting your doctor. Use caution when driving a motor vehicle or operating machinery. Do not use any other products containing diphenhydramine while using this product. As with any drug, if you are pregnant or nursing a baby, seek the advice of a health professional before using this product. KEEP THIS AND ALL DRUGS OUT OF THE REACH OF CHILDREN. In case of accidental overdose, seek professional assistance or contact a Poison Control Center immediately.

Drug Interaction Precaution: Do not use this product if you are now taking a prescription monoamine oxidase inhibitor (MAOI) (certain drugs for depression, psychiatric or emotional conditions, or Parkinson's disease), or for 2 weeks after stopping the MAOI drug. If you are uncertain whether your prescription drug contains an MAOI, consult a health professional before taking this product.

How Supplied: Benadryl Allergy Decongestant Liquid Medication is supplied in 4 fl. oz. bottles.
Store at room temperature 59°–86°F. Protect from freezing.

Shown in Product Identification Guide, page 524

BENADRYL® Allergy Liquid Medication
[bĕ′nă-drĭl]

Active Ingredient: Each teaspoonful (5 mL) contains Diphenhydramine Hydrochloride 12.5 mg.

Inactive Ingredients: Each teaspoonful (5 mL) contains: Citric Acid, D&C Red No. 33, FD&C No. 40, Flavors, Glycerin, Poloxamer 407, Polysorbate 20, Saccharin Sodium, Sodium Benzoate, Sodium Citrate, Sugar, and Water.

Indications: Benadryl temporarily relieves runny nose and sneezing, itching of the nose or throat and itchy, watery eyes due to hay fever or other upper respiratory allergies, and runny nose and sneezing associated with the common cold.

Directions: Follow dosage recommendations below or use as directed by your doctor.

Benadryl® Allergy Liquid Medication

AGE	DOSAGE
Children Under 6 years of age	Consult a Doctor
Children 6 to under 12 years of age	**1 to 2 teaspoonfuls (12.5 to 25 mg.)** every 4 to 6 hours. Not to exceed 12 teaspoonfuls in 24 hours.
Adults and Children 12 years of age and over	**2 to 4 teaspoonfuls (25 to 50 mg.)** every 4 to 6 hours. Not to exceed 24 teaspoonfuls in 24 hours.

Warnings: May cause excitability, especially in children. Do not take this product, unless directed by a doctor, if you have a breathing problem such as emphysema, or chronic bronchitis, or if you have glaucoma or difficulty in urination due to enlargment of the prostate gland. May cause marked drowsiness; alcohol, sedatives, and tranquilizers may increase the drowsiness effect. Avoid alcoholic beverages while taking this product. Do not take this product if you are taking sedatives or tranquilizers, without first consulting your doctor. Use caution when driving a motor vehicle or operating machinery. Do not use any other products containing diphenhydramine while using this product. As with any drug, if you are pregnant or nursing a baby seek the advice of a health professional before using this product. KEEP THIS AND ALL DRUGS OUT OF THE REACH OF CHILDREN. In case of accidental overdose, seek professional assistance or contact a Poison Control Center immediately.

How Supplied: Benadryl Allergy Liquid Medication is supplied in 4 and 8 fluid ounce bottles.
Store at room temperature 59°–86°F. Protect from freezing.
Shown in Product Identification Guide, page 524

BENADRYL® Allergy Sinus Headache Caplets
[bĕ′nă-drĭl]

Active Ingredients: Each caplet contains Diphenhydramine Hydrochloride 12.5 mg, Pseudoephedrine Hydrochloride 30 mg and Acetaminophen 500 mg.

Inactive Ingredients: Candelilla Wax, Croscarmellose Sodium, D&C Yellow No. 10 Aluminum Lake, FD&C Blue No. 1 Aluminum Lake, FD&C Yellow No. 6 Aluminum Lake, Hydroxypropyl Cellulose, Hydroxypropyl Methylcellulose, Microcrystalline Cellulose, Polyethylene Glycol, Polysorbate 80, Pregelatinized Starch, Sodium Starch Glycolate, Starch, Stearic Acid, Titanium Dioxide, and Zinc Stearate.

Indications: For the temporary relief of minor aches, pains, and headache, runny nose and sneezing, itching of the nose or throat, and itchy, watery eyes due to hay fever, and nasal congestion due to the common cold, hay fever, or other upper respiratory allergies. Helps decongest sinus openings and passages; temporarily relieves sinus congestion and pressure.

Action: BENADRYL ALLERGY/SINUS/HEADACHE is specially formulated to provide effective relief of your upper respiratory allergy symptoms complicated by sinus and headache problems. It combines the strength of BENADRYL to relieve your runny nose: sneezing; itchy water eyes; itchy nose or throat with a maximum strength NASAL DECONGESTANT to relieve nasal and sinus congestion and a maximum strength non-aspirin PAIN RELIEVER to relieve sinus pain and headache.

Warnings: Do not exceed recommended dosage. If nervousness, dizziness, or sleeplessness occur, discontinue use and consult a doctor. Do not take this product for more than 10 days. If symptoms do not improve or are accompanied by fever that lasts for more than 3 days, or if new symptoms occur, consult a doctor. Do not take this product, unless directed by a doctor, if you have a breathing problem such as emphysema or chronic bronchitis, heart disease, high blood pressure, thyroid disease, diabetes, or if you have glaucoma or difficulty in urination due to enlargement of the prostate gland. May cause excitability especially in children. May cause marked drowsiness; alcohol, sedatives, and tranquilizers may increase the drowsiness effect. Avoid alcoholic beverages while taking this product. Do not take this

product if you are taking sedatives or tranquilizers, without first consulting your doctor. Use caution when driving a motor vehicle or operating machinery. Do not use any other products containing diphenhydramine while using this product. As with any drug, if you are pregnant or nursing a baby, seek the advice of a health professional before using this product. KEEP THIS AND ALL DRUGS OUT OF THE REACH OF CHILDREN. In case of accidental overdose, seek professional assistance or contact a Poison Control Center immediately. Prompt medical attention is critical for adults as well as for children even if you do not notice any signs or symptoms.

Drug Interaction Precaution: Do not use this product if you are now taking a prescription monoamine oxidase inhibitor (MAOI) (certain drugs for depression, psychiatric or emotional conditions, or Parkinson's disease), or for 2 weeks after stopping the MAOI drug. If you are uncertain whether your prescription drug contains an MAOI, consult a health professional before taking this product.

Directions: Adults and children 12 years of age and over: two (2) caplets every 6 hours while symptoms persist, not to exceed 8 caplets in 24 hours. Children under 12 years of age: consult a doctor.

How Supplied: Benadryl Allergy Sinus Headache is available in boxes of 24 and 48 caplets. Store at room temperature, 15°–30°C (59°–86°F).
Shown in Product Identification Guide, page 525

BENADRYL® Dye-Free Allergy Liqui-gel® Softgels
[bĕ′nă-drĭl]

Active Ingredients: Each softgel contains: Diphenhydramine Hydrochloride 25 mg.

Inactive Ingredients: Gelatin, Glycerin, Polyethylene Glycol 400 and Sorbitol.

Indications: Temporarily relieves runny nose and sneezing, itching of the nose or throat, and itchy, watery eyes due to hay fever or other upper respiratory allergies, and runny nose and sneezing associated with the common cold.

Directions: Follow dosage recommendations below, or use as directed by your doctor.

Continued on next page

This product information was prepared in November 1995. On these and other Warner Wellcome Consumer HealthCare Products, detailed information may be obtained by addressing Warner Wellcome Consumer HealthCare Products, Warner-Lambert, Morris Plains, NJ 07950

Warner Wellcome—Cont.

Benadryl® Dye-Free Allergy
Liqui-Gels® Softgel

AGE	DOSAGE
Adults and Children 12 years of age and over	25 to 50 mg. (1 to 2 softgels) every 4 to 6 hours. Not to exceed 12 softgels in 24 hours.
Children 6 to under 12 years of age See ** symbol below	12.5** to 25 mg. (1 softgel) every 4 to 6 hours. Not to exceed 6 softgels in 24 hours.
Children Under 6 years of age	Consult a Doctor

**12.5 mg. dosage strength is not available in this package. Do not attempt to break softgels. This dosage is available in Benadryl® Dye-Free Allergy Liquid Medication.

Warnings: May cause excitability, especially in children. Do not take this product, unless directed by a doctor, if you have a breathing problem such as emphysema or chronic bronchitis, or if you have glaucoma or difficulty in urination due to enlargement of the prostate gland. May cause marked drowsiness; alcohol, sedatives, and tranquilizers may increase the drowsiness effect. Avoid alcoholic beverages while taking this product. Do not take this product if you are taking sedatives or tranquilizers, without first consulting your doctor. Use caution when driving a motor vehicle or operating machinery. Do not use any other products containing diphenhydramine while using this product. As with any drug, if you are pregnant or nursing a baby, seek the advice of a health professional before using this product. KEEP THIS AND ALL DRUGS OUT OF THE REACH OF CHILDREN. In case of accidental overdose, seek professional assistance or contact a Poison Control Center immediately.

How Supplied: Benadryl® Dye-Free Allergy Liqui-Gels® Softgels are supplied in boxes of 24.
Store at 59°–77°F.

Liqui-Gels is a registered trademark of R.P. Scherer Corporation.
Protect from heat and humidity.
Shown in Product Identification Guide, page 525

BENADRYL® Dye-Free Allergy Liquid Medication
[bĕ′nă-drĭl]

Active Ingredients: Each teaspoonful (5 mL.) contains Diphenhydramine HCL 6.25 mg.

Inactive Ingredients: Each teaspoonful (5 mL.) contains: Carboxymethylcellulose Sodium, Citric Acid, Flavor, Glycerin, Saccharin Sodium, Sodium Benzoate, Sodium Citrate, Sorbitol Solution and Water.

Indications: Temporarily relieves runny nose and sneezing, itching of the nose or throat, and itchy, watery eyes due to hay fever or other upper respiratory allergies, and runny nose and sneezing associated with the common cold.

Directions: Follow dosage recommendations below, or use as directed by your doctor.

Benadryl® Dry-Free Allergy
Liquid Medication

AGE	DOSAGE
Children Under 6 years of age	Consult a Doctor
Children 6 to under 12 years of age	**2–4 Teaspoonfuls (12.5 to 25 mg)** every 4 to 6 hours. Not to exceed 24 teaspoonfuls in 24 hours.
Adults and Children 12 years of age and over	**4–8 teaspoonfuls (25 to 50 mg)** every 4 to 6 hours. Not to exceed 48 teaspoonfuls in 24 hours.

Warnings: May cause excitability especially in children. Do not take this product, unless directed by a doctor, if you have a breathing problem such as emphysema or chronic bronchitis, or if you have glaucoma or difficulty in urination due to enlargement of the prostate gland. May cause marked drowsiness; alcohol, sedatives, and tranquilizers may increase the drowsiness effect. Avoid alcoholic beverages while taking this product. Do not take this product if you are taking sedatives or tranquilizers, without first consulting your doctor. Use caution when driving a motor vehicle or operating machinery. Do not use any other products containing diphenhydramine while using this product. As with any drug, if you are pregnant or nursing a baby, seek the advice of a health professional before using this product. KEEP THIS AND ALL DRUGS OUT OF THE REACH OF CHILDREN. In case of accidental overdose, seek professional assistance or contact a Poison Control Center immediately.

How Supplied: Benadryl Dye-Free Allergy Liquid Medication is supplied in 8 fl. oz. bottles.
Store at room temperature 59°–86°F. Protect from freezing.
Shown in Product Identification Guide, page 525

BENADRYL® Itch Relief Stick Extra Strength
Topical Analgesic/Skin Protectant
[bĕ′nă-drĭl]

Active Ingredients: Diphenhydramine Hydrochloride 2%, Zinc Acetate 0.1%.

Inactive Ingredients: Alcohol 73.5% v/v, Glycerin, Povidone, Purified Water, and Tromethamine.

Indications: For the temporary relief of itching and pain associated with insect bites, minor skin irritations, and rashes due to poison oak, poison ivy or poison sumac. Dries the oozing and weeping of poison ivy, poison oak and poison sumac.

Warnings: FOR EXTERNAL USE ONLY. Do not use on chicken pox, measles, blisters, or on extensive areas of skin, except as directed by a physician. Avoid contact with the eyes. If condition worsens or does not improve within 7 days, or if symptoms persist for more than 7 days or clear up and occur again within a few days, discontinue use of this product and consult a physician. Do not use on children under 6 years of age without consulting a physician. Do not use any other drugs containing diphenhydramine while using this product. KEEP THIS AND ALL DRUGS OUT OF THE REACH OF CHILDREN. In case of accidental ingestion, seek professional assistance or contact a Poison Control Center immediately. Flammable. Keep away from fire or flame.

Directions: Adults and children 6 years of age and older; apply to the affected area not more than 3 to 4 times daily. For children under 6 years of age: consult a physician.
Store at room temperature (59°–86°F).

How Supplied: Benadryl® Itch Relief Stick is available in a .47 oz (14 mL) dauber.
Shown in Product Identification Guide, page 525

BENADRYL® Itch Stopping Cream Original Strength & Extra Strength
[bĕ′nă-drĭl]

Active Ingredients:
Original Strength: Diphenhydramine Hydrochloride 1% and Zinc Acetate 0.1%.
Extra Strength: Diphenhydramine Hydrochloride 2% and Zinc Acetate 0.1%.

Inactive Ingredients: Cetyl Alcohol, Diazolidinyl Urea, Methylparaben, Polyethylene Glycol Monostearate 1000, Propylene Glycol, Propylparaben, and Purified Water.

Indications: For the temporary relief of itching and pain associated with insect bites, minor skin irritations and rashes due to poison ivy, poison oak or poison sumac. Dries the oozing and weeping of poison ivy, poison oak and poison sumac.

Actions: Benadryl Itch Stopping Cream:
- Stops your itch at the source by blocking the histamine that causes itch.
- Provides local anesthetic itch and pain relief in a greaseless vanishing cream. Benadryl gives you the kind of itch and pain relief you can't get from hydrocortisone.

Warnings: FOR EXTERNAL USE ONLY.
Original Strength: Do not use on chicken pox, measles, blisters or on extensive areas of skin, except as directed by a physician. Avoid contact with the eyes. If condition worsens, or does not improve within 7 days or if symptoms persist for more than 7 days, or clear up and occur again within a few days, discontinue use of this product and consult a physician. Do not use on children under 12 years of age without consulting a physician. Do not use any other drugs containing diphenhydramine while using this product. KEEP THIS AND ALL DRUGS OUT OF THE REACH OF CHILDREN. In case of accidental ingestion, seek professional assistance or contact a Poison Control Center immediately.
Extra Strength: Do not use on chicken pox, measles, blisters or on extensive areas of skin, except as directed by a physician. Avoid contact with the eyes. If condition worsens, or does not improve within 7 days or if symptoms persist for more than 7 days, or clear up and occur again within a few days, discontinue use of this product and consult a physician. Do not use on children under 12 years of age without consulting a physician. Do not use any other drugs containing diphenhydramine while using this product. KEEP THIS AND ALL DRUGS OUT OF THE REACH OF CHILDREN. In case of accidental ingestion, seek professional assistance or contact a Poison Control Center immediately.

Directions: Original Strength: Adults and children 2 years of age and older: apply to affected area not more than 3 to 4 times daily. Children under 2 years of age: consult a physician. Extra Strength: Adults and children 12 years of age and older: apply to affected area not more than 3 to 4 times daily. Children under 12 years of age: consult a physician.

How Supplied: Benadryl Itch Stopping Cream is available in ½ oz. (14.2g) Original Strength and ½ oz. (14.2g) Extra Strength tubes.
Store at room temperature 59°–86°F.
Shown in Product Identification Guide, page 525

BENADRYL® Itch Stopping Spray Original Strength & Extra Strength
[bĕ'nă-drĭl]

Active Ingredients:
Original Strength: Diphenhydramine Hydrochloride 1% and Zinc Acetate 0.1%.
Extra Strength: Diphenhydramine Hydrochloride 2% and Zinc Acetate 0.1%.

Inactive Ingredients: Alcohol up to 73.6% v/v, Glycerin, Povidone, Purified Water and Tromethamine.

Indications: For the temporary relief of itching and pain associated with insect bites, minor skin irritations and rashes due to poison ivy, poison oak, or poison sumac. Dries the oozing and weeping of poison ivy, poison oak, and poison sumac.

Actions: Benadryl Itch Stopping Spray
- Stops your itch at the source by blocking the histamine that causes itch.
- Provides local anesthetic itch and pain relief in a greaseless vanishing cream. Benadryl gives you the kind of itch and pain relief you can't get from hydrocortisone. The spray feature allows soothing relief without touching or rubbing the affected area.

Warnings: FOR EXTERNAL USE ONLY.
Original Strength: Do not use on chicken pox, measles, blisters or on extensive areas of skin, except as directed by a physician. Avoid contact with the eyes. If condition worsens, or does not improve within 7 days or if symptoms persist for more than 7 days or clear up and occur again within a few days, discontinue use of this product and consult a physician. Do not use on children under 2 years of age without consulting a physician. Do not use any other drugs containing diphenhydramine while using this product. KEEP THIS AND ALL DRUGS OUT OF THE REACH OF CHILDREN. In case of accidental ingestion, seek professional assistance or contact a Poison Control Center immediately.
Extra Strength: Do not use on chicken pox, measles, blisters or on extensive areas of skin, except as directed by a physician. Avoid contact with the eyes. If condition worsens, or does not improve within 7 days or if symptoms persist for more than 7 days or clear up and occur again within a few days, discontinue use of this product and consult a physician. Do not use on children under 12 years of age without consulting a physician. Do not use any other drugs containing diphenhydramine while using this product. KEEP THIS AND ALL DRUGS OUT OF THE REACH OF CHILDREN. In case of accidental ingestion, seek professional assistance or contact a Poison Control Center immediately.

Directions: Original Strength: Adults and children 2 years of age and older: apply to affected area not more than 3 to 4 times daily. Children under 2 years of age: consult a physician. Extra Strength: Adults and children 12 years of age and older: apply to affected area not

more than 3 to 4 times daily. Children under 12 years of age: consult a physician.

How Supplied: Benadryl Itch Stopping Spray Original and Extra Strength is available in a 2 oz. (59mL) pump spray bottle.
Store at room temperature 59°–86°F.
Shown in Product Identification Guide, page 525

BENADRYL® Itch Stopping Gel Original Strength & Extra Strength
[bĕ'nă-drĭl]

Active Ingredients:
Original Strength: Diphenhydramine Hydrochloride 1% and Zinc Acetate 1%.
Extra Strength: Diphenhydramine Hydrochloride 2% and Zinc Acetate 1%.

Inactive Ingredients: SD Alcohol 38B, Camphor, Citric Acid, Diazolidinyl Urea, Glycerin, Hydroxypropyl Methylcellulose, Methylparaben, Propylene Glycol, Propylparaben, Purified Water, Sodium Citrate.

Indications: For the temporary relief of itching and pain associated with insect bites, minor skin irritations and rashes due to poison ivy, poison oak or poison sumac. Dries the oozing and weeping of poison ivy, poison oak and poison sumac.

Actions: Benadryl Itch Stopping Gel stops your itch at the source by blocking the histamine that causes itch. It provides local anesthetic itch and pain relief and it has added drying action for the oozing and weeping associated with some rashes. The non-runny, clear gel is packaged in a pump dispenser for easy application. Benadryl gives you the kind of itch and pain relief that you can't get from hydrocortisone or calamine.

Warnings: FOR EXTERNAL USE ONLY.
Original Strength: Do not use on chicken pox, measles, blisters or on extensive areas of skin, except as directed by a physician. Avoid contact with the eyes. If condition worsens, or does not improve within 7 days or if symptoms persist for more than 7 days or clear up and occur again within a few days, discontinue use of this product and consult a physician. Do not use on children under 6 years of age without consulting a physician. Do not use any other drugs containing diphenhydramine while using this product. **KEEP THIS AND ALL DRUGS OUT OF THE REACH OF CHILDREN.**

Continued on next page

This product information was prepared in November 1995. On these and other Warner Wellcome Consumer HealthCare Products, detailed information may be obtained by addressing Warner Wellcome Consumer HealthCare Products, Warner-Lambert, Morris Plains, NJ 07950

Warner Wellcome—Cont.

In case of accidental ingestion, seek professional assistance or contact a Poison Control Center immediately.

Extra Strength: Do not use on chicken pox, measles, blisters or on extensive areas of skin, except as directed by a physician. Avoid contact with the eyes. If condition worsens, or does not improve within 7 days or if symptoms persist for more than 7 days or clear up and occur again within a few days, discontinue use of this product and consult a physician. Do not use on children under 12 years of age without consulting a physician. Do not use any other drugs containing diphenhydramine while using this product. **KEEP THIS AND ALL DRUGS OUT OF THE REACH OF CHILDREN.** In case of accidental ingestion, seek professional assistance or contact a Poison Control Center immediately.

Directions: Original Strength: Adults and children 6 years of age or older: apply to affected area not more than 3 to 4 times daily. Children under 6 years of age: consult a physician. Extra Strength: Adults and children 12 years of age or older: apply to affected area not more than 3 to 4 times daily. Children under 12 years of age: consult a physician.

How Supplied: Benadryl Itch Stopping Gel is supplied in 4 fl. oz. bottles in both Original and Extra Strength. Store at room temperature 59°–86°F.

Shown in Product Identification Guide, page 525

BENYLIN® Multisymptom
[bĕ'-nă-lĭn]

Active Ingredients: Each teaspoonful (5 mL) contains Guaifenesin 100 mg, Pseudoephedrine Hydrochloride 15 mg, and Dextromethorphan Hydrobromide 5 mg.

Inactive Ingredients: Caramel, Citric Acid, D&C Red No. 33, Edetate Disodium, FD&C Red No. 40, Flavors, Poloxamer 407, Polyethylene Glycol 1450, Propyl Gallate, Propylene Glycol, Purified Water, Saccharin Sodium, Sodium Benzoate, Sodium Chloride, Sodium Citrate, and Sorbitol Solution.

Indications: For temporary relief of cough due to minor throat and bronchial irritation and nasal congestion as may occur with the common cold. Helps loosen phlegm (mucus) and thin bronchial secretions to drain bronchial tubes and make coughs more productive.

Directions for Use: Follow dosage recommendations below or use as directed by your physician. Dosage may be repeated every 4 hours, not to exceed 4 doses in 24 hours.

Benylin® Multisymptom

AGE	DOSAGE
Adults and children 12 years and over	4 teaspoonfuls
Children 6 to under 12 years	2 teaspoonfuls
Children 2 to under 6 years	1 teaspoonful
Children under 2 years	Consult Physician

Warnings: Do not exceed recommended dosage. If nervousness, dizziness, or sleeplessness occur, discontinue use and consult a doctor. If symptoms do not improve within 7 days or are accompanied by fever, consult a doctor. Do not take this product if you have heart disease, high blood pressure, thyroid disease, diabetes, or difficulty in urination due to enlargement of the prostate gland unless directed by a doctor. A persistent cough may be a sign of a serious condition. If cough persists for more than 1 week, tends to recur, or is accompanied by a fever, rash or persistent headache, consult a doctor. Do not take this product for persistent or chronic cough such as occurs with smoking, asthma, chronic bronchitis, or emphysema, or where cough is accompanied by excessive phlegm (mucus) unless directed by doctor. As with any drug, if you are pregnant or nursing a baby, seek the advice of a health professional before using this product. **KEEP THIS AND ALL DRUGS OUT OF THE REACH OF CHILDREN.** In case of accidental overdose, seek professional assistance or contact a Poison Control Center immediately.

Drug Interaction Precaution: Do not use this product if you are now taking a prescription monoamine oxidase inhibitor (MAOI) (certain drugs for depression, psychiatric or emotional conditions, or Parkinson's disease), or for 2 weeks after stopping the MAOI drug. If you are uncertain whether your prescription drug contains an MAOI, consult a health professional before taking this product.

How Supplied: Benylin Multisymptom is available in 4 oz bottles. Store at 59–86 F.

Shown in Product Identification Guide, page 525

BENYLIN® Expectorant
[bĕ'-nă-lĭn]

Active Ingredients: Each teaspoonful (5 mL) contains Guaifensin 100 mg and Dextromethorphan Hydrobromide 5 mg.

Inactive Ingredients: Caramel, Citric Acid, D&C Red No. 33, Disodium Edetate, FD&C Red No. 40, Flavors, Poloxamer 407, Polyethylene Glycol, Propyl Gallate, Propylene Glycol, Purified Water, Saccharin Sodium, Sodium Benzoate, Sodium Chloride, Sodium Citrate, and Sorbitol Solution.

Indications: Temporarily relieves cough due to minor throat and bronchial irritation occurring with the common cold. Helps loosen phlegm (mucus) and thin bronchial secretions to drain bronchial tubes and make coughs more productive.

Directions: Follow dosage recommendations below, or as directed by a doctor. Dosage may be repeated every 4 hours, not to exceed 6 doses in 24 hours.

Benylin® Expectorant

AGE	DOSAGE
Adults and children 12 years of age and older	Four (4) teaspoonfuls
Children 6 to under 12 years of age	Two (2) teaspoonfuls
Children 2 to under 6 years of age	One (1) teaspoonful
Children under 2 years of age	Consult a doctor

Warning: A persistent cough may be a sign of a serious condition. If cough persists for more than one week, tends to recur, or is accompanied by fever, rash, or persistent headache, consult a physician. Do not take this product for persistent or chronic cough such as occurs with smoking, asthma, chronic bronchitis or emphysema, or where cough is accompanied by excessive phlegm (mucus), unless directed by a physician. As with any drug, if you are pregnant or nursing a baby, seek the advice of a health professional before using this product. KEEP THIS AND ALL DRUGS OUT OF THE REACH OF CHILDREN. In case of accidental overdose seek professional assistance or contact a Poison Control Center immediately.

Drug Interaction Precaution: Do not use this product if you are now taking a prescription monoamine oxidase inhibitor (MAOI) (certain drugs for depression, psychiatric or emotional conditions, or Parkinson's disease), or for 2 weeks after stopping the MAOI drug. If you are uncertain whether your prescription drug contains an MAOI, consult a health professional before taking this product.

How Supplied: Benylin Expectorant is available in 4 oz. bottles. Store at room temperature 59°–86°F.

Shown in Product Identification Guide, page 525

BENYLIN® Adult Formula Cough Suppressant
[bĕ'-nă-lĭn]

Active Ingredient: Each teaspoonful (5 mL) contains: Dextromethorphan Hydrobromide 15 mg.

Inactive Ingredients: Caramel, Citric Acid, D&C Red No. 33, FD&C Red No. 40, Flavors, Glycerin, Poloxamer 407, Polysorbate 20, Purified Water, Saccharin Sodium, Sodium Benzoate, Sodium Carboxymethyl Cellulose, Sodium Citrate, and Sorbitol Solution.

Indication: Temporarily relieves cough due to minor throat and bronchial irritation as may occur with the common cold or inhaled irritants.

Directions For Use: Follow dosage recommendations below, or use as directed by your physician. Repeat every 6 to 8 hours, not to exceed 4 doses in a 24 hour period.

Benylin® Adult Formula

AGE	DOSAGE
Adults and children 12 years of age and over	2 teaspoonfuls
Children 6 to under 12 years	1 teaspoonful
Children 2 to under 6 years	½ teaspoonful
Children under 2 years	Consult Physician

Warnings: A persistent cough may be a sign of a serious condition. If cough persists for more than one week, tends to recur, or is accompanied by fever, rash or persistent headache, consult a physician. Do not take this product for persistent or chronic cough such as occurs with smoking, asthma, emphysema, or if cough is accompanied by excessive phlegm (mucus), unless directed by a physician. As with any drug, if you are pregnant or nursing a baby, seek the advice of a health professional before using this product. KEEP THIS AND ALL DRUGS OUT OF THE REACH OF CHILDREN. In case of accidental overdose, seek professional assistance or contact a Poison Control Center immediately.

Drug Interaction Precaution: Do not use this product if you are now taking a prescription monoamine oxidase inhibitor (MAOI) (certain drugs for depression, psychiatric or emotional conditions, or Parkinson's disease), or for 2 weeks after stopping the MAOI drug. If you are uncertain whether your prescription drug contains an MAOI, consult a health professional before taking this product.

How Supplied: Benylin Adult Formula is supplied in 4 oz. bottles. Store at room temperature 59–86°F. See bottom flap for lot number and expiration date.
Shown in Product Identification Guide, page 525

BENYLIN® Pediatric Cough Suppressant
[bĕ'-nă-lĭn]

Active Ingredient: Each teaspoonful (5 mL) contains: Dextromethorphan Hydrobromide 7.5 mg.

Inactive Ingredients: Citric Acid, FD&C Blue No. 1, FD&C Red No. 40, Flavors, Glycerin, Poloxamer 407, Polysorbate 20, Purified Water, Saccharin Sodium, Sodium Benzoate, Sodium Carboxymethyl Cellulose, Sodium Citrate, and Sorbitol Solution.

Indications: Temporarily relieves cough due to minor throat and bronchial irritation as may occur with the common cold or inhaled irritants.

Directions for Use: Follow dosage recommendations below or use as directed by your physician. Repeat every 6 to 8 hours not to exceed 4 doses in a 24 hour period.

Benylin® Pediatric

AGE	DOSAGE
Children under 2 years	Consult Physician
Children 2 to under 6 years	1 teaspoonful
Children 6 to under 12 years	2 teaspoonfuls
Adults and children 12 years of age and over	4 teaspoonfuls

Warnings: A persistent cough may be a sign of a serious condition. If cough persists for more than one week, tends to recur, or is accompanied by fever, rash, or persistent headache, consult a physician. Do not take this product for persistent or chronic cough such as occurs with smoking, asthma, emphysema, or if cough is accompanied by excessive phlegm (mucus), unless directed by a physician. As with any drug, if you are pregnant or nursing a baby, seek the advice of a health professional before using this product. KEEP THIS AND ALL DRUGS OUT OF THE REACH OF CHILDREN. In case of accidental overdose, seek professional assistance or contact a Poison Control Center immediately.

Drug Interaction Precaution: Do not use this product if you are now taking a prescription monoamine oxidase inhibitor (MAOI) (certain drugs for depression, psychiatric or emotional conditions, or Parkinson's disease), or for 2 weeks after stopping the MAOI drug. If you are uncertain whether your prescription drug contains an MAOI, consult a health professional before taking this product.

How Supplied: Benylin Pediatric is supplied in 4 oz bottles.
Shown in Product Identification Guide, page 525

BOROFAX® Skin Protectant
[bôr'uh-făks]

Active Ingredients: Zinc oxide 15% and white petrolatum 68.6%.

Inactive Ingredients: Lanolin, mineral oil, and fragrance.

Indications: Helps treat and prevent diaper rash. Protects chafed skin due to diaper rash and helps seal out wetness.

Directions: Change wet and soiled diapers promptly, cleanse the diaper area, and allow to dry. Apply ointment liberally as often as necessary, with each diaper change, especially at bedtime or anytime when exposure to wet diapers may be prolonged.

Warnings: For external use only. Avoid contact with the eyes. If condition worsens or does not improve within 7 days, consult a doctor. Keep this and all drugs out of the reach of children. In case of accidental ingestion, seek professional assistance or contact a Poison Control Center immediately.

How Supplied: Tube, 1.8 oz (50 g) Store at 15° to 25°C (59° to 77°F).
Shown in Product Identification Guide, page 525

CALADRYL® Lotion
CALADRYL® Cream For Kids
CALADRYL® Clear Lotion
[că'lă drĭl"]

Active Ingredients: Caladryl Lotion and Caladryl Cream For Kids; Calamine 8%, and Pramoxine Hydrochloride 1%. Caladryl Clear Lotion; Pramoxine Hydrochloride 1% and Zinc Acetate 0.1%.

Inactive Ingredients: Caladryl Lotion —SD Alcohol 38B 2.7% v/v, Camphor,

Continued on next page

This product information was prepared in November 1995. On these and other Warner Wellcome Consumer HealthCare Products, detailed information may be obtained by addressing Warner Wellcome Consumer HealthCare Products, Warner-Lambert, Morris Plains, NJ 07950

Warner Wellcome—Cont.

Diazolidinyl Urea, Fragrance, Hydroxypropyl Methylcellulose, Methylparaben, Polysorbate 80, Propylene Glycol, Propylparaben, Water and Xanthan Gum.
Caladryl Cream for Kids—Camphor, Cetyl Alcohol, Cyclomethicone, Diazolidinyl Urea, Fragrance, Methylparaben, Polysorbate 60, Propylene Glycol, Propylparaben, Sorbitan Stearate, Soya Sterol and Water.
Caladryl Clear Lotion—SD Alcohol 38B 2.5% v/v, Camphor, Citric Acid, Diazolidinyl Urea, Fragrance, Glycerin, Hydroxypropyl Methylcellulose, Methylparaben, Polysorbate 40, Propylene Glycol, Propylparaben, Purified Water and Sodium Citrate.

Indications: For the temporary relief of itching and pain associated with rashes due to poison ivy, poison oak or poison sumac, insect bites and minor irritations. Dries the oozing and weeping of poison ivy, poison oak or poison sumac.

Warnings: For external use only. Avoid contact with the eyes. If condition worsens, or does not improve within 7 days or symptoms persist for more than 7 days or clear up and occur again within a few days, discontinue use of this product and consult a physician. Do not use on children under 2 years of age without consulting a physician. KEEP THIS AND ALL DRUGS OUT OF THE REACH OF CHILDREN. In case of accidental ingestion seek professional assistance or contact a Poison Control Center immediately.

Directions: (Before each application, wash affected area of skin.) Adults and children 2 years of age and older: apply to the affected area no more than 3 to 4 times daily. Children under 2 years of age: Consult a physician.
Additional instructions for only Lotion and Clear Lotion: Shake Well.

How Supplied: Caladryl Cream for Kids—1½ oz tubes
Caladryl Clear Lotion—6 fl. oz. bottles
Caladryl Lotion—6 fl. oz. bottles
Shown in Product Identification Guide, page 525

EMPIRIN® ASPIRIN Tablets
[ĕm′puh-rŭn]

Active Ingredients: Each tablet contains aspirin 325 mg (5 gr).

Inactive Ingredients: Microcrystalline Cellulose and Potato Starch.
For relief of headache, minor muscular aches and pains, toothache, discomfort and fever of colds and flu, pain of the premenstrual and menstrual periods, and temporary relief of minor arthritis pain (see CAUTION below).

Directions: Adults: 1 or 2 tablets with a full glass of water. Repeat every 4 hours as needed, up to 12 tablets a day.
Children: Consult a physician (see WARNINGS).
Caution: In arthritic conditions, if pain persists for more than 10 days or redness is present, consult a physician immediately.
Warnings: Children and teenagers should not use this medicine for chicken pox or flu symptoms before a doctor is consulted about Reye syndrome, a rare but serious illness reported to be associated with aspirin. Keep this and all medicines out of children's reach. In case of accidental overdose, seek professional assistance or contact a poison control center immediately.
High or continued fever, severe or persistent sore throat especially when accompanied by high fever, headache, nausea or vomiting, may be serious. Consult your physician. Do not exceed dose unless directed by a physician. Do not take this product if you are allergic to aspirin, have asthma, a gastric ulcer or its symptoms, or are taking a medication that affects the clotting of blood, except under the advice of a physician. As with any drug, if you are pregnant or nursing a baby, seek the advice of a health professional before using this product.
IT IS ESPECIALLY IMPORTANT NOT TO USE ASPIRIN DURING THE LAST 3 MONTHS OF PREGNANCY UNLESS SPECIFICALLY DIRECTED TO DO SO BY A DOCTOR BECAUSE IT MAY CAUSE PROBLEMS IN THE UNBORN CHILD OR COMPLICATIONS DURING DELIVERY.

How Supplied: Bottle of 50.
Store at 15° to 25°C (59° to 77°F) in a dry place.

---

e·p·t® PREGNANCY TEST

You can find out whether or not you're pregnant by testing any time of day and as early as the first day of your missed period.
With just one easy step **e·p·t** gives you clear results in just 3 minutes. **e·p·t Pregnancy Test.** The name more women trust™

Before You Begin The Test. Please read the instructions carefully. Registered nurses are available to confidentially answer your calls regarding **e·p·t.** If you have any questions about **e·p·t.** call toll-free 1-800-378-1783 (8:30 am to 8:00 pm EST) weekdays.
To Use e·p·t.
For in-vitro diagnostic use. Only for external use (not for internal use). Remove the test stick from the foil pouch just prior to use and throw away the freshness packet.
Slide back the clear splashguard to expose the absorbent tip and protect the results and control windows. [See figure at bottom of page.]
Hold the test stick by the thumb grip with the exposed **absorbent tip pointing downward and directly into your urine stream** for at least 5 seconds until it is thoroughly wet.

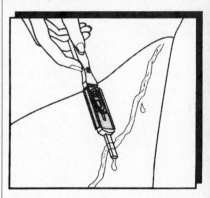

Do not urinate on the windows. (If you prefer, you can urinate into a clean dry cup or container. **Dip only the absorbent tip of the stick** in the urine for at least 5 seconds.)
Lay the test stick down on a flat surface with the windows facing upward while you wait for the test result. (If you wish, you can slide forward the clear splashguard to cover the saturated area.)
As the test begins to work, you may notice a light pink color moving across the windows.
To Read The Results.
Wait at least 3 minutes to read the result. After 3 minutes, a line will appear in the square Control Window to tell you that the test is finished. Once the line

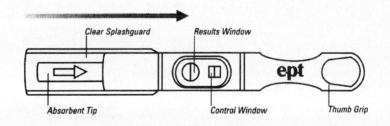

Clear Splashguard   Results Window

ept

Absorbent Tip   Control Window   Thumb Grip

appears in the square Control Window, you may read the result.
Do not read the results after 20 minutes have passed. The round Results Window shows you test results.

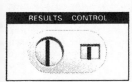

2 LINES—PREGNANT

If you see one line in each window as illustrated, the test has indicated that you are pregnant.

(One line can be darker than the other. The two lines can be any shade of pink and can be lighter or darker than the color picture. However, you should see two clear parallel lines as indicated.)

1 LINE–NOT PREGNANT

If you see a line in the square Control Window but no line in the round Results Window, the test has indicated that you are not Pregnant.

Frequently Asked Questions
How Does e·p·t Work?
e·p·t detects a hormone in your urine that the body produces only during pregnancy (hCG human Chorionic Gonadotropin).

Do I Have To Test in the Morning?
No. You can use e·p·t any time of day. You do not have to use first morning urine.

How Soon Can I use e·p·t?
e·p·t can detect hCG hormone levels in your urine as early as the first day your period is late. e·p·t can be used on the day of your missed period as well as any day thereafter.

What If I Don't Think The Results of the Test are Correct?
If it is hard to tell whether there is a line or not in the round Results Window, repeat the test after 2–3 days with a new e·p·t· if the result is positive, the line should be darker. If you follow the instructions carefully, you should not get a false result. Certain drugs which contain hCG or that are used in combination with hCG (such as Pegnyl, Profasi, Pergonal) and rare medical conditions may give a false result. Alcohol, analgesics, antibiotics, birth control pills, hormone therapies containing clomiphene citrate (such as Clomid, Serophen) or painkillers **should not** affect the test result. If you repeat the test and continue to get an unexpected result, contact your doctor.
The test may give a false positive result if you have had a miscarriage, or have given birth within the past 8 weeks. This is because the test may detect hCG still in your system from a previous pregnancy. You should ask your doctor for help in interpreting the results of your e·p·t test if you have recently been pregnant.

What if the Line in the Round Results Window is Dark but the Line in the Square Control Window is Very Faint?
The result is positive (2 lines).

What Should I Do If the Result is Positive (Pregnant)?
If the result is positive, you should see your doctor to discuss your pregnancy and next steps. Early prenatal care is important to ensure the health of you and your baby.

What Should I do if the Result is Negative (Not Pregnant)?
If the result is negative, no pregnancy hormone (hCG) has been detected and you are probably not pregnant. However, you may have miscalculated when your period was due, especially if you have irregular periods. If your period does not start within a week, repeat the test. If you still get a negative result and your period has not started, you should see your doctor.

What If I Don't Wait the Full 3 Minutes Before Reading the Test Result?
If you read the test result before 3 minutes, you may not give the test enough time to work, and the results may be inaccurate. The appearance of a line in the square control window will tell you that the test is finished and you may read the results.

Shown in Product Identification Guide, page 525

GELUSIL®
Antacid–Anti-gas
Liquid/Tablets
Sodium Free
[jĕl'ū-sĭl"]

Each teaspoonful (5 mL) of Gelusil Liquid contains: Aluminum Hydroxide Gel (equivalent to 200 mg of Aluminum Hydroxide Dried Gel), Magnesium Hydroxide 200 mg and Simethicone 25 mg (an antiflatulent).
Each Gelusil Tablet contains: Aluminum Hydroxide Dried Gel 200 mg, Magnesium Hydroxide 200 mg and Simethicone 25 mg (an antiflatulent).
Also contains: Liquid: Ammonia Solution Strong; Calcium Hypochlorite; Citric Acid; Flavors; Hydroxypropyl Methylcellulose; Menthol; Sodium Saccharin; Sorbitol Solution; Water; Xanthan Gum. Tablets: Flavors; Magnesium Stearate; Mannitol; Sorbitol; Sugar.

Advantages:
- High acid-neutralizing capacity
- Sodium free
- Simethicone for antiflatulent activity
- Good taste for better patient compliance
- Fast dissolution of chewed tablets for prompt relief

Indications: For the relief of heartburn, sour stomach, acid indigestion and to alleviate or relieve symptoms of gas.

Directions for Use: Two to 4 teaspoonfuls or tablets one hour after meals and at bedtime, or as directed by a physician.
Tablets should be chewed.
Liquid: Shake well before use.

Warnings: Do not take more than 12 tablets or teaspoonfuls in a 24-hour period, or use the maximum dosage of this product for more than two weeks, or use this product if you have kidney disease, except under the advice and supervision of a physician.
Keep this and all drugs out of the reach of children.

Professional Warnings: Prolonged use of aluminum-containing antacids in patients with renal failure may result in or worsen dialysis osteomalacia. Elevated tissue aluminum levels contribute to the development of the dialysis encephalopathy and osteomalacia syndromes. Small amounts of aluminum are absorbed from the gastrointestinal tract and renal excretion of aluminum is impaired in renal failure. Aluminum is not well removed by dialysis because it is bound to albumin and transferrin, which do not cross dialysis membranes. As a result, aluminum is deposited in bone, and dialysis osteomalacia may develop when large amounts of aluminum are ingested orally by patients with impaired renal function. Aluminum forms insoluble complexes with phosphate in the gastrointestinal tract, thus decreasing phosphate absorption. Prolonged use of aluminum-containing antacids by normophosphatemic patients may result in hypophosphatemia if phosphate intake is not adequate. In its more severe forms, hypophosphatemia can lead to anorexia, malaise, muscle weakness, and osteomalacia.

Drug Interaction Precaution: Antacids may interact with certain prescription drugs. If you are presently taking a prescription drug, do not take this product without checking with your physician or other health professional.

How Supplied:
Liquid—In plastic bottles of 12 fl oz. (355 mL)
Tablets—White, embossed Gelusil P-D 034—individual strips of 10 in boxes of 100.

Continued on next page

This product information was prepared in November 1995. On these and other Warner Wellcome Consumer HealthCare Products, detailed information may be obtained by addressing Warner Wellcome Consumer HealthCare Products, Warner-Lambert, Morris Plains, NJ 07950

Warner Wellcome—Cont.

Store at Room Temperature 59°–86°F (15°–30°C).

Shown in Product Identification Guide, page 525

LISTERMINT®
Alcohol-Free Mouthrinse
[lĭs ′tər mĭnt]

Ingredient: Water, Glycerin, Poloxamer 335, PEG 600, Flavors, Sodium Lauryl Sulfate, Sodium Benzoate, Sodium Saccharin, Benzoic Acid, Zinc Chloride, D&C Yellow No. 10, FD&C Green No. 3.

Indications: Freshens breath; contains no fluoride.

Directions: Rinse with 30 ml (1 fl. oz.) for 30 seconds to freshen breath in the morning and after meals as needed.

Warnings: Do not swallow. Keep out of reach of children.

How Supplied: Listermint® is supplied to consumers in 18 and 32 fl. oz. bottles and available to professionals in 3 fl. oz. bottles and in gallons.

Shown in Product Identification Guide, page 526

LISTERINE® Antiseptic
[lĭs ′tər ēn]

Active Ingredients: Thymol 0.064%, Eucalyptol 0.092%, Methyl Salicylate 0.060% and Menthol 0.042%.

Inactive Ingredients: Water, Alcohol 26.9%, Benzoic Acid, Poloxamer 407 and Caramel.

Indications: To help prevent and reduce plaque and gingivitis/For bad breath.

Actions: Listerine® Antiseptic has been shown to help prevent and reduce supragingival plaque accumulation and gingivitis when used in a conscientiously applied program of oral hygiene and regular professional care. Its effect on periodontitis has not been determined. Listerine is the only leading nonprescription mouthrinse that has received the American Dental Association's Council on Scientific Affairs Seal of Acceptance for helping to prevent and reduce plaque above the gumline and gingivitis.

Directions: Rinse full strength for 30 seconds with 20 ml (⅔ fl. ounce or 4 teaspoonfuls) morning and night. If bad breath persists, see your dentist.

Warnings: Do not administer to children under twelve years of age. Keep this and all drugs out of the reach of children. Do not swallow. In case of accidental overdose, seek professional assistance or contact a Poison Control Center immediately.

How Supplied: Listerine® Antiseptic is supplied in 250 ml, 500 ml, 1.0 liter and 1.5 liter bottles, as well as 3 fl. oz. bottles. It is also available to professionals in 3 fl. oz. bottles and in gallons.

Shown in Product Identification Guide, page 525

COOL MINT LISTERINE®
[lĭs ′tər ēn]

Active Ingredients: Thymol 0.064%, Eucalyptol 0.092%, Methyl Salicylate 0.060% and Menthol 0.042%.

Inactive Ingredients: Water, Sorbitol Solution, Alcohol 21.6%, Poloxamer 407, Benzoic Acid, Flavoring, Sodium Saccharin, Sodium Citrate, Citric Acid and FD&C Green No. 3.

Indications: To help prevent and reduce plaque and gingivitis/For bad breath.

Actions: Cool Mint Listerine® Antiseptic has been shown to help prevent and reduce supragingival plaque accumulation and gingivitis when used in a conscientiously applied program of oral hygiene and regular professional care. Its effect on periodontitis has not been determined. Listerine is the only leading nonprescription mouthrinse that has received the American Dental Association's Council on Scientific Affairs Seal of Acceptance for helping to prevent and reduce plaque above the gumline and gingivitis.

Directions: Rinse full strength for 30 seconds with 20 ml (⅔ fl. ounce or 4 teaspoonfuls) morning and night. If bad breath persists, see your dentist.

Warnings: Do not administer to children under twelve years of age. Keep this and all drugs out of the reach of children. Do not swallow. In case of accidental overdose, seek professional assistance or contact a Poison Control Center immediately.

How Supplied: Cool Mint Listerine® Antiseptic is supplied in 250 ml, 500 ml, 1.0 liter and 1.5 liter bottles, as well as 3 and 58 fl. oz. bottles. It is also available to professionals in gallon bottles.

Shown in Product Identification Guide, page 526

FRESHBURST LISTERINE®
[lĭs ′tər ēn]

Active Ingredients: Thymol 0.064%, Eucalyptol 0.092%, Methyl Salicylate 0.060% and Menthol 0.042%.

Inactive Ingredients: Water, Sorbitol Solution, Alcohol 21.6%, Poloxamer 407, Benzoic Acid, Flavoring, Sodium Saccharin, Sodium Citrate, Citric Acid, D&C Yellow No. 10 and FD&C Green No. 3.

Indications: To help prevent and reduce plaque and gingivitis/For bad breath.

Actions: FreshBurst Listerine® Antiseptic has been shown to help prevent and reduce supragingival plaque accumulation and gingivitis when used in a conscientiously applied program of oral hygiene and regular professional care. Its effect on periodontitis has not been determined. Listerine is the only leading nonprescription mouthrinse that has received the American Dental Association's Council on Scientific Affairs Seal of Acceptance for helping to prevent and reduce plaque above the gumline and gingivitis.

Directions: Rinse full strength for 30 seconds with 20 ml (⅔ fl. ounce or 4 teaspoonfuls) morning and night. If bad breath persists, see your dentist.

Warnings: Do not administer to children under twelve years of age. Keep this and all drugs out of the reach of children. Do not swallow. In case of accidental overdose, seek professional assistance or contact a Poison Control Center immediately.

How Supplied: FreshBurst Listerine® Antiseptic is supplied in 250 ml, 500 ml, 1.0 liter and 1.5 liter bottles, as well as 3 fl. oz. bottles. It is also available to professionals in gallon bottles.

Shown in Product Identification Guide, page 526

LUBRIDERM®
Dry Skin Care Lotion
[lū brĭ dĕrm]

Composition:
Scented—Contains Water, Mineral Oil, Petrolatum, Sorbitol, Lanolin, Stearic Acid, Lanolin Alcohol, Cetyl Alcohol, Tri (PPG-3 Myristyl Ether) Citrate, Triethanolamine, Methylparaben, Methyldibromo Glutaronitrile/Phenoxyethanol, Fregrance, Ethylparaben, Propylparaben, Butylparaben, Sodium Chloride.
Fragrance Free—Contains Water, Mineral Oil, Petrolatum, Sorbitol, Lanolin, Stearic Acid, Lanolin Alcohol, Cetyl Alcohol, Tri (PPG-3 Myristyl Ether) Citrate, Triethanolamine, Methylparaben, Methyldibromo Glutaronitrile/Phenoxyethanol, Ethylparaben, Propylparaben, Butylparaben, Sodium Chloride.

Actions and Uses: Lubriderm Lotion is an oil-in-water emulsion indicated for use in softening, soothing and moisturizing dry chapped skin. Lubriderm relieves the roughness, tightness and discomfort associated with dry or chapped skin and helps protect the skin from further drying.
Lubriderm's formula smoothes easily into skin without leaving a greasy feeling.

Administration and Dosage: Apply as often as needed to hands and body to restore and maintain the skin's natural suppleness.

Precautions: For external use only.

How Supplied:
Scented: Available in 6, 10 and 16 fl. oz. plastic bottles, and a 2.5 ounce tube.
Fragrance Free: Available in 1, 6, 10 and 16 fl. oz. plastic bottles, and a 2.5 ounce tube.
Shown in Product Identification Guide, page 526

LUBRIDERM® BATH AND SHOWER OIL
[lū brĭ dĕrm]

Composition: Contains Mineral Oil, PPG-15 Stearyl Ether, Oleth-2, Nonoxynol-5, Fragrance, D&C Green No. 6.

Actions and Uses: Lubriderm Bath and Shower Oil is a lanolin-free, mineral oil–based, bath oil designed for softening and soothing dry skin during the bath. The formula disperses into countless droplets of oil that coat the skin and help lubricate and soften. It is equally effective in hard or soft water and provides an excellent way to moisturize the skin and help counterbalance the drying effects of harsh soaps and hot water.

Administration and Dosage: Use one or two capfuls in the bath. For shower, or sponge bath, apply all over your body by hand or with a sponge and rinse.

Precautions: Avoid getting in eyes; if this occurs, flush with clear water. When using any bath and shower oil, take precautions against slipping. For external use only.

How Supplied: Available in 8 fl. oz. plastic bottles.
Shown in Product Identification Guide, page 526

LUBRIDERM® Moisture Recovery Alpha Hydroxy Creme/Lotion
[lū brĭ dĕrm]

Composition: Creme—Contains Water, Isostearic Acid, Stearic Acid, Sodium Lactate, PPG-12/SMDI Copolymer, Lactic Acid, Steareth-21, Steareth-2, Mineral Oil, Cetyl Alcohol, Magnesium Aluminum Silicate, Imidazolidinyl Urea, Fragrance, Potassium Sorbate, Xanthan Gum.
Lotion—Contains Water, Isostearic Acid, Stearic Acid, Steareth-21, Sodium Lactate, PPG-12/SMDI Copolymer, Lactic Acid, Steareth-2, Magnesium Aluminum Silicate, Cetyl Alcohol, Imidazolidinyl Urea, Fragrance, Potassium Sorbate, Xanthan Gum.

Actions and Uses: Lubriderm Moisture Recovery Alpha Hydroxy Formula is ideal for patients with extra dry skin. It accelerates the process of exfoliation, allowing newer, healthier looking skin to emerge. The patented alpha hydroxy delivery system provides long lasting, concentrated healing of severely dry skin.

Administration and Dosage: Apply creme to rough, dry skin areas like feet, knees, and elbows. The lotion is ideal for overall body moisturization.

Precautions: For external use only. Avoid contact in and around the eyes.

How Supplied:
Creme—Available in 4 oz. plastic tubes.
Lotion—Available in .5 and 8 fl. oz. plastic bottles.
Shown in Product Identification Guide, page 526

LUBRIDERM® Moisture Recovery GelCreme
[lū brĭ dĕrm]

Composition: Contains Water, Cetyl Alcohol, Glycerin, Mineral Oil, Cyclomethicone Fluid, Propylene Glycol Dicaprylate/Dicaprate, PEG-40 Stearate, Isopropyl Isostearate, Emulsifying Wax, Lecithin, Carbomer 940, Diazolidinyl Urea, Titanium Dioxide, Sodium Benzoate, BHT, Tri(PPG-3 Myristyl Ether) Citrate, Disodium Edetate, Retinyl Palmitate, Tocopheryl Acetate, Sodium Pyruvate, Iodopropynyl Butylcarbamate, Fragrance, Sodium Hydroxide, Xanthan Gum.

Actions and Uses: Lubriderm Moisture Recovery GelCreme is recommended for patients with extra dry skin. It's patented emollient system contains vitamins, nutrients, and antioxidants to heal and protect dry skin. The unique formulation combines the richness of a creme with the light feel of a gel.

Administration and Dosage: Apply to hands and body.

Precautions: For external use only.

How Supplied: Available in .75, 4, and 7.5 fl. oz. plastic bottles.
Shown in Product Identification Guide, page 526

LUBRIDERM® Seriously Sensitive Lotion
[lū brĭ dĕrm]

Composition: Contains Water, Butylene Glycol, Mineral Oil, Petrolatum, Glycerin, Cetyl Alcohol, Propylene Glycol Dicaprylate/Dicaprate, PEG-40 Stearate, C11-C13 Isoparaffin, Glyceryl Stearate, Tri (PPG-3 Myristyl Ether) Citrate, Emulsifying Wax, Dimethicone, DMDM Hydantoin, Methylparaben, Carbomer 940, Ethylparaben, Propylparaben, Titanium Dioxide, Disodium EDTA, Sodium Hydroxide, Butylparaben, Xanthan Gum.

Action and Uses: Lubriderm Seriously Sensitive Lotion's unique combination of emollients provides sensitive dry skin with the moisture it needs while helping to create a protective layer. It is noncomedogenic, and 100% lanolin free, fragrance free, and dye free so its appropriate for skin that is sensitive to these ingredients. It is lightweight, nongreasy, and absorbs quickly.

Administration and Dosage: Apply to hands and body to help protect and heal sensitive dry skin.

Precautions: For external use only.

How Supplied: Available in 1, 6, 10, and 16 fl. oz. plastic bottles.
Shown in Product Identification Guide, page 526

NEOSPORIN® Ointment
[nē'uh-spō'rŭn]

Each Gram Contains: Polymyxin B Sulfate 5,000 units, Bacitracin Zinc 400 units and Neomycin 3.5 mg in a special White Petrolatum Base.

Indications: First aid to help prevent infection in minor cuts, scrapes, and burns.

Directions: Clean the affected area. Apply a small amount of this product (an amount equal to the surface area of the tip of a finger) on the area 1 to 3 times daily. May be covered with a sterile bandage.

Warnings: For external use only. Stop use and consult a physician if the condition persists or gets worse, or if a rash or other allergic reaction develops. Do not use this product if you are allergic to any of the listed ingredients. Do not use in the eyes or apply over large areas of the body. In case of deep or puncture wounds, animal bites, or serious burns, consult a physician. Do not use longer than 1 week unless directed by a physician. Keep this and all drugs out of the reach of children. In case of accidental ingestion, seek professional assistance or contact a Poison Control Center immediately.

How Supplied: Tubes, ½ oz (14.2 g) (with applicator tip), 1 oz (28.4 g); ¹⁄₃₂ oz (0.9 g) (approx.) foil packets packed 10 per box (Neo To Go™) or 144 per box.

Store at 15° to 25°C (59° to 77°F).
Professional Labeling: Consult *1996 Physicians' Desk Reference®*.
Shown in Product Identification Guide, page 526

NEOSPORIN® PLUS MAXIMUM STRENGTH Cream
[nē"uh-spō'rŭn]

Each Gram Contains: Polymyxin B Sulfate 10,000 units, Neomycin 3.5 mg,

Continued on next page

This product information was prepared in November 1995. On these and other Warner Wellcome Consumer HealthCare Products, detailed information may be obtained by addressing Warner Wellcome Consumer HealthCare Products, Warner-Lambert, Morris Plains, NJ 07950

Warner Wellcome—Cont.

and Lidocaine 40 mg. Also contains: Methylparaben 0.25% (added as a preservative), Emulsifying Wax, Mineral Oil, Poloxamer 188, Propylene Glycol, Purified Water, and White Petrolatum. Pramoxine Hydrochloride will replace Lidocaine starting April 1996.

Indications: First aid to help prevent infection and provide temporary relief of pain or discomfort in minor cuts, scrapes, and burns.

Directions: Adults and children 2 years of age and older: Clean the affected area. Apply a small amount of this product (an amount equal to the surface area of the tip of a finger) on the area 1 to 3 times daily. May be covered with a sterile bandage. **Children under 2 years of age: Consult a physician.**

Warnings: For external use only. If condition worsens, or if symptoms persist for more than 1 week or clear up and occur again within a few days, or if a rash or other allergic reaction develops, discontinue use of this product and consult a physician. Do not use this product if you are allergic to any of the listed ingredients. Do not use in the eyes or apply over large areas of the body. Do not use in large quantities, particularly over raw surfaces or blistered areas. In case of deep or puncture wounds, animal bites, or serious burns, consult a physician. Do not use longer than 1 week unless directed by a physician. Keep this and all drugs out of the reach of children. In case of accidental ingestion, seek professional assistance or contact a Poison Control Center immediately.

How Supplied: ½ oz (14.2 g) tubes. Store at 15° to 25°C (59° to 77°F).

Shown in Product Identification Guide, page 526

NEOSPORIN® PLUS MAXIMUM STRENGTH Ointment
[nē "uh-spō 'rŭn]

Each Gram Contains: Polymyxin B Sulfate 10,000 units, Bacitracin Zinc 500 units, Neomycin 3.5 mg, and Lidocaine 40 mg in a special White Petrolatum Base. Pramoxine Hydrochloride will replace Lidocaine starting April 1996.

Indications: First aid to help prevent infection and provide temporary relief of pain or discomfort in minor cuts, scrapes, and burns.

Directions: Adults and children 2 years of age and older: Clean the affected area. Apply a small amount of this product (an amount equal to the surface area of the tip of a finger) on the area 1 to 3 times daily. May be covered with a sterile bandage. **Children under 2 years of age: Consult a physician.**

Warnings: For external use only. If condition worsens, or if symptoms persist for more than 1 week or clear up and oc-

cur again within a few days, or if a rash or other allergic reaction develops, discontinue use of this product and consult a physician. Do not use this product if you are allergic to any of the listed ingredients. Do not use in the eyes or apply over large areas of the body. Do not use in large quantities, particularly over raw surfaces or blistered areas. In case of deep or puncture wounds, animal bites, or serious burns, consult a physician. Do not use longer than 1 week unless directed by a physician. Keep this and all drugs out of the reach of children. In case of accidental ingestion, seek professional assistance or contact a Poison Control Center immediately.

How Supplied: ½ oz (14.2 g) and 1 oz (28.4 g) tubes. Store at 15° to 25°C (59° to 77°F).

Shown in Product Identification Guide, page 526

NIX® Creme Rinse
Permethrin
Lice Treatment
[nĭks]

Each Fluid Ounce Contains: Permethrin 280 mg (1%). Inactive ingredients are: Balsam Canada, Cetyl Alcohol, Citric Acid, FD&C Yellow No. 6, Fragrance, Hydrolyzed Animal Protein, Hydroxyethylcellulose, Polyoxyethylene 10 Cetyl Ether, Propylene Glycol, and Stearalkonium Chloride. Also contains: Isopropyl Alcohol 5.6 g (20%) and added as preservatives, Methylparaben 56 mg (0.2%) and Propylparaben 22 mg (0.08%).

Product Benefits: Nix Creme Rinse kills lice and their unhatched eggs with only one application. Nix protects against head lice reinfestation for a full 14 days. The unique creme rinse formula leaves hair manageable and easy to comb.

Indications: For the treatment of head lice.

Directions for Use: Nix Creme Rinse should be used after hair has been washed with your regular shampoo, rinsed with water and towel dried. A sufficient amount should be applied to saturate hair and scalp (especially behind the ears and on nape of the neck). Leave on hair for 10 minutes but no longer. Rinse with water. A single application is sufficient. Retreatment is required in less than 1% of patients. If live lice are observed seven days or more after the first application of this product, a second treatment should be given. For proper head lice management, remove nits with the nit comb provided.
Head lice live on the scalp and lay small white eggs (nits) on the hair shaft close to the scalp. The nits are most easily found on the nape of the neck or behind the ears. All personal headgear, scarfs, coats, and bed linen should be disinfected by machine washing in hot water and drying, using the hot cycle of a dryer for at

least 20 minutes. Personal articles of clothing or bedding that cannot be washed may be dry-cleaned, sealed in a plastic bag for a period of about 2 weeks, or sprayed with a product specifically designed for this purpose. Personal combs and brushes may be disinfected by soaking in hot water (above 130°F) for 5 to 10 minutes. Thorough vacuuming of rooms inhabited by infected patients is recommended.
Shake well before using.

Warnings: For external use only. Itching, redness, or swelling of the scalp may occur. If skin irritation persists or infection is present or develops, discontinue use and consult a doctor. Do not use near the eyes or permit contact with mucous membranes. If product gets into the eyes, immediately flush with water. Consult a doctor if infestation of eyebrows or eyelashes occurs. This product may cause breathing difficulty or an asthmatic episode in susceptible persons. This product should not be used on children less than 2 months of age. As with any drug, if you are pregnant or nursing a baby, seek the advice of a health professional before using this product. Keep this and all drugs out of the reach of children. In case of accidental ingestion, seek professional assistance or contact a Poison Control Center immediately.
Store at 15° to 25°C (59° to 77°F).

How Supplied: Bottles of 2 fl oz (50 mL) with special comb and Family Pack of 2 bottles, 2 fl oz (50 mL) each, with special comb.

Shown in Product Identification Guide, page 526

POLYSPORIN® Ointment
[pŏl 'ē-spō 'rŭn]

Each Gram Contains: Polymyxin B Sulfate 10,000 units and Bacitracin Zinc 500 units in a special White Petrolatum Base.

Indications: First aid to help prevent infection in minor cuts, scrapes, and burns.

Directions: Clean the affected area. Apply a small amount of this product (an amount equal to the surface area of the tip of a finger) on the area 1 to 3 times daily. May be covered with a sterile bandage.

Warnings: For external use only. Stop use and consult a physician if the condition persists or gets worse, or if a rash or other allergic reaction develops. Do not use this product if you are allergic to any of the listed ingredients. Do not use in the eyes or apply over large areas of the body. In case of deep or puncture wounds, animal bites, or serious burns, consult a physician. Do not use longer than 1 week unless directed by a physician. Keep this and all drugs out of the reach of children. In case of accidental ingestion, seek professional assistance or contact a Poison Control Center immediately.

How Supplied: Tubes, ½ oz (14.2 g) with applicator tip, 1 oz (28.4 g); 1/32 oz (0.9 g) (approx.) foil packets packed in cartons of 144.
Store at 15° to 25°C (59° to 77°F).
Shown in Product Identification Guide, page 526

POLYSPORIN® Powder
[pŏl 'ē-spō 'rŭn]

Each Gram Contains: Polymyxin B Sulfate 10,000 units and Bacitracin Zinc 500 units in a Lactose Base.

Indications: First aid to help prevent infection in minor cuts, scrapes, and burns.

Directions: Clean the affected area. Apply a light dusting of the powder on the area 1 to 3 times daily. May be covered with a sterile bandage.

Warnings: For external use only. Stop use and consult a physician if the condition persists or gets worse, or if a rash or other allergic reaction develops. Do not use this product if you are allergic to any of the listed ingredients. Do not use in the eyes or apply over large areas of the body. In case of deep or puncture wounds, animal bites, or serious burns, consult a physician. Do not use longer than 1 week unless directed by a physician. Keep this and all drugs out of the reach of children. In case of accidental ingestion, seek professional assistance or contact a Poison Control Center immediately.

How Supplied: 0.35 oz (10 g) shaker-vial.
Store at 15° to 25°C (59° to 77°F). Do not store under refrigeration.
Shown in Product Identification Guide, page 526

REPLENS® Vaginal Moisturizer
[ree 'plenz]

Ingredients: Purified Water, Glycerin, Mineral Oil, Polycarbophil, Carbomer 934P, Hydrogenated Palm Oil Glyceride, and Sorbic Acid.

Description: Replens relieves the discomfort of vaginal dryness for days with a single application. Replens non-hormonal vaginal moisturizer provides natural feeling moisture to continuously hydrate vaginal tissue. Replens is non-staining, fragrance free, non-greasy and non-irritating Estrogen-Free.

Actions: When used as directed, Replens provides long-lasting relief from the discomfort of vaginal dryness by providing continuous hydration to the vaginal tissue.

Warnings: Keep out of the reach of children. Replens is not a contraceptive. Does not contain spermicide. If vaginal irritation occurs, discontinue use. If symptoms persist, contact your physician.

Usage: Use as needed. One single application approximately once every 2 to 3 days is recommended.

How Supplied: Replens is available in boxes containing 3 or 8 pre-filled disposable applicators. Each applicator delivers 2.5 grams.
Store at room temperature (59°–86°F). Avoid exposure to extreme heat or cold.
Shown in Product Identification Guide, page 526

SINUTAB® Non-Drying Liquid Caps
[sîn 'ū tăb]

Active Ingredients: Each liquid cap contains: Pseudoephedrine Hydrochloride 30 mg., Guaifenesin 200 mg.

Inactive Ingredients: FD&C Blue No. 1, Gelatin, Glycerin, Polyethylene Glycol 400, Povidone, Propylene Glycol, and Sorbitol.

Indications: Temporarily relieves nasal congestion associated with sinusitis. Helps loosen phlegm (mucus) and thin bronchial secretions to drain bronchial tubes.

Dosage and Administration: Adults and children 12 years of age and over: swallow 2 liquid caps every 4 hours, not to exceed 8 liquid caps in 24 hours, or as directed by a doctor. Children under 12 years of age, consult a doctor.

Warnings: Do not exceed recommended dosage. If nervousness, dizziness, or sleeplessness occur, discontinue use and consult a doctor. If symptoms do not improve within 7 days or are accompanied by fever, consult a doctor. Do not take this product if you have heart disease, high blood pressure, thyroid disease, diabetes, or difficulty in urination due to enlargement of the prostate gland unless directed by a doctor. Do not take this product for persistent or chronic cough such as occurs with smoking, asthma, chronic bronchitis, or emphysema, or where cough is accompanied by excessive phlegm (mucus) unless directed by a doctor. A persistent cough may be a sign of a serious condition. If cough persists for more than 1 week, tends to recur, or is accompanied by a fever, rash, or persistent headache, consult a doctor. As with any drug, if you are pregnant or nursing a baby, seek the advice of a health professional before using this product.
KEEP THIS AND ALL DRUGS OUT OF THE REACH OF CHILDREN. In case of accidental overdose, seek professional assistance or contact a Poison Control Center immediately.

Drug Interaction Precaution: Do not use this product if you are now taking a prescription monoamine oxidase inhibitor (MAOI) (certain drugs for depression, psychiatric or emotional conditions, or Parkinson's disease), or for 2 weeks after stopping the MAOI drug. If you are uncertain whether your prescription drug contains an MAOI, consult a health professional before taking this product.

How Supplied: Sinutab® Non-Drying supplied in a box of 24 liquid caps.
Shown in Product Identification Guide, page 526

SINUTAB® Sinus Allergy Medication, Maximum Strength Formula, Tablets and Caplets
[sîn 'ū tăb]

Active Ingredients: Each tablet/caplet contains: Acetaminophen 500 mg., Chlorpheniramine Maleate 2 mg., Pseudoephedrine Hydrochloride 30 mg.

Inactive Ingredients:
Tablets contain: Croscarmellose Sodium, Crospovidone, D&C Yellow No. 10 Aluminum Lake, FD&C Yellow No. 6 Aluminum Lake, Microcrystalline Cellulose, Povidone, Pregelatinized Starch, Stearic Acid, and Zinc Stearate.
Caplets contain: Carnauba Wax, Croscarmellose Sodium, Crospovidone, D&C Yellow No. 10 Aluminum Lake, FD&C Yellow No. 6 Aluminum Lake, Hydroxypropyl Cellulose, Hydroxypropyl Methylcellulose, Microcrystalline Cellulose, Polyethylene Glycol, Povidone, Pregelatinized Starch, Stearic Acid, Titanium Dioxide, and Zinc Stearate.

Indications: For the temporary relief of minor aches, pains and headache and nasal congestion associated with sinusitis. Temporarily relieves runny nose, sneezing itching of the nose or throat, and itchy watery eyes due to hay fever or other upper respiratory allergies.

Product Benefits: Sinutab® Sinus Allergy Medication, Maximum Strength Formula, Tablets and Caplets contain an analgesic (acetaminophen) to relieve pain, a decongestant (pseudoephedrine hydrochloride) to reduce congestion of the nasopharyngeal mucosa, and an antihistamine (chlorpheniramine maleate) to help control allergic symptoms.
Acetaminophen is both analgesic and antipyretic. Because acetaminophen is not a salicylate, Sinutab® Sinus Allergy Medication, Maximum Strength Formula, Tablets and Caplets can be used by patients who are allergic to aspirin.
Pseudoephedrine hydrochloride, a sympathomimetic drug, provides vasoconstriction of the nasopharyngeal mucosa resulting in a nasal decongestant effect.

Continued on next page

This product information was prepared in November 1995. On these and other Warner Wellcome Consumer HealthCare Products, detailed information may be obtained by addressing Warner Wellcome Consumer HealthCare Products, Warner-Lambert, Morris Plains, NJ 07950

Warner Wellcome—Cont.

Chlorpheniramine maleate is an antihistamine incorporated to provide relief of running nose, sneezing, itching of the nose or throat, and itchy and watery eyes as may occur in allergic rhinitis.

Dosage and Administration: Adults and children 12 years of age and over: 2 tablets or caplets every 6 hours while symptoms persist, not to exceed 8 tablets or caplets in 24 hours, or as directed by physician. Children under 12 years of age: consult a doctor.

Warnings: Do not exceed recommended dosage. If nervousness, dizziness, or sleeplessness occur, discontinue use and consult a doctor. Do not take this product for more than 10 days. If symptoms do not improve or are accompanied by fever that lasts for more than 3 days, or if new symptoms occur, consult a doctor. Do not take this product, unless directed by a doctor, if you have heart disease, high blood pressure, thyroid disease, diabetes, a breathing problem such as emphysema or chronic bronchitis, or if you have glaucoma or difficulty in urination due to enlargement of the prostate gland. May cause excitability especially in children. May cause drowsiness; alcohol, sedatives, and tranquilizers may increase the drowsiness effect. Avoid alcoholic beverages while taking this product. Do not take this product if you are taking sedatives or tranquilizers, without first consulting your doctor. Use caution when driving a motor vehicle or operating machinery. As with any drug, if you are pregnant or nursing a baby, seek the advice of a health professional before using this product. **KEEP THIS AND ALL DRUGS OUT OF THE REACH OF CHILDREN.** In case of accidental overdose, seek professional assistance or contact a Poison Control Center immediately. Prompt medical attention is critical for adults as well as for children even if you do not notice any signs or symptoms.

Drug Interaction Precaution: Do not use this product if you are now taking a prescription monoamine oxidase inhibitor (MAOI) (certain drugs for depression, psychiatric or emotional conditions, or Parkinson's disease), or for 2 weeks after stopping the MAOI drug. If you are uncertain whether your prescription drug contains an MAOI, consult a health professional before taking this product.

How Supplied: Sinutab® Sinus Allergy Medication, Maximum Strength Formula, Caplets and Tablets are supplied in child-resistant blister packs in boxes of 24 tablets or caplets.

Store at room temperature (59°–86°F).
Shown in Product Identification Guide, page 527

SINUTAB® Sinus Medication, Maximum Strength Without Drowsiness Formula, Tablets and Caplets
[sîn 'ū tăb]

Active Ingredients: Each tablet/caplet contains: Acetaminophen 500 mg., Pseudoephedrine Hydrochloride 30 mg.

Inactive Ingredients:
Tablets contain: Croscarmellose Sodium, Crospovidone, D&C Yellow No. 10 Aluminum Lake, FD&C Yellow No. 6 Aluminum Lake, Microcrystalline Cellulose, Povidone, Pregelatinized Starch, Stearic Acid, and Zinc Stearate.
Caplets contain: Carnauba Wax, Croscarmellose Sodium, Crospovidone, D&C Yellow No. 10 Aluminum Lake, FD&C Yellow No. 6 Aluminum Lake, Hydroxypropyl Cellulose, Hydroxypropyl Methylcellulose, Microcrystalline Cellulose, Polyethylene Glycol, Povidone, Pregelatinized Starch, Stearic Acid, Titanium Dioxide, and Zinc Stearate.

Indications: For the temporary relief of minor aches, pains, and headache, nasal congestion associated with sinusitis.

Product Benefits: Sinutab® Sinus Medication, Maximum Strength Without Drowsiness Formula, Tablets and Caplets contain an analgesic (acetaminophen) to relieve pain, and a decongestant (pseudoephedrine hydrochloride) to reduce congestion of the nasopharyngeal mucosa.
Acetaminophen is both analgesic and antipyretic. Because acetaminophen is not a salicylate, Sinutab® Sinus Medication, Maximum Strength Without Drowsiness Formula, can be used by patients who are allergic to aspirin.
Pseudoephedrine hydrochloride, a sympathomimetic drug, provides vasoconstriction of the nasopharyngeal mucosa resulting in a nasal decongestant effect. The absence of antihistamine in the formula provides the added benefit of reduced likelihood of drowsiness side effects.

Dosage and Administration: Adults and children 12 years of age and over: 2 tablets or caplets every 6 hours while symptoms persist, not to exceed 8 tablets or caplets in 24 hours or as directed by physician. Children under 12 years of age: consult a doctor.

Warnings: Do not exceed recommended dosage. If nervousness, dizziness, or sleeplessness occur, discontinue use and consult a doctor. Do not take this product for more than 10 days. If symptoms do not improve or are accompanied by fever that lasts for more than 3 days, or if new symptoms occur, consult a doctor. Do not take this product if you have heart disease, high blood pressure, thyroid disease, diabetes or difficulty in urination due to enlargement of the prostate gland unless directed by a doctor. As with any drug, if you are pregnant or nursing a baby, seek the advice of a health professional before using this product. **KEEP THIS AND ALL DRUGS**

OUT OF THE REACH OF CHILDREN. In case of accidental overdose, seek professional assistance or contact a Poison Control Center immediately. Prompt medical attention is critical for adults as well as for children even if you do not notice any signs or symptoms.

Drug Interaction Precaution: Do not use this product if you are now taking a prescription monoamine oxidase inhibitor (MAOI) (certain drugs for depression, psychiatric or emotional conditions, or Parkinson's disease), or for 2 weeks after stopping the MAOI drug. If you are uncertain whether your prescription drug contains an MAOI, consult a health professional before taking this product.

How Supplied: Sinutab® Sinus Medication, Maximum Strength Without Drowsiness Formula, Caplets and Tablets are supplied in child-resistant blister packs in boxes of 24 tablets or caplets and in boxes of 48 caplets.
Shown in Product Identification Guide, page 527

SUDAFED® 12 Hour Caplets
[sū 'duh-fĕd]

Active Ingredient: Each coated extended-release caplet contains Pseudoephedrine Hydrochloride 120 mg in a capsule-shaped tablet.

Inactive Ingredients: Hydroxypropyl Methylcellulose, Magnesium Stearate, Microcrystalline Cellulose, Polyethylene Glycol, Povidone, and Titanium Dioxide. Printed with edible blue ink.

Indications: For temporary relief of nasal congestion due to the common cold, hay fever, or other upper respiratory allergies, and nasal congestion associated with sinusitis; promotes nasal and/or sinus drainage.

Directions: Adults and children 12 years and over—One caplet every 12 hours, not to exceed two caplets in 24 hours. Sudafed 12 Hour is not recommended for children under 12 years of age.

Warnings: Do not exceed recommended dosage because at higher doses, nervousness, dizziness, or sleeplessness may occur. Do not take this product if you have heart disease, high blood pressure, thyroid disease, diabetes, or difficulty in urination due to enlargement of the prostate gland unless directed by a doctor. If symptoms do not improve within 7 days or are accompanied by fever, consult your doctor before continuing use. As with any drug, if you are pregnant or nursing a baby, seek the advice of a health professional before using this product.

Drug Interaction Precaution: Do not take this product if you are presently taking a prescription drug for high blood pressure or depression, without first consulting your doctor.
KEEP THIS AND ALL DRUGS OUT OF THE REACH OF CHILDREN. In

case of accidental overdose, seek professional assistance or contact a Poison Control Center immediately.

How Supplied: Boxes of 10 and 20. Store at 15° to 25°C (59° to 77°F) in a dry place and protect from light.
Shown in Product Identification Guide, page 527

SUDAFED® Nasal Decongestant Tablets 30 mg.
[sū 'duh-fĕd]

Active Ingredient: Each tablet contains Pseudoephedrine Hydrochloride 30 mg.

Inactive Ingredients: Acacia, Carnauba Wax, Corn Starch, Dibasic Calcium Phosphate, FD&C Red No. 40 Aluminum Lake, FD&C Yellow No. 6 Aluminum Lake, Magnesium Stearate, Pharmaceutical Glaze, Polysorbate 60, Potato Starch, Povidone, Sodium Benzoate, Stearic Acid, Sucrose, Talc, and Titanium Dioxide. Printed with edible black ink.

Indications: For the temporary relief of nasal congestion due to the common cold, hay fever or other upper respiratory allergies, and nasal congestion associated with sinusitis. Helps decongest sinus openings and passages; temporarily relieves sinus congestion and pressure. Temporarily restores freer breathing through the nose.

Directions: To be given every 4 to 6 hours. Do not exceed 4 doses in 24 hours. Adults and children 12 years of age and over: 2 tablets. Children 6 to under 12 years of age, 1 tablet. Children 2 to under 6 years of age, use Children's Sudafed Liquid. For children under 2 years of age, consult a doctor.

Warnings: Do not exceed recommended dosage. If nervousness, dizziness or sleeplessness occur, discontinue use and consult a doctor. If symptoms do not improve within 7 days, or are accompanied by fever, consult a doctor. Do not take this product if you have heart disease, high blood pressure, thyroid disease, diabetes, or difficulty in urination due to enlargement of the prostate gland, unless directed by a doctor. As with any drug, if you are pregnant or nursing a baby, seek the advice of a health professional before using this product. **KEEP THIS AND ALL DRUGS OUT OF THE REACH OF CHILDREN.** In case of accidental overdose, seek professional assistance or contact a Poison Control Center immediately.

Drug Interaction Precaution: Do not use this product if you are now taking a prescription monoamine oxidase inhibitor (MAOI) (certain drugs for depression, psychiatric or emotional conditions, or Parkinson's disease), or for 2 weeks after stoppping the MAOI drug. If you are uncertain whether your prescription drug contains an MAOI, consult a health professional before taking this product.

How Supplied: Boxes of 24, 48. Bottles of 100. Institutional Pack. Carton of 500 x 2.
Store at 15° to 25°C (59°–77°F) in a dry place and protect from light.
Shown in Product Identification Guide, page 527

SUDAFED® Nasal Decongestant Tablets 60 mg.
[sū 'duh-fĕd]

Active Ingredient: Each coated tablet contains Pseudoephedrine Hydrochloride 60 mg.

Inactive Ingredients: Acacia, Carnauba Wax, Corn Starch, Dibasic Calcium Phosphate, Hydroxypropyl Methylcellulose, Magnesium Stearate, Pharmaceutical Glaze, Polysorbate 60, Pregelantinized Corn Starch, Sodium Starch Glycolate, Stearic Acid, Sucrose, Talc, and Titanium Dioxide. Printed with edible red ink.

Indications: For the temporary relief of nasal congestion due to the common cold, hay fever or other upper respiratory allergies, and nasal congestion associated with sinusitis. Helps decongest sinus openings and passages; temporarily relieves sinus congestion and pressure. Temporarily restores freer breathing through the nose.

Directions: To be given every 4 to 6 hours. Do not exceed 4 doses in 24 hours. Adults and children 12 years of age and over, 1 tablet. Children 6 to under 12 years of age, use Sudafed 30 mg Tablets. Children 2 to under 6 years of age, use Children's Sudafed Liquid. Children under 2 years of age, consult a doctor.

Warnings: Do not exceed recommended dosage. If nervousness, dizziness or sleeplessness occur, discontinue use and consult a doctor. If symptoms do not improve within 7 days, or are accompanied by a fever, consult a doctor. Do not take this product if you have heart disease, high blood pressure, thyroid disease, diabetes, or difficulty in urination due to enlargement of the prostate gland, unless directed by a doctor. As with any drug, if you are pregnant or nursing a baby, seek the advice of a health professional before using this product. **KEEP THIS AND ALL DRUGS OUT OF THE REACH OF CHILDREN.** In case of accidental overdose, seek professional assistance or contact a Poison Control Center immediately.

Drug Interaction Precaution: Do not use this product if you are now taking a prescription monoamine oxidase inhibitor (MAOI) (certain drugs for depression, psychiatric or emotional conditions, or Parkinson's disease), or for 2 weeks after stopping the MAOI drug. If you are uncertain whether your prescription drug contains an MAOI, consult a health professional before taking this product.

How Supplied: Bottles of 100. Store at 15° to 25°C (59°–77°F) in a dry place and protect from light.
Shown in Product Identification Guide, page 527

SUDAFED® CHILDREN'S COLD & COUGH LIQUID MEDICATION
[sū 'duh-fĕd]

Active Ingredients: Each teaspoonful (5 mL) contains Guaifenesin 100 mg, Pseudoephedrine Hydrochloride 15 mg, and Dextromethorphan Hydrobromide 5 mg.

Inactive Ingredients: Caramel, Citric Acid, D&C Red No. 33, Edetate Disodium, FD&C Red No. 40, Flavors, Poloxamer 407, Polyethylene Glycol 1450, Propyl Gallate, Propylene Glycol, Purified Water, Saccharin Sodium, Sodium Benzoate, Sodium Chloride, Sodium Citrate and Sorbitol Solution.

Indications: For the temporary relief of nasal congestion due to the common cold; temporarily quiets cough due to minor throat and bronchial irritation occurring with a cold. Suppresses cough impulses without narcotics. Helps loosen phlegm (mucus) and thin bronchial secretions to rid the bronchial passageways of bothersome mucus and make coughs more productive.

Directions: Follow dosage recommendations below, or as directed by a doctor. Dosage may be repeated every 4 hours, not to exceed 4 doses in 24 hours.

Age	Dosage
Children under 2 years of age	Consult a doctor
Children 2 to under 6 years of age	One (1) teaspoonful
Children 6 to under 12 years of age	Two (2) teaspoonfuls
Adults and children 12 years of of age and over	Four (4) teaspoonfuls

Warnings: Do not exceed recommended dosage. If nervousness, dizziness, or sleeplessness occur, discontinue use and consult a doctor. If symptoms do not improve within 7 days or are accompanied by fever, consult a doctor. Do not take this product if you have heart dis-

Continued on next page

This product information was prepared in November 1995. On these and other Warner Wellcome Consumer HealthCare Products, detailed information may be obtained by addressing Warner Wellcome Consumer HealthCare Products, Warner-Lambert, Morris Plains, NJ 07950

Warner Wellcome—Cont.

ease, high blood pressure, thyroid disease, diabetes, or difficulty in urination due to enlargement of the prostate gland unless directed by a doctor. A persistent cough may be a sign of a serious condition. If cough persists for more than 1 week, tends to recur, or is accompanied by a fever, rash, or persistent headache, consult a doctor. Do not take this product for persistent or chronic cough such as occurs with smoking, asthma, chronic bronchitis, or emphysema, or where cough is accompanied by excessive phlegm (mucus) unless directed by a doctor. As with any drug, if you are pregnant or nursing a baby, seek the advice of a health professional before using this product. **KEEP THIS AND ALL DRUGS OUT OF THE REACH OF CHILDREN.** In case of accidental overdose, seek professional assistance or contact a Poison Control Center immediately.

Drug Interaction Precaution: Do not use this product if you are now taking a prescription monoamine oxidase inhibitor (MAOI) (certain drugs for depression, psychiatric or emotional conditions, or Parkinson's disease), or 2 weeks after stopping the MAOI drug. If you are uncertain whether your prescription drug contains an MAOI, consult a health professional before taking this product.

How Supplied: Sudafed Children's Cold & Cough is supplied in 4 fl. oz. bottles
Store at 15° to 25°C (59° to 77°F) and protect from light.
Shown in Product Identification Guide, page 527

SUDAFED® CHILDREN'S NASAL DECONGESTANT LIQUID MEDICATION
[sū ' duh-fĕd]

Active Ingredient: Each teaspoonful (5 mL) contains Pseudoephedrine Hydrochloride 15 mg.

Inactive Ingredients: Citric Acid, Edetate Disodium, FD&C Red No. 40, FD&C Blue No. 1, Flavors, Glycerin, Poloxamer 407, Polyethylene Glycol 1450, Povidone K-90, Purified Water, Saccharin Sodium, Sodium Benzoate, Sodium Citrate and Sorbitol Solution.

Indications: For the temporary relief of nasal congestion due to the common cold, hay fever or other upper respiratory allergies, and nasal congestion associated with sinusitis. Promotes nasal and/or sinus drainage; temporarily relieves sinus congestion and pressure.

Directions: Follow dosage recommendations below. Dosage may be repeated every 4 to 6 hours, not to exceed 4 doses in 24 hours.

Age	Dosage
Children under 2 years of age	Consult a doctor
Children 2 to under 6 years of age	One (1) teaspoonful
Children 6 to under 12 years of age	Two (2) teaspoonfuls
Adults and children 12 years of age and over	Four (4) teaspoonfuls

Warnings: Do not exceed recommended dosage. If nervousness, dizziness, or sleeplessness occur, discontinue use and consult a doctor. If symptoms do not improve within 7 days or are accompanied by fever, consult a doctor. Do not take product if you have heart disease, high blood pressure, thyroid disease, diabetes, or difficulty in urination due to enlargement of the prostate gland unless directed by a doctor. As with any drug, if you are pregnant or nursing a baby, seek the advice of a health professional before using this product. **KEEP THIS AND ALL DRUGS OUT OF THE REACH OF CHILDREN.** In case of accidental overdose, seek professional assistance or contact a Poison Control Center immediately.

Drug Interaction Precaution: Do not use this product if you are now taking a prescription monoamine oxidase inhibitor (MAOI) (certain drugs for depression, psychiatric or emotional conditions, or Parkinson's disease), or for 2 weeks after stopping the MAOI drug. If you are uncertain whether your prescription drug contains an MAOI, consult a health professional before taking this product.

How Supplied: Sudafed Children's Nasal Decongestant is supplied in 4 fl. oz. bottles
Store at 15° to 25°C (59° to 77°F) and protect from light.
Shown in Product Identification Guide, page 527

SUDAFED® Cold & Allergy Tablets
[sū 'duh-fĕd]

Active Ingredients: Each tablet contains: Chlorpheniramine Maleate 4 mg. and Pseudoephedrine Hydrochloride 60 mg.

Inactive Ingredients: Lactose, Magnesium Stearate, Potato Starch, and Povidone.

Indications: Temporary relieves nasal congestion due to the common cold; dries runny nose and alleviates sneezing, itching of the nose or throat, and itchy, watery eyes due to hay fever or other upper respiratory allergies.

Directions: To be given every 4 to 6 hours. Do not exceed 4 doses in 24 hours, or as directed by a doctor. Adults and children 12 years of age and over, 1 tab-

let. Children 6 to under 12 years of age, ½ tablet. Children under 6 years of age: consult a doctor.

Product Benefits: For the temporary relief of nasal or sinus congestion, sneezing, runny nose, and itchy, water eyes associated with the common cold, hay fever, or other upper respiratory allergies.

Warnings: Do not exceed recommended dosage. If nervousness, dizziness, or sleeplessness occur, discontinue use and consult a doctor. If symptoms do not improve within 7 days or are accompanied by fever, consult a doctor. Do not take this product, unless directed by a doctor, if you have a breathing problem such as emphysema or chronic bronchitis, heart disease, high blood pressure, thyroid disease, diabetes, or if you have glaucoma or difficulty in urination due to enlargement of the prostate gland. May cause excitability especially in children. May cause drowsiness; alcohol, sedatives, and tranquilizers may increase the drowsiness effect. Avoid alcoholic beverages while taking this product. Do not take this product if you are taking sedatives or tranquilizers, without first consulting your doctor. Use caution when driving a motor vehicle or operating machinery. As with any drug, if you are pregnant or nursing a baby, seek the advice of a health professional before using this product. **KEEP THIS AND ALL DRUGS OUT OF THE REACH OF CHILDREN.** In case of accidental overdose, seek professional assistance or contact a Poison Control Center immediately.

Drug Interaction Precaution: Do not use this product if you are now taking a prescription monoamine oxidase inhibitor (MAOI) (certain drugs for depression, psychiatric or emotional conditions, or Parkinson's disease), or for 2 weeks after stopping the MAOI drug. If you are uncertain whether your prescription drug contains an MAOI, consult a health professional before taking this product.

How Supplied: Boxes of 24 and 48. Store at 15° to 25° C (59°–77°F) in a dry place and protect from light.
Shown in Product Identification Guide, page 527

SUDAFED® Cold & Cough Liquid Caps
[sū 'duh-fĕd]

Active Ingredients: Each liquid cap contains: Acetaminophen 250 mg, Guaifenesin 100 mg, Pseudoephedrine Hydrochloride 30 mg, and Destromethorphan Hydrobromide 10 mg.

Inactive Ingredients: D&C Yellow No. 10, FD&C Red No. 40, Gelatin, Glycerin, Polyethylene Glycol 400, Povidone, Propylene Glycol, Purified Water, and Sorbitol. Printed with edible white ink.

Indications: For the temporary relief of nasal congestion, minor aches, pains, headache, muscular aches, sore throat, and fever associated with the common cold. Temporarily relieves cough occurring with a cold. Helps loosen phlegm (mucus) and thin bronchial secretions to drain bronchial tubes and make coughs more productive.

Directions: Adults and children 12 years of age and over, 2 liquid caps every 4 hours, while symptoms persist, not to exceed 8 liquid caps in 24 hours, or as directed by a doctor. Not recommended for children under 12 years of age.

Warnings: Do not exceed recommended dosage. If nervousness, dizziness, or sleeplessness occur, discontinue use and consult a doctor. Do not take this product for more than 10 days. A persistent cough may be a sign of a serious condition. If symptoms do not improve of if cough persists for more than 7 days, tends to recur, or is accompanied by rash, persistent headache, fever that lasts for more than 3 days, or if new symptoms occur, consult a doctor. Do not take this product for persistent or chronic cough such as occurs with smoking, asthma, chronic bronchitis, emphysema, or where cough is accompanied by excessive phlegm (mucus) unless directed by a doctor. If sore throat is severe, persists for more than 2 days, is accompanied or followed by fever, headache, rash, nausea, or vomiting, consult a doctor promptly. Do not take this product if you have heart disease, high blood pressure, thyroid disease, diabetes, or difficulty in urination due to enlargement of the prostate gland unless directed by a doctor. As with any drug, if you are pregnant or nursing a baby, seek the advice of a health professional before using this product. **KEEP THIS AND ALL DRUGS OUT OF THE REACH OF CHILDREN.** In case of accidental overdose, seek professional assistance or contact a Poison Control Center immediately. Prompt medical attention is critical for adults as well as for children even if you do not notice any signs or symptoms.

Drug Interaction Precaution: Do not use this product if you are now taking a prescription monoamine oxidase inhibitor (MAOI) (certain drugs for depression, psychiatric or emotional conditions, or Parkinson's disease), or for 2 weeks after stopping the MAOI drug. If you are uncertain whether your prescription drug contains an MAOI, consult a health professional before taking this product.

How Supplied: Boxes of 10 and 20. Store at 15° to 25°C (59°–77°F) in a dry place and protect from light.
Shown in Product Identification Guide, page 527

SUDAFED® NON-DRYING SINUS LIQUID CAPS
[sū 'duh-fĕd]

Active Ingredients: Each liquid cap contains Guaifenesin 200 mg. and Pseudoephedrine Hydrochloride 30 mg.

Inactive Ingredients: FD&C Blue No. 1, Gelatin, Glycerin, Polyethylene Glycol 400, Povidone, Propylene Glycol and Sorbitol. Printed with edible white ink.

Indications: For the temporary relief of nasal congestion associated with sinusitis. Promotes nasal and/or sinus drainage; temporarily relieves sinus congestion and pressure. Helps loosen phlegm (mucus) and thin bronchial secretions to rid the bronchial passageways of bothersome mucus and make coughs more productive.

Directions: Adults and children 12 years of age and over, swallow 2 liquid caps every 4 hours, not to exceed 8 liquid caps in 24 hours, or as directed by a doctor. Children under 12 years of age should use only as directed by a doctor.

Warnings: Do not exceed recommended dosage. If nervousness, dizziness, or sleeplessness occur, discontinue use and consult a doctor. If symptoms do not improve within 7 days or are accompanied by fever, consult a doctor. Do not take this product if you have heart disease, high blood pressure, thyroid disease, diabetes, or difficulty in urination due to enlargement of the prostate gland unless directed by a doctor. A persistent cough may be a sign of a serious condition. If cough persists for more than 1 week, tends to recur, or is accompanied by a fever, rash, or persistent headache, consult a doctor. Do not take this product for persistent or chronic cough such as occurs with smoking, asthma, chronic bronchitis, or emphysema, or where cough is accompanied by excessive phlegm (mucus) unless directed by a doctor. As with any drug, if you are pregnant or nursing a baby, seek the advice of a health professional before using this product. **KEEP THIS AND ALL DRUGS OUT OF THE REACH OF CHILDREN.** In case of accidental overdose, seek professional assistance or contact a Poison Control Center immediately.

Drug Interaction Precaution: Do not use this product if you are now taking a prescription monoamine oxidase inhibitor (MAOI) (certain drugs for depression, psychiatric or emotional conditions, or Parkinson's disease), or for 2 weeks after stopping the MAOI drug. If you are uncertain whether your prescription drug contains an MAOI, consult a health professional before taking this product.

How Supplied: Sudafed Non-Drying Sinus is supplied in boxes of 24 liquid caps.
Store at 15° to 25°C (59° to 77°F) in a dry place and protect from light.
Shown in Product Identification Guide, page 527

SUDAFED® PEDIATRIC NASAL DECONGESTANT LIQUID ORAL DROPS
[sū 'duh-fĕd]

Active Ingredient: Each dropperful (0.8 mL) contains Pseudoephedrine Hydrochloride 7.5 mg.

Inactive Ingredients: Carboxymethylcellulose Sodium, Citric Acid, Flavors, Glycerin, Poloxamer 407, Purified Water, Saccharin Sodium, Sodium Benzoate, Sodium Chloride, Sodium Citrate and Sorbitol Solution.

Indications: For the temporary relief of nasal congestion due to the common cold, hay fever or other upper respiratory allergies, and nasal congestion associated with sinusitis. Promotes nasal and/or sinus drainage; temporarily relieves sinus congestion and pressure.

Directions: TAKE BY MOUTH ONLY; NOT FOR NASAL USE. Use enclosed calibrated dropper for accurate dosing. Dosage may be repeated every 4 to 6 hours, not to exceed 4 doses in 24 hours. Follow dosage recommendations below.

Age	Dosage
Children under 2 years of age	Consult a doctor
Children 2 to under 6 years of age	2 Dropperfuls (1.6 mL)

Warnings: Do not exceed recommended dosage. If nervousness, dizziness, or sleeplessness occur, discontinue use and consult a doctor. If symptoms do not improve within 7 days or are accompanied by fever, consult a doctor. Do not give this product to a child who has heart disease, high blood pressure, thyroid disease or diabetes unless directed by a doctor. **KEEP THIS AND ALL DRUGS OUT OF THE REACH OF CHILDREN.** In case of accidental overdose, seek professional assistance or contact a Poison Control Center immediately.

Drug Interaction Precaution: Do not give this product to a child who is taking a prescription monoamine oxidase inhibitor (MAOI) (certain drugs for depression, psychiatric or emotional conditions), or for 2 weeks after stopping the MAOI drug. If you are uncertain whether your child's prescription drug contains an MAOI, consult a health professional before giving this product.

Continued on next page

This product information was prepared in November 1995. On these and other Warner Wellcome Consumer HealthCare Products, detailed information may be obtained by addressing Warner Wellcome Consumer HealthCare Products, Warner-Lambert, Morris Plains, NJ 07950

Warner Wellcome—Cont.

How Supplied: Sudafed Pediatric Nasal Decongestant Oral Drops are supplied in ½ fl. oz. bottles.
Store at 15° to 25°C (59° to 77°F).
Shown in Product Identification Guide, page 527

SUDAFED® Severe Cold Formula Caplets
[sū 'duh-fĕd]

Active Ingredients: Each coated caplet contains: Acetaminophen 500 mg, Pseudoephedrine Hydrochloride 30 mg, and Dextromethorphan Hydrobromide 15 mg.

Inactive Ingredients: Carnauba Wax, Crospovidone, Hydroxypropyl Methylcellulose, Magnesium Stearate, Microcrystalline Cellulose, Polyethylene Glycol, Povidone, Pregelatinized Corn Starch, Stearic Acid, and Titanium Dioxide.

Indications: For the temporary relief of nasal congestion, minor aches, pains, headache, muscular aches, sore throat, and fever associated with the common cold. Temporarily relieves cough occurring with a cold.

Product Benefits: Maximum allowable levels of nasal decongestant, cough suppressant, and non-aspirin pain reliever/fever reducer provide temporary relief from symptoms of the common cold and flu. This product contains no ingredients that may cause drowsiness. The **DECONGESTANT** (pseudoephedrine) temporarily relieves nasal and sinus congestion due to the common cold. It temporarily relieves nasal stuffiness; reduces the swelling of nasal passages; shrinks swollen membranes; and temporarily restores freer breathing through the nose. The **COUGH SUPPRESSANT** (dextromethorphan) temporarily relieves cough due to the common cold. The non-aspirin **PAIN RELIEVER/FEVER REDUCER** (acetaminophen) temporarily relieves headache, body aches and pains, minor sore throat pain, and reduces fever due to the common cold.

Directions: Adults and children 12 years of age and over, 2 caplets every 6 hours, while symptoms persist, not to exceed 8 caplets in 24 hours, or as directed by a doctor. Not recommended for children under 12 years of age.

Warnings: Do not exceed recommended dosage. If nervousness, dizziness or sleeplessness occur, discontinue use and consult a doctor. Do not take this product for more than 10 days. A persistent cough may be a sign of a serious condition. If symptoms do not improve or if cough persists for more than 7 days, tends to recur, or is accompanied by rash, persistent headache, fever that lasts for more than 3 days, or if new symptoms occur, consult a doctor. Do not take this product for persistent or chronic cough such as occurs with smoking, asthma or emphysema, or if cough is accompanied by excessive phlegm (mucus) unless directed by a doctor. If sore throat is severe, persists for more than 2 days, is accompanied or followed by fever, headache, rash, nausea, or vomiting, consult a doctor promptly. Do not take this product if you have heart disease, high blood pressure, thyroid disease, diabetes, or difficulty in urination due to enlargement of the prostate gland unless directed by a doctor. As with any drug, if you are pregnant or nursing a baby, seek the advice of a health professional before using this product. **KEEP THIS AND ALL DRUGS OUT OF THE REACH OF CHILDREN.** In case of accidental overdose, seek professional assistance or contact a Poison Control Center immediately. Prompt medical attention is critical for adults as well as for children even if you do not notice any signs or symptoms.

Drug Interaction Precaution: Do not use this product if you are now taking a prescription monoamine oxidase inhibitor (MAOI) (certain drugs for depression, psychiatric or emotional conditions, or Parkinson's disease), or for 2 weeks after stopping the MAOI drug. If you are uncertain whether your prescription drug contains an MAOI, consult a health professional before taking this product.

How Supplied: Boxes of 12 and 24.
Store at 15° to 25°C (59°–77°F) in a dry place and protect from light.
Shown in Product Identification Guide, page 527

SUDAFED® Severe Cold Formula Tablets
[sū ' duh-fĕd]

Active Ingredients: Each coated tablet contains: Acetaminophen 500 mg, Pseudoephedrine Hydrochloride 30 mg, and Dextromethorphan Hydrobromide 15 mg.

Inactive Ingredients: Carnauba Wax, Crospovidone, Hydroxypropyl Methylcellulose, Magnesium Stearate, Microcrystalline Cellulose, Polyethylene Glycol, Povidone, Pregelatinized Corn Starch, Stearic Acid and Titanium Dioxide.

Indications: For the temporary relief of nasal congestion, minor aches, pains, headache, muscular aches, sore throat, and fever associated with the common cold. Temporarily relieves cough occurring with a cold.

Product Benefits: Maximum allowable levels of nasal decongestant, cough suppressant, and non-aspirin pain reliever/fever reducer provide temporary relief from symptoms of the common cold and flu. This product contains no ingredients that may cause drowsiness. The **DECONGESTANT** (pseudoephedrine) temporarily relieves nasal and sinus congestion due to the common cold. It temporarily relieves nasal stuffiness; reduces the swelling of nasal passages; shrinks swollen membranes; and temporarily restores freer breathing through the nose. The **COUGH SUPPRESSANT** (dextromethorphan) temporarily relieves cough due to the common cold. The non-aspirin **PAIN RELIEVER/FEVER REDUCER** (acetaminophen) temporarily relieves headache, body aches and pains, minor sore throat pain, and reduces fever due to the common cold.

Directions: Adults and children 12 years of age and over, 2 tablets every 6 hours, while symptoms persist, not to exceed 8 tablets in 24 hours, or as directed by a doctor. Not recommended for children under 12 years of age.

Warnings: Do not exceed recommended dosage. If nervousness, dizziness, or sleeplessness occur, discontinue use and consult a doctor. Do not take this product for more than 10 days. A persistent cough may be a sign of a serious condition. If symptoms do not improve or if cough persists for more than 7 days, tends to recur, or is accompanied by rash, persistent headache, fever that lasts for more than 3 days, or if new symptoms occur, consult a doctor. Do not take this product for persistent or chronic cough such as occurs with smoking, asthma or emphysema, or if cough is accompanied by excessive phlegm (mucus) unless directed by a doctor. If sore throat is severe, persists for more than 2 days, is accompanied or followed by a fever, headache, rash, nausea or vomiting, consult a doctor promptly. Do not take this product if you have heart disease, high blood pressure, thyroid disease, diabetes, or difficulty in urination due to enlargement of the prostate gland unless directed by a doctor. As with any drug, if you are pregnant or nursing a baby, seek the advice of a health professional before using this product. **KEEP THIS AND ALL DRUGS OUT OF THE REACH OF CHILDREN.** In case of accidental overdose, seek professional assistance or contact a Poison Control Center immediately. Prompt medical attention is critical for adults as well as for children even if you do not notice any signs or symptoms.

Drug Interaction Precaution: Do not use this product if you are now taking a prescription monoamine oxidase inhibitor (MAOI) (certain drugs for depression, psychiatric or emotional conditions, or Parkinson's disease), or for 2 weeks after stopping the MAOI drug. If you are uncertain whether your prescription drug contains an MAOI, consult a health professional before taking this product.

How Supplied: Boxes of 12.
Store at 15° to 25°C (59°–77°F) in a dry place and protect from light.
Shown in Product Identification Guide, page 527

SUDAFED® Sinus Caplets
[sū'duh-fĕd]

Active Ingredients: Each coated caplet contains: Acetaminophen 500 mg and Pseudoephedrine Hydrochloride 30 mg.

Inactive Ingredients: Carnauba Wax, Crospovidone, FD&C Yellow No. 6 Aluminum Lake, Hydroxypropyl Methylcellulose, Magnesium Stearate, Microcrystalline Cellulose, Polyethylene Glycol, Polysorbate 80, Povidone, Pregelatinized Starch, Stearic Acid and Titanium Dioxide.

Indications: For the temporary relief of nasal congestion associated with sinusitis. Helps decongest sinus openings and passages; temporarily relieves sinus congestion and pressure. Temporarily relieves headache, minor aches, and pains. Temporarily restores freer breathing through the nose.

Product Benefits:
- Maximum allowable levels of non-aspirin pain reliever and nasal decongestant provide temporary relief of sinus headache pain, pressure and nasal congestion due to colds and flu or hay fever and other allergies.
- Contains no ingredients which may cause drowsiness.

Directions: Adults and children 12 years and over: 2 caplets every 6 hours, while symptoms persist, not to exceed 8 caplets in a 24 hours, or as directed by a doctor. Not recommended for children under 12 years of age.

Warnings: Do not exceed recommended dosage. If nervousness, dizziness, or sleeplessness occur, discontinue use and consult a doctor. Do not take this product for more than 10 days. If symptoms do not improve or are accompanied by fever that lasts for more than 3 days, or if new symptoms occur, consult a doctor. Do not take this product if you have heart disease, high blood pressure, thyroid disease, diabetes, or difficulty in urination due to enlargement of the prostate gland unless directed by a doctor. As with any drug, if you are pregnant or nursing a baby, seek the advice of a health professional before using this product. **KEEP THIS AND ALL DRUGS OUT OF THE REACH OF CHILDREN.** In case of accidental overdose, seek professional assistance or contact a Poison Control Center immediately. Prompt medical attention is critical for adults as well as children even if you do not notice any signs or symptoms.

Drug Interaction Precaution: Do not use this product if you are now taking a prescription monoamine oxidase inhibitor (MAOI) (certain drugs for depression, psychiatric or emotional conditions, or Parkinson's disease), or for 2 weeks after stopping the MAOI drug. If you are uncertain whether your prescription drug contains an MAOI, consult a health professional before taking this product.

How Supplied: Boxes of 24 and 48. Store at 15° to 25°C (59° to 77°F) in a dry place and protect from light.
Shown in Product Identification Guide, page 527

SUDAFED® Sinus Tablets
[sū'duh-fĕd]

Active Ingredients: Each coated tablet contains: Acetaminophen 500 mg and Pseudoephedrine Hydrochloride 30 mg.

Inactive Ingredients: Carnauba Wax, Crospovidone, FD&C Yellow No. 6 Aluminum Lake, Hydroxypropyl Methylcellulose, Magnesium Stearate, Microcrystalline Cellulose, Polyethylene Glycol, Polysorbate 80, Povidone, Pregelatinized Starch, Stearic Acid and Titanium Dioxide.

Indications: For the temporary relief of nasal congestion associated with sinusitis. Helps decongest sinus openings and passages; temporarily relieves sinus congestion and pressure. Temporarily relieves headache, minor aches, and pains. Temporarily restores freer breathing through the nose.

Product Benefits:
- Maximum allowable levels of non-aspirin pain reliever and nasal decongestant provide temporary relief of sinus headache pain, pressure and nasal congestion due to colds and flu or hay fever and other allergies.
- Contains no ingredients which may cause drowsiness.

Directions: Adults and children 12 years of age and over: 2 tablets every 6 hours, while symptoms persist, not to exceed 8 tablets in 24 hours, or as directed by a doctor. Not recommended for children under 12 years of age.

Warnings: Do not exceed recommended dosage. If nervousness, dizziness, or sleeplessness occur, discontinue use and consult a doctor. Do not take this product for more than 10 days. If symptoms do not improve or are accompanied by fever that lasts for more than 3 days, or if new symptoms occur, consult a doctor. Do not take this product if you have heart disease, high blood pressure, thyroid disease, diabetes, or difficulty in urination due to enlargement of the prostate gland unless directed by a doctor. As with any drug, if you are pregnant or nursing a baby, seek the advice of a health professional before using this product. **KEEP THIS AND ALL DRUGS OUT OF THE REACH OF CHILDREN.** In case of accidental overdose, seek professional assistance or contact a Poison Control Center immediately. Prompt medical attention is critical for adults as well as for children even if you do not notice any signs or symptoms.

Drug Interaction Precaution: Do not use this product if you are now taking a prescription monoamine oxidase inhibitor (MAOI) (certain drugs for depression, psychiatric or emotional conditions, or Parkinson's disease), or for 2 weeks after stopping the MAOI drug. If you are uncertain whether your prescription drug contains an MAOI, consult a health professional before taking this product.

How Supplied: Boxes of 24 and 48. Store at 15° to 25°C (59° to 77°F) in a dry place and protect from light.
Shown in Product Identification Guide, page 527

TUCKS® Clear Hemorrhoidal Gel
[tŭks]

Active Ingredients: Witch Hazel 50% and Glycerin 10.7%.

Inactive Ingredients: Alcohol, Benzyl Alcohol, Carbomer 974 P, Disodium Edetate, Propylene Glycol, Sodium Hydroxide and Water.

Indications: For the temporary relief of external itching, burning and discomfort associated with inflamed hemorrhoidal tissues.

Directions: For External Use Only. Adults: When practical, cleanse the affected area with mild soap and warm water and rinse thoroughly. Gently dry by patting or blotting with toilet tissue or soft cloth before application of this product. Apply externally to the affected area up to 6 times daily or after each bowel movement. Children under 12 years of age: consult a physician.

Warnings: If condition worsens or does not improve within 7 days, consult a physician. Do not exceed recommended daily dosage unless directed by a physician. In case of bleeding, consult a physician promptly. Do not put this product into the rectum by using fingers or any mechanical device or applicator. **Keep this and all drugs out of the reach of children.** In case of accidental ingestion, seek professional assistance or contact a Poison Control Center immediately.

How Supplied: Tucks Clear Gel is supplied in 0.7 oz (19.8g) tubes. Store at room temperature 15°–30°C (59°–86°F).
Shown in Product Identification Guide, page 528

Continued on next page

This product information was prepared in November 1995. On these and other Warner Wellcome Consumer HealthCare Products, detailed information may be obtained by addressing Warner Wellcome Consumer HealthCare Products, Warner-Lambert, Morris Plains, NJ 07950

Warner Wellcome—Cont.

TUCKS®
Pre-moistened Hemorrhoidal/Vaginal Pads
[tŭks]

Active Ingredients: Soft pads are pre-moistened with a solution containing 50% Witch Hazel.

Inactive Ingredients: Water, Glycerin, Alcohol, Propylene Glycol, Sodium Citrate, Diazolidinyl Urea, Citric Acid, Methylparaben, Propylparaben.

Indications: For the temporary relief of external itching, burning and irritation associated with hemorrhoids.

Uses:
Hemorrhoids: Tucks extra-soft cloth pads allow for the gentlest possible care of tender inflamed hemorrhoidal tissue.
Hygienic Wipe: Tucks Pads are effective for everyday personal hygienic use on outer rectal and vaginal areas. Used in place of toilet tissue, Tucks Pads gently and thoroughly remove irritation-causing matter. They are especially handy during menstrual periods.
Moist Compress: For additional relief, Tucks Pads can be folded and used as a compress on inflamed tissue. Tucks Pads are particularly helpful in relieving discomfort following childbirth, rectal or vaginal surgery.

Directions: For external use only. *As a hemorrhoidal treatment* —Adults: When practical, cleanse the affected area with mild soap and warm water, and rinse thoroughly. Gently dry by patting or blotting with toilet tissue or soft cloth before each application of this product. Gently apply to affected area by patting and then discard. Can be used up to six times daily. Children under 12 years of age: consult a physician.
As a hygienic wipe —Use as a wipe instead of toilet tissue.
As a moist compress —For soothing relief, fold pad and place in contact with irritated tissue. Leave in place for 5 to 15 minutes. Repeat as needed.

Warnings: If condition worsens or does not improve within 7 days, consult a physician. Do not exceed recommended daily dosage unless directed by a physician. In case of bleeding, consult a physician promptly. Do not put this product in the rectum by using fingers or any mechanical device or applicator. **Keep this and all drugs out of the reach of children.** In case of accidental ingestion, seek professional assistance or contact a Poison Control Center immediately.

How Supplied: Jars of 40 and 100. Also available as Tucks Take-Alongs®, individual, foil-wrapped, nonwoven 6 Two-Packs) pads..

Shown in Product Identification Guide, page 527

Wellness International Network, Ltd.
1501 LUNA ROAD, BLDG. 102 CARROLLTON, TX 75006

Direct Inquiries to:
Director, Product Development
(214) 245-1097
FAX: (214) 389-3060

BIO-COMPLEX 5000™
Gentle Foaming Cleanser

Uses: BIO-COMPLEX 5000™ Gentle Foaming Cleanser, with alpha-hydroxy acids, aloe vera, and botanical infusions, is an advanced cleansing gel designed for all skin types. BIO-COMPLEX 5000 Gentle Foaming Cleanser protects the skin while gently removing surface impurities, make-up, and pollution.

Inactive Ingredients: Aloe Vera Gel, Infusion of Sage, Infusion of Chamomile, Ammonium Lauryl Sulfate, Lauramidopropyl Betaine, Glycerin, Lauramide DEA, Cetyl Betaine, Tocopherol, Citric Acid, Lactic Acid, Malic Acid, Ascorbic Acid, Methylchloroisothiazolinone, Methylisothiazolinone, Propylparaben, Methylparaben.

Directions: Splash warm water onto face. Place a small amount of gel on fingertips. Apply evenly to face and neck in circular motions, massaging skin gently but thoroughly. Rinse completely and pat dry with a soft towel.

How Supplied: 8 fluid ounce/236 ml. bottle.

BIO-COMPLEX 5000™
Revitalizing Conditioner

Uses: BIO-COMPLEX 5000™ Revitalizing Conditioner, with vitamins, anti-oxidants, and sunscreen, helps restore moisture to dried-out, heat-styled hair. Its nourishing formula contains the essence of awapuhi, a Hawaiian ginger plant extract known for its healing qualities. This advanced conditioner enhances hair with silkening agents and detangles hair after shampooing. Hair is left clean, soft, manageable, and protected against styling aids and environmental elements. BIO-COMPLEX 5000 Revitalizing Conditioner is excellent for all hair types, especially damaged or over-processed hair.

Inactive Ingredients: Water, Stearyl Alcohol, Propylene Glycol, Stearamidopropyl Dimethalymine, Cyclomethicone, Polyquaternium - 11, Stearalkonium Chloride, Cetearyl Alcohol, PEG - 40 Hydrogenated Castor Oil, Citric Acid, Tocopherol, Ascorbic Acid, Retinyl Palmitate, Octyl Methoxycinnamate, Awapuhi Fragrance, Ceteth - 20, Soluble Animal Keratin, Imidazolidinyl Urea, Propylparaben, Methylparaben.

Directions: After shampooing with BIO-COMPLEX 5000™ Revitalizing Shampoo, apply to wet hair. Massage through hair, paying special attention to the ends. Leave on 2–3 minutes. Rinse thoroughly. Towel dry and style as usual.

How Supplied: 12 fluid ounce bottle.

BIO-COMPLEX 5000™
Revitalizing Shampoo

Uses: BIO-COMPLEX 5000™ Revitalizing Shampoo, with vitamins, anti-oxidants, and sunscreen, cleanses and moisturizes hair for excellent manageability. Specially formulated with the essence of awapuhi, a Hawaiian ginger plant extract known for its healing qualities, this formula contains the mildest blend of surfactants and a wealth of natural conditioning ingredients to provide body, luster, and healthier-looking hair.

Inactive Ingredients: Water, Ammonium Lauryl Sulfate, Tea Lauryl Sulfate, Cetyl Betaine, Lauramide DEA, Cocamidopropyl Betaine, Glycerin, Ascorbic Acid, Tocopherol, Retinyl Palmitate, Citric Acid, Hydrolyzed Wheat Protein, Awapuhi Fragrance, Octyl Methoxycinnamate, PEG - 7 Glyceryl Cocoate, Methylchloroisothiazolinone, Methylisothiazolinone, Caramel.

Directions: Apply a small amount to wet hair and massage gently into scalp, creating a generous lather. Rinse and repeat if necessary. For best results, follow with BIO-COMPLEX 5000™ Revitalizing Conditioner.

How Supplied: 12 fluid ounce bottle.

BIOLEAN®
Herbal & Amino Acid Food Supplement

Uses: BIOLEAN® is a unique combination of Chinese herbal extracts and pharmaceutical grade amino acids specifically designed to help raise overall health, participate in individual life extension programs, and enhance athletic performance. It has been shown to be extremely effective in promoting the healthy loss of excess body fat while helping to maintain lean body mass and potent energy levels. BIOLEAN, when used as a daily nutritional supplement, has been shown to stimulate immune function in individuals with blunted sympathetic nervous systems, especially overweight and obese persons. It also acts as a positive stimulator to immune functions involved in protection from environmental and dietary carcinogens. Components in BIOLEAN are known to cause fat loss through thermogenic activity and altered fuel metabolism resulting from sympathomimetic response to stimulation of beta receptors in adipose and muscle cells. The positive immune response, though not completely understood, is at least partially attributable to beta stimulation in adipocytes and the adaptogenic and tonifying activity of certain of the herbal extracts. This has been demonstrated in their long history of use in tradional Chinese herbal medicine as well as current scientific research which points to, among other possibilities, the extremely potent antioxidant properties found in some of the component plants, most notably in the Green Tea and Schizandrae extracts. BIOLEAN may increase athletic performance and endurance through three pathways: 1) increased oxygen uptake in the lungs as a result of expanding bronchial passages; 2) enhanced mental acuity and response resulting from sympathetic nervous system stimulus; and 3) increasing the employment of fatty acids as fuel in muscle mitochondria while simultaneously sparing muscle glycogen and nitrogen.

The herbal extracts in BIOLEAN are produced in a unique and exclusive process which is proprietary to this product. Instead of creating extracts based on a set quantity of one particular active within many which may be present in any particular plant, BIOLEAN components are concentrated to maintain the natural and complete spectrum of biologically active factors, in the same ratio presented by the unprocessed plant.

Directions: Adults take one white capsule and one to three tablets with low-calorie food mid to late morning. If using BIOLEAN for the first time, take one capsule and one tablet on days 1 and 2, one capsule and two tablets on days 3 and 4, and one capsule and three tablets beginning day 5. Needs vary with the individual. Some persons may require less than three tablets daily or wish to spread the taking of the tablets throughout morning and early afternoon to achieve optimum results. Do not exceed recommended daily amounts. It is recommended that you drink at least eight glasses of water daily.

Warnings: Phenylketonurics: Contains Phenylalanine. Not for use by children. Consult your physician before using this product if you are taking asthma medications, appetitie suppressing drugs, antidepressants, or cardiovascular medication. Do not consume if you are pregnant or lactating, or have high blood pressure, cardiovascular disease, diabetes, prostatic hypertrophy, glaucoma, hyperthyroidism, psychosis, or thyroid disease. If symptoms of allergy develop, discontinue use.

Ingredients: *Capsules:* 400 mg. of the following mix: L-Phenylalanine, L-Tyrosine, L-Carnitine. *Tablets:* 650 mg. of the following herbal mix: Ma Huang, Green Tea, Schizandrae Berry, Rehmannia Root, Hawthorne Berry, Jujube Seed, Alisma Root, Angelicae Dahuricae Root, Epemidium, Poria Cocos, Rhizoma Rhei, Stephania Root, Angelicae Sinensis Root, Codonopsis Root, Eucommium Bark, and Notoginseng Root.

How Supplied: One box contains 28 packets. One capsule and three tablets per packet.

BIOLEAN ACCELERATOR™
Herbal & Amino Acid Formulation

Uses: BIOLEAN ACCELERATOR™ is a unique combination of Chinese herbal extracts and pharmaceutical grade amino acids specifically designed to complement BIOLEAN®by extending and accelerating its actions. BIOLEAN is, in the traditional view of Chinese herbal medicine, a strong Yang blend. This means that it is energy or heat-producing at its core, though the addition of the amino acids and certain of the herbal components lends a very definite restorative, or Yin element, as well. BIOLEAN ACCELERATOR is a strong Yin formula, intended to augment the lesser replenishing Yin elements of BIOLEAN. Though the physiological actions of many herbs are complex and not totally understood, the formula in BIOLEAN ACCELERATOR extends the adaptogenic, thermogenic, restorative, and detoxifying results experienced with BIOLEAN, with an emphasis on the restorative and adaptogenic effects. The herbal formula is a combination of tonifiers traditionally used in China for the lungs, liver, and kidneys.

Directions: For maximum effectiveness, use in conjunction with original BIOLEAN. Take one tablet in the morning with original BIOLEAN. BIOLEAN ACCELERATOR™ may also be taken in the afternoon with or without additional BIOLEAN if desired. As with original BIOLEAN, maximum absorption will be attained if taken with low-calorie food.

Warnings: Phenylketonurics: Contains Phenylalanine. Not for use by children. Consult your physician before using this product if you are taking appetite suppressing drugs or antidepressants. If symptoms of allergy develop, discontinue use.

Ingredients: Each tablet contains 250 mg. herbal mix (Black Sesame Seed, Raw Chinese Foxglove Root, Chinese Wolfberry Fruit, Achyranthes Root, Cornelian Cherry Fruit, Chinese Yam, Eclipta Herb, Rose Hips, Privet Fruit, Mulberry Fruit-Spike, Polygonati Rhizome, Cooked Chinese Foxglove Root, Poria Cocos, Cuscuta Seed, Foxnut Seed, Alisma Rhizome, Moutan Bark, Phellodendron Bark, Anemarrhena Rhizome, Schisandra Berry, Royal Jelly), L-Tyrosine, L-Phenylalanine.

How Supplied: One bottle contains 56 tablets.

BIOLEAN Free™
Herbal & Amino Acid Food Supplement

Uses: BIOLEAN Free™ is a strategic blend of herbs, spices, vitamins, minerals, and amino acids specifically formulated to enhance fat utilization and energy production through various metabolic pathways. It has been shown to reduce body fat through its thermogenic effects and to enhance both physical and mental performance.

Thermogenesis refers to the body's ability to convert substrates such as proteins, fats, and carbohydrates into heat energy. This is carried out most efficiently in the Brown Adipose Tissue of our body which uses fatty acids as its preferred fuel. Other fat cells, namely White Adipose Tissue, are concerned primarily with the storage of fat rather than its conversion to energy. The thermogenic pathway is complex and relies upon a series of reactions to occur. BIOLEAN Free utilizes many compounds which act at various locations in this pathway to ensure the maximum efficiency of the thermogenic process. Quebracho is one of these very special compounds. This South American plant contains quebrachine, aspidiospermine, and other alkaloids that possess the ability to block alpha-2 adrenergic receptors in the body. This produces an enhanced sympathetic nervous system effect which, in turn, increases lipolysis (fat breakdown) within fat cells. The fatty acids released by this process can then be transported into the mitochondria to be used as a fuel. Ginger, cinnamon, horseradish, turmeric, cayenne, and mustard are spices that stimulate thermogenesis in different ways. Some stimulate lipid mobilization in adipose tissue; others raise the resting metabolic rate; and some increase cAMP levels by inducing more beta receptors on fat cells and by increasing the concentration of adenylate cyclase. cAMP increases the breakdown of triglycerides to free fatty acids which are later used as fuel by the mitochondria in the cell. Methylxanthines (such as those found in green tea and yerba maté) also increase cAMP levels, but do this by inhibiting the enzyme, phosphodiesterase. These compounds have been noted to increase mental alertness, improve vitality, satisfy the appetite, and increase energy. In addition to its methylxanthine content, green tea has recently been shown to possess strong antioxidant properties. Yerba maté is a plant that has been shown to produce the positive effects above without causing the insomnia seen with other methylxanthine-containing plants (such as coffee and kola nut). BIOLEAN Free also contains vitamin B-3, vitamin B-6, chromium, and vanadium which aid in the proper metabolism of fats, proteins, and carbohydrates. L-Tyrosine also aids in metabolism and promotes satiety through hypothalamic release of CCK. Methionine is a precursor of L-Carnitine which aids in the transport of fatty acids into the mitochondria for thermogenesis. Other herbs have been utilized in BIOLEAN Free. Ginseng and Ho shou wu possess adaptogenic properties. Adaptogens help the body adapt to physiological and environmental stresses. Ginseng accomplishes this through its stabilizing effect on the hypothalamic-pituitary-adrenal-sympathetic nervous system. It

Continued on next page

Wellness International—Cont.

can mediate an increase adrenal response to stress.

Ho shou wu has a stabilizing effect on the endocrine system and has restorative properties. It is also an antioxidant with a high flavonoid content. *Centella asiatica* contains asiaticoside and has been shown to increase activity levels and ease the body's ability to overcome fatigue when taken with ginseng and cayenne. Individually, *centella* has been shown to increase memory and mental acuity in studies abroad. Uva ursi contains the glycoside arbutin and promotes urinary health and body strength through its purifying effects. Ginkgo biloba is a tree whose leaves have been used for centuries as an herbal medicine. It contains flavonoids and is therefore a strong antioxidant. It reduces the tendency of platelets to stick together by inhibiting Platelet Activating Factor. It has been shown to increase blood flow to the heart, brain, and other organs.

Directions: Adults (18 years and older) may take 4 caplets in the mid to late morning with a low-calorie food. Needs may vary with each individual. Some persons may require less than 4 caplets, or may prefer taking 3 caplets mid morning and 1 additional caplet mid afternoon to achieve optimum results. Do not exceed recommended daily amounts.

Warnings: Not for use by children, pregnant women, or lactating women. Consult your physician before using this product if you are taking appetite suppressing drugs or cardiovascular medication. Also consult your physician if you have hypertension, heart disease, arrhythmias, prostatic hypertrophy, glaucoma, liver disease, renal disease, or diabetes. Do not use if you have hyperthyroidism, psychosis, Parkinson's Disease, or are taking Monoamine oxidase inhibitors. BIOLEAN Free should not be taken on the same day as original BIOLEAN®. It is recommended that you minimize your caffeine intake while consuming this product. If allergic symptoms develop, discontinue use. Store in a cool, dry place. Keep out of reach of children.

Ingredients: Each caplet contains the following: Standardized botanical extracts containing 720 mg of the following mixture: Green tea, Yerba maté, Korean ginseng, Uva ursi, and Quebracho. Non-irradiated pure herbs and spices containing 360 mg of the following mixture: Jamaican ginger, Ceylon cinnamon, Chinese horseradish, Alleppy turmeric, Nigerian cayenne, English mustard, *Centella asiatica*, Ho shou wu, Ginkgo biloba. Also included are 125 mg of L-Tyrosine, 25 mg of Methionine, 25 mg of Potassium (citrate), 10 mg of Vitamin B-3, 4 mg of Vitamin B-6, 100 mcg of Chromium Chelavite™, and 100 mcg of Vanadium.

How Supplied: One box contains 28 packets. Four caplets per packet.

BIOLEAN LIPOTRIM™
All-Natural Dietary Supplement

Uses: LipoTrim™ is a highly active, synergistic combination of garcinia cambogia extract and chromium polynicotinate. The method of action is by inhibition of lipogenesis and regulation of blood glucose levels. Serum glucose derived from dietary carbohydrates and not immediately converted to energy or glycogen tends to be converted into fat stores and cholesterol. In individuals with excess body fat stores or slow basal metabolism, this tendency is thought to be higher. The garcinia cambogia extract present in LipoTrim is verified by HPLC analysis to be no less that 50%(-) hydroxycitrate (HCA). HCA inhibits ATP-citrate lyase which retards Acetyl CoA synthesis, severely restricting conversion of excess glucose into fatty acids and cholesterol. Animal studies have shown post-meal fatty acid synthesis reduction of 40–80% for an 8–12 hour period. When glucose to fat/cholesterol conversion is retarded, glycogen conversion continues, increasing liver stores and causing satiety signals to be sent to the brain resulting in appetite suppression. In situations of intense physical exercise, increased glycogen stores have been shown to result in enhanced endurance and recovery. By restricting the activity of insulin, chromium has been shown to exhibit a regulating effect on blood glucose levels thus extending the benefits of HCA.

Directions: As a dietary supplement, take one capsule three times daily, 30 minutes before each meal. LipoTrim should be used in conjunction with a healthy diet and exercise plan.

Ingredients: CitriMax™* (garcinia cambogia), ChromeMate®* (chromium polynicotinate).

How Supplied: One bottle contains 84 easy-to-swallow capsules.

*CitriMax™ is a trademark of InterHealth.
ChromeMate® is a registered trademark of InterHealth.

BIOLEAN MEAL™
Nutritional Meal Replacement Drink

Uses: BIOLEAN MEAL™ is formulated specifically for use with the other products in the BIOLEAN®System. It has a natural chocolate flavor which mixes instantly, without need for blending, to form a creamy drink which is equally delicious in water, milk, or milk substitutes, including rice and soy base. BIOLEAN MEAL is a low-calorie, nonfat, low-lactose powder designed to provide an optimum, alternative blend of protein, carbohydrates, and dietary fiber to individuals who have unhealthy or insufficient dietary habits, are on a fat loss program, or desire to enhance their athletic ability.
BIOLEAN MEAL has been biologically engineered to contain a 1:1 ratio of casein

proteins to whey proteins. This represents a significant improvement in taste, solubility, nutritional content, and BV (biological value) compared to caseinates, soy defatted whole egg, and egg white protein, the latter historically being the standard of comparison for all protein sources. There are several factors contributing to this higher BV. Bovine milk has a ratio of casein to whey of 4:1, whereas human milk is 2:3. The amino acid composition, absorption, and utilization of whey protein is superior to other sources of supplemental dietary protein. This is especially true for individuals with limited or compromised GI function which often accompanies situations involving physical and emotional stress, illness, disease, and trauma. Athletes with increased protein requirements will also benefit from a higher BV protein source. Whey protein has the highest ratio of essential to nonessential amino acids and contains the highest quantity of Branched Chain Amino Acids (BCAA), especially Leucine, which is double that of egg protein. Leucine is consumed in large amounts during periods of exercise, trauma, infection, and caloric restriction. Muscle recovery, fuel production, and immune function are dependent upon adequate supply and replacement of Leucine. Research has also shown that tissues stores of glutathione are increased by the regular intake of whey protein.
The immune enhancing effects of whey protein, combined with the high nutritive value of milk protein isolate, promotes the loss of body fat and the retention and growth of lean body mass (muscle, bone, and internal organs) as well as supporting all other normal physiological processes such as immune function and cellular replacement, especially during periods of added stress brought on by dieting, illness, and athletic activity.

Directions: Add contents to 8 ounces of water or nonfat milk and stir or shake until completely mixed. For a thicker drink, blend for 10 seconds and drink immediately. For pudding, blend for 30 seconds and refrigerate. BIOLEAN MEAL has been formulated specifically for use with the other products in the BIOLEAN System.

Warnings: Phenylketonurics: Contains Phenylalanine.

Ingredients: Myotein (Proprietary bio-engineered protein blend of specially isolated fat and lactose free milk proteins and whey protein concentrate), Fructose, Maltodextrin, Nonfat Milk Solids, Naturally Processed Cocoa, Natural Flavor Complex (Chocolate, Vanilla, and Vanilla Cream), Cellulose Gel, Guar Gum, Corn Starch, Aspartame.

How Supplied: One box contains 14 packets. Serving size equals one packet.

FOOD FOR THOUGHT™
Choline-Enriched Nutritional Drink

Uses: A great-tasting citrus cooler, this choline-enriched nutritional beverage provides nutrients important for mental fitness. Food For Thought™ is ideal for work, school or any time performance is needed. For vigor of body, mind and spirit, this tangy citrus beverage delivers essential minerals and vitamins to the body.

Directions: Add 6 ounces of chilled water or fruit juice to one packet of mix. Stir briskly. Consume 1–2 times per day. Keep in a cool, dry place.

Warnings: Not for use by children, pregnant or lactating women. Persons taking medications should seek medical advice before taking this product. Persons with ulcers or a history of ulcers should consult their physician before using a choline supplement. Do not consume more than four servings per day. Avoid the use of antacids containing aluminum with this product.

Ingredients: Fructose, Choline Bitartrate, Calcium Pantothenate, Natural Flavor, Glycine, Ascorbic Acid, Vitamin E Acetate, Niacinamide, Lysine, Silicon Dioxide, Zinc Gluconate, Chromium Aspartate, Niacin, Magnesium Gluconate, Pyridoxine Hydrochloride, Thiamin Mononitrate, Riboflavin, Copper Gluconate, Vitamin B12.

How Supplied: One box contains 28 packets of drink mix. Serving size equals one packet.

STEPHAN™ BIO-NUTRITIONAL
Daytime Hydrating Creme

Uses: Hypo-allergenic STEPHAN™ BIO-NUTRITIONAL Daytime Hydrating Creme hydrates the skin and maintains the moisture level of the upper layers of the epidermis. It is an excellent day cream for both men and women who wish to combat the visible signs of aging skin, the appearance of wrinkles or lines, and the loss of that firm look of facial features and contours. These light emulsions are absorbed rapidly by the skin and leave an invisible protective film which hydrates the epidermis, regulates the moisture level, and leaves skin feeling supple and soft.

Inactive Ingredients: Water, Stearic Acid, Isodecyl Neopentanoate, Isostearyl Stearoyl Stearate, DEA Cetyl Phosphate, C12-15 Alkyl Benzoate, Squalane, Dimethicone, Aloe Vera Gel, Tocopherol, Cetyl Esters, Carbomer, Fragrance, Benzophenone-3, Triethanolamine, Imidazolidinyl Urea, Propylparaben, Methylparaben, Annatto.

Directions: Apply evenly on a completely cleansed face and neck. May be used around the eye area, avoiding direct contact with the eyes. Suitable for all skin types.

Warnings: For external use only. Avoid contact with eyes.

How Supplied: Net Wt. 1.75 oz.

STEPHAN™ BIO-NUTRITIONAL
Eye-Firming Concentrate

Uses: Hypo-allergenic STEPHAN™ BIO-NUTRITIONAL Eye-Firming Concentrate is specially formulated to revitalize the delicate area around the eyes. This non-oily fluid pampers sensitive eyes, reduces the look of puffiness and dark circles around eyes, and smoothes and softens the appearance of fine lines in the eye area.

Inactive Ingredients: Infusion of Chamomile, Cornflower Extract, Horsetail Extract, Sugar Cane Extract, Citrus Extract, Apple Extract, Green Tea Extract, Methyl Gluceth-20, Panthenol, Cyanocobalamin, Propylene Glycol, Laureth-4, Hydrolyzed Wheat Protein, Tissue Respiratory Factors, Plant Pseudocollagen, Aloe Vera Gel, Triethanolamine, Dimethicone Copolyol, PEG-30 Glyceryl Laurate, Phenethyl Alcohol, Carbomer, Xanthan Gum, Benzophenone-4, Disodium EDTA, Methylchloroisothiazolinone, Methylisothiazolinone, Methylparaben, Propylparaben.

Directions: Apply in the morning, or any time of the day, in small quantities to the skin around the eyes with light, tapping motions, avoiding direct contact with the eyes. In the evening, apply gently to the entire eye contour area.

Warnings: For external use only. Avoid direct contact with eyes.

How Supplied: 1 fl. oz.

STEPHAN™ BIO-NUTRITIONAL
Nightime Moisture Creme

Uses: Hypo-allergenic STEPHAN™ BIO-NUTRITIONAL Nightime Moisture Creme is a heavier, richer cream for mature, dry, or sun-damaged skin. This advanced formula is excellent for dehydrated skin, promoting suppleness and moisture, and improving the appearance of fine lines and wrinkles.

Inactive Ingredients: Water, Caprylic/Capric Triglyceride, Propylene Glycol, Stearic Acid, Polysorbate 60, Cetyl Alcohol, Octyl Palmitate, Beeswax, Sorbitan Stearate, Canola Oil, Avocado Oil, Safflower Oil, Squalane, Liposomes, Soluble Collagen, Dimethicone, Bisabolol, Aloe Vera Gel, Fragrance, C12-15 Alkyl Benzoate, Hydroxyethylcellulose, Octyl Methoxycinnamate, Disodium EDTA, Sodium Borate, Benzophenone-3, Allantoin, Phenoxyethanol, Methylparaben, Propylparaben, Butylparaben, Ethylparaben, FD&C Yellow No. 10, Caramel.

Directions: In the evening, apply by lightly massaging onto a thoroughly cleansed face and neck. Avoid direct con-

tact with eyes. For drier skin, it may be used during the day as a moisturizer, under make-up, or after sun bathing.

Warning: For external use only. Avoid contact with eyes.

How Supplied: Net Wt. 1.75 oz.

STEPHAN™ BIO-NUTRITIONAL
Refreshing Moisture Gel

Uses: Hypo-allergenic STEPHAN™ BIO-NUTRITIONAL Refreshing Moisture Gel is specially formulated to refine pores and promote a clear, clean, and smooth-looking complexion. It is designed to deeply cleanse and super-stimulate the skin. This gel is suitable for all skin types, especially problem areas. A quick "pick-me-up," STEPHAN BIO-NUTRITIONAL Refreshing Moisture Gel immediately restores the radiant, firm, and youthful appearance of the face while acting as a cumulative, revitalizing beauty treatment.

Inactive Ingredients: Water, Propylene Glycol, Glycerin, Hydroxyethylcellulose, Sugar Cane Extract, Citrus Extract, Apple Extract, Green Tea Extract, Hydrolyzed Wheat Protein, Tissue Respiratory Factors, Panthenol, Aloe Vera Gel, Laureth-4, Magnesium Aluminum Silicate, Tetrasodium EDTA, Benzophenone-3, Imidazolidinyl Urea, Methylchloroisothiazolinone, Methylisothiazolinone, Methylparaben, Propylparaben, Phenethyl Alcohol, FD&C Yellow No. 10, FD&C Red No. 40, FD&C Yellow No. 5.

Directions: After thoroughly cleansing in the morning or evening, apply a liberal layer to the face, neck and eye area, avoiding eye contact. Remove after 20–30 minutes with warm water. Suitable for all skin types.

Warnings: For external use only. Avoid contact with eyes.

How Supplied: Net Wt. 1.75 oz.

STEPHAN™ BIO-NUTRITIONAL
Ultra Hydrating Fluid

Uses: Hypo-allergenic STEPHAN™ BIO-NUTRITIONAL Ultra Hydrating Fluid is a complete treatment to help firm the skin, soften fine lines, and preserve youthful-looking, radiant skin. STEPHAN BIO-NUTRITIONAL Ultra Hydrating Fluid helps combat the aged look of the skin.

Inactive Ingredients: Water, Glycerin, Panthenol, Sodium Hyaluronate, Phenethyl Alcohol, Aloe Vera Gel, Methyl Gluceth-20, PEG-30 Glyceryl Laurate, Methylsilanol Hydroxyproline Aspartate, Xanthan Gum, Methylchloroisothiazolinone, Methylisothiazolinone.

Directions: Gently apply all over the face, neck, and eye contour area, prefer-

Continued on next page

Wellness International—Cont.

ably in the morning. Use as a part of a regular daily skin care routine or as an occasional preventive treatment.

Warnings: For external use only. Avoid direct contact with eyes.

How Supplied: 1 fl. oz.

STEPHAN™ CLARITY
Nutritional Supplement

Uses: Designed for both men and women, STEPHAN™ Clarity contains selected tissue proteins supported by vitamins, minerals, amino acids, and herbs regarded as important to memory and concentration.

Directions: Take one to two capsules per day.

Warnings: Phenylketonurics: Contains Phenylalanine.

Ingredients: Lecithin, Bee Pollen, Glutamic Acid, Vitamin C, Ribonucleic Acid, Ginkgo Biloba (as 8:1 extract), Aspartic Acid, Vitamin E, Vitamin B-3, Leucine, Arginine, Lysine, Phenylalanine, Serine, Valine, Proline, Isoleucine, Alanine, Glycine, Threonine, Tyrosine, Vitamin B-5, Vitamin B-1, Histidine, Methionine, Cysteine, Adenosine Triphosphate, Vitamin B-6, Vitamin B-2, Vitamin A, Folic Acid, Biotin, Vitamin D-3, Vitamin B-12.

How Supplied: One bottle contains 30 easy-to-swallow capsules.

STEPHAN™ ELASTICITY
Nutritional Supplement

Uses: A nutritional food supplement for men and women, STEPHAN™ Elasticity contains a scientifically balanced mixture of specific tissue proteins (in the form of nutrients) supported by vitamins, minerals, amino acids, and herbs which are established as important for skin tone, texture, and appearance.

Directions: Take one capsule per day.

Warning: Phenylketonurics: Contains Phenylalanine.

Ingredients: Equisetum Arvense, Protein Isolates (Alanine, Arginine, Aspartic Acid, Cysteine, Glutamic Acid, Glycine, Histidine, Isoleucine, Leucine, Lysine, Methionine, Phenylalanine, Proline, Serine, Threonine, Tyrosine, Valine), Fucus, Vitamine E (Dl-Alpha), Zinc (Amino Acid Chelate), Vitamin C, Ribonucleic Acid, Calcium (Amino Acid Chelate), Magnesium (Amino Acid Chelate), Iron (Amino Acid Chelate), Manganese (Amino Acid Chelate), Selenium (Amino Acid Chelate), Chromium (Amino Acid Chelate), Adenosine Triphosphate, Vitamin A (Acetate).

How Supplied: One bottle contains 30 easy-to-swallow capsules.

STEPHAN™ ELIXIR
Nutritional Supplement

Uses: Formulated with an exclusive blend of specific proteins, STEPHAN™ Elixir is ideal for both men and women. These tissue proteins are supported by vitamins, minerals, amino acids, and herbs recognized as important for general health and well being.

Directions: Take one capsule per day.

Warnings: Phenylketonurics: Contains Phenylalanine.

Ingredient: Soya Isolate (Alanine, Arginine, Aspartic Acid, Cysteine, Glutamic Acid, Glycine, Histidine, Isoleucine, Leucine, Lysine, Methionine, Phenylalanine, Proline, Serine, Threonine, Tyrosine, Valine), Bee Pollen, Vitamin C, Malic Acid, Ginkgo Biloba (8:1 extract), Citric Acid, Ribonucleic Acid, Vitamin E, Vitamin B-3, Zinc (Amino Acid Chelate), Iron (Amino Acid Chelate), Calcium Pantothenate, Vitamin B-1, Vitamin B-5, Adenosine Triphosphate, Vitamin B-6, Vitamin B-2, Vitamin A, Folic Acid, Selenium (Amino Acid Chelate), Biotin, Vitamin D-3, Vitamin B-12.

How Supplied: One bottle contains 30 easy-to-swallow capsules.

STEPHAN™ ESSENTIAL
Nutritional Supplement

Uses: Designed for both men and women, STEPHAN™ Essential is a nutritional food supplement which contains specific tissue proteins supported by vitamins, minerals, herbs, and amino acids which have long been established as being important for the health of the heart and circulatory system.

Directions: Take one to two capsules per day.

Warnings: Phenylketonurics: Contains Phenylalanine.

Ingredients: Bee Pollen, L-Carnitine, Omega 3 Oil, Glutamic Acid, Ribonucleic Acid, Aspartic Acid, Vitamin E, Leucine, Arginine, Lysine, Magnesium (Amino Acid Chelate), Phenylalanine, Serine, Valine, Proline, Isoleucine, Alanine, Glycine, Threonine, Tyrosine, Histidine, Methionine, Cysteine, Adenosine Triphosphate, Selenium (Amino Acid Chelate).

How Supplied: One bottle contains 30 easy-to-swallow capsules.

STEPHAN™ FEMININE
Nutritional Supplement

Uses: Specifically designed for women, STEPHAN™ Feminine contains selected tissue proteins supported by vitamins, minerals, and amino acids regarded as important to the ever-changing female body.

Directions: Take one to two capsules per day.

Warnings: Phenylketonurics: Contains Phenylalanine.

Ingredients: Magnesium Oxide, Glutamic Acid, Ribonucleic Acid, Aspartic Acid, Vitamin E, Leucine, Arginine, Lysine, Phenylalanine, Serine, Valine, Proline, Isoleucine, Alanine, Glycine, Threonine, Tyrosine, Histidine, Methionine, Cysteine, Boron (Amino Acid Chelate), Adenosine Triphosphate, Selenium.

How Supplied: One bottle contains 30 easy-to-swallow capsules.

STEPHAN™ FLEXIBILITY
Nutritional Supplement

Uses: A nutritional supplement for both men and women, STEPHAN™ Flexibility is rich with exclusive proteins which are supported by vitamins, minerals, and amino acids recognized as beneficial to the health of joint and soft tissues.

Directions: Take one to two capsules per day.

Warnings: Phenylketonurics: Contains Phenylalanine.

Ingredients: Vitamin C, Ribonucleic Acid, Vitamin E, Vitamin B-3, Glutamic Acid, Zinc (Amino Acid Chelate), Calcium (Amino Acid Chelate), Aspartic Acid, Bee Pollen, Leucine, Arginine, Lysine, Vitamin B-5, Vitamin B-1, Phenylalanine, Serine, Valine, Proline, Isoleucine, Alanine, Glycine, Threonine, Tyrosine, Histidine, Cysteine, Adenosine Triphosphate, Vitamin B-6, Boron (Amino Acid Chelate), Vitamin B-2, Methionine, Vitamin A, Folic Acid, Selenium (Amino Acid Chelate), Biotin, Vitamin D-3, Vitamin B-12.

How Supplied: One bottle contains 30 easy-to-swallow capsules.

STEPHAN™ LOVPIL
Nutritional Supplement

Uses: STEPHAN™ Lovpil is a nutritional food supplement for men and women of all ages. STEPHAN Lovpil is formulated with vitamins, minerals, herbs, amino acids, and selected proteins recognized as important for general health and vitality.

Directions: Take one capsule per day.

Warnings: Phenylketonurics: Contains Phenylalanine.

Ingredients: Calcium Carbonate, Vitamin C, Damiana Powder, Zinc (Amino Acid Chelate), Ribonucleic Acid, Soya Isolate (Isoleucine, Phenylalanine, Leucine, Threonine, Lysine, Methionine, Valine, Alanine, Glycine, Histidine, Arginine, Proline, Aspartic Acid, Serine, Cysteine, Tyrosine, Glutamic Acid), Manganese (Amino Acid Chelate), Adenosine Triphosphate, Vitamin A (Acetate), Folic

Acid, Vitamin D (Cholecalciferol), Selenium (Methionine), Vitamin B12.

How Supplied: One bottle contains 30 easy-to-swallow capsules.

STEPHAN™ MASCULINE
Nutritional Supplement

Uses: A nutritional food supplement formulated for the adult male, STEPHAN™ Masculine contains a special blend of nutrients with vitamins, minerals, herbs, and amino acids.

Directions: Take one to two capsules per day.

Ingredients: L-Histidine, Calcium (Carbonate), Bee Pollen, Parsley, Ribonucleic Acid, Zinc (Amino Acid Chelate), Magnesium (Amino Acid Chelate), Adenosine Triphosphate.

How Supplied: One bottle contains 30 easy-to-swallow capsules.

PHYTO-VITE™
Advanced Antioxidant, Vitamin, and Chelated Mineral Formulation

Uses: Phyto-Vite is a state-of-the-art nutritional supplement providing chelated minerals, vitamins, and a diverse group of antioxidants. It was formulated to meet the nutritional needs of our society where studies estimate only 9% consume foods in the quantities necessary to protect against the oxidative damage by free radicals.

The antioxidant coverage provided by Phyto-Vite is both comprehensive and diverse. First, it includes optimal amounts of vitamins A, C, and E as well as the pro-vitamins alpha and beta carotene. Vitamin A, in addition to its antioxidant capabilities, is also felt to improve immune function, protein synthesis, RNA synthesis, and steroid hormone synthesis. In this product, vitamin A is derived from two sources: retinyl palmitate and lemongrass. Additional vitamin A activity is provided by the alpha and beta carotene found in *Dunaliella salina*. These carotenoids are strong antioxidants in their own right; however, they can also be converted to vitamin A. This occurs only when the body is deficient in this vitamin. Consequently, vitamin A toxicity cannot be caused by alpha or beta carotene. Vitamin C has long been associated with wound healing, collagen formation, and maintaining the structural integrity of capillaries, cartilage, dentine, and bone. Its antioxidant effects are felt to play a major role in the prevention of cardiovascular disease and some cancers. Phyto-Vite utilizes esterified vitamin C which has been shown to provide a quicker uptake and a decreased rate of excretion when compared with conventional vitamin C. This allows for higher, more sustained levels of this vitamin in the body. Phyto-Vite also contains 400 I.U. of vitamin E, from natural sources. The antioxidant effects of vitamin E have been shown to stabilize cell membranes, increase HDL cholesterol, and decrease platelet aggregation.

Many flavonoids are incorporated into Phyto-Vite. These substances possess antioxidant activity themselves and also potentiate the effects of vitamins C and E. This later effect is produced by decreasing the degradation of vitamin C and E into inactive metabolites. Ginkgo biloba has flavonoid activity as well as other significant effects. Among these are a decrease in platelet aggregation and an increase in vasodilation which appears to increase blood flow to the peripheral arteries and the brain. Some improvement in cognitive abilities has been noted. It also helps to inhibit lipid peroxidation, thereby stabilizing the cell wall against free radical attack.

A Phytonutrient blend has been incorporated into Phyto-Vite to further enhance its antioxidant effects. Phytonutrient is a term given to the thousands of chemical compounds found in fruits and vegetables. Some of these compounds, including sulforaphane in broccoli and isothiocyanate in cabbage, have been shown to inhibit cancer in laboratory animals and human cell cultures. Others have shown great promise in aiding the cardiovascular system. Currently, much research is ongoing to isolate and identify more of these compounds, but it has already been clearly established that phytonutrients work best when the entire plant source is used rather than just the isolated compound. The phytonutrients found in Phyto-Vite are obtained from alfalfa (lutein), broccoli (indoles), cabbage (isothiocyanates), cayenne (capsanthin and capsorubin), green onion (thioallyl compounds), parsley (chlorophyll), spirulina (gamma linolenic acid), tomato (lycopene), soy isoflavones (genistein, lecithin, and daidzein), aged garlic concentrate, and Pure-Gar-A-8000™ (allicin).

The antioxidant minerals copper, zinc, manganese, and selenium have also been incorporated into Phyto-Vite. These minerals have been chelated via a patented process in which the mineral is wrapped within an amino acid. Once inside the body, the minerals can then be utilized in the millions of metabolic reactions that take place in the body. With this process, overall mineral absorption can approach 95% instead of the 5 to 10% absorption seen with other mineral supplements.

Phyto-Vite also provides two antioxidant enzymes (catalase and peroxidase). These help to reduce the body's free radical burden by neutralizing free radicals in the pharynx or stomach.

There are three other features that make Phyto-Vite unique among supplements. First, a small amount of canola oil was included to aid in the proper absorption of fat soluble vitamins, even on an empty stomach. Canola oil also provides essential fatty acids. Second, the product is formed into prolonged-release tablets which allow flexibility in dosing frequency. It can be taken all at once or staggered throughout the day. Dissolution testing has been performed to insure that the product will dissolve properly. Lastly, Phyto-Vite tablets are covered with a Betacoat™. This is a beta carotene coating that is designed to provide antioxidant coverage to the tablet itself. This helps to protect the integrity and activity of the product.

Directions: As a dietary supplement take six tablets per day with eight ounces of liquid. Tablets may be taken all at once or staggered throughout the day.

Warnings: If pregnant or lactating, consult physician before using.

Ingredients: Vitamin A (5,000 IU), Alpha and beta Carotene (20,000 IU), Vitamin C (500 mg), Vitamin E (400 IU), Citrus bioflavonoids with hesperidin (50 mg), Rutin and quercetin (50 mg), Bilberry standardized extract (10 mg), Grape seed proanthocyanidins (5 mg), Red grape polyphenols (5 mg), Ginkgo biloba standardized extract (20 mg), Copper (2 mg), Zinc (15 mg), Manganese (5 mg), Selenium (200 mcg), Catalase and peroxidase enzymes (3,500 units), Phytonutrient blend (800 mg), Vitamin B-1 (15 mg), Vitamin B-2 (17 mg), Vitamin B-3 (100 mg), Vitamin B-5 (75 mg), Vitamin B-6 (20 mg), Vitamin B-12 (60 mcg), Biotin (300 mcg), Folic Acid (400 mcg), Choline (50 mg), Inositol (50 mg), PABA (25 mg), Vitamin D-3 (400 IU), Vitamin K (70 mcg), Boron (1 mg), Calcium (500 mg), Magnesium (400 mg), Phosphorus (250 mg), Chromium (200 mcg), Iodine (150 mcg), Iron (4 mg), Potassium (70 mg), Essential Fatty Acids (100 mg).

How Supplied: One bottle contains 180 Betacoat™ tablets.

STEPHAN™ PROTECTOR
Nutritional Supplement

Uses: STEPHAN™ Protector is a nutritional food supplement that combines specific proteins, vitamins, minerals, and amino acids recognized as important for the health of areas associated with the human immune system. STEPHAN Protector may be used by men and women of all ages.

Directions: Take one capsule per day.

Warnings: Phenylketonurics: Contains Phenylalanine.

Ingredients: Bee Pollen, Astragalus, Kelp, Glutamic Acid, Ribonucleic Acid, Aspartic Acid, Leucine, Arginine, Lysine, Phenylalanine, Serine, Proline, Valine, Isoleucine, Alanine, Glycine, Threonine, Tyrosine, Histidine, Methionine, Cysteine, Adenosine Triphosphate.

How Supplied: One bottle contains 30 easy-to-swallow capsules.

Continued on next page

Wellness International—Cont.

STEPHAN™ RELIEF
Nutritional Supplement

Uses: Designed for both men and women, STEPHAN™ Relief has been formulated with a special combination of nutrients, vitamins, minerals, amino acids, and herbs which are recognized as important to the digestive and excretory systems.

Directions: Take one to two capsules per day.

Ingredients: Fucus, Parsley (extract 4:1), Psyllium, Leucine, Isoleucine, Valine, Bee Pollen, Ribonucleic Acid, Calcium Pantothenate, Adenosine Triphosphate.

How Supplied: One bottle contains 30 easy-to-swallow capsules.

STEPHAN™ TRANQUILITY
Nutritional Supplement

Uses: Designed for both men and women, STEPHAN™ Tranquility is a nutritional food supplement which contains a blend of vitamins, minerals, and amino acids recognized as important to areas involved in stress management.

Directions: Take one to two capsules per day.

Warnings: Phenylketonurics: Contains Phenylalanine.

Ingredients: Lecithin, Choline Bitartrate, Myo-Inositol, Vitamin C, Valerian (As 4:1 extract), Ribonucleic Acid, Vitamin E, Vitamin B-3, Glutamic Acid, Aspartic Acid, Calcium (Amino Acid Chelate), Leucine, Arginine, Lysine, Phenylalanine, Serine, Valine, Proline, Isoleucine, Alanine, Glycine, Threonine, Tyrosine, Vitamin B-5, Vitamin B-1, Histidine, Magnesium, Methionine, Cysteine, Adenosine Triphosphate, Vitamin B-6, Vitamin B-2, Vitamin A, Folic Acid, Biotin (Amino Acid Chelate), Vitamin D-3, Vitamin B-12.

How Supplied: One bottle contains 30 easy-to-swallow capsules.

WINRGY™
Nutritional Drink with Vitamin C

Uses: A delicious, Vitamin C-enriched beverage, WINRGY™ was formulated with a special blend of nutrients designed to offer a nutritional alternative to coffees and colas.

Directions: Add 6 ounces of chilled water or fruit juice to one packet of mix. Stir briskly. Consume 1–2 times per day. Keep in a cool, dry place.

Warnings: Phenylketonurics: Contains Phenylalanine. Not for use by children, pregnant or lactating women. Persons taking medications should seek medical advice before taking this product. Do not consume more than four servings per day. Avoid the use of antacids containing aluminum with this product.

Ingredients: Fructose, L-Phenylalanine, Natural Flavors, Citric Acid, Taurine, Glycine, Ascorbic Acid, Caffeine, Niacinamide, Vitamin E Acetate, Calcium Pantothenate, Silicon Dioxide, Potassium Aspartate, Manganese Aspartate, Chromium Aspartate, Pyridoxine Hydrochloride, Zinc Gluconate, Riboflavin, Thiamin Mononitrate, Copper Gluconate, Folic Acid, Vitamin B12.

How Supplied: One box contains 28 packets. Serving size equals one packet.

Whitehall-Robins Healthcare
American Home Products Corporation
FIVE GIRALDA FARMS
MADISON, NJ 07940

Direct Inquiries to:
Whitehall Consumer Product Information 800-322-3129
Robins Consumer Product Information 800-762-4672
Professional Samples: Whitehall-Robins 800-343-0856

ADVIL®
[ad'vil]
Ibuprofen Tablets, USP
Ibuprofen Caplets
(Oval-Shaped Tablets)
Ibuprofen Gel Caplets
(Oval-Shaped Gelatin Coated Tablets)
WARNING: ASPIRIN-SENSITIVE PATIENTS. Do not take this product if you have had a severe allergic reaction to aspirin, e.g.—asthma, swelling, shock or hives, because even though this product contains no aspirin or salicylates, cross-reactions may occur in patients allergic to aspirin.

Active Ingredient: Each tablet or caplet contains Ibuprofen 200 mg.

Inactive Ingredients: Tablets and Caplets Acetylated Monoglyceride, Beeswax and/or Carnauba Wax, Croscarmellose Sodium, Iron Oxides, Lecithin, Methylparaben, Microcrystalline Cellulose, Pharmaceutical Glaze, Povidone, Propylparaben, Silicon Dioxide, Simethicone, Sodium Benzoate, Sodium Lauryl Sulfate, Starch, Stearic Acid, Sucrose, Titanium Dioxide. Gel Caplets Croscarmellose/Sodium, FD&C Red #40, FD&C Yellow #6, Gelatin, Glycerin, Hydroxypropyl Methylcellulose, Iron Oxides, Lecithin, Pharmaceutical Glaze, Propyl Gallate, Silicon Dioxide, Simethicone, Sodium Lauryl Sulfate, Starch, Stearic Acid, Titanium Dioxide, Triacetin.

Indications: For the temporary relief of minor aches and pains associated with the common cold, headache, toothache, muscular aches, backache, for the minor pain of arthritis, for the pain of menstrual cramps and for reduction of fever.

Dosage and Administration: Adults: Take one tablet or caplet every 4 to 6 hours while symptoms persist. If pain or fever does not respond to one tablet or caplet, two tablets or caplets may be used but do not exceed six tablets or caplets in 24 hours unless directed by a doctor. The smallest effective dose should be used. Take with food or milk if occasional and mild heartburn, upset stomach, or stomach pain occurs with use. Consult a doctor if these symptoms are more than mild or if they persist. Children: Do not give this product to children under 12 years of age except under the advice and supervision of a doctor.

Warnings: Do not take for pain for more than 10 days or for fever for more than 3 days unless directed by a doctor. If pain or fever persists or gets worse, if new symptoms occur, or if the painful area is red or swollen, consult a doctor. These could be signs of serious illness. If you are under a doctor's care for any serious condition, consult a doctor before taking this product. As with aspirin and acetaminophen, if you have any condition which requires you to take prescription drugs or if you have had any problems or serious side effects from taking any nonprescription pain reliever, do not take this product without first discussing it with your doctor. **IF YOU EXPERIENCE ANY SYMPTOMS WHICH ARE UNUSUAL OR SEEM UNRELATED TO THE CONDITION FOR WHICH YOU TOOK IBUPROFEN, CONSULT A DOCTOR BEFORE TAKING ANY MORE OF IT.** Although ibuprofen is indicated for the same conditions as aspirin and acetaminophen, it should not be taken with them except under a doctor's direction. Do not combine this product with any other ibuprofen-containing product. As with any drug, if you are pregnant or nursing a baby, seek the advice of a health professional before using this product. **IT IS ESPECIALLY IMPORTANT NOT TO USE IBUPROFEN DURING THE LAST 3 MONTHS OF PREGNANCY UNLESS SPECIFICALLY DIRECTED TO DO SO BY A DOCTOR BECAUSE IT MAY CAUSE PROBLEMS IN THE UNBORN CHILD OR COMPLICATIONS DURING DELIVERY.** Keep this and all drugs out of the reach of children. In case of accidental overdose, seek professional assistance or contact a poison control center immediately.

How Supplied: Coated tablets in bottles of 4, 8, 24, 50 (non-child resistant size), 72 (E-Z Cap) 100, 165 and 250. Coated caplets in bottles of 24, 50 (non-child resistant size), 72 (E-Z Cap) 100, 165, and 250. Coated tablets in thermoform packaging of 8.
Gel caplets in bottles of 4, 8, 24, 50, 100, 165 and 250.

Storage: Store at room temperature; avoid excessive heat (40°C, 104°F).

Shown in Product Identification Guide, page 528

ADVIL® Cold and Sinus
Ibuprofen/Pseudoephedrine HCl
Caplets* and Tablets
Pain Reliever/Fever Reducer/Nasal
Decongestant

*Oval-Shaped tablets

WARNING: ASPIRIN-SENSITIVE PATIENTS. Do not take this product if you have had a severe allergic reaction to aspirin, eg, asthma, swelling, shock or hives, because even though this product contains no aspirin or salicylates, cross-reactions may occur in patients allergic to aspirin.

Indications: For temporary relief of symptoms associated with the common cold, sinusitis or flu, including nasal congestion, headache, fever, body aches, and pains.

Directions: *Adults:* Take 1 caplet or tablet every 4 to 6 hours while symptoms persist. If symptoms do not respond to 1 caplet or tablet, 2 caplets or tablets may be used, but do not exceed 6 caplets or tablets in 24 hours unless directed by a doctor. The smallest effective dose should be used. Take with food or milk if occasional and mild heartburn, upset stomach, or stomach pain occurs with use. Consult a doctor if these symptoms are more than mild or if they persist. *Children:* Do not give this product to children under 12 years of age except under the advice and supervision of a doctor.

Warnings: Do not take for colds for more than 7 days or for fever for more than 3 days unless directed by a doctor. If the cold or fever persists or gets worse, or if new symptoms occur, consult a doctor. These could be signs of serious illness. As with aspirin and acetaminophen, if you have any condition which requires you to take prescription drugs or if you have had any problems or serious side effects from taking any nonprescription pain reliever, do not take this product without first discussing it with your doctor. IF YOU EXPERIENCE ANY SYMPTOMS WHICH ARE UNUSUAL OR SEEM UNRELATED TO THE CONDITION FOR WHICH YOU TOOK THIS PRODUCT, CONSULT A DOCTOR BEFORE TAKING ANY MORE OF IT. If you are under a doctor's care for any serious condition, consult a doctor before taking this product.
Do not exceed recommended dosage. If nervousness, dizziness, or sleeplessness occur, discontinue use and consult a doctor. Do not take this product if you have high blood pressure, heart disease, diabetes, thyroid disease or difficulty in urination due to enlargement of the prostate gland, except under the advice and supervision of a doctor.

Drug Interaction Precaution: Do not use if you are now taking a prescription monoamine oxidase inhibitor (MAOI) (certain drugs for depression, psychiatric or emotional conditions, or Parkinson's disease), or for 2 weeks after stopping the MAOI drug. If you are uncertain whether your prescription drug contains an MAOI, consult a health professional before taking this product. Do not combine this product with other non-prescription pain relievers. Do not combine this product with any other ibuprofen-containing product. As with any drug, if you are pregnant or nursing a baby, seek the advice of a health professional before using this product.
IT IS ESPECIALLY IMPORTANT NOT TO USE THIS PRODUCT DURING THE LAST 3 MONTHS OF PREGNANCY UNLESS SPECIFICALLY DIRECTED TO DO SO BY A DOCTOR BECAUSE IT MAY CAUSE PROBLEMS IN THE UNBORN CHILD OR COMPLICATIONS DURING DELIVERY. Keep this and all drugs out of the reach of children. In case of accidental overdose, seek professional assistance or contact a poison control center immediately.

Active Ingredients: Each caplet or tablet contains Ibuprofen 200 mg and Pseudoephedrine HCl 30 mg.

Inactive Ingredients: Carnauba or Equivalent Wax, Croscarmellose Sodium, Iron Oxides, Methylparaben, Microcrystalline Cellulose, Propylparaben, Silicon Dioxide, Sodium Benzoate, Sodium Lauryl Sulfate, Starch, Stearic Acid, Sucrose, Titanium Dioxide.

How Supplied: Advil® Cold and Sinus is an oval-shaped tan-colored caplet or tan-colored tablet supplied in consumer bottles of 40 and blister packs of 20. Medical samples are available in a 2's pouch dispenser.

Storage: Store at room temperature; avoid excessive heat (40°C, 104°F).
Shown in Product Identification Guide, page 528

CLEARBLUE EASY®
Pregnancy Test Kit
Clearblue Easy is one of the easiest and fastest pregnancy tests available because all a woman has to do is hold the absorbent tip in her urine stream and in 3 minutes she can read the result. A blue line appears in the small window to show that the test is complete and the large window shows the test result. If there is a blue line in the large window, the woman is pregnant. If there is no line, she is not pregnant.

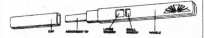

Clearblue Easy is a rapid, one-step pregnancy test for home use, which detects the pregnancy hormone HCG (human chorionic gonadotropin) in the urine. This hormone is produced in increasing amounts during the first part of pregnancy. Clearblue Easy uses sensitive monoclonal antibodies to detect the presence of this hormone from the first day of a missed period.
A negative result means that no pregnancy hormone was detected and the woman is probably not pregnant. If the menstrual period does not start within a week, she may have miscalculated the day her period was due. She should repeat the test using another Clearblue Easy test. If the second test still gives a negative result and she still has not menstruated, she should see her doctor. Clearblue Easy is specially designed for easy use at home. However, if there are any questions about the test or results, give the Clearblue Easy TalkLine a call at 1-800-883-EASY. A specially trained staff of advisors is available to answer your questions.
Manufactured by Unipath Ltd., Bedford, U.K. Unipath, Clearblue Easy and the fan device are trademarks.
Distributed by Whitehall Laboratories, Madison, NJ 07940-0871.
Shown in Product Identification Guide, page 528

CLEARPLAN EASY™
One-Step Ovulation Predictor
CLEARPLAN EASY is one of the easiest home ovulation predictor tests to use because of its unique technological design. It consists of just one piece and involves only one step to get results. To use CLEARPLAN EASY, a woman simply holds the absorbent tip in her urine stream (a woman can test any time of day) for 5 seconds, and after 5 minutes, she can read the results. A blue line will appear in the small window to show her that the test has worked correctly. The large window indicates the presence of luteinizing hormone (LH) in her urine. If there is a line in the large window which is similar to or darker than the line in the small window, she has detected her LH surge.

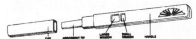

Laboratory tests confirm that CLEARPLAN EASY is over 98% accurate in detecting the LH surge as shown by radioimmunoassay (RIA).
CLEARPLAN EASY employs highly sensitive monoclonal antibody technology to accurately predict the onset of ovulation, and, consequently, the best time each month for a woman to try to become pregnant. The test monitors the amount of LH in a woman's urine. Small amounts of LH are present during most of the menstrual cycle, but the level normally rises sharply about 24 to 36 hours before ovulation (which is when an egg is released from the ovary). CLEARPLAN EASY detects this LH surge preceding ovulation so that a woman knows 24–36 hours beforehand the time she is most able to become pregnant.

Continued on next page

Whitehall-Robins—Cont.

A woman will be most fertile during the 1 to 3 days after an LH surge is detected. Sperm can fertilize an egg for many hours after sexual intercourse. So, if sexual intercourse occurs during the 1–3 days after a similar or darker line appears in the large window, the chances of getting pregnant are maximized.

CLEARPLAN EASY contains 5 days of tests. If, because a woman's cycles are irregular or if for any other reason a woman does not detect her LH surge after 5 days of testing, she should continue testing with a second CLEARPLAN EASY kit. CLEARPLAN EASY offers users the support of a TalkLine (1-800-883-EASY). This service is operated by trained advisors who are available to answer any questions about using the test or reading the results.

Produced by Unipath Ltd., Bedford, U.K. Unipath, CLEARPLAN EASY and the fan device are trademarks.
Distributed by Whitehall Laboratories, Madison, NJ 07940-0871.
Shown in Product Identification Guide, page 528

DIMETAPP Allergy Dye-Free Elixir
[dī'mĕ-tap]

Description: (Brompheniramine Maleate) Antihistamine Dye-Free Elixir

Active Ingredients: Each 5 mL (1 teaspoonful) contains: Brompheniramine Maleate, USP 2 mg.

Inactive Ingredients: Citric Acid, Flavors, Glycerin, Sodium Benzoate, Sorbitol, Water.

Indications: For temporary relief of runny nose, sneezing, itching of the nose or throat, and itchy, watery eyes due to hay fever or other upper respiratory allergies.

Warnings: Do not take this product, unless directed by a physician, if you have a breathing problem such as emphysema or chronic bronchitis, or if you have glaucoma or difficulty in urination due to enlargement of the prostate gland. May cause drowsiness; alcohol, sedatives and tranquilizers may increase the drowsiness effect. Avoid alcoholic beverages while taking this product. Do not take this product if you are taking sedatives or tranquilizers without first consulting your physician. Use caution when driving a motor vehicle or operating machinery. May cause excitability, especially in children.
As with any drug, if you are pregnant or nursing a baby, seek the advice of a health professional before using this product.
KEEP THIS AND ALL DRUGS OUT OF THE REACH OF CHILDREN. IN CASE OF ACCIDENTAL OVERDOSE, SEEK PROFESSIONAL ASSISTANCE OR CONTACT A POISON CONTROL CENTER IMMEDIATELY.

Directions: Adults and children 12 years of age and over: 2 teaspoonfuls every four to six hours, not to exceed 12 teaspoonfuls in 24 hours, or as directed by a physician; children 6 to under 12 years: 1 teaspoonful every four to six hours, not to exceed 6 teaspoonfuls in 24 hours, or as directed by a physician; children under 6 years: Consult a physician.
Store at Controlled Room Temperature, between 20°C and 25°C (68°F and 77°F). Not a USP Elixir.

How Supplied: 4 oz. bottle. Dose cup provided. NDC 0031-2232-12

DIMETAPP® Allergy Sinus
(Previously Cold & Flu)

Description: Nasal Decongestant, Antihistamine, Pain Reliever-Fever Reducer.

Active Ingredients: Each caplet contains Acetaminophen, USP 500 mg, Phenylpropanolamine Hydrochloride, USP 12.5 mg and Brompheniramine Maleate, USP 2 mg.

Inactive Ingredients: Corn Starch, Hydroxypropyl Cellulose, Hydroxypropyl Methylcellulose, Magnesium Stearate, Methylparaben, Microcrystalline Cellulose, Polysorbate 20, Povidone, Propylparaben, Propylene Glycol, Stearic Acid, Titanium Dioxide.

Indication: For the temporary relief of minor aches, pains, and headache; for the reduction of fever; for the relief of nasal congestion due to the common cold or associated with sinusitis; and for the relief of runny nose, sneezing, itching of the nose or throat and itchy and watery eyes due to hay fever (allergic rhinitis). Temporarily restores freer breathing through the nose.

Warnings: Do not take this product if you have a breathing problem such as emphysema or chronic bronchitis or if you have heart disease, high blood pressure, thyroid disease, diabetes, glaucoma, or difficulty in urination due to enlargement of the prostate gland, unless directed by a physician.

Alcohol Warning: Avoid alcohol beverages while taking this product. If you generally consume 3 or more alcohol-containing drinks per day, you should consult your physician for advice on when and how you should take ths product or any other acetaminophen-containing product.
May cause drowsiness; alcohol, sedatives and tranquilizers may increase the drowsiness effect. Do not take this product if you are taking sedatives or tranquilizers without first consulting your physician. Use caution when driving a motor vehicle or operating machinery. May cause excitability, especially in children.
Do not exceed recommended dosage. If nervousness, dizziness or sleeplessness occur, discontinue use and consult a physician. Do not take this product for more than 7 days or for fever for more than 3

days. If pain or fever persists or gets worse, if new symptoms occur, or if redness or swelling is present, consult a physician because these could be signs of a serious condition.
As with any drug, if you are pregnant or nursing a baby, seek the advice of a health professional before using this product.

Drug Interaction Precaution: Do not use this product if you are now taking a prescription monoamine oxidase inhibitor (MAOI) (certain drugs for depression, psychiatric or emotional conditions, or Parkinson's disease), or for 2 weeks after stopping the MAOI drug. If you are uncertain whether your prescription drug contains an MAOI, consult a health professional before taking this product.
KEEP THIS AND ALL DRUGS OUT OF THE REACH OF CHILDREN. IN CASE OF ACCIDENTAL OVERDOSE, SEEK PROFESSIONAL ASSISTANCE OR CONTACT A POISON CONTROL CENTER IMMEDIATELY. PROMPT MEDICAL ATTENTION IS CRITICAL FOR ADULTS AS WELL AS FOR CHILDREN EVEN IF YOU DO NOT NOTICE ANY SIGNS OR SYMPTOMS.

Directions: Adults (12 years and over): Two caplets every 6 hours. DO NOT EXCEED 8 CAPLETS IN A 24-HOUR PERIOD.
Children under 12: Consult a physican.
Store at Controlled Room Temperature, between 20°C and 25°C (68°F and 77°F).

How Supplied: Blister packs of 12 (NDC 0031-2284-46)
Bottles of 24 (NDC 0031-2284-54)

DIMETAPP® Cold & Allergy
[di'mĕ-tap]
Chewable Tablets

Description: Each chewable tablet contains:
Brompheniramine Maleate, USP .... 1 mg
Phenylpropanolamine Hydrochloride, USP .... 6.25 mg

Inactive Ingredients: Aspartame, Citric Acid, Crospovidone, D&C Red 30 Lake, D&C Red 7 Lake, FD&C Blue 1 Lake, Flavor, Glycine, Magnesium Stearate, Mannitol, Microcrystalline Cellulose, Pregelatinized Starch, Silicon Dioxide, Sorbitol, Stearic Acid.

Indications: For temporary relief of nasal congestion due to the common cold, hay fever, or other upper respiratory allergies or associated with sinusitis. Temporarily relieves runny nose, sneezing, and itchy, watery eyes due to hay fever (allergic rhinitis). Temporarily restores freer breathing through the nose.

Warnings: Do not to give this product to children who have a breathing problem such as chronic bronchitis, or who have glaucoma, high blood pressure, heart disease, diabetes, or thyroid disease, without first consulting the child's physician. This product may cause drowiness: sedatives and tranquilizers may increase the drowsiness effect. Do not give this product to children who are taking sedatives or tranquilizers without first consulting the child's physician. May cause excitability, especially in children.

Do not exceed recommended dosage. If nervousness, dizziness, or sleeplessness occur, discontinue use and consult a doctor. If symptoms do not improve within 7 days, or are accompanied by a fever, consult a physician. As with any drug, if you are pregnant or nursing a baby, seek the advice of a health professional before using this product.

Drug Interaction Precaution: Do not give this product to a child who is taking a prescription monoamine oxidase inhibitor (MAOI) (certain drugs for depression, psychiatric or emotional conditions, or for 2 weeks after stopping the MAOI drug. If you are uncertain whether your child's prescription drug contains an MAOI, consult a health professional before taking this product.
KEEP THIS AND ALL DRUGS OUT OF THE REACH OF CHILDREN. IN CASE OF ACCIDENTAL OVERDOSE, SEEK PROFESSIONAL ASSISTANCE OR CONTACT A POISON CONTROL CENTER IMMEDIATELY.
Phenylketonurics: contains phenylalanine, 8 mg per tablet.

Directions: Children 6 to under 12 years of age: 2 chewable tablets every 4 hours. Children under 6: Consult a physician. DO NOT EXCEED 6 DOSES IN A 24-HOUR PERIOD.

Professional Labeling: The suggested dosage for children age 2 to under 6 years, only when the child is under the care of a physician, is 1 tablet every 4 hours, not to exceed 6 doses in a 24-hour period.

How Supplied: Purple tablet scored on one side and engraved with AHR 2290 on the other in bottles of 24 tablets (NDC 0031–2290–54).
Store at Controlled Room Temperature, Between 15°C and 30°C (59°F and 86°F).

DIMETAPP® Cold & Cough Liqui-Gels®
Maximum Strength
[dī'mĕ-tap]

Description: Nasal Decongestant, Antihistamine, Cough Suppressant Liqui-Gels®

Active Ingredients: Each softgel contains: Brompheniramine Maleate, USP 4 mg, Phenylpropanolamine Hydrochloride, USP 25 mg, and Dextromethorphan Hydrobromide, USP 20 mg.

Inactive Ingredients: FD&C Red #40, Gelatin, Glycerin, Mannitol, Pharmaceutical Glaze, Polyethylene Glycol, Povidone, Propylene Glycol, Sorbitan, Sorbitol, Titanium Dioxide, Water.

Indications: Temporarily relieves cough due to minor throat and bronchial irritation as may occur with a cold. For temporary relief of nasal congestion due to the common cold, hay fever or other upper respiratory allergies or associated with sinusitis; temporarily relieves runny nose, sneezing, itching of the nose or throat, and itchy, watery eyes due to hay fever (allergic rhinitis). Temporarily restores freer breathing through the nose.

Warnings: Do not take this product unless directed by a doctor, if you have a breathing problem such as emphysema or chronic bronchitis, or persistent or chronic cough such as occurs with smoking or asthma, or if cough is accompanied by excessive phlegm (mucus). Likewise, if you have heart disease, high blood pressure, thyroid disease, diabetes, glaucoma or difficulty in urination due to enlargement of the prostrate gland, do not take this product unless directed by a physician. May cause drowsiness; alcohol, sedatives and tranquilizers may increase the drowsiness effect. Avoid alcoholic beverages while taking this product. Do not take this product if you are taking sedatives or tranquilizers without first consulting your physician. Use caution when driving a motor vehicle or operating machinery. May cause excitability, especially in children.
Do not exceed recommended dosage. If nervousness, dizziness or sleeplessness occur, discontinue use and consult a physican. A persistent cough may be a sign of a serious condition. If cough or other symptoms persist, do not improve within 7 days, tend to recur, or are accompanied by fever, rash, or persistent headache, consult a physician. As with any drug, if you are pregnant or nursing a baby, seek the advice of a health professional before using this product.

Drug Interaction Precaution: Do not use this product if you are not taking a prescription monoamine oxidase inhibitor (MAOI) (certain drugs for depression, psychiatric or emotional conditions or Parkinson's disease), or for 2 weeks after stopping the MAOI drug. If you are uncertain whether your prescription drug contains an MAOI, consult a health professional before taking this product.
KEEP THIS AND ALL DRUGS OUT OF THE REACH OF CHILDREN. IN CASE OF ACCIDENTAL OVERDOSE, SEEK PROFESSIONAL ASSISTANCE OR CONTACT A POISON CONTROL CENTER IMMEDIATELY.

Directions: Adults and children 12 years of age and over: one softgel every 4 hours. Children under 12: Consult a physician. DO NOT EXCEED 6 SOFTGELS IN A 24-HOUR PERIOD.
Store at Controlled Room Temperature, between 20°C and 25°C (68°F and 77°F). Not a USP Elixir.

How Supplied: Blister packs of 12's NDC 0031-2279-46.
Blister packs of 24's NDC 0031-2279-54.
Liqui-Gels is a registered trademark of R.P. Scherer International Corporation

DIMETAPP Cold and Fever Suspension
[dī'mĕ-tap]

Description: Nasal Decongestant, Antihistamine, Pain reliever-Fever reducer
Alcohol Free

Active Ingredients: Each 5 mL (1 teaspoonful) contains: Acetaminophen, USP, 160 mg; Pseudoephedrine Hydrochloride, USP, 15 mg; Brompheniramine Maleate, USP, 1 mg.

Inactive Ingredients: Carboxymethylcellulose Sodium, Citric Acid, D&C Red 33, Disodium Edetate, FD&C Blue 1, Flavors, Glycerin, High Fructose Corn Syrup, Maltol, Methylparaben, Microcrystalline Cellulose, Polysorbate 80, Potassium Sorbate, Propylene Glycol, Propylparaben, Sorbitol, Sucrose, Water, Xanthan Gum

Indications: For temporary relief of nasal congestion, minor aches, pains, headache and sore throat and to reduce fever associated with a cold or sinusitis. Temporarily relieves runny nose and sneezing, itching of the nose or throat and itchy, watery eyes due to hay fever or other upper respiratory allergies.

Warnings: Do not give this product to children who have a breathing problem such as chronic bronchitis, or who have high blood pressure, heart disease, diabetes, thyroid disease, or glaucoma unless directed by a physician. May cause drowsiness; sedatives and tranquilizers may increase the drowsiness effect. Do not give this product to children who are taking sedatives or tranquilizers without first consulting the child's physician. Use caution when driving a motor vehicle or operating machinery. May cause excitability, especially in children.
Do not exceed recommended dosage. If nervousness, dizziness or sleeplessness occur, discontinue use and consult a doctor. If symptoms do not improve within 7 days or are accompanied by a fever, consult a doctor. If sore throat is severe, persists for more than 2 days, is accompanied or followed by fever, headache, rash, nausea or vomiting, consult a physician promptly. Do not give this product for pain for more than 5 days or for fever for more than 3 days unless directed by a doctor. If pain or fever persists, or gets worse, if new symptoms occur or if redness or swelling is present, consult a physician because these could be signs of a serious condition.

Drug Interaction Precaution: Do not give this product to a child who is taking a prescription monoamine oxidase inhibitor (MAOI) (certain drugs for depression, psychiatric or emotional conditions, or Parkinson's disease), or for 2 weeks after stopping the MAOI drug. If you are uncertain whether your child's prescription drug contains an MAOI, consult a health professional before giving this product.

Continued on next page

Whitehall-Robins—Cont.

Directions: Shake Well Before Using. Children 6 to under 12: two teaspoonfuls every 4 hours (or as directed by a physician). Do Not Exceed 4 Doses in a 24-hour Period. Children under 6 years: consult a physician.
KEEP THIS AND ALL DRUGS OUT OF THE REACH OF CHILDREN. IN CASE OF ACCIDENTAL OVERDOSE, SEEK PROFESSIONAL ASSISTANCE OR CONTACT A POISON CONTROL CENTER IMMEDIATELY, PROMPT MEDICAL ATTENTION IS CRITICAL FOR ADULTS AS WELL AS CHILDREN EVEN IF YOU DO NOT NOTICE ANY SIGNS OR SYMPTOMS.

Storage: Store at Controlled Room Temperature, Between 20°C and 25°C (68°F and 77°F).

How Supplied: 4 oz bottle with dosage cup. NDC 0031-2281-12

DIMETAPP® Decongestant Pediatric Drops
[dī'mě-tap]

Description: Nasal Decongestant (Pseudoephedrine Hydrochloride)

Active Ingredients: Each 0.8 mL (1 dropperful) contains: 7.5 mg Pseudoephedrine Hydrochloride, USP.

Inactive Ingredients: Carmel, Citric Acid, FD&C Blue 1, D&C Red 33, Flavors, Glycerin, High Fructose Corn Syrup, Maltol, Menthol, Polyethylene Glycol, Propylene Glycol, Sodium Benzoate, Sorbitol, Sucrose, Water.

Indications: For temporary relief of nasal congestion due to the common cold, hay fever, other upper respiratory allergies or associated with sinusitis.

Warnings: Do not exceed recommended dosage. If nervousness, dizziness, or sleeplessness occur, discontinue use and consult a physician. If symptoms do not improve within 7 days or are accompanied by a fever, consult a physician. Do not give this product to a child who has heart disease, high blood pressure, thyroid disease, or diabetes, unless directed by a physician.

Drug Interaction Precaution: Do not give this product to a child who is taking a prescription monoamine oxidase inhibitor (MAOI) (certain drugs for depression, psychiatric or emotional conditions), or for 2 weeks after stopping the MAOI drug. If you are uncertain whether your child's prescription drug contains an MAOI, consult a health professional before giving this product.
KEEP THIS AND ALL DRUGS OUT OF THE REACH OF CHILDREN. IN CASE OF ACCIDENTAL OVERDOSE, SEEK PROFESSIONAL ASSISTANCE OR CONTACT A POISON CONTROL CENTER IMMEDIATELY.

Directions: Children 2 to 3 years: Two droppertuls (1.6 mL) every 4–6 hours (or as directed by a physician). Children under 2: Consult a physician. DO NOT EXCEED 4 DOSES IN A 24-HOUR PERIOD. Take by mouth only. Not for nasal use.
Store at Controlled Room Temperature, between 20°C and 25°C (68°F and 77°F).

How Supplied: ½ oz (8 mL) bottle with dropper. (NDC 0031-2283-78)

DIMETAPP® Elixir
[dī' mě-tap]

Description: Each 5 mL (1 teaspoonful) contains:
Brompheniramine
   Maleate, USP ....2 mg
Phenylpropanolamine
   Hydrochloride, USP ....12.5 mg

Inactive Ingredients: Citric Acid, FD&C Blue 1, FD&C Red 40, Flavors, Glycerin, Saccharin Sodium, Sodium Benzoate, Sorbitol, Water.

Indications: For temporary relief of nasal congestion due to the common cold, hay fever or other upper respiratory allergies or associated with sinusitis. Temporarily relieves runny nose, sneezing, itching of the nose or throat, and itchy and watery eyes due to hay fever (allergic rhinitis). Temporarily restores freer breathing through the nose.

Warnings: Do not take this product if you have a breathing problem such as emphysema or chronic bronchitis, or if you have high blood pressure, heart disease, diabetes, thyroid disease, glaucoma, or difficulty in urination due to enlargement of the prostate gland, unless directed by a physician. May cause drowsiness; alcohol, sedatives and tranquilizers may increase the drowsiness effect. Avoid alcoholic beverages while taking this product. Do not take this product if you are taking sedatives or tranquilizers without first consulting your physician. Use caution when driving a motor vehicle or operating machinery. May cause excitability, especially in children.
Do not exceed the recommended dosage. If nervousness, dizziness or sleeplessness occur, discontinue use and consult a doctor. If symptoms do not improve within 7 days, or are accompanied by a fever, consult a doctor.
As with any drug, if you are pregnant or nursing a baby, seek the advice of a health professional before using this product.
KEEP THIS AND ALL DRUGS OUT OF THE REACH OF CHILDREN. IN CASE OF ACCIDENTAL OVERDOSE, SEEK PROFESSIONAL ASSISTANCE OR CONTACT A POISON CONTROL CENTER IMMEDIATELY.

Drug Interaction Precaution: Do not use this product if you are now taking a prescription monoamine oxidase inhibitor (MAOI) (certain drugs for depression, psychiatric or emotional conditions, or

Parkinson's disease) or for 2 weeks after stopping the MAOI drug. If you are uncertain whether your prescription drug contains an MAOI, consult a health professional before taking this product.

Directions: Adults and children 12 years of age and over: 2 teaspoonfuls every 4 hours; children 6 to under 12 years: 1 teaspoonful every 4 hours; DO NOT EXCEED 6 DOSES IN A 24-HOUR PERIOD. Children under 6 years: consult a physician.

Professional Labeling: The suggested dosage for children age 2 to under 6 years, only when the child is under the care of a physician, is ½ teaspoonful every 4 hours, not to exceed 6 doses in a 24-hour period. The dosage for children under 2 years should be determined by the physician on the basis of the patient's weight, physical condition, or other appropriate consideration. Dimetapp Elixir is contraindicated in neonates (children under the age of one month).

How Supplied: Purple, grape-flavored liquid in bottles of 4 fl. oz. (NDC 0031-2230-12), 8 fl. oz. (NDC 0031-2230-18), 12 fl. oz. (NDC 0031-2230-22), pints (NDC 0031-2230-25), and gallons (NDC 0031-2230-29).
Store at Controlled Room Temperature, between 20°C and 25°C (68°F and 77°F). Not a USP elixir.
Shown in Product Identification Guide, page 528

DIMETAPP® DM ELIXIR
[dī'mě-tap]

Description: Each 5 mL (1 teaspoonful) contains:
Brompheniramine
   Maleate, USP .... 2 mg
Phenylpropanolamine
   Hydrochloride, USP .... 12.5 mg
Dextromethorphan
   Hydrobromide, USP .... 10.0 mg

Inactive Ingredients: Citric Acid, FD&C Blue 1, FD&C Red 40, Flavors, Glycerin, Propylene Glycol, Saccharin Sodium, Sodium Benzoate, Sorbitol, Water.

Indications: Temporarily relieves cough due to minor throat and bronchial irritation as may occur with a cold. For temporary relief of nasal congestion due to the common cold, hay fever or other upper respiratory allergies or associated with sinusitis. Temporarily relieves runny nose, sneezing, itching of the nose or throat and itchy and watery eyes due to allergic rhinitis (hay fever). Temporarily restores freer breathing through the nose.

Warnings: Do not take this product if you have a breathing problem such as emphysema or chronic bronchitis or persistent or chronic cough such as occurs with smoking or asthma, or cough that is accompanied by excessive phlegm (mucus) unless directed by a physician. Likewise, if you have high blood pressure, heart disease, diabetes, thyroid disease, glaucoma, or difficulty in urination due to enlargement of the prostate gland, do not take this product unless directed by a physician.

May cause marked drowsiness; alcohol, sedatives and tranquilizers may increase the drowsiness effect. Avoid alcoholic beverages while taking this product. Do not take this product if you are taking sedatives or tranquilizers without first consulting your physician. Use caution when driving a motor vehicle or operating machinery. May cause excitability, especially in children.

Do not exceed the recommended dosage. If nervousness, dizziness or sleeplessness occur, discontinue use and consult a physician. A persistent cough may be a sign of a serious condition. If cough or other symptoms persist for more than one week without improvement, tend to recur, or are accompanied by fever, rash or persistent headache, consult a physician.

As with any drug, if you are pregnant or nursing a baby, seek the advice of a health professional before using this product.

KEEP THIS AND ALL DRUGS OUT OF THE REACH OF CHILDREN. IN CASE OF ACCIDENTAL OVERDOSE, SEEK PROFESSIONAL ASSISTANCE OR CONTACT A POISON CONTROL CENTER IMMEDIATELY.

Drug Interaction Precaution: Do not use this product if you are now taking a prescription monoamine oxidase inhibitor (MAOI) (certain drugs for depression, psychiatric or emotional conditions, or Parkinson's disease) or for 2 weeks after stopping the MAOI drug. If you are uncertain whether your prescription drug contains an MAOI, consult a health professional before taking this product.

Directions: Adults and children 12 years of age and over: Two teaspoonfuls every 4 hours; children 6 to under 12 years: one teaspoonful every 4 hours. DO NOT EXCEED 6 DOSES IN A 24-HOUR PERIOD. Children under 6 years: consult a physician.

Professional Labeling: The suggested dosage for children age 2 to under 6 years, only when the child is under the care of a physician, is ½ teaspoonful every 4 hours, not to exceed 6 doses in a 24-hour period. The dosage for children under 2 years should be determined by the physician on the basis of the patient's weight, physical condition, or other appropriate consideration. Dimetapp DM Elixir is contraindicated in neonates (children under the age of one month).

How Supplied: Red, grape-flavored liquid in bottles of 4 fl. oz. (NDC 0031-2240-12), 8 fl. oz. (NDC 0031-2240-18), and 12 fl. oz. (NDC 0031-2240-22).
Store at Controlled Room Temperature, Between 20°C and 25°C (68°F and 77°F) Not a USP elixir.

DIMETAPP® Extentabs®
[dī' mĕ-tap]

Description: Each **Dimetapp Extentabs**® Tablet contains:
Brompheniramine Maleate,
   USP .... 12 mg
Phenylpropanolamine
   Hydrochloride, USP .... 75 mg

Inactive Ingredients: Acacia, Acetylated Monoglycerides, Calcium Sulfate, Carnauba Wax, Citric Acid, Edible Ink, FD&C Blue 1, Gelatin, Hydrogenated Castor Oil, Magnesium Stearate, Magnesium Trisilicate, Pharmaceutical Glaze, Polysorbates, Povidone, Silicon Dioxide, Stearyl Alcohol, Sucrose, Titanium Dioxide, White Wax. May also contain Wheat Flour.

Indications: For temporary relief of nasal congestion due to the common cold, hay fever or other upper respiratory allergies or associated with sinusitis; temporarily relieves runny nose, sneezing, and itchy and watery eyes due to allergic rhinitis (hay fever). Temporarily restores freer breathing through the nose.

Warnings: Do not take this product, unless directed by a physician, if you have a breathing problem such as emphysema or chronic bronchitis, or if you have high blood pressure, heart disease, diabetes, thyroid disease, glaucoma, or difficulty in urination due to enlargement of the prostate gland.
This product may cause drowsiness; alcohol, sedatives and tranquilizers may increase the drowsiness effect. Avoid alcoholic beverages while taking this product. Do not take this product if you are taking sedatives or tranquilizers without first consulting your physician. Use caution when driving a motor vehicle or operating machinery. May cause excitability, especially in children.
Do not exceed recommended dosage. If nervousness, dizziness or sleeplessness occur, discontinue use and consult a physician. If symptoms do not improve within 7 days, or are accompanied by fever, consult a physician.
Do not give this product to children under 12 years, except under the advice and supervision of a physician. Do not take this product if you are hypersensitive to any of the ingredients. As with any drug, if you are pregnant or nursing a baby, seek the advice of a health professional before using this product.
KEEP THIS AND ALL DRUGS OUT OF THE REACH OF CHILDREN. IN CASE OF ACCIDENTAL OVERDOSE, SEEK PROFESSIONAL ASSISTANCE OR CONTACT A POISON CONTROL CENTER IMMEDIATELY.

Drug Interaction Precaution: Do not use this product if you are now taking a prescription monoamine oxidase inhibitor (MAOI) (certain drugs for depression, psychiatric or emotional conditions, or Parkinson's disease) or for 2 weeks after stopping the MAOI drug. If you are uncertain whether your prescription drug

contains an MAOI, consult a health professional before taking this product.

Directions: Adults and children 12 years of age and over: one tablet every 12 hours. DO NOT EXCEED 1 TABLET EVERY 12 HOURS OR 2 TABLETS IN A 24-HOUR PERIOD.

How Supplied: Pale blue sugar-coated tablets monogrammed DIMETAPP AHR in bottles of 100 (NDC 0031-2277-63), 500 (NDC 0031-2277-70); Dis-Co® Unit Dose Packs of 100 (NDC 0031-2277-64); and blister packs of 12 tablets (NDC 0031-2277-46), 24 tablets (NDC 0031-2277-54) and 48 tablets (NDC 0031-2277-59).
Store at Controlled Room Temperature, between 15°C and 30°C (59°F and 86°F).
Dimetapp Extentabs® Tablets are the A. H. Robins Company's uniquely constructed extended action tablets.
Shown in Product Identification Guide, page 528

DIMETAPP® Tablets and Liqui-Gels®
[dī' mĕ-tap]
Maximum Strength

Description: Each **Dimetapp** Tablet or Liquigel® contains:
Brompheniramine
   Maleate, USP .... 4 mg
Phenylpropanolamine
   Hydrochloride, USP .... 25 mg

Inactive Ingredients: <u>Tablets:</u> Corn Starch, FD&C Blue 1 Aluminum Lake, Magnesium Stearate, Microcrystalline Cellulose. <u>Liqui-Gels:</u> D&C Red 33, Gelatin, Glycerin, Mannitol, Pharmaceutical Glaze, Polyethylene Glycol, Povidone, Propylene Glycol, Sorbitan, Sorbitol, Titanium Dioxide, Water.

Indications: For temporary relief of nasal congestion due to the common cold, hay fever or other upper respiratory allergies or associated with sinusitis. Temporarily relieves runny nose, sneezing, and itchy, watery eyes due to allergic rhinitis (hay fever). Temporarily restores freer breathing through the nose.

Warnings: Do not take take this product, unless directed by a physician, if you have a breathing problem such as emphysema or chronic bronchitis, or if you have high blood pressure, heart disease, diabetes, thyroid disease, glaucoma, or difficulty in urination due to enlargement of the prostate gland. This product may cause drowsiness; alcohol, sedatives and tranquilizers may increase the drowsiness effect. Avoid alcoholic beverages while taking this product. Do not take this product if you are taking sedatives or tranquilizers without first consulting your physician. Use caution when driving a motor vehicle or operating machinery. May cause excitability, especially in children. **Do not exceed the recommended dosage.** If nervousness, dizziness or sleeplessness occur, discontinue use and consult a physician. If symptoms

Continued on next page

Whitehall-Robins—Cont.

do not improve within 7 days or are accompanied by fever, consult a physician. As with any drug, if you are pregnant or nursing a baby, seek the advice of a health professional before using this product.
KEEP THIS AND ALL DRUGS OUT OF THE REACH OF CHILDREN. IN CASE OF ACCIDENTAL OVERDOSE, SEEK PROFESSIONAL ASSISTANCE OR CONTACT A POISON CONTROL CENTER IMMEDIATELY.

Drug Interaction Precaution: Do not use this product if you are now taking a prescription monoamine oxidase inhibitor (MAOI) (certain drugs for depression, psychiatric or emotional conditions, or Parkinson's disease) or for 2 weeks after stopping the MAOI drug. If you are uncertain whether your prescription drug contains an MAOI, consult a health professional before taking this product.

Directions: Tablets: Adults and children 12 years of age and over: one tablet every 4 hours. Children 6 to under 12 years: one-half tablet every 4 hours. DO NOT EXCEED 6 DOSES IN A 24-HOUR PERIOD. Liqui-Gels: Adults and children 12 years of age and over: one softgel every 4 hours. Children under 12 years: consult a physician. DO NOT EXCEED 6 SOFTGELS IN A 24-HOUR PERIOD.

How Supplied: Tablets: Blue, scored compressed tablets engraved AHR and 2254 in consumer packages of 24 (NDC 0031-2254-54) (individually packaged).
Liqui-Gels: Purple Liquigel imprinted AHR and 2255 in consumer packages of 12 (NDC 0031-2255-46) and 24 (NDC 0031-2255-54) (individually packaged).
Tablets and Liqui-Gels: Store at Controlled Room Temperature, between 20°C and 25°C (68°F and 77°F).
Liqui-Gels is a registered trademark of R.P. Scherer International Corporation.

ORUDIS® KT™
[Orūdĭs]

Description: Pain Reliever/Fever Reducer.

Active Ingredients: Each tablet or caplet contains ketoprofen 12.5 mg.

Inactive Ingredients: Cellulose, D&C Yellow #10 Lake, FD&C Blue #1 Lake, Iron Oxide, Pharmaceutical Glaze, Povidone, Silica, Sodium Benzoate, Sodium Lauryl Sulfate, Starch, Stearic Acid, Sugar, Titanium Dioxide, Wax. Contains FD&C Yellow #5 Lake (Tartrazine) as a color additive.

Indications: Temporarily relieves minor aches and pains associated with the common cold, headache, toothache, muscular aches, backache, minor pain of arthritis and menstrual cramps. Temporarily reduces fever.

Warnings: Do not take this product if you have had asthma, hives or other allergic reaction after taking any pain reliever/fever reducer. Ketoprofen could cause similar reactions in patients allergic to other pain relievers/fever reducers. As with any drug, if you are pregnant or nursing a baby, seek the advice of a health professional before using this product. IT IS ESPECIALLY IMPORTANT NOT TO USE KETOPROFEN DURING THE LAST 3 MONTHS OF PREGNANCY UNLESS SPECIALLY DIRECTED TO DO SO BY A DOCTOR BECAUSE IT MAY CAUSE PROBLEMS IN THE UNBORN CHILD OR COMPLICATIONS DURING DELIVERY.
If you generally consume 3 or more alcohol-containing drinks per day, you should talk to your doctor for advice on when and how you should take ORUDIS® KT™ or other pain relievers. Do not use with any other pain reliever/fever reducer, with any other product containing ketoprofen, for more than 3 days for fever or for more than 10 days for pain. **Ask a doctor before use if:** the painful area is red or swollen, you take other drugs on a regular basis, you are under a doctor's care for any continuing medical condition or you have had problems or side effects with any pain reliever/fever reducer. **Ask a doctor after use if** symptoms continue or worsen, new or unexpected symptoms occur or stomach pain occurs with use of this product.
Keep this and all drugs out of the reach of children. In case of accidental overdose, seek professional assistance or contact a poison control center immediately.

Directions: Take with a full glass of water or other liquid. **Adults:** Take 1 tablet every 4–6 hours. If pain or fever does not get better in 1 hour, you may take 1 more tablet. With experience, some people may find they need 2 tablets for the first dose. The smallest effective dose should be used. **Do not take more than:** 2 tablets in any 4–6 hour period; 6 tablets in any 24 hour period. **Children:** Do not give to children under age 16 unless directed by a doctor.
Store at room temperature. Avoid excessive heat 98°F (37°C).

How Supplied: Coated tablets in bottles of 24, 50, 100
Coated caplets in bottles of 24, 50, 100
ORUDIS is a registered trademark of RHONE-POULENC. KT and the appearance of the green ORUDIS KT tablet are trademarks of WHITEHALL-ROBINS HEALTHCARE.
If you have questions or comments, please call 1-800-Orudis2.
Shown in Product Identification Guide, page 528

PREPARATION H®
[prep-e 'rā-shen-āch]
Hemorrhoidal Ointment and Cream
PREPARATION H®
Hemorrhoidal Suppositories

Description: Preparation H is available in ointment, cream and suppository product forms. The **Ointment** contains Petrolatum 71.9%, Mineral Oil 14%, Shark Liver Oil 3% and Phenylephrine HCl 0.25%.
The **Cream** contains Petrolatum 18%, Glycerin 12%, Shark Liver Oil 3% and Phenylephrine HCl 0.25%.
The **Suppositories** contain Cocoa Butter 79% and Shark Liver Oil 3%.

Indications: Preparation H Ointment and Cream temporarily shrink hemorrhoidal tissue and give temporary relief of the itching, burning and discomfort associated with hemorrhoids. Preparation H Suppositories provide temporary relief of the itching, burning, and discomfort associated with hemorrhoids.

Warnings: In case of bleeding, or if condition worsens or does not improve within 7 days, consult a doctor promptly. Do not exceed the recommended daily dosage unless directed by a doctor. Keep this and all drugs out of the reach of children. In case of accidental ingestion, seek professional assistance or contact a poison control center immediately. As with any drug, if you are pregnant or nursing a baby, seek the advice of a health professional before using this product.
Ointment/Cream: Do not use this product if you have heart disease, high blood pressure, thyroid disease, diabetes, or difficulty in urination due to enlargement of the prostate gland unless directed by a doctor.
Ointment: Do not use this product with an applicator if the introduction of the applicator into the rectum causes additional pain. Consult a doctor promptly.
Cream: Do not put this product into the rectum by using fingers or any mechanical device or applicator.

Drug Interaction Precaution: Ointment/Cream—Do not use this product if you are presently taking a prescription drug for high blood pressure or depression, without first consulting your doctor.

Dosage and Administration:
Ointment/Cream/Suppositories—
ADULTS—When practical, cleanse the affected area by patting or blotting with an appropriate cleansing tissue. Gently dry by patting or blotting with toilet tissue or a soft cloth before application of this product.
Children under 12 years of age: consult a doctor.
Ointment—Apply to the affected area up to 4 times daily, especially at night, in the morning or after each bowel movement. Regular application and lubrication with Preparation H Ointment provide continual therapy for relief of hemorrhoidal symptoms. FOR INTRARECTAL USE: Before applying, remove pro-

tective cover from applicator. Attach applicator to tube. Lubricate applicator well, then gently insert applicator into the rectum. Thoroughly cleanse applicator after each use and replace protective cover. Also apply ointment to external area.

Cream—Apply externally to the affected area up to 4 times daily, especially at night, in the morning, or after each bowel movement. Preparation H Cream is to be applied externally or in the lower portion of the anal canal only. The enclosed dispensing cap is designed to control dispersion of the cream to the affected area in the lower portion of the anal canal. Before applying, remove protective cover from dispensing cap. Attach cap to tube. Lubricate dispensing cap well, then gently insert dispensing cap part way into the anus. Thoroughly cleanse dispensing cap after each use and replace protective cover. Regular application and lubrication with Preparation H Cream provide continual therapy for relief of hemorrhoidal symptoms.

Suppositories—Remove wrapper before inserting into the rectum. Insert one suppository into the rectum up to 6 times daily, especially at night, in the morning or after each bowel movement. Regular application and lubrication with Preparation H Suppositories provide continual therapy for relief of hemorrhoidal symptoms.

Inactive Ingredients: Ointment—Beeswax, Benzoic Acid, BHA, Corn Oil, Glycerin, Lanolin, Lanolin Alcohol, Methylparaben, Paraffin, Propylparaben, Thyme Oil, Tocopherol, Water.
Cream—BHA, Carboxymethylcellulose Sodium, Cetyl Alcohol, Citric Acid, Edetate Disodium, Glyceryl Oleate, Glyceryl Stearate, Lanolin, Methylparaben, Propyl Gallate, Propylene Glycol, Propylparaben, Simethicone, Sodium Benzoate, Sodium Lauryl Sulfate, Stearyl Alcohol, Tocopherol, Xanthan Gum, Water.
Suppositories—Ascorbyl Palmitate, Benzoic Acid, BHA, Corn Oil, Edetate Disodium, Glycerin, Methylparaben, PEG-12 Dilaurate, Propylparaben, Tocopherol, Water, White Wax.

How Supplied: Ointment: Net Wt. 1 oz. and 2 oz. **Cream:** Net wt. 0.9 oz. and 1.8 oz. **Suppositories:** 12's, 24's and 48's.
Store at room temperature in cool place but not over 80° F.
Shown in Product Identification Guide, page 528

PREPARATION H®
HYDROCORTISONE 1%
[prep-e 'ra-shen-ach]
Anti-Itch Cream

Description: Preparation H® Hydrocortisone 1% is an antipruritic cream containing 1% Hydrocortisone.

Indications: For the temporary relief of external anal itch and itching associated with minor skin irritations and

rashes. Other uses of this product should be only under the advice and supervision of a doctor.

Warnings: For external use only. Avoid contact with the eyes. If condition worsens, or if symptoms persist for more than 7 days or clear up and occur again within a few days, stop use of this product and do not begin use of any other hydrocortisone product unless you have consulted a doctor. Do not exceed the recommended daily dosage unless directed by a doctor. In case of bleeding, consult a doctor promptly. Do not put this product into the rectum by using fingers or any mechanical device or applicator. Do not use for the treatment of diaper rash; consult a doctor. Keep this and all drugs out of the reach of children. In case of accidental ingestion, seek professional assistance or contact a Poison Control Center immediately.

Directions: Adults: When practical, cleanse the affected area by patting or blotting with an appropriate cleansing tissue. Gently dry by patting or blotting with toilet tissue or soft cloth before application of this product. Apply to affected area not more than 3 to 4 times daily.
Children under 12 years of age: consult a doctor.

Inactive Ingredients: BHA, Cellulose Gum, Cetyl Alcohol, Citric Acid, Disodium EDTA, Glycerin, Glyceryl Oleate, Glyceryl Stearate, Lanolin, Methylparaben, Petrolatum, Propyl Gallate, Propylene Glycol, Propylparaben, Simethicone, Sodium Benzoate, Sodium Lauryl Sulfate, Stearyl Alcohol, Water, Xanthan Gum.

How Supplied: Available in Net Wt. 0.9 oz. tube. Store at room temperature or in cool place but not over 80°F. If cellophane tear strip is missing or if cellophane wrap is broken or missing when purchased, do not use.

PRIMATENE®
[prīm 'a-tēn]
Mist
(Epinephrine Inhalation Aerosol Bronchodilator)

Description: Primatene Mist contains Epinephrine 5.5 mg/mL.

FDA approved uses.

Indications: For temporary relief of shortness of breath, tightness of chest, and wheezing due to bronchial asthma. Eases breathing for asthma patients by reducing spasms of bronchial muscles.

Directions: Inhalation dosage for adults and children 12 years of age and over, and children 4 to under 12 years of age: Start with one inhalation, then wait at least 1 minute. If not relieved, use once more. Do not use again for at least 3 hours. The use of this product by children should be supervised by an adult.

Children under 4 years of age: Consult a physician. Each inhalation delivers 0.22 mg of epinephrine.

Warnings: Do not use this product unless a diagnosis of asthma has been made by a physician. Do not use this product if you have heart disease, high blood pressure, thyroid disease, diabetes, or difficulty in urination due to enlargement of the prostate gland unless directed by a physician. As with any drug, if you are pregnant or nursing a baby, seek the advice of a health professional before using this product. Do not use this product if you have ever been hospitalized for asthma or if you are taking any prescription drug for asthma unless directed by a physician. Keep this and all drugs out of the reach of children. In case of accidental overdose, seek professional assistance or contact a poison control center immediately. **DO NOT CONTINUE TO USE THIS PRODUCT BUT SEEK MEDICAL ASSISTANCE IMMEDIATELY IF SYMPTOMS ARE NOT RELIEVED WITHIN 20 MINUTES OR BECOME WORSE. DO NOT USE THIS PRODUCT MORE FREQUENTLY OR AT HIGHER DOSES THAN RECOMMENDED UNLESS DIRECTED BY A PHYSICIAN.** EXCESSIVE USE MAY CAUSE NERVOUSNESS AND RAPID HEART BEAT AND, POSSIBLY, ADVERSE EFFECTS ON THE HEART.

Drug Interaction Precaution: Do not use this product if you are now taking a prescription monoamine oxidase inhibitor (MAOI) (certain drugs for depression, psychiatric or emotional conditions, or Parkinson's disease), or for 2 weeks after stopping the MAOI drug. If you are uncertain whether your prescription drug contains an MAOI, consult a health professional before taking this product.

Caution: Contents under pressure. Do not puncture or throw container into incinerator. Using or storing near open flame or heating above 120° F (49° C) may cause bursting. Store at room temperature 59° F to 86° F (15° C to 30° C).

Directions For Use of Mouthpiece:
The Primatene Mist mouthpiece, which is enclosed in the Primatene Mist 15 mL size (not the refill size), should be used for inhalation only with Primatene Mist.
1. Take plastic cap off mouthpiece. (For refills, use mouthpiece from previous purchase.)
2. Take plastic mouthpiece off bottle.
3. Place other end of mouthpiece on bottle.
4. Turn bottle upside down. Place thumb on bottom of mouthpiece over circular button and forefinger on top of vial. Empty the lungs as completely as possible by exhaling.
5. Place mouthpiece in mouth with lips closed around opening. Inhale deeply while squeezing mouthpiece and bottle together. Release immediately and remove unit from mouth. Complete taking the deep breath, drawing the medi-

Continued on next page

Whitehall-Robins—Cont.

cation into your lungs and holding breath as long as comfortable.
6. Exhale slowly keeping lips nearly closed. This helps distribute the medication in the lungs.
7. Replace plastic cap on mouthpiece.

Care of the Mouthpiece:
The Primatene Mist mouthpiece should be washed once daily with soap and hot water, and rinsed thoroughly. Then it should be dried with a clean, lint-free cloth.
If the unit becomes clogged and fails to spray, please send the clogged unit to:
Whitehall Laboratories
5 Giralda Farms
Madison, N.J. 07940

Inactive Ingredients: Alcohol 34%, Ascorbic Acid, Fluorocarbons (Propellant), Water. Contains No Sulfites.

Warning: Contains CFC 12, 114, substances which harm public health and environment by destroying ozone in the upper atmosphere.

How Supplied:
½ Fl. oz. (15 mL) With Mouthpiece.
½ Fl. oz. (15 mL) Refill
¾ Fl. oz. (22.5 mL) Refill
Shown in Product Identification Guide, page 528

PRIMATENE®
[prīm 'a-tēn]
Tablets

Description: Primatene Tablets contain Theophylline Anhydrous 130 mg and Ephedrine Hydrochloride 24 mg.

Indications: For temporary relief of shortness of breath, tightness of chest, and wheezing due to bronchial asthma. Eases breathing for asthma patients by reducing spasms of bronchial muscles.

Warnings: Do not use this product unless a diagnosis of asthma has been made by a doctor. Do not use this product if you have heart disease, high blood pressure, thyroid disease, diabetes or difficulty in urination due to enlargement of the prostate gland unless directed by a doctor. Do not use this product if you have ever been hospitalized for asthma or if you are taking any prescription drug for asthma unless directed by a doctor. **DRUG INTERACTION PRECAUTION:** Do not use this product if you are now taking a prescription monoamine oxidase inhibitor (MAOI) (certain drugs for depression, psychiatric or emotional conditions or Parkinson's disease), or for 2 weeks after stopping the MAOI drug. If you are uncertain whether your prescription drug contains an MAOI, consult a health professional before taking this product. Do not continue to use this product but seek medical assistance immediately if symptoms are not relieved within 1 hour or become worse. Some users of this product may experience nervousness, tremor,

sleeplessness, nausea, and loss of appetite. If these symptoms persist or become worse, consult your doctor. As with any drug, if you are pregnant or nursing a baby, seek the advice of a health professional before using this product. Keep this and all drugs out of the reach of children. In case of accidental overdose, seek professional assistance or contact a poison control center immediately.

Directions: Adults and children 12 years of age and over: 1 tablet initially and then one every 4 hours, as needed, not to exceed 6 tablets in 24 hours. For children under 12 years of age, consult a doctor.

Inactive Ingredients:
Croscarmellose Sodium, D&C Yellow No. 10 Lake, FD&C Yellow No. 6 Lake, Magnesium Stearate, Microcrystalline Cellulose, Silica, Starch, Stearic Acid.

How Supplied: Available in 24 and 60 tablet thermoform blister cartons. Store at room temperature, between 20°C and 25°C (68°F to 77°F).
Shown in Product Identification Guide, page 528

ROBITUSSIN® COLD & COUGH LIQUI-GELS®
[ro "bĭ-tuss 'ĭn]

Description: Each Softgel contains:
Guaifenesin, USP .... 200 mg
Pseudoephedrine Hydrochloride, USP .... 30 mg
Dextromethorphan Hydrobromide, USP .... 10 mg

Inactive Ingredients: FD&C Blue 1, FD&C Red 40, Gelatin, Glycerin, Mannitol, Pharmaceutical Glaze, Polyethylene Glycol, Povidone, Propylene Glycol, Sorbitan, Sorbitol, Titanium Dioxide, Water.

Indications: Temporarily relieves cough due to minor throat and bronchial irritation and nasal congestion due to the common cold, hay fever or other upper respiratory allergies, or associated with sinusitis. Helps loosen phlegm (mucus) and thin bronchial secretions to make coughs more productive.

Warnings: Do not take this product for persistent or chronic cough such as occurs with smoking, asthma, chronic bronchitis, emphysema, or if cough is accompanied by excessive phlegm (mucus), unless directed by a physician. Likewise, if you have heart disease, high blood pressure, thyroid disease, diabetes, or difficulty in urination due to enlargement of the prostate gland, do not take this product unless directed by a physician.
Do not exceed the recommended dosage. If nervousness, dizziness or sleeplessness occur, discontinue use and consult a physician. A persistent cough may be a sign of a serious condition. If cough or other symptoms persist, do not improve within 7 days, tend to recur, or are

accompanied by fever, rash, or persistent headache, consult a physician.
As with any drug, if you are pregnant or nursing a baby, seek the advice of a health professional before using this product.
KEEP THIS AND ALL DRUGS OUT OF THE REACH OF CHILDREN. IN CASE OF ACCIDENTAL OVERDOSE, SEEK PROFESSIONAL ASSISTANCE OR CONTACT A POISON CONTROL CENTER IMMEDIATELY.

Drug Interaction Precaution: Do not use this product if you are now taking a prescription monoamine oxidase inhibitor (MAOI) (certain drugs for depression, psychiatric or emotional conditions, or Parkinson's disease) or for 2 weeks after stopping the MAOI drug. If you are uncertain whether your prescription drug contains an MAOI, consult a health professional before taking this product.

Directions: Follow dosage below: DO NOT EXCEED 4 DOSES IN A 24-HOUR PERIOD. Adults and children 12 years of age and over: swallow two Softgels every 4 hours. Children 6 to under 12 years: swallow one Softgel every 4 hours. Children under 6—consult your doctor.

How Supplied: Red Liquigel imprinted AHR and 8600 in consumer packages of 12 (NDC 0031-8600-46) and 20 (NDC 0031-8600-52) (individually packaged).
Store at controlled room temperature, between 20°C and 25°C (68°F and 77°F)
Liqui-Gels and Liquigel are registered trademarks of R.P. Scherer International Corporation.

Note: Guaifenesin had been shown to produce a color interference with certain clinical laboratory determinations of 5-hydroxyindoleacetic acid (5-HIAA) and vanillylmandelic acid (VMA).

ROBITUSSIN® COLD, COUGH & FLU LIQUI-GELS®
[ro "bĭ-tuss 'ĭn]

Description: Pain Reliever, Fever Reducer, Cough Suppressant, Nasal Decongestant, Expectorant.

Active Ingredients: Acetaminophen 250 mg, Guaifenesin 100 mg, Pseudoephedrine HCl 30 mg, Dextromethorphan HBr 10 mg

Inactive Ingredients: D&C Yellow #10, FD&C Red #40, Gelatin, Glycerin, Mannitol, Polyethylene Glycol, Povidone, Propylene Glycol, Sorbitan, Sorbitol, Water

Indications: For the temporary relief of minor aches and pains, headache, muscular aches and sore throat associated with cold or flu, and to reduce fever. Temporarily relieves cough due to minor throat and bronchial irritation and nasal congestion as may occur with a cold. Helps loosen phlegm (mucus) and thin bronchial secretions to make coughs more productive.

Warnings: Do not take this product for persistent or chronic cough such as occurs with smoking, asthma, chronic bronchitis, emphysema, or if cough is accompanied by excessive phlegm (mucus), unless directed by a doctor. Likewise, if you have heart disease, high blood pressure, thyroid disease, diabetes, glaucoma or difficulty in urination due to enlargement of the prostate gland, do not take this product unless directed by a doctor.

Alcohol Warning: If you generally consume 3 or more alcohol-containing drinks per day you should consult your physician for advice on when and how you should take this product or any other acetaminophen-containing product.
Do not exceed recommended dosage. If nervousness, dizziness, or sleeplessness occur, discontinue use and consult a doctor. Do not take this product for more than 7 days (adults) or 5 days (children under 12) or for fever for more than 3 days unless directed by a doctor.
If pain or fever persists or gets worse, if new symptoms occur, or if redness or swelling is present, consult a doctor because these could be signs of a serious condition. If sore throat is severe, persists for more than 2 days, is accompanied or followed by fever, headache, rash, nausea, or vomiting, consult a doctor promptly. A persistent cough may be a sign of a serious condition. If cough or other symptoms persist, do not improve within 7 days, tend to recur, or are accompanied by fever, rash, or persistent headache, consult a doctor.
As with any drug, if you are pregnant or nursing a baby, seek the advice of a health professional before using this product.

Drug Interaction Precaution: Do not use this product if you are now taking a prescription monoamine oxidase inhibitor (MAOI) (certain drugs for depression, psychiatric or emotional conditions, or Parkinson's disease), or for 2 weeks after stopping the MAOI drug. If you are uncertain whether your prescription drug contains an MAOI, consult a health professional before taking this product.

Directions: Follow dosage below: Do not exceed 4 doses in a 24-hour period. Adult Dose (and children 12 yrs. and over): Swallow 2 Softgels every 4 hrs. Child Dose: (6 yrs. to under 12 yrs.): Swallow 1 Softgel every 4 hrs. Children under 6—Consult your doctor. KEEP THIS AND ALL DRUGS OUT OF THE REACH OF CHILDREN. IN CASE OF ACCIDENTAL OVERDOSE, SEEK PROFESSIONAL ASSISTANCE OR CONTACT A POISON CONTROL CENTER IMMEDIATELY. PROMPT MEDICAL ATTENTION IS CRITICAL FOR ADULTS AS WELL AS CHILDREN EVEN IF YOU DO NOT NOTICE ANY SIGNS OR SYMPTOMS.

How Supplied: Blister Packs of 12's, NDC 0031-8602-46

Blister Packs of 20's, NDC 0031-8602-52
Storage: Store at Controlled Room Temperature, Between 20°C and 25°C (68°F and 77°F).

ROBITUSSIN® SEVERE CONGESTION LIQUI-GELS®
[ro "bĭ-tuss 'ĭn]

Description: Each Robitussin Severe Congestion Liquigel® contains:

Guaifenesin, USP .... 200 mg
Pseudoephedrine Hydrochloride, USP .... 30 mg

Inactive Ingredients: FD&C Green 3, Gelatin, Glycerin, Mannitol, Pharmaceutical Glaze, Polyethylene Glycol, Povidone, Propylene Glycol, Sorbitan, Sorbitol, Titanium Dioxide, Water.

Indications: For the temporary relief of nasal congestion due to the common cold, hay fever or other upper respiratory allergies, or associated with sinusitis. Helps loosen phlegm (mucus) and thin bronchial secretions to make coughs more productive.

Warnings: Do not take this product for persistent or chronic cough such as occurs with smoking, asthma, chronic bronchitis, emphysema, or if cough is accompanied by excessive phlegm (mucus), unless directed by a physician. Likewise, if you have heart disease, high blood pressure, thyroid disease, diabetes, or difficulty in urination due to enlargement of the prostate gland, do not take this product unless directed by a physician.
Do not exceed the recommended dosage. If nervousness, dizziness or sleeplessness occur, discontinue use and consult a physician. A persistent cough may be a sign of a serious condition. If cough or other symptoms persist, do not improve within 7 days, tend to recur, or are accompanied by fever, rash, or persistent headache, consult a physician.
As with any drug, if you are pregnant or nursing a baby, seek the advice of a health professional before using this product.
KEEP THIS AND ALL DRUGS OUT OF THE REACH OF CHILDREN. IN CASE OF ACCIDENTAL OVERDOSE, SEEK PROFESSIONAL ASSISTANCE OR CONTACT A POISON CONTROL CENTER IMMEDIATELY.

Drug Interaction Precaution: Do not use this product if you are now taking a prescription monoamine oxidase inhibitor (MAOI) (certain drugs for depression, psychiatric or emotional conditions or Parkinson's disease) or for 2 weeks after stopping the MAOI drug. If you are uncertain whether your prescription drug contains an MAOI, consult a health professional before taking this product.

Directions: Follow dosage below: DO NOT EXCEED 4 DOSES IN A 24-HOUR PERIOD. Adults and children 12 years of age and over: swallow two Softgels every 4 hours. Children 6 to under 12 years:

swallow one Softgel every 4 hours. Children under 6, consult a physician.

How Supplied: Aqua Liquigel imprinted AHR and 8501 in consumer packages of 12 (NDC 0031-8601-46) and 20 (NDC 0031-8601-52) (individually packaged).
Store at controlled room temperature, between 20°C and 25°C (68°F and 77°F). Liqui-Gels and Liquigel are registered trademarks of R.P. Scherer International Corporation.

Note: Guaifenesin has been shown to produce a color interference with certain clinical laboratory determinations of 5-hydroxyindoleacetic acid (5-HIAA) and vanillylmandelic acid (VMA).

ROBITUSSIN®
[ro "bĭ-tuss 'ĭn]
(Guaifenesin Syrup, USP)

Active Ingredients: Each teaspoonful (5 mL) contains:
Guaifenesin, USP .... 100 mg
Alcohol-Free Cough Formula

Inactive Ingredients: Caramel, Citric Acid, FD&C Red 40, Flavors, Glucose, Glycerin, High Fructose Corn Syrup, Saccharin Sodium, Sodium Benzoate, Water.

Indications: Helps loosen phlegm (mucus) and thin bronchial secretions to make coughs more productive.

Professional Labeling: Helps loosen phlegm and thin bronchial secretions in patients with stable chronic bronchitis.

Warnings: Do not take this product for persistent or chronic cough such as occurs with smoking, asthma, chronic bronchitis, emphysema, or where cough is accompanied by excessive phlegm (mucus) unless directed by a physician.
A persistent cough may be a sign of a serious condition. If cough persists for more than one week, tends to recur, or is accompanied by a fever, rash, or persistent headache, consult a physician.
Do not take this product if you are hypersensitive to any of the ingredients. As with any drug, if you are pregnant or nursing a baby, seek the advice of a health professional before using this product.
KEEP THIS AND ALL DRUGS OUT OF THE REACH OF CHILDREN. IN CASE OF ACCIDENTAL OVERDOSE, SEEK PROFESSIONAL ASSISTANCE OR CONTACT A POISON CONTROL CENTER IMMEDIATELY.

Directions: Follow dosage below. Dosage cup provided. **Do Not Exceed Recommended Dosage.** Adults and children 12 years and older: 2–4 teaspoonfuls every 4 hours; children 6 years to under 12 years: 1–2 teaspoonfuls every 4 hours. Children 2 years to under 6 years: ½–1 teaspoonful every 4 hours. Children under 2 years—consult your doctor.

Continued on next page

Whitehall-Robins—Cont.

How Supplied: Robitussin (wine-colored) in bottles of 4 fl. oz. (NDC 0031-8624-12), 8 fl. oz. (NDC 0031-8624-18), pint (NDC 0031-8624-25).
Store at controlled room temperature, between 20°C and 25°C (68°F and 77°F).
Note: Guaifenesin has been shown to produce a color interference with certain clinical laboratory determinations of 5-hydroxyindoleacetic acid (5-HIAA) and vanillylmandelic acid (VMA).

ROBITUSSIN®–CF
[ro "bĭ-tuss 'ĭn]

Active Ingredients: Each teaspoonful (5 mL) contains:
Guaifenesin, USP .... 100 mg
Phenylpropanolamine
　Hydrochloride, USP .... 12.5 mg
Dextromethorphan
　Hydrobromide, USP .... 10 mg

Inactive Ingredients: Citric Acid, FD&C Red 40, Flavors, Glycerin, Propylene Glycol, Saccharin Sodium, Sodium Benzoate, Sorbitol, Water.

Indications: Temporarily relieves coughs due to minor throat and bronchial irritation and nasal congestion as may occur with a cold. Helps loosen phlegm (mucus) and thin bronchial secretions to make coughs more productive.

Warnings: Do not take this product for persistent or chronic cough such as occurs with smoking, asthma, chronic bronchitis, emphysema, or if cough is accompanied by excessive phlegm (mucus) unless directed by a physician. Likewise, if you have heart disease, high blood pressure, thyroid disease, diabetes, or difficulty in urination due to enlargement of the prostate gland, do not take this product unless directed by a physician.
Do not exceed the recommended dosage. If nervousness, dizziness, or sleeplessness occur, discontinue use and consult a doctor. Do not take this product for more than 7 days. A persistent cough may be a sign of a serious condition. If cough or other symptoms persist, do not improve within 7 days, tend to recur, or are accompanied by fever, rash, or persistent headache, consult a physician. As with any drug, if you are pregnant or nursing a baby, seek the advice of a health professional before using this product.
KEEP THIS AND ALL DRUGS OUT OF THE REACH OF CHILDREN. IN CASE OF ACCIDENTAL OVERDOSE, SEEK PROFESSIONAL ASSISTANCE OR CONTACT A POISON CONTROL CENTER IMMEDIATELY.

Drug Interaction Precautions: Do not use this product if you are now taking a prescription monoamine oxidase inhibitor (MAOI) (certain drugs for depression, psychiatric or emotional conditions, or Parkinson's disease) or for 2 weeks after stopping the MAOI drug. If you are uncertain whether your prescription drug contains an MAOI, consult a health professional before taking this product.

Directions: Follow dosage below: Dosage cup provided. DO NOT EXCEED 6 DOSES IN A 24-HOUR PERIOD. Adults and children 12 years and over: 2 teaspoonfuls every 4 hours; children 6 years to under 12 years, 1 teaspoonful every 4 hours; children 2 years to under 6 years, ½ teaspoonful every 4 hours; children under 2 years—consult your doctor.

How Supplied: Robitussin-CF (red-colored) in bottles of 4 fl. oz. (NDC 0031-8677-12), 8 fl. oz. (NDC 0031-8677-18), and 12 fl. oz. (NDC 0031-8677-22).
Store at Controlled Room Temperature, between 20°C and 25°C (68°F and 77°F).
Note: Guaifenesin has been shown to produce a color interference with certain clinical laboratory determinations of 5-hydroxyindoleacetic acid (5-HIAA) and vanillylmandelic acid (VMA).

ROBITUSSIN®-DM
[ro "bĭ-tuss 'ĭn]

Active Ingredients: Each teaspoonful (5 mL) contains:
Guaifenesin, USP .... 100 mg
Dextromethorphan Hydrobromide,
　USP .... 10 mg

Inactive Ingredients: Citric Acid, FD&C Red 40, Flavors, Glucose, Glycerin, High Fructose Corn Syrup, Saccharin Sodium, Sodium Benzoate, Water.

Indications: Temporarily relieves cough due to minor throat and bronchial irritation as may occur with a cold and helps loosen phlegm (mucus) and thin bronchial secretions to make coughs more productive.

Warnings: Do not take this product for persistent or chronic cough such as occurs with smoking, asthma, chronic bronchitis, emphysema, or if cough is accompanied by excessive phlegm (mucus) unless directed by a physician.
A persistent cough may be a sign of a serious condition. If cough persists for more than one week, tends to recur, or is accompanied by a fever, rash, or persistent headache, consult a physician.
Do not take this product if you are hypersensitive to any of the ingredients. As with any drug, if you are pregnant or nursing a baby, seek the advice of a health professional before using this product.
KEEP THIS AND ALL DRUGS OUT OF THE REACH OF CHILDREN. IN CASE OF ACCIDENTAL OVERDOSE, SEEK PROFESSIONAL ASSISTANCE OR CONTACT A POISON CONTROL CENTER IMMEDIATELY.

Drug Interaction Precaution: Do not use this product if you are now taking a prescription monoamine oxidase inhibitor (MAOI) (certain drugs for depression, psychiatric or emotional conditions, or Parkinson's disease) or for 2 weeks after stopping the MAOI drug. If you are uncertain whether your prescription drug contains an MAOI, consult a health professional before taking this product.

Directions: Follow dosage below or use as directed by a doctor. Dosage cup provided. DO NOT EXCEED 6 DOSES IN A 24-HOUR PERIOD. Adults and children 12 years and over: 2 teaspoonfuls every 4 hours; children 6 years to under 12 years, 1 teaspoonful every 4 hours; children 2 years to under 6 years, ½ teaspoonful every 4 hours; children under 2 years—consult your doctor.

How Supplied: Robitussin-DM (cherry-colored) in bottles of 4 fl. oz. (NDC 0031-8685-12), 8 fl. oz. (NDC 0031-8685-18), 12 fl. oz. (NDC 0031-8685-22), pint (NDC 0031-8685-025) and single doses: 6 premeasured doses—⅓ fl. oz. each (NDC 0031-8685-06).
Store at Controlled Room Temperature, between 20°C and 25°C (68°F and 77°F).
Note: Guaifenesin has been shown to produce a color interference with certain clinical laboratory determinations of 5-hydroxyindoleacetic acid (5-HIAA) and vanillylmandelic acid (VMA).
Shown in Product Identification Guide, page 528

ROBITUSSIN®–PE
[ro "bĭ-tuss 'ĭn]

Active Ingredients: Each teaspoonful (5 mL) contains:
Guaifenesin, USP .... 100 mg
Pseudoephedrine Hydrochloride,
　USP .... 30 mg

Inactive Ingredients: Citric Acid, FD&C Red 40, Flavors, Glucose, Glycerin, High Fructose Corn Syrup, Maltol, Propylene Glycol, Saccharin Sodium, Sodium Benzoate, Water.

Indications: Temporarily relieves nasal congestion due to a cold. Helps loosen phlegm (mucus) and thin bronchial secretions to make coughs more productive.

Warnings: Do not take this product for persistent or chronic cough such as occurs with smoking, asthma, chronic bronchitis, emphysema, or if cough is accompanied by excessive phlegm (mucus) unless directed by a physician. Likewise, if you have heart disease, high blood pressure, thyroid disease, diabetes, or difficulty in urination due to enlargement of the prostate gland, do not take this product unless directed by a physician.
Do not exceed the recommended dosage. If nervousness, dizziness, or sleeplessness occur, discontinue use and consult a doctor. Do not take this product for more than 7 days. A persistent cough may be a sign of a serious condition. If cough or other symptoms persist, do not improve within 7 days, tend to recur, or are accompanied by fever, rash, or persistent headache, consult a physician. As

with any drug, if you are pregnant or nursing a baby, seek the advice of a health professional before using this product.
KEEP THIS AND ALL DRUGS OUT OF THE REACH OF CHILDREN. IN CASE OF ACCIDENTAL OVERDOSE, SEEK PROFESSIONAL ASSISTANCE OR CONTACT A POISON CONTROL CENTER IMMEDIATELY.

Drug Interaction Precautions: Do not use this product if you are now taking a prescription monoamine oxidase inhibitor (MAOI) (certain drugs for depression, psychiatric or emotional conditions, or Parkinson's disease) or for 2 weeks after stopping the MAOI drug. If you are uncertain whether your prescription drug contains an MAOI, consult a health professional before taking this product.

Directions: Follow dosage below. Dosage cup provided. DO NOT EXCEED 4 DOSES IN A 24-HOUR PERIOD. Adults and children 12 years and over: 2 teaspoonfuls every 4 hours; children 6 years to under 12 years, 1 teaspoonful every 4 hours; children 2 years to under 6 years, ½ teaspoonful every 4 hours; children under 2 years—consult your doctor.

How Supplied: Robitussin-PE (orange-red) in bottles of 4 fl. oz. (NDC 0031-8695-12), and 8 fl. oz. (NDC 0031-8695-18). Store at Controlled Room Temperature, Between 20°C and 25°C (68°F and 77°F).
Note: Guaifenesin has been shown to produce a color interference with certain clinical laboratory determinations of 5-hydroxyindoleacetic acid (5-HIAA) and vanillylmandelic acid (VMA).

ROBITUSSIN® MAXIMUM STRENGTH COUGH SUPPRESSANT
[ro "bĭ-tuss 'ĭn]

Description: Each 5 mL (1 teaspoonful) contains:
Dextromethorphan
  Hydrobromide, USP .... 15 mg

Inactive Ingredients: Alcohol 1.4%, Citric Acid, FD&C Red 40, Flavors, Glycerin, Glucose, High Fructose Corn Syrup, Saccharin Sodium, Sodium Benzoate, Water.

Indications: Temporarily relieves cough due to minor throat and bronchial irritation as may occur with a cold.

Warnings: Do not take this product for persistent or chronic cough such as occurs with smoking, asthma, emphysema, or if cough is accompanied by excessive phlegm (mucus) unless directed by a physician.
A persistent cough may be a sign of a serious condition. If cough persists for more than one week, tends to recur, or is accompanied by fever, rash, or persistent headache, consult a physician.
As with any drug, if you are pregnant or nursing a baby seek, the advice of a health professional before using this product.

KEEP THIS AND ALL DRUGS OUT OF THE REACH OF CHILDREN. IN CASE OF ACCIDENTAL OVERDOSE, SEEK PROFESSIONAL ASSISTANCE OR CONTACT A POISON CONTROL CENTER IMMEDIATELY.

Drug Interaction Precaution: Do not use this product if you are now taking a prescription monoamine oxidase inhibitor (MAOI) (certain drugs for depression, psychiatric or emotional conditions, or Parkinson's disease) or for 2 weeks after stopping the MAOI drug. If you are uncertain whether your prescription drug contains an MAOI, consult a health professional before taking this product.

Directions: Follow dosage recommendations below or use as directed by a doctor. Repeat every 6–8 hours as needed. DO NOT EXCEED 4 DOSES IN A 24-HOUR PERIOD. Adults and children 12 years and over: 2 teaspoonfuls every 6–8 hours, in medicine cup. Children under 12 years: consult your doctor.

Professional Labeling: Children 6 years to under 12 years, 1 teaspoonful every 6–8 hours; children 2 years to under 6 years, ½ teaspoonful every 6–8 hours. Do not exceed 4 doses in a 24-hour period.
Tamper-Evident Bottle Cap. If Breakable Ring Is Separated, Do Not Use.

How Supplied: Robitussin Maximum Strength (dark red-colored) in bottles of 4 fl. oz. (NDC 0031-8670-12) and 8 fl. oz. (NDC 0031-8670-18). Store at Controlled Room Temperature, between 20°C and 25°C (68°F and 77°F).

ROBITUSSIN® MAXIMUM STRENGTH COUGH & COLD
[ro "bĭ-tuss 'ĭn]

Description: Each teaspoonful (5 mL) contains:
Dextromethorphan Hydrobomide,
  USP .... 15 mg
Pseudoephedrine Hydrochloride,
  USP .... 30 mg

Inactive Ingredients: Alcohol 1.4%, Citric Acid, FD&C Red 40, Flavors, Glycerin, Glucose, High Fructose Corn Syrup, Saccharin Sodium, Sodium Benzoate, Water.

Indications: Temporarily relieves coughs due to minor throat and bronchial irritation and nasal congestion as may occur with a cold.

Warnings: Do not take this product for persistent or chronic cough such as occurs with smoking, asthma, emphysema, or if cough is accompanied by excessive phlegm (mucus) unless directed by a physician. Likewise, if you have heart disease, high blood pressure, thyroid disease, diabetes, or difficulty in urination due to enlargement of the prostate gland, do not take this product unless directed by a physician.
Do not exceed the recommended dosage. If nervousness, dizziness, or sleeplessness occur, discontinue use and con-

sult a doctor. Do not take this product for more than 7 days. A persistent cough may be a sign of a serious condition. If cough or other symptoms persist, do not improve within 7 days, tend to recur, or are accompanied by fever, rash, or persistent headache, consult a physician.
As with any drug, if you are pregnant or nursing a baby, seek the advice of a health professional before using this product.
KEEP THIS AND ALL DRUGS OUT OF THE REACH OF CHILDREN. IN CASE OF ACCIDENTAL OVERDOSE, SEEK PROFESSIONAL ASSISTANCE OR CONTACT A POISON CONTROL CENTER IMMEDIATELY.

Drug Interaction Precaution: Do not use this product if you are now taking a prescription monoamine oxidase inhibitor (MAOI) (certain drugs for depression, psychiatric or emotional conditions, or Parkinson's disease) or for 2 weeks after stopping the MAOI drug. If you are uncertain whether your prescription drug contains an MAOI, consult a health professional before taking this product.

Directions: Follow dosage recommendations below or use as directed by a doctor. Repeat every 6 hours as needed. DO NOT EXCEED 4 DOSES IN A 24-HOUR PEROID. Adults and children 12 years and over: 2 teaspoonfuls every 6 hours in medicine cup. Children under 12 years: consult your doctor.

How Supplied: Red syrup in bottles of 4 fl. oz. (NDC 0031-8671-12) and 8 fl. oz. (NDC-0031-8671-18). Store at Controlled Room Temperature, Between 20°C and 25°C (68°F and 77°F).

ROBITUSSIN® NIGHT-TIME COLD FORMULA
[ro "bĭ-tuss 'ĭn]

Description: Cough Suppressant, Nasal Decongestant, Antihistamine, Pain Reliever-Fever Reducer

Active Ingredients: Acetaminophen 325 mg, Pseudoephedrine HCl 30 mg, Dextromethorphan HBr 15 mg, Doxylamine Succinate 6.25 mg.

Inactive Ingredients: D&C Green #5, D&C Yellow #10, FD&C Green #3, FD&C Yellow #6, Gelatin, Glycerin, Mannitol, Pharmaceutical Glaze, Polyethylene Glycol, Povidone, Propylene Glycol, Sodium Acetate, Sorbitan, Sorbitol, Titanium Dioxide, Water

Indications: For the temporary relief of minor aches and pains, headache, muscular aches and sore throat associated with cold or flu, and to reduce fever. Temporarily relieves cough due to minor throat and bronchial irritation and nasal congestion as may occur with a cold. Temporarily relieves runny nose, and sneezing, itching of the nose or throat, and itchy, watery eyes due to hay fever or

Continued on next page

Whitehall-Robins—Cont.

other upper respiratory allergies (allergic rhinitis).

Warnings: Do not take this product for persistent or chronic cough such as occurs with smoking, asthma, chronic bronchitis, emphysema, or if cough is accompanied by excessive phlegm (mucus), unless directed by a doctor. Likewise, if you have heart disease, high blood pressure, thyroid disease, diabetes, glaucoma or difficulty in urination due to enlargement of the prostate gland, do not take this product unless directed by a doctor.

Alcohol Warning: Avoid alcoholic beverages while taking this product. If you generally consume 3 or more alcohol-containing drinks per day, you should consult your physician for advice on when and how you should take this product or any other acetaminophen-containing product.

May cause marked drowsiness; alcohol, sedatives, and tranquilizers may increase the drowsiness effect. Do not take this product if you are taking sedatives or tranquilizers, without first consulting your doctor. Use caution when driving a motor vehicle or operating machinery. May cause excitability especially in children.

Do not exceed recommended dosage. If nervousness, dizziness or sleeplessness occur, discontinue use and consult a doctor. Do not take this product for more than 7 days or for fever for more than 3 days unless directed by a doctor.

If pain or fever persists or gets worse, if new symptoms occur, or if redness or swelling is present, consult a doctor because these could be signs of a serious condition. If sore throat is severe, persists for more than 2 days, is accompanied or followed by fever, headache, rash, nausea, or vomiting, consult a doctor promptly. A persistent cough may be a sign of a serious condition. If cough or other symptoms persist for more than one week without improvement, tend to recur, or are accompanied by fever, rash or persistent headache, consult a doctor. As with any drug, if you are pregnant or nursing a baby, seek the advice of a health professional before using this product.

Drug Interaction Precaution: Do not use this product if you are now taking a prescription monoamine oxidase inhibitor (MAOI) (certain drugs for depression, psychiatric or emotional conditions, or Parkinson's disease), or for 2 weeks after stopping the MAOI drug. If you are uncertain whether your prescription drug contains an MAOI, consult a health professional before taking this product.

Directions: Follow dosage below: Do not exceed 4 doses in a 24-hour period. Adult Dose (and children 12 yrs. and over): Swallow 2 Softgels every 6 hrs. Not recommended for children under 12 years of age

KEEP THIS AND ALL DRUGS OUT OF THE REACH OF CHILDREN. IN CASE OF ACCIDENTAL OVERDOSE, SEEK PROFESSIONAL ASSISTANCE OR CONTACT A POISON CONTROL CENTER IMMEDIATELY. PROMPT MEDICAL ATTENTION IS CRITICAL FOR ADULTS AS WELL AS CHILDREN EVEN IF YOU DO NOT NOTICE ANY SIGNS OR SYMPTOMS.

Storage: Store at Controlled Room Temperature, Between 20°C and 25°C (68°F and 77°F).

How Supplied: Blister Pack of 12's NDC 0031-8603-46
Blister Pack of 20's NDC 0031-8603-52

ROBITUSSIN® PEDIATRIC COUGH & COLD FORMULA
[ro "bĭ-tuss 'ĭn]

Description: Each 5 mL (1 teaspoonful) contains:
Dextromethorphan
Hydrobromide, USP .... 7.5 mg
Pseudoephedrine
Hydrochloride .... 15 mg

Inactive Ingredients: Citric Acid, FD&C Red 40, Flavors, Glycerin, Propylene Glycol, Saccharin Sodium, Sodium Benzoate, Sorbitol, Water.

Indications: Temporarily relieves cough due to minor throat and bronchial irritation and nasal congestion as may occur with a cold.

Warnings: Do not take this product for persistent or chronic cough such as occurs with smoking, asthma, or emphysema, or if cough is accompanied by excessive phlegm (mucus) unless directed by a physician. Likewise if you have heart disease, high blood pressure, thyroid disease, diabetes, or difficulty in urination due to enlargement of the prostate gland, do not take this product unless directed by a physician.

Do not exceed the recommended dosage. If nervousness, dizziness, or sleeplessness occur, discontinue use and consult a doctor. A persistent cough may be a sign of a serious condition. If cough or other symptoms persist, do not improve within 7 days, tend to recur, or are accompanied by fever, rash, or persistent headache, consult a physician.

As with any drug, if you are pregnant or nursing a baby, seek the advice of a health professional before using this product.

KEEP THIS AND ALL DRUGS OUT OF THE REACH OF CHILDREN. IN CASE OF ACCIDENTAL OVERDOSE, SEEK PROFESSIONAL ASSISTANCE OR CONTACT A POISON CONTROL CENTER IMMEDIATELY.

Drug Interaction Precautions: Do not use this product if you are now taking a prescription monoamine oxidase inhibitor (MAOI) (certain drugs for depression, psychiatric or emotional conditions, or Parkinson's disease) or for 2 weeks after stopping the MAOI drug. If you are uncertain whether your prescription drug contains an MAOI, consult a health professional before taking this product.

Directions: Follow dosage recommendations below or use as directed by a physician. Repeat every 6 hours as needed. DO NOT EXCEED 4 DOSES IN A 24-HOUR PERIOD. Dosage: choose by weight, if known; if weight is not known, choose by age.
[See table below.]

How Supplied: Robitussin Pediatric Cough & Cold formula (bright red) in bottles of 4 fl. oz. (NDC 0031-8609-12) and 8 fl. oz. (NDC 0031-8609-18).
Store at Controlled Room Temperature, Between 20°C and 25°C (68°F and 77°F).

ROBITUSSIN® PEDIATRIC COUGH SUPPRESSANT
[ro "bĭ-tuss 'ĭn]

Description: Each 5 mL (1 teaspoonful) contains:
Dextromethorphan
Hydrobromide, USP .... 7.5 mg

Inactive Ingredients: Citric Acid, FD&C Red 40, Flavors, Glycerin, Propylene Glycol, Saccharin Sodium, Sodium Benzoate, Sorbitol, Water.

Indications: Temporarily relieves coughs due to minor throat and bronchial irritation as may occur with a cold.

Warnings: Do not take this product for persistent or chronic cough such as occurs with smoking, asthma, or emphysema, or if cough is accompanied by excessive phlegm (mucus) unless directed by a physician.

A persistent cough may be a sign of a serious condition. If cough persists for more than one week, tends to recur, or is accompanied by fever, rash, or persistent headache, consult a physician.

Do not take this product if you are hypersensitive to any of the ingredients. As with any drug, if you are pregnant or nursing a baby, seek the advice of a health professional before using this product.

KEEP THIS AND ALL DRUGS OUT OF THE REACH OF CHILDREN. IN CASE OF ACCIDENTAL OVERDOSE, SEEK PROFESSIONAL ASSISTANCE OR CONTACT A POISON CONTROL CENTER IMMEDIATELY.

Drug Interaction Precaution: Do not use this product if you are now taking a prescription monoamine oxidase inhibi-

ROBITUSSIN® PEDIATRIC COUGH & COLD FORMULA

Age	Weight	Dose
Under 2 yrs.	Under 24 lbs.	Consult doctor
2 to under 6 yrs.	24–47 lbs.	1 Teaspoonful
6 to under 12 yrs.	48–95 lbs.	2 Teaspoonfuls
12 yrs. and older	96 lbs. and over	4 Teaspoonfuls

Age	Weight	Dose
Under 2 yrs.	Under 24 lbs.	Consult doctor
2 to under 6 yrs.	24–47 lbs.	1 Teaspoonful
6 to under 12 yrs.	48–95 lbs.	2 Teaspoonfuls
12 yrs. and older	96 lbs. and over	4 Teaspoonfuls

tor (MAOI) (certain drugs for depression, psychiatric or emotional conditions, or Parkinson's disease) or for 2 weeks after stopping the MAOI drug. If you are uncertain whether your prescription drug contains an MAOI, consult a health professional before taking this product.

Directions: Follow dosage recommendations below or use as directed by a physician. Repeat every 6–8 hours. DO NOT EXCEED 4 DOSES IN A 24 HOUR PERIOD. Dosage: choose by weight, if known; if weight is not known, choose by age.
[See table above.]

How Supplied: Robitussin Pediatric (cherry-colored) in bottles of 4 fl. oz. (NDC 0031-8610-12) and 8 fl. oz. (NDC 0031-8610-18).
Store at Controlled Room Temperature, Between 20°C and 25°C (68°F and 77°F).

ROBITUSSIN PEDIATRIC DROPS
[ro "bǐ-tuss 'ǐn]

Description: Nasal Decongestant/ Cough Suppressant/Expectorant

Active Ingredients: Each 2.5 mL contains Guaifenesin, USP 100 mg, Pseudoephedrine Hydrochloride, USP 15 mg, Dextromethorphan Hydrobromide, USP 5 mg in a pleasant tasting berry flavored syrup.

Inactive Ingredients: Citric Acid, FD&C Red 40, Flavors, Glycerin, High Fructose Corn Syrup, Menthol, Polyethylene Glycol, Propylene Glycol, Saccharin Sodium, Sodium Benzoate, Sodium Carboxymethylcellulose, Sorbitol, Water.

Indications: Temporarily relieves cough due to minor throat and bronchial irritation, and nasal congestion due to a cold. Helps loosen phlegm (mucus) and thin bronchial secretions to make coughs more productive.

Warnings: Do not give this product for persistent or chronic cough such as occurs with asthma, or where cough is accompanied by excessive phlegm (mucus) unless directed by a physician. Likewise, do not give this product to a child who has heart disease, high blood pressure, thyroid disease, or diabetes, unless directed by a physician.
Do not exceed recommended dosage. If nervousness, dizziness or sleeplessness occur, discontinue use and consult a physician. A persistent cough may be a sign of a serious condition. If cough or other symptoms persist, do not improve within 7 days, tend to recur, or are accompanied by fever, rash, or persistent headache, consult a physician

Drug Interaction Precaution: Do not give this product to a child who is taking a prescription monoamine oxidase inhibitor (MAOI) (certain drugs for depression, psychiatric or emotional conditions), or for 2 weeks after stopping the MAOI drug. If you are uncertain whether your child's prescription drug contains an MAOI, consult a health professional before giving this product.
KEEP THIS AND ALL DRUGS OUT OF THE REACH OF CHILDREN. IN CASE OF ACCIDENTAL OVERDOSE, SEEK PROFESSIONAL ASSISTANCE OR CONTACT A POISON CONTROL CENTER IMMEDIATELY.

Directions: Follow recommended dosage below or use as directed by a doctor. Repeat every 4 hours. Do Not Exceed 4 Doses in a 24-Hour Period.

Dosage: Choose by weight. (If weight is not known, choose by age):

Age	Weight	Dose
Under 2 yrs.	Under 24 lbs.	Consult doctor
2–under 6 yrs.	24–47 lbs.	2.5 mL

Store at Controlled Room Temperature, between 20°C and 25°C (68°F and 77°F).

How Supplied: 1 oz bottle with dosing syringe (NDC 0031-8679-01)

J.B. Williams Company, Inc.
65 HARRISTOWN ROAD
GLEN ROCK, NJ 07452

Address Inquiries to:
Consumer Affairs: (800) 254-8656
(201) 251-8100
FAX: (201) 251-8097

For Medical Emergency Contact:
(800) 254-8656

CĒPACOL®/CĒPACOL MINT
[sē 'pə-cŏl]
Antiseptic Mouthwash/Gargle

Ingredients: Cēpacol Antiseptic Mouthwash contains: Ceepryn® (cetylpyridinium chloride) 0.05%. Also contains: Alcohol 14%, Edetate Disodium, FD&C Yellow No. 5 (tartrazine) as a color additive, Flavors, Glycerin, Polysorbate 80, Saccharin, Sodium Biphosphate, Sodium Phosphate, and Water.
Cēpacol Mint Mouthwash contains: Ceepryn® (cetylpyridinium chloride) 0.05%. Also contains: Alcohol 14.5%, D&C Yellow No. 10, FD&C Green No. 3, Flavor, Glucono Delta-Lactone, Glycerin, Poloxamer 407, Saccharin Sodium, Sodium Gluconate, and Water.

Actions: Cēpacol/Cēpacol Mint is an effective antiseptic mouthwash/gargle. It kills germs that cause bad breath for a fresher, cleaner mouth.
Cēpacol/Cēpacol Mint has a low surface tension, approximately ½ that of water. This property is the basis of the spreading action in the oral cavity as well as its foaming action. Cēpacol/Cēpacol Mint leaves the mouth feeling fresh and clean and helps provide soothing, temporary relief of dryness and minor mouth irritations.

Uses: Recommended as a mouthwash and gargle for daily oral care; as an aromatic mouth freshener to provide a clean feeling in the mouth; as a soothing, foaming rinse to freshen the mouth.
Used routinely before dental procedures, helps give patient confidence of not offending with mouth odor. Often employed as a foaming and refreshing rinse before, during, and after instrumentation and dental prophylaxis. Convenient as a mouth-freshening agent after taking dental impressions. Helpful in reducing the unpleasant taste and odor in the mouth following gingivectomy.
Used in hospitals as a mouthwash and gargle for daily oral care. Also used to refresh and soothe the mouth following emesis, inhalation therapy, and intubations, and for swabbing the mouths of patients incapable of personal care.

Warning: In case of accidental ingestion seek professional assistance or contact a poison control center immediately. Do not use in children under 6 years of age. Children over 6 should be supervised when using Cēpacol. Keep out of reach of children.

Directions for Use: Rinse vigorously before or after brushing or any time to freshen the mouth. Particularly useful after meals or before social engagements. Cēpacol/Cēpacol Mint leaves the mouth feeling refreshingly clean.
Use full strength every two or three hours as a soothing, foaming gargle, or as directed by a physician or dentist. May also be mixed with warm water.
Product label directions are as follows: Rinse or gargle full strength before or after brushing or as directed by a physician or dentist.

How Supplied: Cēpacol/Cēpacol Mint Antiseptic Mouthwash: 12 oz, 24 oz, and 32 oz. 4 oz trial size.
Shown in Product Identification Guide, page 528

CĒPACOL® Maximum Strength Sore Throat Spray; Cherry and Cool Menthol Flavors.

Ingredients:
Cherry: Active Ingredient: Dyclonine Hydrochloride 0.1%. Also contains: Alcohol 10%, Cetylpyridinium Chloride, D&C Red No. 33, Dibasic Sodium

Continued on next page

J.B. Williams—Cont.

Phosphate, FD&C Yellow No. 6, Flavors, Glycerin, Phosphoric Acid, Poloxamer, Potassium Sorbate, Sorbitol, and Water.
Cool Menthol: Active Ingredient: Dyclonine Hydrochloride 0.1%. Also contains: Alcohol 10%, Cetylpyridinium Chloride, Dibasic Sodium Phosphate, FD&C Blue No. 1, Flavors, Glycerin, Phosphoric Acid, Poloxamer, Potassium Sorbate, Sodium Saccharin, Sorbitol and Water.

Indications: For temporary relief of occasional minor sore throat pain and sore mouth. Also, for temporary relief of pain due to canker sores, minor irritation or injury to the mouth and gums, minor dental procedures, dentures or orthodontic appliances.

Administration and Dosage: Adults and children 12 years of age and older: Spray 4 times into throat or affected area and swallow. Repeat as needed up to 4 times daily or as directed by a physician or dentist. Children under 12 years: Consult physician or dentist.

Warnings: If sore throat is severe, persists for more than 2 days, is accompanied or followed by fever, headache, rash, nausea, or vomiting, consult a physician promptly. If sore mouth symptoms do not improve in 7 days, or if irritation, pain, or redness persists or worsens, see your dentist or physician promptly. Do not exceed recommended dosage. Keep this and all drugs out of the reach of children. In case of accidental overdose, seek professional assistance or contact a Poison Control Center immediately. As with any drug, if you are pregnant or nursing a baby, seek the advice of a health professional before using this product.

How Supplied: Available in Cherry and Cool Menthol flavors in 4 fl. oz. (118 mL) plastic bottles with pump sprayer.
Shown in Product Identification Guide, page 528

CĒPACOL®
[*sē'pə-cŏl*]
Sore Throat Lozenges
Regular Strength Original Mint,
Regular Strength Cherry,
Maximum Strength Original Mint,
Maximum Strength Cherry.
Oral Anesthetic

Ingredients: (per lozenge)

Regular Strength Original Mint:
Active Ingredient: Menthol 2 mg. Also contains: Cetylpyridinium Chloride (Ceepryn®), D&C Yellow No. 10, FD&C Yellow No. 6, Flavor, Glucose, and Sucrose.

Regular Strength Cherry: Active Ingredient: Menthol 3.6 mg. Also contains: Cetylpyridinium Chloride (Ceepryn®), D&C Red No. 33, FD&C Red No. 40, Flavor, Glucose, and Sucrose.

Maximum Strength Original Mint: Active Ingredients: Benzocaine 10 mg., Menthol 2 mg. Also contains: Cetylpyridinium Chloride (Ceepryn®), D&C Yellow No. 10, FD&C Yellow No. 6, Flavor, Glucose, and Sucrose.

Maximum Strength Cherry: Active Ingredients: Benzocaine 10 mg., Menthol 3.6 mg. Also contains: Cetylpyridinium Chloride (Ceepryn®), D&C Red No. 33, FD&C Red No. 40, Flavor, Glucose, and Sucrose.

Actions: Menthol provides a mild anesthetic effect and cooling sensation for symptomatic relief of occasional minor sore throat pain and minor throat irritations. Benzocaine in the Maximum Strength lozenges provides an anesthetic effect for additional symptomatic relief of minor sore throat pain.

Indications: For temporary relief of occasional minor sore throat pain and dry, scratchy throat.

Warnings: If sore throat is severe, persists for more than 2 days, is accompanied or followed by fever, headache, rash, nausea, or vomiting, consult a physician promptly. Do not administer to children under 6 years of age unless directed by physician or dentist. Keep this and all drugs out of the reach of children. In case of accidental overdose, seek professional assistance or contact a Poison Control Center immediately. As with any drug, if you are pregnant or nursing a baby, seek the advice of a health professional before using this product.

Dosage and Administration: Adults and children 6 years of age and older: Dissolve 1 lozenge in the mouth every 2 hours as needed or as directed by a physician or dentist. For children under 6, consult a physician or dentist.

How Supplied:

Trade package:
18 lozenges in 2 pocket packs of 9 each.

Professional package: Regular and Maximum Strength Original Mint: 648 lozenges in 72 blisters of 9 each.
Store at room temperature, below 86°F (30°C). Protect contents from humidity.
Shown in Product Identification Guide, page 528

UNKNOWN DRUG?
Consult the
Product Identification Guide
(Gray Pages)
for full-color photos of
leading over-the-counter
medications

The Winning Combination

For product information, please see **AML Laboratories**

Wyeth-Ayerst Laboratories
Division of American Home Products Corporation
P.O. BOX 8299
PHILADELPHIA, PA 19101

Direct Inquiries to:
Professional Service
(610) 688-4400

For Medically-related Product Information Contact:
Mon-Fri:
(800) 934-5556 (8:30 AM to 4:30 PM Eastern Standard Time)

In Emergencies:
Mon-Fri: 8:30 AM to 4:30 PM Eastern Standard Time only—(800) 934-5556 or (610) 688-4400

Wyeth-Ayerst
Tamper-Resistant/Evident Packaging

Statements alerting consumers to the specific type of Tamper-Resistant/Evident Packaging appear on the bottle labels and cartons of all Wyeth-Ayerst over-the-counter products. This includes plastic cap seals on bottles, individually wrapped tablets or suppositories, and sealed cartons. This packaging has been developed to better protect the consumer.

ALUDROX®
[*al'ū-drox*]
Antacid
(alumina and magnesia)
ORAL SUSPENSION

Composition: *Suspension* —each 5 ml teaspoonful contains 307 mg aluminum hydroxide [$Al(OH)_3$] as a gel and 103 mg of magnesium hydroxide. The inactive ingredients present are artificial and natural flavors, benzoic acid, butylparaben, glycerin, hydroxypropyl methylcellulose, methylparaben, propylparaben, saccharin, simethicone, sorbitol solution, and water. Sodium content is 0.10 mEq per 5 ml suspension.

Indications: For temporary relief of heartburn, upset stomach, sour stomach, and/or acid indigestion.

Directions: *Suspension* —Two teaspoonfuls (10 ml) every 4 hours or as directed by a physician. Medication may be followed by a sip of water if desired.

Warnings: Do not take more than 12 teaspoonfuls (60 ml) of suspension in a 24-hour period or use maximum dosage for more than two weeks except under the advice and supervision of a physician. Prolonged use of aluminum-containing antacids in patients with renal failure may result in or worsen dialysis osteomalacia. Elevated tissue aluminum levels contribute to the development of dialysis encephalopathy and osteomalacia syndromes. Also, a number of cases of dialysis encephalopathy have been associated with elevated aluminum levels in the dialysate water. Small amounts of aluminum are absorbed from the gastrointestinal tract and renal excretion of aluminum is impaired in renal failure. Prolonged use of aluminum-containing antacids in such patients may contribute to increased plasma levels of aluminum. Aluminum is not well removed by dialysis because it is bound to albumin and transferrin, which do not cross dialysis membranes. As a result, aluminum is deposited in bone, and dialysis osteomalacia may develop when large amounts of aluminum are ingested orally by patients with impaired renal function. As with any drug, if you are pregnant or nursing a baby, seek the advice of a health professional before using this product.

Drug Interaction Precautions: Do not take this product if you are presently taking a prescription antibiotic drug containing any form of tetracycline.

Keep at Room Temperature, Approx. 77°F (25°C).

Suspension should be kept tightly closed and shaken well before use. Avoid freezing.

Keep this and all drugs out of the reach of children.

How Supplied: *Oral Suspension* —bottles of 12 fluidounces.

Shown in Product Identification Guide, page 529

Professional Labeling: Consult *1996 Physicians' Desk Reference.*

AMPHOJEL®
[*am'fo-jel*]
Antacid
(aluminum hydroxide gel)
ORAL SUSPENSION • TABLETS

Composition: *Suspension—Peppermint flavored* —Each teaspoonful (5 mL) contains 320 mg aluminum hydroxide [Al(OH)$_3$] as a gel, and not more than 0.10 mEq of sodium. The inactive ingredients present are calcium benzoate, glycerin, hydroxypropyl methylcellulose, menthol, peppermint oil, potassium butylparaben, potassium propylparaben, saccharin, simethicone, sorbitol solution, and water. *Suspension—Without flavor* —Each teaspoonful (5 mL) contains 320 mg of aluminum hydroxide [Al (OH)$_3$] as a gel. The inactive ingredients present are butylparaben, calcium benzoate, glycerin, hydroxypropyl methylcellulose, methylparaben, propylparaben, saccharin, simethicone, sorbitol solution, and water. *Tablets* are available in 0.3

and 0.6 g strengths. Each contains, respectively, the equivalent of 300 mg and 600 mg aluminum hydroxide as a dried gel. The inactive ingredients present are artificial and natural flavors, cellulose, hydrogenated vegetable oil, magnesium stearate, polacrilin potassium, saccharin, starch, and talc. The 0.3 g (5 grain) strength is equivalent to about 1 teaspoonful of the suspension and the 0.6 g (10 grain) strength is equivalent to about 2 teaspoonfuls. Each 0.3 g tablet contains 0.08 mEq of sodium and each 0.6 g tablet contains 0.13 mEq of sodium.

Indications: For temporary relief of heartburn, upset stomach, sour stomach, and/or acid indigestion.

Directions: *Suspension* —Two teaspoonfuls (10 ml) to be taken five or six times daily, between meals and on retiring or as directed by a physician. Medication may be followed by a sip of water if desired. *Tablets* —Two tablets of the 0.3 g strength, or one tablet of the 0.6 g strength, five or six times daily, between meals and on retiring or as directed by a physician. It is unnecessary to chew the 0.3 g tablet before swallowing with water. After chewing the 0.6 g tablet, sip about one-half glass of water.

Warnings: Do not take more than 12 teaspoonfuls (60 ml) of suspension, or more than twelve (12) 0.3 g tablets, or more than six (6) 0.6 g tablets in a 24-hour period or use this maximum dosage for more than two weeks except under the advice and supervision of a physician. May cause constipation. Prolonged use of aluminum-containing antacids in patients with renal failure may result in or worsen dialysis osteomalacia. Elevated tissue aluminum levels contribute to the development of dialysis encephalopathy and osteomalacia syndromes. Also, a number of cases of dialysis encephalopathy have been associated with elevated aluminum levels in the dialysate water. Small amounts of aluminum are absorbed from the gastrointestinal tract and renal excretion of aluminum is impaired in renal failure. Prolonged use of aluminum-containing antacids in such patients may contribute to increased plasma levels of aluminum. Aluminum is not well removed by dialysis because it is bound to albumin and transferrin, which do not cross dialysis membranes. As a result, aluminum is deposited in bone, and dialysis osteomalacia may develop when large amounts of aluminum are ingested orally by patients with impaired renal function. As with any drug, if you are pregnant or nursing a baby, seek the advice of a health professional before using this product.

Drug Interaction Precaution: Antacids may interact with certain prescription drugs. Do not use this product if you are presently taking a prescription antibiotic containing any form of tetracycline. If you are presently taking a prescription drug, do not take this product without checking with your physician.

Keep tightly closed and store at room temperature, Approx. 77°F (25°C).
Suspension should be shaken well before use. Avoid freezing.
Keep this and all drugs out of the reach of children.

How Supplied: *Suspension* —Peppermint flavored; without flavor—bottles of 12 fluidounces. *Tablets* —a convenient auxiliary dosage form—0.3 g (5 grain) bottles of 100; 0.6 g (10 grain), boxes of 100.

Shown in Product Identification Guide, page 529

Professional Labeling: Consult *1996 Physicians' Desk Reference.*

BASALJEL®
[*bā'sel-jel*]
(basic aluminum carbonate gel)
ORAL SUSPENSION • CAPSULES • TABLETS

Composition: *Suspension* —each 5 mL teaspoonful contains basic aluminum carbonate gel equivalent to 400 mg aluminum hydroxide [Al(OH)$_3$]. The inactive ingredients present are artificial and natural flavors, butylparaben, calcium benzoate, glycerin, hydroxypropyl methylcellulose, methylparaben, mineral oil, propylparaben, saccharin, simethicone, sorbitol solution, and water. *Capsule* contains dried basic aluminum carbonate gel equivalent to 608 mg of dried aluminum hydroxide gel or 500 mg aluminum hydroxide [Al(OH)$_3$]. The inactive ingredients present are D&C Yellow 10, FD&C Blue 1, FD&C Red 40, FD&C Yellow 6, gelatin, polacrilin potassium, polyethylene glycol, talc, and titanium dioxide. *Tablet* contains dried basic aluminum carbonate gel equivalent to 608 mg of dried aluminum hydroxide gel or 500 mg aluminum hydroxide. The inactive ingredients present are cellulose, hydrogenated vegetable oil, magnesium stearate, polacrilin potassium, starch, and talc.

Indications: For the symptomatic relief of hyperacidity, associated with the diagnosis of peptic ulcer, gastritis, peptic esophagitis, gastric hyperacidity, and hiatal hernia.

Warnings: Do not take more than 24 tablets/capsules/teaspoonsful of BASALJEL in a 24-hour period, or use this maximum dosage for more than two weeks except under the advice and supervision of a physician. Dosage should be carefully supervised since continued overdosage, in conjunction with restriction of dietary phosphorus and calcium, may produce a persistently lowered serum phosphate and a mildly elevated alkaline phosphatase. A usually transient hypercalciuria of mild degree may be associated with the early weeks of therapy. Prolonged use of aluminum-containing antacids in patients with renal failure may result in or worsen dialy-

Continued on next page

Wyeth-Ayerst—Cont.

sis osteomalacia. Elevated tissue aluminum levels contribute to the development of dialysis encephalopathy and osteomalacia syndromes. Also, a number of cases of dialysis encephalopathy have been associated with elevated aluminum levels in the dialysate water. Small amounts of aluminum are absorbed from the gastrointestinal tract and renal excretion of aluminum is impaired in renal failure. Prolonged use of aluminum-containing antacids in such patients may contribute to increased plasma levels of aluminum. Aluminum is not well removed by dialysis because it is bound to albumin and transferrin, which do not cross dialysis membranes. As a result, aluminum is deposited in bone, and dialysis osteomalacia may develop when large amounts of aluminum are ingested orally by patients with impaired renal function. As with any drug, if you are pregnant or nursing a baby, seek the advice of a health professional before using this product.

Dosage and Administration: *Suspension*—two teaspoonsful (10 mL) in water or fruit juice taken as often as every two hours up to twelve times daily. Two teaspoonsful have the capacity to neutralize 23 mEq of acid. *Capsules*—two capsules as often as every two hours up to twelve times daily. Two capsules have the capacity to neutralize 24 mEq of acid. *Tablets*—two tablets as often as every two hours up to twelve times daily. Two tablets have the capacity to neutralize 25 mEq of acid. The sodium content of each dosage form is as follows: 0.13 mEq/5 mL for the suspension, 0.12 mEq per capsule, and 0.12 mEq per tablet.

Precautions: May cause constipation. Adequate fluid intake should be maintained in addition to the specific medical or surgical management indicated by the patient's condition.

Drug Interaction Precaution: Alumina-containing antacids should not be used concomitantly with any form of tetracycline therapy.

How Supplied: Suspension—bottles of 12 fluidounces.
Capsules—bottles of 100 and 500.
Tablets (scored)—bottles of 100.
Shown in Product Identification Guide, page 529

Professional Labeling: Consult *1996 Physicians' Desk Reference.*

BONAMIL®
[bŏn'ă-mil]
Infant Formula with Iron

- **Powder**
- **Ready-to-Feed Liquid**
- **Concentrated Liquid**

Bonamil is a casein predominant infant formula intended to meet the nutritional needs of infants who are not breastfed and who are not allergic to cow's milk protein and/or intolerant to lactose.

IMPORTANT NOTICE: BREAST MILK IS BEST FOR BABIES. Infant formula is intended to replace or supplement breast milk when breast-feeding is not possible or is insufficient, or when mothers elect not to breast-feed. PROFESSIONAL ADVICE SHOULD BE FOLLOWED ON THE NEED FOR AND PROPER METHOD OF USE OF INFANT FORMULA AND ON ALL MATTERS OF INFANT FEEDING.

Ingredients: NONFAT MILK, LACTOSE, SOYBEAN OIL AND COCONUT OIL, SOY LECITHIN, POTASSIUM BICARBONATE, ASCORBIC ACID, CHOLINE CHLORIDE, FERROUS SULFATE, TAURINE, ALPHA TOCOPHERYL ACETATE, ZINC SULFATE, NIACINAMIDE, CUPRIC SULFATE, VITAMIN A PALMITATE, CALCIUM PANTOTHENATE, THIAMINE HYDROCHLORIDE, RIBOFLAVIN, PYRIDOXINE HYDROCHLORIDE, MANGANESE SULFATE, BETA CAROTENE, FOLIC ACID, PHYTONADIONE, BIOTIN, CHOLECALCIFEROL, CYANOCOBALAMIN.

WHEN DILUTED ACCORDING TO DIRECTIONS, EACH 5 FL. OZ. (150 mL) CONTAINS 100 CALORIES.

NUTRIENTS:	PER 100 Cal	
PROTEIN	2.3	g
FAT	5.4	g
CARBOHYDRATE	10.7	g
WATER	135	g
LINOLEIC ACID	1300	mg
VITAMINS:		
VITAMIN A	300	IU
VITAMIN D	60	IU
VITAMIN E	2.85	IU
VITAMIN K	8	mcg
THIAMINE (VIT. B₁)	100	mcg
RIBOFLAVIN (VIT. B₂)	150	mcg
VITAMIN B₆	63	mcg
VITAMIN B₁₂	0.2	mcg
NIACIN	750	mcg
FOLIC ACID (FOLACIN)	7.5	mcg
PANTOTHENIC ACID	315	mcg
BIOTIN	2.2	mcg
VITAMIN C (ASCORBIC ACID)	8.3	mg
CHOLINE	15	mg
INOSITOL	4.7	mg
MINERALS:		
CALCIUM	69	mg
PHOSPHORUS	54	mg
MAGNESIUM	6	mg
IRON	1.8	mg
ZINC	0.75	mg
MANGANESE	15	mcg
COPPER	70	mcg
IODINE	5	mcg
SODIUM	27	mg
POTASSIUM	93	mg
CHLORIDE	63	mg

Directions For Preparation And Use:
Powder
Carefully measure and mix formula to avoid health hazards.
Always wash hands before mixing. **Wash and rinse can top before opening.** Clean bottles, nipples, caps, and utensils and boil in water for 5 minutes. Boil additional water for formula for no longer than 1 minute, then let cool to lukewarm temperature. For normal dilution (20 calories per fl. oz.), pour required amount of previously boiled water into nursing bottle(s). Using the measuring scoop enclosed in the can, add one level unpacked scoop (8.3 g) of powder for each 2 fl. oz. (60 mL) of water. Always add the powder to the water. Cap bottle and shake well. **Refrigerate prepared formula and use within 24 hours, warming to body temperature and shaking well before use.** After feeding, discard any remaining formula. To ensure freshness, cover opened can with plastic lid and store in a cool, dry place. DO NOT REFRIGERATE OR FREEZE. Use contents within one month after opening.
Warning: Do not use microwave to prepare or warm formula. Serious burns may occur.
Using standard mixing instructions, 1 lb. (453 g) of powder yields approximately 120 fl. oz. of infant formula (20 calories/fl. oz.).
Ready to Feed
Prepare and use as directed to avoid health hazards. Bonamil Ready to Feed is premixed and presterilized—**do not add water.**
Always wash hands before preparing formula. Wash and rinse can top before opening. Shake can before opening. Clean bottles, nipples, caps, and utensils and boil water for 5 minutes. Pour formula into nursing bottle(s). Cap bottle(s). **Refrigerate prepared formula and use within 24 hours, warming to body temperature and shaking well before use.** After feeding, discard any remaining formula. Store unopened can at room temperature. DO NOT FREEZE. Cover opened can and store in refrigerator. Use within 48 hours.
Warning: Do not use microwave to prepare or warm formula. Serious burns may occur.
Concentrated Liquid
Carefully measure and mix formula to avoid health hazards. Always wash hands before mixing. **Wash and rinse can top before opening.** Shake can before opening. Clean bottles, nipples, caps, and utensils and boil in water for 5 minutes. Boil additional water for formula for no longer than one minute, then let cool to lukewarm temperature. For normal dilution (20 calories per fl. oz.), pour equal amounts of formula and previously boiled water into nursing bottle(s). Cap bottle(s) and shake well. **Refrigerate prepared formula and use within 24 hours, warming to body temperature and shaking well before use.** After feeding, discard any remaining formula. Store unopened can at room temperature. DO NOT FREEZE. Cover opened can and store in refrigerator. Use within 48 hours.
Warning: Do not use microwave to prepare or warm formula. Serious burns may occur.

How Supplied:
Powder—1 pound cans, cases of 6 cans.
Ready-to-Feed—32 fluid ounce cans, cases of 6 cans
Concentrated Liquid—13 fluid ounce cans, cases of 12 cans.
Questions or Comments:
1-800-999-9384
W-YETH
Shown in Product Identification Guide, page 529

CEROSE®DM
[se-ros 'DM]
Antihistamine/Nasal Decongestant/ Cough Suppressant

Description: Each teaspoonful (5 mL) contains 15 mg dextromethorphan hydrobromide, 4 mg chlorpheniramine maleate, and 10 mg phenylephrine hydrochloride. Alcohol 2.4%. The inactive ingredients present are artificial flavors, citric acid, edetate disodium, FD&C Yellow 6, glycerin, saccharin sodium, sodium benzoate, sodium citrate, sodium propionate, and water.

Indications: For the temporary relief of cough due to minor throat and bronchial irritation as may occur with the common cold or with inhaled irritants. Temporarily relieves nasal congestion, runny nose, and sneezing due to the common cold, hay fever, or other upper respiratory allergies.

Directions: Adults and children 12 years of age and over: One teaspoonful every four hours as needed. Children 6 to under 12 years of age: One-half teaspoonful every four hours as needed. Do not exceed six doses in a 24-hour period. Consult a physician for use in children under 6 years of age.
Warnings: May cause marked drowsiness; alcohol, sedatives, and tranquilizers may increase the drowsiness effect. Avoid alcoholic beverages while taking this product. Do not take this product if you are taking sedatives or tranquilizers, without first asking your doctor. Use caution when driving a motor vehicle or operating machinery. May cause excitability, especially in children. Do not take this product if you have heart disease, high blood pressure, thyroid disease, diabetes, a breathing problem such as emphysema or chronic bronchitis, glaucoma, or difficulty in urination due to enlargement of the prostate gland unless directed by a doctor. Do not take this product for persistent or chronic cough such as occurs with smoking, asthma, or emphysema, or if cough is accompanied by excessive phlegm (mucus) unless directed by a doctor. A persistent cough may be a sign of a serious condition. If cough or other symptoms persist for more than one week without improvement, tend to recur, or are accompanied by fever, rash, or persistent headache, consult a doctor. **Do not exceed recommended dosage.** If nervousness, dizziness, or sleeplessness occur, discontinue

use and consult a doctor. As with any drug, if you are pregnant or nursing a baby, seek the advice of a health professional before using this product. Keep this and all drugs out of the reach of children. In case of accidental overdose, seek professional assistance or contact a Poison Control Center immediately.

Drug Interaction Precaution: Do not use this product if you are now taking a prescription monoamine oxidase inhibitor (MAOI) (certain drugs for depression, psychiatric or emotional conditions, or Parkinson's disease), or for 2 weeks after stopping the MAOI drug. If you are uncertain whether your prescription drug contains an MAOI, consult a health professional before taking this product.

How Supplied: Cases of 12 bottles of 4 fl. oz.; bottles of 1 pint.
Keep tightly closed—Store at room temperature, below 77° F (25° C).
Shown in Product Identification Guide, page 529

COLLYRIUM for FRESH EYES
[ko-lir 'e-um]
a neutral borate solution
EYE WASH

Description: Soothing Collyrium Eye Wash for Fresh Eyes is specially formulated to soothe, refresh, and cleanse irritated eyes. Collyrium Eye Wash is a neutral borate solution that contains boric acid, sodium borate, benzalkonium chloride (as a preservative), and water.

Indications: To cleanse the eye, loosen foreign material, air pollutants or chlorinated water.

Recommended Uses:
Home—For emergency flushing of foreign bodies or whenever a soothing eye rinse is necessary.
Hospitals, dispensaries and clinics—For emergency flushing of chemicals or foreign bodies from the eye.

Directions: Remove the eyecup from blister. Puncture bottle by twisting threaded eyecup down onto bottle; then remove it from the bottle. Rinse eyecup with clean water immediately before and after each use. Avoid contamination of rim and interior surface of eyecup. Fill eyecup one-half full with Collyrium Eye Wash. Apply cup tightly to the affected eye to prevent the escape of the liquid and tilt head backward. Open eyelid wide and rotate eyeball to thoroughly wash eye. Rinse bottle with clean water after use and recap by twisting threaded eyecup on the bottle for storage.

Warnings: Do not use if solution changes color or becomes cloudy, or with a wetting solution for contact lenses or other eye care products containing polyvinyl alcohol.
This product contains benzalkonium chloride as a preservative. Do not use this product if you are sensitive to benzalkonium chloride.

To avoid contamination do not touch tip of container to any surface. Replace cap after using. If you experience eye pain, changes in vision, continued redness, irritation of the eye, or if the condition worsens or persists, consult a doctor. Obtain immediate medical treatment for all open wounds in or near the eye.
The Collyrium for Fresh Eyes bottle is sealed for your protection. Prior to first use, remove cap and squeeze bottle. If bottle leaks, do not use.
Keep this and all medication out of the reach of children.
Keep bottle tightly closed at Room Temperature, Approx. 77°F (25°C).

How Supplied: Bottles of 4 fl. oz. (118 ml) with eyecup.
Shown in Product Identification Guide, page 529

COLLYRIUM FRESH™
[ko-lir 'e-um]
Sterile Eye Drops
Lubricant
Redness Reliever

Description: Collyrium Fresh is a specially formulated sterile eye drop which can be used, up to 4 times daily, to relieve redness and discomfort due to minor eye irritations caused by dust, smoke, smog, swimming, or sun glare.
The active ingredients are tetrahydrozoline HCl (0.05%) and glycerin (1.0%). Other ingredients include benzalkonium chloride (0.01%) and edetate disodium (0.1%) as preservatives, boric acid, hydrochloric acid and sodium borate.

Indications: For the temporary relief of redness due to minor eye irritations or discomfort due to burning or exposure to wind or sun.

Directions: Tilt head back and squeeze 1 to 2 drops into each eye up to 4 times daily, or as directed by a physician.

Warnings: Do not use if solution changes color or becomes cloudy. Remove contact lenses before using. If you have glaucoma, do not use this product except under the advice and supervision of a physician. Overuse of this product may produce increased redness of the eye. To avoid contamination, do not touch tip of container to any surface. Replace cap after using. If you experience eye pain, changes in vision, continued redness or irritation of the eye, or if the condition worsens or persists for more than 72 hours, discontinue use and consult a physician.
Keep this and all medication out of the reach of children.
Retain carton for complete product information.
Keep bottle tightly closed at Room Temperature, Approx. 77°F (25°C).

How Supplied: Bottles of ½ fl. oz. (15 ml) with built-in eye dropper.
Shown in Product Identification Guide, page 529

Continued on next page

Wyeth-Ayerst—Cont.

DONNAGEL®

[don 'nă-jel]

Liquid and Chewable Tablets

Each tablespoon (15 mL) of **Donnagel Liquid** contains: 600 mg Attapulgite, Activated, USP.

Inactive Ingredients: Alcohol 1.4%, Benzyl Alcohol, Carboxymethylcellulose Sodium, Citric Acid, FD&C Blue 1, Flavors, Magnesium Aluminum Silicate, Methylparaben, Phosphoric Acid, Propylene Glycol, Propylparaben, Saccharin Sodium, Sorbitol, Titanium Dioxide, Water, Xanthan Gum.

Each **Donnagel Chewable** Tablet contains: 600 mg Attapulgite, Activated, USP.

Inactive Ingredients: D&C Yellow 10 Aluminum Lake, FD&C Blue 1 Aluminum Lake, Flavors, Magnesium Stearate, Mannitol, Saccharin Sodium, Sorbitol, Water.

Indications: Donnagel is indicated for the symptomatic relief of diarrhea. It reduces the number of bowel movements, improves consistency of loose, watery bowel movements and relieves cramping.

Warnings: Patients are told that diarrhea may be serious. They are warned not to use this product for more than 2 days, or in the presence of fever, or in children under 3 years of age unless directed by a doctor.
This product should not be taken by patients who are hypersensitive to any of the ingredients. As with any drug, women who are pregnant or nursing a baby should seek the advice of a health professional before using this product.
KEEP THIS AND ALL DRUGS OUT OF THE REACH OF CHILDREN. IN CASE OF ACCIDENTAL OVERDOSE, SEEK PROFESSIONAL ASSISTANCE OR CONTACT A POISON CONTROL CENTER IMMEDIATELY.

Dosage and Administration: Full recommended dose should be administered at the first sign of diarrhea and after each subsequent bowel movement, NOT TO EXCEED 7 DOSES IN A 24-HOUR PERIOD.
[See table below.]

How Supplied: Donnagel Liquid (green suspension) in 4 fl. oz. (NDC 0008-0888-02), and 8 fl. oz. (NDC 0008-0888-04). Donnagel Chewable Tablets (light-green, flat-faced, beveled-edged, round tablets with darker green flecks; one side engraved "W", obverse engraved Donnagel) in consumer blister packages of 18 (NDC 0008-0889-02.)
Store at controlled room temperature, between 20°C and 25°C (68°F and 77°F).

Shown in Product Identification Guide, page 529

NURSOY®

[nur-soy]

Soy protein isolate formula
READY–TO–FEED
CONCENTRATED LIQUID
POWDER

Breast milk is best for babies. NURSOY® milk-free, lactose-free formula is intended to meet the nutritional needs of infants and children who are not breast-fed and are allergic to cow's milk protein and/or intolerant to lactose. It should not be used in infants and children allergic to soybean protein.
NURSOY Ready-to-Feed and Concentrated Liquid are corn free and contain only sucrose as their carbohydrate. NURSOY Powder contains corn syrup solids and sucrose as its carbohydrate. Professional advice should be followed. NURSOY's fat blend provides a fatty acid composition which closely resembles that of human milk. NURSOY has physiologic levels of linoleic and linolenic acid. NURSOY contains beta-carotene, a component of human milk. The estimated renal solute load of NURSOY is relatively low.

Ingredients (in normal dilution supplying 20 calories per fluidounce): 87% water; 6.7% sucrose; 3.4% oleo, coconut, oleic (safflower) and soybean oils; 2.0% soy protein isolate; and less than 1% of each of the following: potassium citrate; monobasic sodium phosphate; calcium carbonate; dibasic calcium phosphate; magnesium chloride; calcium chloride; soy lecithin; calcium carrageenan; calcium hydroxide; L-methionine; sodium chloride; potassium bicarbonate; taurine; ferrous, zinc, and cupric sulfates; L-carnitine; potassium iodide; ascorbic acid; choline chloride; alpha-tocopheryl acetate; niacinamide; calcium pantothenate; riboflavin; vitamin A palmitate; thiamine hydrochloride; pyridoxine hydrochloride; beta-carotene; phytonadione; folic acid; biotin; cholecalciferol; cyanocobalamin.

PROXIMATE ANALYSIS
at 20 calories per fluidounce
READY-TO-FEED, CONCENTRATED
LIQUID, and POWDER

	(W/V)	
Protein	1.8	%
Fat	3.6	%
Carbohydrate	6.9	%
Water	87.0	%
Crude fiber ... not more than	0.01	%
Calories/fl. oz.	20	

Vitamins, Minerals: In normal dilution, each liter contains:

A	2,000	IU
D$_3$	400	IU
E	9.5	IU
K$_1$	100	mcg
C (ascorbic acid)	55	mg
B$_1$ (thiamine)	670	mcg
B$_2$ (riboflavin)	1000	mcg
B$_6$	420	mcg
B$_{12}$	2	mcg
Niacin	5000	mcg
Pantothenic acid	3000	mcg
Folic acid (folacin)	50	mcg
Choline	85	mg
Inositol	27	mg
Biotin	35	mcg
Calcium	600	mg
Phosphorus	420	mg
Sodium	200	mg
Potassium	700	mg
Chloride	375	mg
Magnesium	67	mg
Manganese	200	mcg
Iron	12.0	mg
Copper	470	mcg
Zinc	5	mg
Iodine	60	mcg

Preparation: *Ready-to-Feed* (32 fl. oz. cans of 20 calories per fluidounce formula)—shake can, open and pour into previously sterilized nursing bottle; attach nipple and feed. Cover opened can and immediately store in refrigerator. Use contents of can within 48 hours of opening.
Prolonged storage of can at excessive temperatures should be avoided.
Expiration date is on top of can.
WARNING: DO NOT USE A MICROWAVE TO PREPARE OR WARM FORMULA. SERIOUS BURNS MAY OCCUR.
Concentrated Liquid—For normal dilution supplying 20 calories per fluidounce, use equal amounts of NURSOY® liquid and cooled, previously boiled water.
Note: Prepared formula should be used within 24 hours.
Prolonged storage of can at excessive temperatures should be avoided.
Expiration date is on top of can.
WARNING: DO NOT USE A MICROWAVE TO PREPARE OR WARM FORMULA. SERIOUS BURNS MAY OCCUR.
Powder—For normal dilution supplying 20 calories per fluidounce, add 1 level measuring scoop to 2 fluidounces of previously boiled water, cooled to room temperature.
Note: Prepared formula should be used within 24 hours.
Prolonged storage of can at excessive temperatures should be avoided.
Expiration date is on bottom of can.
WARNING: DO NOT USE A MICROWAVE TO PREPARE OR WARM

DONNAGEL®

	Liquid	Chewable Tablets
Adults	2 Tablespoons	2 Tablets
Children		
12 years and over	2 Tablespoons	2 Tablets
6 to under 12 years	1 Tablespoon	1 Tablet
3 to under 6 years	½ Tablespoon	½ Tablet
Under 3 years	Consult Physician	

Liquid should be shaken well. Tablets should be chewed thoroughly and swallowed.

FORMULA. SERIOUS BURNS MAY OCCUR.

How Supplied: *Ready-to-Feed* —pre-sterilized and premixed, 32 fluidounce (1 quart) cans, cases of 6 cans; *Concentrated Liquid* —13 fluidounce cans, cases of 12 cans; *Powder* —1 pound cans, cases of 6 cans.
Questions or Comments regarding NURSOY: 1-800-99-WYETH.

Shown in Product Identification Guide, page 529

SMA®
Iron fortified
Infant formula
READY–TO–FEED LIQUID
CONCENTRATED LIQUID
POWDER

Breast milk is best for babies. Infant formula is intended to replace or supplement breast milk when breast feeding is not possible or is insufficient, or when mothers elect not to breast feed.
Good maternal nutrition is important for the preparation and maintenance of breast feeding. Extensive or prolonged use of partial bottle feeding, before breast feeding has been well established, could make breast feeding difficult to maintain. A decision not to breast feed could be difficult to reverse.
Professional advice should be followed on all matters of infant feeding. Infant formula should always be prepared and used as directed. Unnecessary or improper use of infant formula could present a health hazard. Social and financial implications should be considered when selecting the method of infant feeding.
SMA® is close in nutrient composition to human milk with its physiologic fat blend, whey-dominated protein composition, and inclusion of beta-carotene and nucleotides.
SMA, utilizing a hybridized safflower (oleic) oil, became the first infant formula offering fat and calcium absorption closest to that of human milk, with physiologic levels of linoleic acid and linolenic acid. Thus, the fat blend in SMA provides a ready source of energy, helps protect infants against neonatal tetany and produces a ratio of vitamin E to polyunsaturated fatty acids (linoleic acid) more than adequate to prevent hemolytic anemia and yields a serum lipid profile close to that of the breast-fed infant.
With a combination of reduced minerals whey and skim cow's milk, SMA has a whey to casein ratio resembling human milk and a physiologic mineral level. The resultant 60:40 whey-protein to casein ratio provides protein nutrition superior to a casein-dominated formula. In addition, the essential amino acids, including cystine, are present in amounts close to those of human milk yielding a protein of high biologic value. SMA is the only infant formula available on the market that is supplemented with five of the thirteen nucleotides found in human milk.

The physiologic mineral content makes possible a low renal solute load which helps protect the functionally immature infant kidney, increases expendable water reserves and helps protect against dehydration.
Use of lactose as the carbohydrate results in a physiologic stool flora and a low stool pH, decreasing the incidence of perianal dermatitis.

Ingredients: SMA Concentrated Liquid or Ready-to-Feed. Water; nonfat milk; reduced minerals whey; oleo, coconut, oleic (safflower or sunflower), and soybean oils; lactose; soy lecithin; taurine; cytidine-5′-monophosphate; calcium carrageenan; adenosine-5′-monophosphate; disodium uridine-5′-monophosphate; disodium inosine-5′-monophosphate; disodium guanosine-5′-monophosphate; *Minerals:* Potassium bicarbonate and chloride; calcium chloride and citrate; sodium bicarbonate and citrate; ferrous, zinc, cupric, and manganese sulfates. *Vitamins:* ascorbic acid, alpha tocopheryl acetate, niacinamide, vitamin A palmitate, calcium pantothenate, thiamine hydrochloride, riboflavin, pyridoxine hydrochloride, beta-carotene, folic acid, phytonadione, biotin, cholecalciferol, cyanocobalamin.
SMA Powder. Lactose; oleo, coconut, oleic (safflower or sunflower), and soybean oils; nonfat milk; whey protein concentrate; soy lecithin; taurine; cytidine-5′-monophosphate; adenosine-5′-monophosphate; disodium uridine-5′-monophosphate; disodium inosine-5′-monophosphate; disodium guanosine-5′-monophosphate. *Minerals:* Potassium phosphate; calcium hydroxide; magnesium chloride; calcium chloride; sodium bicarbonate; ferrous sulfate; potassium hydroxide; potassium bicarbonate; zinc, cupric, and manganese sulfates; potassium iodide. *Vitamins:* Ascorbic acid, choline chloride, inositol, alpha tocopheryl acetate, niacinamide, calcium pantothenate, vitamin A palmitate, riboflavin, thiamine hydrochloride, pyridoxine hydrochloride, beta-carotene, folic acid, phytonadione, biotin, cholecalciferol, cyanocobalamin.

PROXIMATE ANALYSIS
at 20 calories per fluidounce
READY-TO-FEED, POWDER, and
CONCENTRATED LIQUID:

	(W/V)
Fat	3.6 %
Carbohydrate	7.2 %
Protein	1.5 %
60% Lactalbumin (whey protein)	0.9 %
40% Casein	0.6 %
Crude Fiber	None
Total Solids	12.6 %
Calories/fl. oz.	20

Vitamins, Minerals: In normal dilution, each liter contains:

A	2000	IU
D$_3$	400	IU
E	9.5	IU
K$_1$	55	mcg
C (ascorbic acid)	55	mg
B$_1$ (thiamine)	670	mcg
B$_2$ (riboflavin)	1000	mcg
B$_6$	420	mcg
(pyridoxine hydrochloride)		
B$_{12}$	1.3	mcg
Niacin	5000	mcg
Pantothenic Acid	2100	mcg
Folic Acid (folacin)	50	mcg
Choline	100	mg
Biotin	15	mcg
Calcium	420	mg
Phosphorus	280	mg
Sodium	150	mg
Potassium	560	mg
Chloride	375	mg
Magnesium	45	mg
Manganese	100	mcg
Iron	12	mg
Copper	470	mcg
Zinc	5	mg
Iodine	60	mcg

Preparation: *Ready-to-Feed* (8 and 32 fl. oz. cans of 20 calories per fluidounce formula)—shake can, open and pour into previously sterilized nursing bottle; attach nipple and feed immediately. Cover opened can and immediately store in refrigerator. Use contents of can within 48 hours of opening.
Prolonged storage of can at excessive temperatures should be avoided.
Expiration date is on top of can.
WARNING: DO NOT USE A MICROWAVE TO PREPARE OR WARM FORMULA. SERIOUS BURNS MAY OCCUR.
Powder —(1 pound and 2 pound 3 ounce cans)—For normal dilution supplying 20 calories per fluidounce, use 1 level measuring scoop to 2 fluidounces of cooled, previously boiled water.
Prolonged storage of can of powder at excessive temperatures should be avoided.
Expiration date is on bottom of can.
WARNING: DO NOT USE A MICROWAVE TO PREPARE OR WARM FORMULA. SERIOUS BURNS MAY OCCUR.
Concentrated Liquid —For normal dilution supplying 20 calories per fluidounce, use equal amounts of SMA® liquid and cooled, previously boiled water.
Prolonged storage of can at excessive temperatures should be avoided.
Expiration date is on top of can.
WARNING: DO NOT USE A MICROWAVE TO PREPARE OR WARM FORMULA. SERIOUS BURNS MAY OCCUR.
Note: Prepared formula should be used within 24 hours.

How Supplied: *Ready-to-Feed* —pre-sterilized and premixed, 32 fluidounce (1 quart) cans, cases of 6 cans; 8 fluidounce cans, cases of 24 (4 carriers of 6 cans). *Powder* —1 pound and 2 pound 3 ounce cans with measuring scoop, cases of 6 cans. *Concentrated Liquid* —13 fluidounce cans, cases of 24 cans.
Also Available: SMA® lo-iron. Those who appreciate the particular advantages of SMA® infant formula, close in nutrient composition to mother's milk,

Continued on next page

Wyeth-Ayerst—Cont.

sometimes need or wish to recommend a formula that does not contain a high level of iron. SMA® lo-iron has all the benefits of regular SMA® but with a reduced level of iron of 1.4 mg per quart. Infants should receive supplemental dietary iron from an outside source to meet daily requirements.
Concentrated Liquid—13 fl. oz. cans, cases of 12 cans. *Powder*—1 pound cans with measuring scoop, cases of 6 cans. *Ready-to-Feed*—32 fl. oz. cans, cases of 6 cans.
Preparation of the standard 20 calories per fluidounce formula of SMA® lo-iron is the same as SMA® iron fortified given above.
Questions or Comments regarding SMA: 1-800-99-WYETH.
Shown in Product Identification Guide, page 529

WYANOIDS® Relief Factor
[wi'a-noids]
Hemorrhoidal Suppositories

Description: Active Ingredients: Cocoa Butter 79% and Shark Liver Oil 3%. **Inactive Ingredients:** Ascorbyl Palmitate, Benzoic Acid, BHA, Corn Oil, Edetate Disodium, Glycerin, Methylparaben, PEG-12 Dilaurate, Propylparaben, Tocopherol, Water, White Wax.

Indications: Gives temporary relief of the itching, discomfort and burning associated with hemorrhoids and protects irritated areas.

Directions: *Adults*—When practical, cleanse the affected area by patting or blotting with an appropriate cleansing pad. Gently dry by patting or blotting with toilet tissue or a soft cloth before application of this product. Remove wrapper before inserting into the rectum. Insert one suppository into the rectum up to 6 times daily or after each bowel movement. *Children under 12 years of age*—Consult a doctor.

Warnings: In case of bleeding or if the condition worsens or does not improve within 7 days, the patient should consult a doctor promptly. Do not exceed the recommended daily dosage unless directed by a doctor. Keep this and all medicines out of the reach of children. In case of accidental ingestion, seek professional assistance or contact a Poison Control Center immediately. As with any drug, if you are pregnant or nursing a baby, seek the advice of a health professional before using this product.
Do not store above 80°F.
Do Not Use if Cellophane Safety Tear Strip is Missing or Cellophane Safety Wrap is Broken or Missing When Purchased.

How Supplied: Boxes of 12.
Shown in Product Identification Guide, page 529

Audiovisual Programs
The ***Wyeth-Ayerst Audiovisual Catalog***, listing audiovisual programs available through the Wyeth-Ayerst Audiovisual Library or on loan through the local Wyeth-Ayerst representative, can be obtained by writing Professional Service, Wyeth-Ayerst Laboratories, P.O. Box 8299, Philadelphia, PA 19101.

Zila Pharmaceuticals, Inc.
**5227 NORTH 7th STREET
PHOENIX, AZ 85014-2817**

Direct Inquiries to:
Jerry Kaster,
Director of Marketing:
(602) 266-6700

**ZILACTIN® Medicated Gel
ZILACTIN®-L Liquid
ZILACTIN®-B Medicated Gel
with Benzocaine**

Description: Zilactin Medicated Gel stops pain and speeds healing of canker sores, fever blisters and cold sores. Zilactin forms a tenacious, occlusive film which holds the medication in place while controlling pain. Intra-orally, the film can last up to 8 hours, usually allowing pain-free eating and drinking. Extra-orally, the film will last much longer.
Zilactin-L is a non film-forming liquid that treats and relieves the pain, itching and burning of developing and existing cold sores and fever blisters. Zilactin-L is specially formulated to treat the initial signs of tingling, itching or burning that signal an oncoming cold sore or fever blister. Zilactin-L can often prevent developing cold sores or fever blisters from breaking out. If a lesion does occur, Zilactin-L will significantly reduce the size and the duration of the outbreak.
Zilactin-B is a medicated gel containing benzocaine that forms a smooth, flexible and occlusive film on the oral mucosa. It's specially formulated to control pain and shield the mouth sores, canker sores, cheek bites and gum sores that occur from dental appliances from the environment of the mouth. The film can last up to 8 hours.

Clinical studies on the effectiveness of Zila's products are available on request.

Active Ingredients: Zilactin—Benzyl Alcohol (10%); **Zilactin-L**—Lidocaine (2.5%); **Zilactin-B**—Benzocaine (10%);

Application: Zilactin: FOR USE IN THE MOUTH AND ON LIPS. Apply every four hours for the first three days and

then as needed. Dry the affected area. Apply a thin coat of Zilactin and allow 60 seconds for the gel to dry into a film. Outside the mouth, Zilactin forms a transparent film. Inside the mouth, the film is white.

Zilactin-L: FOR USE ON THE LIPS AND AROUND THE MOUTH. Apply every 1-2 hours for the first three days and then as needed. For maximum effectiveness use at first signs of tingling or itching. Moisten a cotton swab with several drops of Zilactin-L. Apply on lip area where symptoms are noted or directly on existing cold sore or fever blister and allow to dry for 15 seconds.

Zilactin-B: FOR USE IN THE MOUTH. Apply every four hours for the first three days and then as needed. Dry the affected area. Apply a thin coat of Zilactin-B and allow 60 seconds for the gel to dry into a film.

Warning: A mild, temporary stinging sensation may be experienced when applying Zilactin, Zilactin-L or Zilactin-B to an open cut, sore or blister. This may be minimized by first applying ice for a minute before application of the medication. DO NOT USE IN OR NEAR EYES. In the event of accidental contact with the eye, flush with water immediately and continuously for ten minutes. Seek immediate medical attention if pain or irritation persists. For temporary relief only. As with all medications, keep out of the reach of children. Do not use Zilactin-L or Zilactin-B if you have a history of allergy to local anesthetics such as benzocaine, lidocaine or other "caine" anesthetics.

How Supplied: Zila products are non-prescription and carried by most drug wholesalers, retail chains and independent pharmacies. Each product is available to physicians and dentists directly from Zila in single use packages.
For further information call or write:

Zila Pharmaceuticals, Inc.
5227 N. 7th Street, Phoenix, AZ 85014-2817, (602) 266-6700

U.S. patent numbers 4,285,934; 4,381,296; and 5,081,158
Shown in Product Identification Guide, page 529

Samples and literature are available to medical professionals on request.

STATE BOARDS OF PHARMACY

Questions on local regulations governing prescription and over-the-counter drugs, controlled substances, and pharmacy licensure can often be answered by your local state board of pharmacy. For your convenience, a contact name, address, and phone number for each state board is listed in the directory that follows.

ALABAMA
Jerry Moore, R.Ph.
Executive Secretary
1 Perimeter Park S.,
Suite 425 S
Birmingham, AL 35243
205-967-0130
Fax: 205-967-1009

ALASKA
Brandi Barger
Licensing Examiner
Dept. of Commerce and
Economic Development
Division of Occupational
Licensing
P.O. Box 110806
Juneau, AK 99811
907-465-2589
Fax: 907-465-2974

ARIZONA
L.A. Lloyd, R.Ph.
Executive Director
5060 N. 19th Ave.,
Suite 101
Phoenix, AZ 85015
602-255-5125
Fax: 602-255-5740

ARKANSAS
Lester Hosto, P.D.
Executive Director
101 E. Capitol Ave.
Suite 218
Little Rock, AR 72201
501-682-0190
Fax: 501-682-0195

CALIFORNIA
Patricia Harris
Executive Officer
400 "R" St., Suite 4070
Sacramento, CA 95814
916-445-5014, Fax:
916-327-6308

COLORADO
W. Kent Mount
Program Administrator
1560 Broadway
Suite 1310
Denver, CO 80202
303-894-7750
Fax: 303-894-7764

CONNECTICUT
Margherita R. Giuliano,
R.Ph.
Board Administrator
State Office Bldg.
Room G-3A
165 Capitol Avenue
Hartford, CT 06106
203-566-3290
Fax: 203-566-7630

DELAWARE
Bonnie Wallner, R.Ph.
Executive Secretary
P.O. Box 637
Dover, DE 19903
302-739-4798
Fax: 302-739-3071

DISTRICT OF COLUMBIA
Barbara Hagans
Contact Representative
614 "H" St., NW
Room 923
Washington, DC 20001
202-727-7832
Fax: 202-727-7662

FLORIDA
John D. Taylor, R.Ph.
Executive Director
Agency for Health Care
Administration
Board of Pharmacy
1940 N. Monroe St.
Tallahassee, FL 32399
904-488-7546
Fax: 904-921-7865

GEORGIA
Gregg W. Schuder
Executive Director
166 Pryor St. SW
Atlanta, GA 30303
404-656-3912, Fax:
404-657-4220

HAWAII
Ruth Gushiken
Executive Officer
P.O. Box 3469
Honolulu, HI 96801
808-586-2698

IDAHO
R.K. Markuson, R.Ph.
Director
P.O. Box 83720
Boise, ID 83720-0067
208-334-2356
Fax: 208-334-3536

ILLINOIS
Ed Duffy, R.Ph.
Executive Administrator
Drug Compliance
Illinois Dept. Of
Professional
Regulation
100 W. Randolph
Suite 9-300
Chicago, IL 60601
312-814-4573
Fax: 312-814-3145

INDIANA
Frances L. Kelly
Director
402 W. Washington St.
Room 041
Indianapolis, IN 46204
317-232-2960
Fax: 317-233-4236

IOWA
Lloyd K. Jessen, R.Ph., J.D.
Exec. Sec./Director
1209 East Court Ave.
Executive Hills West
Des Moines, IA 50319
515-281-5944
Fax: 515-281-4609

KANSAS
Larry Froelich
Director
900 Jackson St.
Room 513
Topeka, KS 66612
913-296-4056, Fax:
913-296-8420

KENTUCKY
Ralph E. Bouvette,
R.Ph., Ph.D., J.D.
Executive Director
1024 Capital Center Dr.
Suite. 210
Frankfort, KY 40601
502-573-1580, Fax:
502-573-1582

LOUISIANA
Howard B. Bolton, R. Ph.
Executive Director
5615 Corporate Blvd., 8E
Baton Rouge, LA 70808
504-925-6496
Fax: 504-925-6499

MAINE
Susan Greenlaw
Board Clerk
Dept. of Professional
and Financial
Regulations
Board of Commissions
Profession of Pharmacy
Augusta, ME 04333
207-624-8603
Fax: 207-624-8637

MARYLAND
Norene Pease
Executive Director
4201 Patterson Ave.
Baltimore, MD 21215
410-764-4755
Fax: 410-358-6207

MASSACHUSETTS
Lori Bassinger
Executive Secretary
100 Cambridge St.
Room 1514
Boston, MA 02202
617-727-7390
Fax: 617-727-2197

MICHIGAN
Patrick Gaven, R.Ph.
Chairman
611 W. Ottawa St.
P.O. Box 30018
Lansing, MI 48909
517-373-9102, Fax:
517-373-2179

MINNESOTA
David E. Holmstrom,
R.Ph., J.D.
Executive Director
2700 University Ave. W.,
Room 107
St. Paul, MN 55114
612-642-0541
Fax: 612-643-3530

MISSISSIPPI
William L. Stevens
Executive Director
P.O. Box 24507
C & F Plaza, Suite D
Jackson, MS 39225
601-354-6750
Fax: 601-354-6071

MISSOURI
Kevin E. Kinkade, R.Ph.
Executive Director
P.O. Box 625
Jefferson City, MO 65102
314-751-0093
Fax: 314-526-3464

MONTANA
Warren R. Amole, Jr., R.Ph.
Executive Director
111 N. Last Chance
Gulch
Helena, MT 59620
406-444-1698
Fax: 406-444-1667

NEBRASKA
Katherine A. Brown
Executive Secretary
Board of Examiners in
Pharmacy
P.O. Box 95007
301 Centennial Mall S.
Lincoln, NE 68509
402-471-2118
Fax: 402-471-0555

NEVADA
Keith W. MacDonald,
R.Ph.
Executive Secretary
1201 Terminal Way
Suite 212
Reno, NV 89502-3257
702-322-0691
Fax: 702-322-0895

NEW HAMPSHIRE
Paul G. Boisseau, R.Ph.
Executive Director
57 Regional Drive
Concord, NH 03301
603-271-2350
Fax: 603-271-2856

NEW JERSEY
H. Lee Gladstein, R.Ph.
Executive Director
124 Halsey St.
6th Floor
P.O. Box 45013
Newark, NJ 07102
201-504-6450
Fax: 201-648-3355

NEW MEXICO
Richard W. Thompson
Executive Director
1650 University Blvd. NE
Suite 400-B
Albuquerque, NM
505-841-9102
Fax: 505-841-9113

NEW YORK
Lawrence H. Mokhiber,
R.Ph.
Executive Secretary
Cultural Education
Center
Room 3035
Albany, NY 12230
518-474-3848
Fax: 518-473-6995

NORTH CAROLINA
David R. Work, R.Ph.
Executive Director
P.O. Box 459
Carrboro, NC 27510
919-942-4454
Fax: 919-967-5757

NORTH DAKOTA
William J. Grosz, Sc.D.,
R.Ph.
Executive Director
P.O. Box 1354
Bismarck, ND 58502
701-258-1535
Fax: 701-258-9312

OHIO
Franklin Z. Wickham,
R.Ph.
Executive Director
77 S. High St.
17th Floor
Columbus, OH 43266
614-466-4143
Fax: 614-752-4836

OKLAHOMA
Bryan Potter, R.Ph.
Executive Director
4545 N. Lincoln Blvd.
Suite 112
Oklahoma City, OK 73105
405-521-3815
Fax: 405-521-3758

OREGON
Ruth Vandever, R.Ph.
Executive Director
State Office Bldg.
Suite 425
800 NE Oregon St., #9
Portland, OR 97232
503-731-4032
Fax: 503-731-4067

PENNSYLVANIA
W. Richard Marshman,
R.Ph.
Executive Secretary
P.O. Box 2649
Harrisburg, PA 17105
717-783-7157
Fax: 717-783-4853

PUERTO RICO
Arnalo LaLuc
President
Call Box 10200
Santurce, PR 00908
809-725-8161
Fax: 809-725-7903

RHODE ISLAND
Mario Casinelli, Jr., R.Ph.
Chairman of the Board
Dept. of Health
Division of Drug Control
Three Capitol Hill
Room 304
Providence, RI 02908
401-277-2837
Fax: 401-277-2499

SOUTH CAROLINA
Joseph L. Mullinax, R.Ph.
Administrator
S.C.L.L.R./Board of
Pharmacy
1026 Sumter St.
Room 209
P.O. Box 11927
Columbia, SC 29211
803-734-1010
Fax: 803-734-1552

SOUTH DAKOTA
Galen Jordre, R.Ph.
Secretary
P.O. Box 518
Pierre, SD 57501
605-224-2338
Fax: 605-224-1280

TENNESSEE
William S. Chance,
D.Ph.
Acting Director
500 James Robertson
Pkwy.
Nashville, TN 37243
615-741-2718
Fax: 615-741-6470

TEXAS
Fred S. Brinkley, Jr., R.Ph.
Executive Director
8505 Cross Park Dr.
Suite 110
Austin, TX 78754
512-832-0661
Fax: 512-832-0855

UTAH
David E. Robinson
Director
Utah Dept. of
Commerce
160 E. 300 S
P.O. Box 48505
Salt Lake City, UT 84145
801-530-6628
Fax: 801-530-6511

VERMONT
Carla Preston
Staff Assistant
109 State Street
Montpelier, VT 05609
802-828-2875
Fax: 802-828-2496

VIRGINIA
Scotti W. Milley, R.Ph.
Executive Director
6606 W. Broad St.
Richmond, VA 23230
804-662-9911
Fax: 804-662-9313

WASHINGTON
Donald H. Williams,
R.Ph.
Executive Director
P.O. Box 47863
Olympia, WA 98504
360-753-6834
Fax: 360-586-4359

WEST VIRGINIA
Sam Kapourales, R.Ph.
President
236 Capitol St.
Charleston, WV 25301
304-558-0558
Fax: 304-558-0572

WISCONSIN
Patrick D. Braatz
Bureau Director
P.O. Box 8935
1400 E. Washington Ave.
Madison, WI 53708
608-266-2811
Fax: 608-267-0644

WYOMING
Marilynn H. Mitchell,
R.Ph.
Executive Director
1720 S. Poplar St.
Suite 5
Casper, WY 82601
307-234-0294
Fax: 307-234-7226

POISON CONTROL CENTERS

Many centers in this directory are certified members of the American Association of Poison Control Centers (AAPCC). Certified centers are marked by an asterisk after the name. They must meet certain criteria: for example, serve a large geographic area; be open 24 hours a day and provide direct dialing or toll-free access; be supervised by a medical director; and have registered pharmacists or nurses available to answer questions from healthcare professionals and the public.

Centers in each state are listed alphabetically by city. "TTY" numbers are reserved for the hearing impaired, and "TTD" numbers reach a telecommunication device for the deaf.

ALABAMA

BIRMINGHAM
Regional Poison Control Center Children's Hospital of Alabama (*)
1600 7th Ave. South
Birmingham, AL 35233
Business: 205-939-9720
Emergency: 205-933-4050
            205-939-9201
            800-292-6678
            (AL)
Fax: 205-759-7994

TUSCALOOSA
Alabama Poison Control Systems, Inc. (*)
408 A. Paul Bryant Dr. East
Tuscaloosa, AL 35401
Business: 205-345-0600
Emergency: 205-345-0600
            800-462-0800
            (AL)
Fax: 205-759-7994

ALASKA

ANCHORAGE
Anchorage Poison Center
Providence Hospital
P.O. Box 196604
3200 Providence Dr.
Anchorage, AK 99519
Business: 907-562-2211
            ext. 3633
Emergency: 907-261-3193
            800-478-3193
            (AK)
Fax: 907-261-3645

FAIRBANKS
Fairbanks Poison Control Center
1650 Cowles St.
Fairbanks, AK 99701
Business: 907-456-7182
Emergency: 907-456-7182
Fax: 907-452-5776

ARIZONA

PHOENIX
Samaritan Regional Poison Center (*)
Good Samaritan Medical Center
1111 East McDowell Rd.
Phoenix, AZ 85006
Business: 602-495-4884
Emergency: 602-253-3334
Fax: 602-256-7579

TUCSON
Arizona Poison & Drug Information Center (*)
University of Arizona Arizona Health Sciences Center
1501 North Campbell Ave. #1156
Tucson, AZ 85724
Emergency: 602-626-6016
            800-362-0101
            (AZ)
Fax: 602-626-4063

ARKANSAS

LITTLE ROCK
Arkansas Poison and Drug Information Center
College of Pharmacy - UAMS
4301 West Markham St.
Slot 522
Little Rock, AR 72205
Business: 501-661-6161
Emergency: 800-376-4766
            (AR)

CALIFORNIA

FRESNO
Central California Regional Poison Control Center (*)
Valley Children's Hospital
3151 North Millbrook
Fresno, CA 93703
Business: 209-241-6040
Emergency: 209-445-1222
            800-346-5922
            (Central CA)
Fax: 209-241-6050

LOS ANGELES
Los Angeles County Regional Drug & Poison Information Center (*)
LAC & USC Medical Center
1200 North State St.
Los Angeles, CA 90033
Business: 213-226-7741
Emergency: 213-222-3212
            800-777-6476
Fax: 213-226-4194

SACRAMENTO
UC Davis Medical Center Regional Poison Control Center (*)
2315 Stockton Blvd.
Sacramento, CA 95817
Business: 916-734-3415
Emergency: 916-734-3692
            800-342-9293
            (N. CA only)
Fax: 916-734-7796

SAN DIEGO
San Diego Regional Poison Center (*)
UCSD Medical Center
200 West Arbor Dr.
San Diego, CA 92103
Business: 619-543-3666
Emergency: 619-543-6000
            800-876-4766
            (San Diego and Imperial counties only)
Fax: 619-692-1867

SAN FRANCISCO
San Francisco Bay Area Regional Poison Control Center (*)
SF General Hospital
1001 Potrero Ave.
Bldg. 80
San Francisco, CA 94110
Business: 415-206-5524
Emergency: 800-523-2222
Fax: 415-821-8513

COLORADO

DENVER

**Rocky Mountain Poison
and Drug Center (*)**
8802 East 9th Ave.
Denver, CO 80220
Business: 303-739-1100
Emergency: 303-629-1123
TTY: 303-739-1127
Fax: 303-739-1126

CONNECTICUT

FARMINGTON

**Connecticut Poison Control
Center (*)**
**University of Connecticut
Health Center**
263 Farmington Ave.
Farmington, CT 06032
Business: 203-679-3473
Emergency: 800-343-2722
(CT)
TTY: 203-679-4346
Fax: 203-679-1623

DISTRICT OF COLUMBIA

WASHINGTON, DC

**National Capital Poison
Center (*)**
3201 New Mexico Ave., NW
Suite 310
Washington, DC 20016
Business: 202-362-3867
Emergency: 202-625-3333
TTY: 202-362-8536
Fax: 202-362-8377

FLORIDA

TAMPA

**Florida Poison Information
and Toxicology
Resource Center (*)**
Tampa General Hospital
P.O. Box 1289
Tampa, FL 33601
Emergency: 813-253-4444
800-282-3171
(FL)
Fax: 813-253-4443

GEORGIA

ATLANTA

Georgia Poison Center (*)
Grady Memorial Hospital
80 Butler St. SE
P.O. Box 26066
Atlanta, GA 30335-3801
Emergency: 404-616-9000
800-282-5846
(GA)
Fax: 404-616-9288

MACON

**Regional Poison
Control Center
Medical Center
of Central Georgia**
777 Hemlock St.
Macon, GA 31201
Poison Ctr: 912-633-1427
Fax: 912-633-5082

ILLINOIS

CHICAGO

**Chicago & NE Illinois
Regional Poison
Control Center
Rush-Presbyterian-
St. Luke's Medical Center**
1653 West Congress Pkwy.
Chicago, IL 60612
Business: 312-942-7064
Emergency: 312-942-5969
800-942-5969
(IL)
Fax: 312-942-4260

NORMAL

**Bro Menn Poison
Control Center (*)**
**Bro Menn Regional
Medical Center**
Virginia at Franklin
Normal, IL 61761
Business: 309-454-0738
Emergency: 309-454-6666
Fax: 309-888-0902

URBANA

**Animal Poison
Control Center (*)**
**University of Illinois
College of Veterinary
Medicine**
Vet Med Basic
Sciences Bldg.
2001 South Lincoln
Room 1220
Urbana, IL 61801
Business: 217-333-2053
800-548-2423
(24-hour
subscribers)
Fax: 217-244-1580

INDIANA

INDIANAPOLIS

Indiana Poison Center (*)
**Methodist Hospital of
Indiana**
1701 North Senate Blvd.
P.O. Box 1367
Indianapolis, IN 46206
Emergency: 317-929-2323
800-382-9097
(IN)
TTY: 317-929-2336
Fax: 317-929-2337

IOWA

DES MOINES

**Variety Club Poison and
Drug Information Center
Iowa Methodist
Medical Center**
1200 Pleasant St.
Des Moines, IA 50309
Business: 515-241-6254
Emergency: 800-362-2327
(IA)
Fax: 515-241-5085

IOWA CITY

Poison Control Center (*)
**University of Iowa
Hospitals and Clinics**
200 Hawkins Dr.
Iowa City, IA 52242
Business: 319-356-2577
Emergency: 800-272-6477
(IA only)

KANSAS

KANSAS CITY

**Mid-America Poison
Control Center
University of Kansas
Medical Center**
3901 Rainbow Blvd.
Room B-400
Kansas City, KS 66160
Business & 913-588-6633
Emergency: 800-332-6633
(KS)
Fax: 913-588-2350

TOPEKA

**Stormont-Vail Regional
Medical Center
Emergency Department**
1500 West 10th
Topeka, KS 66604
Business: 913-354-6000
Emergency: 913-354-6100
Fax: 913-354-5004

KENTUCKY

LOUISVILLE

**Kentucky Regional
Poison Center (*)**
Kosair Children's Hospital
Medical Towers S.
Suite 572
P.O. Box 35070
Louisville, KY 40232
Business: 502-629-7264
Emergency: 502-629-7275
502-589-8222
800-722-5725
(KY)
Fax: 502-629-7277

LOUISIANA

HOUMA

**Terrebonne General
Medical Center
Drug and Poison
Information Center**
936 East Main St.
Houma, LA 70360
Business: 504-873-4067
Emergency: 504-873-4069
Fax: 504-873-4573

MONROE
Louisiana Drug and Poison
Information Center (*)
Northeast Louisiana
University
School of Pharmacy
Monroe, LA 71209-6430
Business: 318-342-1710
Emergency: 800-256-9822
(LA)
Fax: 318-342-1744

MAINE

PORTLAND
Maine Poison Center (*)
Maine Medical Center
22 Bramhall St.
Portland, ME 04102
Business: 207-871-2950
Emergency: 800-442-6305
(ME)
Fax: 207-871-6226

MARYLAND

BALTIMORE
Maryland Poison Center (*)
University of Maryland
School of Pharmacy
20 North Pine St.
Baltimore, MD 21201
Business: 410-706-7604
Emergency: 410-528-7701
800-492-2414
(MD only)
TTY: 410-706-1858
Fax: 410-706-7184

MASSACHUSETTS

BOSTON
Massachusetts Poison
Control System (*)
300 Longwood Ave.
Boston, MA 02115
Emergency: 617-232-2120
800-682-9211
TTY: 617-355-6089
Fax: 617-738-0032

MICHIGAN

DETROIT
Poison Control Center (*)
Children's Hospital of
Michigan
Harper Professional
Office Bldg., Suite 425
Detroit, MI 48201
Business: 313-745-5335
Emergency: 313-745-5711
TTY: 313-993-7152
Fax: 313-745-5493

GRAND RAPIDS
Blodgett Regional
Poison Center (*)
Blodgett Memorial
Medical Center
1840 Wealthy St. SE
Grand Rapids, MI 49506
Business: 616-774-7851
Emergency: 800-764-7661
(MI)
Fax: 616-774-7204

KALAMAZOO
Bronson Poison
Information Center
Bronson Methodist
Hospital
252 East Lovell St.
Kalamazoo, MI 49007
Business & 616-341-6409
Emergency: 616-341-6409
800-442-4112
(MI)
Fax: 616-341-7861

MINNESOTA

MINNEAPOLIS
Hennepin Regional
Poison Center (*)
Hennepin County
Medical Center
701 Park Ave.
Minneapolis, MN 55415
Business: 612-347-3144
Emergency: 612-347-3141
TTY: 612-337-7474
Fax: 612-347-3500

Minnesota Regional
Poison Center (*)
8100 34th Ave. South
Box 1309
Minneapolis, MN 55440
Business: 612-851-8100
Emergency: 612-221-2113
Fax: 612-851-8166

MISSISSIPPI

HATTIESBURG
Poison Center
Forrest General Hospital
400 South 28th Ave.
Hattiesburg, MS 39401
Business: 601-288-4221
Emergency: 601-288-4235

JACKSON
Mississippi Regional
Poison Control (*)
University of Mississippi
Medical Center
2500 North State St.
Jackson, MS 39216
Business: 601-984-1675
Emergency: 601-354-7660
Fax: 601-984-1676

MISSOURI

KANSAS CITY
Poison Control Center (*)
Children's Mercy Hospital
2401 Gillham Rd.
Kansas City, MO 64108
Business: 816-234-3053
Emergency: 816-234-3430
816-234-3000
Fax: 816-234-3421
Emergency 816-234-3039
Department: (Office)

ST. LOUIS
Cardinal Glennon
Children's Hospital (*)
Regional Poison Center
1465 South Grand Blvd.
St. Louis, MO 63104
Emergency: 314-772-5200
800-366-8888
Fax: 314-577-5355

MONTANA

DENVER, CO
Rocky Mountain Poison
and Drug Center (*)
645 Bannock St.
Denver, CO 80204
Emergency: 303-629-1123
800-525-5042
(MT)
Fax: 303-623-1119

NEBRASKA

OMAHA
The Poison Center (*)
Children's Memorial
Hospital
8301 Dodge St.
Omaha, NE 68114
Emergency: 402-390-5555
(Omaha)
800-955-9119
(NE, WY)
Fax: 402-390-3049

NEVADA

LAS VEGAS
Poison Center
Humana Medical Center
3186 Maryland Pkwy.
Las Vegas, NV 89109
Emergency: 800-446-6179
(NV)

RENO
Poison Center
Washoe Medical Center
77 Pringle Way
Reno, NV 89520
Business: 702-328-4129
Emergency: 702-328-4100
Fax: 702-328-5555

NEW HAMPSHIRE

LEBANON
New Hampshire Poison
Information Center (*)
Dartmouth-Hitchcock
Memorial Hospital
1 Medical Center Dr.
Lebanon, NH 03756
Emergency: 603-650-5000
(ask for
Poison
Center)
800-562-8236
(NH only)
TTY: 603-650-6318

NEW JERSEY

NEWARK

New Jersey Poison Information and Education System Newark Beth Israel Medical Center
201 Lyons Ave.
Newark, NJ 07112
Emergency: POISON-1
(800-764-7661)
TTY: POISON-1
(800-764-7661)
Fax: 201-926-0013

PHILLIPSBURG

Warren Hospital Poison Control Center
185 Roseberry St.
Phillipsburg, NJ 08865
Business: 908-859-6768
Emergency: 908-859-6767
800-962-1253
(NJ)

NEW MEXICO

ALBUQUERQUE

New Mexico Poison & Drug Information Center University of New Mexico
Albuquerque, NM 87131
Emergency: 505-843-2551
800-432-6866
(NM)
Fax: 505-277-5892

NEW YORK

BUFFALO

Western New York Regional Poison Control Center Children's Hospital of Buffalo
219 Bryant St.
Buffalo, NY 14222
Business: 716-878-7657
Emergency: 716-878-7654
800-888-7655
(NY & W. PA only)

MINEOLA

L.I. Regional Poison Control Center (*) Winthrop University Hospital
259 First St.
Mineola, NY 11501
Emergency: 516-542-2323
TTY: 516-747-3323
Fax: 516-739-2070

NEW YORK

New York City Poison Control Center (*) NYC Dept. of Health
455 First Ave., Room 123
New York, NY 10016
Business: 212-447-8154
Emergency: 212-340-4494
212-POISONS
(212-764-7667)
TTD: 212-689-9014
Fax: 212-447-8223

NYACK

Hudson Valley Poison Center Nyack Hospital
160 North Midland Ave.
Nyack, NY 10960
Emergency: 914-353-1000
800-336-6997
Fax: 914-353-1050

ROCHESTER

Finger Lakes Regional Poison Control Center (*) University of Rochester Medical Center
601 Elmwood Ave.
Rochester, NY 14642
Business: 716-273-4155
Emergency: 716-275-3232
800-333-0542
(NY)
Fax: 717-244-1677

SYRACUSE

Central NY Poison Control Center SUNY Health Science Center
750 East Adams St.
Syracuse, NY 13210
Business: 315-464-7073
Emergency: 315-476-4766
800-252-5655
(NY)
Fax: 315-464-7077

NORTH CAROLINA

ASHEVILLE

Western North Carolina Poison Control Center (*) Memorial Mission Hospital
509 Biltmore Ave.
Asheville, NC 28801
Emergency: 704-255-4490
800-542-4225
(NC)
Fax: 704-255-4467

CHARLOTTE

Carolinas Poison Center (*)
P.O. Box 32861
Charlotte, NC 28232
Business: 704-355-3054
Emergency: 704-355-4000
(Charlotte area)
800-848-6946

HICKORY

Catawba Memorial Hospital Poison Control Center
810 Fairgrove Church Rd., SE
Hickory, NC 28602
Business: 704-326-3385
Emergency: 704-322-6649
Fax: 704-326-3324

NORTH DAKOTA

FARGO

North Dakota Poison Information Center (*) Meritcare Medical Center
720 North 4th St.
Fargo, ND 58122
Business: 701-234-6062
Emergency: 701-234-5575
800-732-2200
(ND)
Fax: 701-234-5090

OHIO

AKRON

Akron Regional Poison Control Center Children's Hospital Medical Center
1 Perkins Square
Akron, OH 44308
Business: 216-258-3066
Emergency: 216-379-8562
800-362-9922
(OH)
TTY: 216-379-8446
Fax: 216-379-8447

CINCINNATI

Regional Poison Control System Cincinnati Drug and Poison Information Center (*) University of Cincinnati College of Medicine
P.O. Box 670144
Cincinnati, OH 45267
Emergency: 513-558-5111
800-872-5111
(OH)
Fax: 513-558-5301

CLEVELAND

Greater Cleveland Poison Control Center (*)
11100 Euclid Ave.
Cleveland, OH 44106
Emergency: 216-231-4455

COLUMBUS

Central Ohio Poison Center (*)
700 Children's Dr.
Columbus, OH 43205
Business: 614-722-2635
Emergency: 614-228-1323
800-682-7625
TTY: 614-228-2272
Fax: 614-221-2672

Greater Dayton Area Hospital Association (*) at Central Ohio Poison Center
700 Children's Dr.
Columbus, OH 43205
Business: 614-722-2635
Emergency: 513-222-2227
800-762-0727
(OH)

TOLEDO
**Poison Information Center
of NW Ohio (*)
Medical College of
Ohio Hospital**
3000 Arlington Ave.
Toledo, OH 43614
Business: 419-381-3898
Emergency: 419-381-3897
            800-589-3897
            (OH)

ZANESVILLE
**Drug Information/Poison
Control Center (*)
Bethesda Hospital**
2951 Maple Ave.
Zanesville, OH 43701
Business: 614-454-4246
Emergency: 614-454-4221
            614-454-4000
            800-686-4221
            (OH)
Fax: 614-454-4059

OKLAHOMA

OKLAHOMA CITY
**Oklahoma Poison
Control Center (*)
University of Oklahoma and
Children's Hospital
of Oklahoma**
940 Northeast 13th St.
Oklahoma City, OK 73104
Emergency: 405-271-5454
            (Bus.)
            800-522-4611
            (Bus.) (OK)
TTD: 405-271-1122
Fax: 405-271-1816

OREGON

PORTLAND
**Oregon Poison Center (*)
Oregon Health Sciences
University**
3181 SW Sam Jackson
  Park Rd.
Portland, OR 97201
Emergency: 503-494-8968
            800-452-7165
            (OR)
Fax: 503-494-4980

PENNSYLVANIA

HERSHEY
**Central Pennsylvania
Poison Center (*)
University Hospital, Milton
S. Hershey Medical Center**
P.O. Box 850
Hershey, PA 17033
Emergency: 800-521-6110

LANCASTER
**Poison Control Center (*)
St. Joseph Hospital and
Health Care Center**
250 College Ave.
Lancaster, PA 17604
Business: 717-299-4546
Emergency: 717-291-8111

PHILADELPHIA
**The Poison Control
Center (*)**
3600 Market St.
Room 220
Philadelphia, PA 19104
Business: 215-590-2003
Emergency: 215-386-2100
Fax: 215-590-4419

PITTSBURGH
**Pittsburgh Poison Center (*)
Children's Hospital of
Pittsburgh**
3705 Fifth Ave.
Pittsburgh, PA 15213
Business: 412-692-5600
Emergency: 412-681-6669
Fax: 412-692-7497

RHODE ISLAND

PROVIDENCE
**Rhode Island
Poison Center (*)
Rhode Island Hospital**
593 Eddy St.
Providence, RI 02903
Emergency: 401-444-5727
Fax: 401-444-8062

SOUTH CAROLINA

COLUMBIA
**Palmetto Poison Center
College of Pharmacy (*)
University of
South Carolina**
Columbia, SC 29208
Business: 803-777-7909
Emergency: 803-777-1117
            800-922-1117
            (SC)
Fax: 803-777-6127

SOUTH DAKOTA

ABERDEEN
**Poison Control Center
St. Luke's Midland
Regional Medical Center**
305 South State St.
Aberdeen, SD 57401
Business: 605-622-5000
Emergency: 605-622-5100
            800-592-1889
            (SD, MN, ND,
            WY)

RAPID CITY
**Rapid City Regional
Poison Center**
835 Fairmont Blvd.
P.O. Box 6000
Rapid City, SD 57709
Business &
Emergency: 605-341-3333

SIOUX FALLS
**McKennan Poison Center
McKennan Hospital**
800 East 21st St.
P.O. Box 5045
Sioux Falls, SD 57117
Business: 605-339-7873
Emergency: 605-336-3894
            800-843-0505
            (IA, MN, NE,
            ND)
            800-952-0123
            (SD)
Fax: 605-333-8206

TENNESSEE

MEMPHIS
Southern Poison Center (*)
847 Monroe Ave.
Suite 230
Memphis, TN 38163
Business: 901-448-6800
Emergency: 901-528-6048
            800-288-9999
            (TN only)
Fax: 901-448-5419

NASHVILLE
**Middle Tennessee
Poison Center (*)**
501 Oxford House
1161 21st Ave. S.
Nashville, TN 37332
Business: 615-936-0760
Emergency: 615-936-2034
            800-288-9999
            (TN)
TTD: 615-936-2047
Fax: 615-936-2046

TEXAS

DALLAS
**North Texas Poison Center
Texas Poison
Center Network (*)
Parkland Memorial
Hospital**
5201 Harry Hines Blvd.
P.O. Box 35926
Dallas, TX 75235
Business: 214-590-6625
Emergency: 800-Poison-1
            (800-764-7661)
Fax: 214-590-5008

EL PASO
**West Texas Regional
Poison Center (*)**
4815 Alameda Ave.
El Paso, TX 79905
Business: 915-521-7661
Emergency: 915-533-1244
            800-764-7661
            (800-POISON-1)
Fax: 915-521-7978

GALVESTON

**Southeast Texas
Poison Center (*)
University of Texas
Medical Branch**
Trauma Center
Room 3-112
Galveston, TX 77555
Emergency: 409-765-1420
          800-761-7664
          (TX only)
Fax: 409-761-3917

TEMPLE

**Drug Information Center
Scott and White Memorial
Hospital**
2401 South 31st St.
Temple, TX 76508
Business: 817-724-4636
Fax: 817-724-1731

UTAH

SALT LAKE CITY

**Utah Poison
Control Center (*)**
410 Chipeta Way
Suite 230
Salt Lake City, UT 84108
Emergency: 801-581-2151
          800-456-7707
          (UT)
Fax: 801-581-4199

VERMONT

BURLINGTON

**Vermont Poison Center (*)
Fletcher Allen Health Care**
111 Colchester Ave.
Burlington, VT 05401
Business: 802-656-2721
Emergency: 802-658-3456
Fax: 802-656-4802

VIRGINIA

CHARLOTTESVILLE

**Blue Ridge Poison Center
Blue Ridge Hospital**
Box 67
Charlottesville, VA 22901
Emergency: 804-924-5543
          800-451-1428

HAMPTON

**Drug Information Center
Sentara Hampton
General Hospital**
3120 Victoria Blvd.
Hampton, VA 23669
Business: 804-727-7185
Fax: 804-727-7398

RICHMOND

**Virginia Poison Center
Virginia Commonwealth
University**
P.O. Box 980522
Richmond, VA 23298
Emergency: 804-828-9123
Fax: 804-828-5291

WASHINGTON

SEATTLE

**Washington Poison
Center (*)**
155 NE 100th St.
Suite 400
Seattle, WA 98125-8012
Business: 206-517-2351
Emergency: 206-526-2121
          800-732-6985
          (WA)
TTY: 206-517-2394
          800-572-0638
          (WA)
Fax: 206-526-8490

WEST VIRGINIA

CHARLESTON

**West Virginia
Poison Center (*)
West Virginia University**
3110 MacCorkle Ave. SE
Charleston, WV 25304
Business: 304-347-1212
Emergency: 304-348-4211
          800-642-3625
          (WV)
Fax: 304-348-9560

PARKERSBURG

**Poison Center
St. Joseph's Hospital
Center**
19th St. and Murdoch Ave.
Parkersburg, WV 26101
Emergency: 304-424-4222

WISCONSIN

MADISON

**Poison Control Center
University of Wisconsin
Hospital (*) and Clinics**
600 Highland Ave.
E5/238
Madison, WI 53792
Business: 608-262-7537
Emergency: 608-262-3702
          800-815-8855
          (WI)

MILWAUKEE

**Children's Hospital
Poison Center
Children's Hospital of
Wisconsin**
9000 W. Wisconsin Ave.
P.O. Box 1997
Milwaukee, WI 53201
Business: 414-266-2000
Emergency: 414-266-2222
          800-815-8855
          (WI)
Fax: 414-266-2820

Source: Red Book and
POISINDEX® System,
MICROMEDEX, INC.
6200 S. Syracuse Way
Englewood, CO 80111-4740

For more information on the
POISINDEX System, please
contact MICROMEDEX, INC.
at (800) 525-9083 or
(303) 486-6400.